NATIONAL
HEALTH SYSTEMS
OF THE WORLD

NATIONAL HEALTH SYSTEMS OF THE WORLD

Volume One

The Countries

Milton I. Roemer

New York   Oxford   OXFORD UNIVERSITY PRESS   1991

Oxford University Press

Oxford   New York   Toronto
Delhi   Bombay   Calcutta   Madras   Karachi
Petaling Jaya   Singapore   Hong Kong   Tokyo
Nairobi   Dar es Salaam   Cape Town
Melbourne   Auckland

and associated companies in
Berlin   Ibadan

Roemer, Milton Irwin, 1916–
National health systems of the world / Milton I. Roemer.
p. cm.   Includes bibliographical references and index.
Contents: v. 1. The countries.
ISBN 0-19-505320-6 (v. 1)
1. Medical policy.   2. Medical care.
3. Public health.   4. Insurance, Health.   I. Title.
RA393.R593   1991   362.1—dc20

9 8 7 6 5 4 3 2 1

Printed in the United States of America
on acid-free paper

To Ruth

Preface

This comparative study of national health systems has evolved from my experience as a public health worker. Aside from a year in Germany at age six, I had not really visited another country until 1950. In that postwar year, I served as leader of a university-sponsored studytour on "Health Services in Western Europe." The impact on me was stunning. Even superficial examination of the health service programs in four European "welfare states," where the ashes of war were still smoldering, made a profound impression. It was like a flash of light, illuminating problems of health care organization on which I had been working in the United States for some 10 years.

When, a few months later in 1950, the World Health Organization (WHO) invited me to do a health survey of one rural region in El Salvador, in order to plan a "health demonstration area," I seized that opportunity to visit a developing country. Then in 1951, WHO sent me to Ceylon (now Sri Lanka), a newly independent former British colony, to do a similar survey. This led to two years of work in Geneva, Switzerland at WHO headquarters, where it was possible to become acquainted with health conditions in several more countries. In the 36 years since then, I have been invited to serve as a public health consultant in 62 countries on all the continents—countries of all economic levels, every major political ideology, and a great variety of cultural characteristics. (Some countries were visited several times.) This work has been done principally for WHO headquarters and regional offices, but also for the International Labour Organisation (ILO), the Organization of American States, regional divisions of the World Bank, the United Nations Development Program, the United States Agency for International Development (USAID) and numerous groups with which USAID contracts, for the U.S. Peace Corps, the University of California (under various research grants), and in response to the direct invitation of governments and universities of numerous countries.

Such experiences naturally stimulate one's thinking, and pose a challenge to find some order among the countless observations that one can make. Visiting a country and trying to learn about its health activities, however, is only the point of entry to its health system. The study of documents both before and after the visit provides as much or more understanding. And the obligation of a teacher to convey to students a clear picture of any national health system is a further challenge—both intellectually and emotionally. The course I have conducted for graduate students at the UCLA School of Public Health ("Health Care Issues in International Perspective") for some 25 years, and the exchange of ideas inside and outside the classroom, have generated countless thoughts contributing to this book.

From these remarks, it is evident that the methodology behind this work cannot be described as one would recite the protocol of a scientific experiment, even in the social sciences. The facts in these pages have been acquired, and the interpretations reached, in diverse ways. Many have come, of course, from direct observations, and those have inevitably included not only visual perceptions but the responses of various informants to questions, the examination of written records, the perusal of typewritten or processed reports—never to be found in a library—as well as the study of all sorts of published materials. The latter included journals, books, reports, proceedings of conferences, special monographs, and various items that librarians describe as "fugitive."

Much information has also come from correspondence with knowledgeable individuals. Sometimes a crucial point about realities in a health system is disclosed in the midst of casual conversation on a totally different subject.

One problem often encountered in international health studies is receiving conflicting information from different sources. Disparities are encountered between oral accounts of different persons, between such accounts and written reports, or between published documents of different or even the same official agency. When this occurs, one must use the information that seems most consistent with the overall situation or avoid the topic entirely.

These diverse methods of acquiring information on countries and their health systems may explain why exact citations are not indicated in the text of this book. If precise sources for every point were to be cited, the reader would be confronted with an awkward mixture of "personal communications," "unpublished documents," and the like, which would be of very little use. Instead, there are listed alphabetically, at the end of each chapter, the relevant publications that should be available in libraries or other public places—materials that may be consulted by anyone seeking further information or insights on each health system or other subject.

Beyond the references for each chapter, this international or cross-national study has been enormously assisted by several compilations of data published, usually periodically, by official international agencies. Rather than citing these repeatedly at the close of each chapter, they are listed following this preface, along with a few equivalent though nonofficial publications, that are valuable sources of data on many, if not all, countries.

For giving me the opportunity to visit and study the health systems of so many countries, I must express my profound appreciation to the World Health Organization, providing inspired leadership in international health work since 1948. I have been fortunate enough to work on projects under WHO sponsorship for almost 40 years. The numerous other international and national agencies, to which I am also indebted, were noted above. It is not a cli-

ché to stress that the public health and other workers, whom I have met in all these countries, have been my main teachers.

Aside from generally distributed publications, the World Bank was generous in providing me with copies of its "Health Sector Reports," intended for official use. Likewise, the World Health Organization staff gave me access to numerous field reports of their personnel and consultants, often in cases where no publication was intended. I am also indebted to the American Public Health Association, whose Committee on International Health I chaired for six years, for the numerous documents on developing countries that came to my attention through this work.

Support for library research was provided by the UCLA International Studies and Overseas Program (ISOP), for which I am grateful. For their assistance in various literature searches, I thank Erin Kenney, Daniel Barzman, Alice Lim, Maria Chen, and Ruth Roemer. For their amazing skill in transforming reams of old-fashioned handwriting into clear typescript, and their labors far beyond duty, I wish to thank Mary Hunter and Evalon Witt. Finally I must express special appreciation to Henry Ernest Sigerist, whom I had the privilege of knowing from 1936 to his death in 1957, for his enormous intellectual inspiration on medicine and health service as worldwide issues. His unfulfilled plan to prepare a four-volume international "sociology of medicine" served always to goad me to undertake this work.

No one knows better than the author the inadequacies of these analyses of national health systems in 68 countries, selected to illustrate all types of such systems in the world. Deficiencies in these accounts are of several types. Many are due to changes that have occurred after the words were written or after the dates for which explicit data were available. Other deficiencies are doubtless due to the faulty recording of information or the improper interpretation of facts that may have been faithfully provided. Some weaknesses are surely due to the author's failure to probe deeply enough into the meaning of commonplace terms—which, in a certain country, may signify something different from their meaning in most other countries—leading then to faulty conclusions.

I hope that these several latter types of defect are not numerous, and that readers will be good enough to send notes correcting them to the author. As for health system information that has become outdated, I can only appeal to the reader's understanding. The changes in all national health systems are so endless that if one were to aim to publish a *currently accurate* account of the systems in even a few countries—even in a single country—the task would be hopeless; by the time of printing, the account would be out-of-date. One can only try to analyze any social system, in relation to a certain period of time—in this instance, at various points in the decade of the 1980s. Health systems in later periods must be studied at future times.

Every analysis of a social phenomenon, such as a health system, is bound to be influenced by the viewpoint of the writer. I do not think that this need be regarded as a "bias," so long as the facts available are fully and faithfully reported, even if the interpretations assume certain social or ethical values. In this comparative analysis of national health systems, the viewpoint taken is frankly that of the public health discipline. This viewpoint regards the purpose of a health system as attempting to protect and advance the health of total populations, including the recovery of health by treatment when prevention has failed.

This viewpoint may sometimes result in contentious and controversial postures regarding various social issues. Health systems involve interpersonal relationships affecting the place in society of many individuals; some disagreements about this place are inevitable. The interpretation of matters, even within an explicit public health viewpoint, may sometimes be subject to debate. Whatever strengths or weaknesses these analyses may have, I hope that they contribute to an understanding of the dynamics of the national health system in any country.

Los Angeles　　　　　　　　　　　　　M.I.R.
June 1990

Sources of International Data on Health and Social Conditions

Harris, William H., and Judith S. Levey (Editors)
The New Columbia Encyclopedia. New York: Columbia University Press, 1975.

Hoffman, Mark S. (Editor)
The World Almanac and Book of Facts: 1989. New York: Pharos Books, 1989.

Organization for Economic Cooperation and Development (OECD)
Measuring Health Care 1960–1983. Paris: OECD, 1985.

Sivard, Ruth Leger
World Military and Social Expenditures. Washington, D.C.: World Priorities, for 1989 and earlier years.

United Nations Children's Fund (UNICEF)
The State of the World's Children. New York: Oxford University Press, for 1989 and earlier years.

U.S. Social Security Administration
Social Security Programs Throughout the World. Washington, D.C.: U.S. Department of Health and Human Services, for 1987 and earlier years.

World Bank
Financing Health Services in Developing Countries. Washington, D.C.: The World Bank, 1987.

World Bank
World Development Report. Washington, D.C., published by Oxford University Press, New York, for 1988 and earlier years.

World Health Organization
Sixth Report on the World Health Situation 1973–1977, Part II: Review by Country and Area. Geneva: WHO, 1980.

World Health Organization
World Directory of Medical Schools, Sixth Edition. Geneva: WHO, 1988.

World Health Organization
World Health Statistics Annual. Geneva: WHO, for 1988 and earlier years.

Contents

PART ONE

HEALTH SYSTEMS

CHAPTER ONE

Introduction

This book attempts to analyze the national health systems of many types that operate in countries throughout the world. It also examines the main components of systems across countries. In modern times there are some 165 sovereign nations, each with its own history, geography, and social characteristics. No two countries are exactly alike, and accordingly no two national health systems are exactly alike.

The many determinants of the configuration and dynamics of national health systems are explored in Chapter 4. The boundaries, the internal structure, and the functions of health systems—their anatomy and physiology—are analyzed in Chapter 3. Here we may examine the nature of "systems" in general—a subject about which a major body of knowledge and literature has grown in recent years. We then consider the meaning of health systems and the studies that have been made of them. Finally we consider why national health systems should be compared.

SYSTEMS IN GENERAL

In response to the complexity of military operations in World War II, and to the even greater postwar problems of physical and social reconstruction of nations, a scientific discipline called *systems analysis* developed. In all sorts of social situations, it was increasingly found that the solution to problems required considering the nature of each problem in the broadest possible context. A certain intellectual mystique grew around the phrase, but the discipline of systems analysis and a "general systems approach" involve essentially *seeing the situation as a whole.*

More formally, and doubtless more completely, a system may be defined as *a set of in-*terrelated and interdependent parts, designed to achieve a set of goals. An orientation toward the task of analyzing systems leads to defining systems analysis as *the separation of systems into components for further study, which usually consists of examining the influence of one or more components on system performance.*

Virtually every system in nature or society encompasses subsystems. One could, for example, set out to analyze a national system of transportation. Its components might include railroads, airlines, automobiles, bicycles, and other elements. The subsystem of automobile transportation, furthermore, might include vehicle manufacturers, roads, fuel, traffic rules, and drivers. Roads and fuel are further subsubsystems. Fuel encompasses geological explorations, petroleum extraction, refineries, petroleum shipment, gasoline (or petrol) stations, pricing and marketing, and so on. One systems expert has theorized a nine-level hierarchy of system complexity, into which any *open* system—that is, a system functioning in a social or physical environment and interacting with that environment—can be subdivided and analyzed.

In the same way, a national health system's component parts and their interrelationships can be analyzed.

HEALTH SYSTEMS AND THEIR STUDY

The term *health system* or *system of health care* has been used with different meanings. Anthropologists use the terms health systems and systems of medicine to refer to various practices for healing the sick, according to diverse religious, philosophical, magical, and empirical doctrines. Many health observers analyze the prevailing patterns of personal medical care in a country, defining these as the country's *health care system*. Government officials may describe the structure and functions of a country's ministry of health as its health system.

Chapter 3 discusses a more comprehensive approach to national health systems, as the term is used in this book, based on a model with five interacting components: resources, organization, management, economic support, and delivery of services. Thus, personal health services may be the output of a health system, but many other actions and interactions must precede them. Each of the major system components includes many subsystems, which can be explored only superficially. Under *resources,* for example, a large subsystem is health manpower. Within this subsystem is a further sub-subsystem for physicians. Understanding physicians, in turn, requires study of their education, their distribution, specialization, pattern of service, method of remuneration, and so on. The education of physicians is a further microsystem involving procedures for planning medical schools, appointing teachers, constructing classrooms and laboratories, admitting students, designing curricula, evaluating knowledge through examinations, regulating performance through licensure, and much more. Equivalent complexities would concern *social insurance* under economic support or *primary care* under delivery of services.

As we will see, countless studies have been made on the subsystems and sub-subsystems within the health systems of individual countries (or even provinces). Work has been done on certain health system topics across countries, such as (to pursue the preceding example) international medical school curricula or even the design of a course in pediatric surgery. The scope of this book, however, cannot cover all subdivisions of all health systems. The book attempts to analyze only the major components of the health systems in countries demonstrating the principal types of such systems in the world; in some countries only selected aspects of health systems are analyzed. The components are discussed, I hope, in sufficient depth to permit comparison with equivalent features of the health systems of other countries.

This, of course, is not the first attempt to analyze and compare national health systems. Analytical accounts of health services in specific countries have been published for decades. These are sometimes a sort of public relations report by the Ministry of Health—often limited to a review of the ministry's own activities. One of the first comprehensive overviews of a national health system in English was stimulated by the Russian Revolution—*Red Medicine: Socialized Health in Soviet Russia,* published in 1933. In 1934, Henry Sigerist's historically oriented account of *American Medicine* appeared.

Only a few comparative analyses of several countries were published before World War II. The first in English was an extensive analysis by Arthur Newsholme of Western European countries, focusing on "the relation between the private and official practice of medicine," published in several volumes in 1931. This study was supported by a philanthropic foundation in the United States, and the objective was clearly to inform Americans about the experience of European health insurance programs. A similar objective motivated the second multinational study by I. S. Falk, *Security Against Sickness,* which appeared in 1936.

After World War II interest in cross-national studies of health systems mushroomed. Investigations and analyses were made by scholars, as well as journalists and public figures. The war brought Europeans and Americans in touch with countries on other continents, and enormous interest was aroused in the diverse cultures and social orders of the world. The postwar national liberation movements, followed by emancipation of colonies, gave rise to worldwide economic and technical exchanges. The United Nations, founded in 1946, followed by the specialized agencies a few years later, fostered countless relationships among countries.

In this atmosphere, health leaders felt obliged to look to other countries for "lessons." Franz Goldmann's 1946 article on "Foreign Programs of Medical Care and Their Lessons" was typical. John Grant wrote of "International Trends in Health Care" in 1948, and my review of "Rural Health Programs in Different Nations" was also published that year. In 1952, *The Advance to Social Medicine* by René Sand examined worldwide historical developments in every feature of health systems. In 1959, the World Health Organization published its *First Report on the World Health Situation (1954–1956),* presenting synopses of the national health systems of 157 countries—the broadest such compilation prepared up to that time.

These accounts of national health systems were largely descriptive rather than analytical or comparative. In the 1960s, more selective and analytical studies of certain countries and certain subjects appeared. Brian Abel-Smith's *International Study of Health Expenditures* appeared in 1967. Karl Evang published *Health Services, Society, and Medicine* in 1960. John Fry wrote *Medicine in Three Societies* in 1969. E. Richard Weinerman published *Social Medicine in Eastern Europe* (1969). John Bryant published *Health and the Developing World* (1969). Maurice King edited the multiauthored work on *Medical Care in Developing Countries* in 1966.

In 1970 William Glaser published two highly analytical accounts of special aspects of European health insurance programs—the payment of doctors and the organization of hospitals. For the most part, however, the 1970s produced a number of multiauthored collections on national health systems. This was perhaps a response to the growing interest in the subject, combined with recognition of its complexities. With writers from many countries, comparative reviews of national health systems could be produced quite rapidly. Hence there appeared *International Medical Care,* edited by Fry and Farndale (1972); *Health Service Prospects: An International Survey,* edited by Douglas-Wilson and McLachlan (1973); *The Impact of Health Services on Medical Education: A Global View,* edited by Bowers and Purcell (1978); *Health Care: An International Study,* edited by Kohn and White (1976); and others.

Victor and Ruth Sidel's *A Healthy State,* examining health policies in Sweden, Great Brit-

ain, the Soviet Union, China, and the United States (1977), showed special sensitivity to political determinants of health system characteristics. The equivalence of problems in three different national systems was stressed in 1972 by Odin Anderson in *Health Care: Can There Be Equity?* In 1980, Ray Elling stressed political determinism in his *Cross-National Study of Health Systems.* Economic factors were the focus in Robert Maxwell's *Health and Wealth: An International Study of Health Care Spending* (1981) and in Lee and Mills' edited volume on *The Economics of Health in Developing Countries.* Other special topics were comparatively explored in Ingle and Blair's *International Dental Care Delivery Systems* (1978); Bridgman and Roemer's *Hospital Legislation and Hospital Systems* (1973); and Brocklehurst's *Geriatric Care in Advanced Societies* (1975).

The 1980s brought further multiauthored collections reviewing numerous national health systems. In 1984 Marshall Raffel edited *Comparative Health Systems,* which covered 14 countries. Richard B. Saltman in 1988 edited *The International Handbook of Health-Care Systems* dealing with 21 countries. My *National Strategies for Health Care Organization* in 1985 assembled essays on health systems of 12 countries and 13 health care issues.

WHY STUDY HEALTH SYSTEMS?

What accounts for this growing interest in studying and comparing health systems? Why have such efforts been made to analyze health policies and practices at different times and places? Several reasons may be suggested.

First of all, learning about the health systems of other countries can help give us perspective to understand our own. It can be reassuring to find that certain health system problems, which may be very vexing, have been encountered elsewhere and have led to certain solutions. Even if the solutions are not transferrable, the commonality of experience can give confidence that health system problems are to be expected and are manageable.

A second and more concrete reason is that certain features of one health system can offer lessons for another. Ideas on health technology, of course, transmitted across national borders, have been countless—from stethoscopes to x-rays, from vaccines to antibiotics—and they have shaped practices throughout health systems. Ideas on the social organization of health services may take longer to transmit, but they eventually permeate the structure and function of all health systems.

The concept of hospitals arose simultaneously in different societies, but features of their structure and operation were transmitted from place to place; likewise for dispensaries for the sick and health centers providing both preventive and curative service. Organized public health programs for environmental sanitation, communicable disease control, and other purposes were explored in some countries before being developed in others. The same applies to social insurance and its various applications to the financing of medical care. Ideas still too new to have been transmitted and accepted everywhere include regionalization of health facilities, quality surveillance of medical performance, and the participation of community people in formulating health policy.

A third reason for comparative study of health systems is to observe the strategies for achieving health equity under different circumstances. Worldwide political pressures have mounted for the equitable distribution of health service, in response to needs. How have various health systems tried to attain this objective? What balance is assigned between individual and social responsibility, between private and public sectors?

To identify methods of achieving maximum efficiency is a fourth reason for comparative study of national health systems. Efficiency, of course, measures the cost—in both money and resources—of the inputs needed to achieve a certain output. In some countries, health service organization may be very inefficient because of certain social values—for example, insistence that the patient has free choice of personal doctor—for which a high price is paid. In other countries, low costs are important and efficiency comes first, even at the sac-

rifice of some personal freedom. Efficiency may have implications for centralized standards as against localized pluralism. It may favor the maximum use of health care teams, rather than autonomous health care providers. A national health system may demonstrate efficiency in one aspect and relative inefficiency in another, both of which may be explained by societal values.

A fifth reason for studying health systems must be suggested with caution—to learn about their influence on the health status of the population. Caution is necessary because, as we explore in Chapter 2, the health of a population is influenced by much more than the health services that it receives. In fact, for many sections of populations, the health system may be the least important of many factors affecting health. Still, as more knowledge about the determinants of health and disease is acquired, health services—especially the preventive services—become more influential. From comparison of countries in which standards of living are reasonably similar but health system characteristics are markedly different, one may infer something about the influence of health services. Moreover, in countries whose overall economic and social levels are very low and yet the health status record is good, the health systems may deserve special credit.

Thus, health systems may be regarded as an array of experiments in a global laboratory. Numerous different arrangements of resources, activities, and interactions are being tested, and the results can be compared. With careful control of the many variables, judgments can be made on how well one or another system achieves equity or efficiency or improved health status in the population. If conclusions are drawn with care, they may point to the value of specific changes in a system that may increase the probability of enhancing equity, efficiency, or health status. Even if such "results" cannot be assessed, the attitudes and satisfaction of people with their health system could be measured and compared.

A sixth reason for studying national health systems is scientific—to draw generalizations. In any natural or social science one observes many situations—at different times and places—before forming a general conclusion. By carefully examining selected aspects of numerous health systems, one may infer generalizations that apply to all or nearly all systems—even those not directly observed. The allotment of an increasing share of national wealth to health systems over the last century, for example, is one such generalization. With urbanization occurring in virtually all countries, the devotion of an increasing proportion of health expenditures to hospitals is another such generalization. The role of government in health systems, on the other hand, may warrant one generalization in one type of health system and a different one in another.

Generalizations are the bedrock of science. They give us the power to predict. At the end of this volume, after we have reviewed the health systems of numerous countries, we will consider some generalizations that have emerged from the analyses.

THE PLAN OF THIS BOOK

This book on *National Health Systems of the World* is planned in two volumes. The first volume is devoted principally to a study of the diverse health systems in various countries of the world; the second volume is devoted to a cross-national analysis of the major issues within these systems. Information about the health system of Brazil, for example, can be found in Volume One; information about hospitals or about national health insurance in various countries can be found in Volume Two.

Chapter 2 of this first volume provides an overview of world health and its many determinants. Trends in the major diseases of humans are traced, insofar as they obviously influence the nature of health systems. The general structure and dynamics of national health systems are elaborated in Chapter 3, as interpreted by this author. Different observers, of course, may analyze health systems in various ways, and the model formulated here has been found applicable to the circumstances observed in many countries. Chapter 4 classifies the diverse types of national health systems

found in the world. A conceptual matrix or typology is composed by considering systems along two dimensions: the economic level of the country and the social policy of the health system; altogether 14 types of health system can be defined. This completes Part I.

Part II is devoted to analysis of the health systems of 24 industrialized and high-income countries. The systems are clustered around four kinds of social policy, scaled by the degree of government intervention in the health service market. Thus, Chapter 5 considers entrepreneurial health systems in industrialized countries; Chapter 6, welfare-oriented systems in such countries; Chapter 7, their comprehensive systems; and Chapter 8, socialist health systems in industrialized countries.

Part III examines the health systems of 25 transitional and middle-income countries. The health systems are classified according to policies reflecting the same four degrees of market intervention as described in Part II. Chapter 9 examines entrepreneurial systems in four countries. Because welfare-oriented health systems in transitional countries are so numerous, however, they are grouped into Latin American countries (Chapter 10) and Middle East and Asian countries (Chapter 11). Socialist health systems are demonstrated in transitional countries of three continents (Chapter 13).

Part IV is devoted to 18 health systems in very poor countries, also grouped according to the four degrees of market intervention. In spite of the great poverty of these countries, it is worth noting that the social policies shaping their health systems can be classified along a scale similar to that used for systems in the richest countries.

In Part V, Chapter 18 analyzes four oil-rich developing countries that, because of their sudden wealth in recent decades, do not fit into the schema of Parts II, III, and IV. Chapter 19 concludes Volume One, with some general conclusions on national health systems—generalizations that emerge from the study of systems in some 68 countries.

A final *caveat* concerning Volume One is in order. The analyses apply generally to health systems as they were in the 1980s. Like all social systems, health systems change constantly.

They change in response to economic and political forces in the world around them and also to changes in health technology and the demography of populations. One can hardly expect a printed text to be up-to-date on the latest health developments in each country. One can only hope that future scholars will paint a new picture when the time is ripe.

The plan of Volume Two is based on the health system model presented in Chapter 3 of Volume One. It examines the principal components and subdivisions of health systems in various countries around the world. Almost all elements of these system take different forms in various health systems; they differ in quantity, design, and characteristics as they evolve in various national environments. A health center in the entrepreneurial health system of a high-income country, for example, is quite different from such a facility in the socialist health system of a very poor country. The work done by a pharmacist in Belgium differs greatly from that done by a pharmacist in Sri Lanka. Because these matters are often involved in debates concerning the "best" policy, they are considered as issues.

Part I of Volume Two examines the major types of health resources across national health systems—physicians and traditional healers in Chapter 1, other health personnel in Chapter 2, health facilities in Chapter 3, drugs and supplies in Chapter 4, and knowledge and technology in Chapter 5. Each chapter begins with the historic development of the resources, then describing its major points of diversity among systems. Only the highlights of cross-national comparisons can be considered, as they appeared in the 1980s.

Part II examines health care organization in government (Chapters 6 and 7), in nongovernmental agencies, and in the commercial market. The strength of organization in governmental and nongovernmental bodies, in relation to the strength of the private market, are crucial characteristics distinguishing national health systems. Every health system has a central Ministry of Health or its equivalent, but the scope of work of that body varies endlessly. Private markets for personal health care are also universal, but they vary from very strong to very weak.

In Part III the economic support and management of health systems are explored. The spectrum or mixture of various forms of economic support, analyzed in Chapter 10, delineates the profile of a health system in much more than fiscal terms. Perhaps no two national economic support profiles are exactly alike, but certain general configurations fit with certain types of system. The strategies of health planning and administration are explored in Chapter 11, and those of regulation and legislation in Chapter 12; on these issues, systems vary so greatly only the discussion of examples is permitted.

The goal of Part IV is especially ambitious—to summarize the many ways that specific health services are delivered within different types of health system. Ambulatory care patterns are examined in Chapter 13 and hospital care patterns in Chapter 14, both being activities in unusually great ferment in modern systems. Chapters 15, 16, and 17 examine health services for special populations, for special disorders, and for the use of special technical modalities. The relative weights assigned to these categorical services differ greatly among systems, but in every country certain persons, disorders, or modalities summon special attention. This attention may warrant patterns of health care delivery different from that prevailing in the health system as a whole.

Finally, Part V attempts to interpret world trends in all five health system components. Can definable trends along the direction each health system component seems to be moving be found? How are health systems as a whole adjusting to changing values in a changing world?

REFERENCES

Abel-Smith, Brian, *An International Study of Health Expenditures and Its Relevance for Health Planning.* Geneva: World Health Organization (Public Health Paper No. 32), 1967.
Anderson, Odin W., *Health Care: Can There Be Equity? 1 The United States, Sweden, and England.* New York: John Wiley & Sons, 1972.
Bowers, John Z., and Elizabeth F. Purcell, *The Im-

pact of Health Services on Medical Education: A Global View. New York: Josiah Macy, Jr. Foundation, 1978.

Bridgman, Robert F., and Milton I. Roemer, Hospital Legislation and Hospital Systems. Geneva: World Health Organization (Public Health Papers No. 50), 1973.

Brocklehurst, J. C. (Editor), Geriatric Care in Advanced Societies. Lancaster Medical & Technical Publishing Co., 1975.

Bryant, John, Health and the Developing World. Ithaca, N.Y.: Cornell University Press, 1969.

Churchman, C. West, The Systems Approach. New York: Delacorte Press, 1968.

Doan, Bui Dang Ha (Editor), The Future of Health and Health Care Systems in the Industrialized Societies. New York: Praeger, 1988.

Douglas-Wilson, I., and Gordon McLachlan, Health Service Prospects: An International Survey. London: The Lancet and Nuffield Provincial Hospitals Trust, 1973.

Elling, Ray H., Cross-National Study of Health Systems. New Brunswick, N.J.: Transaction Books, 1980.

Evang, Karl, Health Services, Society, and Medicine. London: Oxford University Press, 1960.

Falk, I. S., Security Against Sickness: A Study of Health Insurance. Garden City, N.Y.: Doubleday, Doran & Co., 1936.

Field, Mark G., "The Concept of the 'Health System' at the Macrosociological Level." Social Science and Medicine, 7:763–785, 1973.

Frenk, Julio, and Avedis Donabedian, "State Intervention in Medical Care: Types, Trends and Variables." Health Policy and Planning, 2(1):17–31, 1987.

Fry, John, Medicine in Three Societies. New York: American Elsevier Publishing Co., 1969.

Fry, John, and W. A. J. Farndale (Editors), International Medical Care. Oxford and Lancaster: Medical & Technical Publishing Co., 1972.

Fulcher, Derick, Medical Care Systems: Public and Private Health Coverage in Selected Industrialized Countries. Geneva: International Labour Office, 1974.

Glaser, William A., Social Settings and Medical Organization: A Cross-National Study of the Hospital. New York: Atherton Press, 1970.

Glaser, William A. Paying the Doctor: Systems of Remuneration and Their Effects. Baltimore: Johns Hopkins Press, 1970.

Glisson, T. H., Introduction to System Analysis. New York: McGraw-Hill Book Co., 1985.

Goldmann, Franz, "Foreign Programs of Medical Care and Their Lessons." New England Journal of Medicine, 234:156–160, 1946.

Grant, John B., "International Trends in Health Care." American Journal of Public Health, 38:381–397, 1948.

Ingle, John I., and Patricia Blair (Editors), International Dental Care Delivery Systems. Cambridge, Mass.: Ballinger Publishing Co., 1978.

Kent, P. W. (Editor), International Aspects of the Provision of Medical Care. London: Oriel Press, 1976.

King, Maurice (Editor), Medical Care in Developing Countries. London: Oxford University Press, 1966.

Kohn, Robert, and Kerr L. White (Editors), Health Care: An International Survey. London: Oxford University Press, 1976.

Lee, Kenneth, and Anne Mills (Editors), The Economics of Health in Developing Countries. Oxford: Oxford University Press, 1983.

Leichter, Howard M., Comparative Approach to Policy Analysis: Health Care Policy in Four Nations. New York: Cambridge University Press, 1979.

Levey, Samuel, and N. Paul Loomba, "Systems," in Health Care Administration: A Managerial Perspective. Philadelphia: J. B. Lippincott Co., 1973, pp. 58–104.

Mahajan, Vijay, and C. Carl Pegels (Editors), Systems Analysis in Health Care. New York: Praeger, 1979.

Maxwell, Robert J., Health and Wealth: An International Study of Health Care Spending. Lexington, Mass.: Lexington Books, 1981.

Medical Sociology Research Committee, International Sociological Association, "Comparative Health Systems," Supplement to Inquiry, 12(2), June 1975.

Mountin, J. W., and G. St. J. Perrott, "Health Insurance Programs and Plans of Western Europe." Public Health Reports, 62:369 ff, 1947.

Newsholme, Arthur, International Studies on the Relation Between the Private & Official Practice of Medicine with Special Reference to the Prevention of Disease, 3 Volumes. London: George Allen & Unwin, 1931.

Newsholme, Arthur, and John A. Kingsbury, Red Medicine: Socialized Health in Soviet Russia. Garden City, N.Y.: Doubleday, Doran & Co., 1933.

Pannenborg, P. O., et al. (Editors), Reorienting Health Services: Application of a Systems Approach. New York: Plenum Press, 1984.

Raffel, Marshall W. (Editor), Comparative Health Systems: Descriptive Analyses of Fourteen National Health Systems. University Park: Pennsylvania State University Press, 1984.

Rodwin, Victor G., "Comparative Health Systems: Notes on the Literature," in The Health Planning Predicament. Berkeley: University of California Press, 1984, pp. 239–248.

Roemer, Milton I., "Health Departments and Medical Care—A World Scanning." American Journal of Public Health, 59:154 ff, 1960.

Roemer, Milton I., Health Care Systems in World

Perspective. Ann Arbor, Mich.: Health Administration Press, 1976.

Roemer, Milton I., *National Strategies for Health Care Organization—A World Overview.* Ann Arbor, Mich.: Health Administration Press, 1985.

Roemer, Milton I., *The Organization of Medical Care under Social Security—A Study Based on the Experience of Eight Countries.* Geneva: International Labour Office, 1969.

Roemer, Milton I., "Rural Health Programs in Different Nations." *Milbank Memorial Fund Quarterly,* 26:58–59, 1948.

Saltman, Richard B. (Editor), *The International Handbook of Health-Care Systems.* Westport, Conn.: Greenwood Press, 1988.

Sheldon, Alan, Frank Baker, and Curtis P. McLaughlin (Editors), *Systems and Medical Care.* Boston: MIT Press, 1971.

Shigan, E. N., and R. Gibbs (Editors), *Modeling Health Care Systems.* Laxenburg (Austria): International Institute for Applied Systems Analysis, 1977.

Sidel, Victor W., and Ruth Sidel, *A Healthy State: An International Perspective on the Crisis in United States Medical Care.* New York: Pantheon Books, 1977.

Sigerist, Henry E., *American Medicine.* New York: W. W. Norton & Co., 1934.

Weinerman, E. Richard, *Social Medicine in Eastern Europe.* Cambridge, Mass.: Harvard University Press, 1969.

Weinerman, E. R., "Research on Comparative Health Service Systems." *Medical Care,* 9:272–290, May–June 1971.

World Health Organization, *First Report of the World Health Situation 1954–1956.* Geneva (Official Records of WHO No. 94), 1959.

CHAPTER TWO

Global Health and Its Determinants

The health systems with which this book deals have developed in response to the problems of disease and disability. Health services are provided, of course, because people become sick or injured and they want to be treated. Furthermore, with knowledge about the causes of a disease, much can be done to prevent it. Before exploring the nature of health systems in specific countries, therefore, we should consider the main features of health and disease throughout the world.

In spite of the development of health systems in response to health needs in populations, surprisingly little is known about the extent of physical and mental disorders in most countries. In a few highly developed countries, such as the United States and Great Britain, a great deal has been learned about morbidity, but in most countries health conditions must be analyzed principally from information about mortality. Even these data vary greatly in accuracy and reliability from country to country. Nevertheless, mortality rates—general and specific for age, sex, and certain social characteristics—in various countries provide a rough basis for judgments on the health status of national populations.

MORTALITY AND LIFE EXPECTANCY AMONG COUNTRIES

The general or crude mortality rate in a country is the total number of persons who die during a year, from any cause, per 1,000 population. In 1980 the United States, for example, had a crude death rate of 8.7 per 1,000 people. In that year, the crude death rate in Rwanda—a very low-income country in Africa—was 22.0 per 1,000. Since the crude death rate does not take into account a country's age composition, however, this may be deceptive. If a population has a relatively high proportion of children (e.g., age 1–15 years)—among whom the risk of death tends to be relatively low—its crude death rate may be lower than that in a country with a high proportion of elderly (e.g., over 65 years of age), among whom death rates are typically high. Thus, Colombia had a crude death rate in 1977 of 8.2 per 1,000, while Norway—a much more highly developed country with a lower death rate at each age level examined separately—had a crude death rate in 1980 of 10.1 per 1,000.

A statistical measure that is not affected by the proportions of people at different age levels is the life expectancy. Calculation of this figure at birth (i.e., for a person just born) is based on the mortality rate at each age level, without respect to the proportions of the total population alive at those age levels. Thus, Table 2.1, presents the life expectancies at birth in a number of countries, selected to represent ascending degrees of economic development; the latter is reflected by the gross national product (GNP, the value of all goods and services produced in a year) per capita.

It is evident from the data on 17 countries in Table 2.1 that life expectancies at birth vary from 44 years in an African country (Malawi) to 79 years in a Western European country (Switzerland). In a general way, these variations correspond to the levels of national wealth (as reflected in the GNP per capita), but the deviations from this general relationship are also notable. Bolivia, for example, has an appreciably shorter life expectancy at birth than India, although its per capita GNP is almost twice as high. Japan has a greater life expectancy than the United States, although its GNP per capita is 40 percent lower. Health sta-

Table 2.1. Life Expectancy at Birth and Gross National Product Per Capita, Selected Countries, 1983.

Country	Gross National Product, Per Capita (U.S. dollars)	Life Expectancy at Birth (years)
Bangladesh	130	50
Malawi	210	44
India	260	55
Kenya	340	57
Bolivia	510	51
Egypt	700	58
Thailand	820	63
Colombia	1,430	64
Malaysia	1,860	67
Yugoslavia	2,570	69
Spain	4,780	75
New Zealand	7,730	74
Japan	10,120	77
Sweden	12,470	78
United States	14,110	75
Switzerland	16,290	79
Kuwait	17,880	71

Source: World Bank, *World Development Report 1985,* Washington, D.C., 1985.

tus, in other words, must be affected by factors not reflected in the level of economic development—a subject to be explored later.

Another mortality figure that reveals a great deal about the effect of living conditions on health is the death rate of infants—that is, the number of deaths before one year of age per 1,000 live births during a year. In the first month of life, the survival of infants is likely to be affected very much by the conditions of childbirth—whether or not it is hygienically and appropriately handled, including the prenatal care of the mother. The next 11 months of the first year are bound to be influenced strongly by environmental conditions and the nature of infant nutrition and care. The educational level of mothers has been found to be closely associated with infant mortality rates. The wide range of these rates among countries is shown in Table 2.2. This range is even greater than that for life expectancy, and the close association with the literacy levels of adult women is striking.

The nature of disease problems in countries is reflected in many ways (but not entirely) in the major causes of death. The economically less developed countries are heavily afflicted with diseases that are linked to unsanitary environments, are spread by insect vectors, and

strike infants and small children in large numbers. The more highly developed countries have generally reduced these types of disease, so that most people live on to the later years of life, when degenerative or noncommunicable disorders—principally cardiovascular disease and cancer—become the major killers.

To show these contrasts in a simple form, the World Bank has analyzed mortality data from a number of countries at high and low stages of economic development, as of 1963. The percentage distributions of the causes of death in these two types of country are shown in Table 2.3. The problems to be addressed by health care systems are obviously different in these contrasting environments. In developing countries, where infectious and parasitic diseases are prevalent, strategies for communicable disease prevention and environmental controls must obviously have high priority. In the more developed countries, with their heavy burdens of chronic disorders in later life, effective medical care is clearly important, although the potentialities for prevention of these disorders through behavior modification are also being increasingly recognized.

Many infectious diseases are preventable by immunization, and in nearly all industrialized countries and most developing countries they

Table 2.2. Infant Mortality Rates (1982) and the Literacy Levels of Adult Women (1980) in Selected Countries

Country	Infant Deaths per 1000 Live Births per Year	Percent Literacy of Adult Women
Afghanistan	200	6
Mali	150	8
Niger	140	6
India	120	26
Egypt	110	28
Ghana	100	37
Indonesia	90	64
Brazil	70	73
Thailand	50	83
Sri Lanka	39	82
Yugoslavia	30	81
USSR	25	98
Israel	15	91
Belgium	12	99
United States	11	99
France	9	99
Sweden	7	98

Source: United Nations Children's Fund, *The State of the World's Children 1985.* New York, 1985.

Table 2.3. Major Causes of Death in More Developed and Less Developed Countries: Percentage Distributions, 1963

Cause of Death	Percentage	
	More Developed Countries	Less Developed Countries
Infectious, parasitic, and respiratory diseases	10.8	43.7
Traumatic injury	6.8	3.5
Diseases of circulatory system	32.2	14.8
Cancer	15.2	3.7
Other causes	35.0	34.3
All causes of death	100.0	100.0

Source: World Bank, *Sector Policy Paper—Health.* Washington, D.C., February 1980, p. 13.

have been greatly reduced. These include diphtheria, tetanus, pertussis (whooping cough), measles, and poliomyelitis. Smallpox has been completely eradicated from the earth, as a result of an intensive vaccination campaign carried out in the 1970s, under World Health Organization leadership. Yet there are several parasitic diseases, for which no immunization is currently available, that remain very important causes of disability and death in the developing tropical countries. Recent estimates of their extent in the world—both the numbers infected and those with serious resultant disorders—are given in Table 2.4.

Mortality reports may also shed light on the adequacy of health service in a country. In virtually all countries, deaths are supposed to be registered by formal certificates submitted to health authorities or other officials of government. A statement of the basic or underlying cause of death is theoretically to be recorded, but many death certificates note only symptoms or vague conditions. Such reporting usually means that the person was not seen by a physician at the time of death. In Honduras 32 percent of deaths occurring in 1978 were reported in this way. In nearby Costa Rica, on the other hand (where the health services are more highly developed), the equivalent proportion was only 9 percent. Ill-defined causes were recorded in Jordan on 21.5 percent of the death certificates and on 52.9 percent of the certificates in Thailand (around 1973). One can imagine the deficiencies of health care, when even a terminal illness is not medically attended. In highly developed countries such as Great Britain, Sweden, or Hungary, the corresponding record of ill-defined causes of death (in the early 1970s) was under 1 percent.

Mortality rates reflect sharp differences in the health status of populations not only between countries, but also within countries among various population groups. In Great Britain, the occupation of heads of families has been recorded on death certificates for more than a century. Based on this information, death rates can be calculated for different social classes; Class I, for example, includes professional occupations, Class V comprises unskilled workers. It has been found that, for all

Table 2.4. Important Parasitic Diseases: Estimated Infections, Disorders, and Deaths per Year in Tropical Countries, about 1980

Disease	Infections	Resultant Disorders	Deaths
Malaria	800,000,000	150,000,000 (fever, coma)	1,200,000
Schistosomiasis	200,000,000	20,000,000 (liver & urinary tract fibrosis)	750,000
Trypanosomiasis (South American)	12,000,000	1,200,000 (heart disease)	60,000
Onchoceciasis	30,000,000	350,000 (blindness)	35,000
Trypanosomiasis (African)	1,000,000	10,000 (sleeping sickness)	5,000
Filariasis	250,000,000	2,500,000 (elephantiasis)	?
Leishmaniosis	12,000,000	12,000,000 (sores)	5,000
Amebiasis	400,000,000	1,500,000 (dysentery, liver abscess)	30,000
Hookworm disease	900,000,000	1,500,000 (anemia)	55,000
Ascariasis	1,000,000,000	1,000,000 (intestinal obstruction)	20,000

Source: Bruer, J., "The Great Neglected Diseases." *RF Illustrated* (Rockefeller Foundation), June 1982.

age groups, the death rates in the lower social classes have long been substantially higher than those in the upper classes. (This remains true, in spite of the availability of health service for everyone since 1948.) The differentials are greater for infants and children up to age 15 years than for adult age groups. A study in Chile in 1972–1973 found that the mortality rate of blue-collar workers was 3.2 times higher than that of white-collar workers. Such findings, of course, give important clues to the determinants of health and disease, to be discussed later.

Careful study of mortality in selected age groups may shed light on social conditions that affect health in a country. A 1982 study of mortality rates in young adults (15 to 24 years of age)—among whom the death rate from drug abuse, suicide, homicide, and road accident is relatively high—found two patterns in the more affluent versus the poorer countries. In countries with GNP per capita (in 1978) below $3,000 per year, the rate of young adult mortality rose with *decreasing* wealth. In countries with higher GNP per capita (generally industrialized), the young adult mortality rose with *increasing* wealth. In both sets of countries, high mortality among young adults was significantly associated with lesser per capita expenditures on education and greater diversity of ethnic groups in the population.

Considering the world as a whole, the overall crude rate of mortality in 1980–1984 was 10.6 per 1,000 population. In all developed regions of the world it was 9.6 per 1,000 and in the developing regions it was 11.0 per 1,000—a differential that would doubtless be greater if adjustments were made for age composition (more children being found in less developed regions and more elderly in the more developed regions).

With 4,432,147,000 people in the world in 1980, this means that about 47,000,000 die of all causes each year. Since about three-quarters of the world's population are in developing countries, and the death rates there are higher, about 36 million of these deaths occur in those countries and about 11 million in the developed countries. In spite of this, the rate of population growth in the developing countries is much greater than that in the industrialized

countries, because the birth rates in the former are much higher. Subtracting the crude death rate from the crude birth rate yields the "natural increase." In 1980 this was 6.2 per 1,000 per year in the industrialized countries and 20.4 per 1,000, or three times higher, in the developing countries.

MORBIDITY AND DISABILITY

Much less is known about worldwide morbidity and disability than about mortality. Official notification about sickness is confined essentially to communicable diseases in nearly all countries. In some countries, diseases linked to occupation are reportable, and in a few (where special cancer registries are organized) cancer is reportable. The completeness of all this reporting, however, is extremely uneven, particularly in developing countries.

The most common method of estimating the general burden of morbidity and disability in a population, therefore, is by household surveys. These must be done with great care, they are costly, and they are carried out in relatively few countries. In the United States, periodic household surveys of illness have been done since 1957, and certain general findings for different demographic groups are probably also relevant for other industrialized countries.

Table 2.5 presents the major findings on sickness and disability, derived from interviews of a national sample of about 41,000 households (with 111,000 persons) throughout the United States in 1981. The measurement of "restricted-activity days" is intended to encompass disorders due to all types of sickness or injury; "bed-disability days" presumably reflect more serious disorders—severe enough to confine the person to bed.

Several of the relationships shown in Table 2.5 would be found in virtually all industrialized countries and also in many developing countries. Regarding age level, except for children under age 17 years (among whom disability might be relatively greater in developing countries), the steady rise of disability rates with aging would be expected in all countries. The higher rates of disability for females, com-

Table 2.5. Days of Disability, According to Age, Sex, Race, Urban–Rural Location, and Family Income, United States, 1981

Characteristic	Days per Person per Year	
	Restricted-activity	Bed-disability
Age (years)		
Under 17	10.5	4.8
17–44	15.1	5.4
45–64	27.5	9.0
65 and over	39.9	14.0
Sex		
Male	17.5	6.0
Female	19.6	7.6
Race		
White	18.0	6.4
Black	23.6	10.3
Location		
Urban	18.4	6.7
Rural	19.0	6.9
Family income (per year)		
Under $7,000	32.1	11.9
$7,000–$9,999	23.5	8.5
$10,000–$14,999	18.1	6.3
$15,000–$24,999	16.2	5.2
$25,000 or more	13.6	5.0
TOTAL	18.5	6.8

Source: U.S. National Center for Health Statistics, *Health—United States 1983.* Washington, D.C.: U.S. Government Printing Office, December 1983, p. 127.

pared with males, are also found in almost all countries. (Life expectancies, on the other hand, are longer for females in all but a few countries.)

The higher rates of disability among blacks than among whites in the United States is undoubtedly associated with the generally lower socioeconomic levels of this racial group. The disability differences between urban and rural populations in the United States are minor; in developing countries, however, one would expect considerably higher rates among rural people. Perhaps the most interesting data in Table 2.5 concern the rates of disability according to family income levels. Lower-income families have substantially greater disability rates than those with higher incomes. Comparing the lowest- and the highest-income groups, the differential for both types of measurement is more than 2:1. We have already noted that a similar differential applies to mortality rates in other countries, and it doubtless also applies to morbidity.

Another feature of sickness, not evident from any of these tabulations, has had a substantial impact on most national health systems—its usual unpredictability in an individual. Within a certain age group or income group, at a given time and place, the rate of sickness (episodes or aggregate days of morbidity) may be generally predictable. But no one can be sure which individuals will be affected on a certain day or even during a certain year. In a random year, most individuals may experience little illness or none, while a small fraction accounts for 90 percent of the sickness burden. This basic reality has given rise to insurance in groups of people as a mechanism for financing medical services. The same irregularities do not apply to the needs for education or for nutrition in a population. But the unpredictability of sickness has generated the insurance mechanism for supporting health services, which, in both private and public forms, has come to play a part in most national health systems.

One of the relatively few nationwide household surveys of illness made in a developing country was conducted in Colombia in the 1960s. A national sample of 51,000 persons was interviewed by techniques similar to those used in the U.S. National Health Survey. The findings are reported in Table 2.6, where it may be noted that the upward gradient of disability with age replicates the findings in the United States. The numbers of days of "restricted-activity" as well as "bed-disability" per person in Colombia tend to be higher at all age levels.

The Colombia survey also solicited infor-

Table 2.6. Days of Disability by Age Level, Colombia, 1965

Age Level (years)	Days per Person per Year	
	Restricted-activity	Bed-disability
6–14	8.9	5.8
15–24	10.9	6.3
25–44	19.8	10.9
45–64	29.6	12.7
65 and over	53.6	24.9
All ages, 6 and over	13.6	7.3

Source: Ministry of Public Health of Colombia and Colombian Association of Medical Schools, *Study on Health Manpower and Medical Education in Colombia: II. Preliminary Findings.* Washington, D.C.: Pan American Health Organization, June 1967.

Table 2.7. Selected Chronic Conditions: Prevalence by Urban–Rural Location, Colombia, 1965

Chronic Condition	Chronic Conditions per 1,000	
	Urban	Rural
Asthma	30.6	29.7
Deafness	9.4	15.3
Mental retardation	5.7	6.3
Ulcers	4.4	5.9
Paralysis	3.7	3.0
Deaf-mutism	1.7	3.3
Loss of extremity	1.6	2.3
Epilepsy	0.8	2.2
Other deformities	1.2	1.9
Blindness	1.0	1.6
Defective feet	0.8	1.4
Harelip	0.4	0.3
All conditions	61.3	73.2

Source: Same as Table 2.6.

mation on the prevalence of 12 specific chronic conditions regarded as important at the time. (Findings are based on clinical and laboratory examinations of samples of people.) These findings for urban and rural populations are reported in Table 2.7. The generally higher burden of chronic disorders in the rural population is evident. By age level, chronic conditions increased steadily from 19.6 per 1,000 under the age of 1 year to 240.7 per 1,000 at 65 years and older.

A household survey of chronic diseases was conducted on a national population sample in Egypt in 1979. (The findings are based solely on responses to interview questions, without medical examinations.) For the total sample of 58,000 persons, the data are presented in Table 2.8. Nearly 58 percent of the sample population lived in rural areas, and among these people the prevalence of both forms of schistosomiasis was much higher than that in the total sample. The overall prevalence of chronic diseases reported in rural areas was also higher— 263 compared with 198 per 1,000 for the total. According to rough estimates of the World Bank, illness disrupts normal activities for about 10 percent of people's time in most developing countries, and for about 5 percent of people's time in most developed countries.

Morbidity and disability in populations of both industrialized and developing countries have been determined by countless surveys fo-

cused on detection of specific disorders. Examinations of stool specimens, for example, have shown some 92 percent of children in Bangladesh to suffer from worm infestations. In the rural areas of Thailand, blood examinations have found 40 percent of the population to be anemic. Malnutrition in children has been studied extensively. Basing this diagnosis on a finding of significantly low weight for the child's age, the results of numerous national surveys done from 1973 to 1983 are summarized in Table 2.9. Malnourished children, of course, are highly susceptible to many infectious diseases.

Another reflection of health status is the birth weight of newborns. In all developed countries infants born in 1982 with weights below a minimum standard (2,500 grams) constituted 6.9 percent of the total; in developing countries the figure was 17.6 percent.

Certain communicable diseases of high incidence have been the subject of special studies throughout the world. Tuberculosis, despite substantial declines, is still estimated to strike about 3.5 million people per year, of whom more than half a million die of it. Morbidity from tuberculosis ranges from 300 to 500 per 100,000 population per year in Burma, the Philippines, and South Korea. Rates lower than 20 per 100,000 per year are reported in Australia, Canada, Denmark, the Netherlands, and the United States.

Leprosy, known since biblical times, remains a contemporary problem in many de-

Table 2.8. Chronic Diseases Reported in National Household Survey, Egypt, 1979

Disease	Cases Reported per 1,000
Schistosomiasis (urinary)	76.0
Schistosomiasis (intestinal)	22.5
Hypertension	14.6
Other chest diseases	13.2
Digestive troubles	12.4
Diabetes	8.0
Heart diseases	7.8
Other parasites	5.6
Epileptic fits	1.9
Tuberculosis	1.1
Loss of consciousness	0.9
Other conditions	34.1
All chronic disorders	198.1

Source: Ministry of Health, Arab Republic of Egypt, *Health Interview Survey: Results of the First Cycle.* Cairo, July 1982.

Table 2.9. Estimated Malnutrition among Children in Developing Countries: Percentages by Age, 1973–1983

Region	Age, in Years					
	Under 1	1–2	2–3	3–4	4–5	0–5
Africa	15.1	35.2	29.9	23.9	23.8	25.6
Latin America and Caribbean	9.8	21.9	21.3	17.9	17.9	17.7
Asia (excluding China)	25.9	60.0	61.4	60.2	62.5	54.0
Oceania	3.9	21.3	17.3	5.6	9.0	11.5
All developing regions	——	——	——	——	——	42.3

Source: World Health Organization, Advisory Committee in Maternal and Child Health, *Health Situation Analysis and Trends: The Health Situation of Mothers and Children.* Geneva: WHO/MCH/84.5, 1984.

veloping countries. India is estimated to have 3.2 million cases, or about 5 per 1,000 population. In Africa, leprosy is found in most countries, ranging from 10 to 40 cases per 1,000. Total blindness is caused by many infections; in the Middle East it afflicts 3 percent of the population.

Debilitating diseases, of course, are not confined to the developing countries. Infectious and parasitic diseases, which strike children most extensively, are more prevalent there. But in the industrialized countries, where most people live to 50, 60, and 70 years of age, and beyond, cancer, cardiovascular diseases, diabetes, arthritis, hypertension, cataracts, and mental disorders occur with high frequency. One of the crucial paradoxes about human morbidity is that prevention does not usually reduce the overall need for medical care. Prevention (or even cure) of diseases in childhood, of course, extends life, but the child who lives to adulthood comes to be at risk for the many noncommunicable diseases. Healthful living habits (e.g., with respect to diet, exercise, avoidance of tobacco and other harmful substances, etc.) may postpone the occurrence of disease, but eventually some pathological process occurs. To an increasing extent, medical treatment enables people to live and function for long periods after a disease is first diagnosed.

By way of summary of the world burden of morbidity and disability, one may estimate conservatively that the average person experiences about 16 days of restricted activity per year. (The rate in the United States in 1981 was 18.5 days per person per year; in Colombia in 1965 it was 13.6 days; and in some smaller studies in India it was reported to be 14 to 18 days in 1963–1970.) Accordingly, this would amount to 16,000 days of disability per 1,000 persons per year. This figure, however, omits days spent in hospitals or other health care institutions; roughly these days of sickness would add about 1,000 days per 1,000 persons per year (there are 3.82 hospital beds of all types per 1,000 people in the world, and occupancy of each bed about 260 days a year would amount to around 1,000 bed-days)—or a grand total of 17,000 days of disability per 1,000 per year. In 1980, the global crude death rate was 10.6 deaths per 1,000 persons per year. Thus, the worldwide burden of sickness causing restricted activity or disability amounts to about 1,600 days for each death. For the world population of 4,776 million people in 1984, it meant more than 81 billion days of disability per year, or more than 222 million disabled persons per day.

These ratios may give an idea of how inadequately mortality data reflect the burden of sickness in a population. As noted earlier, survival to the later years of life usually means living *with* sicknesses and disabilities that may be kept under control by medical care. The reduction of deaths, therefore, does not necessarily yield a reduced rate of disability. (The rate of restricted-activity days in the United States was 18.5 per person per year, compared with 13.6 days in Colombia.) Hence, the need for health services, both therapeutic and preventive, continues to be great or greater in countries that have become highly developed socioeconomically than with the less developed countries. This explains why the operation of health systems is a matter of great social concern in countries of all economic levels.

With this background of mortality and morbidity in the world, what can be said about the determinants of health and disease in populations?

DETERMINANTS OF HEALTH AND DISEASE

The higher rates of mortality and lower life expectancies in the less economically developed countries suggest at once that poverty is a major determinant of fatal disease. The similar relationships within countries between upper and lower social classes points to the same conclusion. But "poverty" is a broad concept that encompasses many other features of life and of the physical and social environment.

Poverty implies a great deal about the quality of diet and nutrition in a family or population. It tells much about the type of housing and environmental sanitation (water supply, sewage, waste-disposal, disease vectors, etc.). It may reflect unemployment or the type of employment. Poverty may also reflect the level of education attained (although the relationship is certainly not simple and direct). Poverty usually means crowded and unpleasant living conditions. Psychologically, poverty often means frustration, hopelessness, and fatalism. Poverty usually implies, although to very varying degrees among countries, less access to effective health services.

The relative impacts on health of these social and environmental conditions have long been subjects of study and debate. In 1790, Johann Peter Frank, director general of Public Health in Austrian Lombardy, wrote of "The People's Misery: Mother of Diseases." Writing in 1976, Professor Thomas McKeown of England showed that infant mortality and deaths from tuberculosis began to decline in England in the early nineteenth century, long before the discovery of the microorganisms that caused these deaths and the development of public health and medical strategies to combat them. Improved living and working conditions— housing, nutrition, education—rather than medical intervention accounted for the gains in health.

The issue of causation of disease or the determinants of health has often focused on the question of medical care and its value versus the impact of social and environmental factors. The views of some about the importance for health of "natural" processes, in contrast to medical intervention regarded as artificial, are sometimes extreme. A widely read book written in 1975 by a former priest, Ivan Illich, argued that modern medical technology (even preventive measures such as immunizations) usually did more harm than good.

Another issue has developed with respect to the responsibilities of society or government for ensuring conditions that are conducive to health, as against the individual's responsibility for his or her own behavior. This is well illustrated by the habit of smoking tobacco (cigarettes), which has been convincingly demonstrated to cause lung cancer and to contribute strongly to cardiovascular disease. Although the decision to smoke is, of course, an individual one, it is influenced by national policies to encourage (even to subsidize) the growing of tobacco, to permit glamorous advertising of cigarettes, and so on. Some countries have put legal constraints on cigarette advertising, required cigarette packages to contain warnings that smoking "is dangerous to your health," and prohibited smoking in public places. How much of the cigarette habit, therefore, can be considered an individual rather than a social responsibility?

A former Canadian minister of health articulated in 1974 a balanced position on these issues. Society, he stated, must do the maximum to provide circumstances conducive to health, including socioeconomic conditions, a protected physical environment, and provision of comprehensive preventive and therapeutic health services. Beyond these social measures, it is an individual responsibility to maintain a prudent and healthful life-style. Such behavior, in turn, is subject to social influence through deliberate health education and the promotion of various circumstances that influence behavior.

Modifying human behavior is always difficult, whereas adjusting the environment may be feasible even if expensive. Consider the achievements of sanitary public water systems in reducing enteric diseases in industrialized countries in contrast to a policy that ignores water sources and simply calls on each household to boil its water. The major reductions in typhoid fever, dysentery, and other enteric infections in developed countries, especially in the urban centers, are clearly attributable to water treatment and public water supplies.

In the least developed countries or in the rural areas of transitional and moderately developing countries, such as in Latin America, the potential for health improvement through purely environmental measures is clearly great. Safe water supplies and sanitary sewage disposal have greatly reduced infant moratlity, as well as adult morbidity and mortality, from several enteric diseases. Vector control, through swamp drainage and pesticide spraying of houses, has contributed to vast reductions in malaria and filariasis, even though the development of insect resistance has complicated these programs. Immunizations have enormously reduced the incidence of diphtheria, poliomyelitis, measles, and other infectious diseases in numerous countries, both industrialized and developing.

Urbanization has been increasing in virtually all countries of the world. In the highly industrialized countries, this has meant much deterioration of living conditions in central-city slums, where mortality and morbidity rates are typically greater than elsewhere in the metropolis and in the suburbs. In developing countries, urbanization usually means the accretion of periurban slums and shantytowns, where disease is rampant. Urban life in both types of country usually brings higher rates of trauma, industrial accidents, and occupational diseases and more sexually transmitted disease, alcoholism, and drug abuse. In spite of these negative effects, the advantages of city life tend to outweigh its disadvantages. Improved environmental sanitation brings enormous benefits. Most (though not all) city dwellers have greater access to nutritious food. Resources for education, with all its vaues for

health, are invariably greater. Health services of every sort are more abundant in cities, for the implementation of both treatment and prevention.

Even when the potentials of classical environmental and immunological prevention have been realized, the capacity of preventive action to protect health is still large. Trauma—from road accidents, farm or industrial machinery, and simple falls—is a major cause of disability and death in all types of country, especially among teenage children and young adults. Establishing safe environmental conditions, protected machinery, safely designed vehicles, along with warnings and education, can reduce these hazards. In the United States, the age-adjusted deaths from accidents declined from 57.5 per 100,000 in 1950 to 34.9 in 1983. For motor vehicle accidents alone, the decline over this period was from 23.3 to 18.1 per 100,000 per year. Safe working conditions, especially with respect to the use of toxic substances, can reduce the risk of cancer and other disorders. Proper prenatal care can reduce the maternal risks of childbirth, as well as the risk of defective or low-birth-weight newborns. Elimination of prostitution, in its various forms, can reduce the occurrence of sexually transmitted diseases.

These preventive strategies, of course, imply various causes of disease or injury, that may be modified or eliminated before damage is done. Working and living conditions may be stressful and cause psychosomatic tensions in the individual; these, in turn, may lead to excessive smoking and drinking alcohol, to poor dietary habits, to drug abuse, to inadequate sleep, and other forms of behavior that contribute to disease. In some individuals, external pressures may lead directly to disorders such as psychoneurosis, hypertension, and peptic ulcers. The preventive challenge is to attempt to establish living and working conditions that are not stressful. If this has not been done, education and health services may help susceptible persons to cope more effectively with stress.

Cultural and religious beliefs may contribute to health problems. Sexual and reproductive processes are of concern to many religions, some of which are opposed to "artificial" contraception. As a result, women may bear far more children than is good for their health, and more than the family can economically provide for. This is quite aside from the socioeconomic problems created by excessive population in a country or region. Effective contraceptive methods are widely available throughout the world, but they are not used in most families, especially those of low income, where they are greatly needed. To cope with unwanted pregnancies, millions of women in most countries resort to abortion (legal or illegal), and this may create other health problems.

The many social and environmental factors that cause or contribute to disease or injury do not affect all persons alike. Sputum coughed up by a tuberculous patient may cause tuberculosis in a second nearby person but not in a third. A slippery road may lead to an accident for one vehicle but not for another. A prolonged stressful situation may lead one person to harmful cigarette smoking but not another. In other words, the occurrence of disease or injury depends initially on certain external conditions, but the equation defining causation also requires certain characteristics in the individual. These may be genetic to some extent, or they may be related mainly to social circumstances. Children are more liable to certain disorders than adults; some disorders strike men more often than women, or vice versa. A certain stressful environment may lead to hypertension in one person, alcoholism and liver cirrhosis in a second, severe depression in a third, and no disorders in a fourth.

A model summarizing the whole complex of influences that determine health and disease throughout the world is shown in Figure 2.1. The features that define each of the component cells of this model, of course, differ substantially from country to country. The relative impact of the forces represented by each of the cells, insofar as they contribute to disease, also differs greatly among countries. In the less developed countries the physical environment generally contributes substantially to disease and death. In the more developed countries, the physical environment has been better controlled or counteracted as a pathogenic force,

but the social environment usually contains many harmful influences.

In both types of country, health services play a role of varying importance in preventing disease and the treatment of disorders that have not been prevented. In recent decades, the effectiveness of the health services in promoting health has increased greatly. Immunization against poliomyelitis, developed only in the 1950s, has almost eliminated this once crippling disease from many countries. Antibiotic drugs have enabled doctors and other health care providers to cure patients with many infectious diseases that were once fatal or permanently disabling.

Consider the decline in death rates from certain forms of cancer over recent decades (cervical cancer, Hodgkin's disease, leukemia), which can be attributed only to health care. Even cardiovascular mortality rates have declined significantly in several industrialized countries. In the United States the age-adjusted rate was 308 deaths per 100,000 in 1950, and it fell to 210 per 100,000 in 1977. This 32 percent decline was doubtless a result of many factors—reduction in cigarette smoking, more prudent diets (mainly less animal fat), increased exercise, antihypertensive medication, and treatment of cardiac patients; all of these factors involve health service, preventive or therapeutic.

A great deal of the benefit of health care, furthermore, is reflected in betterment of the quality of life, which may be reflected only faintly in mortality rates. Modern medical care enables countless patients with chronic disorders—such as heart disease, diabetes, arthritis, visual and hearing disorders, paralysis, amputations, and so on—to function in society more effectively and happily, even though the underlying disorder is incurable.

Yet the very availability of health services depends largely on many social factors. The degree of urbanization of a country is highly relevant; medical and sanitation technologies are always more difficult to apply in rural areas. The economic level of a population affects not only the occurrence of disease, but also the resources of the health system to deal with it. The literacy rate determines the appli-

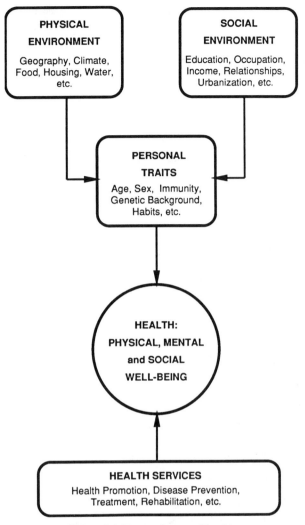

Figure 2.1 Determinants of health.

cability of many sorts of health education. A country's history—for example, as a colony of a European power—invariably influences the amount and type of resources that have been developed, such as health manpower and health facilities. The geographic terrain, the roads, and the means of transportation inevitably affect the logistics of distributing drugs and supplies from cities to rural locations. The position of women in a culture may seriously inhibit their opportunity to obtain medical care from male practitioners.

The entire political structure and ideology of a country, of course, influence the organization and operations of a health system, as we will explore more fully later. Insofar as social and political policies promote egalitarian principles, the distribution of resources and services affecting health obviously affects the well-being of the population.

An index of the equality of distribution of income in a country was developed many years ago by Professor Gini, an Italian economist. A Gini-coefficient close to 1.0 means very uneven distribution of the available wealth, and a Gini-coefficient close to 0 means greater equality in the distribution of wealth. Table 2.10 presents data for around 1973 on three pairs of countries, with each country in a pair having nearly the same GNP per capita.

Table 2.10. Gini-Coefficients (Reflecting Distribution of Wealth) of Selected Countries, with Their Life
Expectancies and Infant Mortality Rates, about 1973

Country	GNP Per Capita ($ U.S.)	Gini-Coefficient	Life Expectancy at Birth (years)	Infant Deaths per 1,000 Live Births
Sri Lanka	100	0.358	67.8	50.3
India	110	0.461	49.2	139.0
Taiwan	430	0.317	61.6	18.0
Iran	450	0.473	51.0	160.0
Yugoslavia	730	0.333	67.5	44.0
Chile	760	0.487	64.3	71.0

Source: Derived from Jaim, S., *Size Distribution of Income—A Compilation of Data.* Washington, D.C.: World Bank, 1975; also World Health
Organization sources.

The Gini-coefficient of the first country in each pair, however, is substantially lower than that of the second country—meaning that income distribution among its people is more equal. It is evident that the figures on life expectancy at birth and the infant mortality rate are significantly better for the three countries with more equalized income distribution, even though by the measure of GNP per capita they are slightly less affluent. In other words, a more egalitarian distribution of wealth in a country more than compensates for lesser overall wealth in the achievement of low mortality rates.

In certain countries or regions the influence of health services on the population's health status has been demonstrated dramatically in recent years. The state of Kerala in south India is one of the poorest among India's 20 states. The employment level has deteriorated over recent decades and the rate of economic growth has been low. The overall consumption of food—calories and proteins—has been below standard, without any significant improvement in recent years. The state government, however, has implemented progressive policies in land tenure, education, and distribution of food grains. Most important, health care programs have had high priority. State government expenditures for health care increased steadily from 1957 to 1981, at a rate greater than that of the gross domestic product. The utilization of ambulatory service in public facilities increased between 1957 and 1977 by 5.06 percent per year, while the population increase was 2.34 percent annually. In-patient hospital cases increased over this period by 6.62 percent. Immunizations were promoted,

and water supplies and sanitation were improved.

As a result of these policies, the crude death rate in Kerala declined by 1979 to 6.8 per 1,000, compared with 12.8 per 1,000 in India as a whole. In 1977 the infant mortality rate in Kerala was 47 per 1,000 live births compared with 130 in India generally. In 1979, life expectancy at birth in Kerala was 65.5 years compared with 52.0 years in all of India. Indian experts studying the Kerala situation refer to "the paradox of economic backwardness and health development." They speak of a "low mortality—high morbidity syndrome." Morbidity levels involving the diseases of poverty (diarrheal disorders, respiratory infections, etc.) have remained high, but the patients survive because of abundant and intensive medical care.

A comparative study by J. Hadley of mortality rates in 400 counties of the United States in 1980 gave striking evidence of the benefits of medical care. After controlling for other factors, such as income level, education, marital status, work experience, cigarette consumption, and prevalence of disability, population cohorts with greater estimated use of medical care were found to have lower mortality rates. A 10 percent increase in medical care expenditures per capita was estimated to reduce mortality rates by an average of 1.57 percent.

On an international level, Samuel Preston has analyzed mortality trends in 43 countries between the 1930s and 1960s. About one-third of the decline in death rates resulted from the control of infectious diseases and about one-quarter from control of respiratory diseases.

Control of diarrheal disease—which might be attributed to improved sanitation—actually lessened in importance. Examining the relationship between income level and life expectancy in the two periods (specifically 1938 and 1963) yielded the conclusion that rising wealth could explain only 16 percent of the extension in life expectancy. Improvements in the distribution of income, in educational opportunities, and in the status of women were considered modest during the 1938–1963 period. Preston concludes, therefore, that most of the gains in health status over these 25 years must be attributed to advances in health care.

Thus, in stressing the social and environmental determinants of health and disease, one should not overlook the impact of specific health services—both curative and preventive—at least in recent decades. Perhaps before 1940 or 1950, when the powerful antimicrobial drugs had not yet been developed and immunizations were available for only a few diseases in the most affluent countries, the effects of health service were quite limited. But in recent decades, it seems clear that *both* socioenvironmental conditions and health services (preventive and therapeutic) have substantially influenced the health of populations.

TRENDS IN MORTALITY AND MORBIDITY

As the world has developed economically and socially, standards of living have improved in most (though not all) countries, and levels of education and health service have advanced, the longevity of people has increased. Information on life expectancy as far back as 1850 is available for only a few countries of Europe and the United States. At that time life expectancy at birth in England, Sweden, and the United States was about 40 years.

Life expectancy data became available by 1870 for a number of Latin American countries and by 1875 for India. The striking improvements in their indices of health are shown in Table 2.11. For all 13 countries shown, the great extension of longevity over the century 1870–1970 was doubtless due

Table 2.11. Trends in Life Expectancy (at Birth) in Years, Selected Countries, 1870–1970

Country	Life Expectancy (years)	
	1870	1970
England Sweden United States	42	72
Chile Brazil Colombia Costa Rica Mexico Panama	25	59
Dominican Republic Guatemala Nicaragua	22	52
India	23 (1875)	49

Source: Basch, P., *International Health.* New York: Oxford University Press, 1978, p. 91.

mainly to the survival of infants and small children. In these age groups, the gains have been largely related to preventive measures—both environmental and personal. Still, some extension of life expectancy has occurred at all age-levels, even in the latest years of life. In the older age groups, it is likely that the extension of life has been principally due to the benefits of medical diagnosis and treatment.

In the United States, life expectancy data on various age groups are available as far back as 1900–1902. At this time, the capabilities of medical science to cure disease were relatively limited. At 65 years of age, the life expectancy of the U.S. population (both sexes and all races) was 11.9 additional years. It was higher for females and for the white race. The extension of life expectancy over the next 80 years in the United States was as follows:

Year	Additional Years of Life Expectancy at 65 Years of Age (United States)
1900–1902	11.9
1950	13.9
1960	14.3
1970	15.2
1980	16.4
1983	16.8

Source: U.S. National Center for Health Statistics, *Health—United States 1984.* Washington, D.C.: U.S. Government Printing Office, 1984.

Thus, in 1983, residents of the United States who had survived to age 65 could expect to live another 16.8 years or 4.9 years (41 percent) longer than they could have expected in 1900–1902. These additional years of life, moreover, would usually be fairly comfortable years, although not free from various ailments. As noted earlier, health services have succeeded in keeping people alive and often functioning reasonably well in society *with* various chronic or even acute disorders.

Indications of life with *higher* rates of disability are not abundant, but the U.S. National Health Survey has shown signs of this over a recent decade. Adjusting for the changed age-composition over time, the U.S. data on various indicators of disease or disability were as follows:

Indicator of Disorder (United States)	Number per Person per Year	
	1970	1981
Restricted activity days	8.5	9.9
Bed-disability days	3.8	4.4
Bouts of acute disorder	2.04	2.27

Source: Same as previous table.

Without exception, the same upward trend is found on examination of each age group separately. A rising volume of disability, over recent years at least, seems to be due not only to the changing age composition of the population (i.e., more people surviving to the older age groups), but also to the survival of people with various physical and mental disorders at every age level.

One medical observer, James Fries, has argued that, with scientific advances, life expectancy will not only increase in all countries but the occurrence of significant disability may also be postponed. According to Fries, robust health and vitality will eventually prevail at all age levels until a very advanced age—perhaps 85 years or more—when over a relatively brief period, terminal illness will set in and life will end. The needs for medical care, therefore, will greatly diminish. This happy hypothesis is based on observation of the extending average longevity in the United States and the reduced

rates of mortality below age 60. It does not seem to be borne out, however, by studies of *morbidity* in the population that survives in both the United States and other countries. With decreasing mortality in the young and adult years, the demands for medical care do not decline, but increase. (Quick death following any significant illness would be the surest way to reduce the needs for health service in a population.)

For Africa, Asia, and other regions of the developing world, data on trends are available only for recent decades. According to the World Health Organization and the Population Division of the United Nations, life expectancy at birth for the entire world rose from 45.9 years in 1950–1955 to 59.6 years in 1980–1985. The details, by region, are shown in Table 2.12. In spite of serious world economic crises, wars, famines, and other social disasters during this 30-year period, the remarkable fact is that health status—insofar as it is reflected by life expectancy at birth—has improved in all regions of the world.

The poorest economic levels, shown clearly in the figures for GNP per capita, are in Africa and South Asia (largely India). These two regions had the lowest life expectancies in 1950–1955, and they remain the lowest today. Their improvements over three decades, nevertheless, have been substantial. Contrary to common assertions, the gap between Africa and the highly developed countries of the world has not been increasing. It has decreased from a differential of 27.7 years in 1950–1955

Table 2.12. Life Expectancy at Birth in Major World Regions, 1950–1985

Region	Life Expectancy at Birth (years)	
	1950–1955	1980–1985
Africa	38.0	49.9
South Asia	38.8	54.4
East Asia	42.7	68.4
Latin America	51.2	64.5
All developing countries	41.0	57.6
All developed countries	65.7	72.3
World total	45.9	59.6

Source: United Nations, Department of International Economic and Social Affairs, *World Population Prospects 1988* (Population Studies No. 106). New York: U.N., 1989, pp. 166–189.

to one of 22.4 years in 1980–1985. Most impressive has been the extension of life expectancy over the three decades in East Asia (largely representing China and Japan). Advancing by 23.7 years or 56 percent, the life expectancy there of 68.4 years in 1980–1985 nearly reached the level of many of the old industrialized countries.

As might be expected from life expectancy trends, infant mortality rates have also declined sharply over recent decades. Examining broad regions of the world, the following data show the trends:

Region	Infant Deaths per 1,000 Live Births	
	1950–1955	1980–1985
Africa	187	116
South Asia	189	113
East Asia	181	36
Latin America	126	63
Oceania	67	31
Northern America	29	11
Europe	62	15
USSR	73	26
World total	155	79

Source: Same as Table 2.12, pp. 190–197.

Trends in selected reportable communicable diseases have not been so encouraging. Malaria is still a major world problem. The number of reported cases of this insect-borne parasitic disease has undulated over the years, as the anopheles mosquito has developed resistance to various insecticides and the parasite in human blood has become resistant to various drugs. The trend in the world total of reported malaria cases in selected years has been as follows.

Year	Malaria Cases Reported Globally
1962	3,290,000
1967	5,855,000
1972	7,686,000
1977	15,590,000
1982	6,460,000

Source: World Health Organization, "The World Malaria Situation," different years.

Much of this irregularity in the trend of malaria cases may be attributable to changes in the thoroughness of reporting. Still, in Latin America, parts of Africa, and elsewhere the disease has clearly been on the increase. In some countries, on the other hand—such as Venezuela, Cuba, the United States, Spain, Italy, Hungary, Bulgaria, Romania, Yugoslavia, and Australia—where malaria was once prevalent, it has now been entirely eradicated.

Cholera is another infectious disease with uneven trends worldwide, as the following data show.

Year	Cases of Cholera Reported
1963	59,600
1968	36,400
1973	112,200
1978	78,700
1982	54,900

Source: World Health Organization.

This bacterial disease is concentrated heavily in certain countries, such as India, the Philippines, Indonesia, Ghana, Bangladesh, and Burma, but in 1981 some cases were reported in as many as 49 countries.

The rising trends of total morbidity and disability over a recent decade were shown earlier for the United States, even when the age composition was adjusted for the two time periods. Age adjustment, however, is a statistical manipulation, and we know that in the real world the age composition of populations is changing with increased life expectancies; higher proportions of people in all regions of the world are living into the older age groups. This means even more that a higher total volume of disease and disability must be expected in virtually all countries. (Table 2.5 showed the higher rate of disability in the older age groups of the United States in 1981.) Lest one suspect a different situation in less developed countries, the relationship of total disability to age level in Colombia for 1965 is shown in Table 2.13. Greater life expectancy clearly means a higher proportion of persons surviving to the later years, when rates of sickness and disability are substantially higher. The United Nations has forecast that in developing countries, where only 6 percent of the population was 60 years of age and over in 1970, this age group will constitute 12 percent of the population by the year 2025.

Table 2.13. Disability and Age Level in a Developing Country: Disability Days per Person per Year by Age-Level, Colombia, 1965

| Age Level (years) | Days per Person per Year | |
	Restricted Activity	Bed-Disability
6–14	8.9	5.8
15–24	10.9	6.3
25–44	19.8	10.9
45–64	29.6	12.7
65 and over	53.6	24.9
All ages	13.6	7.3

Source: Same as Table 2.6.

The same household survey of 1965 in Colombia determined the number of chronic conditions per 1,000 population reported in each age group. These rates were as follows.

Age Group (years)	Chronic Conditions per 1,000
Under 1	19.6
1–4	54.6
5–14	55.1
15–24	48.3
25–44	67.2
45–64	110.0
65 and over	240.7

Source: Same as Table 2.6.

The chronic disorders reported most frequently were asthma, deafness, mental retardation, ulcers, paralysis, deaf-mutism, loss of extremity, epilepsy, and blindness. Noticeably lacking were heart ailments and cancer, but one must recall that this information was drawn from a household survey of a largely rural population in a developing country, where access to education and medical services at the time was sparse.

In the reduction of certain disorders, health services have undoubtedly been decisive in recent decades. Tuberculosis is a disease principally of young and middle-aged adults; thus, changes in the age composition of the population would not markedly affect its rate of incidence or mortality. Between 1948 and 1971, the global rate of tuberculosis mortality declined by 51 percent. This decline can hardly be attributed to improved environmental conditions over this period; it must have been due to health care interventions—to tuberculosis case-finding, contact-tracing, isolation of pa-

tients, treatment of active cases with chemotherapeutic drugs, and BCG vaccination of newborns in developing countries. In the United States, where BCG vaccination is seldom used but other strategies are widely applied, the rate of reported cases of tuberculosis declined from 80.5 per 100,000 in 1950 to 11.0 in 1982. In other industrialized countries, such as Australia, Canada, Denmark, Ireland, and the Netherlands, respiratory tract tuberculosis declined between 1947 and 1967 by more than 90 percent.

For diseases preventable by immunization, the reduced incidence over recent decades, in countries where immunizations are extensively carried out, has been dramatic. In the United States, even though immunizations have not reached 100 percent of children, the trend in reported cases of immunizable diseases has been as follows.

| Disease | Cases Reported per 100,000 | | |
	1950	1970	1982
Diphtheria	8.83	0.21	0.00
Measles	211.01	23.23	0.74
Rubella	———	27.75	1.00
Pertussis	79.82	2.08	0.82
Mumps	———	55.55	2.46
Poliomyelitis	22.02	0.02	0.00

Source: Same as Table 2.5.

In spite of these impressive declines in infectious diseases, which strike mainly the young, the childhood diarrheas and respiratory infections, for which immunizations are not available, are still rampant in developing countries. Among adults, the principal determinant of overall morbidity in the world has been the higher proportions of persons living to the older age groups. Even the prevention of death from cardiovascular diseases and certain forms of cancer in many industrialized countries, since 1950, has not reduced the burden of disability in the population. Patients surviving with these chronic disorders require continuing medical care to live comfortably and function socially.

In the less developed countries, such care is seldom available to the general population, so that these chronic disorders have not yet shown a decline in either mortality or morbidity. In fact, developing countries with the most dramatic reductions of communicable disease, malnutrition, and infant deaths—such as Sri Lanka, Costa Rica, Cuba, the Indian state of Kerala, and the People's Republic of China— report *rising* rates of heart disease and cancer as a reflection of their health accomplishments. In other words, they are becoming more like the highly developed countries (two or three decades ago).

Worldwide trends in fertility have a major bearing on the health of the population, particularly on the needs for health service. Since World War II, international and national agencies have been concerned about the relationships of world population to economic development. With high rates of birth and natural increase (birth rate minus death rate), it is feared that many developing countries might nullify the benefits of economic development with excessive growth of national populations to feed, educate, and care for. While the theoretical issue, long ago posed by Malthus, may be debated, the great majority of developing countries have adopted the principle that population growth should be slowed down. Even if the population issue is set aside, as the World Health Organization does, the principle of enabling families to control their size (i.e., through family planning) warrants the provision of contraceptive measures as an element of health service. Policies along this line have been effective in most countries, to varying degrees.

Considering the world as a whole, the crude birth rate has declined from 34.8 per 1,000 population per year in 1960–1964 to 27.5 per 1,000 in 1980–1984. The differential in rates among different regions, however, is great, as Table 2.14 shows. Although the decline of the birth rate in Africa has been small (5 percent), in all the other developing regions it has been 20 percent or more, and in East Asia (largely China) the birth rate has declined by 41 percent in two decades.

Within countries, birth rates tend to be highest in lower income groups and among rural populations. Reductions in birth rates, through the use of contraception, usually occur first and most consistently in families with higher educational levels, typically urban

Table 2.14. Birth Rate Trends in World Regions 1960–1964 to 1980–1984

Region	Births per 1,000 per Year	
	1960–1964	1980–1984
Africa	47.9	45.6
Latin America	41.0	32.3
South Asia	44.8	34.8
East Asia	32.2	19.1
Oceania	26.7	21.4
Europe	18.7	14.1
USSR	22.3	18.8
North America	22.8	17.3
Total world	34.8	27.5

Source: Same as Table 2.12.

families of higher income. Large numbers of children born to poor families are sometimes "justified" as a form of "social security" for aging parents, but more often they constitute a growing burden—economic, social, and psychological. They are also a drain on the mother's health, both through the stress of repeated pregnancies and the demands of child-rearing.

The achievement of reduced fertility rates in countries requires energetic efforts at disseminating contraceptive knowledge and devices. Generally improved standards of living are equally or more crucial. The benefits of smaller family size and lower rates of population growth, in virtually all countries, must be counted as contributing to the improvement of health status.

These positive trends in the health of populations of virtually all countries should indicate that the countless social efforts applied since World War II have not been in vain. Political rhetoric may stress the differences between rich nations and poor—and these differences, of course, are real—but the many strategies of governments to increase the accessibility of health services have had measurable effects. The substantially better health records of more economically developed countries should not obscure the fact that even in the least developed countries, improvements have been achieved.

The worldwide economic difficulties of the 1980s have slowed the development of organized health programs in many countries. One might expect health status measurements to reflect these deficiencies. Yet, up to the present, significant evidence of declining health in the developing countries is lacking. Thus, in Africa's largest country, Nigeria, between 1982 and 1987 the infant mortality rate declined further from 120 to 106 deaths per 1,000 live births. In Brazil, Latin America's largest country, infant deaths declined over these recent years from 70 to 64 per 1,000 live births. In India, with more than 700,000,000 people, mostly impoverished, the infant mortality rate has gone from 120 in 1982 to 100 in 1987. Some Latin American countries reported evidence of greater childhood malnutrition in the 1980s, but not enough to cause an increase in mortality rates; in some countries supplementary feeding programs were even accelerated.

HEALTH NEEDS AND HEALTH SYSTEMS

Disorders contributing to mortality as well as to morbidity, disability, and even personal pain or anxiety, all constitute health problems or health needs. The burden of disease and death throughout the world is the major reason for health systems. These involve not only the development of techniques to treat disease and their application, but also the discovery and implementation of strategies for prevention and health promotion.

The need for health care of a child with a high fever, for example, is obvious enough. But much health need is not so obvious. An adult with a vague but persistent headache has a serious health need for diagnosis, because the symptom may reflect an underlying hypertension, a brain tumor, or some other condition requiring care. The need for preventive health service is more subtle, insofar as such service is usually required *before* a person becomes sick. Prevention calls for understanding hazards of the environment, the harmful effects of certain types of behavior, the nature of a proper diet, and so on. Prevention also calls for aggressive actions, such as immunizations, prenatal examinations, routine case-detection tests (to discover disease without symptoms), and periodic "checkups" of populations at special risk. The diagnosis of any disorder at an early

stage, when treatment is usually more effective and disability can be averted, is also preventive.

As Hugh Leavell and Gurney Clark pointed out many years ago (in 1953), no sharp line exists between prevention and treatment. Prevention is carried out at four levels (1) health promotion (e.g., good nutrition), (2) protection against specific diseases (e.g., immunization), (3) early case detection (e.g., identifying tuberculosis through a routine chest x-ray), and (4) prompt treatment to prevent disability (e.g., therapy of glaucoma to prevent blindness). With this broad conception of prevention, it is clear that health needs exist in all populations at all times.

The objectives of a health system go even beyond the treatment and the prevention of disease. The dimensions of human well-being go beyond the occurrence of explicit disease entities. Though no specific diagnosis is determined, pain or discomfort may be relieved and mental anguish reduced. In many countries, "tonics" are widely used by elderly and frail individuals to increase their general sense of physical and mental well-being.

The various measures of mortality, morbidity, and disability reviewed in this chapter all indirectly reflect health status. Much remains to be done for nations or international bodies to develop measurements of health in a positive sense. Attempts have been made to quantify the physical and mental prowess in individuals, or even the capacity to cope with various forms of stress. But nowhere have such measurements been accomplished on a national scale. For the present, the various indicators of a *loss* of health must be accepted as evidence of the vast needs of health service, both therapeutic and preventive, throughout the world.

The burden of disease, disability, and death in all countries—from the most disease-ridden to the healthiest—calls for stronger development of comprehensive preventive and curative health services. One need not argue whether health care is more important or less important than general standards of living. Both are obviously important. Health care and the construction of housing, for example, both contribute to the health status of the population. They complement each other in the sense that healthy people can construct better housing, and better housing contributes to the health of people. Good agriculture produces more food, and good nutrition can mean healthier and more productive farmers.

Likewise, within health systems, there should be a reasonable balance between prevention and treatment, or more accurately a balance among environmental control, personal prevention, early medical care, and late medical treatment. Prevention should be emphasized not because it is "cheaper than cure"; it may often be less expensive in an individual, but in a large population it can be very costly. Nevertheless, prevention should have priority because it is more humane. An enormous volume of preventable disease and injury occurs in populations of even the most favored countries. Disorders occur because knowledge of how to prevent them has not been applied. The latter circumstance may be due to negligence, but it is more often due to poverty and lack of sufficient political will.

A pervasive problem in every health system is the achievement of equity in the distribution of resources and services. This is not the same as equality. As we have seen, there are vast differences in the rates of morbidity and disability in different social classes (income groups), age groups, and regional populations. These disparities mean differential needs for health services. Yet all too often services are more abundant where needs are less, and vice versa. Health system equity demands adjustments, through various interventions in market dynamics.

In summary, disease and disability are caused by countless biological, environmental, and social influences, which vary enormously from country to country. Variations are also great within national populations of different age levels, social classes, living conditions, personal behavior, and many other characteristics. Every country has developed a national health system to cope with disease and promote health, with extremely variable results. Mortality data indicate that for at least a century, the health status of populations throughout the world has improved, principally because of advances in socioeconomic development. Since about 1950, however, the benefits of health systems have been substantial.

Great differences in health status persist, of course, between countries with highly developed and weakly developed economies and with health systems of generally corresponding strength. Discrepancies in the survival of infants, children, women, and men among these countries are daily tragedies. The application of current knowledge in Africa, Asia, and Latin America could soon save millions of lives.

Yet improvements have occurred in all countries over the last several decades. Life expectancies at birth are growing longer, because of achievements in both prevention and medical care. Larger proportions of national populations, therefore, live to the older-age brackets, when chronic noncommunicable diseases are more prevalent. The success of health systems in reducing deaths among the young does not relieve them of the tasks of providing health care to the elderly. The dynamics of health create an ever-increasing demand for effective and equitable national health systems.

REFERENCES

Basch, Paul F., *International Health.* New York: Oxford University Press, 1978, p. 191.

Bruer, John, "The Great Neglected Diseases." *RF Illustrated* (The Rockefeller Foundation), June 1982, pp. 26–28.

Crawford, R. "You Are Dangerous to Your Health: The Ideology and Politics of Victim Blaming." *International Journal of Health Services,* 7:663–680, 1977.

Davies, A. M., "Epidemiology and the Challenge of Aging." *International Journal of Epidemiology,* 14(1):9–21, 1985.

Dohrenwend, B. S., and B. P. Dohrenwend (Editors), *Stressful Life Events and Their Contexts.* New York: Prodist, 1981.

Fries, James F., "Aging, Natural Death, and the Compression of Morbidity." *New England Journal of Medicine,* 303:130–135, 17 July 1980.

Goldsmith, John R., "Young Adults Mortality as an Index Reflecting Social and Economic Impacts on Health." Faculty of Health Sciences, Ben Gurion University of the Negev, 1982 (unpublished document).

Grosse, Robert N., and Barbara H. Perry, "Correlates of Life Expectancy in Less Developed

Countries." *Health Policy and Education,* March 1982, pp. 275–304.

Hadley, J., *More Medical Care, Better Health?* Washington, D.C.: Urban Institute Press, 1982.

Illich, Ivan, *Medical Nemesis: The Expropriation of Health.* New York: Random House, 1975.

Kroeger, Axel, "Health Interview Surveys in Developing Countries: A Review of the Methods and Results." *International Journal of Epidemiology,* 12(4):465–481, December 1983.

Lalonde, Marc, *A New Perspective on the Health of Canadians: A Working Document.* Ottawa: Health and Welfare Canada, April 1974.

Leavell, H. R., and E. G. Clark, *Textbook of Preventive Medicine.* New York: McGraw-Hill Book Co., 1953.

McKeown, Thomas, *The Role of Medicine: Dream, Mirage, or Nemesis.* London: Nuffield Provincial Hospitals Trust, 1976.

Ministry of Health, Arab Republic of Egypt, *Health Interview Survey: Results of the First Cycle,* Cairo, July 1982, p. 70.

Ministry of Public Health of Colombia and Colombian Association of Medical Schools, *Study on Health Manpower and Medical Education in Colombia: II. Preliminary Findings.* Washington, D.C.: Pan American Health Organization, June 1967, pp. 25–29.

Musgrove, Philip, "The Impact of the Economic Crisis on Health and Health Care in Latin America and the Caribbean." *WHO Chronicle,* 40(4):152–157, 1986.

Myers, George C., and Kenneth G. Manton, "Compression of Mortality: Myth or Reality?" *Gerontologist,* 24(4):346–353, 1984.

Pan American Health Organization, *Health Conditions in the Americas 1977–1980.* Washington, D.C.: PAHO Scientific Publication No. 427, 1982, p. 23.

Panikar, P. G. K., and C. R. Soman, *Health Status of Kerala: The Paradox of Economic Backwardness and Health Development.* Trivandrum (India): Centre for Development Studies, 1984.

Preston, Samuel H. *Mortality Patterns in National Populations, with Special Reference to Recorded Causes of Death.* New York: Academic Press, 1976.

Rodgers, G. B., "Income and Inequality as Determinants of Mortality: An International Cross-Section Analysis." *Population Studies,* 33(2):343–351, July 1979.

Roemer, Milton I., "The Value of Medical Care for Health Promotion." *American Journal of Public Health,* 74(3):243–248, March 1984.

Roemer, Ruth, *Legislative Action to Combat the World Smoking Epidemic.* Geneva: World Health Organization, 1982.

Sigerist, Henry E, *Landmarks in the History of Hygiene.* London: Oxford University Press, 1956, pp. 47–63.

U.S. National Center for Health Statistics, *Health—United States 1983.* Washington, D.C.: U.S. Government Printing Office, December 1983, p. 127. Same for 1984.

U.S. Public Health Service, *Healthy People: The Surgeon-General's Report on Health Promotion and Disease Prevention.* Washington, D.C.: U.S. Government Printing Office, 1979.

United Nations Children's Fund, *The State of the World's Children.* New York: UNICEF, 1985.

United Nations, Department of International Economic and Social Affairs, *World Population Prospects 1988* (Population Studies No. 106). New York: U.N., 1989, pp. 166–197.

Viel, Benjamin, *The Demographic Explosion: The Latin American Experience.* New York: John Wiley & Sons, 1976.

Wasi, Prawase, "Thailand," in J. Z. Bowers and E. F. Purcell (Editors), *The Impact of Health Services on Medical Education: A Global View.* New York: Josiah Macy, Jr. Foundation, 1979, pp. 279–303.

World Bank, *World Development Report.* Washington, D.C.: World Bank, 1985.

World Health Organization, *World Health Statistics Annual.* Geneva: WHO, 1983.

World Health Organization, *Health Aspects of Family Planning.* Geneva: Report of a WHO Scientific Group (Technical Report Series 442), 1970.

World Health Organization, Advisory Committee in Maternal and Child Health, *Health Situation Analysis and Trends: The Health Situation of Mothers and Children.* Geneva: WHO/MCH/84.5, 1984.

World Health Organization, *Sixth Report of the World Health Situation 1973–1977, Part One.* Geneva, 1980, p. 48.

World Health Organization, *Prevention of Perinatal Morbidity and Mortality.* Geneva: WHO (Public Health Papers No. 42), 1972.

World Health Organization, "World Malaria Situation 1983." *World Health Statistics,* 38(2):193–231, 1985.

World Bank, *Health: Sector Policy Paper.* Washington, D.C.: World Bank, February 1980.

CHAPTER THREE

Health System Components and Their Relationships

In response to the burdens of disease, disability, and death, numerous resources have been developed and social actions taken in every country. The combined structure and functional relationships of these resources and actions contribute to a national health system. Every country has such a system, just as it has systems of agriculture, industry, education, justice, and so on. The diverse concepts of a "system," and the meaning of a "health system" in particular, have been reviewed in the introductory chapter; here we regard a health system as the *combination of resources, organization, financing, and management that culminate in the delivery of health services to the population.*

This does not imply, of course, that health services are the only or even the most important determinants of health. As we already observed, numerous social and environmental factors probably influence health more fundamentally than health services. Yet the intervention of health services, both therapeutic and preventive, can modify the health of a population substantially, in spite of numerous deleterious effects from the general circumstances of living.

THE OBJECTIVES AND BOUNDARIES OF HEALTH SYSTEMS

It may be noted that the preceding definition does not include within a health system all factors that *influence* health. If it did, the scope of health systems would be hopelessly broad; virtually all aspects of nature, society, and human relations influence health. The health system, however, is bound by the phenomena that culminate in health services. Insofar as other social systems or sectors have an impact on health, it becomes necessary to mobilize "intersectoral actions."

National health systems may show varying degrees of complexity and coherence, but it is not reasonable to describe a country's arrangements for health care—as one hears so often about the health situation in the United States—as being a "nonsystem." The U.S. health system happens to be especially complex, but it is still a system that can be analyzed. At the other extreme, the structure and operations that result in health care on a small island-state of the South Pacific may be rudimentary, but they are still analyzable as a health system.

Among the approximately 165 countries in the world, no two health systems are exactly like—for many reasons we explore later. In fact, within any one country, the structure and operations of the health system are continually changing. Yet, at any given time, one can analyze any country's health system according to certain universal components. Just as every automobile has a motor and wheels and a place for passengers, so every health system has definite components even though the characteristics of each component may vary greatly.

The analysis of any system should be comprehensive, and yet it must have boundaries; these are defined by the main objective to which the system is oriented. The primary objective of health systems, almost everyone would agree, is to promote health or recover it if disease or injury has occurred. Obviously, however, a health system may also have other secondary objectives, such as to provide employment for health personnel or to enhance industrial production through maintenance of healthy workers.

One may engage in philosophical arguments about health as an end in itself or as the means to other ends, such as happiness, economic productivity, or military capabilities. Whatever these *ultimate* objectives may be, the immediate and primary purpose of the health system is to advance and protect the health of people. If health services are provided mainly to augment the income of a doctor, or for any other nonhealth purpose, serious ethical and even legal problems are encountered.

Even this restricted definition of a health system—as being devoted *primarily* to protecting or improving the health of people—is not free from ambiguity. Bed care in a hospital, for example, is clearly a health service that falls within the scope of a health system, but what about the care of an elderly person in a custodial institution? Vitamin therapy of a child with rickets is likewise an obvious activity within a health system, but what about a subsidized lunch program for all school children? The custodial institution and the school lunch program manifestly influence the health of the persons served, but this is not their primary purpose. In the housing of the elderly or the feeding or school children, health protection is a by-product but not the main objective.

What then should be included within the boundaries of a health system? Study of the complex of resources and activities that lie behind the provision of health services in any country discloses a number of major clusters of action. In earlier societies, when cities had not yet taken shape and government had hardly developed, the ministrations of a "medicine man" were the totality of health systems. The process of historical development to the current complexities of health systems is explored later, but here we simply note that in the modern world the structure and functions of health systems almost everywhere have become infinitely more complex.

In every national health system today, it is relatively easy to identify five major interconnected component activities: (1) several types of resources (human and physical) must be produced or available in some way; (2) varying greatly among countries, health programs are organized from these resources, and there is also usually an informal free market of medical care; (3) economic support from several different sources is used for financing both the formation of health resources and the provision of the services they offer; (4) to achieve the best feasible services in various organized programs (public and private), management of some sort is necessary; and finally (5) the ultimate delivery of various services to people, sick or well, may follow diverse patterns in different national systems and even for different population groups within one system. Thus, in a few words, the major components of any national health system can be summarized under five simple terms as follows:

1. Production of resources
2. Organization of programs
3. Economic support mechanisms
4. Management methods
5. Delivery of services

The principal interrelationships of these components are shown in Figure 3.1. The health system, it can be noted, is within the broken lines or boundaries; outside these lines are the health problems or needs that feed into the system, on one side, and, on the other side, the health results (hopefully improvements) that come from the operation of the system.

The health system in any country today has developed slowly over the centuries, with inputs from religion, science, industry, urbanization, communication, international trade, war, police power, and many social phenomena. In each country, the level of economic development and the dominant political ideology have decisive effects on the characteristics of each component of the health system, which must be explored in a later chapter.

A complete mapping of the relationship among the five main components of health systems would require many more lines and arrows than appear in Figure 3.1. Likewise, within each of the component boxes are numerous subdivisions, many of which may be regarded as subsystems, and even a further level of sub-subsystems. Within the compo-

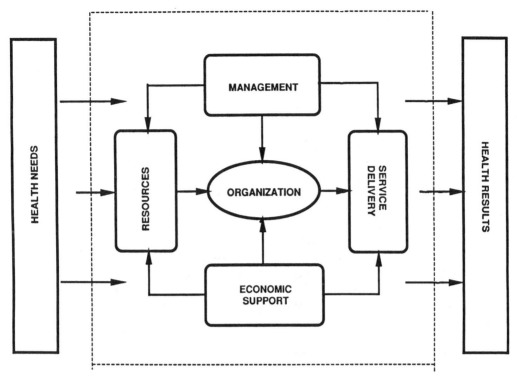

Figure 3.1 Model of a national health system, showing its components and their relationships to health status.

nent "Production of Resources," for example, there is a subdivision for "health manpower development," and the latter includes a further subdivision for "education of nurses." Within the component "Organization of Programs," there is virtually always a subdivision for "voluntary health agencies," and under this might come an "association for tuberculosis." The more profoundly one analyzes the health systems of a country, the more one finds differences from other countries in the content and characteristics of each of the five main components.

Against this general background on the meaning of health systems, we examine in more detail the specific content of each of the five system components in any country.

PRODUCTION OF RESOURCES

Every health system must have resources of several types. There must be persons capable

of providing health services, or *health manpower*. There must be *facilities* in which the health personnel can do their work—even if these are only the homes of traditional healers. There must be *commodities* or supplies of some sort, used in the care of patients, particularly drugs. And finally, there must be a body of *knowl:dge,* applied in the system for various curative or preventive purposes; the application of knowledge is often regarded as technology. (Note that, notwithstanding frequent reference to "financial resources," financing or economic support is not considered here to be a resource. Rather, it is a medium of exchange, which may be converted into resources or health services, and is discussed later.)

Each of these four types of resource must be produced or acquired in some way. Health manpower or personnel are ordinarily trained in a certain manner or they may be acquired by immigration from another country. Health facilities of various sorts must be constructed and the funds necessary to do this—along with the labor, the materials, and so on—must be mobilized. Health commodities, such as drugs or bandages or laboratory equipment, must be manufactured or imported or sometimes collected from the natural environment (e.g., medicinal herbs). Knowledge must be acquired by research or observation or, to a great extent, by dissemination from other places, as well as by accumulation from lessons of the past. The many actions involved in production or acquisition of each of these types of health resource require elaboration.

Health Manpower

As the health sciences have developed, the types and numbers of various kinds of health manpower have multiplied. For many historical reasons physicians play a key role in all health systems, but there are scores of other categories of health personnel everywhere. More highly developed countries usually have a greater variety than do less developed countries. In a very general way, one can classify health manpower as (a) physicians, (b) other personnel with independent health roles, (c) allied health personnel who essentially support the physician or other independent health professionals, and (d) allied personnel who serve people directly, but usually under the nominal supervision of another person.

Physicians. Although physicians play an important part in every national health system, they are not easy to define. Some years ago, the member nations of the World Health Organization attempted to define the *physician* in terms of his or her qualifications and functions, for the purpose of achieving international equality and recognition. After lengthy debate, the best formulation that could be agreed on in 1972 was as follows:

> A physician is a person who, having been regularly admitted to a medical school, duly recognized in the country in which it is located, has successfully completed the prescribed course of studies in medicine and has acquired the requisite qualifications to be legally licensed to practice medicine (comprising prevention, diagnosis, treatment, and rehabilitation),

using independent judgement, to promote community and individual health.

In other words, a physician was defined as anyone trained to be a physician for the "independent" promotion of health, according to the legal standards of each country. The requirements of education and licensure of physicians, in effect, are so variable among countries that it was found quite impossible to establish any universally acceptable international standards.

By such a definition, all countries have professional persons, with certain formal education, who are recognized as the principal experts in the diagnosis and treatment of disease as well as in the prevention of sickness or promotion of health. In most but not all countries, medical schools or medical faculties are established within universities. Typically, medical education begins with the study of natural sciences—chemistry, biology, physics, anatomy, physiology, pathology, and other subjects. Next comes theoretical study of the various components of clinical medicine—pediatrics, surgery, obstetrics, gynecology, psychiatry, internal medicine, and so on. The social and psychological aspects of disease and the strategies for health promotion and disease prevention are getting increasing attention in the preparation of physicians. Finally, the student engages in clinical training by examination and treatment of patients with a wide range of diseases, to learn the practical application of theoretical principles. The exact sequence, duration, and manner of teaching these subjects, of course, differ considerably among countries and often within different medical schools of one country.

The graduate of a medical school is essentially a generalist in human disease, its diagnosis and treatment—often known as a *general practitioner.* As knowledge and technology have expanded, and the human value of medical services has become increasingly appreciated, specialization in medicine developed. In all health systems—more so in the more highly industrialized countries—physicians have come to be trained in a wide spectrum of specialties. The supplemental training is usually undertaken through a *residency* in hospitals, requiring several years. Because of this lengthy training, it is costly to prepare specialists, and their services are typically more expensive than those of general practitioners. Greater supplies and use of specialists, therefore, ordinarily require higher expenditures in a country's health system.

Physicians specialize along several lines. Their work may concentrate on certain organs or organ systems, such as in ophthalmology, cardiology, or neurology. Specialization may be developed around certain technological approaches, such as in radiology, pathology, or anesthesiology. Demographic groups may be the focus, such as in pediatrics or gynecology, and more recently gerontology. Internal (or general) medicine has subspecialties in cardiology, endocrinology, gastroenterology, nephrology, and so on. Surgical specialties, involving cutting, may concentrate on the skeletal system (orthopedics), the brain and nervous system (neurosurgery), or other body parts.

In reaction to the worldwide movement toward specialization many countries have elevated the position of the general practitioner; this has been done through periodic continuing education, higher fees or salaries; provision of personnel support in health centers, and other means. Several countries have introduced a postgraduate residency program in general or family medicine, to recognize general practice as a specialty of medicine.

Other Independent Health Practitioners. The most widespread type of health manpower, to whom patients have direct access throughout the world, is the "traditional practitioner" or *traditional healer.* Historically, of course, these providers of health care are the oldest personnel, long antedating the rise of scientific medicine. In almost all developing countries they still play a significant role, often being much more numerous than trained modern physicians.

There are hundreds of types of traditional healers, whose exact characteristics are reviewed later. Their methods of treatment are based principally on (a) religious or magical concepts of disease, (b) empirical knowledge involving the use of herbal or other natural products, or (c) a combination of these two approaches. Sometimes, particularly in Asia, these practitioners undertake a formal course of study, and sometimes they learn their skills only through apprenticeship to an older practitioner. Traditional healers are usually separate and independent health manpower resources, but sometimes they are absorbed (fully or partially) into the official health program of the government. In certain countries, they are legally prohibited.

Closely related to the traditional healer in nearly all developing countries is the *traditional birth attendant.* Usually a mature woman, who has given birth to many of her own children, she delivers babies or oversees childbirths in the homes of mothers—predominantly in rural areas, but often in the cities as well. (The TBA is not to be confused with the trained midwife or nurse-midwife, discussed later.) She has learned her skills mainly by experience and by becoming familiar with local customs and childbirth practices. TBAs are so extensively used for maternity service in developing countries that many government health authorities have systematically trained them in hygienic practices. Sometimes they are provided devices for cutting the infant's umbilical cord properly and are instructed in how to sterilize the instruments.

In many economically developed countries (as well as in others) there are other providers of health care, not qualified as physicians nor as healers, who trace their practices to an ancient religious or empirical doctrine. These are called sectarian or *cultist practitioners,* and their theory of disease and its treatment has generally arisen within recent times. Such practitioners include the chiropractor, who claims to be able to treat all diseases by manipulating the spinal column, and the homeopath, who treats almost all disorders with extremely diluted drugs. Other such cultists include the naturopath or food faddist, who treats every ailment by special diets, and the Christian Science practitioner, who uses various forms of prayer and religious dialogue. At one time, osteopaths followed a therapeutic doctrine similar to that of chiropractic, but they have gradually broadened their concepts to correspond essentially to those of general modern medicine (sometimes called *allopathy*). The laws of numerous countries protect the right of many of these practitioners to provide services, as long as patients seek their help.

Other independent practitioners are trained to do scientifically grounded work, but applied to certain parts of the human body. Best known are the *dentist,* expert in the teeth and surrounding oral tissues, and the *stomatologist,* specialist in conditions of the mouth. In most health systems, dentists are educated in universities and are required to undertake training nearly as extensive as that of the physician. Like physicians, dentists may specialize—for example, in the care of children, the treatment of gum disorders, of malocclusion (orthodontia), or of other aspects of the teeth.

In the more highly developed countries, and sometimes in the less developed countries, there are independent trained personnel focused on other body organs. *Optometrists* (sometimes called *ophthalmic opticians*) may prescribe eyeglasses for refractive errors of vision, but these practitioners are usually not authorized to treat other eye disorders. *Podiatrists* are trained to treat relatively superficial diseases of the feet, such as bunions or plantar warts. There may be contention in a country over where the line should be drawn between the services authorized for these practitioners and those requiring a physician.

The field of mental disorder is particularly complex, with respect to health manpower; some personnel may legally serve patients directly, while others must work under the supervision of a physician. In some health systems, *psychologists* may treat patients directly and perhaps also *social workers.* Among the latter sometimes only "psychiatric social workers" have this authority. Among psychologists, the right to treat patients directly may be accorded only to those with an advanced academic degree.

The expert on drugs in every health system is the *pharmacist* or chemist, but his or her degree of independence in relation to patients is highly variable. In all countries some drugs (e.g., aspirin) may be dispensed directly by pharmacists "over the counter" to any patient. Many drugs in most countries, however, require a medical prescription under law. In reality, these laws or regulations may not be enforced, and the pharmacist may dispense restricted drugs, such as penicillin or digitalis, without a prescription. This illegal dispensing is sometimes done by personnel who are not qualified pharmacists—often termed *drug-sellers.*

Allied Personnel Supportive to Independent Practitioners. The principal health associate supportive to physicians, and the largest category of health personnel throughout the world, is the *nurse.* There are many types of nurses, varying generally in extent of education and training, and they perform diverse functions, but all of them work directly or indirectly under the general supervision of physicians (and sometimes dentists or other independent practitioners). The nurse originated in hospitals to take care of bed-patients, evolving from religious sisters or nuns. As health systems have become more complex, nurses have been trained for and called on to perform an increasing variety of tasks. Their preparation, though still mainly in hospitals, is now also offered in several other settings, and according to curricula of varied lengths and contents.

A widely adopted schedule for preparing nurses to attend hospital patients calls for three years of training in a hospital, following completion of secondary school (10 to 12 years of basic education). These nursing graduates must pass certain examinations to become entitled to "registration" by the government and to be regarded as "professional." To cope with the expanding needs of hospitals and other types of institution, most national health systems have also prepared large numbers of more briefly trained *"practical"* or *assistant nurses.* Elementary schooling (from 4 to 8 years) and nursing education for only one to two years are a common schedule. Beyond these, some nursing personnel learn to perform their duties entirely on the job, and are often called *nurse's aides* or, if men, *orderlies.*

Outside of hospitals, nurses of the several types may also perform diverse functions. Nurses work in health centers and other facilities intended mainly for ambulatory care.

They work in schools, to be available for serving school children and also for health education. They perform somewhat similar tasks for workers in factories. Nurses are important personnel in public health programs, staffing clinics, giving immunizations, visiting homes, and supervising other personnel. Sometimes nurses work with physicians in private premises or give bedside care to patients at home. The overwhelming majority of nurses, however, are employed in some organized facility, governmental or nongovernmental.

Because hospitals and other organized health programs employ large numbers of health personnel, some supervision is usually required. To prepare nurses for such supervisory responsibilities, as well as for teaching, many countries have developed university-level nursing education. Even though nurses of all levels may come under the ultimate supervision of physicians, in their daily work they usually exercise much independent judgment. The trend everywhere has been to assign to nurses functions that were once reserved for physicians. In some health systems, this has come to include even diagnosing and treating common ailments, for which the professional nurse may receive supplementary training as a *nurse practitioner.*

Nurses in many countries may be trained an extra year or two, to become *nurse-midwives,* doing obstetrical deliveries in hospitals. Special training may also be given in providing anasthesia, to prepare *nurse-anesthetists.* Theoretically, both these types of specialized nurses work under medical supervision, but this may be minimal. The same applies to hospital-based professional *midwives,* who are not nurses but are trained for about the same duration.

Besides nurses, numerous other technical personnel assist or support the physician in the diagnosis and treatment of patients. For diagnostic procedures, there are *laboratory technicians* or technologists, trained to several levels of expertise. They may specialize in examination of blood specimens, biochemical analyses, the study of bacterial cultures, preparation and examination of pathological tissues, or some other area. They may be educated in universities, in polytechnical institutes, in hospitals, and in other settings. They work in hospitals, ambulatory care centers, research institutes, private quarters, and elsewhere.

Similarly, developments in radiology have given rise to many types of x-ray or *radiographic technician.* Electrocardiography has spawned a special technician in larger institutional settings; likewise for electroencephalography and for diagnostic scanning by the computerized tomography (CT) machine.

With respect to the treatment of patients, still other types of allied personnel support physicians in the medical care process. *Dieticians* are the technical experts in food selection, purchase, preparation, and distribution to the sick and the well. Usually women, they are trained in secondary schools in most developing countries, and often at universities in more developed countries. In a public health context, experts in the food needs and dietary habits of populations, in the levels of malnutrition that may exist, and in the development of strategies for improving community nutrition are considered *nutritionists.* These are often specialized physicians, but some nutritionists may be trained exclusively in this field. (Strictly speaking, nutritionists are not auxiliary to the physician.) Records of patients are maintained by *record librarians* or specially trained clerks.

For various modalities in rehabilitation of the physically handicapped there are *physical therapists, occupational therapists,* and *speech therapists.* For testing hearing there may be *audiologists.* A general *medical social worker* may assist any type of doctor in helping the patient to cope with sickness and make proper use of all community resources. Moreover, ancillary to all these health workers is a second echelon of auxiliary personnel, including the *laboratory assistant* and the *physical therapy assistant.*

As new technologies develop, still further classes of health worker are trained. The *inhalation therapist,* a recent example, is trained in the special problems of administering oxygen or doing procedures for treating lung disease. The *hearing aid technician,* the family planning (contraception) specialist, and the emergency ambulance paramedic are further types of personnel who have emerged in response to newly recognized requirements in the health services. Highly sophisticated equipment, such as kidney dialysis machines and heart–lung equipment used during chest surgery, has generated the training of still other specialized technicians.

In connection with mental illness and mental health, we have spoken of independent practitioners besides the physician and psychiatric specialist. In some settings, *psychologists,* social workers, and others may function only as allies or auxiliaries to the physician and as members of a mental health care team. In several countries there are *psychiatric nurses,* whose training is quite different from that of general registered nurses. Mental hospitals may have specially trained *psychiatric aides,* to help in the care of mentally ill patients.

The *pharmacist,* who dispenses many drugs directly to patients, was noted earlier as an independent practitioner. At the same time, pharmacists serve as allies/auxiliaries to the physician, who sends the patient with a prescription. Even in this auxiliary role, the pharmacist may bear a certain legal responsibility, to ensure that the prescription is reasonable and that the doctor has not erred in the dosage prescribed or in some other way. With most compounding of moderns drugs done by the pharmaceutical company, the pharmacist's task is now limited largely to maintaining an appropriate inventory of drugs, storing them properly, and dispensing packages with accurate labels and instructions. (Sometimes an alert pharmacist may advise the physician on certain pharmacological incompatibilities among diverse prescriptions, ordered for a particular patient.)

In either the independent or auxiliary role, pharmacists are frequently assisted by *pharmacy clerks.* Virtually all independent practitioners are supported by allied/auxiliary personnel. To prepare lenses for eyeglasses prescribed by the optometrist (or the medical ophthalmologist), there are *opticians,* optical technicians, and lens-grinders. *Optometry clerks* handle simple adjustments required in eyeglass frames.

The dentist is assisted by a whole spectrum of special personnel. Most numerous is the chairside *dental assistant.* The *dental technician* or dental mechanic fabricates dental prostheses. The *dental hygienist* thoroughly cleans and scales the teeth, either under a dentist's direction or quite separately in schools or workplaces. In some countries, with or without appropriate legislation, *denturists* prepare full upper or lower dental plates for patients directly, without the intervention of a dentist.

Personnel for Direct Service under Nominal Supervision. The fourth general class of health manpower has become increasingly important in contemporary health systems, where recognized needs for direct health service have come to greatly exceed the resources of physicians and other independent practitioners. Worldwide recognition of the health needs of millions of rural people and urban slum dwellers has stimulated the preparation of many types of briefly trained *community health workers,* who provide basic preventive services and treat common ailments. The content and duration of their training have been highly varied, ranging from several years after secondary school to a few weeks after primary school. Their work is under the nominal supervision of a physician or another more fully trained person but is predominantly independent.

Under the influence of the World Health Organization, the scope of health services provided by community health workers (CHWs), even those trained for only a few weeks, has been very broad. It is usually intended to encompass the diverse elements of "primary health care," which is mastered with experience and reinforced by continuing education. Some CHWs, on the other hand, are trained only for single-purpose services, such as immunizations, the control of mosquito disease vectors, or the detection and treatment of eye infections. Whether multipurpose or single-purpose, community health workers are increasingly important members of the health manpower establishment of most developing countries. Although theoretically they work under supervision, the extent of this guidance is often quite tenuous, leading to problems discussed later.

Another example of this type of health personnel is the *school dental nurse* (sometimes called *dental therapist*), who provides virtually complete dental care to school children, under only the occasional supervision of a dentist. Pioneered by New Zealand in 1920, this health care provider is now serving children in about 20 countries. Typically a female secondary school graduate, she is trained for two years to perform almost all dental procedures needed by children, including fillings and extractions. She also gives health education on dental hygiene.

A very important category of health personnel who gives direct service, under only nominal direction, is the *public health worker.* As health systems have matured, organized community efforts have been mounted, for the promotion of health, the prevention of specific diseases, and the efficient organization of medical care. Physicians, sometimes with special graduate training, are usually in positions of leadership—at the national level, at provincial or district levels, and in large municipalities. But at the grass roots level, many types of public health personnel work essentially independently.

Monitoring and controlling the environment so that it does not cause disease demands persons with special knowledge and skills. Broadly speaking, these personnel are *sanitarians* or *environmentalists;* there are many subtypes. The establishment and operation of public water supplies and the proper disposal of human and other waste require sanitary engineers. Surveillance of the environment for its proper sanitary maintenance is done by various sorts of sanitary inspectors of different levels. Some may be trained for several years to carry supervisory responsibilities, while others are trained more briefly to work under supervision. Vector control to eliminate certain insects and other vectors of disease is an environmental health subspecialty. Personnel operating water treatment or sewage disposal plants require special training.

Health education is another special discipline that has developed in recent decades, sometimes oriented toward school children and often the general population. The prevalence of certain diseases has led to the training of personnel such as the venereal disease in-

vestigator or the malariologist. The management of hospitals or other large facilities is often a function of carefully trained *health care administrators,* and specialized tasks in health service management may call for expertise in financial matters, personnel relations, procurement and maintenance of supplies, and so on. Other health administrators deal with the management of health services provided for a geographically defined population. In recent years the overall planning of services to meet needs in the future has evolved as a task for still other special health personnel. The collection, maintenance, and analysis of various types of data in large health jurisdictions require the skills of a *health information specialist.*

The functions of *public health nurses* are highly variable. Ordinarily these personnel receive one year or more of formal training in public health matters, following their completion of professional nursing eduction. Often they supervise many other personnel in a public health agency. They may be in charge of special clinics for patients with tuberculosis, leprosy, sexually transmitted diseases, or even general primary health care. Sometimes they carry out routine clinical examinations of pregnant women and newborn infants or small children—making referrals to a physician only if a serious abnormality is detected. Many public health nurses make home visits, to cope with problems of communicable disease or monitor the care of newborn infants. Closely related is the *visiting nurse,* who gives bedside care to chronically ill patients in their own homes.

This completes a relatively cursory review of the wide spectrum of the health manpower resources in any national health system. To achieve some order in a very heterogeneous field, personnel have been categorized into four groups: (1) physicians, (2) other independent practitioners (to whom people have direct access), (3) personnel allied to or supportive of the first two types, and (4) other personnel giving people direct health service, under only nominal supervision. The lines between these four categories are not sharp, and the placement of a particular personnel type—such as a pharmacist, a public health nurse, or a psychologist—may differ substantially from one health system to another. As noted, the manner of training and the functions performed are also highly variable among systems.

The production and use of health manpower in every health system are in constant flux. The individual medical practitioner of old can no longer render comprehensive health care alone. A whole team of doctors, pharmacists, nurses, dentists, technicians, sanitarians, community health workers, administrators, and many others is needed—whether such a team is deliberately organized or operates only implicitly and informally. As we shall see, the very dynamism of the health manpower panorama in every country is leading increasingly to explicitly organized arrangements for achieving the efficient delivery of services in national health systems.

Health Facilities

The second major type of resource in a health system is the physical facility in which personnel provide their services. Once health care was provided outside the patient's home, it was necessary to establish structures in which health personnel could do their work. Health facilities can be classified into six major types: (1) hospitals, (2) general ambulatory care units, (3) special categorical clinics, (4) long-term care facilities, (5) environmental health protection facilities, and (6) other specialized health units. Within each of these major categories of health structure are several subtypes.

Hospitals. Historically oldest among health facilities are hospitals to shelter and give bed care to the seriously sick. Hospitals are most frequently general, serving patients with a wide range of acute and chronic diseases and also serious injuries. General hospitals may vary greatly in size and technological development—small hospitals usually having limited apparatus and large ones more complex technical resources. Even the term *general* is subject to varying interpretations; in some countries it specifically excludes maternity cases, and in others it may rule out the care of cases of infectious disease.

Special or nongeneral hospitals may be of several types. Almost all health systems have institutions exclusively for the mentally ill. Some general hospitals admit certain mental patients, but mental hospitals are entirely for such cases; they are predominantly large and serve both acute and long-term mental patients. Certain mental hospitals serve mentally retarded as well as disturbed patients, although retarded patients are frequently kept in separate institutions.

Special hospitals may also focus on other types of condition. Some are devoted to maternity cases (childbirth and problems of pregnancy) and sometimes to all disorders of women. Others are entirely for sick children. Special hospitals may be limited to cases of infectious or communicable disease. Because of the once high prevalence of tuberculosis and the formerly long duration of its treatment, many special hospitals or sanataria have treated this disease, although their numbers have sharply declined in recent years. Leprosaria or leprosy colonies serve patients with this chronic disorder in many developing countries. Still other special hospitals may be devoted to patients with disorders of the bones and joints or with conditions requiring orthopedic surgery. Hospitals for rehabilitation of patients with various crippling disorders are another type. Because of the rising prevalence of cancer in many countries, hospitals specialized in the treatment of this disease have been on the increase. The same applies to heart disease.

Some general hospitals may be limited to the care of specific groups of persons, such as active military personnel or military veterans. Special hospitals may serve certain aboriginal inhabitants of a country. In large industrial firms, mines, or agricultural estates (plantations), general hospitals may be established exclusively for employees and their families. Universities may maintain general hospitals for their students, and even prisons may have hospitals for the care of sick convicts.

Irrespective of the type or types of patients they serve, hospitals differ in their sponsorship or ownership. Ordinarily a hospital is sponsored and controlled by the body that constructed it, but sometimes ownership changes by sale or by legislative action. The most widely used differentiation of sponsorship is (a) governmental or public, (b) voluntary and nonprofit, and (c) purely private or proprietary. Each of these types has several subdivisions.

Governmental hospitals include facilities controlled by various levels of government—national, provincial or state, and local, county, or municipal. Voluntary nonprofit hospitals include facilities controlled by various religious groups and others sponsored by nonsectarian bodies. Proprietary hospitals are often owned by physicians (individuals or groups), but they may also be owned and controlled by corporate investors.

Under all three types of sponsorship, hospitals may be single and autonomous institutions or part of a network of many facilities. National governments may control a network of military hospitals or special institutions for aborigines; even municipal governments in large cities may operate a network of general hospitals. Religious bodies, especially in the Catholic Church, may sponsor general hospitals throughout a country or even across national borders. In recent years, private corporations in certain countries have come to own and control large chains of general and special hospitals.

The mix of hospital sponsorships differs markedly among various types of national health system. On a world scale, the supply of hospitals (usually measured by the number of available hospital beds) and the ratio of beds to population have been increasing steadily over the past century. There has also been a general trend toward increasing governmental sponsorship, with notable exceptions in certain countries. The percentage distribution of hospitals under various sponsorships has many implications for the accessibility to needed hospital care. The internal administrative structure of hospitals and their patterns of medical service organization also tend to differ with the various types of sponsorship.

As health systems have developed, the functions of hospitals have become more numerous. Originally limited to the bed care of the seriously sick, hospitals today provide many services to out-patient or ambulatory persons, provide education to health personnel and offer a setting for medical research, sometimes furnish health education and other preventive services, sometimes dispatch personnel to care for sick patients in their homes, and can serve as the administrative center for the management of all personal health services in a geographic area.

General Ambulatory Care Units. Much more recently established than hospitals are health facilities for the organized provision of services to ambulatory patients. As noted, hospitals usually have out-patient departments, but quite apart from these are numerous separate structures devoted entirely to the patient not confined to bed. Most often these facilities are known as *health centers* or community health centers. Sometimes, as satellites to a main health center (serving, for example, 50,000 people), there may be smaller subcenters (serving perhaps 10,000 people), and even peripheral to these may be simple health posts, staffed with only a single health worker.

Health centers and related units are typically sponsored and controlled by government agencies, but sometimes they may be sponsored by voluntary bodies, such as religious missions. Their relative importance in national health systems varies greatly among countries, but they are generally more numerous and have a wider scope of functions in developing countries. The staffing of health centers and subcenters is correspondingly variable; in more affluent countries the staff typically includes several physicians along with nurses and other personnel, while in poorer countries the staff may be composed entirely of allied/auxiliary personnel, or perhaps a single physician with certain other health workers.

In the sense used here, health centers provide general ambulatory care, both preventive and therapeutic. Sometimes the range of services is characterized as consisting of *primary health care.* Preventive services to mothers and children are often emphasized, but the sick are usually treated in accordance with the capabilities of the staff. Some health centers may include a small laboratory for diagnostic examinations. A pharmacy may also be present to dispense drugs for the treatment of common ailments.

In certain health systems, the major facility for general ambulatory care is the *polyclinic,* so designated because its staff includes several types of medical specialist. A polyclinic may have one multispecialty team or be staffed as elaborately as a large complex hospital but with no beds. Conceptually, the polyclinic is a more highly developed health center, and it is extensive mainly in health systems under the overall control of government.

Health centers and polyclinics are striking reflections of the trend toward an increasing organization of health services throughout the world. For the care of bed patients, organized facilities were recognized to be necessary centuries ago. Gradually the same need has come to be recognized for ambulatory care. This has begun to apply to health activities under private as well as government sponsorship.

Finally, with respect to general ambulatory care, one should not overlook the facility in which an individual medical or other health practitioner works. Known variously as offices, surgeries, rooms, private clinics, or by other terms, these quarters play a definite role in nearly all health systems. They may vary greatly in the amount of space and equipment and their accommodations for examining patients. In the large cities of some countries, entire buildings may hold scores of individual medical and allied practitioners; such provision of pharmacies, laboratories, and appliance shops in the same medical arts building is convenient for patients.

Special Categorical Clinics. While the health center and related facilities typically serve general populations, several types of clinic provide ambulatory care of special populations or disorders. As with special hospitals, such facilities for ambulatory care may serve military personnel, industrial workers, or prisoners. Special clinics may also be devoted to the care of selected diseases, or to preventive services with respect to defined health problems. Often these units are called *dispensaries.*

Organized clinics may be classified conveniently according to their sponsorship. Most numerous generally are those sponsored by public health agencies or ministries of health. In virtually every country, these agencies operate clinics to examine infants and children up to 5 years of age, advising the mother on breast-feeding, proper diet, and infant care, giving im-

munizations, following the baby's development for any signs of abnormality, and so on. Variously called *well-baby clinics, infant welfare stations, maternal and child health clinics,* or other terms, these units have played a substantial role in protecting infant health and reducing infant mortality. In most, but not all, countries these infant health units give limited treatment to any disorder detected in the baby. Somewhat less numerous are clinics for prenatal examinations of pregnant women.

The clinics for diseases of public health importance are manifold. They operate for the detection and follow-up of tuberculosis, sexually transmitted diseases, disorders of malnutrition, leprosy, schistosomiasis, crippling disorders (in adults, children, or both), cancer, eye diseases, dental disease, skin disorders, heart disease, mental problems, drug abuse, and other conditions. Special clinics are also held for contraception (family planning) and for various immunizations. Although most of these clinics are sponsored by official public health agencies, some are founded and operated by voluntary bodies or other branches of government, often with subsidy from the ministry of health.

An increasingly important part of hospitals—especially governmental, but also voluntary—are out-patient departments or ambulatory care clinics for various types of patient. These clinics may be scheduled at certain times each week for specialized purposes, such as surgical conditions, gynecology, pediatrics, heart conditions, or orthopedic problems. In addition, most general hospitals maintain a 24-hour emergency or casualty service. Many but by no means all patients seeking emergency care are accidental injury cases. Hospital out-patient departments are attended by a diverse group of people seeking the attention of a medical or surgical specialist.

Still other organized ambulatory clinics are established at industrial plants, particularly those with several hundred employees. At these clinics, the workers may receive preemployment medical examinations, but also first-aid and treatment for any health problem arising at the workplace. In general, larger enterprises offer a more comprehensive scope of services than small ones. The staffing with doctors and nurses corresponds to the clinic size, and certain resource standards may be defined by law.

Schools at all levels may maintain special clinics for the health care of students, staffed principally with nurses. In elementary schools, these clinics give immunizations and are usually on the alert for communicable diseases. Secondary schools often have services for athletic injuries, drug abuse, sexually transmitted diseases, and common respiratory infections. At universities, where students are often living away from their family homes, the clinic services tend to be comprehensively therapeutic and preventive, and doctors are usually available full-time or part-time.

In countries where the medical profession has grown large as a purely private occupation, physicians themselves may organize *group practice clinics.* Sometimes these private clinics bring together doctors of different specialties, in the same manner as in hospitals. Sometimes physicians in a single specialty cluster in a group clinic. When the specialties in a health system are intimately linked to hospital work, private group clinics may consist entirely of general practitioners; each doctor in such group clinics may focus on a special type of patient—women, children, the elderly, and so on.

In a few countries, group practice clinics may be linked to special populations that have purchased insurance for medical costs privately. Before 1959 in Cuba, these were called *mutualistas* or mutual societies, and in the United States they were called *prepaid group practices.* After about 1970, the pattern in the United States became known as the *health maintenance organization* (HMO). Other countries, such as Australia and Indonesia, have shown interest in developing this type of organized ambulatory service for middle-class populations that could afford the private insurance.

Clinic facilities may also be sponsored by voluntary agencies in their field of concentration, such as clinics for mental problems, for cancer detection, for crippled children, or for other specific purposes. Governmental welfare agencies may sponsor special clinics for destitute people or for care of the elderly or the mentally ill. Ministries of agriculture may operate clinics for rural families or for specially disadvantaged people, such as migratory farm workers. Religious missions in many developing countries build and operate clinics for particularly isolated rural people.

Long-term Care Facilities. Several types of hospital, as noted, focus on the care of patients with long-term illness, such as mental disorder, tuberculosis, or leprosy. Beyond these, many countries have health facilities for general chronically ill and disabled persons, most of whom are elderly. These facilities are becoming especially important in the affluent industrialized countries, where high proportions of the population (more than 10 or 12 percent) are living to advanced ages—often defined as more than 65 years. Varying with the type of national health system, these institutions may be under governmental sponsorship or under the control of voluntary nonprofit (usually religious) or proprietary bodies.

There are gradations of health facilities for the aged and chronically ill. Some general hospitals, providing active medical attention at all times, are confined to long-term patients. In some countries a medical specialty of geriatrics has developed for the treatment of these patients. The staffing and equipment of long-term general hospitals put stress on various modalities of physical and mental rehabilitation.

For chronically ill patients, who require no active medical intervention but still need nursing service and bedside care, various other types of health facility are available. In some countries they are known as *nursing homes* or *skilled nursing facilities.* They may be called *convalescent hospitals.* Sometimes they are designated *old people's homes,* though they are meant for *sick* old people. In one facility of this type, some patients may be completely bedridden, while others may need only minimal assistance for activities-of-daily-living (ADL).

Still fewer medically oriented services are provided in facilities for elderly people who are essentially frail but do not require nursing service. Institutions for this purpose may be called *retirement homes, residential hotels,* or *board and care facilities.* The occupants are considered "guests," rather than patients, but they are unable to live alone and they lack a family or friends with whom to reside. Only in the more affluent countries are such custodial facilities found, because their maintenance is more costly than low-income countries could afford.

For patients of any age level, often quite young, another type of long-term care is given at *rehabilitation centers.* Although somewhat like hospitals in the intensity of their service, the rehabilitation center specializes in the techniques of physical medicine. Patients with serious neurological handicaps, such as occur after spinal cord injury, may improve their mobility from prolonged physical and occupational therapy. They learn to use prosthetic braces, artificial limbs, crutches, wheelchairs, and other devices. Some patients reside in the rehabilitation facility full-time, and others may be brought in periodically. The rehabilitation center movement became prominent after the great devastation of World War II, but since then it has come to serve patients with disorders that are not war-connected.

For seriously sick patients, beyond the capabilities of medical treatment and not expected to live very long, the "hospice" has been developed in certain affluent countries. A large proportion of hospice patients are terminally ill with cancer but can be helped through relief of pain. Hospices are also devoted to sympathetic care for the grieving family and friends as well as to providing the maximum possible comfort for the dying patient.

Finally, the most common long-term care facility of all should not be overlooked—the patient's home. As the operational and resource costs of the various formal facilities have mounted, many countries have tried to provide systematic services that will enable frail and disabled persons to remain in their own homes, either with a family or by themselves. Food may be prepared and transported each day, through a program of Meals on Wheels. Visiting nurses may come to the home on a regular schedule, to help the patient with medication, surgical dressings, or simply personal hygiene. Such services may be provided by voluntary or public agencies. In certain large cities, hospitals operate *organized home care* programs for long-term patients, since they have the needed technical personnel and can then release beds for patients who require active in-hospital care.

Environmental Health Facilities. Although they do not constitute personal health services, many forms of physical structure are important for the protection of people against hazards of the environment. Sanitation facilities differ greatly among national health systems, largely in relation to their levels of economic development and urbanization.

A hallmark of modern civilization is the availability of public water supply facilities, to provide safe water for drinking and other purposes. Numerous strategies in sanitary engineering have been designed to bring piped and potable water to urban homes and other buildings. In most national settings, the water must be treated physically and chemically to ensure its purity, depending on the source from which the water comes. No matter how carefully a piped water system has been constructed, the water must be tested periodically for safety.

Most of the world's population is still rural, and the facilities required for potable water in rural settings are quite different from those in cities. Provision of safe water to a village seldom means the convenience of indoor water faucets and sinks; there is usually a well or stand-pipe in the village square, where families go to collect and carry home their daily supply. Rural water may be drawn from a stream, a cistern (rain water), a well, a spring, or another source; in the absence of such a constructed facility, raw water collected from rivers or lakes is usually hazardous.

Equally important are the facilities developed in all health systems for disposal of human excreta. Large cities often have sewage disposal networks, which require constant maintenance. In smaller towns and rural villages, excreta disposal presents continual problems. Before sewage is discharged into a river or sea, in the more economically developed countries, it may be processed through a *sewage treatment plant,* to reduce environmental pollution. Individual households in rural areas, and even in many towns and cities of developing countries, must depend on septic tanks or more often on pit latrines for excreta disposal; the widespread construction of such small facilities usually requires organized social efforts.

Numerous other facilities contribute to environmental sanitation to various degrees in different health systems. Cities everywhere require mechanisms for solid waste (garbage) disposal, which involve vehicles for collection of the waste and some arrangement for its dumping. The latter may simply be an isolated place, a designated area for sanitary landfill, a place for incineration, transportation out to sea, or some other method.

Waste products from industrial production present serious water pollution problems when they are discharged into rivers. The many dangers of toxic industrial wastes have become increasingly recognized, and the disposal of radioactive materials from nuclear power plants presents a crucial challenge in several countries. The control of insect vectors of disease may call for the drainage of swamps and other strategies. Hygienic housing requires construction that will protect residents against rodents and insects. Air pollution control requires equipment to neutralize industrial waste products, automobile exhaust gases, and numerous other volatile substances.

Other Specialized Health Facilities. Still other types of facility must be counted among the resources for all or most national health systems. Most ubiquitous are *pharmacies,* where people can obtain drugs and certain medical supplies. These may be chosen directly by the patient or, depending on the nation's legislation and the rigor of its enforcement, on the basis of a doctor's prescription. When the pharmacy sells many other products beyond drugs—cosmetics, toiletries, tobacco products, candies—it is more properly called a *drugstore.*

In some countries, nearly all shops of either type are individually owned and operated, and in others many are part of large national chains. Predominantly they are small private enterprises, but in some health systems they are public facilities in the same sense as hospitals. Persons of low income in many systems look to the pharmacy or drugstore as a convenient source of medical care on short notice,

when professional medical attention is not available or is too expensive.

Another essential facility is the *medical laboratory,* where various bodily specimens are examined for diagnostic purposes. The great majority of laboratories are simply parts of hospitals or other health facilities. Some, however, are free-standing and operated privately or by an agency. Large clinical laboratories may have separate departments for examining bacteriological specimens, studying pathological tissues, examining blood, carrying out diverse chemical tests, and performing other purposes.

In some national health systems, laboratories are operated as a regionalized network in which simple examinations are performed at small peripheral units, and examinations requiring more complex analytical procedures are referred to larger centralized facilities. Certain countries maintain laboratories specifically for public health purposes (examinations of water, food products, and specimens from cases of possible communicable diseases, etc.), while other laboratories examine specimens from all types of patient. This distinction, however, is gradually breaking down.

Blood banks or repositories for different biological types of human blood and blood products are, like laboratories, usually maintained in larger hospitals. Sometimes, as part of an emergency or disaster relief program, they are maintained in separate facilities. Aside from essential refrigeration, great care must be taken in the proper identification, testing, and transportation of blood if it is to be safe and beneficial. Collecting blood from healthy donors is another activity often performed by blood banks.

For providing various types of *prosthetic appliances,* special facilities may be available under public or private auspices. Orthopedic prostheses are the specialty of certain shops—crutches, corsets, trusses, wheelchairs, and so on. Appliances that must be fitted to the individual—such as braces, artificial limbs—are the province of other special shops. In some health systems, optical shops for spectacles (eyeglasses) exist separately from optometrists, prescribing opticians, or ophthalmologists, who determine the exact corrective lenses required. Other shops fit and provide hearing aids.

Health Commodities

The third basic type of resource in every health system is a constellation of physical or chemical commodities required in treating or preventing disease. Most extensive is the enormous variety of drugs and biological preparations used throughout the world. In addition are medical supplies used for both treating and diagnosing disease. Third is a growing range of increasingly elaborate equipment, developed for the diagnosis and treatment of various disorders.

Drugs and Biologicals. Since ancient times, products of mineral, vegetable, or animal origin have been used in treating disease. With increasing knowledge, medication has been synthesized through various chemical reactions. Drugs developed primarily from herbs, long before the era of modern chemistry, are still widely used in developing countries (and to some extent in all countries). They may be termed *traditional drugs* in contrast to *modern drugs.*

Most traditional drugs are dispensed directly by traditional practitioners, as part of their service to patients. In fact, it is often customary for the healer to charge a fee for the drug while the consultation is free. Traditional medical practice in India and China is backed up by a large literature describing certain compounds for the treatment of various symptoms (such as pain, fever, diarrhea, headache), rather than specific diagnoses. Sometimes traditional practitioners have learned about the value of modern drugs, such as penicillin, and use them in their practice.

Modern drugs have been manufactured in thousands of varieties by pharmaceutical firms throughout the world. The United States, Germany, Switzerland, Great Britain, and a few other countries, however, have developed the largest drug companies, and their products are exported and sold almost everywhere. Many of these companies have established branches in developing countries, to which they send raw materials for conversion into pills or liquids for packaging and sale locally. (The vast multiplicity of drugs is confusing to both physicians and patients, as well as unnecessarily expensive—giving rise to corrective strategies which we discuss later.)

Most industrialized countries have patent laws, which protect the right of the firm that discovers and first produces a new drug to exclusive control over its sale for a certain number of years (20 years in most European countries.) This right is implemented by the use of a special *brand name* to identify the drug. Another company may manufacture and sell the same drug under another name, but only if it pays royalties to the first company for every unit sold. After expiration of the patent period, the drug may be produced by any company, under a *generic* name (designated by government), which describes the chemical composition of the drug. Generic drugs are typically much less expensive than the original brand-name preparation. Much controversy surrounds the marketing of generic-name drugs, but the goal of achieving economies is leading to their maximum use in almost all organized health programs.

Because of competition in drug production, the pharmaceutical industry in nearly all health systems uses a lot of advertising. This is directed mainly to physicians, through advertisements in medical journals, special mailings, and visits from drug sales representatives, usually called *detail men.* For drugs not legally requiring a medical prescription, much advertising is also directed to the general population. Because of the relatively high cost of most imported drugs, many countries have organized governmental agencies to manufacture generic compounds.

The geographic distribution of drugs in national health systems, especially those drugs that are imported, is usually a complex process. In most countries there are governmental networks of health facilities to be supplied, various nongovernmental health facilities, possibly a governmental drug production agency requiring raw materials, and usually hundreds of retail pharmacies. To facilitate this process, wholesale drug distributing firms have been established, and individual foreign plants may also have their own distributing mechanisms. Because drug imports may come in large quantities, central storehouses must be maintained. The storage and distribution of biological products (vaccines and various immunizing agents) require careful refrigeration, and the proper maintenance of a *cold chain* may determine the success or failure of an immunization campaign.

Medical Supplies. The maintenance of hygienic conditions in hospitals, health centers, and all health facilities requires the regular availability of soaps and antiseptic supplies. The care of injuries and postsurgical wounds requires bandages of different types. For surgery, suturing material is essential, and the treatment of fractures or dislocations requires splints and special types of plaster. The operation of laboratories requires various reagents, and x-ray examinations depend on radiographic films.

All of these materials must be produced in a national health system or imported from abroad. Some of the simplest diagnostic and treatment procedures cannot be performed without these essential supplies. In the operation of a hospital, linens for the beds or pesticides to cope with insects in tropical regions might be taken for granted, but purchasing and procuring them require planning so that they will be available in adequate amounts at all times. Paper and writing instruments are needed to keep proper health records.

Medical Equipment. For modern diagnosis and treatment, as well as prevention, countless types of instruments and machines are necessary. For immunizations and many other purposes, syringes are essential. The thermometer is a simple tool, but it must be imported by most countries. The same applies to stethoscopes, blood pressure apparatus, otoscopes, and ophthalmoscopes. Modern laboratories require microscopes, spectrometers, centrifuges, incubators, refrigerators, and hundreds of other types of equipment. The automatic analysis machines, which can perform 12 or 24 different chemical tests on a small sample of blood, would not be expected in most developing countries but may be considered essential in large hospitals of highly developed countries.

With medical advances, more and more equipment has been invented to analyze the workings of the human body. The stethoscope was a great invention in the early nineteenth century, and has almost become the symbol of a modern physician, but no medical examination today would be considered adequate without an electrocardiogram. Observation in bodily orifices requires various types of vaginal specula, cystoscopes, proctoscopes, gastroscopes, and other scopes. The brain is examined with electroencephalographs and muscle function with myelographs.

Modern surgery calls for a galaxy of instruments—tools for cutting, clamping blood vessels, probing organs, retracting operative incisions, and so on. Obstetrics may use forceps and other instruments. Modern ophthalmology has acquired a whole array of elaborate machines for examining and testing the eye. To anesthetize the patient undergoing surgery, increasingly complex equipment for delivering anesthetic agents has been developed. Organ transplants require elaborate heart–lung machines and other types of high technology.

The radiography department of the modern hospital calls for steadily advancing types of machine to examine the inside of the human body in health and disease. The simple one-shot x-ray machine, invented by Roentgen, is being replaced by sophisticated imaging equipment that beams rays from different angles to yield three-dimensional information about internal body structure. This *computerized tomographic* (CT) scanning is being succeeded by equipment that images internal organs through *magnetic resonance.* To avoid the possibly harmful effects of x-ray beams, ultrasound equipment may serve somewhat related diagnostic purposes.

High-technology forms of therapy require still other types of equipment. Laser beams can incise tissue without cutting. Renal dialysis can greatly extend the lives of patients with terminal kidney disease. New forms of blood vessel intubation can open up clotted arteries and extend the life of patients with coronary occlusions. Intravenous infusions of many types and pure oxygen inhalation have become commonplace procedures in modern hospitals. Radiation is standard therapy for cancer and certain other conditions.

In many developing countries these types of advanced technology are found only in a central tertiary hospital or not at all. The simpler equipment, medical supplies, and drugs, however, must be available for a health system to function. Except in the most highly industrialized countries, the great majority of these many commodities must be imported from abroad.

Knowledge

The fourth resource required in any health system is knowledge—a resource often taken for granted, but still requiring deliberate acquisition or production through new research. Much of the store of knowledge on which health systems depend is, of course, handed down from the past and conveyed through literature and the education of health personnel. Most newly acquired knowledge, for the prevention or treatment of disease, is conveyed through current journals and books, and sometimes by the spoken word at scientific conferences.

To some extent, health science research for acquiring new knowledge is conducted in every health system. Some of it may never be reported, but may simply shape the body of "experience" that guides the actions of individual practitioners. No matter how limited it is, health science research is usually conducted in some formal setting—in a university, a ministry of health, a special research institute, a hospital, a clinic, or elsewhere. The research results may be reported only in a local journal.

The greatest volume of medical and related research, and investigations done with the greatest scientific care, come from the most highly industrialized and affluent countries. Fortunately for world health, new findings are usually published as rapidly as possible, so that they are widely spread. The specialization of medical and related sciences has given rise to

hundreds of research institutes, oriented toward specific health problems in national health systems. The focus may be infectious diseases, nutrition, cancer, heart disease, blindness, occupational disorders, mental disease, or scores of other conditions. The institute may also give grants to universities and other bodies to investigate selected problems.

In less affluent developing countries, a major problem is the dissemination of new information from the national center to the periphery. Inadequate communication may deprive residents of isolated rural areas of crucial medical information. In some health systems, deliberate actions are taken by ministries of health or other bodies to ensure the widest possible dissemination of significant new knowledge.

The application of knowledge through drugs or special equipment is often described as technology. Unfortunately much technology for therapeutic or preventive purposes is applied just because it is new, without adequate evaluation of its benefits. Since new technology is often quite expensive, questions have been raised increasingly on the need for careful assessment of its value before it is widely applied. Such evaluation and reporting of results may be done with various degrees of formality.

This completes the account of the major resources in the health system of a country—the manpower, the facilities, the commodities, and the knowledge. The exact characteristics of each of these resources, of course, differ from system to system. The relative proportions of health manpower and facilities of different types that have evolved may influence health system policies along lines different from newly perceived needs. The general amplitude and attributes of each type of resource inevitably influence the adequacy with which the entire health system can protect and advance the health of its national population.

ORGANIZATION OF PROGRAMS

The many types of health resources would have limited impact on populations if they were not organized into various programs. This organizational structure or configuration of activities constitutes the second major component of national health systems. The organizational responsibility may be taken by various social groups (e.g., a government agency, a religious body or a military establishment, a factory or a school) for which the health program essentially supports other objectives. In some health organizations, such as a ministry of health, of course, health is the central objective.

Besides the many organized programs requiring deliberate initiative, there are residual activities in virtually every health system that function as a private health care market. Though not "organized" in the usual sense, these actions are governed to varying extents by the principles of market dynamics—supply, demand, competition, and price. The principal organized structures in a national health system are sometimes considered as subsystems.

The term *organizations* has been defined as the systematic arrangement of various resources, with designated responsibilities and special channels of communication and authority, intended to attain certain objectives. The ultimate objective of organization in a health system is to promote or protect people's health, but this ultimate goal is approached through the intermediary role of many agencies with more focused objectives. Organizations may operate in a small geographic area or span an entire nation.

In very broad terms, the organization of programs in a health system may be either under governmental or public auspices or under nongovernmental or private auspices. Many relationships exist between these two large sectors, and the relative importance of each is a major determinant of the main characteristics of the entire health system. Each sector, of course, has many subdivisions.

In the realm of government, most countries have one agency with major responsibility for health. It may be a discrete body in the central government, concerned exclusively with health, or it may be combined with other agencies responsible for related activities, such as welfare, social security, education, environment, or culture. When health protection of

the population is the sole function, the agency is usually designated as a ministry or department of health. But even in combination with responsibilities for other matters, the top central health authority in government is customarily called the *ministry of health.* Sometimes several social functions are combined with health in the central government, while at the periphery health functions are performed by a separate agency.

Ministries of Health

As the capabilities of the health sciences have increased, and the role of government in health protection has expanded, the range of functions of ministries of health (MOH) has broadened, and MOH organizational structures have become more complex. No two national ministries of health have identical functions and organizational structures, reflecting diverse historical developments. The responsibilities assigned by government to the MOH, in contrast to other public agencies, vary. Any description of the structure and functions of these ministries, therefore, must be in very general terms.

Preventive Services. Having usually originated in an effort to combat epidemics, through various strategies, virtually every MOH carries major responsibilities for disease prevention. On the ministry's organization chart, prevention may constitute one major subdivision or it may fall under several headings. Whatever the administrative arrangement, a prominent place is usually occupied by the control of communicable diseases. Certain disease problems may be of such great importance in a country that special administrative units are devoted to the control of diseases such as malaria, tuberculosis, sexually transmitted diseases, leprosy, vector-borne infections, or other contagious diseases.

The protection of populations against hazards of the environment is nearly always a prominent MOH responsibility. Supplies of safe water and sanitary disposal of human waste are health necessities in every country. Many aspects of environmental sanitation are under the jurisdiction of other public agencies in various countries, although the MOH must usually maintain continuing surveillance on compliance with standards.

Other aspects of prevention may concern several other MOH subdivisions. Preventive services for infants, small children, and school children are usually the focus of a special unit. Either within this unit or closely related to it may be the responsibility for monitoring pregnant women, usually designated as *maternal health.* In many countries this field also includes concern for family planning or contraception—whether this is formulated as promoting the health of mothers or as a strategy for controlling the population growth. In some countries, population control is regarded as such a serious problem, that family planning is assigned to a major MOH subdivision or even to a separate body outside the MOH entirely.

Other preventive or health promotive strategies that often entail separate MOH lines of authority are nutrition and health education. Programs for improving nutrition may play a special role in the organization of meals for school children or in food supplementation for malnourished preschool children. An institute for nutrition research can study the population's nutritional status and find food products that warrant greater emphasis in local diets. Health education responsibilites may concentrate on the production of educational materials about major health problems or they depend on the general promotion of local community participation in activities of the MOH.

Varying with local health conditions, MOH preventive activities may focus on still other special problems. Control of accidents—on the roads, in homes, or in other public places— and injury prevention are often major issues in the more industrialized countries. If trachoma or other eye diseases are endemic, specially organized efforts may be warranted. Prevention of dental disease, through fluoridation of water or other substances and through dental hygiene, constitutes another type of special program.

Curative Services. Most MOHs have a major subdivision concerned with *curative services* or activities for treatment of the sick. Sometimes this is limited to supervision of a national network of ministry hospitals, but it may include a certain amount of regulation over all public and private hospitals in the country. In some health systems, selected large tertiary research and teaching hospitals are controlled by special entities outside the MOH, and the ministry is responsible only for secondary-level facilities. The subdivision for curative services typically stipulates national standards, such as the number of doctors, nurses, and others required per 100 patients, which all hospitals are supposed to follow.

Curative service responsibility sometimes includes supervision of larger facilities for ambulatory care, such as major health centers or polyclinics. Insofar as these facilities also provide immunizations and other preventive services, their administration may come under the wing of preventive services. The staffing and operation of medical laboratories is another function, usually linked to curative programs. This field also includes emergency and ambulance services, sometimes in collaboration with a voluntary agency (the Red Cross). Surveillance of pharmaceuticals is another possible responsibility.

Training. The preparation of numerous types of health personnel requires major efforts in so many countries that it is often the responsibility of a special subdivision of the MOH. Except in certain countries (mainly socialist), this responsibility does not include university education in medicine, dentistry, or sometimes pharmacy; it usually does include training of nurses, medical assistants, laboratory technicians, sanitary inspectors, dieticians, various types of community health workers, and others. The training programs for these personnel are generally conducted within hospitals or health centers controlled by the MOH, but they are sometimes in separate polytechnical institutes.

Training subdivisions may also prepare instructional manuals and various forms of audiovisual material for health personnel education. They may conduct continuing education programs, to keep personnel informed on new scientific developments. They may hold special conferences for physicians and other professionals who were originally university-trained. Sometimes the MOH training unit maintains national registries of physicians, professional nurses, and others, although this licensure function could come under the wing of another unit of the ministry or even be outside it.

The types, numbers, and geographic distribution of health manpower are basic to the overall planning of national health systems. Access of the population to needed health care requires the availability of various types of personnel at virtually all times and places. In most countries, market dynamics are the major determinant of these matters, but planning interventions have come to play an increasing part. Training functions in MOHs are therefore often clearly related to planning responsibilities.

Other Major MOH Line Functions. In one form or another, the three major functions summarized previously play well-defined parts in virtually every ministry of health, but there may be many other line functions as well (i.e., there is a line of responsibility on substantive matters, from center to periphery in both directions). Thus, there is often a separate major branch for environmental sanitation, even though it is conceptually part of preventive services. Pharmaceutical regulation and sometimes production may occupy a discrete unit, although it is theoretically one aspect of curative services. Specialized line activities may focus on mental health service, along with problems of substance abuse (alcoholism and drug addiction). The control of chronic non-communicable diseases also commands special attention (sometimes specifically heart disease and cancer) in industrialized countries, along with general problems of the aged and programs of rehabilitation. The organizational priority that may be assigned to family planning and population control has been noted.

MOH Staff Functions. In contrast to the preceding *line* functions, every MOH has subdivisions for various *staff* functions, intended to support and facilitate activities in all the substantive fields. There is often a major branch for general administration of financing and personnel, on which the performance of all line functions depends. It is this branch that usually maintains channels of communication with the nation's general treasury or the ministry of finance. Insofar as a national authority exists for civil service or government employment, this branch is responsible for compliance with general regulations. All government ministries typically operate according to an annual budget, which must be overseen by the general administrative branch. If some line program finds, during the year, that it requires more funding than was originally anticipated, the administrative branch might be permitted to make certain financial adjustments. This subdivision may also be responsible for the purchase or procurement of all supplies and equipment, and for the maintenance of necessary transportation.

Another important staff function in most MOHs is for health planning. Even though most countries today have a general agency for national planning—often in the office of the prime minister or the president—the more detailed aspects of health system planning are usually handled by the MOH. Closely related to this staff function is a unit for health research and statistics or its equivalent. The maintenance of vital statistics on births, deaths, and certain notifiable diseases is one of the oldest MOH functions.

Finally, most MOHs have a unit for international or external relations. In developing countries, this may play the important role of handling relationships involved in foreign aid. In all countries, it manages relationships with other countries on health matters and also with international bodies such as the World Health Organization (WHO) or the United Nations Children's Fund (UNICEF). In more affluent countries, this office may oversee foreign health aid from the viewpoint of the donor nation.

Local Health Service Relationships. The preceding analysis of MOH activities has concerned mainly the central or top level of national government. In almost all countries, however, except perhaps the very smallest, government has found it necessary to subdivide the national territory into smaller political jurisdictions. Depending on the national population and history, of course, the manner and the echelons of subdividing a country vary greatly, but a common arrangement is three levels below the top. Although they are designated by various terms, we may describe these levels generically as (a) provinces, (b) districts, and (c) communes. (Provinces may be called *states* or *regions;* districts may be called *counties* or *areas;* communes may be called *municipalities* or *communities.*) Moreover, a *province* in one country may be the same as a *county* or even a *republic* in another.

In certain countries, the governmental level just below the top—that is, the province, state, or republic—may have considerable autonomy in its governance. In these federated nations, the fields of education and health are often sectors under substantially local control. In all countries, however, subdivision of the territory into smaller jurisdictions endows these units with some degree of decision-making power. Likewise, some partial degree of centralized power is exercised in the most locally federated countries. In other words, the actual functioning of hierarchical structures of government is always complex, and should not be oversimplified as completely centralized or decentralized in day-to-day operations.

Because of these complexities, many MOHs have a major subdivision for maintaining relationships between the headquarters and all the lower echelons where health functions are carried out. It is the responsibility of this unit to ensure, or help to ensure, that the provinces are staffed as completely as possible and performing their functions properly. Problems that arise in the field are first brought to the attention of this unit and then, if necessary, referred elsewhere for advice. If a nationwide campaign is to be launched or a change in policy to be made, the central MOH unit on local relationships must play the vanguard role.

The administrative relationships between the several MOH echelons are often conceptualized as a *pyramidal framework.* The range of responsibilities delegated to each echelon, of course, varies greatly among countries. Often functions in certain preventive spheres, such as maternal and child health service, are fully del-

egated, while in the curative services, the control of large hospitals is retained mainly at the central headquarters.

As a general principle, the scope of public responsibilities at the first echelon below the top (typically, the province) replicates the scope at the top. As one moves to lower or more peripheral echelons—*district* and *commune*—the range of functions usually becomes somewhat narrower. Still, the spectrum of functions may not be identical in all provinces or districts in the same country. This is especially true in federated countries, but even in highly centralized ones, the initiative of one provincial health director may lead to a wider scope of health functions than is customary.

Much may also depend on the character of the general government in a province, district, or commune. One provincial governor, for example, may have great political prestige and feel free to encourage innovative health activities. The nature of leadership at the MOH headquarters, furthermore, will affect the type of work done in the provinces, as will provincial leadership affect activities in the districts. In one health system, communications between the several echelons may be effective, while in another they may be sporadic, so that both leadership and *espirit de corps* are weak.

It is obvious that ministries of health cannot be described by any single model for all countries. Quite aside from the categories of service they provide, an MOH may be strong and have a great impact in one system, rather weak in another, and quite mixed in a third, with great influence on some functions and little on others. The relative strength of a ministry depends largely on the role played by other entities in the health system structure, particularly by the dimensions of the private health care market. When the private market for medical care is substantial, as it is in many countries, many MOH functions are oriented essentially to the poor. Only certain preventive service may then have a major impact on the general population.

The structure of ministries of health, of course, changes continually. It changes as new health problems arise or new capabilities develop for the prevention or treatment of disease. This has been dramatically illustrated by the worldwide epidemic of AIDS in the 1980s. The WHO/UNICEF 1978 Conference on Primary Health Care led to MOH reorganizations everywhere. A change of political power in a country, or even new personalities within the same power group, generally lead to changes in the arrangement of divisions and subdivisions and the lines of responsibility in a ministry. Difficulties may occur in ministry operations under one long-established arrangement, so that another is tried. Changes may be horizontal in the distribution of responsibilities at a given jurisdictional level, or vertical if responsibilities are altered between different levels.

Other Government Agencies with Health Functions

Whatever the scope of the ministry of health, in every health system other governmental agencies also carry certain health responsibilities. These tend to be more numerous where MOH responsibilities are relatively restricted, but even where they are broad some health functions are intrinsically linked to other branches of government.

The overall roster of ministries or departments varies greatly, of course, among countries. A societal function—transportation, for example—may have ministerial (or cabinet) status in one country and simply be a subdivision of another ministry in another. In this account, the term *ministry* is used in a generic sense, to mean a locus of public responsibility for a stated function, whether or not this function holds official ministerial status.

Social Security Programs. The insurance mechanism under law is used to finance or provide general medical care for all or part of national populations in almost half the countries of the world. In the great majority of these countries, these health responsibilities are vested in a branch of government other than the ministry of health. The most frequent locus of control is in ministries of labor, since historically social insurance programs originated in groups of industrial workers. Sometimes, however, they are linked with public health

under a ministry of health and social security, sometimes with programs of social welfare (not supported by statutory insurance), sometimes they are independent bodies, and sometimes they occupy another place in the arena of government.

In many health systems, social security programs are essentially a mechanism for economic support, but in other systems (especially in developing countries) they are engaged in the direct provision of health services to defined beneficiaries. Under either arrangement, these programs play a substantial role in the overall operation of national health systems. Even if social insurance simply finances services in a private medical market, it exerts many influences on the functioning of that market. The terminology describing these programs is often confusing, insofar as several phrases may describe the same process—sickness insurance, health insurance, compulsory health insurance, prepaid medical care, social security, and so on.

A special type of social security that is actually more extensive than that for general medical care involves medical services solely for work-connected injuries and sometimes occupational diseases. Commonly called *worker's compensation,* this type of program may be administered along with general social security for medical care or in a separate governmental setting. It is usually a responsibility of ministries of labor, even if general health insurance is operated elsewhere. Sometimes special public commissions carry responsibility. The definition of *work injuries* and the arrangements through which the worker receives medical care have countless variations.

In most programs for socially insured medical care, the beneficiary also receives monetary compensation for his or her loss of earnings due to inability to work. This is often called *disability insurance* (short-term or long-term), which also has important implications for health; money is obviously needed for food, shelter, and other essentials of living. Similarly, there are clear health implications in other forms of social security that compensate eligible persons for various human difficulties, such as unemployment and old age. Such compensation obviously helps the individual live a healthier life in times of adversity, not to mention providing money to obtain medical care.

Occupational Health and Safety Programs. Maintaining safe and healthful conditions in factories and other places of work is another governmental function often vested in ministries of labor. Since this involves inspecting workplaces and enforcing certain technical standards, rather than awarding specified benefits, it is usually separate from the administration of social security. Rarely this responsibility may be vested in the ministry of health, or sometimes in an agency concerned with the general surveillance of industrial enterprises.

This essentially preventive health work may be done with varying degrees of rigor. As industrialization and mechanization have increased throughout the world, the hazards for workers have inevitably multiplied. Even in agriculture, the use of farm machinery, fertilizer, and pesticides entail health hazards. In many situations—in both developed and developing countries—there are contentions about the relative benefits of using various procedures or substances versus their human hazards.

Ministries of Education. Schools at all levels are relevant to health systems. In the elementary grades, children are usually taught something about personal hygiene. In many of the more affluent countries, both elementary and secondary schools are staffed with health personnel (often nurses) for first-aid and regular observation of the children. These personnel are sometimes assigned from the ministry of health, but often they are simply part of the school workforce like teachers.

In universities and other institutions of higher education the students may be provided with comprehensive personal health care. Higher educational programs, of course, may include faculties for training physicians, dentists, pharmacists, clinical psychologists, and other health personnel. This control of the output of doctors by ministries of education, in fact, creates a need for coordination with authorities overseeing general health services, to properly meet national health needs.

Environmental Agencies. In some countries, a special ministry or other public authority may have general responsibility for environmental quality. Although this may involve the protection of wild life and certain purely aesthetic aspects of the environment, most of the activities have a direct bearing on health. Reducing the pollution of water and air has become more important, as the world's population and its urbanization have increased.

Environmental protection authorities may have direct responsibility for public water or sewage disposal programs. They may also be concerned with the disposal of solid waste (garbage) from large cities. They may have special authority for control of the waste products of industrial production. The development of nuclear power and the extreme health hazards of nuclear waste disposal or nuclear plant accidents are further concerns of environmental authorities in certain countries.

Ministries of Agriculture. The production of food, of course, has enormous meaning for health, but agricultural agencies in government may also be directly involved in providing health services. In the more affluent countries, these ministries often conduct educational programs for farm families, and among other things disseminate information about health and nutrition. In agricultural areas, where cash crops are the major output, farmers may be educated about the value of small vegetable gardens for the family's personal use. Branches of ministries of agriculture are often devoted to promoting proper animal husbandry, which includes maintaining healthy livestock. The control of animal diseases that may be spread to humans (e.g., brucellosis or tuberculosis in dairy cattle) is an important public health function.

In many developing countries, the ministry of agriculture has concern for the general social development of rural communities. It may promote community development programs, which include the construction of health centers or health posts. In some countries, these ministries have the main statutory responsibility for helping villages to drill deep wells or to obtain safe water in other ways. Developing sources of water to irrigate crops may also be useful in acquiring water for household purposes.

Ministries of Public Works. In many countries, one major ministry is responsible for all sorts of major construction projects, ranging from roads and bridges to schools, hospitals, and health centers. Even when a ministry of health or social security issues the specifications for a health facility, and provides the necessary capital funds, the actual construction may be carried out by the government agency specialized in such matters. Sometimes a facility is constructed by a private firm, under contract, but the ministry of public works has the ultimate responsibility. Sometimes these ministries may also construct major water supply and sewage disposal networks in larger cities.

Ministries of Interior. Among the many agencies in national governments, ministries of interior or their equivalent (sometimes ministries of local government or of internal affairs) often have the most diversified responsibilities. In several countries, before public health functions were deemed important enough to warrant ministerial status, national responsibilities for health protection were vested in a subdivision of the ministry of interior. These ministries typically supervised local police functions to maintain law and order, and the maintenance of a sanitary environment, including prevention of epidemics, was regarded as a matter for police action. Even after separate ministries of health were established, some of these "medical policing" functions have been retained in the ministries of interior.

Ministries of interior may conduct factory inspections for health purposes in countries where industrial development is too limited to warrant a ministry of labor. For the same reason, they may have a subdivision for such social welfare activities as housing of the aged and homeless, physical restoration of seriously disabled workers, treatment of drug addicts, or the rehabilitation of prostitutes.

In some countries, major cities do not come under the jurisdiction of the province or state in which they are located. Correspondingly, the public health activities in those cities are not under provincial jurisdiction, with the line of authority leading up to the ministry of health. Under these circumstances, public health functions in these cities come wholly or partly under the control of the ministry of interior.

Ministries of Commerce. The several commodities required in health systems, especially drugs, are traded commercially to varying extents. Accordingly pharmacies or drugstores must often be registered with a ministry of commerce. The same applies to shops for prosthetic appliances, hearing aids, or eyeglasses. The objective of this registration is usually purely commercial and not oriented to health, but it may provide the only general information on these types of health resource.

Advertising may have many health implications, and this often comes under the supervision of a ministry of commerce. Insofar as the advertising of drugs is subject to regulation, this ministry is often responsible for enforcement. Likewise, many countries have enacted legislation to restrict the advertising of tobacco products or liquor, which may be harmful to health, and enforcement rests with the ministry of commerce.

Social Welfare. Protective services for the aged, orphans, refugees, and others often come under the general rubric of *social welfare.* Sometimes this function is combined in the same ministry as health or labor. In any event, social welfare services have obvious health aspects. Institutions for the aged or for orphan children always require some provision for medical services. Millions of persons throughout the world are political or economic refugees from their native lands; they reside in refugee camps, where some type of health service is always needed. The ministry of social welfare usually provides this, although sometimes the ministry of health is asked to do it.

In the most affluent countries, persons who are impoverished or seriously handicapped may receive financial assistance enabling them to live in a personal home. Social welfare agencies may then pay for needed medical services, furnished in the mainstream of the private medical market. General hospitals may even be maintained by social welfare authorities, exclusively for the care of the very poor.

Transportation and Public Utilities. The maintenance of large public transportation resources, such as railroads, fleets of ships, or airlines has stimulated the organization of special health care programs. In many countries, these transport services are governmental, even when the general economy is dominated by private enterprise. The same applies to public utilities, such as telephone and telegraph communications, electrical power, and piped networks of water and natural gas—all of which likewise usually operate special health programs for their employees.

When these resources are initially constructed, massive engineering problems often must be overcome in very isolated places. Provision of medical services is, therefore, crucial at this stage. As countries develop economically, an infrastructure of transportation and utilities usually grows correspondingly, and these special health programs may also expand.

Ministries of Justice. Every country has some type of judicial system to deal with crime and other offenses against the law. As part of this, prisons and prison camps, and in the more developed countries, certain medical services, are provided for prisoners. For obvious reasons, such services seldom have high priority, but when they are offered the responsibility generally rests with the prison authorities.

Military and Veterans Affairs. With one or two notable exceptions, every country maintains a military establishment, although it may be called a ministry of defense or security, or some other name. There are usually separate branches for military actions on land, at sea, and in the air. To maintain these soldiers and sailors in good health, a well-developed health service nearly always functions in times of both peace and war.

Since almost all countries attach great importance to their military strength, these medical services are typically very fully staffed and provided with the best equipment and supplies available. Developing countries may have massive deficiencies in general urban or rural health service while the health resources for the army and navy are abundant. If some new and expensive type of technology is invented in Europe, for example, and only of one of these machines can be imported, it is often put in the major military hospital.

Because of their typically high quality, military medical facilities are often accessible to important leaders from any branch of the government. Sometimes wealthy individuals not in the government can also obtain care in these facilities, for which they pay. Military physicians usually have the rank of officers; allied health personnel of many types hold different ranks. The major military hospital in most countries is generally located in the national capital, and other health facilities are typically wherever military garrisons are located. In numerous countries, the dependents of military personnel are also entitled to medical care at the official installations. Sometimes they may be authorized to obtain services elsewhere, at the expense of the military department.

The veteran or former military person commands great respect in most countries, especially if he has been engaged in combat. In recognition of military service, therefore, he may be entitled to medical care after retirement from active duty. Usually this applies to care for a health condition attributable to military service, but for higher officers it may apply to any medical problem. In a few countries, military veterans are served by special programs for almost any health problem, whether connected with military service or not, for the rest of their lives.

Ministries of Finance. The collection of taxes and allocation of funds to various ministries are generally functions of a ministry of finance, a treasury, or the equivalent. Since revenues are always limited, and official budgets often exceed the money available, this ministry may have ultimate powers of decision affecting governmental health programs. Sometimes this ministerial role is attached to the office of the president or the prime minister, and authority comes from the highest level. There are also occasions when revenues are delayed in reaching the government, and the ministry of finance decides which public program (perhaps temporarily) will be deprived. The ministry of health and all the other branches of government ordinarily submit their annual budgets to the ministry of finance before they can be finalized.

National Planning. Since World War II, almost every country has, to varying degrees, engaged in national planning of economic and social affairs. There may not be an explicit "planning agency," and the functions will be divided among several ministries, often linked to financing. In developing countries and, of course, all the socialist countries, a central planning body is very likely to be explicit and very influential. In these circumstances, a subdivision of planning is usually concerned with the health sector or sometimes with broadly conceived social welfare, which includes health. This planning unit typically works closely with the equivalent planning body in the ministry of health. The general planning agency may attempt to coordinate MOH activities with relevant functions of other ministries, such as health facility construction carried out by the ministry of public works or physician training under the ministry of education.

As long as this review of "other government agencies with health functions" is, it is doubtless not complete. Certain countries may have a ministry of national minorities, which provides health services, among its functions. In socialist countries, a ministry of light industry may be responsible for drug production. Women's affairs or the elderly may be the subjects of major governmental branches, in which health services play an integral part. Most important, it should be clear that health functions permeate government, at the center and locally, in scores of ways beyond the jurisdiction of ministries of health.

Voluntary Bodies

Quite outside the sphere of government, scores of organized voluntary programs relevant directly or indirectly to the health system are almost everywhere. These tend to be more numerous and stronger in affluent industrialized countries, where a large middle class has developed, and family members (often women) have surplus time and money to devote to various social causes. Yet all countries have nonofficial groups of people whose activities bear on some aspect of the health system.

Voluntary organizations are formed for many reasons. Often groups of citizens wish to promote action toward a certain objective they believe is not getting adequate attention from government. This applies to many agencies focused on a specific disease. Some voluntary groups are formed to focus attention on and advance the well-being of certain sections of the population, such as the elderly. Still other voluntary groups are actually promoted by government, to mobilize private energies for a task that government hesitates to undertake. Certain voluntary organizations are concerned mainly with advancing their own self-interests.

Humanitarian and religious objectives, of course, also play a part. Funds needed to support various activities are always raised in part from voluntary donations, but in many countries voluntary agencies are substantially subsidized by government; public authorities regard them as fulfilling an essential role. Ingenious methods of voluntary fund-raising have been devised, such as widespread sale of Christmas seals for holiday mail.

First we consider voluntary bodies with various specific health objectives. Then we examine organizations in which a health role is one among many.

Disease-Specific Voluntary Agencies. Tuberculosis was one of the first diseases against which extensive voluntary efforts were mobilized. Scores of countries formed associations to help the victims of consumption, long before its bacteriological cause was discovered. Sanatoria were built and special clinics organized by private societies before governments took action along the same lines. The care of patients has often been the initial purpose of a voluntary health agency; then, when this function has been assumed by governmental bodies, other objectives take precedence, such as the support of scientific research, the education of the general population, or the improved training of physicians in treatment of the targeted disease. In some countries where tuberculosis has been greatly reduced, the energy of tuberculosis associations is directed against other disorders.

Voluntary efforts have been mobilized against many serious diseases of long duration. Societies for *social hygiene* have tackled venereal infections. In very poor countries leprosy may be an object of assistance from private groups. Poliomyelitis, described as *infantile paralysis,* has attracted much voluntary initiative. The many tragic aspects of cancer have stimulated voluntary assistance to patients and support of research. In more economically advanced countries, the voluntary battles against heart disease have attracted widespread private support.

Certain relatively uncommon but grave diseases have also summoned voluntary action. This applies to neurological orders, such as multiple sclerosis and epilepsy. Cystic fibrosis and hemophilia are quite rare congenital disorders that have generated voluntary action in certain countries. Mentally retarded children have summoned a great deal of voluntary energy. Crippled children, disabled congenitally or from some other cause, attract the sympathies and voluntary donations of many people. It is often the parents of patients with these conditions who initiate the program. A major objective of these groups is to draw greater government attention to the plight of these patients.

Blindness and deafness have long generated voluntary initiatives. Agencies devoted to these problems may organize schools to instruct blind children in reading Braille and deaf children in lip-reading or sign language. Voluntary transportation services may be organized, dogs may be trained as guides for blind persons, and legislation may be promoted to grant privileges to persons whose blindness is identified by white canes.

For certain disorders, voluntary organizations are essentially self-help initiatives. Best known is Alcoholics Anonymous, which has accomplished a great deal in many countries in rehabilitating chronic alcoholics, through various psychological and spiritual strategies. Similar efforts have been made with victims of drug dependence, without great success. Orga-

nizations for hemophilia, noted earlier, and for epilepsy may have a self-help character.

Agencies for Certain Types of Person. Probably the most universally appealing demographic category is the child, especially the poor and disadvantaged child. In almost all countries, even the least developed, voluntary efforts are extended, usually by mothers who are better off, to help small children. Supplemental feeding is a common strategy, but day care nurseries, essential clothing, and country camps for urban children may also be provided. Activities of this sort have such widespread appeal that in some countries it has become customary for the wife of the nation's president to serve as the titular head of this movement.

In the more industrialized countries, where the proportion of persons living to the later years of life has been gradually rising, many voluntary agencies promote the health and welfare of the aged. A central strategy has been to develop programs that enable the elderly to keep active and occupied. Such activity can help prevent the premature onset of frailty and disability. For aged persons, who are already frail and require help in activities of daily living, voluntary agencies organize programs for meals and other forms of assistance.

Disabled military veterans are another special group that summon voluntary efforts, especially if government programs are weak. The same applies to aboriginal populations, who may live in extremely humble circumstances, and to some ethnic or racial minorities. The dominant culture in any country is often negligent about the health needs of these minorities, so that voluntary bodies come forward. Generally, of course, poor persons of any age may be objects of much charity.

Agencies with Other Special Health Functions. For providing help, including health service in serious emergencies, almost all countries have a Red Cross or sometimes a Red Crescent Society. Though they often start in times of war, these agencies typically continue their work in peacetime. They may operate ambulances, maintain blood banks, and be prepared to render all sorts of assistance in natural disasters. Red Cross Societies often conduct education on safety in swimming, on fire prevention, and for other such prevention purposes. In some countries ambulance services are also operated by a unique organization of ancient origin, the St. John's Ambulance Brigade.

Family planning or the extension of contraception is another frequent object of voluntary action. In some countries, the subject is still controversial for religious reasons, but most countries have come to recognize the overriding importance of reproductive control. More than most health-related fields, family planning or *planned parenthood* services under voluntary sponsorship are heavily subsidized by government. Authorities want this work to be done but often much prefer the responsibility to be carried outside official channels. Family planning programs may or may not include assistance to women who seek abortions.

Another voluntary agency function in many countries is the provision of bedside nurses to visit the homes of chronically ill or convalescent patients. These visiting nurse associations (VNAs) usually work in large cities of the more affluent countries. Although they have typically been founded by private citizens, in time the VNAs are usually asked to render services to indigent government beneficiaries, for which they are reimbursed. Visiting nurse services to patients' homes have become increasingly important as a less costly substitution for the care of patients in hospitals or nursing homes.

Professional Health Associations. In most countries, the major professional groups engaged in health service have formed national or regional associations. Their objectives have been primarily to advance the interests of the profession, but at the same time, the groups may have a general impact on the national health system.

Associations of physicians tend to be the most highly developed, and they may play a large role in the continuing education of doctors. They may also represent all physicians in negotiations with government on medical fees or salaries payable under various health care programs. Or they may serve as the professional guardians of medical ethics, in the event that a doctor is charged with unethical behavior. In some countries, the medical association carries insurance to protect its members from malpractice suits.

In certain countries, a separate medical organization, often called a "college," is responsible for ethical surveillance of physicians. National law may require that all new medical graduates become enrolled in the medical college and that continued membership be a condition of official registration or licensure. Then, if a physician is found by his peers to be guilty of some unethical behavior, he may be dismissed from the college and thereby lose his legal right to practice medicine.

Somewhat similar associations usually function for dentistry, nursing, pharmacy, laboratory technology, and other professions. In certain fields, for example, optometry or podiatry, what sphere health service is legally authorized in is under contention. When does treatment of the eyes or the feet go beyond the scope defined in law and infringe on the domain of medicine? The various associations naturally advocate the broadest possible interpretation of their scope of practice. In countries that license osteopathy or chiropractic, as well as homeopathy or acupuncture, similar contentions over the authorized sphere of practice may become quite bitter.

Hospitals, nursing homes for the chronically ill, and other types of facility also form professional associations for both educational and political purposes. When negotiations are necessary between hospitals and government or even nonpublic agencies, the professional association represents its members. These associations have done much to advance managerial efficiency in health facilities.

As medicine has become increasingly specialized, voluntary associations have been formed in the numerous specialties, largely for educational purposes. Aside from holding meetings and publishing journals, these societies may attempt to explain to the general population the capabilities of each discipline. In certain specialties, such as pediatrics, the association proposes standards for child health that are adopted by government. Unfortunately, serious controversies have sometimes developed between professional groups and government, over the terms of contracts for medical service or even over the provisions of duly enacted legislation; the associations have then sometimes spearheaded work stoppages or strikes. The same has happened in the relationships between hospitals and nurses or other health employees.

Religious Bodies. In almost all countries, as we noted earlier, religious organizations may sponsor hospitals. In addition, religious sects from Europe and North America have long sponsored medical missions in developing countries throughout the world. Thousands of hospitals, health centers, and dispensaries have been built in isolated areas of low-income countries; after the liberation of colonies in Africa and Asia, many of these have become integrated with the governmental health programs. Even though these missions have usually charged patients private fees for the services rendered, the original capital costs typically came from the foreign religious charity.

Almost every religious denomination conducts certain health-related programs domestically. Whether Buddhist, Christian, Hindu, Jewish, Moslem, or other, these groups support various humanitarian programs for the poor and the sick. Drug addiction, for example, is treated at Buddhist temples. Christian and Jewish groups sponsor social service agencies, among the functions of which medical care for needy families can be included. The Salvation Army, a largely Christian charity, extends help to exceptionally destitute persons— usually in the slums of large cities. The ultimate goal may be religious conversion, but health services are rendered as a means to this end.

Philanthropic Foundations. In the most affluent countries, wealthy individuals have endowed philanthropic foundations which, among other things, support health programs. The work of the Rockefeller Foundation in public health and medical education is known around the world. This philanthropy originated in the United States, but similar initiatives have come from Great Britain, continental Europe, Japan, and elsewhere.

Most foundations support diverse humanitarian objectives, but some are focused specifically on health. This is illustrated by the Nuffield Provincial Hospitals Trust in England, the Sasakawa Foundation in Japan, and the Robert Wood Johnson Foundation in America. The Milbank Memorial Fund in the United States is a relatively small foundation, that has long been concerned exclusively with the improvement of health services.

Foundations depend on great individual wealth, but throughout the industrialized countries are community organizations that collect small donations from large numbers of individuals and businesses. This is done through community chests, United Ways, consolidated charities, and the like. All sorts of voluntary health agencies can be supported by these group efforts, but it is then understood that the agencies assisted will refrain from separate fund raising.

General Social Organizations. Beyond all these voluntary activities, every country has numerous other general social organizations that include health work among their efforts. These are usually based on demographic groupings, such as women, youth, workers, farmers, and the like.

Women's organizations may range from elite women's clubs, in wealthy neighborhoods, to mass organizations of working women or the wives of working men. In different ways, these women's groups may participate in the support of services for maternal and child health, immunizations, family planning, or nutritional education. They may give volunteer services in hospitals, to help lonely patients, or participate in programs for the elderly. In the more developed countries, parents (usually mothers) may unite with school teachers in parent–teacher associations to improve health services in the schools.

Organizations of industrial workers, especially in labor unions, may try to improve factory working conditions or to educate workers about occupational safety. Unions have played a significant part in the worldwide movement for extension of social security. In developing countries, workers may volunteer their labor for construction of roads or buildings to advance local health resources.

Rural and farm organizations have been especially active in promoting improved sanitation and water supplies in rural communities.

They may mobilize labor for digging wells, along with agricultural irrigation. They may build health posts to provide primary health care and organize cooperatives to finance primary health care.

Organizations of youth are of many types. In the more industrialized countries, there are troops of Boy Scouts and Girl Scouts, organized by age levels, with numerous educational programs, including activities that can advance health. In the developing countries, youth groups may participate in environmental clean-up campaigns, in mobilizing families for participation in immunization programs, and so on.

Cutting across all demographic groups in many countries are political associations, usually intended to advance a particular political objective. Among their efforts may be support for certain types of health legislation. To fortify the group's general spirit and enthusiasm, the members may cooperate in a concrete project, such as the construction of a health center.

Enterprises

Of much smaller proportions than the health activities of voluntary bodies are health care functions of business enterprises. Either because of legal requirements or simply personnel policy, many large enterprises operate health programs for their employees. The circumstances of urban and rural enterprises are generally different.

Urban Enterprises. The great majority of productive establishments in either affluent or developing countries are small. Most countries regard a workpalce with fewer than 100 workers as small, and little health service is expected in such workplaces. A factory with 100 to 500 workers is considered of moderate size, and those with over 500 may be regarded as large.

Moderate-sized establishments often have someone trained in first-aid on the premises to handle injuries or sudden illness. In more developed countries this is likely to be a nurse, but in less developed countries it may be an office clerk or a manual worker who has learned some primary care essentials. Perhaps arrangements have been made with a nearby facility to have a physician on call in case of emergency.

In large factories or other enterprises (e.g., a transportation network), a physician may be on the premises for a limited period each day. His time might be spent in examining workers with a health problem, in doing preemployment examinations, and so on. Ideally, such an industrial physician inspects working conditions and identifies any hazards to health, but in reality few plant physicians have such skills, outside of very large enterprises (with several thousand employees) in highly developed countries. If a worker in an urban enterprise needs extensive medical care, he is most likely to be referred to a local hospital.

Rural Enterprises. Most numerous among rural enterprises are large estates or plantations for growing certain crops or extractive operations for mining or petroleum. If these have fewer than 100 workers, organized health services are unlikely. For organizations with more than 100 workers, and especially more than 500, some planned health facility is likely to be available, especially because the families of the workers are probably entitled to service as well.

If a governmental health facility in a developing country is nearby, it may meet the needs, but this is not likely. Large rural enterprises are generally expected to take care of their own employees, so that governmental facilities are usually constructed elsewhere. For the workers and their families, therefore, isolated rural enterprises frequently operate their own medical care programs. Since these enterprises are often quite profitable—especially if owned by foreign corporations—their medical and nursing personnel may be paid relatively high salaries and are easily recruited.

In very large rural enterprises, such as those for oil extraction, rubber tapping, or extensive cultivation of tea or sugarcane, a network of health facilities may be maintained. Small dispensaries may be widely available, to be close to the working locales, and a central hospital may function for referral of cases. The degree to which occupational health services are provided, of course, depends on the economic development and the political ideology of the country. In more welfare-oriented countries, the legal requirements are more rigorous for both private and public enterprises.

The Private Proprietary Market

With the multiplicity of organized programs in a country for health service or other health activities—under both governmental and nongovernmental auspices—one might conclude that little is left for purely private commercial initiative. The reality, however, is far from this. Few health systems completely meet all the needs and demands for health care, curative or even preventive, with organized health programs. Almost all countries, to greatly varying extents, have a residual field of purely private for-profit initiative for health care. This private market can be analyzed under the main categories of service.

Traditional Healing. Nearly all traditional medical practitioners are engaged in private practice. Their fees are generally quite low, and sometimes they accept payment by barter. They are widely distributed in the rural villages of most developing countries, and tend to be culturally and psychologically close to the people. Most healers are engaged principally in farming or some other occupation, giving traditional treatments only part-time. Occasionally a healer acquires a reputation for great curative powers; he may then do this work full time, settle in a city, and charge high fees. In certain countries, traditional healers are appointed on salary in the official program of the ministry of health, but their numbers are typically small (except in China).

The traditional birth attendant (TBA) was described earlier. She too is engaged in private practice, usually on a part-time basis. Her fees are relatively low, and often accepted in the form of barter. In developing countries, almost every village has its local TBA, and there are many in the cities as well. While general traditional healers are occasionally integrated into official ministry of health services, hygienic training for and formal recognition of TBAs are extensive. Ministries recognize the widespread popularity and use of TBAs, usually deeming it more prudent to train and use them than to ignore them.

The unlicensed drug-seller is still another form of practitioner in the private medical market of developing countries. He may sell traditional herbal preparations along with modern medications he has purchased from some wholesale source. He makes no attempt to diagnose disorders but simply sells drugs according to the patient's request or his guess on the appropriate remedy for the symptoms reported. The prices charged by drug-sellers, frequently itinerant, are often quite high, since their supply of drugs may have been bought largely through a *black market.*

Physician's and Dentist's Care. Almost all countries have modern physicians and dentists engaged exclusively in private for-profit practice. This may be their lifetime pattern of work, or it may be undertaken after a practitioner is retired from service in a public agency. The purely private medical or dental practitioner functions in his office or clinic with great autonomy, with auxiliary staff and equipment and freqently the mindset of an independent small businessman.

In many affluent industrialized countries, the economic support for medical care may come through social security or another organized source, but the services are still rendered by doctors in private practice. When financial coverage is not forthcoming in some such way, patients consulting private doctors are generally of high or moderate income; even a poor family, however, will consult a private doctor if desperate enough about an illness, especially in a child.

In many developing countries, and in some developed ones, physicians and dentists employed in governmental or other organized services may do this work for perhaps 4 to 6 hours a day. The balance of the time, they are free to go to a private setting—perhaps shared with other doctors—to see private patients. Since official government salaries in developing countries are typically quite low, the private earnings are usually considered important to support a proper standard of living for the doctor and his family. Ministries seldom object to this policy, since they regard it as necessary for recruitment of doctors and their placement in various unattractive locations. Yet the divided loyalties from these two types of medical practice generate problems—hasty service on the public side in order to maximize the time available for more lucrative work on the private side.

Pharmacies and Drugstores. Aside from drug shops in the socialist countries or the units attached to public hospitals and health centers elsewhere, the great majority of pharmacies and drugstores are privately owned and operated. They may sell both medically prescribed and over-the-counter (nonprescribed) drugs; in many developing countries, however, little distinction is made between the two, and almost any drug the patient requests is dispensed. For a prescribed drug, payment may come from an organized health program or the patient directly.

Private pharmacies are often open for long hours every day, and accessible when physicians are not. Patients may therefore go directly to a pharmacy for help from the pharmacist or sometimes from an unqualified pharmacy clerk. Even if a doctor is available, the patient may do this to save the expense of a medical consultation. It is often said that "the drugstore is the poor man's doctor." Like pharmacies, retail shops for prosthetic appliances, hearing aids, optical supplies, and the like are predominantly privately owned, and operated for profit.

Private Hospitals. Many hospitals, of course, are owned and operated by religious and other nonprofit bodies, but in this context are hospitals operated as for-profit commercial enterprises. Often they are owned by a physician or a group of physicians, sometimes by other investors. They are typically small and cater to relatively wealthy patients who can afford their prices. They are located mainly in cities, where wealth is concentrated. Sometimes private hospitals accommodate patients insured by a third-party payment program, such as industrially injured workers.

A special characteristic of private proprietary hospitals is their attention to amenities

for patient comfort. Nursing service is usually abundant, the food served is carefully prepared, most beds are in private rooms, and every patient may have a television set. Since these amenities are costly, less may be spent on diagnostic and therapeutic equipment, so that the tendency is to serve relatively easy cases, such as normal maternity patients, simple appendectomies, or minor injuires. For more serious conditions, the wealthy patient generally seeks care in a larger, more sophisticated hospital.

To provide extra amenities for affluent or socially "important" persons, large public or nonprofit hospitals often maintain a small number of private rooms. These rooms are accessible only by payment of an incremental charge. Whether or not public hospitals should provide such elegant private rooms has been a subject of political debate.

In recent years, a new issue has arisen in the commercial hospital field. Certain large corporations have built or purchased large chains of proprietary hospitals. This has been done predominantly in the United States and Western Europe, where ample capital funds are available from selling shares to investors on the stock market. Studies have shown these for-profit hospitals to render good quality service, but for charges that are significantly higher. The economies-of-scale derived from the operation of many small hospitals, in other words, have been converted into profits rather than lower charges.

Comment. The overall private commercial market for health service calls for general comment. The proportions of this market, in general, are inversely related to the strength of the ministry of health, social security, and other organized programs described here. If these are weak, relative to the population's needs, a large private market is likely to develop. If these socially supported services are strong and well distributed, the private market will be relatively small. Even in the most highly organized health system with a strong public medical service, it may well be prudent to allow a small private market to exist—if only to accommodate individuals not satisfied with the public service and with the money to pay for private care. Without this safety valve for accommodating the rich, political difficulties may arise out of all proportion to the nature of the problem. The relative magnitude of private resources is the issue.

The private proprietary market, of course, is not an organized program in the usual sense of the term. Its characteristics, however, are shaped by economic processes of supply and demand, price and competition. These processes, of course, seldom operate perfectly, especially with respect to a complicated matter like health care. The patient is often unable to exercise sound judgment about service that he may need and therefore should "demand." Most of the decisions on medical care, in fact, are made by the doctor, or supplier, rather than the patient, or demander. The nature of sickness, furthermore, seldom permits the patient to "shop around" to compare prices for a given procedure, nor to judge the relative quality of work done by one doctor or dentist compared to another.

For these and many other reasons, most national health systems, with a few notable exceptions, are moving in the direction of increasing organization along lines intended to ensure quality standards and effective management of resources and services. This has meant gradual replacement of the private medical market with socially organized health programs, even though the gradient of the social change curve undulates. In the late 1980s, political forces in several countries encouraged *privatization* of health services, but—judging from long-term social trends—this will probably prove to be a transitory phase.

ECONOMIC SUPPORT

The many diverse programs reviewed lead to various patterns for the delivery of health services, but before we examine this ultimate system component, we must consider two crucial supportive activities: economic support and management.

The economic support of health programs, as well as of resource production and the final delivery of services, comes from several sources. The relative proportions of these sources vary greatly among countries. Some, such as general tax revenues, are found to some extent in all countries. Others, such as voluntary insurance or foreign aid, are prominent in some countries and nonexistent in others. We start with the type of health support that is ancient and well-established everywhere: general tax revenues.

General Tax Revenues

Economic support for most of the health programs under ministries of health and also other government agencies is derived principally from general tax revenues. Such revenues everywhere support community preventive services—environmental and personal—with somewhat less extensive application to treatment services. This mechanism also supports the training of many types of personnel and the construction of health facilities.

General revenues encompass tax money collected at any level of government—national, provincial, or local. Taxes are levied in many different forms. They may apply to personal incomes and to the incomes of businesses or corporations. Such tax rates are often *progressive,* in that high-income persons or businesses pay a greater percentage of their net earnings than those of lower income. In the economically less developed countries, the collection of income taxes is often difficult; thus, greater use is made of taxes on land and sales taxes. Special taxes are also levied on imports and on the purchase of major types of equipment, such as automobiles or refrigerators. Liquor and tobacco are widely taxed, along with other relative luxuries, such as hotels and restaurant charges. There may be taxes on agricultural and mineral products at the point of marketing or on export. All sorts of special licensing fees yield government revenues, such as fees for operating a business, practicing a profession, driving a car, or showing a theatrical performance.

Most of this tax revenue goes into the general treasury of the central government or some lower jurisdiction. Its use for health purposes must, of course, compete with demands from all the other branches of government.

Countless political forces influence the allocation of tax funds among various ministries. For this reason, health leaders often favor taxes that are earmarked and may be used only for certain health-related purposes; this is true for social security revenue.

Social Security

The legal requirement that periodically (e.g., monthly) all employers of a certain type (e.g., in industrial enterprises with more than 20 workers) and their employees must pay a stated percentage of wages or salaries into a special fund for health or other social purposes is usually called social insurance or social security. Since the money does not go into the general government treasury, the payments are usually called *contributions* rather than taxes. The wages on which contributions are payable by workers may be up to a certain ceiling, such as "5 percent of wages up to $1,000 per month." A similar ceiling may or may not apply to the employer's payments or *payrolls.* In some countries, the social security law also requires a certain proportionate allotment from government.

These mandatory contributions may all go into a central social security fund. In some countries, however, for historical reasons the law simply requires that contributions be made to an independent local insurance fund, which is subject to various regulations. For example, the local fund might be required to pay doctors for specified medical services, according to a schedule of fees negotiated nationally. In federated countries, such as Canada and the United States, social insurance contributions may be levied separately by each province or state. There may be several other variations in the application of this social insurance concept.

The health services financed by social insurance contributions may be of many different kinds and rendered under diverse conditions. Sometimes the insured person must pay a share of the costs for each service, or a copayment. Sometimes the patient must pay the provider an entire fee, and then apply to the insurance fund for reimbursement of 80 or 90 percent of it. Sometimes the doctor is paid a per capita monthly amount for each person who has chosen him for regular care, so that no money changes hands for a service rendered. In many developing countries (and a few others), social security bodies maintain their own polyclinics and simply pay doctors and others a salary. Because of these diverse arrangements, the payments made by social insurance are often described generically as *benefits.*

Voluntary Insurance

Long before insurance for health purposes became required under law or statutory, groups of people pooled their money voluntarily into insurance funds, to help in times of hardship. In most countries these voluntary funds for insurance against the costs of sickness (both the loss of earnings and medical expenses) evolved into statutory insurance; in a few countries—notably Australia, South Africa, and the United States—voluntary insurance remained a significant source of financing medical care into the 1980s. It has been linked largely to employment, with insurance premiums being paid partially or mainly by employers.

Voluntary insurance carriers are of several types. Commercial insurance companies, dealing in life insurance and coverage for accidents and other casualties, are important. Special insurance organizations sponsored by physicians, hospitals, or other professional groups are involved. Relatively fewer, but often more comprehensive in their benefits, are insurance funds sponsored by consumer groups. In several countries where a social security program or even a general tax-supported health service is in effect, private voluntary insurance is sold to higher-income people who want access to private medical and hospital care.

Charitable Donations

Most of the voluntary health agencies discussed earlier are financed by charitable donations. Individuals make donations not to gain entitlement to a specific benefit, as with insurance, but to be helpful. Such donations may be numerous in affluent countries, with a large middle class that has money beyond family needs. Support from philanthropic foundations also belongs in this category.

Money for various charities in health and other humanitarian fields is required so frequently that in many industrialized countries fund raising has become a specialized occupation. These businesses compile computerized lists of people who might donate to certain causes. The overhead required for this money raising may absorb a high proportion of the funds brought in. Yet charitable donations seldom constitute a very large percentage of a country's overall health system costs. Although they are the principal source of support for voluntary health agencies, they may also go to selected hospitals or universities, some of which may even be government-owned.

In the less affluent developing countries, charitable donations may come principally from a handful of wealthy persons or a royal family. Probably more important are the donations of unpaid labor by men and women in small communities, for health purposes.

Lotteries. Charitable organiztions and even governments sometimes sponsor lotteries or games of chance to raise money to support hospitals or health programs. The cost of selling the lottery tickets and awarding the prizes is usually substantial in relation to the funds raised for the heath objective.

Foreign Aid. A special form of charitable donation, prominent in many developing countries, is foreign aid for health purposes. The oldest form comes from foreign religious missions that developed hospitals and clinics, which still operate throughout the world. Since World War II, health assistance and advice have been transmitted to the developing countries, along two general lines: multilateral and bilateral. In both types of foreign support, the aid is rarely in the form of money but through the provision of skilled personnel, equipment, supplies, consultation, and various activities constituting a *health project.*

Principal multilateral programs are the World Health Organization (WHO) and United Nations Children's Fund (UNICEF), but certain health activities are also sponsored by the UN Development Program, the World Bank, and the UN Fund for Population Activities. These organizations represent the governments of nearly all nations in the world, and thousands of projects explore various strategies to improve health. The work is usually described as "collaboration" rather than assistance.

Bilateral programs consist of specific projects in which one country helps another. Within the country, the agent may be governmental or private. Japan builds a hospital in Burma or the United States organizes a family planning project in Kenya. Beneath the surface, the donor may have some ulterior motive, but this need not negate the value of a project in advancing health objectives. Privately sponsored projects may originate from scores of different charitable agencies within the donor country.

Individuals and Families

In every health system, no matter how large a percentage of costs is covered by government revenues and other social mechanisms, some expenditures are made by individuals and families. Because illness and accidents are unpredictable, a family not protected by social financing of some type may suddenly be confronted with large health care costs.

Substantial expenditures are made by individuals in most countries for day-to-day health-related items, such as self-prescribed drugs, insurance copayments, or the charges of private health practitioners. The amounts spent privately on medical care tend to be proportional to family income, with wealthy families spending the most. Severe illness, on the other hand, is more prevalent in low-income families. To compound the inequities, the proportion of earnings spent on health care has generally been found to rise as family incomes decline.

In some countries, social policy dictates that government health expenditures be kept to a minimum, and private expenditures be maximized. Even the use of public hospitals and health centers requires payment of fees. In some very poor countries, patients in government hospitals are provided a bed and little more; private payments must be made for drugs, laboratory tests, and x-rays. Families are expected to provide food, unless the patient has no family.

Comment

The mix or relative proportions of these several sources of economic support is very different from country to country. Exact data are often difficult to get, but if available, this information can shed a great deal of light on the general nature of a health system. It reflects the degree to which a nation has taken social responsibility for the health of its people.

Another indicator of economic support is the percentage of overall government expenditures that are attributable to the health sector. Often military outlays increase the total government budget while the proportion devoted to health declines.

If total health expenditures, public and private, are related to a country's wealth or gross national product (GNP), an important index is derived on the national importance attached to the health system. For many reasons—in the health sciences, in the population, and in society—this percentage has been rising throughout the twentieth century in almost all countries, both the developing and the industrialized. The net percentage of GNP spent for health purposes has also long been higher in wealthy countries than in poor countries; despite the overall elevation this differential persists. In a later chapter, we explore the nature of and reasons for these changes in different types of country.

MANAGEMENT

The second major form of support for health resources, programs, and services in national health systems, after economic support, is management. This term encompasses several managerial processes: (a) planning, (b) administration, (c) regulation, and (d) legislation.

Except for certain socialist states, few countries have an integrated and coherent health system that would permit a unitary analysis of these four processes for the system as a whole. Instead, as we have seen, most health systems consist of an aggregation of "programs" or subsystems, in each of which the management characteristics are somewhat different. The general culture or ideology of a country tends to influence all subsystems, but the precise implementation of management policies is bound to vary in, for example, a government ministry, a voluntary agency, and a private enterprise.

Planning

Health system planning may be carried out with very different degrees of thoroughness. It may be fully centralized and govern practices in every facet of the system, or it may apply only to the ministry of health. The object of planning may be limited to the production of human and physical resources, or it may also include detailed standards for the performance of all health services—personal and environmental.

A centralized national planning body may influence all major health activities, such as autonomous social security health programs, the universities training health professionals, and water supplies constructed by a ministry of interior, as well as the programs of the ministry of health. When the planning applies only to the ministry of health, it may be done by the planning unit of the ministry itself. The locations and activities of health practitioners in the private market (physicians, dentists, pharmacists, etc.) may be left entirely outside the sphere of planning; alternatively, certain restrictions may be imposed on the private market to achieve equitable geographic distribution of health personnel.

Different methods of health planning may be employed. Planners may try to estimate the objective health needs of a population through surveys and other research. The planning approach may set out aggressively to respond to the needs, or simply passively adjust to the capabilities of resources that happen to be available. Decisions on the location of new health centers or hospitals may be made according to some objective formula that estimates varying needs, or simply adjust to the political preferences of influential leaders. Although planning may be the responsibility of a central government agency, nongovernmental experts could be called on to advise on policies, such as the proper schedule of examinations of a newborn infant.

To what extent are planning functions decentralized in a large country? If substantial responsibilities are delegated to peripheral bodies, are standards or guidelines posed by the central body? Do the plans of peripheral bodies require central approval before being implemented? Are certain nongovernmental groups incorporated in the planning process? Such questions must be answered to characterize fully the planning aspects of management.

Administration

Sometimes the terms *administration* and *management* are used interchangeably, but here administration is meant to include the decision making of program leaders and the supervision, controls, and other actions necessary to ensure satisfactory performance and to attain certain goals. Administrative policies applied in one program of a health system, of course, may differ from those in other programs.

Administrative "style" has been described as varying between authoritarian at one extreme and democratic at the other, with several stages in between. Some political settings tend to favor an authoritarian or autocratic approach; others favor the opposite. Furthermore, in some historical periods, more autocratic decisions are fully accepted because of a crisis situation. At other times, administration is not successful unless extensive democratic discussion precedes every major decision. The administration of a health program, large or small, involves to some extent at least eight processes.

Organization. The work in any program must ordinarily be divided into smaller sets of tasks, to be performed by persons with appropriate skills. There is usually a time as well as a physical or spatial dimension; one task must be completed before another can be started. Organization may require the deployment of personnel in a certain geographic area. Various types of equipment may be necessary to perform certain tasks. The organization of resources, of course, is intended to achieve efficiency, so that the goal is attained with the least expenditure of time, resources, and energy. How are these organizational processes carried out?

Staffing and Budgeting. To carry out the intended program, personnel must be recruited. They can already be qualified or they may be trained for the jobs to be done. Selection of personnel usually considers not only technical qualifications, but also how well and enduringly the individual will work in the organization. Proper personnel administration, of course, takes account of salaries, working conditions, and job relationships. How are these matters handled?

When staffing is settled, and other expenses—such as equipment and supplies, communication, and travel—are estimated, the budget may be prepared. This is usually subject to review by some higher echelon in the overall program. Only when a final budget is approved can the program proceed. Does the budget contain contingency funds for unanticipated problems?

Supervision. When an organized staff is in place, its work must be supervised to the extent necessary and feasible. Some individuals may perform so diligently that little supervision is needed. Others require careful surveillance. Supervision may be supportive or intimidating. It may encourage or discourage the worker. Analysis of a national health system should attempt to characterize these features of the administrative process.

Consultation. Closely related to supervision is consultation offered to staff members. Problems may arise on which a health worker (regardless of his or her qualifications) needs advice. The administrator may be able to help, or an outside consultant may be called in. Sometimes a colleague elsewhere has faced a similar problem and can offer helpful advice. If a particular problem occurs frequently, does it signal the need for a staff conference?

A special form of consultation is the participation of community people in the operation of a health program. Any program can benefit from councils of citizens who convey the reactions of local residents to the services being provided. Are there suggestions for improvement? This sort of community participation can serve as continuing consultation from the people. Does it help ensure the accountability of a program to the people being served?

Procurement and Logistics. Most organized health programs require a dependable flow of drugs and other supplies. This can be arranged in various ways. Often there is a central warehouse, from which supplies are sent to facilities periodically. The specific items may depend on a prearranged annual list or may be based on orders submitted by field units. In developing countries, which must import most products, difficulties often arise from shortages of foreign exchange to purchase the imports.

Certain health facilities may be free to acquire supplies on the local market. Eliminating transportation problems may permit needs to be met promptly and efficiently, even though the net costs are higher. The logistics of transporting medical supplies may or may not be integrated with the distribution of supplies for schools, agriculture, or some other program.

Records and Reporting. For a program's administration to be alert to day-to-day performance and to recognize changing needs, it is generally necessary to maintain some form of regular records, summarized by periodic reporting. Health programs usually require records on the persons served, diagnoses, services provided, drugs dispensed, and the like. Sometimes financial data are necessary. For certain activities, such as a meeting for health educational purposes, the number of persons attending can be recorded. Are records of this sort kept?

On the basis of records, reports may be sent periodically to higher levels of administration. Aside from quantitative data on services, a re-

port might indicate any problems encountered or suggest modifications of policy to improve the program. A sophisticated administrator may be able, through a report, to identify problems that are not stated explicitly.

Channels for rapid communication are other essential tools of administration. Telephone, telegraph, and postal systems cannot be taken for granted. Are they kept in operative condition, which is often difficult?

Coordination. Another task of administration is to coordinate programs coming under different administrative directions. Coordination may be required between different health programs or between programs in health and those in other sectors. Conflicts sometimes arise that simple discussion could resolve. The programs in a health system may or may not be well coordinated with those in other sectors. Intersectoral collaboration, in other words, depends on two-way relationships between administrative personnel in various social sectors.

Evaluation. Finally, health programs require evaluation. This may be made at several levels—within a particular health unit or hospital, for an entire health district or province, for a certain category of program such as tuberculosis control or family planning, or for an entire country. As health expenditures have risen throughout the world, evaluation of program accomplishments has become increasingly appreciated.

Numerous methods of health program evaluation can be applied with different degrees of sophistication. Perhaps the method most commonly used is simply to determine the mortality rates—usually the infant mortality and the life expectancy at birth—of a country or region and observe trends over time. These data reflect a great deal about a country or region, but by themselves they cannot be properly interpreted to reflect the value or the performance of a health system. It is well known that total environmental and social conditions—employment, housing, education, income levels, agricultural conditions, and so on—influence mortality rates as much as or probably more than the health system.

Mortality rates are an *outcome* measure of health, along with many other social sectors; only if proper research conditions are set up, can they serve as sound indicators for health program evaluation. Other measures are *input* and *process*. The training and deployment, for example, of 1,000 nurses in a certain province is an input measure; one assumes that the nurses will be rendering some services beneficial to health.

A process measure may be illustrated by the performance of immunizations on 80 percent of the children in one district. This would presumably mean a better quality health program than an immunization rate of 40 percent of the children in another province, granting that the vaccines were of equal potency. It is assumed, of course, that the immunizations will be effective in preventing a certain infectious disease; the final rate of cases of the disease occurring would provide an outcome measure of the effectiveness of the immunization program, again assuming that other conditions in the two provinces were equal.

Countries differ in the extent to which they conduct useful evaluative studies of their health systems. To heighten reliability, such studies are often done by persons outside the program or activity being evaluated. In the management of certain health programs, evaluative data may be built into normal record-keeping, so that administrators get regular feedback on the process, if not the outcome, of the program. Such feedback may also concern expenditures, so that the program leadership can keep track of costs in relation to the funds available.

Regulation

Part of management in any health system is the stipulation of various standards and their enforcement. Regulation is commonly regarded as applying to the surveillance of private activities by governmental authorities. Much regulation is of this type, but it also applies to the inspection of governmental performance at one level by some higher level of authority or by some government body from another sector. Regulatory processes may be classified in many ways. Here we consider the

chief objects of regulation within four principal categories.

Environmental Conditions. Perhaps the earliest form of regulation affecting health was the establishment and intended enforcement of standards for the physical environment. There are many standards for the purity of water consumed, especially for drinking. The disposal of human excreta is subject to much regulation, principally in cities. If sewage is discharged into a river or other body of water, regulations may require some type of physical and chemical treatment to reduce the extent of pollution. The same may apply to industrial waste.

In recent decades, many countries have made regulations to reduce pollution of the air with waste products discharged from industries or even homes. The exhaust from automobiles has come to be recognized as a major cause of air pollution in large cities, and regulations may be imposed on the manufacturers of vehicles. Simple outdoor bonfires or incineration of garbage is sometimes restricted to protect the purity of air.

In societies using animal milk (mainly from cows, but sometimes from other animals), its collection and processing entails many hazards of contamination. Milk sanitation, therefore, is subject to regulation in many countries. Likewise the butchering, storage, and handling of animal meats call for standards and regulation. Restaurant inspection is a common regulatory practice in most developed countries, but not in many developing countries except perhaps in the largest cities.

The various forms of inspection to enforce these sanitary regulations require skilled staff, in adequate numbers. In many countries, even some of the most affluent, the enforcement resources are deficient. Without enforcement or with weak enforcement, regulations are of little value.

Pharmaceuticals. The regulation of drugs is an integral part of the management of most health systems. Since the vast majority of the world's drugs are produced by private firms, in business for profit, the history of pharmaceutical manufacturing has been marked by repeated tragedies from the sale of unsafe or poisonous drugs. In addition, claims made for the benefits of various compounds have been deceptive.

Over the years, therefore, many countries have enacted legislation and issued regulations on drug production and sale. These are intended to ensure the safety of drugs and honesty in claims about the benefits of various preparations. As pharmacological science has advanced, regulations have required that drugs be proven effective with respect to the disorders they are meant to treat. In some countries, regulations restrict the types of drugs that may be imported.

Enforcement of these regulations may require inspection of pharmaceutical manufacturing plants, as well as extensive reports on preliminary drug experimentation. The labeling of packaged drugs is usually subject to careful regulation, as well as the content of advertising. Are the inspection resources adequate?

Health Personnel and Facilities. The registration or licensure of health personnel is another key form of system regulation. Physicians are subject to licensure in every country. In most, proof of the completion of prescribed education and perhaps some practical training (internship, rural service, etc.) is the usual basis for licensure. Membership in a professional "college" for ethical surveillance may be mandatory, and this may call for certification of *moral character.* In some countries, an additional examination by government authorities is required. There are often special requirements for graduates from a foreign medical school. Specialty status in medicine may also be regulated, but often by professional associations rather than government.

Registration is usually required for fully trained nurses, pharmacists, dentists, and several other types of health personnel. Great differences prevail among countries in the classes of personnel licensed, and the criteria applied. For many auxiliary health workers, trained by public health authorities, completion of the prescribed training may be the only requirement. It is expected that such persons will always be employed in an organized setting, even though some may illegally engage in private practice later.

Most registration or licensure is permanent, unless the individual has been found guilty of some crime or serious misbehavior. For a few health disciplines in certain countries, however, some type of periodic relicensure may be required. Often a stipulated amount of continuing education is required, or the individual may have to pass a new examination.

Countries may also establish standards for hospitals. These may apply to physical structures, space per bed, fire safety, provisions for a surgical operating theater, a laboratory, or something else. They may also govern certain practices, such as the maintenance of sanitary conditions, the proper operation of an x-ray department, the employment of qualified health personnel, and so on. In some countries, these standards apply to all hospitals and in others only to public facilities.

In the regulation of hospitals, governmental standards may be supplemented by nongovernmental. An association of hospitals may promulgate standards that, in some ways, go beyond those of government—for example, in the maintenance of patient records, the rules of the medical staff, or the proper procedures for surgical operations. Designation of this nongovernmental approval or *accreditation* is usually intended to reassure the population of the qualifications of some hospitals and perhaps the hazards of others.

Similar governmental and voluntary regulations may be applied to other facilities, such as those for long-term care or for rehabilitation. Certain departments of institutions, such as laboratories or blood banks, may be subject to separate standards and review by voluntary or governmental bodies.

Personal Health Services. By implication, the licensure of health personnel establishes standards for their performance. If a person has been properly trained, it is assumed that he or she will work according to certain principles. Beyond this input standard, however, most health systems have other forms of regulation over performance, though they may be informal.

This informal regulation is probably best developed in hospitals. When doctors, nurses, and other members of the medical care team work together, a certain self-discipline tends to develop. Each member of the team is conscious of being observed by all the others, and presumably wants to win the respect of colleagues. The extent to which such dynamics develop is bound to vary with the nature of the hospital leadership and the morale throughout the entire health system. Similar self-regulatory discipline may exist in health centers or polyclinics.

Under insurance programs for medical care, when practitioners are paid on a fee-for-service basis, the review of professional claims constitutes a type of regulation. Statistical tabulations may show certain doctors to be ordering excessive laboratory procedures or prescribing too many drugs. Certain types of surgical operation may be performed much more frequently than seems reasonable. Although this sort of statistical inference can never be conclusive, it can lead to further investigation of a doctor's performance. Similar surveillance may apply to dental service.

The judicial system, which permits a patient to bring a lawsuit against a doctor for malpractice, is another indirect form of regulation. The laws and practices on this procedure differ greatly among countries; malpractice litigation is easily undertaken in some and difficult in others.

Legislation

Every health system is supported, directly or indirectly, by a body of legislation. Laws permeate all five components of a health system, whether they are explicitly evident or not. They must be regarded ultimately as part of the management of the health system. Much regulation, as noted, is clearly based on law, but the same applies to many other aspects of health systems.

Broadly considered, law supports health system functions in at least six principal ways.

Facilitating Resource Production. Laws may authorize and provide funds for training physicians, nurses, and other types of health personnel. Laws may also require that professional graduates serve in a rural area before licensure. New categories of health personnel

for certain functions may be authorized under legislation. Quality standards may be mandated for licensure.

Hospitals and health centers may be constructed under legislative authorization, and the funds required may be appropriated. Under the concept of regionalization, various types of service may be legally restricted to facilities of certain sizes and capabilities.

Authorization of Programs. Most of the organized programs of health service, reviewed earlier, rest on some legal foundation. A ministry of health is ordinarily established by law, although its scope of activity may be defined in very general terms. Under an objective such as "protection of the public health," a very wide range of activities may be carried out. The same applies to health authorities of ministries of labor for protecting the safety and health of workers.

Legal requirements of countries on financial matters differ greatly. Under parliamentary democracies, legislative authorization of funding may be required each year; other forms of government may simply allow broad spending powers to be exercised by the executive authority. In one way or another, health programs in government, and sometimes even under private auspices, depend on legislative authorization. Programs for communicable disease control, environmental sanitation, access to family planning service, water fluoridation for preventing dental caries, and countless other purposes may rest on legislation.

Social Financing of Health Care. The several methods of economic support for health service rest partially or wholly on legal foundations. For social security programs, mandating periodic employer and employee contributions, legislation is obviously required. Even for voluntary insurance, the general operations of nongovernmental insurance carriers are usually subject to various official constraints. Likewise charitable organizations must often function within certain legal boundaries.

The taxing power, on which most governmental health work depends, is granted by various laws. Rates of taxation on personal incomes, the value of land, the purchase of commodities, and so on are typically defined in laws. When taxes are levied by public jurisdictions below the national level, special legal authorization may be necessary.

Quality Surveillance. The several forms of regulation of personnel and facilities, reviewed earlier, rest largely on law. Their ultimate purpose is to protect the population against health service of poor quality. Laws are necessary to protect people from worthless or injurious services that might be provided for purely pecuniary motives. Various procedures for *peer review* of technical performance may be legally mandated.

Prohibiting Injurious Behavior. Most of the regulations concerned with environmental sanitation rest on laws that restrict the behavior of individuals or groups. Laws may prohibit discarding garbage in the streets or disposing of raw sewage or toxic waste into a stream furnishing drinking water. Laws may establish the speed limits for automobiles or require persons using motorcycles to wear protective helmets.

Such legislation is intended to protect the well-being of the community as well as the individual. Because these laws, and the regulations under them, often restrict individual freedom, contention may arise over their enforcement. This has applied to laws restricting the advertising of tobacco products or smoking of cigarettes, which may be harmful to the individual as well as others. Judicial courts must often decide if and when the protection of public health takes precedence over individual rights, under the constitution and legal structures of various countries. The proper scope of the *police power* of government undergoes continuous reinterpretation, as knowledge about the social determinants of health and disease is extended.

Protecting Individual Rights. Finally, laws in many countries are intended to ensure the protection of individual rights in the operations of a health system. The patient, on whom surgery is to be performed, may be entitled to know the risks entailed and to give *informed consent* to the procedure. Industrial workers may be entitled to know the hazards of substances used in their daily work. Such rights can be guaranteed by law.

DELIVERY OF SERVICES

The endpoint of national health systems, as conceived here, is the delivery of health services to people. The production of resources, their organization, the economic support, and the process of management are all means to an end—to provide health care in order to promote or restore health. The exact manner of delivery of service, however, may take many forms among countries and within countries.

Health services may be analyzed and classified in several ways. A method oriented to the biological character of disease might classify services for the prevention, diagnosis, and treatment of infectious disease, metabolic disorders, mental disorders, trauma, and so on. If therapeutic modalities were the criterion, health services might be classified by their use of drugs, surgery, physical techniques, and so on. A method that is widely considered appropriate to the *organizational* features of health systems categorizes services as primary, secondary, and tertiary care. These rubrics are based mainly on consideration of the complexities of health resources and services of all types and to a lesser extent on the time sequence of disease and patient care.

Before considering the content of primary, secondary, and tertiary health service, we must emphasize that in no country is the pattern of delivery of these services identical for everyone. We have observed the numerous organized programs or subsystems, including a private market, in most national health systems. The manners in which services of all types are provided vary greatly among these programs and especially for different classes of person served in one health system. The diagnosis and treatment of a sprained ankle, for example, are likely to be very different in most countries for an impoverished village dweller, a wealthy urban executive, a soldier in uniform, an industrial worker on his job, and a patient in a mental hospital. All countries may have a predominant pattern for each category of care, but certain population subgroups are nearly always likely to obtain health services in a special way.

Primary Health Care

Primary care embodies most health promotion and disease prevention, including both environmental and personal services. The World Health Organization (WHO) has defined primary health care to encompass at least eight elements: (1) education concerning health problems and the methods of preventing and controlling them; (2) promotion of food supply and proper nutrition; (3) an adequate supply of safe water and basic sanitation; (4) maternal and child health care, including family planning; (5) immunizations against the major infectious diseases; (6) prevention and control of local endemic diseases; (7) appropriate treatment of common diseases and injuries; and (8) provision of essential drugs. Although this definition appears to be oriented largely toward conditions in developing countries, logically it applies everywhere. In affluent countries, an adequate food supply and safe water may be taken for granted, but they are still fundamental to health maintenance. In all countries WHO intends primary health care to embody equity and efficiency in the health services available to total populations.

Preventive Services. The first six of the eight WHO elements of primary health care (PHC) obviously concern the prevention of disease and the promotion of health. The strategies and techniques for each of these elements clearly differ for different social classes within countries and for the same social class (e.g., manual workers in a city) between countries. We consider just two examples of PHC elements: safe water and maternal health care.

The delivery of safe water in one developing country may vary between the use of a drilled well in a village square, where women bring large jugs carried home on their heads, and the use of a gold-plated kitchen faucet in an urban mansion, from which water is drawn and served in a graceful goblet with ice cubes. In some affluent countries, even the average village-dweller has an indoor water faucet; a wealthy city-dweller might consider it a holiday to go camping in the country and get his water from a plastic bottle carried in a knapsack. The variations among countries and population groups are obviously enormous.

For maternal health care, the range of delivery patterns within one health system could be even wider. The low-income slum dweller might have a prenatal examination by an assistant midwife in a crowded outpatient department of a deteriorated public hospital; the examination might be done in a slightly more cheerful prenatal clinic of the local public health agency, or in a community health center operated by a local religious group. The wife of a skilled worker might have a similar examination in the social security agency polyclinic, staffed by an obstetrician, or in the private office of a general medical practitioner. A wealthy woman would visit her private obstetrician in his elegantly appointed suite of offices; this prenatal examination would be conducted on a comfortable examining table, while the patient was carefully draped with clean linens and the doctor was efficiently assisted by a registered nurse. The examining personnel in each situation would be paid somewhat differently: full-time salary from tax revenues, part-time salary from social security funds, or a private fee from personal family income. The training of the personnel and the equipment and supplies used would likewise differ in each setting. These variations apply to maternal health care in one national health system, and across systems they would doubtless be even greater.

Preventive services of the several other types within primary health care can exhibit similarly diverse patterns of delivery. Dietary practices, health education, immunizations, and malaria control could each have different characteristics in various social settings of a single health system and, of course, across systems. Understanding delivery of services in a national health system calls for recognizing these diversities. Within some systems the disparities are greater than in others, but some degree of pluralism is found everywhere. Many analyses of national health systems tend to oversimplify their characteristics and portray the predominant features as uniform and universal.

Therapeutic Services. The last two services in WHO's listing of eight elements, comprising the essential minimum package of services in primary health care, are mainly therapeutic. The "appropriate treatment of common diseases and injuries" is disarmingly simple in its formulation, but extremely wide and diversified in its possible meanings. Perhaps only a dozen diagnostic entities are "common" in the average community, but primary service for them may require a variety of resources, plus careful organization, financing, and management. The patterns of delivery can be correspondingly varied among and within countries.

Within one health system the treatment of a common cold, for example, may vary from self-care at home (with rest in bed and hot tea) to visiting a community health worker at a village post or at the side of a UNICEF truck with the paraphernalia of a *mobile clinic,* to the services of a general medical practitioner at a small urban health center, to the care of a specialist in otorhinolaryngology in a private group practice clinic, to treatment by a uniformed physician at a military post, to care by a trained graduate nurse at a large industrial clinic, to service by a private specialist in internal medicine, and to still other medical care delivery patterns. The drugs used, the tests made (to be certain of the diagnosis), the time absorbed in the examination, the period that the patient was required to wait for attention, the degree of warmth and sensitivity shown by the provider, the payment transaction, if any, for this simple ailment all vary in the pattern of health care delivery even in one national health system.

In certain locales of any one system, of course, one can identify a predominant delivery pattern for primary care. In cities of many industrialized countries, general medical practitioners in private quarters constitute the predominant pattern. In rural villages of very poor developing countries, traditional healers visiting the patient at home may be the most common pattern. In other countries, both developing and industrialized, a team of medical and auxiliary personnel in a health center or polyclinic is the customary arrangement. In all these national settings, primary care for a common ailment is sometimes sought at the out-patient department of a general hospital.

The decision where primary health care leaves off and secondary care begins is subject to debate. Perhaps the definition itself should differ among countries or among different social groups within one country. To facilitate comparisons between countries, however, it is probably wisest to accept the WHO definition, given earlier, as the essential minimum scope of services for PHC. To these eight services we might add (9) simple prophylactic and therapeutic dental care (perhaps already included among "common ailments," but calling for certain special technical procedures) and (10) identification of potentially serious physical or mental conditions that require prompt referral for secondary or tertiary care.

Secondary Health Care

There is little consensus on the meaning and scope of secondary care. In this book, to permit intercountry comparisons of various delivery patterns, we consider secondary health care to consist of four types of service: (1) specialized ambulatory medical service, (2) commonplace hospital care, (3) care by nonmedical specialists, and (4) general long-term care.

Specialized Ambulatory Medical Service. Many disorders require skills for their diagnosis or treatment that cannot be expected to be within the competence of primary health care personnel, whether they are community health workers or general medical practitioners. The conclusive diagnosis of a case of pulmonary tuberculosis and the plan for a precise regimen of treatment illustrate this; cases of diabetes in an adult or epilepsy in a child are other examples. The diagnoses of all three conditions demand certain special types of examination not likely to be feasible at the PHC level, and the proper choice and dosage of medications require specialized training.

If patients with symptoms of such disorders are identified by a PHC worker, they should properly be referred to secondary-level care. This might be available in a well-staffed health center or in the out-patient department of a district general hospital at the first referral level. In a developing country, where the social security program has its own facilities, it could be provided at an urban polyclinic. In larger cities of an industrialized or some developing countries, it might be obtained (for higher income patients) at the premises of a private medical specialist.

The treatment of disorders requiring secondary-level care may demand costly drugs. If only because of the long duration for which therapy is necessary in the preceding examples, the costs might be higher than most families could afford. Accordingly, the delivery of appropriate secondary care often requires the provision of drugs from a socially financed program. It may require adjustments in diet, occupation, or housing that would be feasible only for persons in a moderately comfortable socioeconomic position.

Commonplace Hospital Care. Hospitalization for any condition, even in a small rural or urban facility, should be regarded as secondary care. The objective of in-patient service is to give care and make observations that are feasible only in institutions with appropriate staffing and equipment. One might argue that a normal obstetrical delivery, performed by a midwife, constitutes part of primary health care; in a hospital rather than the mother's home, however, the midwife has medical backup, equipment, supplies, and drugs, not available in her portable midwife bag. The resources of even the humblest hospital, therefore, should be regarded as delivering secondary health care.

The patterns of delivery of commonplace hospital care, of course, also exhibit a wide range. In many developing countries, hospitals of this type may have only 20 beds or fewer and staffs of just one full-time doctor, a few assistant nurses, perhaps a laboratory technician, a cook, a janitor, and little more. At the other extreme, a local hospital might have 100 to 200 beds, a staff of 10 to 20 well-trained specialists, fine apparatus for laboratory, radiological, and other diagnostic studies, full surgical and obstetrical equipment, and much more. In most countries the hospital's medical staff is composed of full-time salaried physicians, but in a few affluent countries there is an *open-staff*

policy; under this, community specialists and generalists visit the hospital a few hours per day, to see only their own private patients. Other hospital characteristics—such as the nursing service, record-keeping, diet, drug therapy, departmental organization, and so on—may affect the delivery of this form of secondary health care in different ways.

Nonmedical Specialist Care. The services of several types of special personnel who are not physicians must also be counted under the rubric of secondary health care. The prescription of eyeglasses, for example, by an optometrist or the equivalent, and the preparation of the proper corrective lenses, is one such service. The care of superficial conditions of the feet by a podiatrist is another example. Various forms of rehabilitation by a physical therapist, occupational therapist, or speech therapist constitute secondary health care. The services of dentists for elaborate prosthetic replacement of teeth or other specialized dental therapy must also be counted as types of secondary health care.

These categories of personnel do not exist in all countries, but where these types of service are available the delivery patterns may differ. The care may be provided in an organized setting, such as a hospital out-patient department or in a polyclinic for ambulatory care. In such settings the health practitioner would typically be on salary and working under some sort of medical direction. Alternatively, some or all of these personnel might be engaged in private practice, serving patients independently, whether the care is paid for privately or by some organized financial source.

General Long-term Care. As we reviewed earlier, long-term care may be provided in a range of facilities. While much of this service involves only a modest level of skill, it is clearly beyond the scope of primary health care. The important attributes in the staff of a long-term care facility may be primarily attitudinal—sensitivity to the feelings of chronically ill and elderly patients—rather than technological. Yet those attitudes are essential for good patient care.

Health care in the home of a chronically ill

patient may or may not be supported by visiting nurse service, transported meals, or other types of organized service. The nature of a personal home differs, of course, with family wealth, just as the delivery of long-term institutional care depends on the staffing and equipment of the facility.

In certain countries, the operation of long-term care facilities has attracted the sponsorship of private entrepreneurs. With the rapid aging of the population in industrialized countries, the demand for such institutional service has steadily increased, permitting high prices to be charged. For wealthy persons or families, therefore, high quality and attractive services may be offered, whereas patients of average or low income must manage with care in very modest facilities or stay at home.

Tertiary Health Care

Health care at the tertiary level refers mainly to medical and related services of extreme complexity and usually very high cost. For many countries, resources for tertiary care are available only in one central location or perhaps just a few. The physicians, technicians, and others qualified to provide such care have typically spent many years in highly specialized training. Equipment required may be so expensive that some developing countries cannot afford to purchase and maintain it. Fortunately, only a very small percentage of persons ever require tertiary care.

Some tertiary care may be only for diagnostic purposes, such as the use of computerized tomography (CT) scanning or magnetic resonance imagery (MRI). Therapeutic types of tertiary care are illustrated by renal hemodialysis, brain or open-heart surgery, and most organ transplants. Inevitably, such services require a great deal of planning and teamwork. Whether financial support is public or private, and whether the institutional setting is governmental or voluntary, the pattern of delivery of tertiary care is inevitably highly organized.

This high-technology service is the usual conception of tertiary care, but another type of service also belongs to this category. Rehabilitation programs for very severely handicapped patients involve services of a cost, duration, and level of sophistication that must be regarded as tertiary. Some very affluent countries have institutions devoted mainly to the rehabilitation of patients in whom spinal cord injury has caused paralysis of all four limbs. These quadriplegics may, through painstaking efforts and ingenious equipment, be taught to master a great many skills with the muscular power remaining only in their fingers and jaws. Of course, skillful nursing service is necessary at almost all times.

Another relevant type of tertiary service is that provided in highly developed psychiatric hospitals. Patients with severe mental illness may receive lengthy and sophisticated care that combines psychotherapy, psychopharmaceutical treatment, and *therapeutic community* service. Because duration of such treatment may be long and the aggregate costs high, it is seldom available in developing countries and may be accessible in affluent countries only to the very rich.

Special Relationships

With respect to all three levels of health care delivery, it has been noted that the patterns differ greatly not only between countries, but also for different social groups within countries. In almost all national health systems, in fact, one can identify certain social groups whose pattern of health care delivery at all three levels differs from that for the general population.

Consider an army officer, whose family lives under the protective wing of the military establishment even after retirement. A child born into that family who also enters the army as a permanent career experiences a highly structured pattern of health care delivery from birth to death. The great bulk of families in the same country may have to use a variety of patterns of health care delivery, depending on changing socioeconomic conditions, the nature of illnesses suffered, the geographic areas in which they live, and so on. The same exceptional delivery pattern might apply to a family that inherits great wealth.

From another perspective, an infant born with severe mental retardation might be admitted to a public institution for the retarded at an early age. He may spend his entire life in this setting, and any health service required at the primary, secondary, or tertiary level would be provided under the sponsorship of the institution. The experience, whether favorable or not, certainly differs markedly from that of the rest of his family or the population at large.

These accounts of primary, secondary, and tertiary care are inevitably somewhat oversimplified; distinctions among the three types are seldom clear-cut. They are useful, nevertheless, to suggest the feasibility of organizing health systems in an appropriate manner, so that resources are used most effectively and efficiently. They should also facilitate analysis of actual practices in different health systems.

Many health systems designate health facilities with a role explicitly labeled as primary, secondary, or tertiary in purpose. This policy is usually defined as *regionalization,* and it tends to be most fully applied in systems where social financing of services is most highly developed. Principles of regionalization can provide guidance for health planning and policy making that is especially valuable where resources are very limited.

HEALTH SYSTEM DYNAMICS

This completes our review of the five major components of health systems. It is possible to find and analyze these components in every national system, and understanding them is essential if any enduring changes or improvments are to be made in a country. By seeing the whole picture, one becomes sensitive to the many effects of an intervention attempted in any one part of it.

The contours of each system component, of course, are continually changing, in response to political, economic, and social developments. A change in one component—for example, a major new mechanism of economic support—is bound to influence the nature and functioning of some or all of the other components. A new discovery, an addition to medical knowledge, may radically change priorities in the organization of ministries of health and in the delivery of certain preventive services. A much increased output of medical manpower resources may modify the patterns of delivery of primary health care. Any deliberate attempt to change a health system must take these dynamics into consideration.

The interplay of sources of economic support and patterns of delivering service is an especially significant reflection of sociopolitical forces in a national health system. One might expect funds from public sources to be spent on service delivered by public providers, and private funds to support services from private providers. In reality, the relationships are seldom this simple. Figure 3.2 illustrates the various combinations of economic support and service delivery. In many national health systems, one finds health services provided in ways conceptualized by all four cells of this matrix. In other words, public money may support services by public providers (as in cell A) or by private providers (as in cell B). Private

Source of Money	Health Care Provider	
	Public	Private
Public	A	B
Private	C	D

Figure 3.2 Possible relationships between source of money (economic support) and health care provider (service delivery) in a national health system.

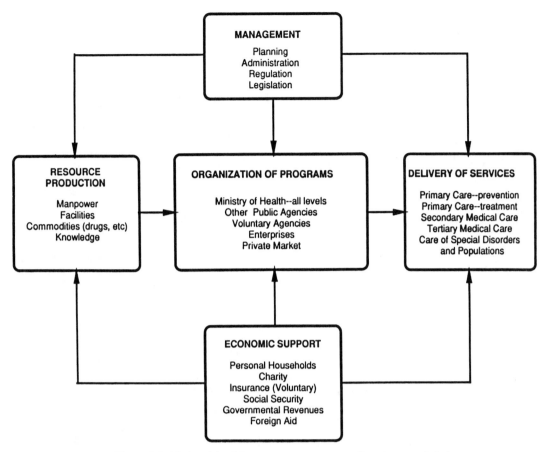

Figure 3.3 National health system: components, functions, and their interdependence.

money may be paid for services by public providers (as in cell C) and, of course, for services by private providers (as in cell D). Examples of all four of these arrangements are found throughout the accounts of national health systems.

At the outset of this chapter, it was claimed that a health system constitutes a constellation of activities designed *primarily* to advance and protect the health of people. It should now be clear how many other objectives must be pursued to reach that end. The production of resources requires fulfillment of objectives in the fields of education, structural engineering, pharmaceutical chemistry, and scientific research. Program organization entails politics, religion, free enterprise, and more. Economic support requires tax collection, charity, insur-

ance, personal wages, and other factors. Management requires forecasting, decision making, interpersonal wisdom, the exercise of power, and so on. Health service delivery requires the matching of technology with the health needs of people in diverse social settings. All five health system components, and their principal subdivisions and relationships, are summarized and modeled in Figure 3.3.

In the course of pursuing these numerous subobjectives, it is easy for the actors to lose sight of the ultimate goal. The private practitioner may be heavily motivated by the desire for a luxurious automobile, and the public servant may be most interested in political advancement. The pharmaceutical company may be most concerned about providing higher dividends to its stockholders, and the public hospital administrator may be less concerned about the treatment of his patients than about the bottom line of his financial statement and the impact of this figure on his promotion in the bureaucracy.

The circumstances prevailing today in all five components of national health systems are the result of long historical developments. Each country's history, of course, is different. The result is a different configuration of all five components in each national health system. Within broad limits, however, certain general commonalities permit the clustering of systems in the world's 165 countries into a relatively small number of types. Such an analysis of health systems, as a whole, is attempted in the next chapter.

REFERENCES

Badgley, Robin F., and Samuel Wolfe, *Doctor's Strike: Medical Care and Conflict in Saskatchewan.* New York: Atherton, 1967.

Bannerman, Robert H., John Burton, and Ch'en Wen-Chieh (Editors), *Traditional Medicine and Health Care Coverage.* Geneva: World Health Organization, 1983.

Banta, H. David, and K. B. Kemp (Editors), *The Management of Health Care Technology in Nine Countries.* New York: Springer Publishing Co., 1982.

Bodenstein, J. W., "Africanization in Mission Hospitals." *Contact* (Geneva: Christian Medical Mission), 21:4–10, June 1974.

Bosch, Paul F., *International Health.* New York: Oxford University Press, 1978.

Bullough, Vern, and Bonnie Bullough, *The Emergence of Modern Nursing.* New York: Macmillan Co., 1969.

Burrell, Craig D., and Cecil G. Sheps, *Primary Health Care in Industrialized Nations.* New York: New York Academy of Sciences, 1978.

Canadian Association of Medical Clinics, *New Horizons in Health Care: Proceedings of First International Congress on Group Medicine.* Winnipeg, Manitoba: Wallingford Press, 1970.

Davis, Karen, "Aging and the Health Care System: Economic and Structural Issues." *Daedalus,* 115:227–246, 1986.

Donabedian, Avedis, *Explorations in Quality Assessment and Monitoring: Vol. II The Criteria and Standards of Quality.* Ann Arbor, Mich.: Health Administration Press, 1982.

Ehlers, V. M., and E. W. Steel, *Municipal and Rural Sanitation,* 4th Edition. New York: McGraw-Hill Book Co., 1950.

Elling, Ray, *The Struggle for Workers' Health.* Farmingdale, N.Y.: Baywood Publishing Co., 1985.

Engel, Arthur, *Perspective in Health Planning.* London: Althone Press, 1968.

Etzioni, Amitai, *Modern Organizations.* New York: Prentice-Hall, 1964.

Fair, G. M., J. C. Geyer, and D. A. Olrun, *Elements of Water Supply and Wastewater Disposal.* New York: John Wiley, 1971.

Fendall, N. R. E., *Auxiliaries in Health Care: Programs in Developing Countries.* Baltimore and London: Johns Hopkins Press, 1972.

Flexner, Abraham, *Medical Education in Europe.* New York: Carnegie Foundation, 1912.

Freeman, Hugh, and James Farndale (Editors), *New Aspects of the Mental Health Services.* Oxford: Pergamon Press, 1967.

Fulop, Tamas, and Milton I. Roemer, *International Development of Health Manpower Policy.* Geneva: World Health Organization (Offset Pub. No. 61), 1982, p. 53.

Fulton, J. T., *Experiment in Dental Care: Results of New Zealand's Use of School Dental Nurses.* Geneva: World Health Organization (Monograph Series No. 4), 1951.

Gray, Bradford H. (Editor), *For-Profit Enterprise in Health Care.* Washington, D.C.: Institute of Medicine, 1986.

Gunn, Selskar M., and Philip S. Platt, *Voluntary Health Agencies: An Interpretive Study,* New York: Ronald Press, 1945.

Hall, Thomas L., and A. Mejia (Editors), *Health Manpower Planning: Principles, Methods, Issues.* Geneva: World Health Organization, 1978.

Hirsch, Monroe, and Ralph E. Wick, *The Optometric Profession,* Philadelphia: Chilton, 1968.

Hoare, Geoff, and Anne Mills, *Paying for the Health Sector: A Review and Annotated Bibliography of the Literature on Developing Countries.* London: London School of Hygiene and Tropical Medicine, 1986.

Howard, Lee M., *A New Look at Development Cooperation for Health: A Study of Official Donor Policies, Programmes, and Perspectives in Support of Health for All by the Year 2000.* Geneva: World Health Organization, 1981.

Huber, John B., *Consumption: Its Relation to Man and His Civilization, Its Prevention and Cure.* Philadelphia: J. B. Lippincott Co., 1906.

Ingle, John I., and Patricia Blair (Editors), *International Dental Care Delivery Systems.* Cambridge, Mass.: Ballinger Publishing Co., 1978.

International Union of School and University Health and Medicine, *School Health Symposium,* Stockholm, Sweden, 1975.

International Social Security Association, "Development and Trends in Social Security 1978–1980." *International Social Security Review,* 23:267–336, 1980.

Jelliffe, D. B., *The Assessment of Nutritional Status of the Community*. Geneva: World Health Organization (Monograph Series No. 53), 1966.

Katz, F. M., and T. Fulop, *Personnel for Health Care: Case Studies of Educational Programmes* Geneva: World Health Organization (Public Health Papers No. 70), 1978.

King, Maurice, et al., *Nutrition for Developing Countries*. Nairobi, Kenya: Oxford University Press, 1973.

Koontz, H. (Editor), *Toward a Unified Theory of Management*. New York: McGraw-Hill, 1964.

Landy, David (Editor), *Culture, Disease, and Healing: Studies in Medical Anthropology*. New York: Macmillan Co., 1977.

Last, John M. (Editor), *Maxcy-Rosenau Public Health and Preventive Medicine*, 12th Edition. Norwalk, Conn.: Appleton-Century-Crofts, 1986.

Lee, Kenneth, and Anne Mills (Editors), *The Economics of Health in Developing Countries*. Oxford: Oxford University Press, 1983.

Levin, Lowell S., et al., *Self Care: Lay Initiatives in Health*. New York: Prodist, 1976.

Likert, R., *New Patterns of Management*. New York: McGraw-Hill, 1961.

Little, Virginia C., *Social Services for the Elderly, International*. Philadelphia: Temple University Press, 1982.

MacEachern, Malcolm T., *Hospital Organization and Management*, Revised Third Edition. Berwyn, Ill.: Physician's Record Co., 1962.

Mangay-Maglacas, A., and H. Pizurki (Editors), *The Traditional Birth Attendant in Seven Countries*. Geneva: World Health Organization (Public Health Papers No. 75), 1981.

March, J. G. (Editor), *Handbook of Organizations*. Chicago: Rand McNally and Co., 1965.

Newell, K. W. (Editor), *Health By the People*. Geneva: World Health Organization, 1975.

Nichols, P. J. R. (Editor), *Rehabilitation Medicine: The Management of Physical Disabilities*. London: Butterworth, 1980.

Pannenborg, C. O., et al. (Editors), *Reorienting Health Services: Application of a Systems Approach*. New York and London: Plenum Press, 1984, pp. 47–59.

Reed, Louis S., *The Healing Cults*. Chicago (Committee on the Costs of Medical Care, No. 16): University of Chicago Press, 1932.

Roemer, Milton I., "General Hospitals in Europe," in J. K. Owen (Editor), *Modern Concepts of Hospital Administration*. Philadelphia and London: W. B. Saunder Co., 1962, pp. 17–37.

Roemer, Milton I., *The Organization of Medical Care under Social Security: A Study based on the Experience of Eight Countries*. Geneva: International Labour Office, 1969.

Roemer, Milton I., *Evaluation of Community Health Centers*. Geneva: World Health Organization (Public Health Papers No. 48), 1972.

Roemer, Milton I., *Ambulatory Health Services in America: Past, Present, and Future*. Rockville, Md.: Aspen Systems Corp., 1981.

Roemer, Milton I., and Ruth J. Roemer, *Health Care Systems and Comparative Manpower Policies*. New York: Marcel Dekker, 1981.

Roemer, Milton I., and John E. Roemer, "The Social Consequences of Free Trade in Health Care: A Public Health Response to Orthodox Economics." *International Journal of Health Services,* 12:111–129, 1982.

Roemer, Ruth, C. Kramer, and J. E. Frink, *Planning Urban Health Services: From Jungle to System*. New York: Springer Publishing Co., 1975.

Roemer, Ruth, and George McKray, *Legal Aspects of Health Policy: Issues and Trends*. Westport, Conn.: Greenwood Press, 1980, pp. 437–446.

Rosen, George, *A History of Public Health*. New York: MD Publications, 1958.

Rosen, George, *From Medical Police to Social Medicine: Essays on the History of Health Care*. New York: Science History Publications, 1974.

Rothkopf, Carol Z., *Jean Henri Dunant, Father of the Red Cross*. New York: Watts, 1969.

Shanas, E., et al., *Older People in Three Industrial Societies*. New York: Atherton, 1968.

Shilling, R. S. F., *Occupational Health Practice*. Toronto: Butterworth, 1973.

Shryock, Richard H., *The Development of Modern Medicine*, 2nd Edition. New York: Knopf, 1947.

Silverman, Milton, and P. R. Lee, *Pills, Profits, and Politics*. Berkeley: University of California Press, 1974.

Somers, Herman M., and Ann R. Somers, *Doctors, Patients, and Health Insurance*. Washington, D.C.: Brookings Institution, 1961.

Sydenstricker, Edgar, *Health and Environment*. New York: McGraw-Hill Book Co., 1933.

Trease, George Edward, *Pharmacy in History*. London: Bailliere, Tindall and Cox, 1964.

Wallace, Helen M. (Editor), *Health Care of Mothers and Children in National Health Services*. Cambridge, Mass.: Ballinger, 1975.

Williams, Cicely D., and D. B. Jelliffe, *Mother and Child Health: Delivering the Services*. London: Oxford University Press, 1972.

World Health Organization, *Hospitalization of Mental Patients*. Geneva: (Reprint from the International Digest of Health Legislation), 1955.

World Health Organization, *University Health Services*. Geneva: WHO (Technical Report Series No. 320), 1966.

World Health Organization, *The Training of Health Laboratory Personnel*. Geneva (Fourth Report of the WHO Expert Committee on Health Laboratory Services, Technical Report Series No. 345), 1966.

World Health Organization, *The Planning and Organization of a Health Laboratory Service*. Geneva: WHO (Technical Report Series No. 491), 1972.

World Health Organization, *Organization of Local and Intermediate Health Administrations.* Geneva: WHO (Technical Report Series No. 499), 1972.

World Health Organization, *Guidelines for Evaluation of Drugs for Use in Man.* Geneva: WHO Technical Report Series No. 563, 1975.

World Health Organization, *The Selection of Essential Drugs.* Geneva: WHO (Technical Report Series No. 615), 1977.

World Health Organization, *Alma Ata 1978: Primary Health Care.* Geneva: WHO, 1978.

World Health Organization, *Financing of Health Services.* Geneva: WHO (Technical Report Series No. 625), 1978.

World Health Organization, *Evaluation of Occupational Health and Industrial Hygiene Services.* Copenhagen: Euro Reports and Studies No. 56, 1982.

World Health Organization, *Rapid Assessment of Sources of Air, Water, and Land Pollution.* Geneva: WHO (Offset Publication No. 62), 1982.

World Health Organization, *Strengthening Ministries of Health for Primary Health Care.* Geneva: WHO (Offset Publications No. 82), 1984.

World Health Organization, *Intersectoral Action for Health.* Geneva: WHO, 1986.

CHAPTER FOUR

Types of Health Systems and Their Determinants

The orderly structure of national health systems, analyzed in the last chapter, has seldom come about from deliberate planning. It is really only in retrospect that one can identify the five components and how they relate to each other. Examining a national health system today, one sees the outcome of long historical developments that have led to certain attributes for each system component. The combination of these components, each with defined characteristics, permits identification of a certain *type* of health system in any country.

DETERMINANTS OF NATIONAL HEALTH SYSTEM TYPES

Analysts of the determinants of any social situation is necessarily artificial, for we are forced to abstract various causative influences as if each operated independently. In fact, the whole process of social development is a complex mixture of many different influences, which interplay with each other as well as on the phenomenon we are studying—in this case, health systems. Moreover, the influences impinging on one system component, such as health manpower resources, might have been very different from those affecting other components, such as economic support or regulatory policies.

To simplify the analytical task, one can conceptualize a great multiplicity of social influences under three broad headings: (a) economic, (b) political, and (c) cultural. In back of each of these social forces are several complex developments that must be recognized. The attributes of the current situation, how-

ever, may be accepted as embodying the net results of a long and complex past.

The world today may be regarded as a great laboratory in which experiments are being conducted on many methods of organizing and providing health services. If we study these diverse experiments objectively, we can learn a great deal about the workings, the problems, and the effects of various kinds of health system.

Economic Determinants

The most pervasive impact of economic development on national health systems is its fundamental determination of the country's health situation—its spectrum of disease problems—that gave rise to its health system. An impoverished country, burdened with rampant infectious diseases of children and malnutrition, naturally develops a health system quite different from that of an affluent country, concerned largely with chronic disorders of the elderly. Even if health system design is not always perfectly attuned to a population's health needs, it is inevitably influenced by them in countless ways.

The level of economic development of a country has other obvious influences on its health system. Very conspicuous is its impact on the supply and quality of health resources—manpower, facilities, commodities, and knowledge. Training physicians, for example, is costly, so a country's wealth should be expected to influence its capabilities in medical education and its output of doctors.

The conventional measure of economic level in a country is the gross national product (GNP) per capita per year. The GNP is the value at current prices of all goods and services produced in the country during the year. To permit international comparisons, it is customary to convert the national currency figures into U.S. dollars (at the current international exchange rate). If we relate the GNP per capita of five countries, selected simply to illustrate different levels of national wealth, to the national stock of physicians in 1983, the relationships are as follows:

Country	GNP per capita	Physicians per 100,000
Zaire	$ 174	7
Tunisia	1,285	27
South Korea	1,978	64
Mexico	2,154	71
Italy	6,549	333

It is clear that as the nation's wealth increases, its supply of doctors (ratio to population) rises, although not at exactly the same pace. If we listed all the countries in the world in this way, a number of discrepancies would be observed, since certain countries have attached great political importance to training doctors beyond the numbers that most countries of that level of wealth might consider "affordable."

Similar relationships are found between a nation's wealth and its supply of other resources, such as hospital beds. Examining another series of five countries, for which hospital bed data were available for the year 1980, the ratios of beds to population were as follows:

Country	GNP per capita	Hospital beds per 100,000
Sudan	$ 393	92.1
Colombia	1,378	164.2
Malaysia	1,876	270.3
Greece	3,932	617.3
Sweden	12,444	1,470.6

It is also a common observation that the quality of hospital resources in a national system usually corresponds to the quantity. Thus, the staffing, equipment, amenities, and general maintenance of hospitals are much better in the systems of relatively affluent countries (Sweden and Greece) than in those of the low-income countries (Sudan and Colombia).

National wealth determines more than the quantity and quality of health resources; it also affects the patterns of work of health personnel. Thus, a wealthy nation is likely to have a robust free market economy. This can provide medical and related practitioners with a substantial market for their services. This is true, whether payment is made largely from private sources (out-of-pocket or through voluntary insurance), as in the United States, or through social insurance, as in France or Japan. In the latter affluent countries, even though nearly the entire populations are covered by social insurance for health care, doctors remain mainly in private practice.

In Latin American countries such as Ecuador or Peru, on the other hand, the great majority of doctors cannot earn a satisfactory income in purely private practice. Insofar as possible, they take salaried positions, usually for 4 to 6 hours a day in the social security system, the ministry of health, the armed forces, private industries, or other organized health programs. The balance of their time (and for some few doctors, all of their time) is devoted to private patients, but there are not enough people who can afford private medical fees to support a greater volume of private practice.

In certain affluent countries, public revenues pay private doctors and hospitals to care for the poor at designated rates. These charges are paid by special public agencies, with the poor being served in private facilities. In less prosperous countries, the poor are usually served, if at all, in public facilities where the doctors work on salary. Lesser wealth induces concern for maximum efficiency in the use of governmental funds. Either way, it is the economic level of the country that determines the pattern of providing health care.

To a large extent a nation's wealth depends on its degree of industrialization, and this has multiple influences on health care patterns. The economically more developed countries are more urbanized, their transportation and communication systems are better, and the people are better educated. These social conditions affect both the demand for medical services and the supply. Urban hospitals can be larger, with more sophisticated staff and equipment. A large proportion of rural people in a nation such as India or Nigeria means less demand for scientific medicine, as well as greater difficulties in providing it. Urban concentration generates its own health problems, but it also facilitates the application of both preventive and therapeutic measures to cope with them. Within any single country, a major determinant of the geographic distribution of all health resources is the economic level of each local area.

The level of economic development of a country determines the extent to which it must depend on other countries for drugs, medical equipment, and even scientific knowledge. Few of the less developed countries have chemical industries to produce modern medications; typically, they must import these at relatively high costs. Even if pills or capsules are locally produced, their ingredients are usually imported. One of the first actions of India after its independence was to develop, with foreign advice, its own plants for producing drugs. The same occurred in China and Cuba after their social revolutions (1949 and 1959).

Research to produce new scientific knowledge requires a large investment in the education of scientists as well as the production of elaborate equipment. It is small wonder that most, though of course not all, scientific discoveries for prevention and treatment of disease have come from the highly developed nations of Europe and North America. This is not to overlook certain achievements of ancient Indian Ayurvedic or Chinese traditional medicine, discussed in later chapters. Fortunately, international ethics ensure the dissemination of scientific knowledge through worldwide publication and in other ways.

Finally, it has been found that even the *share* of a nation's total resources devoted to the health sector depends on its wealth. The more affluent countries spend around 5 to 10 percent of their GNP on all health-related purposes; in poorer countries the comparable share is typically 2 to 5 percent. The developing countries must spend so large a share of their available funds for essentials like food and shelter that relatively little is left for the entire health system; the latter gets a smaller slice of a smaller economic pie.

The GNP per capita, it should be noted, tells us nothing about the *distribution* of wealth in a country. In India, for example, a survey in 1975–1976 found that the poorest 20 percent of households earned 7.0 percent of the national income, while the richest 20 percent earned 49.4 percent of the total income. Based on a 1972 survey, the income distribution in Brazil was even more uneven—2.0 percent of national income going to the poorest 20 percent of the households and 66.6 percent going to the richest 20 percent. These inequalities are the result of political policies, however, and are relevant to the next section.

Political Determinants

Of equal or greater importance than economic factors in shaping the health system of a country are its political policies. Interwoven with economic and other factors, and often altering the operation of economic forces, the exercise of political power is crucial. In accordance with one or another ideology, politics has a pervasive impact on the quantity and delivery patterns of health services in a country.

Political determinants mean much more than the nature of the political party in power or the legal form of the current national government. Political events that are long past exercise continuing influence on many features of a health system. Even when a social revolution suddenly alters the whole structure of society, previous formulations of authority (e.g., the boundaries of provinces and cities) remain in place. In the ordinary course of events, history inevitably influences the policy decisions of today. The past is prologue to the present.

Consider the birth of the United States as an independent nation after a revolution against the British crown starting in 1776. A crucial aspect of the ideology of that American Revolution was opposition to centralized power, whether represented by a distant monarch in London or any other authority. To minimize such power, the Constitution emerging from this revolution incorporated all sorts of "checks and balances" in the executive, legislative, and judicial branches of the central government. It also established the sovereignty of the component states—originally 13 British colonies—in most matters of government, re-serving for them all responsibilities not specif-ically assigned to the federal government. Among the many matters kept under the au-thority of the states was the protection of health. Thus, the licensure of doctors, the op-eration of public health programs, the plan-ning of hospital construction, and countless other aspects of health care are still, more than 200 years after the nation's birth, state (i.e., not national) responsibilities.

Consider also the French Revolution of 1789. The rebellion was against not only the monarchy, but also its allies—the great feudal landowners and the Catholic Church. The Church, among other things, owned and op-erated most hospitals in France at the time. When a parliamentary National Assembly was set up in the first French Republic, it was nat-ural that the hospitals should be transferred to secular authorities. France was divided even-tually into some 90 *departements* or provinces, each of which was assigned responsibility for the church hospitals within its borders. Under the Napoleonic laws, promulgated after the Revolution, quite strong central controls were established; a Prefect or governor was centrally appointed to preside over each province. Among other things, he was responsible for public properties, including the hospitals. The Prefect appointed a Health Officer to handle these responsibilities, with advice from an elected council of citizens, representing the several *arrondissements* in the province. To this day, the French public hospitals are con-trolled by the local governments, under laws and regulations issued by the national govern-ment—all an outgrowth of the French Revo-lution.

It took the practical demands of the British war in the Russian Crimea (1853–1956) to in-spire an English lady, Florence Nightingale, to organize teams of nonclerical young women to go overseas and nurse the wounded soldiers. On her return, realizing the need for proper skills to nurse the sick effectively, Miss Night-ingale founded the first nonreligious school of nursing at St. Thomas' Hospital in London in 1860. Perhaps this professional discipline would have eventually developed anyway, but surely the political circumstances of the Cri-mean War had much to do with the origins of modern nursing at this time and place. And the development of nursing also doubtless con-tributed to the growth and the characteristics of hospitals.

The Industrial Revolution of the late eigh-teenth and nineteenth centuries had vast polit-ical consequences. Wage workers concentrated in the cities and formed cooperative sickness funds; they also gave rise to socialist parties that might improve their lot. In Germany, the conservative Chancellor Otto Bismarck re-sponded by launching the first statutory health insurance laws in the 1880s to "steal the thun-der" of the socialists. At the same time these laws strengthened the workers' sickness funds, which play an important role in the West Ger-man health system to this day.

Consider the influence of colonialism on the organization of health services in the depen-dent lands of Africa and Asia. While the first actions of the European colonial powers were to protect their own overseas armies and set-tlers, eventually the effective exploitation of natural resources required a minimal frame-work of public health and medical services. The British-controlled Indian Medical Service (IMS), for example, established a hierarchy of authority to operate hospitals and dispensaries and to maintain some regulation over urban sanitation in the nineteenth century. The sem-imilitary style of the IMS was an outgrowth of the colonial government, and after India's in-dependence in 1947 it naturally influenced the framework of the new Indian Ministry of Health. As in a military establishment, all doc-tors in India's government health service were full-time civil servants—a policy not seen, for example, in Latin American countries, where the health ministries developed without these political antecedents.

In Africa, colonial authorities could not at-tract many doctors or nurses from Europe. The only practical solution for the staffing of hospitals was to train native men, and to a lesser extent women, to assist in the medical work. Hence, the African "dresser" was taught by apprenticeship and became the most com-mon type of health worker in these colonies. When most African countries were liberated after World War II, the major workforce base of the new health systems was the relatively large number of dressers and other medical assistants. Under the new political authorities, however, these personnel were given more systematic training, along with the establishment of domestic medical schools. The current concept of auxiliary health manpower in Africa was clearly an outgrowth of the nineteenth-century political scene.

In the late nineteenth and early twentieth centuries, the explosion of industrialization, organization of workers, and political labor parties in Western Europe brought a cascade of social insurance programs, including provisions for medical care. With organization, public health expanded, but the private medical markets throughout Europe were most affected by the ever-broadening schemes of governmental health insurance, such as Bismarck had pioneered in Germany. After 1900 health systems began to figure significantly in the policy agendas of most political parties. World War I ushered in the Russian Revolution, and the birth of the first thoroughly socialized health system, departing radically from market dynamics in the distribution of health service.

After World War I, the famous Dawson Report in Great Britain—calling for all health services to be delivered through a network of government health centers—showed how far political events were driving the design of capitalist health systems. In 1922, political forces in Japan made that the first non-European country to enact mandatory health insurance for its employed workers. In 1924, a labor movement in Chile caused the enactment of the first such health insurance legislation in a developing country, eventually to be followed by every other Latin American nation.

Recent political developments have influenced health systems as clearly as those of past decades. Political reaction to the worldwide Depression of the 1930s accelerated the enactment of statutory health insurance programs in countries throughout the world. In the United States, the major legislative response to the Depression was probably the Social Security Act of 1935, which led to great expansion of state and local public health services and laid the groundwork for Medicare for the aged in 1965. The political aftermath of World War II, of course, brought such enormous health care changes as the National Health Service in Great Britain and the very innovative socialist health system of China.

In Southeast Asia, after World War II the British rulers of the Malay Peninsula had turned over authority to the conservative sultans, in spite of their well-known role as collaborators with the Japanese during the war. Understandably this led to a guerilla opposition movement, based in the villages and rural areas. Unlike the French in Vietnam, the British armies effectively repressed this movement by 1952. But in the new Malaysian Parliament, the political question was raised: "After all this bloodshed in the countryside, must we not do something beneficial to gain the support of the rural people?" Thus began the Malaysian Rural Health Services Scheme in 1953, a program that brings hundreds of health centers and greatly improved preventive and treatment services to millions of village people.

Consider the origins in Canada of social insurance for hospitalization and then for physician's care since the end of World War II. The concepts had been discussed by the conventional political parties since 1919, but it took the victory in 1944 of a semisocialist Cooperative Commonwealth Federation (CCF) Party in Saskatchewan to lead to the first social insurance program for hospital care of a total provincial population in 1947. Within 10 years, all of Canada had adopted the same idea. Then in 1962 Saskatchewan again pioneered doctor's care insurance. Despite a traumatic doctor's strike to usher it in, by 1968 the Canadian national government had passed a law financing physician's care insurance, and by 1971 it covered all 10 provinces.

Consider the impact of politics on health services in Latin America. From the first statutory health insurance program in Chile in 1924 to the most recent one in Uruguay in 1958, the political maturation and demands of the urban workers who voted in elections required attention. Many economic purposes were likewise fulfilled, but these health programs, providing greatly improved services in the main cities, would hardly have been launched without the growing political strength of industrial workers. The political revolution in Cuba in 1959, of course, not only brought a total change in the health system of that country, but also stimulated national health planning throughout Latin America.

The development of health systems in Western Europe has been, in large part, a story of the battle for votes in parliamentary democracies. The continuous extension of health benefits in social security programs has paralleled the growth of Social Democratic and Labor Parties. So politically popular have these programs been that, even under conservative parties, the changes have been minor for fear of losing votes. When the Tories regained power, after the British Labour Party had launched the National Health Service in 1948, the only significant change they made was to raise slightly the personal copayment for prescribed drugs. The revolutions in Eastern Europe after World War II led inevitably to adoption of the socialist model of health system, first developed in the USSR after World War I.

For political reasons, the *declared* objective of the leadership of virtually all countries is to ensure a certain minimal level of health service for all citizens. The precise level considered proper or equitable varies, of course, with economic capabilities, but it also varies with political ideology. The latter determines the priority, in access to resources, that will be assigned to the health sector, compared with other sectors such as military affairs, transportation, agriculture, industrial development, or something else. But even within a given priority determination, the accomplishments that may be expected of a health system must vary with the structure and policies of the system— its efficiency and effectiveness.

Many of the examples of major political events shaping health systems concerned wars and revolutions. When revolutions are motivated by a goal of socialism, their impact on health systems are obvious. But even a war for other purposes, if it is large and lasts long, is bound to affect the health systems of countries. Massive military conflicts usually lead to mobilization of society on both sides. With a sense of national purpose, people become motivated and resources organized in countless ways, including the provision of health services. The

strong regional organization of British hospitals in response to the bombings of World War II dramatically demonstrated such an effect. In other ways, conflicts in the Middle East heightened organizational efforts in the health systems of Israel and Egypt. (This is not to mention purely technical developments in emergency care, blood transfusion, nursing, surgery, or ambulance service coming from military field experience.) The energies required for effective social action may lie dormant in a country until a national crisis—unfortunately associated with war—awakens them. War, of course, is the extension of political negotiation that has failed, but it may also strengthen political will for other purposes.

Examples could be multiplied, but it is obvious that political events of many sorts have had great impact on national health systems. If one searches for a *single* common theme, it would be hard to find just one in earlier centuries. The French and American revolutions, the practices of colonialism, the early development of industry and urbanization, the rise of organized labor and socialist movements— all these shaped the configuration of governments and variously influenced the distribution of authority between the state and the individual.

If we think of social events as constituting a chain of causation, however, a more clearly consistent theme can be identified. Political pressure may originate from many causes, but the force of politics has been directed largely to enhancing *government intervention in the free market* of health care, to make services available to people who need them. Market intervention has meant the gradual conversion of health care from being a market commodity to being a public good. This concept requires much further elaboration, but before undertaking this we must consider a third set of determinants of health system characteristics— those that can be identified as *cultural.*

Cultural Determinants

Beyond economic and political factors, health systems are influenced by numerous other social and environmental factors. We consider these *cultural* determinants, not in the precise anthropological usage of that term, but in a sense that includes various social institutions and customs of a society. Important among these cultural determinants are technological development, religion, community structure, language, and the family. For each of these cultural features, certain examples of their impact on health systems can be offered.

Technological developments in society have been countless, and they affect all components of health systems. Drugs, for example, are the basis for vast realms of medical therapy. They gave rise to the discipline of pharmacy, call for special management policies in health programs, have spawned large pharmaceutical enterprises, have generated the enactment of much regulatory legislation, and have led to new forms of insurance protection.

Major technological advances may change the character of all health systems by enlarging the availability of resources or the potential for disease control. Consider the therapeutic effects of streptomycin and isoniazid on the treatment of tuberculosis and the occupancy of sanatoria throughout the world; the reduction of tuberculosis made sanatoria available for other purposes, such as general hospitals or institutions for the aged and chronic sick. Consider the impact of DDT spraying of houses on the control of mosquito vectors of malaria. Technical advances of this type have not only strengthened the potential of health service, but elevated the role of organization and planning in the entire use of resources within a system as well.

The development of hospitals has been profoundly influenced by the discovery of pathogenic microorganisms and their control through aseptic techniques. The discovery of anaesthesia made possible the whole development of surgical departments in hospitals. Equivalent changes came from the discovery of X-ray machines, biochemical and pathological analyses, electrocardiographs, variousforms of physiotherapy, renal dialysis, and much more.

Bacteriology and related fields (virology, parasitology, immunology) contributed importantly to the development of the public health movement. Public health organization, of course, long antedated the work of Pasteur 1860–1890, but the explosion of knowledge following the identification of disease-causing bacteria gave an enormous boost to public health work. Immunizations were extended far beyond smallpox vaccination (which had been known since 1798). Promotion of enviromental sanitation achieved a firmer foundation. The whole concept of personal and community hygiene flowered. Strategies for the control of tuberculosis, veneral disease, and other infectious diseases could be refined. In later years, the maturation of the field of epidemiology beyond the infectious diseases, to encompass chronic noninfectious diseases (such as cancer and heart disease), added further scope to public health work.

Technological developments outside the health sector also determine several features of health systems. Consider the impact of rapid and efficient methods of communication and transportation on health services. Communication has greatly facilitated contacts between the patient and health care provider. Consultations are possible across long distances. Emergency medical services throughout the world depend on the technology for rapid communication and transportation, including ambulance travel by ground, water, and air.

Transportation has changed the whole accessibility of resources in health systems. Where it is well developed, people's access to the system is increased. In the main cities of most countries, both developed and developing, transportation is generally available to enable patients to visit a health facility; as a result, home calls by the physician (once very common) have become infrequent in most countries. In many developing countries, drugs and other supplies are purchased in large quantities and kept at a central depot; they are then sent to health facilities by vehicles. The entire concept of regionalizing the functions of health facilities can be implemented only because of suitable transportation.

Technology relating to information has permeated all aspects of health systems. Printing, of course, and mass distribution of literature have greatly accelerated the diffusion of scientific information. In more highly developed countries, the rapid processing of statistical information by computer has vastly facilitated health program management, and especially evaluation.

Religion and religious organizations have played crucial roles in the development of health systems from the earliest times. In ancient Egypt, the doctor was a priest, and most schools of traditional medicine include concepts from religion (with or without some elements of empiricism). As we discuss later, the modern hospital has been derived largely from the places of refuge of the medieval Christian church. Christianity taught pity for and kindness to the poor and the sick; hospitals were a practical way of implementing this philosophy. Somewhat equivalent policies of compassion for the sick and the poor, with hospitals and even physicians visiting patient homes, were found in the early years of Buddhism and later of Islam.

In the modern world, religious bodies still play a major role in the sponsorship of hospitals. They operate institutions for long-term care of the aged and chronically ill as well. Religious doctrines also affect the provision of certain types of health service. Judaism calls for circumcision of male infants. The Roman Catholic Church has long been opposed to any "artificial" method of contraception, as well as to any type of abortion (except if the mother's life is endangered). These doctrines naturally influence the behavior of Catholic physicians and patients.

The Moslem faith, along with Hinduism, teaches the subordinate role of women; the wife is the property of her husband, and it is sacrilegious for her to be touched, even viewed, by another man. While these ideas are changing, they still influence the organization of health services in India and in many Moslem countries. A woman is supposed to be medically attended by another woman, not by a male doctor or medical assistant. Health centers in rural India are officially supposed to be staffed by a "lady doctor" as well as a male doctor, although the former are often difficult to recruit for this work. The married woman is expected to spend most of her time at home, so as not to be seen or tempted by men on the streets—hence the veiled face outdoors. These attitudes and practices doubtless inhibit the use of health services by women in societies following these religions.

The sacred cow, to outsiders, is a virtual symbol of the Hindu faith. Though this is changing, its influence on the nutritional level of the people of India has been profound. Cows consume grain and other food, yet the beef they could provide people may not be consumed. By an opposite logic, but with similar consequences, the pig is "unclean" and unacceptable as food in both Jewish and Moslem faiths. Hinduism teaches the sanctity of all animal life, along with the cow, even that of the smallest insect. Malaria control programs unfortunately require the destruction of mosquitoes. It is said that only when the great leader, Mahatma Gandhi, developed the formulation that spraying DDT led to the killing of mosquitoes not by man, but by a chemical were these preventive campaigns fully accepted in India.

Perhaps the most pervasive effect of religion on health systems is the influence of efforts to spread the gospel, especially in developing countries. In almost all faiths, the priesthood offers solace to the sick. Religious ideals are invoked to raise funds for constructing health facilities and for other health-related purposes. Hospitals all over the world are still sponsored by religious groups—Catholic, almost every Protestant denomination, Jews, Moslems, and others. Even as late as the nineteenth century, throughout Latin America the the first important hospitals were founded by the Catholic Church. In modern Africa and Asia, religious missions from Europe and North America have established hundred of health facilities and continue to staff them with missionary health personnel.

Religion has also influenced health systems in a general ideological sense. Many countries have an offical state religion, whose doctrines influence government policy on all matters. The policy in the United States of separating church and state is exceptional. In Canada, for example, government funds support religious schools, and this practice is also common in Latin America. The 1980 Islamic revolution in Iran created an extreme example of religious domination over every aspect of a nation. Even when religious affairs are quite divorced from government, they may be important in political parties. Most European countries, for example, have a Christian Democratic Party. Generally speaking, religious influence on public policy tends to be on the conservative side, stressing individual and family obligations more than social responsibility.

Community structure is part of the cultural environment, with influences on the health system that are sometimes taken for granted. The regionalization of hospital and ambulatory services, being applied in almost all countries, rests fundamentally on the geographic arrangement of large cities, small towns, and rural areas. For efficient medical services to be rendered, channels of communication and transportation must be used among various communities in a region. City life may create special disease hazards, but it also makes possible the mobilization of resources to serve large populations.

Consider the whole development of cities as an aspect of the Industrial Revolution. Crowded housing around factories was the basis for the spread of infectious disease, both person-to-person and through media such as food and water. Problems generated corrective actions. Even ancient Rome had recognized the necessity of a system of public sewage disposal, with its *cloaca maxima.* Today, the best developed safe water systems everywhere in the world are found in the largest industrialized cities. At the same time, industrialization led to accidents from hazardous machinery, generating the *employer's liability* laws; then came the industrial injury compensation acts, providing socially insured medical care for the worker injured on the job.

In the modern world almost all large cities have neighborhoods of different social class composition, and in many cities the lower-income neighborhoods become miserable slums. In the industrialized countries these are usually in the center of the city, where housing is old and deteriorated. Slums in the developing countries are typically periurban, occupied by rural people searching for employment, often unsuccessfuly, who settle in shacks at the city's edge. Both types of slum have many impacts on health systems. They are obvious breeding places for infectious disease and therefore require special public health surveillance. Many organized programs for primary health care are developed first in slum areas and later extended elsewhere. This sequence has been common in industrialized countries, where private interests oppose governmental health initiatives. For example, after a community health center, has been launched in a slum area, other such centers can be more readily established in less blighted areas.

Language and cultural identity have still other types of impact on health systems. In many developing countries, such as India or Indonesia, hundreds of different languages are spoken; there may be one official national language, but millions of people do not speak it. Extension of health services throughout such nations is handicapped by elementary problems of communication. Health educational materials, for example, must be prepared in several languages, not to mention the difficulties of oral communication. In most African countries, language problems are complicated by tribal differences. Tribalism often involves long-standing hostilities, which obviously limit cooperation in health care; regionalized relationships among hospitals, for example, may be obstructed.

Even in highly developed countries, such as Belgium or Canada, linguistic differences affect health policy implementation. In Belgium, all public documents must be written in both French and Flemish; in Canada the two national languages are English and French. The stresses between the populations speaking different languages are based, of course, on deeper cultural distinctions. A particular language may be identified with a certain religious and philosophical tradition. All these differences can affect health policy. In Canada, for example, though English is predominant, any national health legislation must still be formulated in a manner acceptable to the French-speaking and proudly independent province of Quebec.

Family structure has still other cultural effects on health systems. Families, of course, can provide the most profound social support to members who are sick. Studies of adult hospitalization rates show them to be highest among people outside intact families—the unmarried, the divorced, or the widowed. Adjusting for age level, the adult without close family ties may lack social support in time of illness and is more likely to require care in a hospital. A society that promotes strong family bonds is therefore likely to have less need for hospitals and other protective institutions.

For essentially the same reason, family culture has great influence on the health care of the elderly. The honoring of the aged in oriental societies means that grandparents remain part of a nuclear family with three generations. This may help explain why China and other developing countries have so few custodial institutions for the aged, quite aside from their low economic level. In the more mobile societies of Europe and America, the family is less stable. Aged parents are more likely to be living independently; old-age pensions under social security programs help them do this. When aged persons become frail, care in an institution is more frequently sought.

These diverse social determinants of national health systems are obviously intermeshed. Economic, political, and cultural forces influence each other, as well as determine the various characteristics of the health system. Furthermore, they change constantly at different times and places. Discovery of a valuable economic resource, such as petroleum, may lead to rapid expansion of all components of the country's health system. More often the dynamics are gradual, so that the health system tends to evolve along a path somewhat parallel with overall national development.

The economic, political, and cultural forces vary greatly, of course, from country to country, and they combine to shape the scores of different health systems in the world. Even within one country substantial differences may exist as already noted, in the patterns of health services in different social classes. The nation-state, however, plays so crucial a role in world affairs and in the daily lives of people that it is appropriate to analyze health systems according to their national identities.

NATIONAL TYPES OF HEALTH SYSTEMS

The many nations of the world can be categorized in various ways. Long before the current era, with 165 nation-states, statesmen as well as scholars divided the world in different ways. The criteria for making subdivisions depended on the objectives. In the period of the Roman Empire, leaders saw the regions of the world that they controlled as "civilized" and all the rest "barbarian." With the rise of Christianity, the globe was divided between the realms of that faith and all the rest—the *pagans.* When, in the nineteenth century, competition for control of the earth's resources was prominent, Europeans spoke of the "have" and the "have-not" nations.

More recently, in the strategy to form a United Nations after World War II, political realists spoke of the "great powers" and the remainder of smaller nations. Later, when colonies were emancipated and the inequalities among people became extremely visible, demanding corrective actions, it was customary to distinguish the *underdeveloped* (later the *developing*) countries form the *developed* ones. As a Cold War of political conflict grew more intense in the 1950s and 1960s, leaders of Western Europe and North America spoke of the "free world", with all other countries hidden behind an "iron curtain" (or "bamboo curtain") in totalitarian bondage. More recently, some speak of a capitalist world, a communist world, and all the rest—a vast unsettled "third world." All of these typologies are obviously great oversimplifications, designed to influence how people think and act, and ultimately to shape political decisions on war and peace.

Turning to our objective—analysis and understanding of the diverse national health systems of the world—we can classify countries less crudely. We can recognize the influence on each country's health system of the economic, political, and cultural determinants reviewed earlier. Insofar as these factors can be be scaled or ranked along theoretical dimensions, it should be possible to classify health systems, or the countries in which they exist, in an orderly typology. On what sort of information can we base the scaling of systems along these dimensions?

An Economic Dimension

Of the three influences, the economic can be most readily quantified and scaled. The gross national product (GNP) per capita is reported each year by the World Bank. Countries that are highly industrialized tend to have a high figure—typically $5,000 or more per capita per year in the mid-1980s. Of course, as in any classification, there are borderline cases, and a country with GNP per capita of $4,800 per year might be quite affluent. These industrialized and affluent countries usually have a large middle class, and the level of living of the majority of people is comfortable, hygienic, and enriched by many labor-saving devices. With certain major exceptions, resulting from political rather than economic factors, these countries have mobilized their national wealth to support modern health services for the great majority of their residents. Even advanced medical technology is widely available, although some degree of rationing of the use of costly equipment may be necessary.

Countries with less than the annual GNP dividing line of $5,000 (in the mid-1980s) are generally regarded as "developing," and their economic output usually depends mainly on agricultural production. Agriculture, of course, produces food for their domestic consumption and, to varying extents, for export earnings. Rather than clustering all the world's nonindustrialized nations into one huge group, however, we can speak of those with GNPs from $5,000 to $500 per capita per year as "moderately developing" or transitional, recognizing that they are usually moving toward a higher economic level. The principal urban population in these countries has often achieved a good standard of living, while most rural people are still quite poor. The GNPs of most of these countries actually cluster around $2,000 per capita per year. Their health systems have typically shown a substantial expansion of resources in recent decades—for the urban, if not the rural, population.

The least developed countries, with GNPs per capita of less than $500 per year (mid-1980s), are considered "very poor." These countries also typically depend on agriculture for their survival, but this usually means *subsistence agriculture.*. In other words, there is barely enough production to meet domestic needs, and relatively little to export for earning money. The level of living for the great majority of people in these very poor countries is extremely low. The health system has many grave deficiencies, and most of the people have limited if any access to modern health service.

Finally, a relatively few countries are not highly industrialized but, because of exceptionally great natural resources (usually petroleum) that are exported, have acquired a very high GNP per capita. They are primarily in the Middle East and have small populations. Their GNPs per capita generally exceed $5000 or even $10,000 per year; the level of living of the upper classes is typically very high, while even the lower classes are moderately well off. Their health systems have developed remarkable physical resources, giving them a unique character.

A Political Dimension

Nations are much more difficult to scale or classify along a political dimension. The general role of government, compared with that of private enterprise, might be a significant indication of political ideology, but measuring this relationship is not easy.

International agencies, such as the World Bank and the International Monetary Fund (IMF) publish tabulations of central government spending, and also of its relationship to GNP, but the meaning of these data is not always clear. Countries differ in how they calculate the public sector. In some countries tranfer payments (e.g., social security benefits) are counted, but not in others. Local government expenditures may be included in some countries and not in others. Military expenditures may have substantial effects but are of highly variable reliability. In some countries, such as in the Middle East, large expenditures are counted in the public sector which are considered in the private sector elsewhere. All sorts of variations in political policy and practice, in other words, affect statistical reports on public versus private activities in a country.

Focusing on health systems and numerical tabulations about health expenditures raises other difficulties. For countries of Western Europe and a few other industrialized nations, excellent data are avaiable on overall national health expenditures and the proportions derived from public and private sources. These data come from the Organization for Economic Cooperation and Development (OECD), but similar data are available for only a handful of the nonindustrialized countries of the world, and these apply to different years and have been derived through varying methods. In some developing countries, for example, provincial health expenditures are not counted in the public sector, since only the central ministry of health budget is deemed to be "governmental."

Beyond these problems are difficulties that stem from a country's historical background. In countries that were formerly colonies, for example, government may still play a very large role in all national affairs, even though the newly independent nation is dedicated to maximizing free private enterprise. At the other end of the political spectrum, the socialist countries use very different methods of economic analysis, which make many of their "national accounts" noncomparable with other countries. A military dictatorship may be staunchly dedicated to private enterprise and to favoring the interests of the national power elite yet take pains to leave undisturbed the comprehensive health system established by a prior democratic government. Health services can be a powerful tool for winning popular support for governments of very diverse ideologies.

Because of all these difficulties, it seems best to conceptualize the political dimension of countries in terms of the policies characterizing the health system itself. To what extent is the national system controlled, organized, and managed by government, in contrast to the laissez-faire principles of the private market? To what extent have organized initiatives from other sources, such as labor unions, religious groups, or even the health professions, modified the process of buying and selling health care as a commerical transaction? In effect, one can characterize a health system according to the degree of *market intervention* by government or other social entities, along a spectrum from minimal to maximal intervention.

Health systems with minimal market interventions may be considered highly entrepreneurial and permissive. Those with maximal intervention are centrally planned and socialist. Between these extremes, one can conceptualize two gradation of moderate and strong market intervention, launched to change health services in various degrees from market commodities to social entitlements.

The reasons behind government or other forms of intervention in the commercial medical market of earlier centuries are many. The basic unpredictbility of illness in any individual has generated insurance (voluntary or government), which provides purchasing power at times of need to all members of an insured group. The initiative for health care insurance or *sickness funds* was taken originally by groups of workers, later by insurance businesses, and eventually (and in many different manners) by governments. Interventions giving merciful care to the poor came initially from religious bodies that mobilized charitable donations to build hospitals, and later from local governments. To protect populations against epidemic disease, it was necessary for government to undertake many public health actions that could not be remotely expected in a commerical market.

In almost all countries, market forces have led to serious maldistribution of health personnel between cities and rural areas. Only through deliberate government interventions has it been possible to allocate more doctors and other health resources to meet the needs of rural populations. All sorts of deception and quackery prevailed in the sale of healing services, until standards of training and knowledge could be established and enforced by government through licensure requirements. Such regulation obviously restricted the entry of sellers into the medical market, but every country has found this necessary to protect people from deception and possible harm. In most countries the government quality controls imposed on the production and distribution of drugs and related substances involve a vast body of law, all of which means intervention in the pharmaceutical market.

As the economic support of health services has become increasingly collectivized, concerns about the quality of care have mounted. Every program of insurance or revenue support for personal medical care has some strategies for professional review built into it. Within hospitals, the dynamics of group discipline have replaced the sovereignty of the individual practitioner in virtually every national health system. Cost-control objectives have imposed schedules of negotiated fees, in place of market prices (responding to changing supply and demand), in most countries. Health care teams, with liberal use of auxiliary personnel, are rapidly replacing individual practitioners because of the efficiency achieved. Competition among hospitals in most countries is being replaced by cooperative regionalized relationships, so that services can be based on scientific planning, rather than market dynamics. Health planning, in fact, has come to permeate every health system in varying degrees, although political rhetoric may define the process with other terms.

All these actions illustrate types of intervention in the health care market. As we examine the several components of national health systems, the various ways that interventions occur in different systems will be evident. It is in their aggregate impact on health system structure and function that these market interventions enable us to scale national health systems along a political dimension.

Cultural Characteristics

If scaling health system characteristics along a political dimension is difficult, such an effort at quantification along a cultural dimension would be quite overwhelming. The embodiment of a country's technological development, dominant religion, community structure, prevailing language, and patterns of family life in a single measurement presents a formidable task. Even if discrete measurements could be determined for each of the five cultural characteristics, their value in formulating a typology of health systems is doubtful. Whatever might be gained in accuracy would be lost in complexity.

Instead, we can achieve a reasonable understanding of national heath systems by classifying them along two basic dimensions: the economic level of the country and the political attributes, as reflected in the extent of market intervention, of the health system itself. The several cultural characteristics, identifiable in each national environment, will be discussed whenever relevant to the understanding of the health system.

A MATRIX OF HEALTH SYSTEMS

Combining the two basic dimensions, economic and political, yields a matrix of cells that depends on the refinement with which each dimension is scaled. The economic dimension can be readily scaled according to the annual GNP per capita. As noted earlier, four levels constitute a useful scaling: (1) the affluent, (2) the transitional, and (3) the very poor, plus the exceptional developing countries that are (4) resource-rich. The quantitative figures defining these levels change from year to year, and they are indicated earlier for the mid-1980s.

The political or health policy dimension, as reflected in the extent of market intervention by government or other forces on the health system, can also be scaled according to four steps. These policies are designated as (1) entrepreneurial, (2) welfare-oriented, (3) comprehensive, and (4) socialist. It is difficult to be absolutely precise about the meaning of these four policy types, but certain general characteristics are suggested.

In entrepreneurial-type health systems, the private market is very strong. Intervention by government or other organized entities has been minimal. When economic data on the total health system are available, it is usually found that a high percentage of expenditures—typically more than half—derives from private sources (individual and family outlays). Private medical practice is strong, and a substantial proportion of hospital beds are usually sponsored by private bodies. Government health programs tend to be weak, meeting only a fraction of the population's needs. Health planning may exist in theory, but it is ineffective in practice. Regulation of drugs, health personnel, and other resources is meager. In spite of frequent use of political rhetoric about "health as a right," accessibility to health care is uncertain and largely an individual responsibility.

In welfare-oriented health systems, government and certain other entities have intervened in the private health care market in many ways. Among the more industrialized countries, this intervention has focused largely on the process of financing personal medical care; the financing has often been collectivized without any disturbance of conventional patterns of health service delivery. Among the less affluent transitional countries, collectivized financing can be linked to organized patterns of health care delivery, but only a fraction of the population is affected. The transitional and very poor countries with welfare-oriented ideology usually undertake major efforts to bring health services to rural people through networks of health centers and extensive training and use of auxiliary personnel. There are numerous initiatives to improve environmental sanitation, provide immunizations, allocate health manpower to rural areas, and generally to extend health service coverage.

In comprehensive-type health systems the welfare-oriented stage of market intervention has been carried still further. It has been extended to the point that all or virtually all of the country's population are entitled to complete health service. (Full implementation of the entitlement may be impeded by limited resources, but all existent resources are equally available to everyone.) In the affluent industrialized countries, this type of health system has typically evolved from the welfare-oriented type, and it is found in numerous countries. In countries of all the other economic levels, comprehensive-type health systems are relatively few. This degree of market intervention is found only where exceptional political will has established health service as a very high priority. Funds have been mobilized to make

health centers and hospitals reasonably staffed and accessible without charge to the entire population.

In socialist health systems, market intervention has been carried to the furthest point. In theory, these health systems have set out to eliminate the private health care market completely and replace it with system control through central planning. In practice, they have all found it necessary to retain certain free market operations within their overall socialist health systems. In every case, however, the socialist systems have collectivized not only the financing of all services, but they have also taken over virtually all human and physical resources providing services. All health personnel and facilities come under direct government control, pharmaceuticals are produced by government, professional education is done by government, and so on. Even with the many deviations from this model in recent years, the socialist health systems, in countries of all economic levels, represent the maximum degree of free market intervention.

From these two dimension—the economic level of the country and the policies of the health system—each scaled in four steps, we derive a matrix of 16 cells. Such a matrix has been prepared as Figure 4.1, and in each cell the names of one to three countries have been placed as *examples* of countries with the designated type of national health system. Theoretically the health system of every country in the world would fit into one of these 16 cells, although it may be noted that two of the cells are empty, as of the 1980s. In some cells only a few nations belong, and many in other cells. As of the late 1980s, the greatest proportion of countries probably fit in the four cells of the "welfare-oriented" column.

The lines between these conceptual cells in both directions cannot be drawn too sharply. As in any scaling, there are borderline cases along both dimensions. Moreover, the economic level of countries and the policies of health systems change continually, so that a national health system might fit in one cell today and in another few years later. Placement of a national health system in a particular cell, if it is done properly, can help us un-

ECONOMIC LEVEL (GNP per Capita)	HEALTH SYSTEM POLICIES (Market Intervention)			
	Entrepreneurial & Permissive	Welfare-Oriented	Univeral & Comprehensive	Socialist & Centrally Planned
Affluent & Industrialized	United States 1	West Germany Canada Japan 2	Great Britain New Zealand Norway 3	Soviet Union Czechoslovakia 4
Developing & Transitional	Thailand Philippines South Africa 5	Brazil Egypt Malaysia 6	Israel Nicaragua 7	Cuba North Korea 8
Very Poor	Ghana Bangladesh Nepal 9	India Burma 10	Sri Lanka Tanzania 11	China Vietnam 12
Resource-Rich	13	Libya Gabon 14	Kuwait Saudi Arabia 15	16

Figure 4.1 Types of national health systems: classified by economic level and health systems policies.

derstand many aspects of that system. Such knowledge can be helpful in providing perspective on problems encountered in the health system. Any strategies for system changes can be formulated with greater assurance, if done in light of experience in other countries of the same type.

With the inadequacy of health and social data in most countries and the incomparability of data across countries (due to different methods of calculation), it is very difficult to quantify exactly the positions of the countries used as examples in Figure 4.1. We may, however,

pose a question about government health expenditures that possibly reflects the commitment of a country to health service as a social right. Data are available for 1986 on the expenditures by government for all aspects of the health system, as a percentage of total GNP. As noted earlier, the overall health system expenditures are higher, as a share of GNP, in the higher income countries. Examining countries at a given economic level, however, with the four types of health policy (degrees of market intervention), one finds interesting gradations.

For the most affluent countries, government

health expenditures as shares of GNP in 1986 are illustrated by the following percentages:

Entrepreneurial (United States)	4.48%
Welfare-oriented (West Germany)	6.31%
Comprehensive (Sweden)	8.00%
Socialist (Czechoslovakia)	4.16%

Except for the socialist system, where health expenditures are minimized by extremely low salary levels (compared with other affluent countries), the sequence reflects increasing government intervention to make health care a social right.

Among countries at a transitional economic level, government health expenditures as shares of GNP in 1986 are illustrated by the following percentages:

Entrepreneurial (Philippines)	0.74%
Welfare-oriented (Malaysia)	1.81%
Comprehensive (Costa Rica)	5.41%
Socialist (Cuba)	3.20%

Among countries of a very poor economic level, the equivalent percentages in 1986 were as follows:

Entrepreneurial (Ghana)	0.30%
Welfare-oriented (India)	0.93%
Comprehensive (Sri Lanka)	1.28%
Socialist (China)	1.40%

In the developing but resource-rich countries, where only two types of health system exist, the percentages in 1986 were as follows:

Welfare-oriented (Gabon)	2.0%
Comprehensive (Saudi Arabia)	4.03%

The countries shown as examples previously were not chosen randomly, but rather to illustate the dynamics of health system operation under various political conditions. The complexities of health systems, with their components and subsystems analyzed in Chapter 3, are so great, and the economic and political forces impinging on systems are so numerous, that no simple quantitative index is available to characterize them. One must, instead, examine each health system as a whole—as an anthropologist would study a certain tribe—to understand how it all works.

On the theoretical foundation of health system content in Chapter 3 and the major types of system conceptualized in this chapter, we proceed to examine the main national health systems of the world. For each of the 14 types found in the 1980s, we analyze at least one in its overall scope. Regarding other systems of the same type, we examine selected features that seem to have special meaning in international health developments. At the end of this volume, we offer estimates about the general direction in which national health systems seem to be moving.

REFERENCES

Abel-Smith, Brian, *An International Study of Health Expenditure and Its Relevance for Health Planning.* Geneva: World Health Organization (Public Health Papers No. 32), 1967.

Blanpain, Jan et al., *National Health Insurance and Health Resources: The European Experience.* Cambridge Mass.: Harvard University Press, 1978.

Bosch, Paul F., *International Health.* New York: Oxford University Press, 1978.

Brockington, C. Fraser, *World Health.* London: Penguin Books, 1958.

Brockington, C. Fraser, *Public Health in the Nineteenth Century.* Edinburgh: E. & S. Livingstone, 1965.

Bryant, John, *Health in the Developing World.* Ithaca, N.Y.: Cornell University Press, 1969.

Croizier, R. C., "Medicine Modernization, and Cultural Crisis in China and India," in *Comparative Studies in Society and History,* 12:275–291, 1970.

deFerranti, David, "Strategies for Paying for Health Services in Developing Countries." *World Health Statistics Quarterly,* 37(4):428–450, 1984.

Douglas-Wilson, I., and G. MacLachlen (Editors), *Health Service Prospects: An International Survey.* London: The Lancet, 1973.

Elling, Ray H., "Medical Systems as Changing Social Systems." *Social Services & Medicine,* 12 (28):490–499, 1978.

Elling, Ray H., *Cross-National Study of Health Systems: Political Economics and Health Care.* New Brunswick, N.J.: Transaction Books, 1980.

Evans, John R., K. L. Hall, and J. Warford, "Shattuck Lecture—Health Care in the Developing World: Problems of Scarcity and Choice." *New England Journal of Medicine,* 305(19):1117–1127, 5 November 1981.

Fry, John, *Medicine in Three Societies: A Comparison of Medical Care in the USSR, USA, and UK.* New York: American Elsevier Co., 1970.

Fry, John, and W. A. J. Farndale (Editors), *International Medical Care: A Comparison and Evaluation of Medical Care Services Throughout the World.* Oxford: Medical & Technical Publishing Co., 1972.

Fulcher, Derick, *Medical Care Systems: Public and Private Health Coverage in Selected Industrialized Countries.* Geneva: International Labour Office, 1974.

Kleczkowski, Bogdan M., M. I. Roemer, and A. van der Werff, *National Health Systems and Their Reorientation Towards Health for All.* Geneva: World Health Organization (Public Health Papers No. 77), 1984.

Lasker, Judith N., "The Role of Health Services in Colonial Rule: The Case of The Ivory Coast." *Culture, Medicine, & Psychiatry,* 1:277–297, 1977.

Maxwell, Robert J., *Health and Wealth: An International Study of Health-Care Spending.* Lexington Books, 1981.

Mesa Lago, Carmelo, *Social Security in Latin America.* Pittsburgh: Univeristy of Pittsburgh Press, 1978.

Raffel, Marshall W. (Editor), *Comparative Health Systems: Descriptive Analyses of Fourteen National Health Systems.* University Park: Pennsylvania State University Press, 1984.

Roemer, Milton I., *Health Care Systems in World Perspective.* Ann Arbor, Mich.: Health Administration Press, 1976.

Roemer, Milton I., "Market Failure and Health Care Policy." *Journal of Public Health Policy,* 3(4):419–431, December 1982.

Roemer, Milton I., "Analysis of Health Service Systems—A General Approach," in Charles O. Pannenborg et al. (Editors), *Reorienting Health Services: Application of a Systems Approach.* New York: Plenum Press, 1984, pp. 47–59.

Rosen, George, *From Medical Police to Social Medicine: Essays on the History of Health Care.* New York: Science History Publications, 1974.

Shryock, Richard H., *The Development of Modern Medicine.* New York: Alfred A. Knopf, 1947.

Sigerist, Henry E., "From Bismarck to Beveridge: Development and Trends in Social Security Legislation." *Bulletin of the History of Medicine,* 13:365–388, 1943.

Sigerist, Henry E., "War and Medicine." *Centaur,* 49:211–217, March 1944.

Sigerist, Henry E., *On the Sociology of Medicine* (Edited by M. I. Roemer). New York: MD Publications, 1960.

Silverman, Milton, and P. R. Lee, *Pills, Profits, and Politics.* Berkeley: University of California Press, 1974.

Sivard, Ruth Leger, *World Military and Social Expenditures,* 11th edition, Washington, D.C.: World Priorities, 1986.

Sivard, Ruth Leger, Ibid, 13th edition, 1989.

Taylor, Malcolm G., *Health Insurance and Canadian Public Policy: The Seven Decisions that Created the Canadian Health Insurance System.* Montreal: McGill-Queen's University Press. 1978.

World Bank, *World Development Report 1986.* New York: Oxford University Press, 1986.

World Bank, *Health Sector Policy Paper.* Washington, D.C.: The Bank, 1980.

World Health Organization, *Financing of Health Services.* Geneva: WHO (Technical Report No. 625), 1978.

World Health Organization, *Sixth Report of the World Health Situation 1973–1977: Part II* (Review by Country and Area). Geneva: WHO, 1980.

World Health Organization, *World Health Statistics Annual 1983,* Geneva: WHO, 1983.

Zschock, Dieter K., *Health Care Financing in Developing Countries.* Washington, D.C.: American Public Health Association, 1979.

PART TWO

INDUSTRIALIZED COUNTRIES

CHAPTER FIVE

Entrepreneurial Health Systems
in Industrialized Countries

In accordance with the typology of national health systems outlined in Chapter 4, the combined features of an affluent and industrialized economic level and entrepreneurial health system policies are not common in the modern world. A few decades ago, before the vast extension of national programs of health insurance, several countries might have belonged in this cell of the health system matrix. In 1988, only one country fitted into this category: the United States. And, as we shall see, even this country is gradually changing its health policies toward a more social orientation in many features of its national health system.

MAJOR FEATURES OF THE
U.S. SYSTEM

The national health system of the United States embodies several major features. First, as an affluent industrialized country, the United States has abundant resources, and it spends a great deal of money in its health system. Second, as a federated nation, it governs its system in a highly decentralized manner through numerous states, counties, and communities. Third, as a nation with a free market economy, it incorporates very permissive laissez-faire concepts throughout its health system. These features are apparent in the forms taken by all five of the system components.

These three general characteristics are all relative—that is, relative to the policies and practices of other countries. There are, of course, other affluent and industrialized nations, other federated republics, and other laissez-faire economies. The degree of these attributes in the U.S. health system, however, is especially

great, resulting in a system that is remarkably pluralistic and complex, with very different meanings for various sections of its population.

The federated political structure can be traced to the American Revolution against the British monarchy, and a determination to avoid strong central government. Even within the national government there are checks and balances among the executive, legislative, and judicial branches that restrain governmental actions of all types. The free market economy was emerging in Europe of the early nineteenth century, just when the new world was beginning to develop. Inevitably the American health system was influenced by these dynamic economic processes around it.

Yet the U.S. health system, like that of all countries, is not static. Despite the dedication of national and health professional leaders to free market principles, many interventions in the operation of the market have been found necessary. As the expectations of people for recovery from disease and for the maintenance of good health have mounted, more initiatives have arisen to change the contours of all five system components. Social actions have been taken to increase the quantity and quality of resources produced, to plan and modify system management, to alter the overall system structure, to strengthen mechanisms of economic support, and to rationalize and improve the delivery of services.

Located in the temperate middle zone of North America, the United States had a population, as of 1986, of about 240,000,000. Its GNP per capita was $17,480—exceeded among the industrialized countries that year only by Switzerland. Income distribution has been uneven; in 1980, the families with the highest one-fifth of household incomes earned 39.9 percent of the total, while those with the bottom one-fifth earned only 5.3 percent of the total. This very uneven distribution of wealth, of course, has many implications for the operation of the national health system.

THE ORGANIZATIONAL STRUCTURE

To analyze the U.S. health system today, it is helpful to begin with an account of its organizational structure. This component stands at the center of the system model, pictured earlier, like the trunk of a tree. Then we consider the four other components that contribute to or support this organizational structure, and how the whole combination of relationships differs from those in other national systems.

In the United States, as in many countries, five major types of health program operate to some degree: (1) a principal government health authority, (2) other agencies of government with health functions, (3) voluntary health agencies, (4) enterprises with health functions, and (5) the private health care market. The size, shape, and proportions of these programs define the organizational structure of the U.S. health system.

Principal Government Health Authority

As in most countries, a central governmental authority carries major responsibility for the health protection of the population. This responsibility can be carried along with other major responsibilities, and this is the arrangement in the United States. Until recently, the U.S. government's equivalent to a ministry of health was combined with authority for other major fields in a Department of Health, Education, and Welfare. Responsibility for education was withdrawn, but the Department of Health and Human Services became responsible for the nation's massive programs of social security and public assistance, as well as for most aspects of health. Within this department is a vast organizational structure to handle the programs of the U.S. federal government in health resource development, health services, health research, health care financing, epidemiological surveillance, health planning and regulation, and other governmental functions within the national health system.

In the U.S. Department of Health and Human Services, many responsibilities are fulfilled by allocating money and delegating authority to numerous other public and private entities throughout the nation. The U.S. Constitution grants the states a great deal of autonomy and responsibility in all social affairs, including health. Relatively few health functions are carried out directly at the national level (principally by the U.S. Public Health Service within the DHHS); these include such tasks as the health examination of immigrants, regulation of drugs that move in interstate commerce, special epidemiological investigations, compilation of national health statistics, or medical services to American Indians. Health functions carried out by the states, for which the federal DHHS gives financial grants, include communicable disease control, environmental sanitation, preventive maternal and child health services, health manpower training, health facility construction, medical care of the poor, health science research, and several other fields.

Below the national level, each of the 50 states likewise has a major health agency, although sometimes it is combined with authorities for social welfare or other functions. The administrative configuration and scope of functions of the state health agencies are highly variable. The heads of these agencies are ordinarily appointed by an elected governor; they are responsible entirely to the state governor and not at all to the national health authority. Only insofar as certain standards must be met, as a condition for receipt of national grants, must the state accept national direction. Federal grants for hospital construction, for example, require that the state must have a law on licensure of hospitals; wide leeway is allowed, however, in providing such laws.

Similarly, below the level of state government are units of local government—about 3,100 counties and many more cities or sometimes special districts—that also have major health agencies, also with much autonomy. On certain health matters, the local health department carries out functions delegated by the state agency, but on most matters it has full authority within the constraints of the general local government.

Other Government Agencies with Health Functions

Most governmental structures are determined by historical developments. Public health agencies grew out of recognition of the need to protect people from hazards of the environment and of epidemic diseases—dangers to the entire population. The social insurance movement, however, was intended to protect the economic position of low-paid workers, who could be ruined by the costs of sickness. In almost all countries, therefore, the place of social insurance in the structure of government has been different from that of public health.

In the United States, we have noted the federal Department of Health and Human Services, and within it the U.S. Public Health Service. The first national social insurance program to finance medical care, however, was placed administratively in the Social Security Administration, not the Public Health Service—that is, *Medicare* insurance for the aged, enacted in 1965. When the Medicare program was later withdrawn from the Social Security Administration, and combined with the *Medicaid* public assistance program for health care of the poor, it was placed in still another organizational setting, the Health Care Financing Administration.

Several other agencies of the federal government in the United States also adminster important health programs. The Department of Labor, with its Occupational Safety and Health Administration, has the main responsibility for protecting the health of workers at their places of work. The health and safety of miners, however, is a concern of the Bureau of Mines in the Department of the Interior. Many aspects of the health of agricultural families and farm workers, including control of diseases of animals, are a concern of the Department of Agriculture. For certain historical reasons, the control of narcotic drugs has long

been in the Department of Treasury. The Veterans Adminstration is an independent federal authority which, among other things, is responsible for operating the nation's largest network of public hospitals—those for military veterans, whether or not their disorders are connected with military service. The separate branches of the armed forces, as in nearly all countries, operate their own large subsystems of health services in time of peace as well as war, under the federal Department of Defense. Even the Department of Justice is responsible for health facilities in a network of federal prisons.

At the state and local levels in the United States, the multiplicity of government agencies concerned with health is even greater. The organizational layout is not the same in any two states. In most states, the medical care programs for the poor, defined in various ways, come under departments of social welfare or public assistance. Factory inspection for accident or disease hazards is usually a function of state departments of labor or industry. Worker's compensation programs, to help workers who incur work-connected injuries or diseases, provide support for much medical care and rehabilitation; they are generally under the control of other special commissions or agencies. Programs of vocational rehabilitation are often found within state departments of education, although a major part of their task is medical. Special state authorities are usually concerned with the licensure and sometimes surveillance of doctors, nurses, pharmacists, and other health personnel. Public water supply and sewage disposal systems are the responsibility of separate departments of public works in many states, and in most states special environmental authorities are established for the control of air and stream pollution. Even the overall planning of health services has often been assigned by governors to a special agency other than the state department of health.

At the local level, the dispersion of governmental health responsibilities in the United States is generally as great. Local boards and agencies concerned with welfare (of the poor and disabled), public schools, garbage disposal, water and sanitation, local government hospitals, first-aid in emergencies, mental health services, parks and recreation, and other programs with health aspects function separately from the local department of health. Only a handful of America's 3,100 counties have integrated these many health functions under one major local health agency.

Voluntary Agencies

In the United States, the permissive and entrepreneural character of the health system is vividly demonstrated in the enormous multiplicity of voluntary health agencies. Hundreds of agencies raise funds and carry out programs for fighting certain diseases—cancer, tuberculosis, mental illness, and others. One society may function at national, state, and local levels. Other agencies focus on the health of certain population groups—children, the elderly, American Indians, war veterans, and others. Still other voluntary agencies are concerned with certain types of health service, such as visiting nurse care, emergency care, hospitalization, or blood donations. The voluntary agency may be devoted exclusively to health purposes, or health services may be incidental to certain larger purposes, such as those of ethnic groups or religious missions (domestically or abroad).

Most numerous in the United States are the disease-specific voluntary agencies that mobilize the interest and financial contributions of millions of citizens. The American Cancer Society is illustrative. As cancer has come to affect more people and to become the second highest cause of death, large numbers of people have become deeply concerned about solving the riddle of this complex disease and helping its victims. Although initiated in a few large cities, a national organization was formed soon with branches in every state of the nation. Below the state level, are city and county chapters. Funds are raised locally from individual donors, and a percentage of the money is passed along to the national headquarters. A large share of the national funds is used to support research projects. Funds kept at the local level are sometimes used to support "cancer detection clinics" or to provide compassionate services to terminal cancer patients. The local, state, and national units of disease-specific vol-

untary agencies in the United States number in the tens of thousands. The initiative taken by voluntary health agencies, furthermore, has often stimulated governmental bodies to do similar work.

Nongovernmental associations of professional health personnel must be counted as another type of voluntary agency. Their funds are raised by membership dues, rather than donations, and their activities are focused largely on advancing the interests of their members. This may be through programs of continuing education and various strategies to elevate professional standards. At the same time, much of the effort of bodies like the American Medical Association or the American Dental Association may be devoted to opposing legislative proposals, regarded as threatening the independence and economic positions of these professional groups.

Enterprises with Health Functions

In the United States, in-plant health services are generally of limited scope, except in large establishments (with 500 workers or more). In smaller factories, services are usually limited to first-aid by an industrial nurse or perhaps only a medicine chest available to the workers. Large plants or mines may maintain a staff of physicians and nurses who perform periodic and preplacement examinations, treat any intercurrent illness, whether or not job-connected, and promote education for healthful living. Enterprises in isolated locations such as mines, railroad junctions, or lumber mills, sometimes operate comprehensive medical care programs for workers. Industrial firms of larger size are obligated by law to protect workers from accidents and occupational diseases, although enforcement may be weak.

The Private Market

As the residual part of the organizational structure of any health system, the arrangements of a private market for medical care are important in most countries. One can regard the private sector in social systems from the vantage point of the buyer or the seller or, in the context of health services, from the vantage point of the financing source or that of the provider of services. Here, in considering the system's organizational structure, we take the viewpoint of the seller, or how the services are provided. (Later, in discussing economic support, we will consider financing from the viewpoint of the buyer.)

From the vantage point of health care provision, the U.S. health system is overwhelmingly dominated by a private market. The great majority of providers of health service were in private business in the 1980s, even though system trends were changing many of these relationships. Ambulatory medical care (both general and specialist), dental care, pharmacy services, medical and surgical services in hospitals, optical services, fitting of prosthetic appliances were all services furnished predominantly by private practitioners. The personal preventive services were often financed by government or other organized entities, but a substantial share of these was still given by private providers. It is especially noteworthy that, even when the financial support for health services was collectivized, as in the various public or voluntary health insurance programs or in the tax-supported Medicaid program for the poor, providing services remained substantially in the private market. For care in the doctor's private office, this was quite obvious, but even in a hospitalized case, the service was like that rendered to a private patient, and any responsible *third-party* agency paid essentially a *private fee*.

Over recent decades a prominent trend for U.S. physicians has been to join together in groups of different sizes for many technical, economic and professional reasons. Nearly half of the American physicians who practice outside of institutions are in groups of three or more, working with nurses and numerous allied personnel. The solo practitioner is gradually disappearing. The vast majority of these group-practice doctors nevertheless function as private physicians, even though they share their incomes in some way. Dental care is similarly provided from a private market setting, for the vast bulk of services rendered. The same applies to the dispensing of drugs and other services at pharmacies.

Hospital care of short-term patients, on the other hand, is provided principally by nonprofit or government facilitates. An important fraction of hospital care, however, is given in private for-profit facilities. Insofar as certain physicians work full time in hospitals, as residents in training or as full-time specialists in certain fields, mainly pathology and radiology, they may be salaried employees and not in private practice. This pattern has also been growing, but the lion's share of medical or surgical services to patients in American hospitals is still provided by private practitioners.

PRODUCTION OF RESOURCES

The U.S. health system is especially well supplied with health resources of all types—health manpower, health facilities, various commodities (including drugs), and knowledge.

Health Manpower

Everywhere physicians are trained in special schools or institutes, which usually play a general policy role in health systems, beyond their educational functions. The United States has numerous medical colleges—about 127 in 1985, or one per 1,920,000 people, or 142 if osteopathic schools are counted. All but a few are attached to universities as separate colleges, sometimes loosely linked with other professional schools as health sciences centers. Just over half of these institutions are sponsored by state governments, as part of state public universities, and the balance are under private auspices. All of the schools, however, have received substantial financial support from the federal government for many years. Entry to U.S. medical schools usually requires a university bachelor's degree (taking 4 years of study), and medical schooling requires another 4 years, for a total of 8 university years. Virtually all 50 states also mandate an internship in a hospital for at least one year, which means medical qualification involves a total of 9 years beyond secondary school. Admission to medical schools is selective, and only about half of those who apply are accepted.

The vast majority of medical students in the United States must pay high tuitions, although they tend to be lower in the public than in the private schools; for a small percentage of students there are fellowships and loan programs to help meet the costs of tuition and living expenses. For a very small fraction of students, federal or state public subsidy programs finance the entire cost of medical schooling, on the condition that the graduate serves in a designated area of doctor shortage (usually rural) for a period equivalent to the years of subsidy. After academic training, when the young doctor is interning, all his or her living expenses are met by the hospital plus a modest salary. The vast majority of interns proceed to further training for qualification as specialists, and as specialty residents they are usually paid salaries. Some 85 percent of active U.S. physicians currently have such specialty credentials.

The optimal supply of physicians required to meet the health needs of a country has long been a subject of discussion and debate. In a period of economic difficulties, such as during the worldwide depression of 1929–1939, there was widespread opinion about a "surplus" of doctors in the United States. Then, when economic conditions are favorable and social insurance facilitates financial access to medical care, physicians become very busy and a "shortage" is perceived. Thus, in the entrepreneurial U.S. health system, there were about 150 doctors per 100,000 population in 1900–1910. This ratio declined or remained stationary until World War II. By the end of the war (1945) a serious shortage was felt, and both federal and state governments gave grants for strengthening the medical schools, both public and private. By 1986 there were 218 active physicians per 100,000 and the supply was continuing to increase. In the early 1980s, it was again widely believed that too many doctors were being produced (although this view was debated). For each U.S. physician, there were 12 or 13 other personnel, the most numerous being nurses.

In the affluent United States, there were 660 registered nurses per 100,000 population in 1986, plus about 300 per 100,000 vocational nurses. Until about 1965, the vast majority of these young women were prepared in hospital-based nursing schools requiring three years of training. Then a different educational pattern, which had started earlier, gained momentum—the preparation of professional nurses through 2 years of academic study in community colleges; by 1980 the vast majority of registered nurses in the United States were being trained through these 2-year academic courses; practical experience was acquired after they became employed. As in several other professions in this country, nursing leadership sought continuous upgrading, and many university-based programs also developed, turning out nurses with a bachelor's degree.

The heterogeneity of the U.S. health system has created a need for nurses in many types of service. Although the majority of registered nurses worked in hospitals (61 percent in 1977), some 39 percent worked in nursing homes for the chronically ill, public health agencies, schools, industrial clinics, nursing education, private medical or dental offices, private duty patient care, and other settings. The turnover among registered nurses is very high in the United States, since many leave nursing service after a few years for other types of employment or marriage.

In some countries, pharmacies are devoted almost exclusively to the sale of drugs, so that the numbers of pharmacists produced are relatively smaller than in countries where the "drugstore" also sells candy, tobacco products, and many other commodities. Thus, in the United States there were 55 pharmacists per 100,000 people in 1986. In Great Britain, where the chemist shop dispenses solely drugs, there were only half as many pharmacists per 100,000.

The numbers and functions of dental personnel in the various health systems is an interesting reflection of system policies. In the entrepreneurial system of the United States, there were 57 dentists per 100,000 population in 1986. There are numerous dental hygienists and dental assistants, but their functions are restricted essentially to preventive work or assisting the dentist at the chairside; publicly financed clinics for dental care are scarce.

Health Facilities

In the United States, with its entrepreneurial health system, the total hospital bed supply in 1981 was 6 beds per 1,000 population, of which 4.4 beds per 1,000 were in short-stay general hospitals. In the welfare-oriented health systems of Western Europe, the hospital bed supplies are usually greater.

The volume of hospitalization provided to people depends on how fully the available beds are used (the occupancy rate), the average length-of-stay per case, and other factors. Thus, although the United States has a lesser supply of general hospital beds than several other countries, the rate of admissions to general hospitals in the United States in 1982 was quite high—158.5 per 1,000 persons per year—and the average length-of-stay quite short—about 8 days per case.

The ownership or sponsorship of the nation's 6,500 hospitals is another important characteristic, reflecting how the institutions function. In general, hospitals owned by government serve patients according to their health needs, often without charge, while those under nongovernment ownership usually must impose charges. In the United States, as of 1986, only 25 percent of the general short-stay hospital beds were institutions owned by government agencies; this excluded mental hospitals, which are mainly controlled by state governments. Among the 75 percent of general hospital beds that were privately sponsored, 65 percent were under the auspices of nonprofit bodies (both religious and nonsectarian), and 10 percent were proprietary (for profit). In the late 1980s, however, a growing proportion of hospitals came under the control of for-profit corporations. This increasing "corporatization" or commercialization of American health services has been a source of mounting concern, to be discussed later.

The hospital out-patient department (OPD) in the United States, unlike that in most other countries, is limited to the care of the poor. Beyond the OPD, however, a major organized resource for the provision of ambulatory care is the health center. Beyond the general hospital, a major resource for long-term care of chronically ill and usually elderly patients is the nursing home.

Since the 1930s, nursing homes for long-term nursing and personal care of chronically ill patients have multiplied rapidly in the United States. They are classified as providing skilled nursing care, intermediate care, and in other ways. In 1986, there were more than 16,000 such facilities, with 1,616,000 beds—a greater capacity than in all general hospitals. With an average size of about 100 beds, their occupancy rates were over 90 percent. In relation to the U.S. population over age 65 (their principal occupants), they had 52 beds per 1,000.

The ownership and operation of U.S. nursing homes are predominantly private. As of 1980, only 4 percent of the facilities were government owned, 15 percent were sponsored by religious and other nonprofit groups, and 81 percent were proprietary. (Since proprietary units were generally smaller, they had 68 percent of the total beds.) In spite of this ownership pattern, financial support for nursing home care has come increasingly from public sources, changing from 20 percent such support in 1960 to 56 percent in 1982. With the steadily rising proportion of elderly in the U.S. population, nursing homes are expected to continue expanding. Widespread criticism of the quality of patient care in proprietary nursing homes has generated many pressures to increase their financial support, strengthen their regulation, or both. At the same time, many efforts have been made to strengthen organized *home care programs* for chronic patients in their own homes.

In the entrepreneurial and permissive setting of the United States, health centers were first established in the 1920s as facilities for coordinated provision of preventive services—often by separate agencies for promotion of maternal and child health, the control of tuberculosis, hygienic education, and so on. They later came to house official public health agencies. Attempts to extend health center scope to provide medical treatment of the poor were successfully resisted by private physicians, on the ground that this would constitute improper invasion of the sphere of private medicine. Not until the 1960s was the role of the health center in the United States broadened to include general ambulatory medical care for selected population groups. Very poor families in urban slums were the main beneficiaries, but special units—often simply called clinics—were established for migratory farm workers, residents of ʾblighted Appalachian areas, low-income children and youth, American Indians, and others. Special government subsidies supported these health centers under various federal laws, about 1,000 such centers in 1980.

The health centers under public auspices confined their services essentially to primary health care, including both its preventive and its curative aspects. Another important type of free-standing facility in the United States is the private group practice clinic, in which a number of doctors, usually of different specialties, join together as a team to provide a broad range of ambulatory services. Other facilities for organized ambulatory care are focused on industrial workers (supported by management) and on school children (supported usually by educational authorities), but these are devoted essentially to prevention and case detection. Public health agencies, of course, also sponsor clinics for prenatal and infant health care, venereal disease control (including treatment), dental care of children, and other specialties, and in recent years some of these clinics have broadened their scope to general primary care.

Health Commodities

Pharmaceutical products are the most important of a wide variety of commodities. Drugs in most economically developed countries are, with few exceptions, produced by pharmaceutical companies on a large scale, and then distributed to the people through numerous pharmacies or general health care facilities (hospitals, nursing homes, and health centers). In the entrepreneurial health system of the United States, the pharmaceutical industry contains hundreds of firms, although about 20 major ones sell most of the products. Because

newly discovered or invented drugs are protected by patents (which endure for 17 years), they are sold under *brand names,* which may command high prices. After a patent expires, the drug's nonpatented or *generic name* may be used to identify the product sold by any qualified manufacturer.

With many companies engaged in drug manufacturing, there is much competition and a great deal of advertising to win the preferences of physicians. There may be, for example, scores or hundreds of drugs to combat insomnia and induce sleep, often with very little difference, sometimes no differences except their names and perhaps their color or packaging. It has been estimated that more than 25 percent of the price paid by the pharmacist for drugs is referable to the manufacturer's advertising costs. On top of this, the patient must pay the middleman costs of the pharmacist and sometimes a wholesale distributor. Although competition may breed extravagant claims for a particular drug, on several occasions drug firms have been found guilty of collusion to fix prices at a specified high level, in violation of the U.S. antitrust laws.

Regulations in the United States indicate which drugs may be dispensed only with a doctor's prescription, and which can be sold over-the-counter directly to patients. In 1930, three-quarters of the U.S. expenditures on drugs were for the latter type, often called patent medicines, but by 1980 these relationships were reversed; that is, most expenditures went for prescribed drugs. Drug therapy over the years has become increasingly effective, and prescription prices have risen steeply, though not as steeply as hospital charges. The development of antibiotic drugs that can effectively combat most infectious diseases (including pneumonia, tuberculosis, syphilis, and gonorrhea), drugs to reduce hypertension, to combat the most serious manifestations of psychosis, to treat diabetes, to eliminate the pains of gout and arthritis, to reduce the eye pressure that leads to glaucoma, and to extend the life of patients with cancer have greatly advanced the effectiveness of medical service in affluent countries like the United States. Even greater benefits have probably come from the many vaccines discovered and produced for the prevention of infectious diseases, such as diphtheria, poliomyelitis, or measles.

Yet the enormous multiplicity of drug preparations in a permissive free enterprise setting has also created problems. The large expenditures on advertising that have been noted include both prescription or *legend* drugs advertised to doctors and nonprescription drugs advertised directly to the general population. The numbers and attributes of different drugs are so great that the average physician could not possibly be expected to remember them all, especially as hundreds of new products appear on the market each year. American pharmacies, which try to respond to the prescription orders of numerous doctors, must keep on hand enormous stocks of diverse products, which is very costly. To get around this problem, many hospitals or health programs prepare a *drug formulary,* which lists only a few hundred drugs that are regularly available in the hospital or program.

With the freedom of hundreds of pharmaceutical companies to manufacture drugs, and in former years the freedom to make grandiose claims about their benefits, there were bound to be abuses that sometimes led to serious tragedies. As a result, the U.S. government has been stimulated to enact a sequence of "pure food and drug control" laws and regulations, which have greatly restricted the freedom of drug manufacturers. The requirements of these laws are discussed later, but here it may simply be noted that the abuses arising in a very entrepreneurial health system have led to legal constraints, sometimes more sweeping than in more socially organized health systems.

There has also been virtually complete freedom to establish pharmacies in the United States. As a result there were some 51,000 drugstores in 1980, or one for every 4,700 population—a ratio greatly in excess of needs. (Each drugstore normally has several pharmacists.) To survive economically, the average drugstore must sell many products other than drugs. This may offer certain conveniences for people, but it means that much of the pharmacists's education is wasted, and other functions that might be performed by pharmacies, such as health education or certain routine screening tests, are not done.

Health Knowledge

Every health system depends on knowledge about health and disease, and the application of knowledge through various technologies. Books, journals, and conferences to disseminate biomedical knowledge are especially abundant in the United States.

Biomedical research is extensive and extremely varied. In the entrepreneurial setting of the U.S. health system, research on countless medical problems is done at every medical school and many other university departments related to the health sciences. The topics investigated have customarily been determined by each scientist, according to his personal interests. In the early decades of the twentieth century, philanthropic bodies such as the Rockefeller Foundation gave grants to universities for medical research and conducted such research itself. The federal government operated a relatively small hygienic laboratory for investigating selected problems of communicable disease.

Since about 1940, these research policies have changed. To encourage research on problems of special public interest, the federal government has provided an increasing volume of research grants in selected fields. At the same time, national research institutes have been established for government work in these fields. The National Cancer Institute, for example, conducts research on a wide range of problems relevant to cancer and, in addition, it makes hundreds of grants each year to investigators throughout the United States and even in other countries. Applications must be submitted for these grants, and they are reviewed by committees of scientists, appointed by the government, who evaluate them for support or rejection. No scientist is compelled to work on the cancer problem, but the relatively great availability of financing in this field obviously has an influence. In this way, government shapes medical research indirectly. A more direct strategy is the posing of certain specific research questions by government, with solicitation of proposals; many proposals (e.g., on the relationship between coffee drinking and pancreatic cancer) may be submitted, but usually only one or a few are chosen and finalized by research contracts.

Aside from government-funded research, conducted mainly (but not solely) by universities, pharmaceutical companies conduct a substantial amount of research on drugs and their effects on disease. These companies also give grants to medical scientists and clinicians, who are asked to investigate new products. Clinical research (i.e., on patients) must be carried out under strictly prescribed conditions, to protect the welfare of all "human subjects." With respect to sociomedical (as distinguished from biomedical) research, many government grants go to nonacademic firms devoted to health care management or administration.

SOURCES OF ECONOMIC SUPPORT

Quantitative data on the various sources of economic support for a health system or on health expenditures are not easily collected. It happens that in the United States, where problems of health economics have been debated for decades, such data are relatively abundant. These have been gathered both from household surveys and by directly soliciting information from major sources, such as voluntary insurance programs and government agencies.

In 1985, the U.S. population spent directly or indirectly about $425,000,000,000 on the health system. This included expenditures for all components of the system discussed in this chapter, except the education of health manpower (in the U.S. national accounts, these expenditures are included as part of the education sector). The total included both recurrent and capital expenditures that year—recurrent ones, of course, being far greater than capital. This large outlay amounted to 10.7 percent of GNP, a percentage that has been rising steadily for the last half-century. In 1988 it was 11.2 percent of GNP, or about $2,000 per person per year.

The sources of these large health expenditures reflect a great deal about the sociopolitical characteristics of the U.S. health system. The great bulk of them are for personal health services, accounting for 96.4 percent of the total (the balance of 3.6 percent being for medical research and construction of health facilities). The multiple sources of these large health expenditures, for the year 1980, were as follows:

Source	Percent
Personal individuals and families	28.5
Charitable donations	1.0
Management of enterprises	0.2
Voluntary health insurance	30.7
All private	(60.4)
Social insurance	14.4
Federal government revenues	14.2
State and local government revenues	11.0
All public	(39.6)
All sources	100.0

In very broad terms, it is evident that more than 60 percent of all U.S. health expenditures come from private sources (or the private sector), and less than 40 percent come from all public or public sector sources. These relationships epitomize the entrepreneurial character of the U.S. health system and help explain many aspects of its delivery patterns. As we will see, the United States is the only affluent industrialized country in which less than half of health expenditures comes from government sources and more than half from private sources. The trend, nevertheless, has been clearly toward a diminishing role for private household spending and an enlarging role for the major collective mechanisms: voluntary insurance, social insurance, and government revenues.

The seven sources of economic support listed here require some elaboration. The "individuals and families" source refers to out-of-pocket expenditures, including repayment of personal loans, but not the payment of insurance premiums. A large share of out-of-pocket expenditures goes to payment for ambulatory medical and dental care and for drugs, which are not very well buffered by either voluntary or social insurance. Personal expenditures include the cost-sharing requirements under insurance (e.g., deductible amounts or copayments), as well as the payment of charges not protected by insurance at all.

The very small percentage of funds derived from charitable donations may appear surprising, particularly insofar as it includes money spent by large philanthropic foundations (Rockefeller, Ford, Johnson, etc.) on health projects, as well as the donations of small sums to voluntary health agencies by millions of people. In absolute terms, the voluntary donations and charitable support for health purposes have risen over the years, but the rise of expenditures from the other sources has been much greater—hence, the small percentage. The same applies basically to expenditures by the management of enterprises for health services to workers (not counting insurance premiums).

The source of funds identified as voluntary health insurance is composed of hundreds of separate organizations. Commercial insurance companies selling policies for health care number around 1,000, and nonprofit Blue Cross and Blue Shield insurance plans paying for hospital and doctor's care number about 120. Other insurance organizations—variously characterized as *prepaid health plans* or *health maintenance organizations* or by other terms—amount to about another 700 entities. The great majority of people protected by these insurance programs are covered through their employment, and the premiums payable are typically shared between employee and employer, the latter usually paying the greater share or the entire amount. Many large employers carry their own insurance or are *self-insured*. The percentages of persons covered by different types of nongovernment insurance organizations in the United States in 1982 were approximately as follows:

Commercial insurance companies	46%
Self-insured firms	10%
Blue Cross and Blue Shield	30%
Prepaid health plans	14%
All types of insurance	100%

Social insurance in the U.S. health system has three major components. One is the mandatory hospital insurance for the elderly beneficiaries of the social security program. Second is the nonmandatory but government insurance for doctor's care and certain other medical services for the same population of elderly persons. Together these two are known as *Medicare,* which is administered by the federal government, with the assistance of about 150 private *fiscal intermediaries.* The latter make direct payments to hospitals, doctors, and others on behalf of the government. Much smaller in their total expenditures are the 50 state programs of *worker's compensation* for occupational injuries or illnesses; each of these state programs is different, but a common feature is the payment of insurance premiums only by employers. The relevant expenditures here are those made for medical purposes, and not for wage replacements during disability.

General U.S. government revenues, as a source of health expenditures, include taxation levied at several political levels. The breakdown in 1980 was roughly 56 percent from federal government sources and 44 percent from state and local government sources. The major health function, on which both federal and state revenues are spent, is for medical care of the poor, principally through *Medicaid.* Federal taxation revenues are derived mainly from individual and corporate income taxes. State revenues come mainly from income and sales taxes. Local government revenues are derived mainly from taxes on property (real estate). The long-term trends have been toward an increase in the federal share of government health expenditures, although in the 1980s (under the Reagan administration) this trend has changed.

The health purposes for which the funds from these several sources are spent are very varied. Hospital care, for example, is supported predominantly by voluntary insurance and by social insurance; drugs and dental care are supported predominantly by individuals and families; public health activities (largely preventive) are supported predominantly by government revenues. Physician's care is supported by significant shares from all major sources of funding. The total matrix of economic sources and health purposes in the U.S.

health system is extremely complex, but the distribution of overall expenditures for different health purposes (from all economic sources) in 1985 was as follows:

Health Purpose	Percent of Expenditure
Hospital care (all types)	39.2
Skilled nursing home care	8.3
Physician's care (ambulatory and in-patient)	19.5
Dental care	6.4
Drugs and supplies	6.7
Eyeglasses and appliances	1.8
Other personal health care	5.6
Health care insurance administration	6.2
Public health services	2.8
Medical research	1.7
Health facility construction	1.9
All purposes	100.0

Trends in these percentages have been toward increasing shares to care in hospitals and nursing homes. As a share of the total, expenditures for public health services have stayed about constant.

MANAGEMENT OF THE SYSTEM

In the entrepreneurial United States, all four aspects of management stress local responsibility and private sponsorship. The role of government, in general, is kept to a minimum. In the United States, planning for health or any other purpose was so long identified with Soviet communism that it did not appear in any national health legislation until the end of World War II. In 1946, the national Hospital Survey and Construction Act (Hill–Burton) required that federal grants to the states for hospital construction be conditional on the preparation by the state of a master plan, in which each hospital would theoretically have a designated role in a regionalized scheme. Not until 1967 did health planning go beyond this to consider other resources and services, through a program of federal grants to some 200 local "comprehensive health planning"

agencies. These bodies were mainly advisory, and in 1974 legislation was enacted to give local health planning agencies greater powers, particularly with respect to hospital construction. Very significantly, however, these local agencies were almost entirely nongovernmental, and very few of them had any connections with local departments of health.

The U.S. comprehensive health planning law of 1967 was passed as a sequel to the first national social insurance program for medical care of the aged (Medicare) and the large public medical care program for the poor (Medicaid). Significantly, the need for general health planning was not appreciated until a substantial amount of health money was to pass through government channels. With such public visibility of health expenditures, one can appreciate that there would be political concern that the funds be wisely spent, greater than such concern for purely private expenditures.

Any deliberate government or nongovernment action in which resources are allocated in some systematic way (outside the mechanisms of the free market) constitutes planning. In this sense, health planning in the United States can be traced to the establishment of the first hospital or the organization of the first department of public health. As customarily used, however, health planning applies to the actions of an agency that functions over and above the health resources and organizations themselves, exerting an influence on them. Accordingly, health planning in the United States has been very weak, indeed. Insofar as it has had any noticeable influence, it has been confined to the construction of hospitals, and the decisions have been local and nongovernmental. Insofar as the national government has played a part, it has been to issue guidelines, not regulations or official standards.

General health administration in the United States, like health planning, is characterized by decentralization and voluntarism. This goes beyond the constitutional requirements of state sovereignty. In the Medicare program, for example, the law might have authorized payments to health care providers through branch offices of the federal government; instead, payments are made to (and relationships maintained with) providers by numerous *fiscal in-*

termediaries, which are not only local bodies but, in every instance, nongovernmental. Likewise, many federally authorized and financed health programs are implemented by grants to local agencies, below the level of the 50 state governments. In addition to the county and municipal governments, to which health grants may be made, a major share of grants go to voluntary nongovernment bodies. This applies, for example, to grants for mental health services and for various types of community health center. It also applies to federal grants for hospital construction or renovation.

To underscore the emphasis on local and nongovernment decision making, almost all federally supported health programs must be governed or advised by a board of local citizens. Sometimes law requires that a majority of the governing board must be "consumers," rather than "providers" of health care. When some health program standard is issued at the state level, it is typically applied at the local level with great leeway. Policies on the education of doctors and other health personnel are essentially up to each educational institution. Within the structure of state governments, the distribution of authority for health matters is extremely variable. Likewise within local governments, there are nearly always departments of health, but the exact scope of activities is hardly ever the same in two such departments of the same state or another state. Because of the multiplicity of health agencies at local and state levels, coordinating councils of various sorts abound, sometimes for health as a whole and sometimes in special fields, such as care of the aged or promotion of mental health.

Insofar as health administration may be characterized by its style it is mainly participatory rather than autocratic. In both the private and the public sectors, rewards and advancement go to the supervisor who seeks everyone's opnion before reaching a decision. Meetings are held frequently to permit maximum discussion of problems. Though some of this democratic style of administration may be more apparent than real, there is no question about the theoretical preferences. National tradition in the United States opposes bureaucracy and glorifies pragmatism and informality. In health program administration, this means delegation of great authority from higher to lower levels, and relatively limited accountability through reporting back to the top. Yet information systems on health services rendered in a program are relatively well developed, to a great extent because such information serves as a basis for financial support.

Regulation in the U.S. health system, somewhat paradoxically, is highly developed. In part because of the easygoing style of administration, many problems and abuses develop; in response, regulations are imposed to prevent further abuses. This is seen in the licensure of physicians which, before about 1870, was extremely loose and permissive; scores of poor-quality medical schools graduated physicians of very limited competence. As a result, the state governments developed their own examinations that had to be passed, over and above the academic examinations. Somewhat similar has been the development of regulatory legislation on drugs. In the nineteenth century, hundreds of uncontrolled pharmaceutical companies made extravagant and false claims about their products. New drugs were put on the market, without proper testing of their safety (not to mention their efficacy), resulting in tragic deaths of patients. In response, drug control legislation, first enacted in 1906, has become progressively more rigorous.

With respect to specialization in medicine, regulation in the United States was initiated entirely outside of government. Starting with ophthalmology in 1916, *specialty board certification* was developed in one specialized medical or surgical discipline after another. Soon all the specialty boards came under the general jurisdiction of the nongovernment American Medical Association—more than 50 fields, counting main specialties and subspecialties. Specific schedules of postgraduate training are required in each field, culminating in examinations. Although entirely private in its management, specialty board certification is recognized fully by government, for purposes of reimbursement or eligibility to participate in certain public programs. Regarding basic medical licensure by the states, it is significant that the first action to simplify procedures, through a nationally uniform examination, was also taken by a nongovernmental body, the National Board of Medical Examiners.

Regulation by nongovernment bodies has shown similar development in other fields. In the U.S. "open staff" hospital before 1920, each doctor was theoretically his own master, free to do almost anything he wished. As a result, some extremely poor medical and surgical work was done. In reaction, the hospital medical staffs, themselves, set up bylaws to govern practices within the hospital. In 1917, the American College of Surgeons, a private society, formulated standards for granting its approval of a hospital's policies (especially the medical staff procedures), and in 1952 the nongovernmental Joint Commission on Accreditation of Hospitals (JCAH) was organized. JCAH accreditation has come to be recognized by the government.

Similarly, professional associations have established *codes of ethics.* Health insurance organizations set their own rules and regulations. These were all outside the sphere of government, but their control over individual behavior is great. Often such nongovernment initiative has been taken deliberately to forestall government regulation. Sometimes a regulatory strategy may itself be abused, as in the case of professional ethics, which have been invoked to inhibit sound innovations in health care delivery.

Finally, the judicial system provides a certain type of regulation in the U.S. health system. The patient who believes that a physician or hospital has caused him harm may bring suit in a court of law. Because the outcomes of such lawsuits are unpredictable (especially since they are usually tried by juries, and lawyers may be very skillful in their pleading), the great majority of cases are settled out-of-court by the doctor's insurance company. Whether settled or tried in court, lawsuits are costly; thus, nearly all practicing physicians carry *malpractice insurance,* which has become increasingly expensive. Regardless of the merits of most malpractice claims, they have served to induce physicians and hospitals to discipline themselves—another form of self-regulatory response to the very permissive character of the U.S. health system.

Health legislation has been quite highly developed in the United States. Because the free market in health service is so firmly established, almost any intervention calls for legislative action at the federal, the state, or even the local level. Programs noted previously for the subsidy of professional education or construction of hospitals were subjects of law. Programs for venereal disease control, for preventive care of small children, or for treatment of mental illness were legislatively based. Social insurance for medical care of the elderly and medical assistance to the poor are based on amendments to the Social Security Act. Likewise, government appropriations for various health programs each year must be made by acts of Congress; the same applies at the state level.

Regulatory controls over professional licensure or over standards for drug production and distribution are matters of legislation. Environmental protection to prevent hazards to health is legally stipulated. The public discussion and legislative debate that usually precedes these legislative actions have important effects in educating the population about issues in the operation of the national health system. In many aspects of health policy, court decisions have the effects of law, for example, the civil rights of patients of any race to be treated in hospitals. Changing judicial decisions on the legality of contraception and abortion have had great influence on these aspects of health service concerning human reproduction.

DELIVERY OF HEALTH SERVICES

The several major components of the U.S. health system we have received culminate in the encounter between the provider and the recipient of health service.

Primary Health Service

In the United States primary health service is delivered predominantly by private physicians in their private offices. As noted earlier, however, increasing proportions of doctors are joining together in small medical groups or group practices (three or more doctors working together and sharing their income in some way), particularly doctors in various specialties. There were about 15,000 such private clinics in 1984. Nevertheless, the majority of community doctors (not based in hospitals or other organizations) were still in individual practice. The patient frequently pays for this service out of pocket; although most people have some health insurance protection, it may not pay for ambulatory primary care. In fact, even with third-party payment for ambulatory services, as under Medicare, preventive services are specifically excluded. Nevertheless, most immunizations are given by private pediatricians, most prenatal examinations by private obstetricians, and general medical checkups by private internists.

There are, indeed, organized public health clinics for these personal preventive services, but they tend to serve only 15 to 20 percent of the population, mainly the poor. Children are sometimes immunized in schools, and industrial workers may get routine medical examinations in larger-size plants. Multiple screening tests may be done at workplaces or elsewhere, and the patient with any positive finding is typically referred to a private physician.

The treatment aspects of primary health service are also most often rendered in private medical offices, typically those of specialists; general practitioners or family practice specialists constitute only a small fraction of the doctors. Low-income patients, however, frequently seek primary medical care in the outpatient department of hospitals, most often in the *emergency room.* Scheduled clinics in various specialties are held only in a small proportion of hospitals, usually in large cities. Since about 1965, various types of community health center have been established in poor sections of large cities and some rural areas. At these units, a wide range of primary services is offered by salaried doctors and allied staffs; only a small fraction of overall ambulatory care encounters, however, occurs in these settings.

Secondary and Tertiary Health Services

Well-developed secondary and tertiary health services are particularly characteristic of the United States. Until quite recent times, any community or group that could raise the money to build a hospital was free to do so and to furnish the facility with whatever sophisticated diagnostic or treatment equipment it could afford. The same freedom applied to physicians who could specialize in whatever field they could undertake postgraduate training, so more than 85 percent of physicians became specialists.

An approach to regionalization of hospital facilities was made in 1946, with the Hospital Survey and Construction Act, and again in 1966, with the Act for Regional Medical Programs on Heart Disease, Cancer and Stroke, but the regionalization concept remains largely a theoretical idea. In reality, almost any patient is free to consult any high-powered specialist for a minor problem (provided he can pay the fee), and almost any doctor is free to hospitalize his private patient for diagnosis and treatment that might well be given in the office of a general practitioner.

The concept of a pyramidal framework of health service, in which the patient is seen by primary care personnel before access to secondary or tertiary care, is used in government programs like those of the Veterans Administration or the Indian Health Service. It is also implemented in certain *health maintenance organizations* (HMOs) in the United States. HMOs, however, covered less than 15 percent of the U.S. population in 1987. The freewheeling pattern noted earlier characterizes health care delivery in the average community. Patients have direct access to specialists in private practice, and only a minority of the average specialist's patients are referred from another doctor.

In general hospitals, medical staff organization is typically "open," that is, almost any qualified physician applying for staff affiliation is granted it. A general hospital of 100 beds in a moderate-size city might have 100 physicians and surgeons on its medical staff, although only 10 or 20 of them might have patients hospitalized at any one time. Each doctor is responsible for his own patients, and seeking consultation from another staff member is entirely up to him. Because of this great permissiveness, and the hazards of improper care, the medical staffs of most American hospitals have established numerous self-disciplinary committees—on surgery, drug therapy, length-of-stay of patients, record-keeping, and so on—to monitor each other.

Most general hospital patients in the United States are protected by voluntary insurance, and hospitals have customarily been paid their charges for each case. Insurance also typically pays the doctor his private fees for in-patient service. Nevertheless, a slowly increasing proportion of hospital doctors are based in the hospital full time, and paid by salary. This has long applied to pathologists and radiologists, but it is becoming more common for internists, surgeons, and other specialists who serve as the full-time heads of clinical departments, out-patient services, continuing medical education, medical rehabilitation, and other fields.

There are also some HMO hospitals, with entirely full-time salaried medical staffs, similar to those in governmental general hospitals, like the network of the Veterans Administration. Government legislation in the 1980s also led to a shift in the methods of paying for hospital services under Medicare from retrospective charges to prospective rates based on the diagnostic category (the diagnosis-related group or DRG) of each case. With the modification of hospital incentives in care of Medicare patients, the rise in government Medicare expenditures was slowed.

In spite of medical staffing trends, the "open-staff" general hospital remains the norm in America; only for mental hospitals, some special government and HMO general hospitals, and institutions attached to medical schools is the full-time salaried "closed staff" of physicians the usual pattern. Very large tertiary hospitals, attached to medical schools, are highly developed in almost all large U.S. cities.

Secondary health care, as defined in Chapter 3 is highly developed in the United States. Medical and surgical specialists, not employed in hospitals, see many patients on an ambulatory basis, usually in private offices. Nonmedical specialists in private practice are numerous—optometrists who test vision and prescribe eyeglasses and podiatrists who diagnose and treat superficial disorders of the feet. Secondary-level hospitals for treatment of relatively commonplace conditions are widely distributed, providing a great deal of maternity

care, treatment of trauma, respiratory infections, simple abdominal surgery, and so on. Long-term care in nursing homes is provided extensively; as noted, there are more beds in long-term care nursing facilities than in general hospitals. The great majority of these beds are in privately owned and operated facilities, and many difficulties are encountered in the attempt of state governments to maintain proper standards of long-term care.

Finally in the United States the large urban public hospital, limited essentially to serving the poor, is an important component of the pattern of delivery of secondary and tertiary care. It is a hangover of the late nineteenth and twentieth centuries, when programs such as Medicaid were not available to finance care of the poor in the ordinary community hospital. With such financial support programs in the mainstream hospital system, these special public hospitals now serve principally low-income patients who are not eligible for Medicaid or other third-party support. Because of the rising costs of hospital maintenance and restrictions in local revenues (on which most of these hospitals depend), public hospitals for the poor face chronic financial difficulties.

Care of Special Populations and Disorders

In the U.S. health system, where private buying and selling of health service is the norm, it is noteworthy that, as in virtually all countries, military personnel are served by a highly structured and comprehensive health care program, financed entirely by government funds. The army, navy, air force, and marines each has its own network of health facilities including hospitals, clinics, and field posts. All personnel are public employees, salaried according to their military ranks. The same basic structure prevails in times of war or peace. Health promotion and prevention are emphasized and integrated with the delivery of treatment services. Even after retirement, high-ranking officers continue to be entitled to these comprehensive services, without personal costs. If service of a highly specialized type is needed, but available only at a distant place, the patient will be transported there promptly; if this resource is private, the bill is paid by the military establishment.

After military service, the U.S. veteran is entitled to a remarkably broad range of medical care. If a disorder is connected with military service, its care is a responsibility of the federal Veterans Administration for life. For any other disorder suffered by the veteran, hospital care is provided through a nationwide network of VA facilities (usually affiliated with medical schools to ensure high quality), as long as the veteran states it would cause him financial "hardship" to obtain the care privately. Normally, about 75 percent of VA hospital beds are occupied by veterans with such conditions, unrelated to military service. The United States is unique in supporting so broad a scope of health services for veterans—a fact probably related to the lack of a national health insurance program for the general population. After World War I, the political demands of veterans for such special benefits led to public action.

Another favored population in the United States is that of American Indians, who are provided a comprehensive range of services through hundreds of special clinics and hospitals in or near Indian reservations throughout the nation. For years these public services were managed by the Bureau of Indian Affairs of the Department of Interior, but in the 1950s they were transferred to administration by the U.S. Public Health Service.

Other health programs for special populations in the United States include those for railroad workers, for employees of special projects such as the Tennessee Valley Authority, and for migratory farm workers. Merchant seamen are another group for whom a special network of federal hospitals was long operated at major port cities. Special programs for industrial workers and school children have already been noted, and in colleges and universities the scope of health services for students is typically comprehensive. In contrast to customary U.S. patterns of health care delivery, through private medical and allied practitioners, services in all these programs are furnished by salaried personnel working in organized frameworks.

Among disorders for which special subsystems of health care delivery are organized in the United States, mental illness is probably the most important. Although much ambulatory psychiatric care is provided by individual psychiatrists in the mainstream of private medical practice, a substantial amount of such care is furnished to low-income patients through thousands of special mental health clinics, under public or voluntary auspices. These clinics are staffed typically by teams of psychiatrists, psychologists, social workers, nurses, and others—all working on a salary basis. Hospitalization for mental illness is predominantly in large mental hospitals, financed and operated by state governments. General hospitals, however, have increasingly been admitting short-term psychiatric patients and state mental hospitals have been discharging large proportions of their patients, relying on psychotherapeutic drugs to help them get along in communities. Tuberculosis, before its steep decline in incidence and prevalence after 1950, also warranted a nationwide network of clinics and hospitals (sanitaria) for its detection and care.

NEW PROBLEMS: EXCESSIVE COMMERCIALIZATION

The highly permissive and entrepreneurial character of the U.S. health system suggests the type of problems increasingly encountered. Although explanations inevitably vary among different observers, there is a broad consensus that health care costs have been rising excessively. The free market in medical care has been so uncontrolled, even for services paid for by government programs, that prices have spiralled to levels much higher than the general consumer price index. The Medicare program for care of the aged, for example, permits the doctor (by not "accepting assignment") to charge the patient any fee he wishes. Hospital charges have been mounting to especially towering heights, as hospital technology has increased, hospital personnel per patient have multiplied, and salaries have risen.

With the escalation of costs, access of the lower-income groups to needed care has become more difficult. Government programs to finance care for the poor, like Medicaid, have been cut back at both the federal and state levels. Even in the social insurance Medicare program, copayments required from the patient have increased, so that the heavy burden of illness in the aged is getting attention only with increasing difficulty. The whole political environment of the Reagan administration in the 1980s has led to reduction in public expenditures for all human services, and much greater reliance on private sector financing.

A special aspect of this ideology has been enhanced privatization of the U.S. health system. More and more voluntary nonprofit hospitals have been bought out by commercial hospital chains. Voluntary and even public hospitals have been turned over to management by private corporations, in the expectation that this will enhance efficiency and productivity. Up to this writing, evidence of such effects has not been shown, and several studies have shown higher costs associated with the commercialization of hospital service.

Other sections of the health care field have shown various signs of commercialization. Nursing homes for long-term care have long been predominantly under proprietary ownership, but in the 1980s an enlarging fraction have come under the control of large corporations. Agencies operating home care programs have traditionally been offshoots of nonprofit hospitals or charitable associations for visiting nurse service, but all this has been changing. About 10 large corporations have bought up or established hundreds of these agencies and have come to control an expanding share of the field. Clinical laboratories are still another health resource numbering in the thousands, and about one-third of these have been acquired by for-profit corporations. Most are independent laboratories, using the mails or messenger services, but some are even in hospitals.

Still other health services have become the basis of for-profit businesses. There are mobile CT scanners (computerized tomography), cardiopulmonary testing machines, dental care programs, weight-control clinics, and alcohol treatment programs. Hemodialysis for end-stage renal disease (a service financed by Medicare) has been especially attractive to private investors, and in 1980 about 40 percent of this service was provided by a handful of large for-

profit corporations. Staffing and operating emergency rooms in hospitals has even been taken up as a corporate activity, with several large companies selling complete "E.R. packages" to hundreds of hospitals.

To stem the tide of rising medical and hospital costs, major reliance has been on promoting competition among providers. The *preferred provider organization* (PPO) has been spawned, as a mechanism by which groups of doctors and hospitals agree to serve certain public or private beneficiaries at competitively lower prices. For some years the prepaid health maintenance organization (HMO) has shown the economies achievable by modification of physician incentives, especially in hospital use, and now a number of variations on the HMO theme are being explored. Although competition is politically favored in preference to regulation, a very great innovation in public medical care policy has been essentially regulatory. This is as noted earlier, the introduction of prospective payment to hospitals for the *diagnosis-related group* (DRG) of each patient under Medicare (and in some states for all insurance payers), rather than for retrospective charges for each unit of service.

The enthusiastic promotion of prevention and sound life-style, which have come to occupy center-stage in recent years, is bound to continue. To expect this policy to result in less need for medical care, however, is questionable. As men and women live longer because of the prevention or postponement of both communicable and noncommunicable disease, they live on to the age when cancer or other disorders strike. Moreover, they live on with diseases under control—hypertension, diabetes, glaucoma, arthritis, cardiovascular problems, and other disorders that are not cured but are controlled by good medical care. Maintenance of the quality of life in the company of chronic disease is quite possible, but it has its costs.

Why, one may ask, should this increasing commercialization of the U.S. health system be a matter of concern? Entrepreneurial advocates argue that selling stock is a sound means of raising money for capital expansion, and large operations yield economies of scale and other efficiencies. Moreover the profit motive has long fueled the pharamaceutical industry and, for that matter, the ordinary private practitioner of medicine or dentistry is engaged in a small for-profit enterprise. But there are differences.

The drug industry, by reason of its entire entrepreneurial history, has generated a large body of regulation at the federal and state levels. Much human tragedy lies in back of that legislation, which has ameliorated the industry's worst abuses. Medical and dental practice is to some degree controlled by ethical codes that have evolved over the centuries. In hospitals, medical staff bylaws impose many constraints on the physician's behavior, and numerous government agencies or insurance programs review the work for which a doctor seeks payment. Even so, the private practice of medicine is replete with problems, ranging from extravagant and unnecessary procedures to faulty performance sufficiently serious to generate malpractice suits.

Commercialization of hospitals, nursing homes, home care programs, clinical laboratories, and so on introduces the profit motive on a much larger scale. Each of these involves a complex series of activities, in which the potential abuses to aggrandize earnings are tremendous. The array of services that might be rendered to a hospital or nursing home patient, each for a price, is almost endless. The incentives to a home care program or any facility serving patients is to accept the "easy" case, on which profits can be high, and reject the case—simple or complex—on which payment is questionable. If dividends are to be paid to stockholders, what incentive is there for a hospital to operate an out-patient clinic for the poor, to conduct continuing education for doctors, or to carry out clinical research? Such nonremunerative activities are, indeed, very rare in for-profit hospitals. The entire role of the health services as a social function for the improvement of human welfare is frontally challenged by the profit motive.

LONG-TERM TRENDS IN THE U.S. HEALTH SYSTEM

These trends in the commercialization of the U.S. health system have caused dismay among many who view health care as a social right, the access to which should not depend on market dynamics. Greater perspective on recent developments, however, can be gained by considering health system trends over a longer period, such as 50 or 60 years.

If we examine a number of keys issues in the system, over a half-century span, we can appreciate how even the entrepreneurial U.S. health system has been evolving. Major developments from about 1935 to 1985 may be noted, according to the same structural components as were used for analyzing the U.S. health system in this chapter.

Production of Resources

Over the last half-century, enormous expansions have occurred in both the human and physical resources of the U.S. health system. In 1930, at the depth of the economic depression, the U.S. had about 126 physicians per 100,000 people. With weak economic demand, the talk was about a "doctor surplus," but by 1940, with economic prosperity, people spoke of a doctor shortage. After the war, the shortage had become *severe*. Government came to the rescue with substantial federal and state support of medical education. The ratio rose from 141 active physicians per 100,000 in 1950 to more than 210 in 1983. Then, one heard again of a surplus of physicians, although critics pointed to continued unmet needs for health care in rural areas, urban slums, nursing homes, and mental hospitals. The spiraling of the supply of graduate professional nurses from 170 per 100,000 in 1930 to nearly 600 in 1985 has been spectacular. This has obviously meant a great deal for patient care, in both health facilities and the community.

In the late 1980s, it was customary to decry the excessive use of hospitals, but in 1940 the U.S. health system was marked by a critical shortage of short-term general hospital beds. In central cities, the buildings were deteriorated, and in many rural regions they were totally absent. Thanks to strong rural demands and effective health planning, the Hill–Burton Hospital Survey and Construction Act was passed in 1946. This not only improved the bed supply from 3.2 per 1,000 people in 1940 to 4.5 per 1,000 in 1980, but it essentially equalized the hospital resources between urban and rural states, led to the construction of health centers for public health purposes, renovated decrepit facilities, and introduced the basic concept of hospital regionalization.

Organizational Structure

In the half-century from 1935 to 1985, government responsibilities in the health system were enormously expanded. The greatest effects were on health care for the poor and the aged. In 1930, when President Roosevelt spoke of "one-third of a nation as ill-fed, ill-housed, and ill-clothed," it was an understatment. Well over one-third had no access to decent health service. What little medical care the poor could get depended on local governments and their county or municipal hospitals. In 1935, the Social Security Act provided the first federal grants to the states for public assistance—a crucial turningpoint in American social welfare. This led several state governments to improve health services for the poor with state funds. In 1950 the *cash-grant rule* was changed to permit use of federal funds for direct medical care for the poor. This led eventually to the vastly expanded Medicaid program in 1965.

The 1960s also brought a "rediscovery of poverty" in America, and with this the U.S. Office of Economic Opportunity; under the OEO, *neighborhood health centers* were developed for general ambulatory medical care for low-income families, even if they were not eligible for formal public assistance. The whole "community health center" idea spread to several other public agencies, with establishment of about 1,000 such facilities. Medicaid protected 22 million poor people in 1986, which was still not all of the poor but most of them.

Health care of the aged was improved by other strategies. Health insurance had grown in the United States mainly as a fringe benefit of employment; when working people retired they lost their insurance protection. With age, furthermore, the burden of sickness inevitably increases. This dilemma was recognized prominently in the mid-1950s, and federal legislation was proposed to correct it. Some 10 years of contention with the private medical profession and insurance companies followed, before statutory health insurance for the aged was en-

acted in 1965. Medicare had plenty of shortcomings, but it was clearly beneficial for millions of Americans aged 65 and over.

Soon the severely disabled were included under Medicare, and then patients with end-stage kidney disease, for a 1986 total of more than 31 million beneficiaries. Medicare, furthermore, gave a great boost to programs of organized home health care. Nursing home regulations were tightened up by the states, and the federal government has been drafting much tougher standards to evaluate the quality of care in the nation's 1.6 million nursing home beds. Almost every state now has a commission of some sort on the elderly, and the whole senior citizen movement has advanced.

Economic Support

Economic support for the U.S. health system has been greatly strengthened, principally through the wider use of insurance to finance medical care. The unpredictability of illness and economic barriers to needed service had been known for years, and the Committee on the Costs of Medical Care showed this dramatically in 1932. It took the courage of some school teachers in Texas, and later some labor groups and innovative hospital adminstrators in Michigan and New Jersey, to demonstrate that small periodic payments or voluntary insurance could finance hospital services effectively. Depsite early attacks on the Blue Cross movement as "socialized medicine," it grew rapidly. By 1940 about 9 percent of the U.S. population was enrolled, and with the entry of commercial insurance companies into the field, coverage expanded to more than 80 percent of Americans by 1980. Benefits for physician's care and other services were less, and there are plenty of inadequacies even in hospital cost protection, but the progress in health insurance has been enormous.

The very growth of voluntary health insurance and the enactment of Medicare and Medicaid created the social expectation in America that everyone should have economic protection against the costs of medical care. In the early 1980s, when unemployment increased and cuts were made in Medicaid funding, the number of unprotected people began to rise.

By the mid-1980s, attention was focused on "the uninsured," hospitals complained of "uncompensated care," Blue Cross plans decried "cost-shifting," and advocates of the poor spoke of "patient dumping." Studies in 1986 found some 15 percent of the national population or 37 million people unprotected by health insurance, Medicare, or Medicaid. Two-thirds of these, moreover, were members of families with an employed breadwinner working in a small shop or part-time, without employer fringe benefits. Around 11 million people were below the very frugal federal poverty line, but still not eligible for Medicaid.

In response to this mounting issue, state governments began to take action. Bills have been introduced or study commissions established in at least 15 states to extend some type of economic protection for health care to the uninsured. Hawaii passed a law in 1975 mandating health insurance for all employed persons and their dependents. Massachusetts passed a similar law in 1988. Less comprehensive laws were enacted in Washington and Oregon, and debate was active in the legislatures of several other states. Federally, a proposed bill would require all employers in the nation to pay at least 75 percent of health insurance premiums for their employees. Once again, social insurance for health care was back on the political agenda at both state and federal levels.

Health System Management

Several problems in the U.S. health system have led to changes in management—health planning, greater regulation, and more democratic policies toward providers and patients.

The combination of widespread insurance for hospital care, the expansion of medical technology, and the aging of the population contributed to the steady escalation of medical care costs, particularly for hospitalization. By the 1950s, the most common allegation was that "hospitals are overutilized." This gave rise to studies demonstrating that a community's hospital bed supply largely determined its rate of hospital utilization, and therefore its costs. In 1964, New York state enacted the first health planning law to limit the construction of hospital beds, and soon several other states

followed. By 1966, the federal Comprehensive Health Planning law was enacted, and in 1975 a stronger law in the National Health Planning and Resources Development Act. Hospital planning, through requirement of *certificates of need* (CON) before any new hospital beds could be contructed, became national policy. Even though the federal administration terminated support for this health system planning around 1985, it is significant that many of the states continued it in modified form under state financing. With this constraint, plus DRGs and HMOs, U.S. hospital use rates (in days per 1,000 per year) have at last begun to decline.

Regulation has become increasingly aggressive with respect to environmental hazards. The industralization and urbanization of America led to increasing pollution of water and air. Widespread reactions occurred in the 1960s, culminating in two major federal actions in 1970. In that year, the federal Environmental Protection Agency (EPA) and the Occupational Safety and Health Administration (OSHA) were established. Soon after, several laws were passed establishing national requirements for maintenance of the purity of water and air, and the safety of the work environment. Before these laws, virtually all environmental and occupational controls had been left entirely in the hands of the states, with very uneven effectiveness. Serious hazards to health, of course, persist in the general environment and at thousands of workplaces, but one may note just two sets of figures. Regarding air pollution, U.S. national sampling has shown improved air quality between 1970 and 1984 by five measures out of six. Regarding occupational diseases, the deaths due to asbestosis and the "outrageous misconduct" of several large corporations have risen substantially. For coalworker's pneumoconiosis, however, deaths have declined in all age groups. For silicosis, the decline from 1970 to 1984 has been by two-thirds, from 702 to 220 deaths, in spite of an increased number of workers.

The extension of democratic principles in system management has occured in many ways. In the 1930s, it was taken for granted that the U.S. medical profession was reserved essentially for white males, preferably Anglo-

Saxon, native-born Protestant males. After World War II and revelations on the bestiality of Fascism, attitudes changed in America. Urban riots in the early 1960s also played a part, as did the civil rights movement personified in Rev. Martin Luther King, Jr. Discrimination in university admissions for medical education on the basis of race, creed, color, or gender became recognized as obscene.

The injection of civil rights principles into the health system was dramatic. Enrollment of black students in U.S. medical schools between 1968 and 1982 rose from 1.4 to 6.0 percent. Women students accepted for medical studies in 1950 constituted 5 percent, but leaped to 33 percent in 1983. The same applied in dentistry, pharmacy, and other previously discriminatory professional schools. Probably more important was the judicial decision in 1963 that the racial segregation of patients in hospitals (so-called separate but equal accommodations) was unconstitutional under the Hill–Burton Act. Civil liberties in the U.S. health system are still far from completely won, but progress has been real. *Affirmative action* to advance the place of ethnic minorities and women has become standard policy in all the top American universities.

Delivery of Health Services

Modified patterns for delivery of health services have been especially great in the U.S. health system. Stimulated by costs, concern for equity, or simple rationality, the mode of providing services has become better attuned to the capabilities of health care technology.

The limitations of services covered by voluntary insurance became an issue in the 1940s. Pioneering consumer groups therefore started insurance plans for comprehensive health services, under the banner of *prepaid group practice.* Incentives of salaried doctors changed from the maximum use of hospitals to maximizing out-of-hospital care. It took 25 years for the federal government to learn that this reduced health expenditures and to support comprehensive prepaid health plans under the new label of *health maintenance organizations* in the HMO Act of 1973. By 1987, HMOs grew to a membership of 28 million (12 per-

cent of the national population) and constituted strong competition to traditional patterns. The cost-control features of HMOs have spawned other strategies, such as *preferred provider organizations* (PPOs) and prospective methods of hospital reimbursement through *diagnosis-related groups* (DRGs). A great deal of comparative health services research has been stimulated, and conventional American patterns of private fee-for-service medical care are no longer accepted as immutable.

The rapid growth of specialization in American medicine led gradually to a severe shortage in the availability of general practitioners for day-to-day primary health care (PHC). Hospital emergency rooms became the standard source of PHC for increasing millions of people. Superfluous surgical specialists performed superfluous surgery. But in the 1960s a wholesome reaction set in. Medical corpsmen, back from Vietnam, were trained as physician assistants (PA), and soon after nurses took supplemental training to became nurse practitioners (NP). By 1985 thousands of PAs and NPs were providing primary health care predominantly in organized settings of hospital out-patient departments, HMOs, private group practices, and community health centers. In 1969 *family practice* was established as a full-fledged specialty of medicine, attracting thousands of new medical graduates. Basic primary health care was regaining a proper position in the American health system.

American social progress has long been based on incrementalism. The Social Security Act of 1935 and Medicare/Medicaid of 1965 were great leaps forward, but most advances have come in small steps. A problem is identified, political attention is mobilized, and finally action is taken. As a result the United States has a patchwork health system, but the gains achieved for special groups should not be overlooked. After World War II, improvements in the medical services of the Veterans Administration (most of whose patients have conditions unrelated to military service) were tremendous. In 1956, the dependents of active military personnel (CHAMPUS) became entitled to publicly supported medical care. In 1957, transfer of the Indian Health Service to the U. S. Public Health Service brought enormous improvements to that program of comprehensive health care for some 900,000 Native Americans. Despite cutbacks by the Reagan administration, nutritional assistance still went in 1985 to 3,140,000 poor women with small children (WIC) and to 21,400,000 other low-income recipients of food stamps. In the late 1980s a group attracting attention for public medical care was the homeless. Outside of government, the Johnson Foundation was providing support for innovative health programs to help school children, the elderly, the uninsured, rural families, and others.

In the 1930s, the U.S. rural population was regarded as the country's most disadvantaged. A dozen or more special programs were launched to improve the economic and social conditions of farm families. Among others were the innovative prepaid health care plans of the Farm Security Administration and the farm labor health program of the War Food Administration. Despite rural improvements in the 1940s and 1950s, associated partly with the migration of rural families to the cities, many problems persisted and generated new health care initiatives. In the 1960s, the Appalachian Regional Commission set up about 100 rural health centers and, under the Migratory Worker's Act of 1962, some 112 rural clinics were established for these depressed families. In 1970, the Emergency Health Personnel Act launched a program to send new medical, dental, and other health professional graduates to underserved areas, most of which were rural. The magnitude of none of these programs was equal to the needs, but they all were steps in the direction of improving health care for rural people.

In the 1960s and 1970s, popular reactions mounted against the supertechnology of American medicine. We have noted one reaction in the training of physician extenders (PAs and NPs) in the 1960s; in 1975 Ivan Illich's muckraking attack on everything medical *(Medical Nemesis)* struck a respondent chord in million of people. A major response was the rediscovery of prevention in the 1970s.

After 1976 President Carter and the U.S. Public Health Service assigned top priority to health promotion through improved personal life-styles. One may point to the inconsisten-

cies between agricultural subsidy of tobacco crops and exhortations about the harmful effects of smoking, but a great many social actions were taken to reinforce healthful living. Cigarette packages and advertisements were required to contain warnings to consumers about the health hazards of tobacco. Many states and cities barred smoking in public places. To encourage prudent dietary habits, state laws required the labeling of food products with respect to their fat and salt content. Seat belts became mandatory in automobiles, and in many states laws requried that they be fastened. Motorcyclists were required to wear helmets. To encourage exercise, cities marked out bicycle lanes on their streets. Salt almost everywhere had to be iodized and water in more and more cities became fluoridated. On a voluntary basis, many industrial firms established exercise periods for their workers.

These are only a sampling of the strategies of the health promotion movement, but the decline achieved in heart disease mortality must be noted. From an age-adjusted death rate of 308 per 100,000 in 1950, U.S. cardiac deaths declined to 184 per 100,000 in 1984. Improved medical care undoubtedly deserved part of the credit, but the substantial reduction of smoking by men and of fat consumption by all adults must share the credit for this remarkable health achievement.

Everyday patterns of personal medical care have changed radically in America. In 1935 the solo medical practitioner, charging private fees for each office or home call, was the norm. Today the solo office-based doctor is a dying breed. Even in 1975, of all licensed U.S. physicians, only 37.7 percent were in this category; the balance were in organized group practices, full-time hospital posts, administration, medical teaching or research, or some other type of work. In 1985 the solo medical practitioner constituted a much smaller fraction of the total. A recent analysis of American Medical Association data showed that in 1979, about 50 percent of American doctors earned most of their income through salaries. Salaries provide very different work incentives from the mercantile motives of patient fees; most important, they mean professional performance in a team setting, where group self-discipline is the normal guardian of health care quality. Similar organizational trends have occurred, of course, within the walls of hospitals, where state licensure laws, the accreditation movement, specialty board standards, and even the epidemic of malpractice suits have induced more and more rigorous medical staff organization.

Documentation of other long-term trends in the U.S. health system could be offered, but these indications of change in all major components of the system should make the point. In spite of the evidence of commercialism and corporate profiteering in the U.S. system in the 1980s, these tendencies do not reflect the long-term trends. The treatment of health care as a market commodity is found to some degree in every national health system. The degree has doubtless been higher in the United States. But the long-term trend in America, as elsewhere, has been to diminish the importance of the market, replacing it with strategies to ensure health service as a social right for everyone.

REFERENCES

American College of Preventive Medicine, *Preventive Medicine USA*. New York: Prodist, 1976.

Anderson, Odin, with J. Feldman, *Family Medical Costs and Voluntary Insurance: A Nationwide Survey*. New York: McGraw-Hill, 1956.

Ashford, Nicholas A., *Crisis in the Workplace: Occupational Disease and Injury*. Cambridge, Mass.: MIT Press, 1976.

Birnbaum, R. W., *Health Maintenance Organizations—A Guide to Planning and Development*. New York: Spectrum Publications, 1976.

Bryant, J. H. et al. (Editors), *Community Hospitals and Primary Care*. Cambridge, Mass.: Ballinger, 1977.

Bunker, John P., "Surgical Manpower." *New England Journal of Medicine*, 282:137, January 1970.

Cambridge Research Institute, *Trends Affecting the U.S. Health Care System*. Washington, D.C.: U.S. Government Printing Office, 1976.

Clark, Duncan, and Brian MacMahon (Editors), *Preventive Medicine*. Boston: Little, Brown and Co., 1967.

Commission on Medical Education, *Final Report*. New York, 1932, pp. 7–11.

Commission on the Survey of Dentistry in the United States, *The Survey of Dentistry*. Washington, D.C.: American Council of Education, 1962.

Committee on the Costs of Medical Care, *Medical Care for the American People*. Chicago: University of Chicago Press, 1932.

Cray, E., *In Failing Health: The Medical Crisis and the A.M.A.* Indianapolis: Bobbs-Merril, 1970.

Davis, Michael, *Medical Care for Tomorrow*. New York: Harper and Brothers, 1955.

Davis, Karen, *National Health Insurance—Benefits, Costs and Consequences*. Washington, D.C.: Brookings Institution, 1975.

DeGroot, L. J. (Editor), *Medical Care—Social and Organizational Aspects*. Springfield, Ill.: Charles C Thomas, 1966.

Donabedian, Avedis, *Benefits in Medical Care Programs*. Cambridge, Mass.: Harvard University Press, 1976.

Donabedian, Avedis, et al., *Medical Care Chartbook, 8th Edition*. Ann Arbor: Health Administration Press, 1986, pp. 231–234.

Eisner, Victor, and L. B. Callan, *Dimensions of School Health*. Springfield, Ill.: Charles C Thomas, 1974.

Ellwood, Paul M., "Health Maintenance Organizations: Concept and Strategy." *Hospitals*, 16 March 1971, pp. 53–56.

Ermann, Dan, and Jon Gabel, "Multihospital Systems: Issues and Empirical Findings." *Health Affairs*, 3:50–64, Spring 1984.

Fein, Rashi, *The Doctor Shortage: An Economic Diagnosis*. Washington, D.C.: Brookings Institution, 1967.

Feingold, Eugene, *Medicare: Policies and Politics*. San Francisco: Chandler, 1966.

Freidson, E., *Professional Dominance: The Social Structure of Medical Care*. New York: Atherton Press, 1970.

Freyman, J. G., *The American Health Care System: Its Genesis and Trajectory*. Baltimore: Williams & Wilkins, 1974.

Georgeopoulos, B. (Editor), *Organization Research on Health Institutions*. Ann Arbor.: University of Michigan Press, 1971.

Goldmann, Franz, *Public Medical Care: Principles and Problems*. New York: Columbia University Press, 1945.

Goodman, L. J., T. H. Bennett, and R. J. Oden, *Group Medical Practice in the United States, 1975*. Chicago: American Medical Association, 1976.

Goodman, L. J., and A. R. Mason, *Physician Distribution and Licensure in the U.S.* Chicago: American Medical Association, 1978.

Grad, Frank P., *Public Health Law Manual*. Washington, D.C.: American Public Health Administration, 1975.

Hanlon, J. J., and G. E. Pickett, *Public Health Administration and Practice, 7th edition*. St. Louis: Mosby, 1979.

Harmer, Ruth, *American Medical Avarice*. New York: Abelard-Schuman, 1975.

Harrington, Charlene et al., "Nursing Home Bed

Capacity in the States, 1978–87." *Health Care Financing Review,* 9(4):81–97, 1988.

Harris, Richard, *A Sacred Trust.* New York: New American Library, 1966.

Harris, Seymour E., *The Economics of American Medicine.* New York: Macmillan, 1964.

Hetherington, R. W. et al., *Health Insurance Plans: Promise and Performance.* New York: Wiley, 1975.

Hollingshead, A. B., and F. C. Redlick, *Social Class and Mental Illness.* New York: Wiley, 1958.

Institute of Medicine, *For-Profit Enterprise in Health Care.* Washington, D.C.: National Academy Press, 1986.

Jaco, E. Gartly (Editor), *Patients, Physicians, and Illness, 2nd edition.* New York: Free Press, 1972.

Joint Commission on Mental Illness and Health, *Action for Mental Health.* New York: Basic Books, 1962.

Jonas, Steve, *Health Care Delivery in the United States.* New York: Springer, 1977.

Kane, Robert L. et al. (Editors), *The Health Gap— Medical Services and the Poor.* New York: Springer, 1976.

Klarman, Herbert, *The Economics of Health.* New York: Columbia University Press, 1965.

Knowles, John H. (Editor), *Doing Better and Feeling Worse: Health in the United States.* New York: Norton, 1977.

Kovner, A. R., and D. Neuhauser (Editors), *Health Services Management—Readings and Commentary.* Ann Arbor, Mich.: Health Administration Press, 1978.

Lalonde, Marc, *A New Perspective on the Health of Canadians.* Ottawa: Department of National Health and Welfare, 1974.

Lander, Louise, "Licensing of Health Care Facilities" in Roemer, Ruth and George McKray, *Legal Aspects of Health Policy: Issues and Trends.* Westport, Conn: Greenwood Press, 1980.

Law, Sylvia A., *Blue Cross: What Went Wrong?* New Haven, Conn.: Yale University Press, 1974.

Lerner, Monroe, and O. W. Anderson, *Health Progress in the United States 1900–1960.* Chicago: University of Chicago Press, 1963.

Levin, Arthur (Editor), *Regulating Health Care— The Struggle for Control.* New York: Academy of Political Science, 1980.

Lewis, Charles E., R. Fein, and D. Mechanic, *A Right to Health: The Problem of Access to Primary Medical Care.* New York: Wiley, 1976.

Marmor, Theodore R., *The Politics of Medicare.* Chicago: Aldine Publishing Co., 1973.

Mechanic, David, *Medical Sociology.* New York: Free Press, 1978.

Mejia, Alfonso et al., *Physician and Nurse Migration: Analysis and Policy Implications.* Geneva: World Health Organization, 1979.

Merritt, Richard, "Washington State Enacts Landmark Health Law." *The Nation's Health,* August 1987.

Moore, Harry H., *American Medicine and the People's Health.* New York: D. Appleton and Co., 1927.

Mott, Frederick D., and M. I. Roemer, *Rural Health and Medical Care.* New York: McGraw-Hill, 1948.

Munts, Raymond, *Bargaining for Health: Labor Unions, Health Insurance, and Medical Care.* Madison: University of Wisconsin Press, 1967.

Mustard, Harry S., *Government in Public Health.* New York: Commonwealth Fund, 1945.

Myers, Robert J., *Medicare.* Bryn Mawr, Pa.: McCahan Foundation, 1970.

Nader, Philip (Editor), *Options for School Health.* Germantown, Md.: Aspen Systems Corp., 1978.

National Center for Health Statistics, *Health United States 1986.* Washington, D.C.: DHHS Pub. No. (PHS) 87-1232, 1987.

National Advisory Committee on Health Manpower, *Report.* Vols. I and II, Washington, D.C.: U.S. Government Printing Office, 1967.

Orris, Peter (Editor), *The Salaried Physician* (A Physicians Forum Monograph). Chicago: Academy Professional Information Service, 1982.

Pattison, Robert V., and Hallie M. Katz, "Investor-Owned and Not-for-Profit Hospitals." *New England Journal of Medicine,* 309:347–353, 11 August 1983.

Reiser, S. J., A. J. Dyck, and W. J. Curran, *Ethics in Medicine: Historical Perspectives and Contemporary Concerns.* Cambridge, Mass.: MIT Press, 1977.

Relman, Arnold S., "The New Medical–Industrial Complex." *New England Journal of Medicine,* 303:963–970, 23 October 1980.

Reverby, Susan, and D. Rosner (Editors), *Health Care in America: Essays in Social History.* Philadelphia: Temple University Press, 1979.

Roemer, Milton I., *Ambulatory Health Services in America—Past, Present, and Future.* Germantown, Md.: Aspen Systems Corp., 1981.

Roemer, Milton, I., *Social Medicine: The Advance of Organized Health Services in America.* New York: Springer Publishing Co., 1978.

Roemer, Milton I., and J. W. Friedman, *Doctors in Hospitals: Medical Staff Organization and Hospital Performance.* Baltimore: Johns Hopkins Press. 1971.

Roemer, Milton I., and Max Shain, *Hospital Utilization Under Insurance.* Chicago: American Hospital Association, Monograph No. 6, 1959.

Roemer, Milton I., *Rural Health Care.* St. Louis.: C. V. Mosby, 1976.

Roemer, Ruth, C. Kramer, and J. E. Frink, *Planning Urban Health Services—From Jungle to*

System. New York: Springer Publishing Co., 1975.

Roemer, Ruth, and George McKray (Editors), *Legal Aspects of Health Policy: Issues and Trends.* Westport, Conn.: Greenwood Press, 1980.

Sadler, Alfred, B. L. Sadler, and S. R. Webb, *Emergency Medical Care: The Neglected Public Service.* Cambridge, Mass.: Ballinger, 1977.

Saward, E. W. (Editor), *The Regionalization of Personal Health Services,* Revised Edition. New York: Prodist, 1976.

Shanas, E., *The Health of Older People.* Cambridge, Mass.: Harvard Univeristy Press. 1963.

Shonick, William, *Elementary Planning for Area-Wide Personal Health Service,* St. Louis: C. V. Mosby, 1976.

Sidel, Victor W., and Ruth Sidel, *A Healthy State— An International Perspective on the Crisis in United States Medical Care.* New York: Pantheon Books, 1977.

Sigerist, Henry E., *American Medicine.* New York: W. W. Norton Co., 1934.

Silver, George, *A Spy in the House of Medicine.* Germantown, Md.: Aspen Systems Corp., 1976.

Silver, George A., *Child Health—America's Future.* Germantown, Md.: Aspen Systems Corp., 1978.

Silverman, Milton, and P. R. Lee, *Pills, Profits, and Politics.* Berkeley: University of California Press, 1974.

Somers, Anne R., *Health Care in Transition: Directions for the Future.* Chicago: Hospital Research and Education Trust, 1971.

Somers, Herman M., and Anne R. Somers, *Doctors, Patients, and Health Insurance.* Washington, D.C.: Brookings Institution, 1961.

Somers, Herman M., and Anne R. Somers, *Work-men's Compensation: Prevention, Insurance, and Rehabilitation of Occupational Disability.* New York: Wiley, 1954.

Starr, Paul, *The Social Transformation of American Medicine.* New York: Basic Books, 1982.

Stern, Bernhard J., *American Medical Practice in the Perspective of a Century.* New York: Commonwealth Fund, 1945.

Stewart, Jane, *Home Health Care.* St. Louis: C. V. Mosby, 1979.

Stevens, Rosemary, *American Medicine and the Public Interest.* New Haven, Conn: Yale University Press, 1971.

U.S. Department of Commerce, *Statistical Abstract of the United States 1987.* Washington, D.C.: Bureau of the Census, p. 343.

U.S. Public Health Service, *Medical Care in Transition* (Reprints from the American Journal of Public Health 1949–1966). Volumes I, II, and III, Washington, D.C., 1964–67.

U.S. Public Health Service, *Healthy People: The Surgeon General's Report on Health Promotion and Disease Prevention.* Washington, D.C.: DHEW (PHS) Pub. No. 79-55071, 1979.

Wallace, Helen M., *Health Services for Mothers and Children.* Philadelphia: W. B. Saunders Co., 1962.

Williams, Stephen J. (Editor), *Issues in Health Services.* New York: Wiley, 1980.

Wilner, Daniel L., R. P. Walker, and E. J. O'Neill, *Introduction to Public Health,* 7th edition. New York: Macmillan Co., 1978.

Wilson, F. A., and D. Neuhauser, *Health Services in the United States.* Cambridge, Mass.: Ballinger, 1974.

Zubkoff, Michael (Editor), *Health: A Victim or Cause of Inflation.* New York: Prodist, 1976.

CHAPTER SIX

Welfare-Oriented Health Systems in Industrialized Countries

In contrast to the United States, with its highly individualistic and entrepreneurial health policies, many other industrialized countries have established statutory programs to support the costs of medical care for the total or nearly the total national population. This broad population coverage has seldom been achieved all at once, but has typically developed gradually over several decades. National health insurance, as it is ordinarily called, is usually part of a general program of social security, also including old-age pensions, maternity benefits, unemployment compensation, disability insurance, and children's allowances.

WELFARE-ORIENTED HEALTH SYSTEMS

These health systems originated in Western Europe, but the national health insurance (NHI) idea spread to Japan in 1922 and later to New Zealand, Australia, and Canada. (It also spread to many nonindustrialized countries, considered in later chapters.) The term *welfare state* is frequently used to describe all these countries, but a distinction between two subtypes of such health system is made in this book. In the first type, discussed in this chapter, are the welfare-oriented systems, in which a high proportion, but not 100 percent, of the population is economically protected for medical care. The support program, however, is limited essentially to payment of health care bills, while the medical and other practitioners remain largely in private practice. In the second type of health system, 100 percent of the resident population is medically protected, without any special requirements for eligibility

or entitlement. Furthermore, major modifications have usually been made in the customary patterns for providing health service. This type of health system, considered universal-comprehensive, is discussed in the next chapter.

The welfare-oriented health systems, in contrast to the U.S. entrepreneurial system, are also characterized by the derivation of well over half of their total health-related expenditures from governmental sources. This is evident in Table 6.1, presenting data on welfare-oriented systems in nine countries, along with comparable data on the United States for 1982. These percentages have implications far beyond taxes and money; they reflect a great deal about the governance of a health system and the degree of equity in its distribution of health services.

On the other hand, the patterns of provision of medical care remain quite traditional in the welfare-oriented systems. Most physicians and dentists remain in private practice. The ownership of hospital beds in seven of these countries on which data are available is shown in Table 6.2. It may be noted that in 1982 more than 25 percent of the beds were in nongovernment (voluntary nonprofit or proprietary) facilities in all seven countries, and in two of these countries—Belgium and Japan—as well as the United States—the majority of beds were in such nonpublic hospitals.

We may now examine in more detail several of these welfare-oriented health systems in industrialized countries. As the pioneer country in developing social insurance to cover the costs of medicare care—a cornerstone of many national health systems—we should first consider the Federal Republic of Germany.

Table 6.1. Health Expenditures as a Proportion of Gross Domestic Product (GDP) and Percentage from Public Sources in Welfare-Oriented Systems and the United States, 1982

Country	Total Health Expenditures as Percentage of GDP	Health Expenditures, Percentage Governmental
France	9.3	71.0
Netherlands	8.7	79.3
West Germany	8.2	80.5
Ireland	8.2	93.9
Canada	8.2	74.4
Switzerland	7.8	60.3
Australia	7.6	63.2
Japan	6.6	66.7
Belgium	6.2	93.5
United States	10.6	42.5

Source: Organization for Economic Cooperation and Development, *Expenditures on Health under Economic Constraints.* Report of the Directorate for Social Affairs, Manpower, and Education. Washington, D.C.: OECD, 1984.

FEDERAL REPUBLIC OF GERMANY

As an outcome of its defeat in World War II, Germany was divided into east and west. The eastern part, coming under the influence of the Soviet Union, became the German Democratic Republic (GDR) and adopted a socialist form of government. The western part became the Federal Republic of Germany (FRG) and carries on the policies identified with prewar Germany.

The FRG had a population in 1984 of 61,200,000 and a GNP per capita of $11,130.

The country is divided into nine provinces or *lander,* which have a great deal of autonomy in matters of health and education. In the central government there is a Ministry of Youth, Family Affairs and Health, which promulgates standards for designated health functions, such as the operation of maternal and child health centers, examination of school children, regulation of the medical and related professions, pharmaceutical and foodstuff regulation, and consumer protection. A Federal Office of Health is responsible for technical advice on standards for communicable disease control, epidemiological research, and environmental sanitation. More crucial for medical care in the central government is the Federal Ministry of Labour and Social Affairs, which supervises social insurance, medical care under sickness insurance, hospitals, rehabilitation, and occupational health. The Ministry of Interior controls water supply, sewage disposal, and other environmental matters. Several voluntary health agencies are subsidized by government to conduct programs in health education.

Greater authority on all these matters is vested in the *lander.* Various federal laws are implemented by the health board of each *land* or province. The province, in turn, contains city health departments and district health departments, which perform the diverse preventive and regulatory activities noted at the federal level. Organizing and financing medical care, on the other hand, are the ultimate responsibilities of the provincial office of the Ministry of Labour and Social Affairs or its

Table 6.2. Hospital Ownership in Welfare-Oriented Systems: Percentage of Beds in Government and Non-government Facilities, 1976–1981

Country	Hospital Beds per 1,000	Percent Government	Percent Nongovernment
Australia	12.0	73.3	26.7
Japan	11.6	32.9	67.1
West Germany	11.5	52.3	47.6
Switzerland	11.2	62.3	37.7
Ireland	9.7	66.3	33.8
Belgium	9.3	37.1	62.9
France	7.2	69.0	31.0
United States	5.8	38.3	61.7

Source: Adapted from World Health Organization, *World Health Statistics Annual 1983.* Geneva: WHO, 1983.

equivalent. The detailed administration of these medical and related services, however, is in the hands of *sickness funds,* financed by social insurance—a complex program that doubtless plays the largest organized role in the German health system.

German Health Insurance and Its Development

The cornerstone of the German health system, like that in many welfare-oriented systems, is the program of social insurance or social security for medical care. Since Germany was the first country to develop such a program on a national level, it warrants special discussion.

Central Europe was the site of the world's greatest industrial development in the early nineteenth century. As working people left agriculture to become wage-earning workers in urban factories, they lost their sense of security. Unemployment or serious sickness meant a total loss of earnings. To protect themselves, therefore, they formed mutual aid societies; workers made regular contributions, and then if sickness struck they received compensation for lost wages and for the costs of medical care. In 1854, Prussia (one region of Germany) passed a law making membership in such mutual aid societies compulsory for low-wage workers, also requiring a matched contribution from employers. Contributions were a stated percentage of wages, and the funds were administered jointly by workers and employers.

Because several other regions established local workers' sickness insurance funds in the 1860s and 1870s there were already hundreds of voluntary and compulsory local sickness insurance funds throughout Germany when Otto von Bismarck became Chancellor in 1871. Bismarck was a member of the Prussian landed aristocracy and a staunch leader of the Conservative Party. The rise at this time of a working class movement, represented politically in the Social Democratic Party, was seen as a threat. In 1878, Bismarck succeeded in getting the Parliament *(Reichstag)* to restrict the freedom of socialist parties, but he was still concerned about the attitudes of the workers. In 1881, therefore, he introduced a bill that

would have established a single national sickness insurance fund for all low-wage workers. Government would make contributions along with employers.

The Social Democrats, representing the workers, opposed the bill because they did not trust Bismarck, they favored 100 percent support by employers, and they objected to governmental paternalism. They described the proposal as *beggar's insurance,* a program that would prevent the worker from becoming poor while compelling him to pay for the tactic. They said insurance did not attack the causes of misery but only their results. After debate for one year, both sides compromised. The Sickness Insurance Act, which became law on 15 June 1883, required that workers, in listed (low-wage) occupations be insured by one of the existing private sickness benefit societies or by new ones created for the purpose. The societies must provide a minimum set of benefits, both monetary and medical, must submit annual reports, and must invest their funds prudently. Workers were to pay two-thirds of the premiums and employers one-third, with corresponding administrative control. A year later, in 1884, another German law was enacted on insurance for industrial accidents, for which contributions were to be made only by employers. Work accidents were recognized as a proper cost of industrial production.

This was the birth of the concept of social security, which eventually spread throughout the world. In Germany and elsewhere, it was soon extended to other risks—especially old age (pensions), invalidity, unemployment, death and widow's benefits, maternity, children's allowances, and more. Applied to medical care, usually along with wage-loss compensation, the idea had spread to 70 countries by 1985.

The course of development in Germany is especially interesting. At the time of the original law 22,000 private sickness funds were estimated, covering about one-sixth of the population. The sequence of coverage and related features was as follows:

1883	—industrial workers with low wages
1889	—all manual workers of any

income plus other workers earning less than 2,000 marks a year

1903 —coverage of office and transport workers

1911 —coverage of domestic workers; sickness funds consolidated to 13,500

1914–1918—coverage of all dependents of the insured

1927 —coverage of seamen

1934–1939—regulation and supervision of hospitals, public health, cost-control data, and financial auditing shared with provinces; further reduction to 4,600 funds

1941 —coverage for pensions; no time limits on medical care

1951 —sickness funds down to 1,992

1957 —employer contributions increased for wage-loss compensation

1961 —waiting period eliminated for wage-loss compensation

1970 —coverage of all employees of any income

1972 —coverage of farmers; sickness funds down to 1,751

1980 —approximately 1,500 funds covering 90.2 percent of the population.

Over this period of about one century, many more developments occurred in German health insurance than are shown in this chronology. The sickness funds are of several types, depending on whether membership is based on geographic location, type of enterprise, or type of occupation. Relevant to occupation, "white-collar" employees who were not compulsorily insured could enroll in "substitute" sickness funds, thereby enjoying certain benefits (such as free coverage of dependents) not available from private insurance. The latter, sold by purely commercial companies, and providing financial reimbursement for medical care rather than direct medical services, could be purchased from about 50 companies.

Thus, taking account of persons protected by this diversity of insurance arrangements, the coverage in Germany in 1974 was as follows:

Insurance Status	Percentage of Population	
Mandatory members	30.75	
Substitute fund members	9.53	
Retired pensioners	12.82	
Dependents of above members (statutorily covered)	37.04	(90.14)
Private insurance coverage	7.20	
Police officers and students	1.29	
Public assistance recipients (other coverage)	1.07	(9.56)
Unprotected	0.30	(0.30)
Total population	100.00	(100.0)

It may be noted that within the mandatory or substitute members would be a small percentage of unemployed persons who are covered by unemployment compensation. Also the 1.07 percent of persons covered under public assistance may be obtaining medical care through different arrangements. In some communities, the welfare authorities may simply pay their premiums for enrollment in an established sickness fund; in others they may be served by doctors and other providers who are paid directly by the welfare agency. Altogether, it is evident that all but a fraction of 1 percent of the German population have some insurance protection for medical care; more than 99 percent have economic access to care, one way or another.

In a sense, the population coverage is even more than 100 percent, because the "private insurance coverage" indicated (7.20 percent) applies only to persons who rely completely on this protection. In addition, several million persons with protection by a statutory scheme have *supplemental* private insurance, to pay for the services of a private physician during hospitalization or for a first-class hospital room.

The scope of benefits provided as a minimum under the German health insurance legislation has gradually been broadened. Initially only the services of community physicians and drugs were required; hospitalization, dental care, eyeglasses, rehabilitative care, and so forth were optional. Soon all of these services came to be included in the typical benefit package, along with cash compensation for loss of wages due to sickness. Because the cost of medical services, furthermore, has gradually increased, cash benefits in the 1980s amounted to less than 10 percent of the total. Some of the more innovative sickness funds offered preventive services such as immunizations and prenatal care and also early case detection (for tuberculosis and venereal disease) back in the 1920s. These services were discontinued in the 1930s, but in the 1970s they were being resumed by selected funds, along with other special benefits such as home nursing and spa therapy.

With this long and complex developmental background, the coverage and administrative arrangements of German health insurance in the 1980s were highly irregular and fragmented. The precise benefits and conditions for medical service vary greatly for the members of different sickness funds. The premiums payable may also vary widely, in accordance with the benefits as well as the risk-composition (age, sex, occupation, etc.) of the fund's membership.

The relationships between the sickness funds and the providers of care have been especially complex. At the turn of the twentieth century, German physicians became concerned about being dominated by the sickness funds. In 1900, therefore, they organized a "Union of German Physicians for the Defense of Their Economic Interests." There were numerous physician strikes, and by the end of World War I (about 1920) the arrangements for medical remuneration had been greatly modified. The sickness funds were required to transmit to regional associations of community doctors quarterly amounts per capita, based on their memberships. The physicians were then paid fees by their own medical association, rather than directly by the sickness funds. Any adjustments of fees necessary to stay within the quarterly allotment were made by the medical body.

Arrangements for hospital care and its payment were different. In Germany, as in most of the world (outside the United States and Canada), medical service in hospitals is quite separate from that in the community. Basically, hospitals are staffed by full-time salaried specialists, whose work is entirely devoted to in-patients. German hospitals have no out-patient departments, since ambulatory care is the prerogative of community doctors. In fact, more than half of nonhospital community doctors in Germany are qualified specialists. For hospital care the sickness funds make payments directly to the hospital on a per diem basis; these per diem amounts are negotiated between each hospital and a federation of the sickness funds, but they are subject to the approval of the provincial social insurance (Labour Ministry) authority. The hospital payments include the costs of not only all hospital services, drugs, diagnostic tests, and so on, but also the salaries of hospital physicians. (They do not include payment for capital costs, which are regarded as an obligation of government or philanthropy.)

German Health Resources and Other Features

Despite its complexities, the German health insurance program clearly makes accessible to almost every resident—even "guest workers" from Turkey and other countries—a virtually complete range of medical and related services. It is noteworthy that neither the health professions nor the sickness societies have found it necessary to introduce any copayment restrictions on access to medical care. (There is only a small copayment for prescribed drugs.) Nor is there any "deductible" in the health insurance process, such as commercial health insurance carriers have often considered essential. Physicians, pharmacists, dentists, and others can be paid on a fee-for-service basis for ambulatory care by skillful management of the funds allotted on a periodic per capita basis. The number of physicians who are free to make contracts with any particular fund (for service to its members) may be restricted, in the interest of cost controls.

The defeat of Germany in two world wars has not prevented the country from developing an ample supply of health resources. Soon after World War II, Germany had 131.5 physicians per 100,000 population, and this had increased to 241.0 per 100,000 by 1984. There were 354.6 professional nurses per 100,000 in 1980 and many auxiliary nursing personnel. There were 29 medical schools in 1984, all of which were parts of public universities, under the control of the ministry of education in each province. As in most of the world, the medical curriculum lasts 6 years after secondary school. Admission may be selective, but if admitted the student usually pays no tuition.

Hospitals are also numerous, with a total of 11.5 beds per 1,000 population in 1980. We have already noted that only slightly more than half of these beds are in governmental institutions. The distribution of overall hospital bed ownership in 1980 was as follows:

Ownership	Percent
Government	52.3
Voluntary nonprofit	35.1
Proprietary	12.5
Total	100.0

Of the 11.5 hospital beds per 1,000, 7.9 were for general short-term care, in which the average stay was 17 days (much longer than in the United States). The remaining beds in "special" hospitals were principally for long-term patients. Hospital accommodations for insured persons are normally at the third-class level (in open wards), which constitute about 80 percent of all beds. Any patient, however, may use a first- or second-class bed by paying the difference in price. Germany has an especially robust private pharmaceutical industry (some 460 companies) that floods the market every year with hundreds of new products which are difficult for the average physician to evaluate.

The years of domination by the Nazi (National Socialist) Party in Germany, 1933 through 1945, were bound to have an impact on the entire health system. Despite the violence of World War II and the horrors of the Nazi holocaust, the general national health system and the health insurance program in particular continued to operate, although not without serious disturbances.

The hundreds of German sickness funds were defiled by bitter anti-Semitism. "Non-Aryans, communists, and socialists" were ex-cluded from the funds, as either physicians or administrators. At first, Jews who had fought in World War I were permitted to hold contracts with the funds, but after 1938 they too were banned. At the same time, the Nazi Party, along with very supportive associations of private physicians, set out to destroy the entire labor leadership of the sickness funds. These experienced union officials were replaced by unqualified old Nazi Party members, and fund administration for a period was in shambles. Before the Nazis came to power in 1933, many sickness funds had established clinics with salaried doctors to provide ambulatory medical care at low cost. These socially oriented clinics were terminated. The associations of sickness funds, which had developed certain public health programs, were broken up. All sickness fund administrators were replaced by appointees of the Ministry of Labour. The National Association of Sickness Fund Physicians was endowed with much greater power to bargain with individual sickness insurance funds.

After the war and the defeat of Nazism, German health insurance continued, but with a much stronger voice for physicians and a weaker voice for workers. Sickness funds, for example, could no longer establish clinics without the approval of a medical association. Physicians could not employ other physicians, thus safeguarding solo private medical practice. Professional associations have mandatory membership and control all payments to physicians. Physicians in public health or industrial work are not permitted to treat patients. Sickness fund boards—previously two-thirds workers and one-third employers—were changed to half workers and half employers. In only one respect does a postwar change correspond with sound health policy in many countries: access to specialists and hospitals was required to depend on referral from a general primary physician.

In the 1970s, a great deal of federal legislation was enacted in Germany to protect the population against environmental hazards. As noted earlier, the ministry of interior has primary jurisdiction over this field, along with corresponding authorities in the provinces. Legislation on drug safety has also been stimulated by such tragic episodes as the serious deformities the German drug Thalidomide caused in babies when it was taken by pregnant women. Other legislative measures in recent years have been directed to cost containment both in hospitals and in ambulatory medical care.

German medical research was noteworthy in the nineteenth and early twentieth centuries. The contributions of Rudolf Virchow, Robert Koch, Wilhelm Roentgen, Karl Landsteiner, and Paul Ehrlich were milestones in the evolution of modern medical science. This leadership role of German science declined after 1930, but after 1980 high priority was again given to medical research. Grants from the federal government and the provinces were made to universities and autonomous research institutions. Since 1978, research objectives have focused on improved methods of prevention, techniques for early disease detection, and validation of concepts relating to diagnosis and therapy.

This account of the health system of the Federal Republic of Germany has emphasized the national health insurance program for several reasons. In the total German system dynamics, sickness insurance funds play a central role. Their policies and behavior have had major effects on the practice of medicine and the performance of hospitals. Second, as the world pioneer in social insurance or social security, Germany has had a great influence on the planning of health insurance programs in other countries. Third, Germany has demonstrated how a mechanism for financing health services can be developed to achieve nearly 100 percent coverage, with little disturbance to the traditional patterns of health care delivery.

It is this third attribute that endows Germany, along with a few other industrialized countries, with its special characteristics in the world spectrum of health systems. Starting with small groups of workers in communities, hundreds of sickness insurance societies arose to become, in effect, local agents of national and provincial governments. Physicians, on the other hand, showed mounting resistance to economic domination by working-class patients, until the conflict was resolved by establishing fiscal "middlemen," controlled by doctors, to manage the actual payment of fees. Customary principles, such as free choice of doctor, private practice, and payment on a fee-for-service basis, were retained. Within the medical profession, the lines between hospital specialist care for in-patients and community care (by both generalists and specialists) for ambulatory patients were carefully maintained. As in most welfare-oriented health systems, the reluctance to make any extensive modification of patterns of medical practice or delivery of other kinds of health care has made it difficult to control the steadily mounting costs.

Another industrialized country with a welfare-oriented health system illustrating somewhat different dynamics is Belgium. Similar in its use of hundreds of local mutual aid societies to handle the economic aspects, Belgium's health system illustrates the preservation of professional autonomy, along with collectivized financing, even more profoundly than Germany.

BELGIUM

Occupying a small territory on the coast of northwest Europe, Belgium had a population in 1985 of 9,900,000. With a GNP that year of $8,280 per capita, it is highly industrialized and generally prosperous. Belgium's king performs a largely ceremonial role within a parliamentary democracy. When the nation took shape in 1830—carved out of the kingdom of the Netherlands—its boundaries were demarcated along religious rather than linguistic lines. This crucial decision made Belgium predominantly Catholic and the Netherlands Protestant; the northern half of Belgium, however, is occupied by people who speak Dutch (or Flemish) and the southern half by people who speak French. Despite the religious homogeneity, the linguistic and associated cultural differences create many problems in the country's governance, including its health system.

Before World War II, the French southern half of Belgium (known as Walloon) was heavily industrialized and dominant. After the war (with much destruction in the south), the Flemish northern half (Flanders) became industrialized and seemed to acquire national dominance. The Christian Democratic Party, a conservative group, has become the principal political force—usually in coalition with other parties—since the end of the war in 1946. Officially the country is divided into nine provinces that contain, for administrative purposes, 44 *arrondissements,* and these contain more than 2,300 communes. Provincial governments, however, have rather limited authority. The governors are not elected, but appointed by the central government. The operation of public hospitals and certain public health functions, nevertheless, are decentralized.

Organization of Health Programs

If the control of money were the criterion, Belgium's health insurance program would clearly be the nation's major health activity, but since its function is to provide economic support for largely private health services it is considered separately. In its scope of authority, the Ministry of Public Health and the Family is Belgium's major health agency; its powers, however, are more indirect than direct.

Ministry of Public Health and the Family. The functions of the Ministry of Public Health and the Family are principally to establish health standards, research, administration of grants, supervise health services carried out by other organized entities, and only to a limited extent to provide direct health services itself. Units in the ministry are concerned with various aspects of environmental protection, with health education, the health of school children, tuberculosis, venereal disease, statistics, medicolegal problems, the control of pharmacies, hospital affairs, mental illness care, and many other health fields. The staffs of these units, however, are not large because the duties are primarily consultative and supervisory, whereas most health services are actually rendered—often through the support of national grants—by other organizations.

In spite of the tradition of local sovereignty in Belgium, the authority of the Ministry of Public Health has become very broad. This policy of centralization has been implemented through various grant-in-aid programs, in which the grants are conditional on compliance of local entities with national standards. Another development with many implications for health service is a law (effective January 1977) that consolidated the numerous local communes from 2,359 into 600. On the other hand there is a parallel movement toward decentralization, but at a higher level, through the formation of three major regional councils for the Flemish (Flanders), the French (Walloon), and the Brussels areas of Belgium. Many public health functions are being delegated to these regional bodies, including the implementation of laws on environmental sanitation, grants for health care facilities, and supervision of activities (such as child and maternal health services) for preventive purposes.

An important program of the Ministry of Public Health and the Family is the control of drugs and pharmacies. In this field, most functions are carried out directly, rather than through delegation to local governments or private agencies. A computerized Information Center operated by the ministry responds to about 25 drug inquiries per day; it also sends a monthly bulletin about new drugs to every pharmacist and doctor in the country. While the MOPHF registers all drugs that may be sold in Belgium (about 11,000 types in 1980), the National Institute of Health and Invalidity Insurance (INAMI) decides which drugs will be financed by the health insurance system. The Ministry of Economy is also involved in monitoring the prices of drugs.

Another aspect of health care that the central MOPHF has certain direct responsibility for is psychiatric service. Of the 76 mental hospitals in Belgium as of 1980, facilities with 78 percent of the beds were under private auspices. Policies in all mental hospitals, however, are subject to control by the ministry, under laws and decrees that determine methods of patient care much more specifically than is done for treatment of somatic disease. Thus, legislation calls for gradual modification of all mental patient wards into two types: one for acute cases requiring intensive care, and the other for long-term cases requiring intermediate or rehabilitative care. The large mental hospitals (with more than 800-bed capacity) must be reduced to a maximum size of 500 beds, discharging patients to community mental health centers.

A unique and interesting approach to care of the mentally ill has been applied in the town of Geel, in the Flemish part of Belgium, since around the year 1400. Starting with religious inspiration, families in this town took retarded and mentally ill patients into their homes. Disturbed patients came to Geel in search of help as to a shrine for divine healing. After 1800, the religious aspects of the work evolved toward a medical approach. A mental hospital was eventually built in the town, to admit some patients if their families could not handle them. This hospital had 250 patients in 1980, but 1,500 patients—essentially quiet and long-term schizophrenics and also mentally retarded—were living in private homes. The health insurance system pays these guardian families just as it supports care in the mental hospitals.

Below the level of the national government, official public health activities in Belgium are largely concentrated in the field of environmental sanitation. Preventive personal health services are principally furnished by private health organizations, supported by grants from the MOPHF.

Each of the nine provinces has a small health department. The provincial health officer is usually part-time, engaging also in private practice or in some other administrative role, such as being an advisory doctor for one of the health insurance federations. He is appointed not by the province, but by the king, on advice of the Ministry of Health. He serves essentially as a provincial representative of the national ministry in the field of "public hygiene." Aside from enforcing sanitation codes, the health officer is responsible for receiving reports and taking necessary actions on cases of acute communicable diseases, for registration of births and deaths, and for doing the administrative work of the Provincial Medical Coun-

cil. The latter is the statutory agency for registration of physicians and certain other health personnel.

There are other health-related functions at the provincial level, although not connected with the Provincial Health Department. To conduct the inspection and approval of pharmacies, a provincial pharmacist is responsible directly to the national unit for this work in the MOPHF. For inspection of meat, there is a corresponding provincial veterinarian. Two provincial physicians are also responsible for liaison with the private agencies devoted to control of tuberculosis, venereal disease, cancer, and other "social diseases" (as defined in Belgium). These physicians conduct a program of general health education, and they may also directly treat cases of venereal disease.

At the municipal or commune level, larger cities have a local health department, concerned essentially with environmental protection. A part-time city physician is in charge, aided by one or two sanitary inspectors. In small communes, the mayor plays this public health role, along with his other duties. Local communities often construct health centers in which maternal and child health clinics are conducted (see later), as well as examinations of school children.

Also at the municipal level are commissions of public assistance (CAP), which are largely responsible for public hospitals. Through hospital out-patient and in-patient services, they provide medical care for the poor who cannot afford the copayments required in the health insurance program. They also serve persons not covered by health insurance, among whom workers immigrating from other countries (before official citizenship is attained) are important. The CAPs are responsible for emergency medical services in their communities. A single telephone number throughout Belgium summons an ambulance, the police, firefighters, or other forms of emergency service.

Preventive health services for school children are also provided at the local level under a variety of arrangements. Screening examinations are done by a doctor four times during elementary school (6 through 12 years of age) and four times during secondary school (12 through 18 years). General practitioners do this work, and they are paid a fee by the MOPHF for each child examined.

Ministry of Labor and Employment. Belgium, along with France, has very advanced standards in occupational health. A law of 1965 specifies that every work establishment must have the service of an industrial physician, either by direct appointment (if the plant has more than 50 workers) or through a multiplant medical service (for smaller enterprises). These arrangements must be approved by the Ministry of Labor. The standard requires the equivalent of one full-time physician for each 2,000 workers. Unfortunately, hundreds of plants in Belgium, as of 1980, were not yet in compliance with this law. A factory inspection program also surveys conditions that might contribute to occupational injuries or diseases.

Approximately 1,200 physicians in Belgium in 1980 were doing some occupational health work, of whom about 300 were full-time. These physicians did preemployment and periodic health examinations of the workers, and they were supposed to be alert to health hazards at the workplace. The examinations were done more frequently on young workers, women, and persons exposed to special hazards. To the extent feasible, first-aid for injury or illness is given by the industrial doctor, but for any continuing medical care the worker must be referred to a private physician. The multienterprise health programs may serve scores of small plants in an area. These programs may be sponsored by physicians, private insurance companies, by universities (schools of public health), or the businesses themselves. In all of these arrangements, the firms pay the costs; there is an annual charge per worker for the service, plus an additional fee for each medical examination.

Compensation for job-related injuries or diseases comes under a special program of mandatory insurance, different from that for general illness. The insurance for both wage replacement and medical care of injuries is generally carried by private insurance companies, based on a law of 1903, as modified in 1971. (An interesting sidelight is that the administrative expenses for these private insur-

ance arrangements are said to be about 35 percent, compared to 7.5 percent in the government health insurance system.) The injured worker has free choice of doctor, except where the firm operates its own medical service. Since 1927, there has been a separate social insurance program for occupational diseases. It is noteworthy that, unlike the insurance for work accidents or for general illness, this is provided through a single national fund in the Ministry of Social Security. The rationale is that an occupational disease can rarely be attributed to work for a single employer, thus maximum pooling of the insurance money is necessary.

The Ministry of Labor and Employment also operates a nationwide program for rehabilitation of the physically handicapped. A national rehabilitation fund has been maintained for the purpose since 1963. Rehabilitation counselors are stationed throughout Belgium to advise disabled workers about medical services needed, vocational training, and job placement.

Voluntary Health Organizations. With its strong tradition of free private enterprise, it is not surprising that Belgium should have an especially large role for voluntary or private health organizations. After starting with private initiative, most of these agencies have become heavily subsidized—for more than 90 percent of their costs—by government, to carry out functions that would otherwise be a direct public responsibility.

The voluntary organization with the greatest nationwide role is the *Oeuvre Nationale de l'Enfance* (ONE or National Work for Children). Founded in 1919 after World War I, ONE has hundreds of local councils throughout Belgium. The planning and administrative work is done by volunteer middle-class women, but 1,200 nurses were employed full-time and paid salaries in 1980. The principal activity is operation of several types of preventive clinics for children and expectant mothers. For support of its entire program, ONE gets 90 percent of the necessary funds from the national Ministry of Health and the Family.

The ONE program has very wide impact. It is estimated that 80 percent of newborns in

Belgium are seen during their first year, although this figure has declined somewhat, as more preventive work is being done by Belgium's expanding supply of private doctors. Hospitals usually notify the social nurses, attached to the local ONE councils, of each childbirth. Although young doctors, both general practitioners and pediatricians, benefit from their appointments in ONE clinics—becoming better known in the community through this work—controversies still exist within the medical profession about the scope of ONE services. These clearly do not include treatment since any sick child is promptly referred to a private physician, but there has been much contention about immunizations.

The ONE also operates camps for handicapped or debilitated children, and provides foster homes for orphans. Day care centers are maintained for the children of working mothers. ONE even conducts programs in West Germany for the children of military personnel stationed there. Since national authorities obviously entrust the entire maternal and child health program to this organization, it is often described as a "paragovernmental" agency. Public health nurses from the Provincial Health Departments, in fact, monitor the ONE program to ensure that proper standards are being met.

Another very important voluntary organization in Belgium is the Yellow and White Cross. This is essentially a home visiting nurse service that employed 1,600 nurses, as of 1980, in virtually every community of the country. Each province has a somewhat autonomous branch, all coordinated by the national office in Brussels. The nurses cover the population of assigned districts, working under the orders of a general practitioner. All the nurses are trained to the *gradué* (3-years training) or *breveté* (2-years training) level, but not always with the supplemental training of a social nurse. In contrast to the preventive service of the ONE nurses, the Yellow and White Cross nurses do mostly bedside care for convalescent or chronically ill patients.

Fees for each nursing visit, paid by the health insurance program, meet 80 percent of the costs of this service. The insurance organization pays the fees directly to the Cross agency, which then pays the nurses by salary. In addition, the Yellow and White Cross receives a small subsidy for each nurse from the Ministry of Public Health and the Family. Also, families who wish to be served by this program pay a small membership fee each year. Most families in Belgium are members.

Equivalent voluntary health agency services are provided in the field of tuberculosis control. The National League Against Tuberculosis runs a network of local TB clinics and mobile chest X-ray surveys. Some of the local health insurance societies may also conduct chest clinics, as may certain hospitals. With the decline in tuberculosis, the National League in Belgium, as elsewhere, has been seeking new roles.

In the mental health field there are several voluntary organizations—at least seven major ones. These bodies have taken the lead in promoting and establishing facilities for ambulatory psychiatric care in the community. They have operated clinics for child guidance, adults, patients discharged from mental hospitals, and a few special *day hospitals* or *night hospitals.* With the legislation of 1974, the mental health organizations are focusing their efforts on setting up comprehensive mental health centers. Most of the financial support for psychiatric clinics comes from fees paid by the health insurance program.

Further voluntary health bodies work in the field of cancer treatment and prevention, poliomyelitis, cerebral palsy, and other areas. Venereal disease control activities are shared between a voluntary society and the provincial liaison physicians. All of these agencies are subsidized to some extent by the MOPHF. In fact, there are numerous *public hygiene councils* under the ministry to coordinate policies between these private and public entities.

The Private Health Care Market. More important than all the organized health activities described so far is Belgium's private market of personal health services. The economic support of these services is provided almost entirely by the program of mandatory health insurance. The historical background and mode of operation of this program is so complex, and also so central a part of Belgium's national health system, that it requires special elaboration.

Health Insurance and the Private Medical Market

Every aspect of Belgium's health system is influenced by the operation of its several health insurance programs. Although these mechanisms for financial support of nearly all types of health service are defined by law, the providers of service are largely private and independent agents.

Historical Development. As in Germany, by the early nineteenth century, there were many mutual aid societies in the towns and cities of the territory that is now Belgium. Most of them gave money to a member who became sick or injured, to help him cope with both his loss of earnings and the costs of medications and doctor's care. (Hospitalization, if needed, was available without charge in public or charitable institutions.) A few of the societies reimbursed members specifically for the fees of doctors or apothecaries. As industrialization grew, the mutual aid societies were joined increasingly by factory workers, who depended on their wages for survival. Sometimes, mutual societies were encouraged and even financially assisted by socially minded employers.

The amount of contributions and the exact benefits of a mutual aid society were decided at general meetings of the members. The administrative work required in collecting contributions and paying out benefits was done by unpaid volunteers. Each community had its own society, and one can understand how local adversities such as a business failure causing high unemployment, an epidemic, or mismanagement of the funds could lead to collapse of a whole mutual society. In 1851, therefore, the Belgian Parliament enacted a law permitting incorporation of the mutual societies, thereby protecting their executives from personal liability in case of economic reverses.

To become incorporated, the law required that the mutual societies had to meet certain standards of operation and come under the supervision of local public authorities. These re-

quirements were so great, however, that only a small fraction of the societies applied for approval (and incorporation). In 1853, 200 sickness funds were estimated, with 68,000 members under mutual societies in Belgium. Of these, only 13 funds with 2,063 members had applied for recognition by the government. As another basis for achieving stability, some funds sought support from labor unions. Since various unions represented differing political viewpoints, this led to ideological differences among the mutual societies—a pluralism that is still prominent in the Belgian health insurance field.

As the mutual societies grew, along with industrialization and urbanization, it was observed that elderly members became sick more often and more seriously. Hence, some societies required higher contribution to the sickness fund from older members. While this may have been inequitable (contrary to the sharing of risks), it showed recognition of principles of sound financial management, necessary for sickness fund survival.

After Germany's pioneer social insurance legislation in 1883 and the rapid advances of medical science in the late nineteenth century, there was a new appreciation of the value of medical care. In this environment, Belgium enacted its law of 1894, which reflected increased trust in the sickness funds and served to strengthen the health insurance movement. Besides providing the advantage of incorporation, this law exempted the sickness funds from various taxes, it entitled them to receive gifts and legacies, and even authorized subsidies from local and national governments.

With greater understanding of the requirements for financial stability, several local societies in a region began to assemble in federations. Since the societies by then had become ideologically identified, those with similar philosophies would band together, so that in the same region several federations were formed. These regional federations, in turn, soon became interested in forming national alliances—that is, groupings of federations from several regions of Belgium. The first of these to take shape was the National Alliance of Christian Mutual Funds in 1906. This was followed by the National Union of Neutral Mutualists

Federations (1908), the National Union of Socialist Mutual Funds (1913), the National League of Liberal Mutualist Federations (1914), and the National Union of Occupational Mutualist Federations (1920). These five national associations of federations of mutual societies, and a sixth Auxiliary Fund formed later, have come to play a crucial role in the administration of Belgian health insurance.

After 1900, subsidies from the central government were increased to encourage the growth of the mutual societies. An act of 1912 then provided for systematic subsidy of all local funds, intended specifically to support the costs of long-term disability (wage replacement). Benefits for the coverage of doctor's fees in this period were purely monetary indemnification of the member; no agreements were made with physicians to accept designated fees for certain services.

After World War I and with continued advances in medical science, the costs of medical care rose rapidly, and governmental subsidies to the funds focused more on sustaining these costs. Subsidies were also intended to support coverage of medical care for family dependents, in addition to the employed worker; this, of course, greatly increased society memberships. An especially heavy financial burden on the sickness funds was the cost of long-term hospital care for tuberculosis, a major scourge in the early twentieth century. To cope with this problem the societies took their first action to establish health care facilities themselves, building a tuberculosis sanitarium in 1918 and another one in 1920.

In spite of the encouragement of the Belgian sickness funds through government subsidies, population coverage remained voluntary and reached only 74 percent by the end of World War II. With the influence of the International Labour Organization, the British Beveridge Report, and the general spirit of the postwar period, a law of 28 December 1944 and a royal decree of 21 March 1945 (even before the war was over) made membership compulsory for all private employees in Belgium. Not until 1963, however, was compulsory enrollment authorized for self-employed persons and their dependents. Under the same law, in 1965 government employees were also covered by royal

decree. The 1945 and 1963 laws brought more than 90 percent of the Belgian population under mandatory health insurance protection, and most of the remaining 10 percent were enrolled in the same mutual societies on a voluntary basis.

The law of 1963 brought many changes in Belgian health insurance. Financial subsidies became based on the expenditures required, rather than the contributions of mutual society members, as was done originally. All six of the health insurance organizations were brought under the general supervision of the National Institute for Sickness and Invalidity Insurance (*Institute National d'Assurance Maladie-Invalidité,* or INAMI). The INAMI is controlled by a board of directors representing the mutual societies, workers, employers, self-employed, hospitals, physicians, and the allied health professions. The institute negotiates with doctors and others over the fees payable for services, it regulates the general policies of all the component health insurance associations, and it provides various advisory, training, and legal services to the national associations, regional federations, and local mutual health insurance societies.

When social insurance was made compulsory for all employees in 1945, a crucial administrative decision had to be made. After the disruption of the war, the left-of-center political parties in Belgium proposed that the entire system be unified under a national authority, with conversion of the numerous local mutual societies into branch offices of this authority. The Christian Democrats, however, opposed this, and their view prevailed; the various local funds, federations, and associations kept their sovereignty. Only the collection of insurance contributions was centralized, through a National Office of Social Security (*Office National de Sécurité Sociale,* or ONSS), that originally came under the Ministry of Labor (though later under the Ministry of Social Welfare). The ONSS then distributes money to various agencies concerned with old-age pensions, unemployment, family allowances, and other issues, and for medical care and disability to the INAMI. The INAMI, in turn, transmits money to the six national associations, from which it is passed down to the federations and ultimately reaches the local mutual aid societies. It is at this local level that benefits are paid to patients or health care providers. The local fund, if it is able to meet the costs, is free to provide supplementary benefits or services to its members.

Health Insurance Operations. From this historical background, one can understand why Belgium's health insurance program is highly pluralistic and complicated. Program operations involve responsibilities at four distinct levels:

1. The central government—including the National Office of Social Security (ONSS) and the National Institute for Sickness and Invalidity Insurance (INAMI).
2. The national associations—five non-government unions or alliances of regional federations of mutual aid societies, plus the sixth quasi-governmental Auxiliary Fund.
3. Federations of local societies—about 150 regional groupings of small mutual aid societies with sickness funds.
4. Local mutual aid societies—about 2,000 organizations at the local level, where sickness funds receive claims and idemnify their members for medical care expenses, or make certain payments directly to health care providers.

The distribution of members among the six national associations is quite uneven. The National Alliance of Christian Mutual Funds has about half the national population, with different memberships under each of the other five groups. The general attitude in Belgium is that the great pluralism of the whole health insurance program yields competition, which stimulates each local fund to work hard to attract and satisfy members. The multiplicity of agencies, moreover, promotes widespread consumer participation in the operations of the whole program. From the local funds to the national associations, councils of elected members make policy decisions, within the constraints of the law.

Monies are derived from insurance contri-butions paid to the National Office of Social Security (ONSS) by employers, workers, and the self-employed, supplemented by subsidies from the national government. Theoretically, the subsidies help finance services for the poor, the unemployed, the aged, and other disadvantaged persons; also theoretically, they support the care of certain "social diseases" such as tuberculosis, mental disorder, or cancer. The overall contribution of government revenues to the health insurance program amounts to about 30 percent of the costs. The percentage of earnings or income payable is, of course, determined by law but may be changed periodically by the Parliament in accordance with the costs of benefits. The health insurance benefits include both partial replacement of earnings during disability and support for most of the costs of medical care. Disability benefits are payable to the employee after only a one-day waiting period, and generally amount to 60 percent of wages up to a defined maximum. Physicians must certify a person's disability periodically; much of the surveillance exercised by "control doctors," attached to the federations of mutual funds, relates to this disability certification process.

The medical care benefits are broader for employees than for self-employed persons. Considering first the worker and his dependents—who constitute four-fifths of the insurance population—the insurance reimburses or indemnifies the patient for 75 percent of designated charges by a physician. This applies to either general practitioners or specialists, for service in the office or at the patient's home. Thus, the patient must pay 25 percent of the fee personally, except for the poor, the aged, and certain others, for whom the insurance pays 100 percent. This fee is indicated on a *nomenclature* or fee schedule established nationally by the INAMI after consultation with representatives of the medical profession. A major contention, however, has long beclouded the degree to which the doctor is legally obligated to abide by this schedule of fees for all his patients. In certain districts, in fact, the doctor may charge any fee he wishes, but is reimbursed by his local society only for 75 percent of the official fee. In practice, with "free choice of doctor" in a competitive market, the great majority abide by the negotiated fee schedule. One inducement for doctors to observe the negotiated fees is a policy of the INAMI to make an annual contribution to a retirement fund for each doctor agreeing to abide by the schedule.

The Belgian patient not only has free choice of any doctor, but (in contrast with the patterns in several other European countries) he may go directly to a specialist without referral. Furthermore, the patient is free to "shop around" among different doctors for treatment of the same ailment, but the obligation of copayment (the *ticket moderateur*) is expected to discourage this. On the other hand, for highly specialized services in a hospital or even on an ambulatory basis, the patient is not required to copay 25 percent of the official fee.

For services rendered in hospitals, moreover, the doctor often sends his or her bill directly to the local sickness fund, rather than bill the patient who must then seek indemnification later. The whole indemnity process is defended in Belgium as a form of protection against fraud by the doctor. Although it is stated that claims for services not actually rendered would be rare, the requirement that the patient pay the doctor and seek reimbursement later is deemed to be a safer procedure.

Beyond physician's service, the most frequently used insurance benefits in Belgium are prescribed drugs. The proportion of prescription costs reimbursed by the insurance program has been quite variable. For drugs compounded by the pharmacist, the patient received 75 percent reimbursement. For those prepared entirely by the pharmaceutical manufacturer, the patient paid a greater share of the costs. This share, however, was less if a brand name or proprietary drug was included on an "approved list" prepared by the INAMI (with the advice of a committee of consultants). For proprietary drugs not on this list—usually because they were considered unduly expensive or ineffective—no insurance reimbursement is made.

Hospitalization in a general ward is supported fully by the insurance program plus the Ministry of Public Health and the Family (with no cost-sharing), whether in public or private hospitals. The ministry's share is 25 percent of approved costs, although this is usually a lower percentage of the charges in private hospitals. If the patient chooses a semiprivate (two beds) or private room, he must pay extra personally, unless such accommodation is ordered by the doctor for medical reasons. The insurance fund to which the patient belongs usually pays hospitals directly, rather than indemnifying the patient.

The rate of payment per-day-of-care is based on the MOPHF's calculation of each hospital's costs, done with the advice of a Hospital Council representing the private and public hospitals. These costs may include amortization of capital debt and education of personnel in hospitals as well as all aspects of patient care, but not the services of doctors, who are paid by separate health insurance fees. Since laboratory and X-ray services are regarded as medical rather than hospital services, their costs are also excluded from the per diem hospital payments. This per diem system of financing, of course, gives the hospitals incentives to maximize bed occupancy, even though this may mean excessive and costly patient-days. To prevent or reduce such wastage, the health insurance *control doctors* perform a monitoring role. A "prior authorization" is theoretically required for admission of any patient, but in practice this is given automatically.

Dental care is also covered by the Belgian health insurance program, with various limitations. Ordinary preventive and restorative services, but not prostheses (full or partial dentures), are benefits up to age 50; after this prosthetic replacements are covered. The patient copays 25 percent of the officially negotiated fee, except that this is waived for pensioners, invalids, and other disadvantaged persons. Free choice of private dentist is unlimited, as is the care of physicians.

The health insurance program finances various other ancillary health services when they are ordered by a physician. These include home nursing care, physiotherapy, speech therapy, eyeglasses, hearing aids, and certain other items. It should be noted, however, that a doctor's prescription is always necessary; thus, eyeglasses prescribed by an optometrist or "dispensing optician" would not be covered. Foot care by podiatrists is likewise not a benefit, nor is occupational therapy. Preventive examinations or immunizations, on the other hand, are insured when they are given in a private office. Virtually the only service workers for whom remuneration is entirely by salary are social workers who serve on the staffs of the insurance organizations; they usually work out of the office of a regional federation.

If patients have a complaint about any medical service, they may bring it to the attention of their local mutual fund. The advisory doctor of the federation can then investigate the matter and, if he believes a physician to have performed improperly, he may refer the matter to the provincial Order of Physicians, a professional body concerned with medical ethics.

As noted, the scope of mandatory health insurance benefits is less for the self-employed than for employees. For the former, mandatory insurance covers essentially "catastrophic" services—that is, hospitalization and expensive specialist care inside or outside the hospital. For day-to-day ambulatory medical care, it is expected that the self-employed person and his family can ordinarily afford to pay private fees without insurance. Nevertheless, most such persons voluntarily purchase insurance for general ambulatory care from the same mutual society in which they are enrolled for the obligatory benefits. Each local mutual society or a regional federation of societies may offer its members supplemental benefits, such as transportation expenses, camps for children, or health resorts for adults.

The independence and sovereignty of the "liberal professions" in Belgium—especially physicians, dentists, and pharmacists—as well as the hospitals are so great they cause many social difficulties. One cannot avoid noticing the sustained tension in Belgium between the health insurance organizations and the providers of service, especially physicians. A doctor strike in 1964 was only one dramatic chapter in a story of persistent strained relationships that go back a half-century or more. Among other things, the 1964 crisis led to the demise of the previous Belgian Federation of Physicians (which had been prepared to accede to governmental proposals) and to the birth of the *medical syndicates* with their very antagonistic posture.

In negotiations on fee schedules between the

health insurance program, through the INAMI, and the medical profession, the doctors are represented by two medical syndicates or unions. These negotiations and the continuing dialogues involve not only the level of fees in the official agreements, but also the degree to which individual doctors are obligated to abide by the fee schedule and to inform patients of their charges in advance. They are also concerned with the whole question of preserving unrestricted free choice of doctor, including direct access of patients to specialists without referral.

With its strict insistence on independence and sovereignty, the Belgian medical profession has resisted almost all types of surveillance over the quality or costs of care. The objection to all systematic review procedures is based largely on the argument that any disclosure of medical records, which would usually be necessary, would constitute a breach of confidentiality or *le secret professionel.* The ordinary filing of insurance payment claims, by either patient or provider, involves some invasion of privacy, which has been reluctantly accepted.

The fees doctors charge for medical service are rarely challenged. Yet a field survey made in 1975 by *Test Achats,* a consumer's organization magazine, caused a great sensation. In this study, a man visited the offices of 65 general practitioners throughout Belgium, stating that his wife "had a cough, and could the doctor help?" In 52 of the offices, the doctor prescribed an antibiotic, without examining the patient, in 10 another drug was prescribed, and in only 3 offices was no prescription given without seeing the patient. Moreover, 56 of the doctors charged for a "consultation"—which, under the health insurance rules, must include a medical examination—7 made no charge at all, and only 2 charged for "advice," which was correct (although the fee payable is much less than for a consultation). The medical association (Ordre des Médecins) responded that the prescriptions given were all reasonable and intended to be helpful and that, furthermore, the whole study was "deceitful." There was little defense, however, for the improper charges levied.

The problems of fee-for-service remuneration are illustrated also by the statement of an official of one of the national insurance associations that 48 percent of childbirths in Belgium are claimed to be "abnormal" in some way; such deliveries command higher insurance fees. Yet we know that the percentage of truly abnormal obstetrical cases is much lower than this. The same official pointed out that when the use of obstetrical forceps commanded higher fees, forceps deliveries were very common. When the fee schedule was changed to eliminate such financial differentials, the rate of use of forceps promptly declined.

The continuous pressure for higher medical fees and greater hospital per diem payments has led, of course, to steadily rising costs in the health insurance program of Belgium, as in most countries. The constantly increasing rates of diagnostic laboratory and X-ray procedures done per case also elevate costs. Because these costs have been rising faster than the mandatory insurance contributions that are politically acceptable, the INAMI, which must finance the whole program, has been in great debt.

Finally, we may take note of one interesting and successful strategy of the health insurance societies, designed to control costs for their members. This has been through the establishment of *polyclinics,* in which specialists explicitly agree to abide by the official fee schedule. The federations or local funds under all six of the national alliances have set up such polyclinics, built mainly in the 1920–1930 period, and about 265 of them were operating in cities throughout Belgium in 1980. Doctors in the polyclinics are usually paid small basic salaries, but most of their earnings come from the insurance fees; they return a share (e.g., 25 percent) of these fees to the polyclinic administration as a form of rental. The polyclinic pattern has brought specialist services into some smaller towns, where they might not otherwise be available. Also, by their competitive effect, they have induced many private specialists to abide by the official schedule.

Patterns of Health Care Delivery

In spite of the collectivized methods of most health care financing in Belgium, through mandatory insurance and general revenue support, the patterns of service delivery remain quite individualistic. Unlike the case in most other European countries, in Belgium specialists, as well as general medical practitioners, are predominantly engaged in private solo practice. The same applies to dentists and pharmacists. The hospitals, both general and special, are predominantly under nongovernmental sponsorship. In these respects, Belgium resembles the entrepreneurial United States more than other countries of Europe.

Ambulatory Health Care. The typical Belgian physician, whether a generalist or a specialist, is engaged in private individual practice. Nearly all specialists have staff appointments in hospitals, but only a small fraction do all their professional work there. Even those specialists who are full-time in hospitals earn their incomes predominantly from individual patient fees rather than from salaries. The general practitioner spends virtually all his time in private office service or on home calls, since he seldom has any hospital affiliation.

The typical general practitioner not only works independently, but is seldom aided even by an office nurse. He often has a medical secretary, to help with the paperwork and receiving patients; for male doctors, this role may be played by his wife. The office is frequently located in the doctor's home. He makes a high rate of calls to patient homes, which yield higher insurance fees than office consultations.

Private group practice is rare in Belgium, although in the 1980s it was beginning to grow. One of the reasons for group practice—coverage of a patient by colleagues when the doctor is away—is obviated through arrangements by the Order of Physicians for such coverage among individual practitioners in a community. To the extent that private grouping or even sharing of certain office facilities occurs, it applies only to general practitioners. Specialists work together to provide ambulatory care in hospital out-patient departments or in the polyclinics of health insurance funds, but not privately.

Occasionally general practitioners (GPs) attend normal childbirths in a hospital. Ordinarily a patient judged to need hospitalization must be referred by the GP to a specialist, who makes the final decision on hospital admission. On discharge of a patient from the hospital, a summary report is customarily sent to the patient's family doctor, whether or not he has referred the case. Few general practitioners or specialists indicate to patients in advance whether they observe the official fee schedule. Inflated fees, beyond the level for insurance reimbursement of 75 percent, are more often attributed to specialists.

Dental service and other forms of ambulatory care in Belgium are provided essentially along similar lines. Dentists tend to work alone, with only a chairside dental assistant. Although dentists are in very short supply, they must perform even simple prophylaxes, since there are no dental hygienists. Without dental clinics in the schools, they must handle children as well as adults. Since the demand for dental services is much greater than the supply, dentists nearly always charge fees higher than the official schedule.

Drugs are dispensed from private pharmacies, which must limit their business to selling drug products. With 5,000 pharmacies in Belgium (one for every 2,000 people in 1975) and regulation to control their locations, the country has been well covered, and in the cities competition is keen. This may explain the damaging findings of a consumer association survey of 80 pharmacies in 1972. The surveyor requested a drug requiring medical prescription, and yet 42 of the pharmacies gave the drug without a prescription. Another surveyor visited the same 80 pharmacies, complaining of back pain; all 80 gave him a drug and only 6 mentioned that a doctor should be consulted.

Health Centers. In Belgium the term *health center* has customarily been reserved for units that provide solely preventive services. Several developments, however, have led to discussion of health centers as facilities for both preventive and curative services. The enactment of a law providing for a network of mental health centers has brought about psychiatric facilities for ambulatory care of mental patients. Experience with the small number of group medical practices has been favorable, and there has been discussion about transforming the poly-

clinics of specialists (set up by the health insurance societies) into private group practices, pooling income and sharing equipment and personnel. Also under discussion are integrated health centers, which would have not only physicians but also a range of paramedical personnel to provide comprehensive health services to a defined population.

The National Program for Children (Oeuvre National de l'Enfance, or ONE), operates health centers with well-baby clinics in hundreds of municipalities, plus more comprehensive children's clinics, and also prenatal clinics. All of these clinics provide only preventive services—immunizations and physical examinations. The comprehensive clinics were developed because it was thought preferable to see fewer children but provide more thorough service, including attention to psychological problems. All ONE clinics are staffed by a physician and a nurse, and in the comprehensive clinics the physician is always a pediatrician. Doctors are paid a basic amount per session plus a fee for each child seen. If a child is sick, he is referred to a private doctor.

Another type of ambulatory care facility in Belgium is the school health center, which also provides only preventive services. School health centers are not located within schools but in separate buildings belonging to the municipality, the Ministry of Health, or the Catholic jurisdiction. The examinations include measurement of height and weight, testing of vision and hearing, urinalysis, and a general clinical examination. About 90 percent of the children are examined by general practitioners, who are paid a fee for each child seen.

In spite of this traditional preventive focus, consideration has been given to establishing health centers in Belgium for preventive and curative services. In addition to preventive examinations, health education, home nursing, and social services, they would offer general physician's care. One commentator called such a pattern of integrated services "group medicine new style" but thought it was still utopian. Yet the interest in preventively oriented and comprehensive care, manifested in Belgium as elsewhere, has led to consideration of alternatives to private, solo, fee-for-service medical practice.

Hospital Care. Belgium has an abundant supply of hospitals. In 1981, 521 facilities had more than 92,000 beds, a ratio of 9.35 beds per 1,000 population. Of these beds, 58 percent were in short-term general hospitals, which account for the vast majority of patient admissions.

Unlike the ownership pattern in other European countries, most of the hospital beds (about 63 percent) were in private facilities, predominantly sponsored by the Catholic Church. A small proportion of the private beds (about 5 percent) were owned and operated by the health insurance societies. Especially unusual is the fact that mental hospital beds, which in most countries are mainly in government facilities, are more heavily private (about 80 percent) than general hospital beds in Belgium.

Public hospital beds are nearly all in facilities operated by local municipalities through their Public Assistance Commissions (*Commissions d'Assistance Publique,* or CAP). The elected city council typically appoints members of the CAP, which serves as a hospital board and selects the administrator. Private hospitals are also headed by a board of directors, usually linked to the Catholic Church; this board appoints an administrator—usually nonmedical—to manage the facility. Sometimes a senior member of the religious nursing order is in charge. A medical director may also be appointed by the hospital board, or the hospital doctors may elect a chief-of-staff. Belgium has no proprietary hospitals, since profit-making from hospital operation is illegal, in spite of other entrepreneurial aspects of the health system.

Hospitals are established by local bodies, religious or public, but construction costs are subsidized by the central government. Public hospital subsidies usually amount to 75 percent of construction costs, and private hospital subsidies are 60 percent. The remaining 40 percent of costs, moreover, may be met through loans from the government, paid back over a 30-year period. Since health insurance payments to hospitals include amortization of capital debts, these loan settlements come from operating income.

Belgian hospitals are staffed with relative frugality. In 1980 they had about 1.0 to 1.5 staff members per bed (varying with hospital size), not counting physicians. Around 60 to 70 percent of hospital personnel are nurses of various grades. Great use is made of assistant nurses, whose training is entirely on the job. Higher-level nurses have been trained for 2 or 3 years in formal programs. Private hospitals are generally better staffed, they contain many private and semiprivate rooms, and they cater to more affluent patients. Public hospitals still have large open wards and serve patients of lower income. Their doctors typically abide by the official fee schedules.

As noted, the per diem costs of each hospital are calculated by the MOPHF, with the advice of a Hospital Council. Since 1965, a uniform accounting procedure has been followed by all hospitals in submitting their budgets to the ministry. Each hospital naturally defends its costs as reasonable. Since 1970 the government review has generally accepted 90 to 95 percent of the hospital annual cost estimates, so that many hospitals are said to have accumulated deficits.

The patterns by which doctors work in Belgian hospitals are especially complex. The independence and autonomy of the physician are greater in private than in public hospitals, but even in the latter the doctor is mainly a private practitioner rather than a salaried hospital employee (as in most of Europe). The free choice concept for patients carries over from ambulatory care to in-patient care. Thus, in the great majority of cases in both public and private hospitals, medical care is given by a specialist selected by the patient. The specialist is ordinarily paid by the insurance program on a fee basis. In a few public hospitals, however, the fees may be paid to the institution and used for engaging certain doctors on a full-time salary. Sometimes a small basic salary is paid, with supplementation from fees of patients using semiprivate or private rooms. These salaried arrangements, however, are exceptional, and even those doctors who work full-time in public hospitals (and to a much lesser extent in private ones) are usually paid entirely by fees for each patient they serve. This applies not only to surgeons or internists, but also to doctors in supportive specialties such as pathology, radiology, or anesthesiology. Although the latter types of specialist may have exclusive control of certain hospital departments, they ordinarily receive insurance fees for each specific act.

Physician services in hospitals and the hospitalization charges, as noted, do not require statutory copayments from the patient. The specialist attending a patient in a semiprivate room, however, may levy a charge about 50 percent more than the official insurance fee; in a private room the surcharge may be 100 percent. The general opinion in Belgium seems to be that higher fees summon better service from the doctor.

Another influence on the selection of a hospital by the specialist is the rate of sharing the medical fee required in his agreement with the hospital. The latter policy is a striking reflection of the "business" aspects of Belgian medicine. On appointment to the staff of a hospital, whether public or private, the specialist must agree to remit to the hospital a designated percentage of each fee earned. The percentage varies with the doctor's specialty and the degree of his dependence on hospital equipment and facilities for providing service. Thus, for pathologists and radiologists, the share of fees going to the hospital is as high as 60 percent. In fact, the costs of pathology or radiology services are not even included in the per diem payments that hospitals collect from the insurance program.

For clinical specialties, such as medicine, pediatrics, and surgery, the percentage of fees payable to the hospital is much lower, but it is always at least 2 percent. For surgeons the share may be from 10 to 30 percent of fees. If the hospital collects doctors' fees, it usually retains 6 percent for the administrative service. All of these percentages are subject to negotiation between the individual doctor and the hospital. For work in the out-patient department, the specialist often pays the hospital not a percentage of his insurance fee, but rather a more explicit "rental"; as in commercial enterprise, this is a monthly amount per square meter of OPD space. For assisting its hospitals in these negotiations, the Federation of Catholic Hospitals issues guidelines, and the medical syndicates advise their members corre-

spondingly. This bargaining process naturally varies with the reputation of the doctor and the prestige of the hospital. Even in mental hospitals, doctors seldom receive a flat salary.

Another reflection of the entrepreneurial features of Belgian medicine is the method by which young doctors-in-training (interns and residents), known usually as assistant physicians, are paid in teaching hospitals. Although they receive salaries, these come not from the hospitals, but from the specialists under whom they work. Thus, the specialist in a teaching hospital is like a small businessperson; he or she pays a percentage of insurance fees to the hospital as a sort of "rental" and a portion for assistant physician salaries for their service to the patients. In past years, Belgian surgeons often brought their own nursing assistants into the operating room, but surgical nurses are now considered a "socially acceptable" hospital expense.

Medical staff surveillance to control the quality of care is not well developed in Belgian hospitals. There are few tissue committees, infection committees, or other mechanisms to review medical performance. Each physician is regarded as autonomous and responsible for his or her own work. Probably the most important activity for quality assurance is the inspectional service of the national MOPHF. On inspection, the hospital must be found to meet specifications in architectural structure, organization (including the staffing), and the provision of patient care. The surveillance does not, however, include review of medical care quality as such.

Another important aspect of hospital service in Belgium is the program of regionalization and planning launched in 1973. To improve the distribution of hospital facilities, and the various specialized services within them, the country was mapped out into 48 hospital regions of about 200,000 population each. Each hospital has been assigned a functional role according to three levels, so that in every region the institutions are designated as belonging to the local or the regional level; for the highest level, only one university hospital is authorized in each of the nine provinces. These three levels of hospital are intended to have average capacities of about 200 beds, 500 beds, and 900 beds, respectively. Whenever a hospital wishes to modify or enlarge its structure or when a new hospital is planned, approval must be obtained from a National Commission on Hospital Planning under the MOPHF.

The hospital legislation of 1973 was also intended to limit the total supply of hospital beds, as well as to improve bed distribution. The planning assumed a total need for 6.2 hospital beds per 1,000 population; these would be composed of 4.7 general short-term beds, 1.0 bed for long-term care, and 0.5 bed for active rehabilitation service. To keep within these limits and to carry out the regionalization scheme, it was expected that some small, inefficient hospitals would be closed down.

With Belgium's high proportion of old people—around 15 percent were over 65 years of age in 1980—there has been a major need for institutional and other types of care for the aged and chronically ill. Aside from hospitals for chronic disease, many custodial institutions for the aged, without any special medical or nursing services, exist. Unlike hospitals, some of these are operated for profit, although most are sponsored by religious groups and others by the local governments (communes). If the latter two types are approved, about 50 percent of their operating costs may be subsidized by the national MOPHF; yet only about 40 percent of these nonprofit or communal institutions have met the standards for approval. If medical care is needed by residents of a custodial facility, a general practitioner is usually called in.

Home care of the aged and chronically ill has also been expanding in Belgium, but not under hospital sponsorship. The principal resource is the home-nursing program of the Yellow and White Cross. These services are financed in large part by payments from the health insurance funds. In addition, through their Public Assistance Commissions, many communes employ visiting nurses for the aged poor.

Summary and Comment

In summary, the Belgian health system epitomizes a highly permissive and individualistic pattern of health services, in which the financial support has been collectivized to make all essential care economically accessible to people. The medical profession is composed of thousands of small autonomous entrepreneurs, who exchange services for fees in both community practice and hospitals. Even voluntary teamwork in private group practices is relatively rare.

The major physical resources of the health system are also predominantly private, in contrast to resources in other welfare-oriented systems of European countries. A substantial majority of hospital beds are in nongovernment facilities, counting short-term general hospitals and even mental institutions. Pharmacies are numerous and entirely private. Medical schools number 11, of which 3 are private and 2 have combined public–private sponsorship; admission is usually open to every secondary school graduate, with high attrition rates after the first and second year.

As elsewhere in industrialized countries, health expenditures have been rising rapidly in Belgium. As a share of gross domestic product (GDP), overall health expenditures (public and private) rose from 3.4 percent in 1960 to 6.5 percent in 1983. This escalation is attributable mainly to government expenditures (including, of course, the national health insurance program), since the 1960 expenditure from public sources was 62 percent and the 1983 expenditure was 92 percent.

Because of these rising health costs, various cost-containment strategies have been introduced in the health insurance program. The schedule of official fees has been modified to discourage expensive and overused procedures. Standards for qualification of specialists have been upgraded and the equipment in a general practitioner's office has become subject to inspection. Maximum prices have been established for drugs. Hospital acquisition of expensive equipment requires prior approval. Copayments, long required for ambulatory care, were imposed in the 1980s for each day of hospital care.

Thus, in spite of its staunch devotion to permissive free market principles, the Belgian health system has been compelled by economic forces to introduce and strengthen regulatory strategies. The system dynamics reflect the continual conflict between the principles of individual freedom and the social demands for economy, along with equity, in a welfare-oriented society.

FRANCE

The highly individualistic and free-market ideology evident in the Belgian health system is seen, perhaps even more vividly, in the health system of France. The French Revolution (1789–1793), followed by a period of domination by Emperor Napoleon Bonaparte (1804–1815), left France with a unique combination of devotion to individual personal freedom and government under highly centralized authority. Both of these attributes are evident in the country's complex health system.

France had a population in 1986 of 55,400,000 people, of which 73 percent were urban. The GNP per capita that year was $10,720. Roman Catholicism is the dominant religion, but this has not decisively influenced health policies; both contraception and abortion are entirely legal and supported by public funds. The crude birth rate in 1987 was only 14 per 1,000 population.

Below the central government in Paris the principal local authorities are 95 *dèpartements,* which might be translated as provinces; each of these is headed by a prefect, who is not elected but appointed by the central government. In 1977 the 95 provinces were grouped into 21 regions—also under centrally appointed prefects—for greater administrative efficiency. At the most local level, are 37,000 communes and municipalities, in which mayors and other officials are elected by the residents. Sometimes several small communes combine for more efficient management.

Social Security for Health Care

Starting in the nineteenth century as a mechanism for spreading the costs of medical care, the French program of national health insurance (NHI) has grown to be the major eco-

nomic and political force in the overall health system. As in Germany and other European countries, industrial workers and miners formed hundreds of local sickness funds *(caisses de maladie),* which applied principles of insurance to compensate for wages lost and medical expenses due to sickness. Not until 1928—later than in other European countries—was membership of low-paid workers made compulsory, and then only in certain types of industry. Gradually coverage was broadened, with major amendments to the law in 1945, 1967, 1971, 1974, 1978, and 1984. Soon after the initial 1928 law, the sickness funds in each *dèpartement* were grouped together in federations, and in 1967 a further consolidation was brought about under the general social security reforms of President Charles de Gaulle.

Since 1967, the great majority of the French people have been covered through the National Health Insurance Fund for Salaried Workers (CNAMTS), which enrolls 76 percent of the population. Agricultural workers (9 percent of the population) come under another fund and self-employed people (7 percent) under a third fund. These funds are somewhat autonomous and regarded legalistically as nongovernment agencies, but they are completely regulated by the Ministry of Social Affairs and Employment. Another 6 percent of the population come under special welfare programs administered by the Ministry of Health. The remaining 2 percent of the French population were unprotected until the scheme of *Assurance Personnelle* in 1978 brought them into the program through certain voluntary arrangements. Local sickness insurance fund offices still administer the insurance benefits.

The insurance contributions payable and the benefit entitlements differ under each of these funds and between certain social groups within each fund. Typically the patient must pay the doctor or other provider for services rendered, and then seek reimbursement for 75 percent of an officially negotiated fee from the local branch of his or her sickness fund. (This indemnification process was a political compromise made in 1928 to win the cooperation of the medical profession.) Until 1971, physicians were free to charge patients any fee they wanted, though reimbursement was only 75 percent of the official fee. Since 1971, NHI regulations have required doctors to conform to the official fee schedule ("nomenclature"), but certain exceptions are still allowed; if the doctor is very prestigious or the patient's demands are "exceptional," larger fees may still be charged.

Substantial copayments by the patient are also required for hospitalization. The patient must pay 20 percent of per diem rates up to a 30-day maximum, although the hospitals bill the NHI sickness funds directly for the 80 percent. Copayments are also waived for old-age pensioners and indigent patients. Financial arrangements differ for public and private hospitals, as they do for the payment of physicians for hospital in-patient care (see following). To meet these copayment expenses, a majority of the French people subscribe to supplementary voluntary insurance through local *mutual aid societies* or commercial companies.

Persistent controversy has characterized the relationships between the various sickness funds and the medical profession. Rival medical federations have taken shape as part of the intense bargaining between the funds and the doctors. To heighten their bargaining position and help their members, many local sickness funds have set up health centers, where primary care may be obtained from salaried physicians; such centers are also operated by municipalities and labor unions—592 facilities in 1977. In spite of the contentions, specialists on the full-time medical staffs of public hospitals are paid by salary. In 1980, it was estimated that 30 percent of French physicians were on full-time salary, and perhaps half of the remaining 70 percent had part-time salaried positions.

In defense of fee-for-service remuneration, the French physician stresses its importance for development of a proper patient–doctor relationship. The direct payment of a fee, in contrast to third-party financing, is claimed to forge a bond between the patient and doctor. Confidentiality, also greatly stressed as an aspect of the relationship, has been used to thwart any attempt by the NHI authorities to examine medical records for the purpose of quality or cost controls.

Health System Organization and Resources

Aside from the Ministry of Social Affairs and Employment, which regulates the sickness funds and the NHI program, the Ministry of Health is the major public authority in the French health system. At the center it includes principal directorates for health (essentially prevention), hospitals, and pharmaceuticals. A number of national research programs (such as the Pasteur Institutes) and a school of public health also come under the direct control of the central MOH.

Below the top are regional health offices in each of the 21 regions, which provide consultation and guidance to the health directors of each of the 95 provinces (or *départements*). Each provincial health director is generally responsible to the local prefect, but he must abide by the general health policies of the MOH, as transmitted by the Regional Health Office.

MOH responsibilities in the *départements* include the control of acute communicable diseases, tuberculosis, venereal infections, and the promotion of maternal and child health. The latter field is especially well developed in France, where the concept of the "well-baby clinic" was first developed in the late nineteenth century. In 1980, there were 6,800 such clinics for infants and 2,000 for children 3 to 6 years of age. In addition the MOH program offers preventive services to all school children from the first year through secondary school. Health services for university students are a responsibility of the Ministry of Education.

One aspect of health protection—the promotion of health and safety in the workplaces—has had exceptional development in France. In 1946, after World War II, legislation was enacted to mandate occupational health and safety service in all factories and other workplaces; large firms had to engage full-time medical and nursing staffs, but even the smallest firms were required to have part-time services through cooperative multiplant arrangements. Workplaces with more than 50 employees were also required to have hygiene and safety committees of the workers to monitor the company's conformity to national regulations of the Ministry of Labor. This ministry along with the MOH is expected to enforce these requirements. While the diligence of enforcement, especially in smaller plants, has been reported to be inadequate, the health protection of French industrial workers (who are highly unionized) has been relatively strong.

The MOH program at the provincial level also includes health education and other activities for the control of cancer, heart disease, and health problems of the elderly. Environmental health controls are functions of the MOH, along with the Ministry of Environment, the Ministry of Housing, and the Ministry of Agriculture (regarding food hygiene). Certain environmental protection activities are delegated to the office of the mayor in the communes. Towns with populations of more than 20,000 are required to have a public health agency with full-time staff.

Surveillance of all hospitals in a *dèpartement,* with respect to MOH technical standards, is another responsibility of the provincial health director. Regarding any public hospital in the jurisdiction, the health director is routinely a member of its governing board. MOH responsibilities for hospitals have increased greatly since 1970, when a groundbreaking Hospital Law was enacted. This legislation called for sweeping reorganization of all French hospitals, public and private.

The Hospital Law of 1970 considered each of the country's 21 administrative regions as a *hospital service region,* in which the specific functions of each facility were defined. To facilitate planning of the bed supply and the institutional functions, each region was subdivided into health sectors—284 in all. For each region there would be a regional hospital center, usually connected with a medical school, and in each sector local hospitals for short-term cases and other institutions for medium-term convalescence and for long-term care. The plan for each region encompassed the public, as well as the private nonprofit and proprietary hospitals.

Public hospitals were required to provide a minimum range of services and to form cooperative agreements with other hospitals for sharing the use of specialized personnel and technology. Nationally stipulated norms for hospital bed-to-population ratios with different types of service were to be adjusted to the needs and conditions in each region. Representatives of public and private hospitals, health insurance funds, the health professions, local government, and other groups were included on regional commissions making decisions on hospital resources. As in many other countries, however, regional hospital planning in France has not been as successful as was hoped. Some superfluous hospital construction has been curbed, but great inequities between regions persist. Some cooperation has been developed between public and nonprofit voluntary hospitals, but not with proprietary *cliniques.* Costs have continued to escalate.

The sponsorship of French hospitals has long been diversified. Most of the beds are in public hospitals, operated by the government of the commune or the *dèpartement,* but almost one-third of the beds are in nongovernment facilities. In 1977, there were altogether about 644,000 hospital beds in France, which amounted to 12.2 beds per 1,000 people. (This high ratio was due to inclusion as hospitals of many units that, in other countries, would be counted as long-term convalescent or nursing homes.) The sponsorship of these beds was 69.0 percent by public authorities, 14.4 percent by voluntary nonprofit groups, and 16.6 percent by private proprietors.

Public hospitals are usually of much larger capacity than others and have more technologically advanced equipment and staff. The large open wards in these hospitals, inherited from a previous era, were gradually being replaced in the 1970s and 1980s by smaller multibed rooms, with various amenities for comfortable patient care. An MOH report for 1973 listed public hospitals as having an average of 240 beds, proprietary *cliniques* 38 beds, and voluntary nonprofit hospitals about 100 beds. Medical staffing differs among the three types. Public hospitals are staffed by full-time salaried medical and surgical specialists, and they have many young assistant physicians in training. They may also have some beds for private patients, whose insurance (with copayment) pays private medical fees to the hospital specialist. Proprietary hospitals may be used for private patients by almost any qualified local community physician, paid on a fee basis. Voluntary nonprofit hospitals are partly staffed by salaried physicians and partly open to other community doctors.

Hospital construction costs come from various sources in France. Public hospital capital comes mainly from local and central governments, and about one-third comes from the NHI program. Voluntary hospital construction must depend on philanthropic and church financing, with some government grants. Proprietary hospitals are built with loans and investments from banks and other private sources. Operating costs, however, are financed mainly by the NHI program in essentially the same way for all three types of hospital.

NHI funds have customarily paid all hospitals on the basis of a negotiated flat rate for each day of care, with extra fees payable for certain ancillary diagnostic and treatment services. This rate was negotiated separately for each hospital, but was heavily influenced by the rate paid to the public hospital in the same area or sector. This payment method inevitably gave hospitals, especially the private *cliniques,* the incentive to multiply various tests, as well as days of care; private hospitals also catered to the less complex surgical and obstetrical cases. After prolonged discussion, in 1984 the payment of public hospitals was finally changed to a prospective global budgetary amount, transmitted each month (with certain deviations allowed). Steps were also under way to negotiate prospective global budget contracts with nonprofit and proprietary hospitals. Such budgetary payment methods were expected to eliminate incentives for superfluous hospital services. Since hospitalization absorbs more than 50 percent of total NHI expenditures, this fiscal issue has obvious importance.

Physicians in France numbered about 120,000 in 1984, or a ratio of 220 per 100,000 population. This ratio had been rising rapidly, but was deliberately slowed down in the late 1970s as a strategy for cost control (similar to the constraint on new hospital construction). Enrollment in the country's 37 medical schools was simply frozen or even reduced. Outside of hospitals, the pattern of individual

private practice is still the norm in France, and only about 5 percent of doctors are working in small medical groups.

As a proportion of gross domestic product (GDP), overall expenditures in the French health system were 9.3 percent in 1983. This was an increase from 4.3 percent of GDP in 1960. Over this same period, the share of total expenditures coming from the public sector rose from 58 percent to 71 percent. Thus, in spite of the strong role played by the private medical and other health professions, nongovernment hospitals, private pharmacies, and other institutions, an increasing proportion of the economic support in France has come from public sources—principally the NHI program. Moreover, a portion of the 29 percent derived from private sources constituted organized financing through voluntary insurance.

Because of this steady increase of health expenditures in France, various strategies have been mobilized for cost containment. The adoption of global budgetary methods for paying hospitals has been noted, as well as the constraints on the expansion of hospital beds and the training of doctors. The development of health centers and dispensaries for prevention and primary care, with staffing by salaried physicians, has also been designed to reduce expenditures. The local sickness funds, paying medical claims, have intensified their reviews of *physician practice profiles* to identify abuses. The regulation of drug prices has also been made more rigorous, and the reimbursement of patients for prescribed drugs considered nonessential has been reduced. All in all, the pressures for cost-control seem to be driving the French health system from its staunchly individualistic to a more socially organized and regulated character.

JAPAN

Japan was the first country of Asia to become industrialized, following the crucial transformation from feudalism to capitalism in 1868, known generally as the Meiji Restoration. For centuries, this island nation off the east coast of China had been isolated from the West, but in the mid-1850s, ships from America and Europe came to invade Tokyo Bay. In 1868 an alliance of landowners, military officers, and mercantile capitalists overthrew the feudal system, by restoring to the throne the Emperor Meiji, who was committed to modernization. In the 1870s, the new rulers sent hundreds of young Japanese to Europe and America to learn scientific technology and modern methods of production. Regarding medicine, ideas were sought from Germany, and in 1870 the German model of medical education was established in Japan by an imperial edict.

Japanese technology and industry developed with remarkable rapidity. By 1875, government had matured to the point of establishing a Bureau of Health in the Ministry of Home Affairs. As had happened often in the West, in 1893 public health services at the local level were made the responsibility of local police authorities. As urbanization grew, Japan followed closely European public health patterns, with organization of maternal and child health services (prevention oriented), communicable disease control, environmental sanitation, health education, and so on.

After World War I in the West, one of the lessons of industrialization was earnestly adopted by Japan. The International Labour Organization was founded in 1919 with the slogan "Peace through social justice"—in other words, decent benefits for working people to prevent misery and preserve peace. Learning from Germany, Japan introduced its first Health Insurance Law in 1922 to protect workers (in plants of five or more employees) and their families. By 1930, Japan felt itself to be a significant imperial power and in 1931 invaded northern China (Manchuria), launching the Asiatic phase of World War II.

This devastating worldwide conflict involved almost all major countries of the world until August 1945. Along with Germany and Italy, Japan was defeated. The next month, the U.S. Army of Occupation came to Japan, and its activities played a major role in the organization or reorganization of health services in the country. While the private market for medical care, as we shall see, plays a major part in Japanese health services, a large government framework is crucial in the economic support and the day-to-day management of the system. As of 1984, Japan had a population of 120,000,000 and an economic level of $10,300 GNP per capita.

Organization of Programs

Overseeing and, in large measure, managing the entire health system of Japan is the Ministry of Health and Welfare. It has a broader scope of functions than are found in most equivalent government agencies elsewhere.

Ministry of Health and Welfare. Established first in 1938, the ministry was reorganized in the postwar period of occupation. Many of its functions concern welfare, pensions, and social activities, and in the health field its scope is extensive. To name only a selection of technical activities, it covers nutrition, tuberculosis prevention, communicable disease control, mental health, environmental sanitation, food chemistry, quarantine, and planning. A medical bureau encompasses hospital guidance, supplies and equipment, nursing, dental health, sanitation affairs, and other functions. A pharmaceutical bureau is concerned with drug manufacturing, biologics and antibiotics, narcotics, pharmaceutical affairs, and so on. A major agency within the ministry is responsible for health insurance and seamen's insurance. Numerous research and training centers are also under this ministry, including the National Institute of Public Health and the National Institute of Hospital Administration.

Much of the work of the Ministry of Health and Welfare (MOHW) is carried out through peripheral government agencies, which it supervises. Japan is divided into 46 prefectural governments and 26 larger municipal governments. Many of the preventive health services are provided through a nationwide network of health centers, staffed by physicians, pharmacists, public health nurses, midwives, health educators, sanitary inspectors, and others. The first health center law was enacted in 1937, and by 1980 these facilities had grown to 855. The costs of construction and operation of health centers are shared between the central and local governments. Since these facilities provide a full range of preventive services without charge, private physicians—paid under various health insurance programs, usually with substantial copayments required—are seldom called on for preventive work.

Japan has had a very low birth rate, only 12 per 1,000 population in 1983. Until recently, however, this rate was achieved largely by extensive use of abortions. In recent years the MOHW has devoted great efforts to disseminating information on contraceptive methods. With the considerable aging of the population, public health strategies have also come to include the early detection of cancer and efforts to influence behavior with respect to smoking, diet, and exercise.

Other Government Agencies. The major government agency with some health responsibility, aside from the MOHW, is the ministry of Education, Science, and Culture. Health promotion and health education in school children is conducted in association with sports and physical education.

Protection of workers against occupational disease and accidents is stipulated in the Labor Standards Act of 1947, administered by the Ministry of Labor. Several specific laws have been enacted on lead, silicosis, radiation, accidents, and other hazards. Each of the prefectural governments has labor standards inspection offices, from which occupational health doctors and others make periodic factory inspections.

The large social insurance program for medical care is, strictly speaking, an agency within the Ministry of Health and Welfare. It operates quite separately from the rest of the ministry, however. Because of its special importance in the Japanese health system, it is discussed later.

Voluntary Health Agencies. The most prominent nongovernment organizations concerned with health in Japan are the several professional associations. The Japan Medical Association plays a large part in shaping public policy on health, as well as in promoting the continuing education of doctors. The Japan Nurses Association, the Japan Hospital Association, the Federation of Health Insurance Societies, and many others speak on behalf of their members in implementing health insurance and other laws.

Since about 1960, multipurpose voluntary organizations have been promoted in both cities and rural areas throughout Japan. They attempt to contribute to recreation, community festivals, environmental sanitation, and specific health service programs. Each household acquires membership with a small contribution. Women's organizations, clubs for the aged, children's association, and parent–teacher associations are also focused on the problems of each demographic group.

Citizen participation has become increasingly active in environmental protection, maternal and child health, family planning, tuberculosis control, parasite control, and nutrition. Guidance is often sought from health center staffs. At the prefecture level, there may be a federation of all the local voluntary associations. The Ministry of Health and Welfare encourages these local bodies to strengthen their programs; since the Alma Ata Conference on Primary Health Care of 1978, voluntary action has been considered a central part of national health policy for "community health development."

The Private Market. The national resources for treatment of the sick in Japan belong mainly to a private market of medical care. There are thousands of physicians, dentists, and allied health personnel, hundreds of hospitals, clinics, pharmacies, and other facilities that provide services, even though nearly everyone is insured under various statutory programs.

The numbers and distribution of these health resources are reviewed next. For ambulatory care, private arrangements are predominant. For a large portion of hospital care, however, physicians serve as institutional employees, the same as technicians, nurses, and others. In either case, the health insurance organization pays for the service on an itemized fee basis.

Pharmaceutical products are also part of the private market. They are most often dispensed by a private physician, but may be sold and purchased in a pharmacy. The drugs are manufactured by large pharmaceutical companies in Japan or imported from companies abroad. If laboratory tests or x-rays are required by an ambulatory patient, they also must be obtained from a private facility for a charge.

Health Resources

Since the end of World War II, Japan has built up its supply of health manpower, facilities, and technology very rapidly. It is still in the process of expanding resources, since the demands for health service tend to be exceptionally high.

Health Manpower. In 1980, Japan had 156,215 active physicians; with a national population of about 117,000,000 at that time, this was a ratio of 133.5 doctors to 100,000 people (not as high as in most countries of Europe). The distribution of these physicians, as between self-employed and employed (salaried) status was as follows:

Status	Number	Percent
Self-employed in hospitals	3,468	2.2
Self-employed in private clinics	61,646	39.5
Employees in hospitals	50,075	32.1
Employees in private clinics	8,747	5.6
Employees in medical schools	28,523	18.3
Administrative and other	3,756	2.4
Total	156,215	100.0

Although the great majority of physicians in private clinics (medical offices) are self-employed, it is noteworthy that the great majority of hospital-based physicians, as well as medical school teachers and researchers, have the status of salaried employees.

Virtually all of Japan's physicians are trained at domestic medical schools. In 1981, there were 80 medical schools with an annual enrollment of 8,360 students. Of these schools, 51 were government (national or prefectural) and 29 were private. Enrollment in a private school is extremely expensive. Medical education in Japan is similar to that in Europe, requiring 6 years of university study, following 12 years of basic schooling.

The following were other health personnel in Japan in 1981:

Pharmacists	95,300
Dentists	52,370
Dental hygienists	23,000
Midwives	25,500
Graduate nurses	285,300
Assistant nurses	251,300
Laboratory technicians	29,160
Acupuncturists	48,700

The vast majority of the nurses (78 percent), both graduate and assistant, are employed in hospitals. About 20 percent of the nurses are employed in private medical clinics, many of which have accommodations for beds (as we shall see). The surprisingly large number of acupuncturists reflects the persistence in Japan of traditional medicine, despite its noncoverage by the health insurance program.

Health Facilities. Hospitals are abundant in Japan, and the availability of beds is enhanced by a unique principle in the Japanese health system. By definition, a hospital is an institution with 20 or more patient beds. Physicians who own and operate a private clinic are free to maintain a complement of up to 19 beds. In 1980, nearly 29,000 private clinics maintained beds, with an average of nearly 10 per clinic. Under the law, patients are supposed to remain in a private clinic bed for no more than 48 hours, unless there are compelling reasons for a longer stay. In practice, however, this rule is seldom observed, and there is little difference between the care provided in a private clinic and in a small general hospital.

As of 1980, the distribution of hospital and clinic facilities in Japan, by ownership, was as follows:

Ownership	General	Special	Total	Percent
National government	437	16	453	1.2
Prefectural government	259	44	303	0.8
Municipality	740	32	772	2.0
Other public unit	292	2	294	0.8
Social insurance	139	1	140	0.4
Private hospital	6136	957	7093	18.7
Private clinic	28,956	—	28,956	76.2
Total	36,959	1,052	38,011	100.0

It is evident that hospital and clinic facilities in Japan are overwhelmingly under private ownership and control. Even if we examine the hospitals separately from the private clinics, about 79 percent are privately owned. The average bed capacity of the public hospitals, however, is larger than that of the private hospitals; public facilities contain 40 percent of the beds and private facilities about 60 percent. With a total hospital bed supply in Japan of 1,319,406 beds, in 1980, 60 percent amounted to 791,644 private beds. The private clinics contain a total of 287,000 beds, which, added to the private hospital beds, makes a total of 1,078,644. As a share of both hospital and clinic beds (1,606,406 beds), private control applies to 67.1 percent of Japan's beds.

Japan's overall ratio of hospital and clinic beds to population in 1980 was 1,606,406 for 117,000,000 people. This means 13.7 beds per 1,000, which is about the same number as in many European countries and much more than in the United States. About three-fourths of these beds were in general facilities, and the rest in mental and other specialized institutions. Except for the latter, Japan has few institutions devoted exclusively to long-term care; therefore, general hospitals accommodate many elderly and chronically ill patients. As a result, their average length of patient stay is very long—38.3 days in 1980.

Regarding pharmaceuticals, Japan has an expanding productive capability. In earlier years, most drugs were imported or produced domestically on the basis of foreign formulas. As of 1980, 40 percent of Japanese drug production was based on compounds developed in Japan. These included antibiotics, cardiovascular preparations, biologicals, gastrointestinal agents, and many others. Many of these drugs are also exported, particularly to other countries of Asia, but numerous drugs must still be imported. The pharmaceutical industry has been very profitable, although its rate of earnings is highly dependent on the prices paid by the health insurance programs.

Traditionally, Japan has acquired new knowledge and technology by seeking ideas and guidance from abroad. Since the 1970s, however, the Ministry of Health and Social Welfare has established several research institutes in which Japanese scientists can explore their own ideas. Among these are a Research Institute for Infectious Disease, a National In-

stitute of Hygienic Sciences, a National Institute of Nutrition, and a National Cancer Center.

Japan has also been making rapid progress in the production of medical equipment. Just as Japanese engineering and industrial management have gained a large share of the world market for automobiles and television sets, they have been increasing their share of the world market for x-ray machines, microscopes, autoanalyzing laboratory equipment, computerized tomography (CT) scanners, and the like.

Economic Support

The total national health system of Japan required an expenditure of 6.7 percent of gross domestic product (GDP) in 1983. This was an increase from 3.0 percent of GDP in 1960—an increase similar to that found in virtually all industrialized countries. In 1983, some 75 percent of this expenditure was derived from public sources and 25 percent from private sources. Much the greater part of the public expenditure comes from Japan's multifaceted program of social insurance for health care, which requires some elaboration.

In 1922, with some collaboration from the International Labour Organization, Japan enacted its first Health Insurance law. Since it applied to all employees of industry, with five or more workers, plus their dependents, it may be called Employees Health Insurance (EHI). The administration of EHI could be handled in either of two ways. If the plant had 300 or more employees and more than half of them agreed, the employer could establish a health insurance society; about 1,800 such company-based societies were established. People in firms with fewer than 5 employees could enroll in a health insurance society voluntarily. Second, for employees in enterprises with between 5 and 300 workers, the EHI was administered directly by the government through a unit of the Ministry of Health and Welfare. In addition, the MOHW later administered a casual worker's health insurance program and a program for seamen, based on legislation enacted subsequently.

In 1938 a second major health insurance law, the National Health Insurance, was enacted to cover farmers and the self-employed. Coverage was initially voluntary, through enrollment in a private insurance society. Then in 1958 the law was substantially revised to require coverage for everyone not under the EHI program or in a voluntary society. Responsibility was assigned to local authorities, cities, towns, or villages. In the 1950s, still other occupational categories—civil servants, schoolteachers, agricultural workers—had been enrolled in MOHW-supervised mutual aid associations.

Outside the social insurance umbrella in Japan are public assistance medical care programs for needy persons and persons with selected disorders. The Daily Life Security Law of 1950 provides various cash benefits plus medical care to needy persons who pass a means test. There are also several special assistance programs for patients with tuberculosis, mental disorders, the elderly, and others.

Altogether it is estimated that as of 1960, some 99 percent of the Japanese population were accessible to medical care through one of the two major health insurance programs, one of the programs for special occupational groups, or public assistance.

Entitlement to services, however, is not uniform in the different programs. Under the EHI program, the employee pays a small first consultation fee. Dependents must pay 30 percent of the cost of all health service. The NHI program is less generous. Here both the primary workers and the dependents must pay 30 percent of the charges. In 1974, these laws were amended to put a ceiling (30,000 yen) on the total annual amount payable by dependents under the 30 percent copayment requirement. Among the 1,700 health insurance societies, competition is great to attract members; some offer rebates on copayments made by members or stipulate lower copayments under various circumstances. Large health insurance societies sometimes provide extra benefits for their members, such as the costs of transportation or holidays in rest homes.

The sources of insurance premiums also vary in the diverse programs. The original EHI law required 50–50 sharing of premium costs, but some health insurance societies were able to obtain more than 50 percent from the employer, especially in very large firms. The worker's premium is theoretically a stated percentage of wages—between 3 and 8 percent. Under NHI, the premium was calculated to cover 70 percent of medical care costs, since the beneficiaries have to pay 30 percent of all charges. Local governments are obliged to pay this 70 percent, but they receive a subsidy of 45 percent from the national government. The remaining 25 percent of premium costs is then collected from each household, in proportion to its resources; around 1980, this contribution amounted to 2.6 percent of taxable household income.

Every few years after World War II, further amendments were made to the several health insurance programs in Japan. Each change usually extended population coverage, health care benefits, or both. The varying percentages of cost-sharing, however, especially for persons employed by small firms, in agriculture, or in casual employment, still meant intergroup inequities. In the 1980s, furthermore, financial pressures led to imposition of small copayments on primary workers.

The several types of health insurance in Japan, of course, provide extensive purchasing power for physician's care, drugs, hospitalization, and other health services. Virtually all of these services are paid for by fee-for-service patterns, even for the services of full-time hospital-based specialists, who receive salaries. (The hospital collects the fees into a fund, from which the salaries are paid.) As a result, the delivery of medical care in Japan is subject to a great deal of abuse from overservicing.

It is evident that much of the funding of health insurance, as well as public assistance, in Japan is derived from the general revenues of national and local governments. One of the great ironies of our time is that the countries defeated in World War II should have great financial capability for such expenditures, while the winners of the war are more constrained by continuing military expenditures. Thus, we can examine the government health expenditures of Japan and also the Federal Republic of Germany in relation to the military expenditures of those countries in 1984. As winners of World War II, we may note the equivalent data for the United States and Great Britain.

Table 6.3. Government Expenditures for Military Purposes, for Health, and Their Relationship, 1984

Country	Health (H) (million $)	Military (M) (million $)	Ratio H:M
Japan	56,874	12,364	4.6:1
West Germany	54,482	21,956	2.5:1
Great Britain	26,525	26,525	1.0:1
United States	159,500	237,052	0.7:1

Source: R. L. Sivard, *World Military and Social Expenditures 1987–88.* Washington, D.C.: World Priorities, 1987.

The figures are shown in Table 6.3. It appears that Japan's public expenditures for health were 4.6 times greater than its military expenditures, and West Germany's were 2.5 times greater. Great Britain, on the other hand, spent the same amount for health as for military purposes and the United States government spent much less.

Management

After the devastation of World War II, the resumption of normal community life in Japan was difficult for at least a decade. The health centers, which were built up relatively quickly throughout the country, served somewhat as nuclei for local health planning. From these units, plans were made for communicable disease control, maternal and child health services, health education, and so on. In 1960, the Ministry of Health and Welfare launched a program of *integrated health planning* at the local authority level. In the 1970s, the functions and scope of the health centers were broadened, and each came to oversee the planning activities of three or four local authorities. These included health screening examinations, vaccinations, basic environmental surveillance, and the administrative functions necessary for national health insurance at the local level. In 1978, the MOHW provided national grants to all local governments, to strengthen their "national health development" efforts.

The local focus in health planning stresses many advisory committees, with representatives of professional groups, voluntary organizations, schools, and the local health center. Although the scope of these local planning efforts is broad, it is still confined to the traditional objectives of public health. It does not include concern for general health personnel or facilities. Thus, the planning of hospitals, which plays a large role in other countries, is lacking in Japan. To establish a new private hospital requires the approval of the prefectural governor, but this depends simply on meeting construction and staffing standards, not on the local need for beds. The Japanese assumption appears to be that any excessive hospital construction will be controlled by competition.

Regulation of medical clinics or hospitals is relatively weak in Japan, because of the great strength of the medical profession. The Japan Medical Association has great political influence and has been successful in averting any significant inspections and surveillance by the Ministry of Health and Welfare or other public agencies. Prefectural medical associations are expected to monitor their own members.

Health legislation, especially since the end of World War II, has played a significant part in spelling out health policy, especially in the sphere of environmental sanitation. Counting only national laws enacted since 1947, statutes have been passed in the following aspects of the health system: administration—2; preventive medicine—5; environmental sanitation—24; health statitics—2; other aspects of public health—7; medical care—14; pharmaceutical affairs—1; social welfare—6; and social insurance—3. Such legislation not only establishes principles and policies for all to see, but also provides a basis for popular education on new health policies.

Delivery of Health Services

The relatively complex combination of mechanisms for health insurance that has evolved in Japan results in a robust flow of money to pay for medical care. This service is furnished mainly by private providers, but procedures differ for ambulatory care and hospitalization.

Ambulatory Care. Of the 149,000 doctors in clinical practice (i.e., not in administration, teaching, research, or the like) in Japan as of 1980, 47 percent were engaged in ambulatory care and 53 percent in full-time hospital work. This meant 70,400 community-based doctors, of whom 88 percent were self-employed and 12 percent were professional employees. The great majority of physicians in ambulatory practice are general or family practitioners, but a minority are specialists in internal medicine, pediatrics, and occasionally other fields (usually former hospital specialists who have left the hospital for outside work). Moreover, most of the generalists have had supplementary hospital training in some special field.

It is conventional in Japan to describe the setting of private community practice as a *clinic.* The great majority of private clinics are staffed by a single physician, and 10 percent or fewer have engaged a second or third physician on salary. A nurse or a clerk or both may also help in the clinic.

About 37 percent of the private clinics include accommodations for beds. As noted, the law permits up to 19 beds (20 beds or more being a hospital) and the average complement is around 10 beds. With or without beds, however, the physician's service to ambulatory patients is paid for directly by the insurance program (not by the patient). Payment is made on a fee-for-service basis, according to a schedule of fees issued by the Ministry of Health and Welfare. Since 1948, the fees submitted by each clinic are reviewed by a "middleman," known as the Social Insurance Medical Fee Payment Fund—actually by one of its prefectural branches. A reviewing committee of the prefectural fund contains representatives of the medical care providers, the insurance carriers, and the consumers. After review, the bill is transmitted to the appropriate insurance carrier and paid. In fact, only a small fraction of 1 percent of the claims is ever challenged.

It is customary in Japan for the physician to keep on hand a supply of his frequently used drugs and to dispense them directly to the patient. Accordingly, it is often claimed that physicians customarily dispense only a small supply of drugs, so that the patient must return soon to be reexamined to receive an additional supply, as well as to yield a further fee. The rate of utilization of ambulatory services has been rising steadily in Japan. In spite of the medical school output of more doctors, the average number of patients seen per day in a clinic has risen from 34.2 in 1955 to 62.6 in 1975. The

belief is widespread in Japan that physicians are abusing the health insurance program to enhance their earnings. The rate of appendectomies, for example, is extremely high—three times the rate performed in England; more than 60 percent of appendices removed were found not to be inflamed. Japanese physician incomes are regarded as exceptionally high.

Hospital Care. The abundant supply of hospital beds in Japan has been noted, as well as the exceptionally long average patient stay. The staffing of these hospital beds is not very high. In general hospitals, which are better staffed than the others, the overall staffing comes to only 82.2 personnel per 100 beds. This includes the physicians (11.5), nurses (38.9), laboratory technicians (8.9), and 23.1 others per 100 beds.

Virtually all hospital physicians, in both public and private hospitals, are appointed on full-time salaries. Hospitalization is also paid on a fee-for-service basis, through the health insurance, but the professional fees are simply paid to the hospital and not to the doctor. The hospital pays the doctor's salary from its general earnings.

As Japan's health achievements have mounted, with dramatic reductions in the infant mortality and extension of the life expectancy at birth to 77 years (in 1984), the proportion of the population living beyond 65 years has increased. By 1980, this was more than 10 percent, so that the health problems of the elderly have become a prominent issue. Even with National Health Insurance, retired elderly people had to pay 30 percent of the charges. In 1973, the law was amended to provide for national government assumption of all medical and hospital costs for persons 70 years old and over. Naturally, utilization rates rose, so that in 1982, the law was again amended to require small copayments by the elderly.

Financial support, of course, has been only part of the problem. Because of the greater prevalence of chronic illness among elderly patients, they occupy beds in hospitals and also in medical clinics for long periods of time. Of all institutionalized patients over age 65, these medical facilities service 73 percent of them.

Japan's supply of nursing homes and even custodial places for the aged is relatively small. Likewise, welfare centers in prefectures and cities are just beginning to provide home care services for the elderly living in their own homes.

In spite of its complexities, the national health system of Japan is based on principles that are not difficult to describe. In a rapidly developing industrialized economy, Japan has produced a large stock of health manpower, facilities, pharmaceuticals, and advanced technology. To promote environmental and personal prevention, it has developed a large national network of well-staffed health centers. To ensure that medical and hospital services are economically accessible, it has gradually built up a many-faceted program of social insurance. Yet to control utilization and limit expenditures, numerous copayments are required. Despite all the collectivized financing, the delivery of medical services is largely by private providers—physicians, dentists, pharmacists, hospitals. In the interests of efficiency, hospitals are staffed by full-time salaried personnel, including physicians. Yet the payment for both ambulatory and hospital care is entirely on a fee-for-service basis. Government regulation is quite limited, and public medical services are confined to prevention. The Japan Medical Association is politically very influential at the national level, as well as in the prefectures, cities, and towns. For reasons that are doubtless related to the total socioeconomic setting of the country, the people's personal life-styles and culture, as well as the health system, the population of Japan has achieved a remarkably good record of health and long life.

CANADA

North America was colonized in the seventeenth century by the British, the French, and the Spanish. After the American Revolution of 1776 through 1783, people loyal to the British crown settled in the northern part of the continent. British settlers formed several provinces in the east (New Brunswick, Nova Scotia, and Prince Edward Island), and the large land mass west of the St. Lawrence River was occupied by both British Protestants and French Catholics. Clashes between these two ethnic groups were resolved in 1791 by dividing this territory into Upper Canada (now Ontario) and Lower Canada (now Quebec). In the nineteenth century, *territories* or provinces took shape in the west, but not until 1867 did the British Parliament enact the British North American Act, establishing a federation, known generally as the Dominion of Canada.

In the early twentieth century, several territories became self-governing provinces, and after World War II, in 1949, the separate British colony of Newfoundland joined the Dominion as its tenth province. The British North America Act granted autonomy to the provinces, each of which was symbolically governed by a lieutenant-governor responsible directly to the British monarch. In this act, health was made a provincial responsibility, and a federal Department of National Health and Welfare was not established until 1944. The British North America Act served as a sort of constitution for more than a century, although World Wars I and II (in which Canada participated fully on the side of the Allies) resulted in a much greater sense of nationhood. In 1964 a new national flag was adopted, symbolizing separation from the British, and in 1984 a completely self-determined Canadian Constitution was proclaimed by Parliament; it included a bill of rights, which was important for health services.

General Features of the Health System

The development and current operations of the entire health system of Canada reflects strikingly the provisions of the Canadian Constitution. Policies on the control of communicable diseases, licensure of professional personnel, the establishment and operation of hospitals, the management of medical care of the poor, and virtually every aspect of the system are provincial responsibilities. Still, when the Department of National Health and Welfare was set up, a certain uniformity of health programs was achieved after 1948 through a series of national health grants to the provinces for specified purposes. In 1968, the most important of these purposes were hospital construction, general public health, mental health, tuberculosis control, and cancer control.

These earmarked grants are dwarfed by the subsequent provincial and federal expenditures for general hospitalization and physician's care, identified generally as *national health insurance*. The evolution and administrative mechanisms of this program are unique and warrant special analysis later.

The resources of Canada's health system are abundant, as would be expected in an affluent country with a per capita GNP of $13,250 in 1984. The national population of 25,200,000 was served in 1984 by more than 49,000 physicians, or 194 per 100,000. Slightly more than half of these are specialists and the balance are generalists; the great majority are engaged in private medical practice. Nearly all have been trained in one of Canada's 16 medical schools, all but two of which are sponsored by provincial governments; even the two private schools are heavily subsidized by the government, and student tuitions are low. The supply of nurses in Canada is especially high, with more than 830 per 100,000 population (in 1981), the great majority of whom are fully qualified.

Considering all types of hospitals, Canada had 186,470 hospital beds as of 1986, amounting to 7.4 beds per 1,000 population. The majority of these beds are in short-term general hospitals, but 44 percent are in mental or long-term care hospitals. Of the total beds, 35 percent are in government institutions—predominantly at the municipal and provincial levels. Slightly over 65 percent are under nongovernment sponsorship; of these about 20 percent are religious and 80 percent are nonsectarian. Only a handful of beds are under proprietary control, mainly for long-term care. There are some 200 community health centers for organized ambulatory care, to be discussed later.

Aside from the Department of National Health and Welfare, and equivalent bodies in each of the provinces, there are other federal agencies with health functions. The Department of Veterans Affairs operates a number of hospitals for military veterans with serious war-connected disabilities, requiring extended rehabilitation services. The federal Depart-

ment of Manpower supports vocational rehabilitation programs, through grants to the provinces—principally to the welfare departments. Other specialized health functions are performed by the Department of Agriculture, the Department of Justice, and the Department of National Defense. Under the Department of National Health and Welfare is a program of health services for people in the far northern territories. This department also runs the Canada Assistance Plan, which has provided grants to the provinces since 1966 for support of the indigent. This includes payment for medical care not provided under the provincial health insurance programs, and this is usually administered by provincial departments of welfare.

At the provincial level, there is usually a Workmen's Compensation Board (under the Department of Labor); in addition to replacing wages for work-connected disabilities, it finances medical care. In Ontario and a few other provinces, these boards operate highly developed rehabilitation programs directly. Some provinces have had commissions for the control of certain diseases such as cancer or tuberculosis. Each province has licensing bodies for medicine, nursing, and the other major health professions.

Voluntary agencies concerned with health problems are also numerous in Canada. The Canadian Red Cross has branches in every province, to provide emergency services, collect and distribute blood, and operate outpost nursing stations in the far north. There are voluntary associations for cancer, heart disease, diabetes, and many other serious disorders. The Victorian Order of Nurses provides visiting nurse services to the home-bound chronically ill, usually with financial support from the provincial governments. Correspondingly, ambulance transportation is provided by the nongovernmental St. John's Ambulance Service. In a few provinces, the Department of Health even operates an Airplane Ambulance Service to transport patients to hospitals from very isolated locations.

National Health Insurance

Statutory health insurance had been discussed in Canada at the Federal level since 1919, but no action was taken. Then, the election to power of a semisocialist government in one prairie province in 1944 led to action, which soon changed the entire national health scene.

Evolution of Hospitalization Insurance. The enactment of the Saskatchewan Hospital Services Plan (SHSP) in 1946 (to take effect in 1947) had its roots in events occurring over the preceding 30 years. Tax-supported *municipal doctor plans* had originated in this sparsely settled prairie region in 1916 as a mechanism for attracting and holding physicians, on modest salaries, in low-income rural areas. The concept of using a cooperative or collective economic process for solving a key health problem in this context made sense, and the idea spread. In the 1920s, funds for hospital construction were raised by the combined efforts of adjacent rural municipalities, which formed *union hospital districts.* In the larger economic environment, cooperatives of wheat farmers for marketing their produce, purchasing fertilizer, and other purposes were found to be similarly effective.

After the years of economic depression that drove down the world price of wheat in the 1930s, compounded by serious drought in the early 1940s, election to power of the Cooperative Commonwealth Federation (CCF) party came as no surprise in Saskatchewan. In its campaign for election in 1944, a key objective was to introduce a program of "socialized health services." With an overwhelming electoral victory, the new government lost no time in acting on its promise.

As the trailblazer in this field, to implement the SHSP Saskatchewan had to solve many problems not faced before in North America. More hospitals had to be built to provide beds for people wherever they lived. Economy dictated a planned scheme of regionalization, with common conditions being treated in a nearby facility while more complex cases were referred to a district hospital, and the most difficult cases were sent to large base hospitals in one of the province's two main cities. Many more nurses, technicians, and other personnel had to be trained to staff the beds. After hospital insurance took effect in 1947, rates of hospital admission rose rapidly. It was soon realized that the conventional system of per

diem remuneration gave both hospitals and doctors incentives to maximize hospital occupancy at all times, and even to set up additional beds in the corridors whenever feasible.

After a few years, it was recognized that more judicious planning was needed. On the basis of initial experience, the provincial health leadership concluded that 7.5 general hospital beds for 1,000 people would be adequate to meet all needs; these beds were to be distributed among local, intermediate, and base hospitals. To staff the bed complement in each facility and meet all the other expenses for serving patients at an estimated 90 percent average occupancy, a certain annual budget would be reasonable. The hospital could be paid one-twelfth of this amount each month, regardless of the actual patient load. Thus, there was no incentive to overcrowd. If the budgeted allotment was not fully spent, the hospital could keep the surplus at the end of the year; if there was a deficit because of an epidemic or some other justifiable cause for high utilization, the provincial SHSP would make it up.

This whole process required careful review of all hospital operating budgets and the stipulation of reasonable standards for the nurses and other staff members, laboratory supplies, food, and all items necessary for hospitals of given sizes. Nationally recommended standards (such as specified nursing hours per patient per day) were applied. Salary scales were left up to each hospital to decide; but, with unionization of hospital employees developing rapidly, provincewide collective bargaining for different categories of employees soon followed. Budgets had to be resubmitted and reevaluated each year, as costs of living, wages, and prices of commodities—as well as proper standards for patient care—changed.

This SHSP method of payment for hospital services came to be known in Canada as *prospective global budgeting.* The process is more complex than described here, and its application requires uniform hospital accounting procedures and a competent staff of administrative consultants. These consultants are not only in the field of general hospital administration and accounting, but also in nursing, laboratory and x-ray technology, dietetics, and the other key aspects of hospital operations.

This staff carefully reviews hospital budgets; more important, it consults with hospitals on recommended policies. Their advice might be to engage additional laboratory technicians, for example, or to hire fewer kitchen helpers, and the advice was backed up by assurance that necessary costs would be met by the hospital insurance program.

An important side benefit of the SHSP was a steady flow of information on every patient hospitalized; when the patient was discharged, the hospital was required to send a one-page summary report to the SHSP. These reports included basic information (name, address, diagnosis, attending doctor, surgical operations if any, condition on discharge, and so on) on all patients, even the occasional nonresident served in a Saskatchewan hospital or the occasional resident hospitalized outside the province (for which the external hospital would be paid on an indemnity basis). From these data, analyses could be made to indicate whether the residents of a particular area (rural municipality, town, or city) were being hospitalized at a rate substantially higher or lower than the provincial average. Such information permitted rational decision-making on whether additional hospital construction or enlargement was justified in an area or, indeed, whether the number of beds was excessive and should be reduced (or budgeted for a lower occupancy level).

Initially there were no limits on admissions or the duration of hospital stay, except the doctor's decision, but it was soon found prudent to introduce certain kinds of surveillance. Short stays (1 to 2 days), which might suggest admission only for some diagnostic tests that could properly be done outside the hospital, were scrutinized, and if they were found excessive for a particular doctor or area, an explanation was required. Likewise, long stays (over 30 days) required periodic medical reports. If the hospital use could not be justified, further abuse was deterred first with a warning and then, if necessary, with a reduced monthly payment to the hospital. On the other hand, any extra funds raised by the hospital through voluntary donations, extra charges for use of private rooms, and so on could be kept without reduction of the global budget allotments.

Over the years, details of these administrative procedures changed, but basically the strategies worked out in Saskatchewan were adopted by British Columbia when its hospital insurance plan was enacted in 1949. The British Columbia plan imposed a $1 per day copayment charge on the patient (designed to discourage overuse) and modified the reporting procedures in certain ways. When the solvency and qualitative improvements of hospitals in Saskatchewan and British Columbia, as well as the great general popularity of the programs, became evident throughout Canada, interest was naturally kindled at the national level. By 1956, the success of the idea and the political dynamics of the time led the national Parliament, under Liberal Party control, to enact the national Hospital and Diagnostic Services Act. Its provision for about 50 percent support of any provincial program meeting certain standards was consistent with the British North America Act. Out-patient diagnostic services were included in the act to pay for work that could avert unnecessary hospital admission. By 1957, conditions for the act to become operative had been met (participation of at least half the provinces with half of the national population), and by 1961 the program had been implemented in all 10 provinces. The general administrative and accounting strategies designed in Saskatchewan were adopted throughout Canada.

Other provinces learned from Saskatchewan's experience. This included planning for a general hospital bed supply lower than 7.5 per 1,000 (the Saskatchewan ratio), since it was found that, under conditions of universal insurance coverage, whatever beds were provided tended to be used. The bed supply ultimately determined the staffing needed (75 percent of hospital operating costs), the supplies consumed, and virtually all the costs. All the provinces found that budget reviews permitted rational planning of hospital functions according to some type of regionalized scheme. Additional training programs for nurses and other personnel were needed. With heavy hospital costs being met through a social mechanism, people had more money to enable them to see doctors, so physicians' incomes rose. With the federal sharing of costs out of general revenues, provincial government expenditures declined, whether these funds were raised through earmarked insurance premiums, a sales tax, general revenues, or a combination of methods. Each year, the overall hospital costs rose, mostly as a result of elevated standards (more staffing, shorter work weeks, better supplies, and so on). Governments and political parties were not greatly concerned, however, because easy access to hospital care was extremely popular with the voters.

Within the broad national criteria were many variations among the provinces in hospital insurance programs. Administrative responsibility was assigned to the Department of Health in some provinces and to special commissions in others, though always under the general control of government through the Minister of Health. The provincial funds were raised in different ways. Periodic payment for "readiness to serve" on a global budgeting basis was applied everywhere, but the budget review criteria differed in details. The optimal bed supply also differed, as did salaries. In a few provinces, the government bargained directly with professional associations or unions on salary scales. Small extra charges were permitted in some provinces, as long as they did not constitute a barrier to hospital use.

Thus, the Canadian strategy achieved a nationwide program of hospital insurance within a few years, without invading provincial prerogatives. By confining benefits to hospitalization, Canada took a first step toward comprehensive health insurance that was politically acceptable, offered important leverage for health service planning, was agreeable to both hospitals and doctors, and yet met a deeply felt need in the general population. At the same time, the problems in this categorical hospital-linked approach generated further actions to broaden the health benefits and correct inequities.

Insurance for Physician's Care. Only a few years after Saskatchewan's hospital cost burden was cut in half by the federal matching legislation, the provincial government, still under control of the CCF (renamed the New Democratic Party), began to think of extending the

scope of socialized health services. Insurance for doctor's care was the obvious next step. The rate of hospital use was high compared with that in other affluent nations, and rigorous controls were not politically feasible. If complete physician's care could be economically supported, hospital abuse might be eliminated at the same time early and more prevention-oriented medical attention was promoted.

As is customary in democratic societies, a study commission was appointed; it recommended further social insurance, and in 1962 the Saskatchewan Medical Care Insurance Act was passed. Despite its provision of free choice of doctor and fee-for-service remuneration, physicians objected to direct payment by the government with a fixed schedule of fees, even though this would be negotiated. As a result, the Saskatchewan Medical Association called the first strike by doctors, withholding all services except for emergency care, in North American history. The strike settlement, after 23 days in July 1962, retained the basic principles of universal coverage and government control, but permitted use of private fiscal intermediaries and allowed doctors to charge patients beyond the officially scheduled fees if they chose a doctor who made such extra charges. Initially, supplemental charges were made by doctors serving 12 percent of the patients, but market competition brought this down to barely 2 percent of the patients by 1974.

Once again all of Canada looked to Saskatchewan's experience—doctors, political leaders, and other citizens. The sudden spurt of average Saskatchewan medical incomes, from the lowest of the 10 provinces to the highest within 2 years, did not escape notice. Despite the bruised relationships left by the strike, the general popularity of the program was clear to both politicians and voters everywhere. A federal Royal Commission on Health Services that was deliberating at the time called for a national medical care insurance program as its principal recommendation. And this time, instead of a 10-year gap between provincial pioneering and national legislation, only 4 years lapsed. In 1966, the national Medical Care Act was passed along essentially the same lines as the Hospital Act of 1956, but with a formula for federal–provincial financing more generous to the poorer provinces. It took a few years for all provinces to take up the "medicare" offer, but by 1971 it had become a nationwide program.

Variations in the provincial medicare administrative mechanisms were somewhat greater than under the hospital insurance program. Commissions separate from the Health Department were more frequently assigned administrative responsibility, and various forms of fiscal intermediaries were used more often. Despite the trauma of the Saskatchewan battle over the doctors' right to levy extra charges on the patient, some provinces were tougher in restricting this practice than Saskatchewan. They called this practice "opting out" and required that a doctor wishing to do so for any of his patients must do so for all of them. As a result, only a small percentage of doctors in these provinces engaged in extra-billing. None of the provinces required copayments from the patient or imposed deductibles. British Columbia was sufficiently confident of the program's popularity that under its law enrollment was theoretically voluntary; the "buy" for the consumer was so good (50 percent federal subsidy, and the province covering the indigent) that the minimum federal requirement of 95 percent coverage was readily met.

Utilization and costs under a nationwide medical insurance program naturally rose, and greater controls by the provincial authorities followed. In some provinces, only one complete medical examination per year would be paid for. Practice profiles, by specialty and diagnosis, were statistically compiled, and deviant physicians were asked for an explanation. Services deemed clearly excessive or unjustified were remunerated at a 50 percent rate or not at all. With insurance of out-of-hospital ambulatory services, however, hospital admission rates did not decline, but rose—evidently because of the increase in available hospital beds and the greater number of cases coming to medical attention, some requiring hospitalization. Now that Saskatchewan was no longer the only province to have insurance, physicians' incomes soared throughout Canada, and

Saskatchewan's rank among the 10 provinces again took a place near the bottom. Doctors and consumers almost everywhere found the program highly agreeable.

Just as hospital insurance generated construction of more hospital beds, the very anticipation of medicare led to a rapid increase in the supply of doctors. New medical schools were started, and the established schools increased their enrollments. Immigration of doctors also increased, not only because immigration restrictions were lowered (medicine was declared a needed occupation), but because the word spread that Canada was a country where medical earnings were high. By 1975, the doctor–population ratio was approaching 167 per 100,000. This ratio was greater than the idealistic recommendation of the Royal Commission on Health Services in 1964. Furthermore, the average number of hours of medical work per week or per year was declining; if a doctor could earn enough to satisfy himself and his family in 40 hours per week, why work 50?

In response to the growing consensus that the supply of physicians was adequate, steps were taken to limit immigration of foreign medical graduates. This not only dealt with the problem that foreign medical graduates were likely to be less well trained than graduates of a Canadian medical school, but helped correct two inequities: qualified Canadian applicants for medical school, now rejected, could be accepted, and the "brain drain" from other nations needing doctors more than Canada would be reduced. It was decided that foreign medical graduates could immigrate to Canada only if they were willing to settle for some years in an area with a shortage of doctors (usually in a northern rural region).

Extended Benefits and Cost Controls. The steadily climbing costs of the two federal–provincial health insurance programs led to further national legislation in 1977. In that year the Federal–Provincial Fiscal Arrangements and Established Programs Financing Act was passed. This reduced the federal sharing of hospital and medical care expenditures from 50 to 25 percent, so that (with 75 percent of the fiscal responsibility) the provinces would have stronger incentives to control costs. At the same time, the law gave new block grants to the provinces to enable them to provide long-term care, as well as other types of health service. It also modified federal taxation policies, giving greater taxing powers to the provinces.

The provinces have devoted the federal block-grant funds to diverse special services. Some provide dental care for children, others support the cost of prescribed drugs for the elderly, others furnish prosthetic appliances, including hearing aids. To some extent additional types of medical care are provided in the more prosperous provinces entirely at provincial expense.

The reduced federal support for basic hospital and medical benefits in the 1977 act put pressures on the provinces to achieve economies in these services. The supply (ratio to population) of hospital beds was kept from rising, and hospital budgets were constrained even below the general rate of inflation. Physician fee schedules were held almost constant. Physicians responded by increasing their volume of services to patients (e.g. multiplying return visits) and adding on special "registration" or administrative fees payable by the patient. Then in the early 1980s, physicians in several provinces opted out of the health insurance program by charging fees higher than those in the official fee schedule; the patient could be reimbursed by the provincial government only for the approved amount.

This "extra billing" by physicians caused great resentment and led to another major legislative action. The Canada Health Act of 1984 replaced and consolidated the three previous national health insurance laws. To discourage or eliminate extra billing, it provided that federal allotments to the provinces would be reduced by the estimated amounts that physicians collected for extra billings or *user charges*. Very soon, all provinces had passed legislation prohibiting such noninsured payments by patients. (Under the Canadian Constitution, of course, the federal government could not make such a prohibition.)

The 1984 act also authorized allotments to the provinces of federal funds for diverse types of long-term care, including services in nursing homes, adult residential facilities (homes for the aged), and organized home care. The use of these funds also varies greatly among the provinces. Copayment requirements, daily payment amounts, durations-of-stay that are covered, and so on differ. Some provinces (such as Ontario) have special supplemental programs for care in residential facilities for the aged, financed solely by provincial funds. Quality standards for long-term care are highly variable. Unlike Canada's southern neighbor, the majority of nursing homes are under voluntary nonprofit or local governmental auspices; only a minority are proprietary.

The conditions stipulated in the two original laws for provincial receipt of federal allotments were also tightened in 1984: (a) the program must be administered by a public authority accountable to the provincial government; (b) the program must cover all necessary hospital and medical care and surgical–dental services rendered in hospitals; (c) 100 percent of the provincial residents (formerly 95 percent were adequate) must be entitled to insured services; and (d) reasonable access to insured services must not be impeded directly or indirectly by charges or other mechanisms.

As Canadian NHI has evolved, the predominant mechanism of financial support has changed gradually from social insurance to general revenues. Although it is described as "national health insurance," the federal input comes entirely from general revenues. Ontario, the most industrialized province, still collects premiums from employer–employee contributions, but additional funds come from provincial revenues. Most other provinces depend entirely on provincial general revenues, sales taxes, or other general taxes.

The various administrative strategies have been relatively successful in controlling health expenditures in Canada. In 1985 the total health system absorbed about 8.6 percent of GNP, compared with 11 percent in the neighboring United States. Of Canadian health expenditures about 75 percent are from public sources (divided between federal and provincial governments) and 25 percent from private. Although rising costs have been a political issue, they do not seem to be of great popular concern, and the entire health program enjoys popularity.

Patterns of Health Care Delivery

In spite of the extensive collectivization of health care costs, the delivery of most health services in Canada has changed little from conventional patterns. Medical services are still predominantly provided in the private offices of private physicians, paid on a fee-for-services basis. Even private medical group clinics are less common than in the United States, and not many of them involve the sharing of income and truly cooperative professional work.

The insurance payment mechanisms have, however, led to more rigorous types of regulation of the quality of medical practice. Negotiated fee schedules are, of course, basic. Most provinces generate statistical "profiles" of practice patterns of each physician. If the health insurance data reveal poor performance by an individual doctor or improper or unsound patterns of practice (such as excessive appendectomies or hysterectomies), the insurance authorities turn to the medical profession for remedial action. Either the provincial registration agency or the provincial medical association is then responsible for investigating the problem and taking appropriate action. Since the health insurance authorities have the power to disallow all or part of the reimbursement to a doctor, or to reduce the fee for a particular procedure deemed unjustified, these agencies are in a position to promote a cooperative attitude in the profession. This integration of controls by the health insurance scheme with the functions of the registration agencies and professional associations has a broad impact on all medical practice in Canada.

In contrast to the experience in the United States, Canada has a very low incidence of malpractice actions, which may be regarded as a method of influencing quality of practice through judicial channels. The reasons are complex and are probably related not only to the beneficial effects of the NHI programs and the more rigorous quality controls on medical performance, but also to the absence of contin-

gency fees in legal practice and other factors. Also in contrast to the United States, the hospital insurance program in Canada has generated relatively strong government surveillance of hospital performance; accordingly, a voluntary accreditation program is less important.

The predominance of nongovernment hospitals in Canada has been noted, and in all general hospitals the prevailing medical care pattern has remained "open staff." Each patient is the responsibility of one private physician. Medical staff privileges are highly permissive and, except in medical school teaching hospitals, almost every local physician is accepted on the medical staff. Self-regulation of quality performance by various control committees is conventional, and it has become quite rigorous.

Probably the most innovative effort to change and rationalize health care delivery patterns in Canada was the movement in the early 1970s to develop community health centers. By 1971, all Canadian provinces were covered by hospital and medical care insurance, and the Ministry of National Health and Welfare was ready to take action to improve delivery patterns. Provision of ambulatory care by teams of medical and allied personnel in health centers could be expected to reduce costs, shift the emphasis away from hospitals, and strengthen health promotion and preventive services. The Conference of Provincial Health Ministers set up a Community Health Center Project, which issued its report in 1973. The report recommended "the development . . . of purposeful reorganization and integration of all health services . . . into a system to ensure basic health service standards for all Canadians."

Soon most of the provinces established planning committees for health centers and a number were constructed in Quebec, Ontario, British Columbia, and elsewhere. After a few years, however, the Canadian Medical Association (which had initially supported the Health Center Report) changed its posture and looked on these facilities, with community boards and salaried physicians, as competitive and alarming. Except in the Province of Quebec, where the provincial government was determined to move ahead, health center construction slowed down or stopped. Units already constructed were limited essentially to the poor.

By 1986, there were about 200 community health centers in all Canada, of which 150 were *community local service centers* (for social service and legal advice as well as health care) in Quebec. Ontario had 37 units, but mostly sponsored by physicians (essentially group practices) without community boards; the remaining provinces altogether had fewer than 20. Canadian health centers have been compared to health maintenance organizations (HMOs) in the United States, but only a few of them are supported by periodic capitation payments in the HMO manner. There seem to be certain legal but mainly cultural objections in Canada to "locking in" a population to a particular clinic or even a medical group for all its health services.

The costs of Canadian health insurance have continued to rise. Quite visible in the public sector, they are of concern to political leaders, who search continually for more rigorous cost controls. It is noteworthy, nevertheless, that the general phenomenon of rising costs is not regarded as a "crisis" among the Canadian people as it is in the United States. As far as the average citizen is concerned, his costs for medical and hospital care are met by government programs, and he is pleased with them. The general taxes he must pay to support these progams do not seem troublesome. One wonders whether the relatively lower share of Canada's GNP devoted to military purposes (2.3 percent in 1984, compared to 6.4 percent in the United States) contributes to this attitude. Put another way, a much larger share of health service costs can come from the public sector, without noticeable complaints from citizens about high taxes.

The relatively large sums invested in hospitals have increased their stability and quality of performance. In just the first 8 years of nationwide hospital insurance, from 1958 to 1966, hospital personnel in Canada nearly doubled, from 135,000 to 256,000 (the majority are registered nurses and other professional personnel). Hospital boards of directors and administrators have been able to devote more of their time to program content and less to fundraising.

The many shibboleths that have long marred discussions of health insurance—both government and voluntary—in some countries have been dispelled by the Canadian experience. Doctors did not leave the country; greater numbers came in and were trained. Medical school applications did not decline, but rose. Doctors' incomes, already high, grew higher. Doctors were not swamped with work; instead their numbers rose and their work week was shortened. The quality of medical care did not deteriorate; by all the evidence, it improved. Free choice of doctor did not disappear but was enhanced since everyone, no matter what their income, could see the doctors of their choice. Copayment was not necessary to control excessive use or abuse; in the limited trial of deterrent fees for ambulatory service in one province, their impact was found to be discriminatory against the poor, and they were soon dropped.

Far from causing a deadly uniformity throughout Canada, the national matching of provincial health expenditures has heightened diversity. With basic hospital and doctor services ensured, each province has been free to develop further its own ideas. Even within the nationwide programs, provincial variations in administration are great. Provincial government responsibilities for health service have not been weakened, but strengthened. Even when responsibilities were assigned to agencies other than the health department, the latter agency acquired new functions, so that its role was not reduced. The trend, moreover, is toward unification of the several health administrative functions at the provincial level.

Thus, the welfare-oriented model of the Canadian health system demonstrates very well how a country can collectivize the financing of most of its health care costs and make essential services available to everyone, while still doing relatively little to modify the basic organizational patterns by which services are delivered. Not that medical and hospital practices are completely unchanged. Surveillance of the quality of medical care has been significantly strengthened, and a modest beginning was made in the development of health centers for health care teamwork.

In the late 1980s, the inherently commercial incentives of fee-for-service medical remuneration and the conspicuous greed of many Canadian doctors gave rise to a certain amount of resentment. High physician incomes, excessive rates of elective surgery, multiplication of office visits, and suppression of the health center movement—problems along recognized by Canadian health leaders—were highlighted again. Some people questioned whether the compromise with conventional patterns of private medical practice, built into Canadian NHI legislation, was sound. A more common attitude, however, was to accept medical commercialism as a price for social progress and take political action to correct its defects. If only to control costs, government is continually driven toward greater organization and regulation of the entire health system.

In 1974, when both basic health insurance programs were nationwide, the Health Minister of Canada issued a report calling for a "new perspective on the health of Canadians." This policy document drew worldwide attention because it called for much greater concern for preventive services and health promotion. Now that treatment services were generally available to everyone, Minister Marc LaLonde called for reexamination of how human behavior could contribute to better health or disease. The message was rapidly conveyed to the United States and then to Europe and elsewhere. *Healthful life-style* became a household term, and educational campaigns on the harmfulness of smoking cigarettes, the benefits of a low-fat diet, prudent use of alcohol, regular exercise, and other strategies for health promotion were launched in most industrialized countries. Much was done, of course, to influence behavior through legislative action (for example, prohibiting the advertising of tobacco products), but it is significant that this great "rediscovery" of prevention was launched by a welfare-oriented country only *after* substantial progress had been made in meeting the population's needs for medical care.

AUSTRALIA

The shaping of national health policies by political forces has been quite evident in the welfare-oriented systems of the five countries already considered. In Australia, these dynamics have been especially conspicuous. The changing positions of private and public sectors over the years, as expressed in the ideologies of major political parties, have caused enormous turbulence in the operation of the Australian health system in general and of a national program of insurance for medical care, in particular.

Like Canada, the Australian continent was colonized by Great Britain in 1788. It was settled as six semiautonomous states, each reporting separately to the British crown—also like the Canadian provinces. Federation of the six states and two centrally governed territories into one parliamentary nation occurred in 1901. The Constitution, established that year, endowed the states with great authority in education, health, and other social matters. In 1984 the national population of Australia was 15,500,000, and the GNP per capita was $11,740.

Voluntary Health Insurance

Friendly societies for cooperative voluntary health assistance had functioned in Australia since the nineteenth century. In 1927, a National Insurance Bill, including sickness and maternity benefits, was introduced into the federal or Commonwealth Parliament, but opposition from the employers, the state governments, and also the friendly societies killed it. Again in 1938 another National Health and Pension Bill was introduced. In spite of opposition by the Labour Party (which favored general revenue rather than social insurance financing), this bill was enacted in July 1938. Before the implementation could be planned, however, World War II began, and the bill never took effect. All this occurred under national administrations of the relatively conservative Liberal Party.

In October 1941, the Australian Labour Party gained power and soon launched Australia's first nationwide health benefit program. In 1944, a Pharmaceutical Benefits Bill was passed to finance high-cost and life-saving drugs for every resident. It was funded not by employer and employee contributions, but by an earmarked part of the federal general revenues. As they did with more bitterness in later years, physicians boycotted the program, leading to court litigation and a constitutional amendment. Not until 1950, when the Liberal Party was returned to power, did the doctors cooperate. Minor procedural changes were made in the law, but it was clear that, under a Liberal Party government, the doctors shed their anxiety that the drug benefits might be the prelude to "fully socialized medicine." Over the years the list of approved drugs gradually extended, and although a copayment charge was introduced, the drug program became very expensive.

In 1945, after the drug benefits program was obstructed in 1944, the Labour Party enacted a modest Hospital Benefits Act, which granted small subsidies (about 60 cents a day) for every patient in a public or private hospital that did not charge for use of its public beds. Over subsequent years, these subsidies were increased, eventually leading to a uniquely Australian scheme for governmental support and encouragement of voluntary health insurance. This was accomplished by the Liberal Party in 1951, by adding a second federal grant to hospitals for each patient who was covered by voluntary health insurance. In 1953, the federal government gave still another hospital subsidy for patients covered by voluntary insurance schemes financing physician services, to encourage membership in these programs. Also in 1953, the Liberal Party government enacted the Pensioner Medical Service, which financed the total cost of general practitioner and public ward hospital service for low-income elderly, the totally disabled, and certain other needy persons.

During the post-World War II years, voluntary health insurance schemes in Australia grew in number and enrollment. Physician fees and hospital charges, however, continued to rise, leading to various copayments, limitations on services, and other restrictions. In 1968, therefore, while the Liberal Party was still in power, a Committee on Enquiry into Health Insurance was appointed. Its report, issued the next year, concluded the following:

1. The health insurance scheme is unnecessarily complex and beyond the comprehension of many.
2. There is often a wide gap between financial benefits received by patients and the costs of hospital and medical care that they must pay.
3. Premiums have become so high that a significant proportion of people cannot afford to enroll in the voluntary funds, and for others they are a hardship to pay.
4. The rules of many funds permit disallowance or reduction of claims in too many cases.
5. Administrative expenses of some funds are unduly high.
6. The financial reserves held by numerous funds are unnecessarily large.
7. Allied health services, like podiatry, optometry, or dentistry, while important, are not included among any of the fund benefits.

In the next 2 years government regulations responded to many of the committee recommendations, such as eliminating exclusion of care for "preexisting conditions" after 6 months' membership in a fund, setting a ceiling on doctor's fees, simplifying hospital benefit procedures, placing top limits on health fund administrative expenses and reserves, increasing the subsidies for low-income families, and so on. Nevertheless, some 90 voluntary funds continued their autonomous operation, and indemnification remained the pattern for covering doctor's fees. As long as a doctor notified the patient in advance that he did not observe the "common fee," the patient could frequently end up paying much more than the statutory 20 percent copayment.

By mid-1972, around 15 to 20 percent of the Australian population remained uninsured. Many of the balance were covered by the Pensioner Medical Services, but with restricted benefits (e.g., no ambulatory specialist service or hospitalization outside of large public wards). Also federal revenues financed the Australian Pharmaceutical Benefits Scheme, which has covered everyone since 1950 for almost all necessary prescribed drugs. The Labour opposition, however, could still point to more than one million uninsured and unprotected persons, and numerous other deficiencies.

National Health Insurance— Come and Gone

In 1972, after 22 years out of power, the Labour Party was reelected. It promptly set to work planning a national health insurance program that would cover everyone under a unified fund, with equal benefits for all (i.e., no restrictions for the aged or indigent). Free choice of doctor was still assured, along with some copayment, but this was limited to 15 percent of the official fee, or a maximum of $5.00 (regardless of the charge, even for a complex surgical operation). There was no cost-sharing in hospitals, if the patient used "standard ward" service. The existing voluntary funds were still free to sell supplemental benefits. In August 1974, the new National Health Act was passed, but by a very slim majority; even this was achieved only by invoking a special constitutional provision under which both houses of Parliament were assembled to vote together. In fact, a further vote required to finance the program, through an intended annual 1.35 percent levy on all individual taxpayers' incomes (up to a $150 ceiling), failed narrowly to pass; as a result, the whole program was financed from general or consolidated revenues.

Of long-term importance were the deliberate steps taken by the Labour government in 1973 to modify traditional Australian health care delivery patterns. Private medical practice had long predominated, but there was concern that the declining proportion of general practitioners (less than 40 percent of the total) was unsound. One strategy to stregthen general practice was the encouragement of group practice among GPs. Another was establishing a specialty College of General Practice and a dynamic Family Medicine Program subsidized by the government to provide a rich schedule of continuing education courses. Third was a movement to develop community health centers for primary care, provided by GPs and several allied health personnel.

A long-recognized problem in Australian medical service has been the sparsity of doctors in the thinly settled rural areas, especially in the vast interior of the outback. One solution has been the renowned Flying Doctor service, with physicians at airplane terminals connected by radio to hundreds of posts in the interior. Another approach has been to send young residents to isolated stations, visited periodically by their teaching hospital chiefs. Bursaries (fellowships) have also been given to Australian medical students, who would agree to serve for a corresponding number of years in rural locations. In Tasmania, rural district doctors on relatively high salaries have long been employed by the health department. Probably most important is the *bush nurse* who is trained to handle minor ailments, give preventive services, and call for medical help when she considers it necessary.

General hospitals in Australia are predominantly under government sponsorship, mainly at the state level. As of 1981, 73.3 percent of the beds were in public hospitals, 13.9 percent in voluntary nonprofit institutions, and 12.8 percent in proprietary units. In 1972, when the Labour Party regained power, the average hospital under either public or nonprofit sponsorship derived its support 53 percent from a state government, 14 percent from the federal government, 23 percent from voluntary insurance, and 10 percent from private payments or other special services.

In this setting, the majority of patients were served in public hospitals on the open wards. They were treated by young doctors in training or by specialist consultants, who received only an annual or monthly honorarium. (The consultant's principal reward was the prestige of the hospital appointment and the right to admit private patients to one of the small number of private beds.) This "charity care" pattern was just beginning to change to a pattern of paying sessional fees for specialist's service to ward patients. Under the 1974 National Health Insurance legislation, such sessional payments became general, and many public hospitals found it more economical and efficient to engage physicians on full-time salaries.

We have noted the strategy to improve health care delivery patterns in Australia through the establishment of community health centers. To minimize controversy with the medical profession, most of these were limited to low-income persons, but some were open to everyone. Some health centers stressed preventive services to mothers and children, some concentrated in geriatric care, and some were truly comprehensive. Doctors were paid either by fee-for-service or by salary, whichever they preferred. It was expected that, with the new health insurance legislation, these health centers would eventually become a common model for providing ambulatory services.

The major administrative mechanism for promoting these and other changes in Australian health services was the Hospitals and Health Services Commission set up in 1972. Although under the Minister for Health, the commission was independent of the traditional public health structure and had a free hand to develop new ideas. Of course, it had to work through the state health authorities in this federated republic, and the configurations for management of hospitals, public health services, mental hygiene, and other fields differ in each of the six states. The commission promoted innovations through relatively generous grants to local bodies.

As scheduled, on 1 July 1975 the *Medibank* program of Australia, as it was called, came into operation, funded entirely from general revenues. But the battle for universal health cost protection was far from won. The mechanism of general revenue financing forced by the opposition's defeat of the earmarked *social insurance levy,* led to a further crisis later the same year. Controlling, as it did, the Senate chamber of the Australian Parliament, the Liberal Party successfully blocked appropriation of general revenue funds for the operation of Medibank, as well as for all other government operations.

To solve this obvious crisis, the governor-general of Australia—previously little more than a ceremonial figure head—invoked an authority given in the Australian Constitution

but never before used. On 11 November 1975, he dismissed the Labour government from office and called a new national election a few weeks later. In December 1975 a coalition of the Liberal and Country parties won and took control of the national government. No time was lost in appointing a Medibank Review Committee, and in May 1976 several key changes in the health insurance programs were announced, to take effect in October 1976.

Consistent with the anti–public sector philosophy of the new government, the major 1976 changes in the Medibank program were as follows:

1. Any individual or family could opt out of the entire program by arranging for private medical and hospital insurance with equivalent benefits.
2. Private health insurance programs (numbering 85 in late 1976) became subject to somewhat greater public regulation, to ensure that they would meet government standards on enrollment and services.
3. Financing was reversed once again to an earmarked levy on taxable income up to a dollar-ceiling; instead of the earlier Labour government proposal of a 1.35 percent tax rate, however, it was made 2.5 percent. (Pensioners and certain veterans were exempted from the tax.)
4. Federal support of public hospitals was modified to permit less than 50 percent subsidy.
5. The national Health Insurance Commission was authorized to operate a competitive Medibank Private program, in addition to its government health service fund.

Less than 2 years later, in July 1978, as medical care prices rose, the conservative government made further changes in the Medibank program:

1. The private health insurance programs were permitted to introduce *deductibles* in their payments for medical and hospital services.
2. The standard medical benefit was reduced from 85 to 75 percent of sched-

uled fees, and the maximum supplemental charge to patients allowable beyond this was raised. The fee schedule was also modified upward.

3. Physicians were authorized either to charge patients directly (compelling them to seek indemnification from the government) or to send their bills to the insurance fund for payment—known as *bulk billing.*

4. National standards for public hospital management were relaxed, to permit greater variations in policy among the states.

The effect of these two sets of Medibank changes in 1976 and 1978 was, as intended, to greatly strengthen the role of private health insurance programs in Australia. With the social insurance tax raised to 2.5 percent of taxable income (even with a dollar ceiling) and with permission to opt out through private insurance coverage, persons and families of higher income (and usually lower sickness risk) usually found private insurance premiums lower. Hence, more and more of the affluent and lower-risk population opted for private insurance coverage, leaving the public Medibank Fund with higher risk people, paying relatively inadequate insurance levies. Hence, by late 1978, about 57 percent of the Australian population—mainly middle- and upper-class families—were insured under private carriers.

The next step in the Australian health care saga was only to be expected. In November 1978, the principle of mandatory social insurance for health care was abandoned entirely. The specific further modifications in the Medibank program were as follows:

1. The requirement that everyone must have health insurance protection at a specified level—through either government or private coverage—was ended.

2. The earmarked government levy of 2.5 percent of taxable income was abolished.

3. Whether or not a person was enrolled in a private insurance program, the federal government would subsidize medical charges at a level of 40 percent

of scheduled fees, with maximum patient obligation of $20 per service. (This subsidy was derived from general revenues but transmitted through private insurance carriers.) The definition of a *service,* furthermore, permitted charges well over the $20 limit; thus, an appendectomy was interpreted to include three services (those of the surgeon, the assistant, and the anaesthetist) aggregating to charges of nearly $60 payable by the patient.

4. Direct payment of physicians by government (rather than by the patient who would later seek indemnification) was applicable only to pensioners and indigent or disadvantaged persons.

5. As a backstop for the noninsured population, *standard ward* care in a public hospital was made available to anyone without charge.

Thus, through the initial opposition strategy in 1975 of rejecting social insurance financing for medical care in Australia and compelling dependence on general revenues, the provisions of the National Health Act of 1974—universal coverage for nearly comprehensive benefits—were gradually eroded, to the point of complete abandonment. A survey in March 1979 showed that private health insurance coverage was protecting 62.4 percent of the Australian population for medical care costs. Of the remainder, 13.2 percent were protected as pensioners or veterans (repatriation beneficiaries), leaving 24.4 percent of the Australian people unprotected by either private or public medical care programs. By April 1980 an estimated 40 percent of the population had abandoned voluntary health insurance—the young and healthiest people. With the highest-risk members left behind, voluntary insurance premiums rose higher than ever. Soon the federal government subsidy of 40 percent of scheduled fees (for both insured and noninsured persons) was abandoned.

Hence, the wheel of health insurance in Australia had turned full circle. Social insurance was abandoned and the essential feature of the old 1953 legislation, subsidized voluntary insurance, was reinstated. Data on Australian health expenditures from 1960 to 1983 reflect the undulation very well:

Thus, from 1960 to 1975, total health expenditures rose steadily from 5.1 to 7.6 percent of gross domestic product (GDP); in 1983 after the erosion of the 1974 law, there was a slight decline to 7.5 percent of GDP. More important, governmental health expenditures, as a percentage of the total, increased steadily from 47.1 in 1960 to 73.7 percent in 1975. Then, with the dismantling of the 1974 law, they declined to 65.3 percent in 1983. Equivalent figures for the later 1980s would doubtless show a resurgence of the public sector.

Year	Total as Percentage of GDP	Government as Percentage of GDP	Government as Percentage of Total
1960	5.1	2.4	47.1
1965	5.3	2.8	52.8
1975	7.6	5.6	73.7
1983	7.5	4.9	65.3

National Health Insurance— Returned

In March 1983, the Australian Labour Party was once again returned to national power. The political debate made it clear that the central government had a strong mandate to reintroduce universal health insurance. This was done in February 1984 and the new law was significantly called *Medicare* rather than Medibank. The Medicare program was financed by a 1.0 percent tax on all income tax payers, although this covered only a share of the full costs; there were large inputs from federal and state general revenues. Medicare provided a rebate of 85 percent of all medical fees, according to official fee schedules. Patients were encouraged, however, to visit physicians who bulk bill, that is, submit to the insurance office charges for numerous patients at one time. In this way, the doctor was paid directly by the government and the patient was relieved of the 15 percent balance; by 1987 some 52 percent of all physician services were paid for in this manner.

Attendance at public hospital out-patient and casualty clinics was free. If hospital admission was required, the patient could opt to be either a hospital or a private case. The former meant treatment by a salaried (full-time or part-time) hospital doctor with no charges; the latter meant free choice of doctor on the visiting staff and payment of both hospital and medical fees. The doctor fees were rebatable (up to the scheduled amount) by Medicare, but hospital charges were payable by the patient or by voluntary insurance. Only a small percentage of people could afford supplemental private insurance to pay for private hospital care; the vast majority had to use public hospitals, with salaried doctors assigned to them. As a result, there were long waiting lists for admission of nonemergency patients to public hospitals while private hospitals had many unoccupied beds.

There were many more aspects of the Australian Medicare program of 1984, especially with regard to hospital specialists and their right to engage in private practice in a public or private hospital. These requirements were largely responsible for some bitter disputes between specialists and the government Health Insurance Commission at the very outset. Surgeons in the state of New South Wales essentially went on strike for well over a year, refusing to do elective surgery (they did treat emergencies), until matters were settled by late 1985. The settlement allowed all hospital specialists (full-time or sessional) to engage in private practice in both public and private hospitals, and physician remuneration was broadly increased. In effect, Australian doctors would get richer, but universal entitlement of the people to medical care prevailed.

The Australian health insurance saga illustrates the difficulties encountered in a health system with a welfare-oriented ideology, where improvements are sought mainly in mechanisms of financing, but only slightly in the manner of delivering health services. From 1951, when the conservative Liberal Party introduced subsidies of voluntary health insurance, up to the 1980s, the vendettas between government and the private medical profession have been almost endless. Under the Labour Party, it is true, hundreds of health centers have been established to serve the poor, and public hospitals have organized their medical staffs in ways more favorable to low-income people. The persistent opposition of doctors to almost any regulation, however, and medical demands for higher financial rewards could only aggravate relationships with patients, and escalate health system costs that had to be met by the population.

GENERAL COMMENTS

This review of major highlights in the welfare-oriented health systems of several countries may warrant certain general conclusions. In affluent industrialized countries, the mechanism of insurance, initially voluntary and later compulsory or social, has proven effective in rendering medical care accessible to the general population. In six major countries of this type—Federal Republic of Germany, Belgium, France, Japan, Canada, and Australia—these dynamics have been clear, though they have taken different routes. The process has never been simple and placid. The following summarizes the development of these systems:

1. Legislative action to achieve social insurance for health services typically follows from a long period of experience with voluntary insurance and many forms of debate.
2. Social insurance for health care has been a popular strategy with parliamentary government of diverse political viewpoints, because it draws funds from a source other than general revenues and is not competitive with various other governmental functions. In contrast to public assistance or charity, it is organized self-help.
3. At the outset, socially insured health care programs simple furnish funds to pay for medical and related services traditionally offered in the country—usually the attention of private doctors paid on a fee-for-service basis.
4. Most often these programs start with coverage of industrial workers of relatively low income. Gradually cover-

age is extended to higher-income workers and also to workers engaged in commerce, agriculture, and other types of occupations. Dependents not covered at the outset are usually included later.
5. The scope of services financed under insurance programs may start with only general doctor's care and prescribed drugs, but it tends gradually to widen to hospital and specialist services, dental care, prostheses, and other health-related benefits.
6. Insurance contributions have customarily come from workers and employers, as a stated percentage of wages and payrolls. Employer contributions are ordinarily passed on to the consumers of a firm's products, through the costs of production; there are also usually increasing inputs from general government revenues, making the impact of funding more progressive.
7. In enacting national health insurance, political parties representing organized labor are usually crucial, either as the party in power or as a threatening opposition.
8. The increased funding provided by health insurance programs typically leads to devotion of a rising percentage of gross national product (GNP) to the health system. This, in turn, increases attention to the entire health system in national political agendas.
9. Enlarged economic support for health services always results in an increased rate of provision or utilization of those services. Some of these services suggest abuse by patients or, more often, by doctors, and stimulate various types of control or cost containment.
10. Health insurance programs are inherently a form of market intervention, through basic modification of the demand side of the supply-and-demand interaction. Therefore, they typically induce further market intervention on the supply side—that is, the supply of health personnel and facilities.
11. Because of heightened demand, health insurance initially tends to stimulate an increased output of per-

sonnel, construction of hospitals, and so forth. Later, constraints are often put on this process.

12. Eventually the rising costs of health insurance programs induce modifications of the conventional patterns of delivering services, if only to control expenditures and increase efficiency. The extent of these modifications varies greatly among countries, but it nearly always involves some form of organization of ambulatory services, through teams working in health centers, and some type of regionalization among hospitals.

13. A common strategy for achieving greater efficiency in the health system is to institute measures for surveillance of the quality of health services. These measures are applied most frequently in hospitals, whereas various forms of statistical identification of deviance are developed for ambulatory services.

14. Another response to rising health care costs has been increased emphasis on prevention and health promotion. Strategies for this purpose usually require greater collaboration with and support from ministries of health.

15. When many local agencies are used to operate a health insurance program, the administrative costs are relatively high; countries are evidently willing to pay these higher costs for the sake of pluralism, involving many social groups and interests.

16. Once started by governments, health insurance programs tend to survive and expand. Technical and administrative problems generate various reforms. Significantly, the unusual reversal of health insurance legislation in Australia in the 1970s was followed by legislative reinstatement in the 1980s.

17. Many different scenarios exist for national health insurance in industrialized and affluent countries, varying with time and place. Methods of implementation differ greatly between federated and centralized governmental structures. A great deal obviously depends on historical background and the relative power of various social forces.

Other affluent countries with welfare-oriented health systems, to which these conclusions also generally apply, are the Netherlands and Switzerland. Local mutual aid societies of various types play a large part in both of their health systems, and nearly the entire population has economic protection (through health insurance) for medical care costs. In the Netherlands, great importance is attached to voluntary agencies, and many government health functions are delegated to them, with major public subsidies. In 1983, of the 8.8 percent of GDP spent for health, 78 percent came from public sources. Switzerland has 24 highly autonomous cantons; public health and health insurance policies differ in each of them. In both of these countries, as in the six analyzed in this chapter, the private medical profession is politically strong, and relatively little has been done to alter patterns of private medical care delivery, in spite of the predominantly social financing.

REFERENCES

General

Fulcher, Derick, *Medical Care Systems: Public and Private Health Coverage in Selected Industrial Countries.* Geneva: International Labour Office, 1974.

Glaser, William, "Health Politics: Lessons from Abroad," in T. J. Litman and L. S. Robins (Editors), *Health Politics and Policy.* New York: John Wiley & Sons, 1984, pp. 305–339.

Maxwell, Robert J., *Health and Wealth: An International Study of Health-Care Spending.* Lexington, Mass.: Lexington Books, 1981.

Navarro, Vicente, "The Public/Private Mix in the Funding and Delivery of Health Services: An International Survey." *American Journal of Public Health,* 75:1318–1320, November 1985.

Organization for Economic Cooperation and Development, *Measuring Health Care 1960–1983.* Paris: OECD, 1985.

World Health Organization, *Health Services in Europe: Vols. I and II.* Copenhagen: WHO Regional Office for Europe, 1981.

Germany

Federal Minister of Labour and Social Affairs, *Survey of Social Security in the Federal Republic of Germany.* Bonn: The Federal Minister, 1972, pp. 123–139.

Goldmann, Franz, and Alfred Grotjahn, *Benefits of the German Sickness Insurance System from the Point of View of Social Hygiene.* Geneva: International Labour Office, 1928.

Iglehart, John K., "Health Policy Report: Canada's Health Care System." *New England Journal of Medicine,* 315(3):202–208, 17 July 1986.

International Hospital Federation, *Report of Study Tour of Hospitals in the German Federal Republic.* London: The Federation, 1958.

Light, Donald W., Stephen Liebfried, and Florian Tennstedt, "Social Medicine vs. Professional Dominance: The German Experience." *American Journal of Public Health,* 76(1):78–83, January 1986.

Light, Donald W., and Alexander Schuller (Editors), *Political Values and Health Care: The German Experience.* Cambridge: Massachusetts Institute of Technology Press, 1986.

MacLeod, Gordon K., "National Health Insurance in the Federal Republic of Germany and Its Implications for U.S. Consumers." *Public Health Reports,* 91(4):343–348, July–August 1976.

McLachlan, Gordon, and Alan Maynard (Editors), *The Public–Private Mix for Health: The Relevance and Effects of Change.* London: Nuffield Provincial Hospitals Trust, 1982.

Reinhardt, Uwe E., "Health Insurance and Health Policy in the Federal Republic of Germany." *Health Care Financing Review,* 3(2):1–14, December 1981.

Schulenberg, J.-Matthias Graf, "Report from Germany: Current Conditions and Controversies in the Health Care Systems." *Journal of Health Politics, Policy, and Law,* 8(2):320–351, Summer 1983.

Sigerist, Henry E., "From Bismarck to Beveridge: Developments and Trends in Social Security Legislation." *Bulletin of the History of Medicine,* 8:365–388, April 1943.

Stone, Deborah A., *The Limits of Professional Power: National Health Care and the Federal Republic of Germany.* Chicago: University of Chicago Press, 1980.

World Health Organization, "Federal Republic of Germany," in *Sixth Report on the World Health Situation: Part Two—Review by Country and Area.* Geneva: WHO, 1980, pp. 191–196.

World Health Organization, Regional Office for Europe, "Federal Republic of Germany," in *Health Services in Europe,* 3rd edition. Copenhagen: WHO/Europe, 1981, pp. 71–79.

Belgium

Déjardin, Jerome, *Monograph on the Organisation of Medical Care Within the Framework of Social Security in Belgium.* Geneva: International Labour Office, 1968.

Engles, J., *L'Evolution de l'Assurance Maladie-Invalidité Obligatoire 1945–1970.* Bruxelles: In stitut National d'Assurance Maladie-Invalidité, 1971.

Glaser, W., *Health Insurance Bargaining: Foreign Lessons for Americans.* New York: Gardner Press, 1978.

International Social Security Association, "Belgium: Creation of a National Hospital Programming Commission." *International Social Security Association Review,* 26:313–314, 1973.

Ministère de la Santé Publique et de la Famille, *Organization Sanitaire de la Belgique: Promotion et Protection de la Santé.* Bruxelles, 1973.

Nys, Herman, and Paul Quaethoven, "Health Services in Belgium," in Marshall W. Raffel (Editor), *Comparative Health Systems.* University Park: Pennsylvania State University Press, 1984, pp. 55–81.

Roemer, Milton I., and Ruth J. Roemer, "The Belgian Health Care System," in *Health Care Systems and Comparative Manpower Policies.* New York: Marcel Dekker, 1981, pp. 129–171.

France

Cassou, Bernard, and B. Pissarro, "Workers' Participation and Occupational Health: The French Experience." *International Journal of Health Services,* 18(1):139–152, 1988.

Glaser, William, Health Insurance Bargaining. New York: Gardner Press, 1978.

Jallade, Jean-Pierre, "Redistribution and the Welfare State: An Assessment of the French Socialists Performance." *Government and Opposition,* 20(3):348 ff. (London), Summer 1985.

Lacronique, Jean-Francois, "Health Services in France," in M. W. Raffel (Editor), *Comparative Health Systems: Descriptive Analyses of Fourteen National Health Systems.* University Park: Pennsylvania State University Press, 1984, pp. 258–285.

Ministère de la Santè Publique, *Annuaire des Statistiques Sanitares et Sociales,* Paris, 1979.

Rodwin, Victor G., "The Marriage of National Health Insurance and 'La Mèdecine Libèral' in France: A Costly Union." *Milbank Memorial Fund Quarterly,* 59(1):16–43, 1981.

Rodwin, Victor G., *The Health Planning Predicament: France, Quebec, England, and the United States.* Berkeley: University of California, 1984.

Stephan, J. C., *Economie et Pouvoir Mèdical.* Paris: Economica, 1978.

Weise, Robert W., "Medical Care Agreement with French Doctors." *Social Security Bulletin,* July 1972, pp. 32–35.

World Health Organization, "France," in *Health Services in Europe,* 3rd edition, Vol. II. Copenhagen: WHO Regional Office for Europe, 1981, pp. 55–62.

Japan

Campbell, John Creighton, "Medical Care for the Japanese Elderly." *Pacific Affairs,* 57(1):53–64, Spring 1984.

Fisher, Paul, "Major Social Security Issues: Japan, 1971." *Social Security Bulletin,* March 1973, pp. 26–38.

Hashimoto, Masami, "Health Services in Japan," in M. W. Raffel (Editor), *Comparative Health Systems.* University Park: Pennsylvania State University Press, 1984, pp. 335–370.

Iwasa, Kiyoshi, "Hospitals in Japan: History and Present Situation." *Medical Care,* 4(4):241–246, October–December 1966.

Jonas, Steven, "The District Health Center in Japan: History, Services and Future Development." *American Journal of Public Health,* 65:58–62, 1975.

Kiikuni, Kenzo, "Health Insurance Programs in Japan." *Inquiry,* 9(1):16–23, March 1972.

Maeda, Nobuo, "Long-term Care for the Elderly in Japan," in Teresa Schwab (Editor), *Caring for an Aging World.* New York: McGraw-Hill Information Services Co., 1988, pp. 246–264.

Matsuura, Toshiro, "Some Recent Problems of Medical Services under the Health Insurance System in Japan." *Asian Medical Journal,* 14(12):791–818, December 1971.

Ministry of Health and Welfare, *Health Services in Japan.* Tokyo, September 1974.

Ministry of Health and Welfare, *Health and Welfare Services in Japan.* Tokyo, 1977.

Ministry of Health and Welfare, Japanese Government, *A Brief Report on Public Health Administration in Japan.* Tokyo, 1970.

Ohtani, F., *One Hundred Years of Health Progress in Japan.* Tokyo: International Medical Foundation of Japan, 1971.

Social Insurance Agency Japanese Government, *Outline of Social Insurance in Japan.* Tokyo, 1971.

Steslicke, William E., "Development of Health Insurance Policy in Japan." *Journal of Health Politics, Policy and Law,* 7(1):197–226, Spring 1982.

Steslicke, William E., "The Japanese State of Health: A Political-Economic Perspective," in E. Norbeck and M. Lock (Editors), *Health, Illness, and Medical Care in Japan: Cultural and Social Dimensions.* Honolulu: University of Hawaii Press, 1987, pp. 24–65.

Steslicke, William E., "Medical Care in Japan: the Political Context." *Journal of Ambulatory Care Management,* November 1982, pp. 65–76.

Steslicke, William E., and Rihito Kimura, "Medical Technology for the Elderly in Japan." *International Journal of Technology Assessment in Health Care,* 1(1):27–39, January 1985.

Steslicke, William E., "Japan," in J. P. DeSario (Editor), *International Public Policy Sourcebook: Vol. 1, Health and Social Welfare.* New York: Greenwood Press, 1989, pp. 89–116.

Yamamoto, Mikio, "Primary Health Care and Health Education in Japan." *Social Science and Medicine,* 17(19):1419–1431, 1983.

Yoshida, Yoichi, and Katsumi Yoshida, "The High Rate of Appendectomy in Japan." *Medical Care,* 14(11):950–957, November 1976.

Canada

Advisory Planning Committee on Medical Care to the Government of Saskatchewan, *Final Report.* Regina: Queen's Printer, 1962.

Badgley, Robin F., and Samuel Wolfe, *Doctor's Strike: Medical Care and Conflict in Saskatchewan.* Toronto: Macmillan of Canada, 1967.

Blishen, B. R., *Doctors and Doctrines: The Ideology of Medical Care in Canada.* Toronto: University of Toronto Press, 1969.

Canadian Hospital Association, *Canadian Hospital Directory,* Ottawa, 1987.

Community Health Centre Project Committee, *The Community Health Centre in Canada.* Ottawa: Health and Welfare Canada, 1972.

Evans, Robert G., and G. L. Stoddart, *Medicare at Maturity: Achievements, Lessons, and Challenges.* Calgary: University of Calgary Press, 1986.

Hastings, John E. F., "Organized Ambulatory Care in Canada: Health Service Organizations and Community Health Centers." *Journal of Public Health Policy,* 7:239–247, Summer 1986.

Hatcher, G. H., "Canadian Approaches to Health Policy Decisions—National Health Insurance." *American Journal of Public Health,* 68:881–889, 1978.

Iglehart, John K., "Canada's Health Care System." *New England Journal of Medicine* (in 3 parts), 17 July 1986, pp. 202–208; 18 September 1986, pp. 778–784; 18 December 1986, pp. 1623–1628.

Lalonde, M., *A New Perspective on the Health of Canadians: A Working Document.* Ottawa: Health and Welfare Canada, 1974.

LeClair, M., "Historical Perspective: The Canadian Health Care System," in S. Andreopoulos, Editor, *National Health Insurance: Can We Learn from Canada?* New York: John Wiley & Sons, 1975, pp. 11–93.

Lee, Sidney S., *Quebec's Health System: A Decade of Change, 1967–77.* Montreal: Institute of Public Administration of Canada, 1979.

Mott, F. D., "Government-Sponsored Care in Saskatchewan." *Hospitals,* 1950, no. 24, p. 58.

Panel on Health Goals for Ontario, *Health for All Ontario.* Toronto: Ontario Ministry of Health, 1987.

Roemer, Milton I., and Ruth Roemer, "The Canadian Health Care System," in *Health Care Systems and Comparative Manpower Policies.* New York: Marcel Dekker, 1981, pp. 3–77.

Royal Commission on Health Services, *Report, Volume 1.* Ottawa: Queen's Printer, 1964.

Schwenger, Cope W., "Health Care for the Elderly in Canada." *Journal of Public Health Policy,* 7:222–240, Summer 1987.

Taylor, Malcolm G., *Health Insurance and Canadian Public Policy: The Seven Decisions that*

Created the Canadian Health Insurance System. Montreal: McGill-Queen's University Press, 1978.

Vayda, Eugene, "The Canadian Health Care System: An Overview." *Journal of Public Health Policy,* 7:205–210, Summer 1986.

York, Geoffrey, *The High Price of Health: A Patient's Guide to the Hazards of Medical Politics.* Toronto: James Lorimer & Co., 1987.

Australia

Adams, A. I., "The 1984–85 Australian Doctor's Dispute." *Journal of Public Health Policy,* 7:93–102, Spring 1986.

Adams, A. I., "The State of Health Services—International Comments: Developments in Australia's Health Services." *International Journal of Epidemiology,* 3:5–7, 1974.

Anderson, N. A., "Primary Care in Australia." *International Journal of Health Services,* 16:199–212, 1986.

Australian Public Health Association, *An Examination of Australian Health Policy Issues.* Melbourne, 1974.

Bates, Erica M., "A Consumer's View of the Australian Experience in Health Insurance." *The Lancet,* 5 July 1980, pp. 26–28.

Committee on Health Careers of the Hospitals and Health Services Commission, *Australian Health Manpower.* Canberra: Australian Government Publishing Service, 1975.

Deeble, J. S., "Health Care Under Universal Insurance: The First Three Years of Medicare." Canberra (Australia): Department of Community Services and Health, 1987 (processed).

Deeble, J. S., and I. W. Scott, *Health Expenditures in Australia: 1960–61 to 1975–76.* Canberra: Australian National University, 1978.

Deeble, J. S., and R. B. Scotton, *Health Care Under Voluntary Insurance: Report of a Survey.* Melbourne: University of Melbourne, September 1968.

Dewdney, J. E. H., *Australian Health Services.* Sydney: John Wiley & Sons Australasia, 1972.

Hetzel, Basil S., *Health and Australian Society.* Middlesex, England: Penguin Books, 1974.

Last, John M., "The Organization and Economics of Medical Care in Australia." *New England Journal of Medicine,* 272:293–297, 11 February 1965.

Minister for Social Security, *The Australian Health Insurance Program.* Canberra: Australian Government Publishing Service, November 1973.

Munro, Ian, "An Unsteady Balance Between Private and Public: Historical Foundations and Economic Realities in Australia." *The Lancet,* 28 February 1976, pp. 467–470, and 6 March 1976, pp. 525–529.

National Hospitals and Health Services Commission, *A Community Health Program for Australia.* Canberra: Australian Government Publishing Service, 1973.

Roemer, Ruth, and Milton I. Roemer, *Health Manpower in the Changing Australian Health Services Scene.* Washington, D. C.: Public Health Service (DHEW Pub. 76-58), 1976.

Sax, Sidney, *Medical Care in the Melting Pot: An Australian Review.* Sydney: Angus and Robertson, 1972.

Scotton, R. B., *Medical Care in Australia: An Economic Diagnosis.* South Melbourne: Sun Brooks, 1974.

Scotton, R. B., "Medibank 1976." *The Australian Economic Review,* First Quarter 1977.

Scotton, R. B., and J. S. Deeble, "The Nimmo Report." *Economic Record,* 45:258–272, June 1969.

CHAPTER SEVEN

Comprehensive Health Systems in Industrialized Countries

In the last chapter, we reviewed the national health systems in six industrialized countries with welfare-oriented health policies. In essence, these policies have collectivized the financing of health services, to make them economically accessible to all or nearly all of the population. The patterns of service delivery, however, have been only slightly modified. While the organized financing has provided political leverage for certain limited modifications of delivery patterns—designed to make them more efficient and effective—the predominant methods of providing both ambulatory and institutional health service have remained essentially unchanged (that is, as under private market conditions). Moreover, the population coverage has been extended incrementally, so that numerous separate agencies finance the care of various population groups, resulting in very complex administrative processes.

In this chapter we analyze the health systems of a number of industrialized countries that have gone further in their intervention in the free medical market and the organization of the several components of the health systems. Although most of these systems have evolved from the welfare-oriented type, they have made substantial modifications in the patterns of delivery of health services, as well as in their financing. Although they usually extend coverage incrementally, they have come to achieve universal population entitlement to health care, and abandoned the complex aggregation of several separate sources of financing. We speak of these as *comprehensive health systems* in a double sense: they provide comprehensive scopes of health services and cover the population comprehensively or universally.

As a prototype of this model of national health system, we selected a Scandinavian country. All of these countries—Norway, Sweden, Finland, Denmark, and Iceland—started social insurance programs for employed workers, enrolled in mutual aid societies around 1910. They gradually extended to universal population coverage after World War II. With their universality, the patterns of health care delivery were gradually modified toward more organized forms. In each of the five Scandinavian countries, health system characteristics differ slightly; the most extensive literature is on Sweden, the largest of the group both in its population and its land area. Our account focuses on Norway, which is closer to the median in its major attributes.

NORWAY

Among the countries of Europe, Norway has a relatively large land area, with 324,000 square kilometers, just west of Sweden on the Scandinavian peninsula, and extending north of the Arctic Circle. Much of its population of only 4,140,000 (in 1984) is thinly dispersed, 43 percent rural and 57 percent urban—a distribution of people that has considerable bearing on its health system. The GNP per capita was $14,344 in 1984, higher in that period than previously, because of the discovery of oil in the North Sea.

Following the Napoleonic Wars in the early nineteenth century, Norway became a satellite of Sweden from 1814 to 1905, when it achieved autonomy. Then in World War II, Norway (unlike neutral Sweden) joined the Allies and was occupied by the Germans (1942–1945) under the rule of the Norwegian Fascist leader Vidkun Quisling. After the war, the constitutional monarchy was restored, and political control was exercised principally by the Labour Party. Most of the significant health legislation reviewed here was enacted during Labour Party rule from 1945 to 1963, but even under periods of Conservative Party control relatively little was changed in the health system.

The long narrow territory of Norway is divided into 19 *filkes,* or provinces (although the word is sometimes translated as "counties"). Each province is further divided into communes, or municipalities. There are 454 communes, 90 percent of them rural and 10 percent urban, including Oslo, the capital. Government authority is much more centralized in Norway than it is in the United States or other federated nations such as Canada, Australia, or Switzerland. The provincial health officers, for example, are appointed by the central government's Directorate of Health Services.

The Norwegian health system may be analyzed readily according to the five major components described in Chapter 3, starting with its basic organizational structure.

Organizational Structure

The basic organizational structure of the Norwegian health system is relatively simple. The most important functions by far come under the authority of the central government's Ministry of Social Affairs. These include the operation of the Directorate of Health Services and the National Insurance Institute. Certain other health functions are performed by other government agencies. Voluntary (nongovernmental) agencies also contribute to the national health system, as do many commercial and industrial enterprises. Finally, there is a private market in which personal health services are bought and sold.

The official responsibilities of the Directorate of Health Services are very large; they are much broader than the purely preventive services often identified with public health. At the national level, for example, there is a Division of Medical Services, which is responsible for the registration of physicians and certain other personnel and for the indirect supervision of a national network of district doctors. Other divisions are responsible for psychiatric services, dental services, the control of drugs, the planning and approval of hospitals, hygiene (virtually all organized environmental and other preventive services), and so on.

At the provincial level is a provincial health office, whose head is appointed by the national directorate. He is essentially the representative of the Directorate of Health Services in the province. His duties include administration of all basic preventive health services; supervision of the work of the district doctors, who also serve as commune health officers; membership on the provincial hospital board; and various other duties. As a member of the hospital board, he is in a position to see that national standards are being met.

At the commune level, principal health responsibilities are vested in a Commune Health Officer, known widely as the *district doctor.* Legislation going back to 1860 authorized establishment of a Board of Health for each municipality (commune), elected partly from members of the overall Municipal Council and partly from the general community. The local health officer serves as chairman of that board and is expected to carry out policy decisions of the board. From 1945 until 1983, local health officers were appointed by the central Directorate of Health Services, but after 1983 were selected by the elected local board. This constitutes greater self-management of local health affairs, but general public health policies of the central government, transmitted through the provincial health officers, are still followed.

The commune health officer, especially in the extensive rural areas, has a double function: administrative and clinical. As the administrative public health official he is responsible for all local preventive services, including the examination of expectant mothers and small children, immunizations, school health services, and environmental sanitation. In the great majority of communes, which have small populations, the commune health officer also serves as a clinical general medical practitioner—hence the former term *district doctor.* Clinical work takes more than half the doctor's time, and he is paid for it by the health insurance system. For official public health work, he is paid a salary by the municipality, the funds for which come mainly from the province and central government. A community nurse assists in the public health work, and an office nurse in the clinical work. Sometimes the communal health team includes a sanitarian. In larger cities, of course, there are larger and more diversified public health staffs. In large municipalities, a second district doctor may carry out purely clinical work.

The National Insurance Institute, also in the Ministry of Social Affairs, is responsible for various social insurance programs (old-age pensions, unemployment protection, and so forth), including health insurance. Its health insurance functions are carried out through a network of 445 local offices throughout the country. These offices reimburse patients for the cost of ambulatory services (hospital costs are paid directly) and maintain relationships with patients, doctors, and other health care providers.

Among other government agencies with health functions is the Ministry of Labour and Local Affairs; this ministry has a factory inspection service that enforces standards for safety and health protection in the workplace. It also operates facilities for vocational rehabilitation of workers. The Ministry of Church and Education maintains schools for the blind and deaf and, of course, oversees the provision of health education in the public schools. (Personal health services for school children, however, are provided by the public health authorities.) Health services for the military establishment, under the appropriate ministry, are another part of the structure of the Norwegian health system.

Norway has several voluntary health agencies devoted to specific disorders or working in certain local areas. These agencies are fewer in number than in other industrialized countries, but they are larger. Many voluntary health activities, for example, have been consolidated into the large Norwegian Women's Public Health Association (NKS). This organization in 1975 had 1,300 local branches, and it operated 670 facilities. Its program included home care of the chronically ill, rehabilitation of the disabled, care of the mentally retarded, operation of nursing homes, nurses' training, and supplemental feeding for children. NKS members spend little time and effort in raising money, since nearly all costs are met by national government grants. The NKS primarily provides voluntary labor and leadership. With the government subsidy, NKS services are well coordinated with those of the public agencies. The same applies to the Norwegian Red Cross and other voluntary bodies.

Industrial enterprises must also be counted as part of the Norwegian health care structure, insofar as on-the-job health services are provided to workers, particularly in large plants. Private health insurance carriers, which play a large part in the health systems of the United States or Australia, are virtually nonexistent in Norway.

Finally, a private sector for medical care must be included in the structure of Norway's health system. Compared with the United States, and even many welfare-oriented countries, the private market for health services has been quite small in Norway. In the mid-1980s, however, in response to waiting lists for care at major hospitals in Oslo, private practice by specialists increased, along with a few small private hospitals. As a share of the national health system, however, the private sector remains very small. Probably the greatest private sector health service is dental care for adults, which is not covered under social insurance.

Dental services for children are provided under two nationwide public dental programs—the School Dental Service and the Public Dental Service. The school-based program provides complete dental care to school children in the larger cities; it is financed principally by local governments, with about 25 percent subsidy from the national government. This program has operated since 1917, but since 1949, the Public Dental Service has provided larger subsidies (about 60 percent of costs) to provinces (rather than to municipalities) for services to rural children not reached by the school program. In both programs, the care is rendered by full-time salaried dentists.

Adults are theoretically entitled to services in the clinics of the Public Dental Service, but they seldom attend. In 1984, the administration of these two dental programs was integrated.

The national health insurance scheme, as noted, does not finance dental services for adults; thus, both the delivery and financing of this care is in the private health care market. A large share of the work done for adults is prosthetic dentistry, and private dentists earn relatively high incomes.

Drugs approved for health insurance benefits are limited to a few hundred considered essential, especially for the treatment of serious disease and disorders of long duration (such as heart disease, diabetes, or cancer). A small copayment is required for all these prescriptions. Medication not included on the approved list must be purchased entirely in the private market, as would apply to all self-prescribed drugs.

Aside from the recent increase in privately practicing medical specialists, noted earlier, a few such specialists have always practiced privately. The vast majority of specialists, however, are employed on full-time salaries in hospitals. Permission for these specialists to engage in private practice for a few hours a week has been granted occasionally under Conservative governments but is usually prohibited under Labor governments.

The 50 to 60 percent of general practitioners who are not appointed as district doctors are also in private medical practice. Both types of practitioners, however, are still paid fees for their services by the health insurance program, with some copayment by the patient. A small proportion (about 10 percent) of Norwegian hospital beds are in nongovernmental hospitals; even their costs are partially covered by the insurance program.

Production of Health Resources

The resources of Norway's health system are relatively abundant, and they seem to be growing in both quantity and quality.

Health Manpower. Norway has a large supply of doctors, with a doctor-to-population ratio of 203 to 100,000 as of 1981. Nearly all of these are trained by one of the four government-sponsored medical schools, located in the country's four main cities. (These schools and their associated teaching hospitals serve as the base centers for the five principal health service regions into which the country is divided.) Some 40 percent of the physicians are general practitioners (including generalists who have become qualified as "specialized"), and 60 percent are specialists.

The supply of dentists in Norway is particularly great. There was one dentist to 1,177 people in 1981, or 85 dentists per 100,000 population—probably the greatest supply of these professionals found in any country. Explanation of this large supply of dentists cannot be found in any exceptionally high incidence of dental disease. It may be due to the generous government support of dental programs for children and also to the ample private market for dental service for adults (in light of the social insurance protection for other health services). Norway has very few dental hygienists, since their typical functions are performed by dentists.

Professional nurses are also abundant in Norway, with 695 per 100,000 population in 1981, plus an approximately equal ratio of auxiliary nurses. Other allied personnel are not as numerous. There are far fewer pharmacists than in most welfare-oriented countries or in the United States, perhaps because of Norway's rigorous control of imported drugs and the limitation of pharmacies to dispensing drugs (and not the sale of various other products permitted in drugstores of many other countries). Because technicians of all sorts are also less numerous, nurses in Norwegian hospitals are often expected to perform functions done by laboratory or x-ray technicians elsewhere. Social workers are likewise relatively few. Among allied health personnel, physical therapists are conspicuously numerous. They work not only in almost all hospitals, but also in health centers, schools, spas, industrial enterprises, and elsewhere.

Higher education, like elementary education, is state-supported in Norway. The universities that train physicians, dentists, pharmacists, and psychologists are all governmental, supervised by the Ministry of Church and Education. This means that no tuition is charged and qualified students in financial need may receive scholarship support for living expenses. The same applies to nearly all schools for training allied health personnel. The training of nurses is largely hospital-based, although the nursing school administration is ordinarily independent of the hospital.

Considering the great proportion of Norwegian territory that is thinly settled, the geographic distribution of doctors and other health personnel is relatively equitable. Coverage by general practitioners is greatly facilitated by the district doctor scheme (even though some of these posts in the very remote far north are occasionally unfilled). Distribution of specialists is linked to hospital beds, which have been established in a planned relationship to the distribution of population. A certain number of beds for eye diseases, for example, determines the appointment of an ophthalmologist. Even private pharmacies are reasonably well distributed, since new pharmacies are established only where they are needed and barred from localities already well covered; this is accomplished through a requirement that all pharmacies must be registered with the Directorate of Health Services.

Health Facilities. Norway, like other Scandinavian countries, is especially well supplied with hospitals, and they are quite evenly distributed throughout the nation. Counting all types of hospital, in 1981 there were more than 900 facilities with beds, amounting to nearly 15 beds per 1,000 people. About half of these were hospitals for the chronically ill and mental patients, but about 7.0 beds per 1,000 could be classified as general (including hospitals for maternity, cancer, orthopedic disorders, etc.). Most of the hospitals have been built in recent years, and stand out with their very functional architectural design.

The ownership and management of Norwegian hospitals are overwhelmingly governmental, principally at the provincial (county) level. Considering only the general hospitals, for which data are available, government units contain 91 percent of the beds. The public facilities, of course, serve the entire population,

and are not limited to the poor. Hospital services are evidently becoming more intensive in Norwegian hospitals, judging by the average length of patient stay. In 1971 this was about 15 days per patient in general hospitals, which declined to 10 days in 1981. The ratio of nurses per 100 beds increased appreciably over this decade.

Norway's population, like that of most industrialized countries, has a high proportion of aged persons, which means a substantial need for long-term hospitals, skilled nursing care units, and custodial institutions for the aged and chronically ill. This need is well met by hundreds of relatively small facilities throughout the country. Unlike the pattern of private nursing homes in the United States, for example, these units are predominantly owned and operated by local municipalities. About 84 percent of the beds were in such public facilities in 1981. The average capacity of either public or private units was 45 beds. The cost of staying in these long-term care facilities, however, is not borne by the national health insurance. Municipally owned units are financed mainly by local revenues, with some assistance from the province. Care in the nongovernment units (with 16 percent of the beds) is financed by the individual families, with some support from charitable or religious groups.

Another type of health facility is the *health center* built by municipalities for combined public health and ambulatory treatment functions. Because of its growing importance in recent years it is discussed later.

Commodities: Drugs. Norway has private pharmaceutical firms that produce about 25 percent of the drugs needed in the country, and this percentage has been declining. Three-quarters of the drugs consumed are imported from abroad. To control both quality and costs, Norway strictly regulates drugs that may be sold in the country, whether manufactured domestically or imported. Only about 1,100 products may be registered (in 2,000 dosage forms), which is much less than in most industrialized countries. All drug importation is done through a central Norwegian Medicinal Depot.

Drug regulation includes the control of wholesale prices, which are negotiated with manufacturers, and even the control of pharmacy profits by setting maximum retail prices. Of total drug expenditures in 1983, about 60 percent were made by the National Insurance Institute or by government health facilities. To ensure that pharmacies are accessible to people, even in remote and thinly settled regions, a special scheme has been organized to subsidize these units from the profits of pharmacies in lucrative urban centers. Periodic inspection of pharmacies is made by public officials, to ensure that they are complying with standards.

Drug advertising in Norway is also subject to review, whether it is aimed at physicians or at patients. It must be objective and moderate, and must not encourage unnecessary or nonmedical drug consumption.

Knowledge. Norway's production of new scientific knowledge through research has not been very great. It is a small country, and its resources have been devoted essentially to the application and equitable distribution of health knowledge, acquired largely through the world medical literature. Most basic science research conducted in Norway is supported by the Ministry of Cultural and Scientific Affairs. In the 1980s, support for scientific research was strengthened by the establishment of five national research councils. The Council for Science and Humanities is the largest, providing grants to universities, research foundations, and independent laboratories for health-related studies.

In recent years, the Ministry of Social Affairs has tried to stimulate research relevant to health policy problems. This has been done mainly through grants to special institutes, established to determine the most effective and efficient methods of applying medical knowledge. Thus, there is an Institute of Public Health, which does a good deal of health services research on issues such as primary health care or the management of handicapped children. There is an Institute for Hospital Research, devoted to finding ways to improve the efficiency of hospital operation and the rationality of hospital use for patient care. Other national institutes focus on alcoholism, gerontology, and general living conditions for children and adults.

To ensure the application of new knowledge in everyday health service, Norway emphasizes the continuing education of physicians. Special attention is given to general practitioners, who lack the regular stimulation of a hospital setting.

Economic Support

As is true of most Western European countries, Norway has had a long history of social action to simplify and equalize economic access to personal health care. In the early nineteenth century, many local mutual aid societies were organized by workers or the residents of rural communities; among other things, these societies paid for doctors' services. A law enacted in 1911, required every low-income worker to belong to such a society—the concept initiated by Germany in 1883. For most of the population, health insurance coverage remained voluntary until 1952, when legislation required that every wage earner plus dependents must be insured, covering 95 percent of the population. In 1956, health insurance protection in Norway was made universal. All Norwegian residents were thus automatically protected. As is sometimes remarked, what was the sense of having complex administrative procedures, to withhold health care benefits from 5 percent of the population? No separate health programs exist for the poor or the aged, who are simply covered the same way as other residents.

In 1930, the local benefit societies had been converted into branch offices of the National Insurance Institute, a component of the Ministry of Social Affairs. In 1967, the collection of all insurance premiums was centralized, with the money then being allocated to the local branches. In 1971, even this task was integrated with general income tax collection.

The national health insurance scheme supports the great bulk (about 65 percent) of all personal health care costs in Norway. For the first two visits to a doctor, however, the patient customarily had to copay 33 and 20 percent, respectively, of the officially negotiated fee; after that, and for in-hospital care, the patient paid nothing. In the mid-1980s, however, economic constraints led the government to increase the copayments required for ambulatory care—especially for initial consultations. Low-income patients (pensioners, widows, and so on) have no copayment obligations, and no one needs to make copayments for diagnostic tests or physiotherapy ordered by the doctor.

Drugs for about 35 serious chronic diseases are paid for entirely by the insurance, but other drugs (accounting for about 40 percent of drug expenditures) must be purchased privately. Visual refractions for children up to age 15 are covered completely by the insurance, but after this age there are various limitations. Seventy-five percent of hospitalization cost was customarily paid for by the insurance program and 25 percent by the local county government; the patient paid nothing to either the hospital or the doctor. (Around 1976 this fiscal relationship was changed to 50–50.) Even travel costs, beyond a certain minimum, are reimbursed by the insurance system. Dental services for adults, as noted before, are not included in Norway's health insurance benefits.

In addition to these medical services, Norwegian social insurance has long paid "sickness allowances" or cash disability benefits to workers absent due to illness. Payments were equal to 100 percent of gross earned income from the first day of disability; for the first 2 weeks the money came from employers, and after this from the National Insurance Institute. Even self-employed persons were entitled to these benefits, although at a lower rate—at 65 percent of their estimated income after the fifteenth day of disability. These payments could continue for up to 260 days. The relevance of this economic support for nutrition, living conditions, and health maintenance is obvious. Charges of abuse of these generous benefits, however, led to some cutbacks in the 1980s.

Altogether, Norway spent 6.8 percent of its GDP on the health system in 1986, rising from about 3 percent in 1950. Around half of the total expenditures is for hospitalization (including the doctor's inpatient services), nearly all of which comes from public sources. More than 95 percent of overall Norwegian health expenditures come from public sources, compared with about 40 percent in the United States. Of the public sources of health expenditures in Norway, about half come from national social insurance and the balance from general revenues—central, provincial, and local; the trend has been toward an increasing share from general revenues. (Some three-quarters of all these public outlays are for institutional services.) Of the approximately 5 percent of total health expenditures coming from private sources, about half is for the dental care of adults.

Management

Historically, the determination of policy and management of the health system in Norway has been highly centralized. Since the 1960s, however, as greater managerial competence has developed at provincial and also municipal levels, along with a stronger desire for self-determination at the local level, decentralized responsibilities have gradually increased.

Planning of the basic governmental jurisdictions (the 19 provinces and 454 communes), with which all the main components of the health system are linked, is a central responsibility. The national Directorate of Health Services in the Ministry of Social Affairs is also responsible for general health policy, such as the standards for environmental sanitation and the establishment of hospitals. The scope of health services at the provincial and communal levels is also planned by the central Directorate of Health Services.

Within these broad definitions of responsibilities and standards, however, the provincial and communal governments are also expected to formulate health plans. These are necessary to permit preparation of health budgets for capital and operating expenses. Expansion or modification of a hospital, for example, requires planning at the provincial level, and establishment of a health center in a municipality requires planning at that level. Programs of health education on conspicuous health problems require local planning. Organized health services for the elderly and chronically ill, both inside and outside institutions, have demanded much planning at the municipal level, as persons over 65 years have come to exceed 15 percent of the population.

Responsibilities for health system administration are correspondingly shared among the three levels, although the central government has the major policy-making power. The organizational structure of the Directorate of Health Services reflects the range of its authority. Since its reorganization in 1983, it has five large departments:

1. The Primary Health Care Department handles general planning, acute treatment and preventive services, and long-term care and rehabilitation.
2. The Hospital Care Department handles hospital planning, general curative services, and dental care.
3. The Pharmaceutical Department handles all functions related to drug regulation and distribution.
4. The Environmental Health Department handles epidemiology and statistics, general preventive environmental services, and nutrition and food hygiene.
5. The Administrative Department handles financial and personnel matters.

Attached to each of these departments are administrative lawyers to consult on actions the law requires (or restricts).

In each of these five broad fields, the central Directorate of Health Services provides guidance and qualitative standards to the provincial authorities. At the provincial level is an elected County (Provincial) Council, under which is an appointed Health and Social Services Committee. The provincial health director or chief health executive officer (appointed by the Central Ministry) reports to this committee.

These provincial authorities are responsible for the construction and operation of hospitals and other health institutions with in-patients. They also appoint and supervise personnel for medical and surgical specialty services (typically in hospitals), for services in clinical psychology, and for laboratory and radiological services (including those for ambulatory patients). Provincial authorities are also responsible for dental services, both prophylactic and restorative. For all these functions, if full-time salaried health personnel are not available or necessary, the provincial government may contract with appropriate private professionals or voluntary agencies.

To carry out these functions, the provinces receive allotments from the central government on a 50–50 matching basis. Thus, the province must raise from its own taxes an amount equal to the funds available from the top. The magnitude of the central government grant to each province varies with demographic, mortality, and geographic factors, to equalize health resources.

At the most local level, the commune or municipality, the highest authority is the Commune Council, elected by the local citizens. This council appoints a local board of health, chaired by the commune health officer (sometimes called commune medical officer). This physician, as noted earlier, is responsible for both the preventive and therapeutic aspects of primary health care. Public health nurses, who serve patients in their homes, may be engaged directly by the commune or by the commune doctor, under contract. To support the costs of commune health services, the national government and the province give grants, which cover some 75 percent of the costs. The balance must be raised by the commune. It must be recalled that for ordinary medical treatment, the national health insurance scheme pays the commune physician's fees.

Health system regulation is less explicit in Norway than in countries with large private medical sectors. Professional licensure, for example, is very simple. Since all the medical schools are governmental and are supervised by the Ministry of Church and Education, the graduate has only to present proof of his graduation and to meet certain other requirements (such as hospital training and evidence of good character) to be "registered" by the central government. He need not take a second state examination, as in the United States. In nursing and certain other fields, the final examinations in the schools contain questions issued by the national ministry (beyond which the school may include its own questions); registration is automatic upon graduation.

Specialty certification in most European countries is supervised by the Ministry of Health, but Norway entrusts this function to the private Norwegian Medical Association. Requirements for hospital training are by nongovernmental committees of specialists, although the final certification is official.

The major regulation of ambulatory medical care in Norway is through the insurance system. Statistical profiles are usually kept on doctors, so that deviant peformance is readily identified; physicians suspected of rendering excessive or improper service (presumably for monetary gain) are contacted by consultant, or *control doctors,* employed by the local insurance offices. If no satisfactory explanation of the services is offered, the practitioner is ordinarily given a warning; if the unjustified performance continues, he may be penalized by reduced payments or even suspension from the insurance program for a period. Patients may also bring complaints to the insurance agency for investigation. The regulation of drugs in Norway, as noted earlier, is quite rigorous, including consideration of price as well as safety and efficacy.

In Norwegian hospitals, regulation is built into day-to-day work by the general structuring of medical staffs. The use of salaries, rather than fees, eliminates any financial incentive for unjustified surgical operations. Even in the few nonpublic hospitals, where private doctors may serve patients for insurance fees, the highly selective policy of staff appointments and the referral of nearly all patients to specialists by a primary care practitioner seem to protect quality standards. It is small wonder, therefore, that malpractice lawsuits, which have reached crisis proportions in America, are rare in Norway or elsewhere in Europe. Differences in the judicial systems and in the customs of law practice also doubtless play a part, as does the fact that malpractice insurance is typically carried by the medical profession itself (rather than by commerical insurance companies) for small, uniform premiums.

Medical associations in Norway, as in many countries, are expected to monitor the ethical behavior of physicians; the same applies to dentists, pharmacists, and nurses. The offical registration unit in the Directorate of Health Services may take action against a doctor found guilty of unethical behavior, but this is rarely done. The Norwegian Medical Association also handles economic matters, such as the negotiation with government on health insurance fee schedules.

Delivery of Health Services

Both ambulatory care and hospital services are more extensively organized in Norway than in either entrepreneurial or welfare-oriented countries. Perhaps this is the other side of the coin in a health system where, except for the dental care of adults, purely private practice plays a very small part.

Ambulatory Medical Care. The comprehensive role of the commune health or medical officer, combining preventive public health with clinical care functions, has been discussed. As the importance of primary health care has become increasingly appreciated, the number of these official posts has increased. For the 454 communes in Norway in the 1980s, there were about 1,000 commune physicians; all of them are paid a salary for their preventive services, but most of their income is derived from insurance fees. Of course, the establishment of these posts throughout the rural areas helps make medical care accessible to rural people, along with preventive services.

The commune physician is inevitably one of the most educated persons in most rural communities. Therefore, he usually becomes a general community leader in all social matters, not only health services. Since many of these doctors are relatively young, this social role is a source of pride, and helps to attract young medical graduates to primary care. It is noteworthy that, except for a 6-month period during medical training, Norway imposes no mandatory rural service on its medical or other graduates.

Teamwork among groups of general practitioners and various allied health personnel—nurses, physiotherapists, clinical pathologists, and others—is encouraged by a policy of central government grants to municipalities for the construction of health centers. In Oslo, health centers had been built since the early 1970s—mainly in satellite suburbs, where private practitioners would not settle. Later they were built throughout the country. In 1982, the Parliament passed a Municipal Health Act requiring municipalities to assure all residents complete primary health care, preventive and therapeutic. These obligations could be fulfilled by appointing doctors and other personnel to salaried posts or entering into agreements with private practitioners. By either method of remuneration, the national health insurance carried most of the costs.

Salaried posts seem to be increasingly preferred by municipalities, and these typically require the organization of primary health services in health centers. In 1986, it was estimated that outside the main cities of Norway 60 percent of general practitioners worked in government health centers. Even in the cities, where private practice predominated, most GPs worked in small group practice clinics.

Aside from the preventive services provided through health centers and commune health officers, Norway has numerous specialized public health clinics for pregnant women and small children. These are attended by mothers and babies from virtually all families, not solely the poor. The insurance system does not pay fees to doctors for routine examinations, so that at least 90 percent of newborns are examined in these public clinics. Many well-baby clinics are operated entirely by nurses, who summon a physician only for special problem cases.

Other personal preventive services in Norway include medical examinations of school children and first-aid services by school nurses, public clinics for tuberculosis and venereal disease, health education activities, and immunizations. Case detection for noncommunicable, chronic diseases is not promoted as much by public health agencies in Europe as in the United States, mainly because of less confidence in the value of such screening procedures. On the other hand, public health nursing services are very highly developed, with home visits made for bedside care as well as for preventive purposes.

Hospital Care. Norwegian patterns of medical care in hospitals are strikingly different from those in the entrepreneurial health system of the United States or even in the hospitals of several welfare-oriented countries, such as Canada, Belgium, and Japan. With very few exceptions, all medical staffs in Norwegian hospitals—general as well as long-term special facilities—are composed entirely of full-time salaried specialists. Appointments to these hospital posts are made by the provincial hospital boards, but, to ensure quality standards, they must be made from a list of three qualified candidates submitted by the national Directorate of Health Services. Admission to a hospital bed can be made only by a hospital physician; when a general practitioner refers a patient to the hospital, he temporarily "gives up the case," and only the hospital doctor decides whether admission is necessary. (On discharge, a report is supposed to be sent to the referring primary care physician.)

Hospital specialists serve both in-patients and out-patients in a framework that puts the most competent and experienced doctors in supervisory positions. Patients are assigned to doctors whose training and experience are appropriate to the particular case. There is much competition for these hospital posts, and the doctors selected (by the provincial governments that control the hospitals) have great prestige, typically greater than that of private practitioners in general practice. Senior hospital specialists may be permitted to spend a few hours per week in private practice.

Normal childbirths (about 80 percent of the total) are customarily attended in hospitals by trained midwives; obstetricians serve only in complicated cases. Anesthesia is given mainly by nurse-anesthetists, under the supervision of medical anesthesiologists. Each hospital has a medical director, who usually does some clinical work as well, and a full-time business manager. Since the funds for hospital operation come almost entirely from two sources (the insurance program and local government), the business tasks are relatively simple and the management staff is small.

The overall staffing of general hospitals in Norway is relatively modest, at least compared with equivalent institutions in the United

States. A Norwegian short-term general hospital of 400 beds, for example, in 1980 would have about 800 personnel (or 2.0 per occupied bed), including physicians; an equivalent American general hospital would have about 4.0 or 5.0 personnel per occupied bed, not counting attending physicians. In very large Norwegian hospitals (e.g., with 1,000 beds or more), the relative frugality of hospital staffing is even greater.

Norwegian hospital functions are regionalized. The central government's approval is required for the staffing and equipping of all hospital facilities; thus, small rural hospitals are not staffed or equipped to handle complex cases that should be sent to appropriate central hospitals. Hospital budget review is done by the Directorate of Health Services, although the insurance program makes large payments to hospitals. The regionalization, in fact, involves hospitals at three levels: in municipalities for hospitals that can handle relatively simple disorders, at provincial urban centers for more complicated conditions, and at one of the five regional teaching medical centers for the most difficult conditions requiring tertiary care.

All in all, it is clear that Norway's general health care system is highly organized, in both its financial support and its patterns of delivery. It is also continually changing in response to changing conditions. In the 1980s, the rising costs of health service, as in most industrialized countries, became a prominent issue in Norway. To reduce the demands on national revenues, actions were being taken or contemplated to shift a greater share of the costs of medical and hospital service to provincial and local units of government, as well as to private individuals. Such a policy was defended as consistent with the general movement for decentralization in government, stimulated by the pressures for greater responsibilities to be borne at the local level.

GREAT BRITAIN

Much larger in population than Norway or any of the Scandinavian countries is Great Britain. Once the center of a worldwide empire, on whose colonies "the sun never set," Great Britain has perhaps had a greater cultural influence globally than any other single country. For this reason, the British health system has attracted widespread attention for many years. Especially after World War II, when a radical transformation in the organization of the system was launched—the British National Health Service, as it was called—Britain became in many ways a health model for the entire world. In 1984, Great Britain had a population of 56,400,000 (in England, Wales, Scotland, and Northern Ireland) and a GNP per capita of $8,570, actually among the lowest in Western Europe.

Rather than attempting to describe every facet of the British system, we could more profitably trace the historic development of the National Health Service (NHS) and some of its recent problems. Its very structure and the evolution of its component parts have helped elucidate the structure and functions of health systems, in general. Moreover, the course of development of the British health system over the last century or more may clarify much of the political dynamics that determine the evolution of health systems in many countries.

To understand the British NHS and its several organizational changes, one must appreciate that it did not arise de novo in 1948. Its origins date back more than a century before.

Health Insurance for Workers

As in all of Europe, trade unions, fraternal associations, and "friendly societies" had been providing sickness and medical care insurance since the early nineteenth century. Germany and several other central European countries had made enrollment in such protective bodies compulsory since the 1880s, and that influence was bound to be felt in other Western European countries and the British Isles. In the 1840s, upper-class employers had encouraged and assisted the mutual aid societies as a means of getting low-paid workers to look after themselves when they were sick; otherwise, they would have become the objects of charity and a burden on the church or local public revenues.

The first National Health Insurance Act was passed by the British Parliament in 1911, under the moderate political leadership of the Liberal Party's Lloyd George. Only the doctors opposed the idea, favoring (as in some countries today) continuation of the voluntary health insurance programs for the self-supporting, coupled with a strengthened public medical service for the very poor.

The 1911 act required certain insurance protection to meet the costs of ambulatory medical care and wage loss during sickness for all manual workers earning less than 160 pounds (about $780 U.S.) per year. Although membership in an approved society was not specifically mandated, all but a small percentage of workers met the law's requirements through such membership. The worker's dependents did not have to be insured but could purchase protection voluntarily through the same mutual aid societies or other insurance carriers. Payment of insurance contributions was required from both workers and employers, and the government provided funds for the support of administration and the coverage of very low-income or indigent persons. The benefits were limited to the services of general practitioners (GPs) and prescribed drugs. Specialization was, in any event, not highly developed at the time. If the GP thought his patient required a specialist, the case could be referred to a hospital out-patient department, where such services were free. Hospitalization was not insured under the law, since open ward service in most public hospitals and some large voluntary ones was provided anyway through local government support or charity. If specialist care in a private office was desired, it had to be obtained privately. Dental or other special services were not covered at all.

Under the original law, GPs were not paid for their services directly by the approved societies, but rather by insurance committees set up by statute in each county or county borough; these committees had to contain a majority of elected representatives of insured workers, with the balance representing the local doctors, local government, and the health authorities. The approved societies were responsible for the enrollment of workers and for the payment of cash disability benefits, but not

for the basic medical and pharmaceutical services; if they accumulated surplus funds, these could finance supplemental benefits, such as part of hospitalization costs.

Under the law, the doctors in each insurance committee area could decide how they wished to be paid—on the basis of attendance (fee-for-service), capitation (according to the number of persons who chose to be on each doctor's list), or a combination of the two. It is not always understood that the British doctors themselves increasingly chose the straight capitation method; by 1927, this pattern had become universal. Capitation was preferred because it involved less red tape and was least subject to competitive abuse among the insurance doctors in each area. It was only later, with the NHS, that capitation remuneration of GPs became mandatory.

Approved societies could sell insurance for other benefits, such as dental care, or for voluntary medical coverage of persons who did not come under the social insurance law, such as dependents or employees with higher incomes. Many approved societies had been set up by commercial insurance companies as nonprofit subsidiaries, and they enrolled several million persons on a voluntary basis; attendance by specialists in hospitals might be covered. GP services in small private hospitals (often called *nursing homes*) were also sometimes covered, especially for maternity cases and relatively simple surgery.

A study in 1923 showed that the average insured person in Great Britain received 3.5 attendances per year. At about the same time (1928–1931), the Committee on the Costs of Medical Care showed that at average person of equivalent income in the United States without insurance was receiving 2.2 physician services per year. Thus, the British doctor gave 50 percent more service under capitation insurance arrangements than did the U.S. doctor, who was paid fees for each service by noninsured patients.

Prelude to the National Health Service

Over the years, the income threshold for mandatory insurance coverage in Great Britain was gradually elevated, covering more workers. Additional persons and benefits were also insured on a voluntary basis. By 1935, the qualifying income was 250 pounds (about $1,250) per year or less, which included about 15 million workers. With a total British population at the time of some 40 million, this meant mandatory health insurance for about 37.5 percent of the population. The number of dependents and others with voluntary health insurance coverage was not clear, though it was doubtless in the millions.

On the eve of World War II, however, the health insurance protection of the British population was obviously far from complete, as to both persons covered and benefits provided. It was not surprising, therefore, that during the war—among whose goals was "freedom from want"—an Inter-Departmental Committee on Social Insurance and Allied Services was set up under the chairmanship of Sir William Beveridge to "survey the existing national schemes of social insurance and allied services . . . and to make recommendations." In late 1942, under Winston Churchill's Conservative government, the famous Beveridge Report was issued.

This classic document explored the deficiencies and need for expansion of all the branches of social insurance, including old-age pensions, unemployment benefits, and disability benefits, as well as health services. Regarding the latter, in summary the Plan for Social Security recommended the following:

> Medical treatment covering all requirements will be provided for all citizens by a national health service organized under the health departments (of England and Wales, Scotland, and Northern Ireland), and post medical rehabilitation treatment will be provided for all persons capable of profiting by it.

The Beveridge Report further elaborated on this goal:

> A comprehensive national health service will ensure that for every citizen there is available whatever medical treatment he requires, in whatever form he requires it, domiciliary or institutional, general, specialist, or consultant, and will ensure also the provision of dental, ophthalmic and surgical appliances, nursing and midwifery and rehabilitation after accidents.

The report explicitly avoided discussion of "the problems of organisation of such a service" as falling outside of its scope.

These were the objectives recommended under a wartime British Conservative Party government in 1942. It remained for a Labour Party government, elected after the war, to implement them through the National Health Service Act in 1946. Allowing a tooling-up period of almost 2 years, the act took effect in July 1948.

As with any sweeping social legislation, debate was intense in the period between the introduction of draft legislation and enactment of the final law. The Minister of Health was Aneurin Bevan, a rugged Welsh former coal miner, who soon found himself at loggerheads with the British Medical Association. The association, anticipating the postwar mood, had set up its own medical planning commission, which had recommended achievement of the Beveridge goals by extending the existing national health insurance to cover higher-income persons, providing government grants to voluntary hospitals to enable them better to serve the poor, and retaining the private medical market for many higher-income persons. Bevan's bill, on the other hand, would not only cover all residents of the nation for comprehensive services, but would have provided a basic salary for all GPs (to be supplemented by capitation payments) and a network of health centers from which both preventive services of local health authorities and primary services of GPs would be furnished—as the Dawson Report proposed in 1920. Moreover, all beds in public hospitals would be solely for NHS patients; specialists could continue private practice on a part-time or full-time basis, but they would have to hospitalize their patients solely in private institutions.

In the ensuing debate, which involved a threat to strike by the doctors, many compromises were naturally made by both sides. Universal population coverage was retained, but basic salaries, which GPs had opposed for fear they would gradually be extended to full government employment, were abandoned. Public hospitals were authorized to maintain about 5 percent of their beds for the private patients of consultants. The network of health centers was not to be established, except for a few experimental facilities. On the other hand, financing was to be derived mainly from general revenues, and only a small fraction from social insurance contributions. Top authority was vested in the Ministry of Health, and nearly all hospital beds were put under the control of the national government.

The most important compromises—or perhaps adjustments to the forces at play would be more accurate—in defining the administrative lines of the National Health Service were in the design of its tripartite structure. The embodiment of historical forces and relationships in the planning and design of future programs is very strikingly illustrated in the original overall structure of the British NHS. It was clear, however, that the program would institute a quantum leap from the former limited health insurance for low-paid workers. The entire population would be covered, the services would be comprehensive, and the financial support would not depend on insurance— hence a National Health *Service.*

Organization of the National Health Service

Past developments in Britain up to 1948 had given rise in the health services to several principal sets of vested interests: (1) the general practitioners, (2) the community hospitals with their staffs of specialists, (3) the medical-school affiliated teaching hospitals, and (4) the local public health authorities. Achieving an operational program, adapted suitably to these distinct clusters of power, required an administrative structure in which each of these groupings retained substantial sovereignties. Coordination among the interests, for the sake of good patient care and efficiency, was a secondary consideration, to be tackled deliberately only later.

Ambulatory Services and Executive Councils. The first interest group, general practitioners,

was already represented, and its remuneration handled, by the insurance committees operating since 1911 under the National Health Insurance Act. These committees generally had subcommittees for prescribed drugs. It was a relatively smooth transition, under the NHS, to establish a network of executive councils— 138 of them in England and Wales—that would assume the functions of the former insurance committees; in the new program, these functions would be broadened to administer services for the total population and also to handle dental care and optical services.

The average executive council administered these ambulatory services for about 350,000 people, although the range was highly variable; one council for part of London covered 3 million people. Most important were the council's responsibilities for capitation payments to and monitoring of the GPs. Each month the GP was paid a fixed amount for every person on his list, whether or not the person used the services. The person could change to another GP at any time, whereupon his or her name would be transferred to the other doctor's list. To protect quality, the maximum number of persons permitted on a GP's list was 3,500, although in the 1970s the average was about 2,200. Furthermore, the rate of capitation payment depended on a slightly descending scale, to discourage excessively long lists. In many ways, the GP, or family doctor, as the primary point of entry into the service, underwent many changes in his mode of work, as we discuss later.

Also part of the responsibility of the executive councils were the dental services. Unlike the GPs, dentists were paid on a fee-for-service basis, but not all procedures were covered by the NHS. For partial dentures, bridgework, crowns, and certain other prostheses, the patient had to pay extra fees personally, although complete dentures were fully covered. The supply of dentists in Great Britain, as in most of Europe, was relatively low in relation to the needs; the demands for care were high, and dentists' incomes in the early years of the NHS were greater than those of the GPs. (Later, adjustments in GP remuneration changed this.) Priority was accorded to children through a free, public dental service, furnished by salaried dentists under the local health authorities.

Prescribed drugs, obtained at local chemist's shops or pharmacies, were another benefit administered by the executive councils. At first, these were entirely covered through NHS fees, calculated by a formula (accounting for the wholesale drug cost, overhead, dispensing service, and so on), paid to the pharmacist. When the Conservatives were returned to power in 1952, they imposed a copayment charge of 1 shilling ($0.14 U.S.) on each prescription, and later this was raised to 2 shillings. With the generally rising consumption of drugs and higher costs per item, certain constraints were introduced around 1960. The Ministry of Health issued a "recommended list," and doctors could order products not on it only if they were specifically justified; otherwise, the patient had to pay the full cost. The deterrent effect of copayments was transitory, and when the Labour Party was reelected these charges were dropped. All the while, over-the-counter products remained available to the British people, at their personal expense, and great quantities were purchased. With advertising and old wives' tales, self-medication did not disappear, even under a publicly financed health service program.

Finally, the executive councils were responsible for optical services. These included vision examinations by prescribing opticians (the equivalent of optometrists elsewhere) and eyeglasses furnished by dispensing opticians. Fees for standard frames were paid by the councils, but the patient was charged extra for unusual fancy frames. Hearing aids, prosthetic limbs, wigs (when medically ordered), and other special medical devices were further benefits.

Regional Hospital and Specialist Services. The second major pillar of the NHS structure was a network of regional hospital boards (RHBs)—15 of them covering England and Wales. Just as the executive councils had evolved from the former insurance committees, the RHBs had antecedents, though more recent, in the system of emergency services set up during World War II, when Britain was being bombed. The wartime experience obviously educated British hospitals about the feasibility of communications and teamwork among institutions in a region.

For some years before the war, British gen-eral hospitals had been confronted with financial difficulties. The public hospitals, depending mainly on local revenue for support, were chronically underfinanced. The voluntary hospitals, despite the long and distinguished traditions of many of them, were likewise hard pressed by the dwindling of charitable contributions and the difficulty of private patients to meet the ever-rising charges. When the Minister of Health took over control of all but a handful (mainly religious) of British hospitals in 1948, therefore, there were no significant objections. With nationalization, the government acquired all of the property of the hospitals and assumed all their debts and obligations. Overnight, Britain's 2,700 hospitals, with some 480,000 beds (about 80 percent municipal), attained financial stability. The nationalization included all mental, tuberculosis, and other chronic disease facilities, as well as the general hospitals, but it did not include old people's homes or convalescent facilities.

The hospital regions were mapped out to contain about 2 million to 3 million people each, and roughly 30,000 hospital beds of all types. The regional hospital boards were appointed by the minister to represent the general population, the medical profession, and the former hospital owners or sponsors. To actually administer the hospitals, the RHB appointed hospital management committees, which were typically responsible for institutions containing a total of between 1,000 and 2,000 beds; this might mean two or three large facilities or as many as 15 or 20 small ones. The funds for both operation and capital costs of all hospitals in a region were allotted by the central government to the RHB, which in turn distributed them to the management committees. Because of Britain's postwar financial difficulties and competing obligations for housing construction, schools, roads, military purposes, and so on, no new hospital construction was undertaken for many years, and capital expenditures went almost entirely for renovating the old structures. As a result, many observers comment on the antiquated physical features of most British hospitals; the dedication of their staffs and the efficiency of their operations, however, have been equally noteworthy.

British specialists in all fields of medicine and surgery are attached mainly to the hospitals. Leaving aside the younger doctors in training (registrars, junior registrars, and so on) about 60 percent are on full-time salaries, and 40 percent spend part of their time (typically 20 to 30 percent) in outside private practice. General practitioners, however, who constitute about half of Britain's doctors, seldom have hospital appointments under the NHS, nor did they have such appointments before. In other words, the GP refers the patient requiring hospitalization (except in emergencies) to a hospital out-patient department, where the examining specialist decides if he or she should be admitted. Sometimes the patient is referred to the hospital out-patient department simply for a diagnostic workup. In either case, whether the patient is admitted to a bed or not, a report is sent back to the referring physician on the specialist's findings.

This separation of community general practice from the hospital has been the subject of criticism from doctors accustomed to "open staff" hospitals. Though it means the community GP is deprived of the stimulation of hospital experience and is temporarily separated from his patient, it also ensures technically high quality service within the hospital walls. Moreover, under the NHS the GP was brought closer to the hospital through direct access to the hospital's laboratory and x-ray services for diagnostic tests (without necessarily sending his patient through the out-patient department), the chance to participate in the hospital's educational programs, and sometimes an appointment to work in the out-patient department or other sections of the institution.

Initially, the salaries of specialists in hospitals were much higher than the earnings of community doctors in general practice. Then in the 1970s, as the importance of good primary health care became better appreciated, and the capitation payments to GPs were raised; additional fees were paid also for preventive services, house calls, and special procedures. Annual GP earnings became similar to those of full-time hospital consultants.

Specialists and consultants (the highest rank) were appointed by the regional hospital boards, and competition has always been great for these positions. When an opening occurs, it

is widely advertised in the medical journals, and the specialist appointed usually acquires permanent tenure. Those not appointed may be frustrated and must face the decision of going into general practice or emigrating. (Some of the ex-British doctors in North America, who denigrate the NHS, are those who failed to win a specialist appointment.) Periodically, specialist salaries are raised, with increased tenure or responsibility, and merit awards are granted for outstanding performance. Thus, the most prestigious and coveted positions in Britain's NHS are those offering salaried hospital employment.

The Teaching Hospitals. Usually associated with a long tradition and exceptionally qualified medical staffs, teaching hospitals in England and Wales objected to coming under the control of regional hospital boards. All 36 of them (26 in London) each with its board of governors, were therefore made directly responsible to the Minister of Health. The teaching hospitals in Scotland, however, were integrated into their respective RHBs. (In the reorganization of 1974, this integration was achieved nationwide.)

Medical education, invariably associated with a teaching hospital falls simultaneously under the wing of a university. As in most of the world, medical students in Great Britain take a continuous 6-year course. Contrary to some forebodings, after the NHS was initiated the volume of applicants to British medical schools did not decline but rose. The majority of medical and other health science students are supported by government scholarships.

Local Health Authorities. The fourth major branch of the British NHS was the network of local health authorities—146 in England and Wales. These were responsible for traditional preventive public health services and several other activities as well. While the NHS withdrew from local authorities their responsibilities for public hospitals (which, in a sense, weakened their role), it assigned them new functions for ambulance transport, visiting nurse services (bedside care at home, which had been traditionally offered by voluntary agencies), homemaker care for the chronically ill, and the operation of long-term facilities for the aged or chronically ill who did not need hospitalization.

Preventive services had long emphasized maternal and child health. The vast majority of pregnant women and infants in Great Britain have been periodically checked by health department clinics. This applies to all social classes, not only lower-income families. One must recall that the GP, being paid on a capitation basis, is happy to have his patients so attended; he loses no fee, it saves him time, and the mother and child are seen by experts in this preventive work. At the child welfare stations, as they are called, infants and small children receive all necessary immunizations, and the mothers are advised on child-rearing practices. Sick children are referred back to their GP. To lighten the load on these health department clinics and promote integrated care, in later years GPs were offered supplementary fees for immunizations and certain other preventive services.

Local health authorities also conducted special clinics for tuberculosis and venereal diseases. Health services for schoolchildren were still financed by the educational authorities, but the local medical officer of health in most jurisdictions was also appointed school health officer. Environmental sanitation has been another major responsibility of the local health authorities. In the water supply and sewage disposal schemes of Britain, which are often quite antiquated, close surveillance is necessary. Housing inspections to enforce minimum standards were another responsibility of the local medical officer and his sanitation staff, and these duties occupied a good deal of time.

Other Special Services. Separate large hospitals for the mentally ill and retarded had evolved in Great Britain, as in most of the world, but with the NHS they were brought under the supervision of the regional hospital boards, along with other hospitals. Commitment to a mental hospital was changed from a judicial to a medical procedure. The vast majority of admissions became voluntary, and in the minority that were mandatory, two doctors (one of whom had to be a psychiatrist) were required for certification, rather than a court of law. After admission, the patient was entitled to a judicial review, but most mandatory admissions were later converted to informal ones. Increasing emphasis was placed on community care for mental illness—through mental health clinics of many types under the local authorities, mental sections in general hospitals, day care centers, and a variety of other special arrangements. The average length of stay in mental hospitals, as well as the total census, greatly declined in the 1950s and 1960s.

Worker's compensation for on-the-job injuries was also modified under the NHS. The payment of cash benefits for wage loss, financed solely by employers, was continued as before, under the social security system. All medical services, however, were simply integrated with and provided by the NHS. Since medical care for all illness was fully covered, there was no reason to attribute a worker's symptoms to an employment-related cause to gain financial protection. Great emphasis was put on rehabilitation, and a special center was developed to treat those few workers, often called malingerers, whose disability was mainly psychosomatic.

Medical inspection of factories for safety and occupational disease hazards was one of the few health-related activities not integrated into the NHS; it was retained as a function of the Department of Labour. First aid in the factories, preplacement examination of workers, safety standards, and the like were enforced through periodic factory inspections, and these imposed a responsibility on industrial management. Medical treatment of sick or injured workers, of course, was through the NHS.

Public assistance for the poor, in its financial aspects, was administered by welfare authorities, but medical care was provided through all the normal procedures of the NHS. No special enrollment or identification of the recipients of public aid was necessary. Likewise, any visitor to Great Britain who became ill or injured was treated by the resources of the NHS, exactly as the police force would be expected to protect a visitor against crime.

These were the main organizational features of the NHS as it was set up in 1948; they were attainable only through the assumption of substantial financial responsibility by the Exchequer, or general treasury of the nation. Because contributions by employer and worker to the old national health insurance had become customary, however, and because the Social Security fund was set up to cover many other cash benefits (old-age pensions, unemployment compensation, disability allowances, and so forth), a share of these funds was assigned to help support the NHS, along with monies from certain other sources.

Economic Support

The intention of the NHS legislation of 1946 was to convert health service from a predominantly market commodity, purchased by individuals and families, to a basic social entitlement of everyone, financed principally from public sources. Although the amount of this public support may fall short of total needs, the intention has been substantially achieved.

The exact proportions of NHS funds derived from different sources were not identical over the years. At the time of the NHS reorganization, discussed later, the funds for running the NHS (both capital and operating expenditures) were derived from sources shown in Table 7.1. Clearly the overwhelming bulk of support has come from the general exchequer or treasury of the nation. In fact, this source is even greater than shown, since a major part of the funds attributed to local authorities actually comes from national grants to those bodies. Patient payments included charges for prescribed drugs, prosthetic dental services, private beds in NHS hospitals, special spectacles, and other miscellaneous purposes.

Altogether in 1982 the British population spent about 510 dollars (U.S.) per capita in the entire health system; this included a relatively small amount spent outside the NHS for private care or self-medication. This amounted to about 5.9 percent of gross domestic product, which may be compared with 10.1 percent in the United States for that year. Since the GDP in the United States was much higher than the British, the American expenditure per capita in 1982 was $1,390, or 2.7 times greater than the British. The remarkable fact is that the

Table 7.1. British National Health Service: Sources of Financing, 1974–1975

Source	Percentage
Central government	78.75
Local authorities (including national grants)	12.25
Social insurance (workers + employers)	4.75
Patient payments	4.00
Others	0.25
All sources	100.00

Source: Levitt, Ruth. *The Reorganized National Health Service.* London: Croom Helm, 1976, p. 170.

British NHS can provide so much health service to its entire population for so modest a percentage of its national wealth. But difficulties have resulted from these frugal expenditures, which we discuss later.

Trends in Services

Patient–physician contacts in the NHS have, of course, risen over the years, but at a relatively slow rate. With Britain's modest expenditures on the health system, the supply of both general practitioners and specialists has increased only slowly. In 1985, Great Britain had 147 physicians per 100,000 which was fewer than the supply in any other European country, east or west. In-patient hospital care was likewise lower than in any other European country, except Denmark, at 2,400 days per 1,000 persons annually.

A propos of services, it is significant that the rate of elective surgery in Great Britain has been much lower than in the United States. It has been pointed out that the ratio of surgeons to population in England and Wales is about half that in the United States, and the rate of elective surgery is correspondingly about half. There can be little doubt that this finding relates to the methods of paying surgeons in the two countries: high fees for each operation in the United States and fixed salaries based on merit in Great Britain. The abundance of unnecessary surgery in the United States has been frequently demonstrated, but it is arguable whether there is too little surgery in Britain. Long waiting lists for elective surgery also dramatize the shortage of beds in Britain, which generated a significant private hospital sector in the 1980s.

The rise in services and corresponding expenditures, after the NHS had been operating for 10 years, aroused political concern, resulting in the Guillebaud investigation. The surprise finding was that, though absolute expenditures had risen over the decade, the outlay for health as a percentage of the GNP had actually declined, from 3.9 percent in 1947–1950 to 3.6 percent in 1958–1959. By 1982, as we have noted, this proportion had risen to 5.9 percent (of gross domestic product), although the comparable percentages were much higher in every other West European country.

The low ceiling on British health expenditures has been attributed to the unitary source of funds, in contrast to the multiple sources in most other countries. Yet, with the aging of the population, advances in technology, and the people's mounting confidence in medical science, demands for health care are clearly increasing every year. In the 1980s, political constraint on expenditures in the public sector led to enlargement of the private sector in the British health system.

Trends in the NHS over the years have involved many developments besides overall health services and money. As in all industrialized nations, the relative importance of hospitals has increased in tandem with the expansion of medical and surgical specialization. As a reflection of this, the expenditures for hospital care in the NHS rose from 55.7 percent of the total in 1951–1952 to 62.6 percent in 1970–1971. In the face of tight caps on new hospital construction, this has meant increased crowding of ancient hospital buildings.

Probably more significant are the major changes occurring in British community general practice. At the time the NHS was enacted, most GPs held forth in their private one-man surgeries. The Ministry of Health, however, gave financial inducements to medical grouping. The quality of isolated general practice had been criticized in several studies, and it was believed that group practice could upgrade it; engaging office assistants to do many simple tasks would be more feasible, and a team of doctors would facilitate consultation and general professional stimulation. Government policy was successful, and the grouping of GPs increased steadily. By 1970, more than

65 percent were in offices of two or more and most in groups of three or more. In such settings, each practitioner would usually develop skills in some special aspect of general practice, such as child care, minor surgery, gynecological problems, emotional difficulties, and the like. Furthermore, to help form a "primary health care team," many local authorities assigned to group practices public health (district) nurses to visit patient homes at local government expense.

Another government objective was to improve the geographic distribution of doctors. This was done principally through a ban against settlement of new graduates in areas designated as "overdoctored" (for purposes of payment under the NHS); the result, of course, was to channel physicians to areas where they were needed. The British population in underdoctored areas was reduced from about 50 percent in 1948 to 20 percent in 1963. Moreover, the sale of medical practices—a traditional custom in Britain, through which a retiring doctor acquired money to live on—was prohibited and replaced with a social insurance pension scheme for doctors. Accordingly, the high price of buying a practice no longer inhibited the young doctor from spending money on modern medical equipment.

Improvement in the quality of general practice was also encouraged by government grants for engagement of allied health personnel, higher capitation payments for aged patients, supplemental fees for various office procedures and for house calls, and other methods. There was a serious pay dispute between GPs and the government in 1965, resulting in a major boost in their earnings and making the whole field of general practice more attractive. By 1970, nearly half of GP incomes came from the various special fees and grants rather than capitation. A Royal College of General Practitioners endowed specialist status to general practice, and this was associated with an intensified program of continuing education and establishment of professorial chairs for general practice in the medical schools.

Perhaps the most significant trend affecting general practice, indeed all ambulatory health care in the NHS, has been the movement that started about 1965 to establish health centers.

As noted earlier, such centers figured prominently in the early planning of the system, but it could not be implemented except in a few experimental projects. In the mid-1960s, first in connection with the development of "new towns" and later in most large cities, buildings were constructed or redesigned to accommodate groups of GPs, complemented by public health nurses, social workers, practice nurses, sometimes laboratory technicians, psychologists, dieticians, clerks, or other allied health personnel. Usually built by local health authorities, the quarters were rented by GPs who had regular lists of patients, but most of the ancillary personnel were furnished at local government expense.

By 1971, 475 such health centers were operating or under construction, housing about 1,500 GPs with space available for about 1,000 more. The centers in full operation had an average of five or six GPs, and these doctors tended naturally to consult with each other, cover the practices of colleagues who were away, and make much greater use of the allied health workers than they would have if these personnel were stationed in the traditional health department. By 1978, in England alone there were 815 health centers, accommodating some 20 percent of the English general practitioners.

Some Consequences and Problems

The first 25 years of the NHS after 1948 can be seen as a prelude to its reorganization in 1974. What were some of the general consequences and problems that led to this restructuring?

Among the population as a whole, the NHS was probably the most popular program that had been launched by any political party. A British Gallup opinion poll in 1964 found 89 percent of the population generally satisfied with the NHS. In 1967, a survey by another organization found that 95 percent of the people approved; of these, 60 percent rated the service as very good or excellent.

Large bureaucratic structures like the NHS are often charged with discouraging local initiative and any incentive for volunteer work to strengthen the program. Yet British voluntary agencies did not decline. Hospital administrators pointed out that their committees of volunteer workers were as busy as ever. However, they devoted their energies to helping the patients and lightening the work of the staff instead of spending time on fundraising as they had in the past.

The charge of "deadly uniformity," often leveled against large governmental systems, does not stand up to scrutiny in the British setting. The diversity of hospitals and health departments in Britain is striking. Though each hospital is administered by a sort of trio—the hospital secretary (or administrator), the matron (or director of nurses), and medical chief—who must work closely together, countless variations in style and emphasis exist among the different hospital services and departments. There is plenty of room for innovation, as long as minimum standards are met.

In terms of resources generated by the NHS, the effect has clearly been to yield an increased supply of physicians—from about 105 per 100,000 people in 1948 to 120 per 100,000 in 1968 and 152 per 100,000 in 1977. The availability of about 25,000 midwives for obstetrical services (both inside and outside hospitals) must be noted if one is to compare this supply with the U.S. ratio of 168 doctors per 100,000 in 1976. Medical incomes, meanwhile, for both GPs and specialists, have risen substantially, and doctors' incomes now fall in the upper 2 or 3 percent of the British income scale.

The general hospital-bed-to-population ratio has not increased significantly in Britain, but since lengths of stay have steadily shortened, rates of admission have arisen. They rose from about 67 admisions per 1,000 annually in 1949 to 92 in 1960 and to about 110 in 1970. This rate is associated with greater use of hospital out-patient departments, admission of more serious cases (clearly in need of hospital care), and a much lower rate of elective surgery in Great Britain than in the United States. Waiting lists for hospital treatment of some elective conditions are still difficult, but there is no problem with admission of emergency cases.

One of the best reflections of the general adequacy of the NHS was the relatively small percentage of people seeking care through private arrangements before 1974. Voluntary health insurance schemes to finance private care have been free to operate, and although they were intensely promoted by private carriers, by 1969 enrollment had grown to only 883,000, or less than 2 percent of the population. In fact, between 1965 and 1967, the rate of disenrollment exceeded that of new enrollments. Fewer than 5 percent of NHS beds were reserved for private patients, but in the 1970s this arrangement for "breaking the queue" with affluence was intensely debated in Labour Party circles. In any event, it seems that few patients were displeased with the limitations of the NHS to the point of paying for private medical care.

Despite this generally favorable picture of achievements, the NHS was not without problems. There were controversies concerning medical remuneration; constraints on the construction of new hospital beds have resulted in waiting lists for elective conditions; some patients complained about the brevity of their visits to the GP; and costs have risen (although more slowly than in other countries). Nevertheless, the basic concepts of the NHS—a strong primary doctor providing convenient entry to the system and overseeing his patient's use of qualified specialists and hospital services, a preventive program, and several other features—have remained a basis of pride for its architects.

If any feature of the NHS was continually vexing to the responsible authorities, it was the persistently segmented administrative model. A pregnant mother, for example, would get prenatal care from a local health authority clinic, treatment of illness from her GP, and delivery of the baby by a hospital midwife. Patient care was similarly fragmented for children, many chronic disease patients of all age groups, those with mental disorders, and other cases. Moreover, economic trends in the NHS showed a gradual escalation of the resources allotted to the hospital services, while primary care made only modest progress through GP group practices and health centers.

Since its beginning in 1948, the NHS had

various coordinating committees attempting to integrate activities among the executive councils, regional hospital boards, local health authorities, and the teaching hospital boards of governors. Some overlapping of board or committee memberships was designed for the same purpose. As early as 1962, the Porritt Committee, under the British Medical Association, had advocated unification of all the vertical components at the local community level. Politically, however, in light of the several pressures responsible for the original divided structure, the time did not seem ripe. Not until 1968 did the national government, then under the Labour Party, issue its first green paper (for discussion) advocating integration; it proposed merging the three main sectors of the service at the local level, through 40 to 50 *area health authorities.*

Responses were quick, and the proposal was criticized as still vesting responsibility too remotely from the local areas, while not making adequate provision for larger regional planning. A Conservative government was elected in 1970, and a second green paper was issued in 1971, responding to the criticisms of the first. Then a government white paper laid out the party's final official plans.

The NHS Reorganization of 1974

Even the careful planning of two green papers and one white paper, to solicit reactions and permit refinement of strategies, could not anticipate all developments. The reorganization was to occur essentially in two stages—establishment first of *area health authorities* and then of *health districts.* Also, larger political forces were to lead to the enhancement of a private sector in the overall British health system.

Area Health Authorities. In recognition of demands for greater local controls, 90 area health authorities (AHAs) were contemplated, with a second tier (largely for planning purposes) of 14 regional health (not hospital) authorities. The AHAs would range in size from 250,000 to 1,500,000 people and would be congruent with (but independent of) simultaneously reorganized general local government bodies. The regional health authorities would have from 1 million to 5 million population; thus, each regional authority would contain from one to 11 AHAs, and usually more than 3. The larger AHAs would be further subdivided into districts of about 250,000 population—or the catchment area of a district general hospital. The law putting this general plan into action took effect 1 April 1974.

The reorganization still took account of past realities. The AHA is responsible for all types of service—ambulatory, hospital, and preventive—within its borders, but it would be advised by a family practitioner committee, the successor to the executive council. The AHAs took over the functions of the former hospital management committees, and the regional authorities took over the responsibilities of the regional hospital boards (planning the construction of facilities). The teaching hospitals were absorbed into the system, but they got especially strong representation on the AHA boards in their areas. The school health services, formerly controlled by educational officials, were also made a responsibility of the AHAs. Only the industrial health services remained separate.

Nonmedical representation on governing bodies, although its meaning is debated, was to be somewhat greater than before. A majority of members of AHA boards are not health professionals, but in the interests of improving efficiency, they are required to have managerial experience. Each area health authority is staffed by an AHA administrative team, consisting of an area administrator, an area treasurer, an area nursing officer, and an area medical officer.

The area medical officer is a new type of medical leader—a *community medicine specialist,* who replaces the old medical officer of health. His duties are not only to administer the preventive services (communicable disease control, environmental hygiene, etc.), but also to consult with the AHA and evaluate the efficacy and efficiency of all health services in local hospitals and doctors' offices. He is expected to provide health education to the people and epidemiological information to the doctors. He is to offer planning guidance to

other local government authorities, particularly in education and social services, as well as to voluntary bodies.

Consumer representation would be ensured through community health councils at the health district level within the AHAs. These councils are to advise the district management team, composed of the community medicine specialist, a district nurse, a chief administrator, and two clinicians (a GP and a specialist), elected by their peers. An ombudsman, called the health services commissioner, is to be employed specifically to hear patient complaints.

Local health centers were expected to continue to be built and, along with extension of group practices, to provide a setting for linking district public health nursing, social work, and other local government personnel with the GPs. Indeed, to some observers the overriding objective of the NHS reorganization was to enhance the importance of the ambulatory and primary care services as a reaction against the growing role assumed by hospitals. The elevated status and strengthened educational support for general practice, with the same objective, were noted earlier.

To other observers, the major purpose of the NHS reorganization was to achieve greater managerial efficiency. A single hierarchy of authorities—from health districts, to area health authorities, to regional health authorities, up to the central Ministry of Health—was deemed more efficient and administratively economical than three or four separate vertical bureaucracies. Strengthened administrative responsibilities at the local level through AHAs, staffed by teams with area administrators, community medicine specialists and others—with backup by various advisory committees of both providers (family practitioner committees) and consumers (community health councils)—would presumably ensure more effective execution of policies formulated at the national level.

Health Districts. In the late 1970s, a great deal of attention was paid to the uneven distribution of resources (doctors, hospital beds, and so on) around the nation, in spite of the entitlement of people everywhere to equal service. In the Ministry of Health and Social Security, therefore, steps were taken to allocate to the regional health authorities on the basis of a formula that would reflect the extent of local needs. A Resource Allocation Working Party (RAWP) undertook careful studies, which showed very wide disparities throughout Great Britain in mortality, morbidity, health care utilization, and other indicators of need. The formula for budgetary allocations from the central government, which resulted from RAWP deliberations, included not only measurements of existing resources, but also indicators of health care requirements, such as the percentage of aged persons in the region and the infant mortality rate.

Experience with NHS administration through the 90 AHAs showed that even at this level there was insufficient adjustment to varying local health needs. The viewpoint therefore developed that the principal local jurisdictions should be the 200 health districts, which had around 250,000 people each. Such districts already operated within most AHAs, and they were quite sensitive to local needs. A major purpose of the 1974 reorganization had been to attain greater managerial efficiency, but the creation of both area and district-level authorities in effect introduced a fourth echelon in the NHS structure. The health districts could achieve greater integration of services than had been possible previously. The AHA administrative level, therefore, was essentially eliminated, and responsibility was vested in the 200 districts. The local authorities remain responsibile for environmental sanitation and social services, but not for personal health services (such as child health clinics). At the district level, the management teams bring together for the first time representatives of GPs and specialists, as well as the community medicine specialist, the district nursing officer, and the district administrator.

As of 1981, the reorganized NHS faced problems of rising costs similar to those of other industrialized countries. Margaret Thatcher's Conservative government, however, saw the remedy for this as greater constraint in the public sector along with enlargement of the private sector. By holding the line on salaries of specialists, the government encouraged them to spend more time in their private practices. At the same time, more people were growing impatient with the waiting lists for service in the public system, and therefore sought medical care privately. The government encouraged the growth of private health insurance and the construction of small private hospitals. The policy of the previous Labour Party government to reduce the number of private beds in NHS hospitals was halted, and these beds were slightly increased.

Private Health Services

Outside of hospitals, one must appreciate that health service providers in Britain are predominantly private agents; general medical practitioners, dentists, pharmacists (chemists), opticians, and others are mainly in private practice, usually owning and controlling their own places of work. (The major exception was found in the salaried staffs of the health centers.) It is the source of their payments that is governmental and, of course, they are subject to various public rules and regulations. In such a context, expansion of "private health services" in the British health system refers to their private financing as well as the private delivery of care.

By 1982, the continued constraints on public spending by the Conservative Party government created still greater pressures in the NHS and longer waiting lists for hospital care. As was to be expected, this stimulated the further growth of the private sector, particularly through expansion of voluntary health insurance for private medical care. The government deliberately encouraged this by allowing tax concessions to management and labor for private insurance premiums. Coverage reached 3.5 million people by 1980—about 6.3 percent of the national population. Since the NHS still provided general practitioner care, drugs, dental, and other services, the private sector was estimated to account for only about 5 percent of total British health expenditures in 1982.

To accommodate these privately insured patients, strictly private hospitals were constructed in London and in a few other main cities, many by U.S. hospital corporations. Under existing law, no approval by hospital planning authorities was required for any new facility with fewer than 120 beds or for the expansion of any existing facility by less than 20 percent. The previous Labour Party government had reduced private pay beds in NHS hospitals, which heightened the demand for such beds in wholly private hospitals. Although the approximately 7,500 beds operated in private hospitals by 1982 constituted less than 2 percent of the total supply, their impact was inevitably to increase competition. By offering higher salaries and more attractive working conditions, private hospitals drew medical and other health manpower resources from NHS hospitals. Moreover, like proprietary hospitals everywhere, they served mainly low-risk, elective surgical cases, leaving the more difficult chronic and elderly patients to the public hospitals. All of these developments were bound to injure the morale of NHS professional personnel.

The Royal Commission on the National Health Service in 1979 had taken note of the growth of a private medical sector, but concluded that its minor proportions "could have, at most, a marginal and local effect on the NHS . . . it is clear that the private sector is too small to make a significant impact on the NHS except locally and temporarily." A few years later, however, some observers disagreed and, anticipating the further growth of private medical and hospital care, called for actions that would deliberately integrate the private sector into the NHS. They advocated including all private hospital construction and technology within the orbit of official health planning, requiring private hospitals to accept all types of patients, establishing uniform salary scales for health personnel in all public and private hospitals, and other measures.

By 1985, enrollment in private health insurance did, indeed, level off at about 10 percent of the population. Private hospital construction, however, continued, and in 1985 there were 198 private facilities with 9,760 beds— about 3 percent of the total.

As elsewhere in the world, in both industralized and developing countries, some people welcomed the growth of a private sector in British health care, on the ground that it brought more health resources (especially hospitals) into the system and lightened the burden on the public sector. Others pointed to its aggravation of public sector problems, by withdrawing scarce medical and allied personnel for service to a favored minority. No one could deny that the private sector would increase access to medical care on the basis of personal wealth rather than need for health care. The ultimate question posed by these British developments was: How could resources (health personnel, facilities, and so on) in a national health system be augmented to meet all health needs? One way to do this is by increased private spending, which naturally benefits those who can spend. The other way is to increase public spending, which benefits everyone. By any criterion of social justice, the answer is manifest; but political decisions in the health sector, as in other sectors, are often based more on other criteria.

In 1985, Great Britain was still spending only 6.1 percent of its GNP on health, compared with 9.5 percent in Sweden and over 11 percent in the United States. Private insurance was reported in 1987 to cover 5.5 million people, or 10 percent of the population. Many hospital consultants, well aware of this private market, reduced their NHS hospital hours, to lengthen the patient queues for elective surgery. Predictably the privately insured or more affluent patients on the queue then sought private care. Beds in private hospitals were serving an estimated 15 percent of all elective surgical cases in the country.

By 1988, the British Medical Association, which over the years had become a strong supporter of the NHS, was declaring it to be in a state of "terminal decline." An Assocation of Community Health Councils stated that "unless there is action now, some parts of the NHS, already on the brink of collapse, will simply fall apart during 1988." These cries of alarm were obviously appeals for greater public expenditures for the NHS, in the face of a government policy for expansion of private spending. Political trends in Britain will determine whether public expenditure will increase to enable the NHS to achieve its original goal of equity or greater private expenditures will create a two-tier system—an elegant one for the affluent and a mediocre one for the rest of the population.

In January 1989, the Thatcher government issued a sweeping proposal that would introduce market principles into the operation of the NHS. The basic regionalized health planning would be replaced by competition among hospitals. General practitioners would get budgetary allotments to finance all the services for which their patients were referred; thereby creating incentives to minimize referrals. Several other market features were advocated. Both physicians and patients, however, reacted to the white paper with great hostility. By late 1989, central policies in the British NHS were in serious turmoil, but future strategies were not clear.

One more observation about the British NHS has general significance for organized health programs in any country. In the late 1970s, the Department of Health and Social Security (DHSS) appointed a working group on Inequalities in Health, chaired by Sir Douglas Black; the report, issued in 1980, became known as the Black Report. The working group set out to examine whether the National Health Service had reduced the inequalities in health that had long prevailed among different social classes in Great Britain. (For more than a century the British Registrar-General had required the reporting of occupation on all death certificates, and this provided the statistical basis for calculating mortality rates for each of five social classes.)

Over the first 30 years of the NHS, 1948 to 1978, the mortality rates of all five social classes had declined. The rates of decline of the upper classes, however, were substantially greater than those of the lower classes. As a result, after 30 years of NHS benefits, the degree of inequality between classes was actually greater than at the outset. Did this mean that the NHS had done little good? This question provoked a great deal of discusison among the health professions, the government, and the general population of Great Britain.

It became widely recognized, as we stressed in Chapter 2 of this book, that health status is determined by far more than medical and related services. As the Black Report states, the "material conditions of life" probably play the greatest part, and of course these differ enormously among the five social classes. Differences prevail in working conditions, housing, nutrition, frequency of unemployment, level of education, family stress, and other features of the physical and social environment. The improvement in health services brought by the NHS was not matched by similar improvements in the material conditions of life for the several social classes. One might say, in fact, that the persistent disparities in the living conditions among classes makes the improved health status of all five social classes all the more remarkable, in spite of the greater degree of material gain among the elite.

In a word, the message of the Black Report is an old and simple one. Organized health services can benefit health, but favorable living and working conditions can benefit health even more.

NEW ZEALAND

Considering its small population, the two islands in the South Pacific Ocean known as New Zealand have earned a remarkable reputation for progressive social legislation, including provisions for health care. After control by Great Britain for nearly a century (since 1840), the British granted independence to the colony in 1931, but full self-government was acquired only in 1947. As early as 1898, New Zealand had begun a social security system with old-age pensions. In 1893, it granted women the right to vote—the first country in the world to do so.

The population of New Zealand in 1984 was 3,266,000 and its GNP per capita that year was $7,730. With great dependence on the export of wool, meat, and dairy products, New Zealand was severely affected by the economic depression of the 1930s. In 1935, the Labour Party was elected to power for the first time, and in 1938 the Parliament enacted a greatly expanded Social Security Act, including provision for medical, hospital, and related benefits. Because of opposition from the medical profession and general political debate, the medical provisions of the act were not implemented until 1941, but when they were, the new program had several unique features among the world's health systems.

First, it covered the total population; this was the first country with a free-market economy to do so. (Britain and the Scandinavian countries made coverage universal later, and the Soviet Union—with universal entitlement to health services in the 1920s—did not have a free-market economy.) Second, though it was originally intended to be financed by an earmarked insurance tax, kept in a separate trust fund, it was finally supported directly from general revenues. No proof of tax payment was required for access to health services. Third, administration was assigned entirely to the Department of Health, not of Labor. Health insurance had not been identified with industrial workers and labor unions, as in Europe, nor was there a background of mutual aid societies or sickness funds. Cash benefits (for old age, unemployment, etc.) were administered by the Department of Social Welfare in the Ministry of Health and Social Security.

In spite of the original intention, the scope of health services provided under the New Zealand Health Service was not comprehensive at the outset. It has generally expanded over the years, although in some ways, especially the copayments required form the patient, it has contracted. Because their methods of organization and funding are very different, we consider hospital care separately from primary health care and other services.

Hospital Care

New Zealand has had a long tradition of public hospitals and a more recent array of private hospitals. Of the total hospital beds—amounting in 1983 to some 10 per 1,000 people—79 percent were in public facilities and 21 percent in private. The latter are mainly of nonprofit sponsorship, but 36 percent of these beds are under proprietary control. The private hospitals principally accommodate medical and long-stay geriatric patients, but some are mainly surgical.

Since the Hospitals Act of 1957, all hospitals—public and private—are periodically monitored, with respect to national standards, by the central Department of Health. The public hospitals come under the immediate management of 29 regional hospital boards, whose members are elected. After 1983 policy changed to encourage coalescence into fewer hospital boards, encompassing larger populations, and conversion into "area *health* boards" that would be responsible for all health services in their territory. This included local public health districts, as well as the public hospitals. By 1987, three such area health boards had been established.

The medical staffing of public hospitals is by carefully chosen salaried specialists, most of whom are also free to engage in private practice outside their official hours. Typically they see patients in the private hospitals, where a great deal of uncomplicated elective surgery is done. General practitioners and some specialists, who are not appointed in the public hospitals, may also admit patients to the private hospitals, following an open staff pattern. Private hospitals provide little out-patient or emergency care, while such ambulatory service is a major function of the network of public hospitals.

The public hospitals are financed in a rather unusual way. Allotments are made by the national Department of Health to each area health board, based largely on the population served by that board, with certain adjustments. The formula used takes account of the age and sex composition of the local population, death and birth rates, and other reflections of health needs. Allowances are also made for the movement of patients across regional lines, for training programs in a hospital, and so on. In addition, the national government subsidizes private hospitals. In short-stay private hospitals, public funds contribute about 40 percent of costs, and in long-stay facilities about 70 percent. The balance must come fom private health insurance or simply from individuals and families.

As in so many other countries, both affluent and poor, the largest share of public money in New Zealand goes to support institutional services. This amounted to 66.2 percent of the total in 1985. Ambulatory care, including pharmaceuticals, accounts for 29.8 percent of the total. All formal public health activities plus administration absorb only 3.9 percent of total health expenditures. Efforts are being made to alter these proportions, to put greater stress on primary health care.

Primary Health Care

The provision of primary health care in New Zealand by general practitioners, as well as by pharmacists, is very different from that for hospital services. At the outset in the 1930s, the Labour Party had wanted to pay general practitioners by capitation, as in the former British mother country. Objections from the GPs were extreme and, when the national program went into full operation in 1941, general practitioners were paid on a fee-for-service basis. After a few years, physicians began to charge patients an extra personal fee, on top of the payments receive from the government program. By the early 1950s, these supplemental charges amounted to about 40 percent of the official fee. With general inflation, these copayments gradually increased; by the 1980s they amounted to 50 percent or more of the government reimbursements.

The general practitioner's *rooms,* as they are called, were meagerly equipped and staffed in the 1940s, but with higher incomes their resources and quality have improved. Individual general practice has been gradually replaced by medical groups, with greater use of ancillary personnel and more equipment. Some years ago the regional hospital boards had been authorized to construct health centers, in which general practitioners would work on salary along with allied personnel financed by the board; however, these units were established in only a few areas.

Development of further area health boards is expected to provide the impetus to establish more organized arrangements for ambulatory service. An instrumentality to this end has been the formation, at the level of area boards (or even more local communities), of *Service Development Groups* (SDG) to strengthen services in various fields. These have included primary health care, mental health, child health, internal medicine, or surgery.

Voluntary agencies play a significant part in certain aspects of primary health care in New Zealand. Most influential is the Plunket Society. Since 1907, this organization of women has been arranging preventively oriented services for mothers and children throughout the country. More than 600 branches employ nurses to conduct the necessary clinic sessions and to advise families through home visits. About 50 percent of the costs are covered by grants from the government, and the services are closely integrated with the official district public health services. Other voluntary health agencies, cooperating with the government and subsidized by public funding, are the Family Planning Association, the St. John Ambulance, and the Crippled Children Society.

Special note should be taken of the New Zealand approach to dental care for children. During the First World War, when young men were examined for military service, a shockingly high rate of untreated dental disease was discovered. It was realized that the national supply of professional dentists was woefully inadequate, so that the dean of the dental school made a completely innovative proposal—to train young women, secondary school graduates, as auxiliary dental workers. The course would last for 2 years and would prepare the students, not only in preventive dental hygiene, but also in simple restorative procedures (drilling and filling teeth) and extractions. Graduates were designated as *school dental nurses* and stationed only in the schools. Their work was supervised by professional dentists in the local public health agency, and difficult cases were referred to fully qualified dentists for treatment. The idea was supported by the New Zealand Dental Assocation and the first training course began in 1921.

Although this basic dental concept has been contended and opposed by dental associations in many countries, it was fully accepted in New Zealand, and has spread, in one form or another, to some 20 nations, mainly developing countries in the British Commonwealth. Studies have shown the quality of work done by these personnel to be good, and the general oral health of New Zealand school children has been much better than that of children in most other countries. To prevent dental caries, New Zealand has also fluoridated most of its public water supplies, so that the incidence of new dental disease has declined. This health manpower innovation strikingly illustrates the worldwide impact of an idea, originating in a very small country, that helps meet health needs found everywhere.

Economic Aspects

The high priority accorded to health by New Zealand governments, after the first bold action of the Labour Party in 1938, is well reflected in data on the country's health expenditures. The government reports that in 1950 New Zealand was spending 4.5 percent of its GDP in the health system (and it was doubtless less before 1940). By 1982, this share had risen to 6.9 percent, although it declined to 6.4 percent in 1985; this reduction reflected rigorous government controls on hospital budgets.

These overall health expenditures were derived about 80 percent from public sources and 20 percent from private over the period 1960 to 1982. In 1985, the public share was down slightly to 78 percent, because of governmental cutbacks. Public support is still much more generous for institutional services than for primary health care. In 1985, for all short-stay in-patient hospital care, more than 95 percent of expenditures came from governmental sources. Only 52 percent of the costs of general practitioner services, on the other hand, were met by public sources, and only 37 percent for total dental care.

Medical care for accidental injury is financed by a remarkable and unique government program in New Zealand. Unlike the usual work-injury compensation program of virtually all industrialized countries, the New Zealand law gives economic protection for medical care and earnings lost in connection with *all* types of accident. Work-injury costs are met by a social insurance tax on employers, but traffic accident costs come from an assessment on all vehicle owners, and the balance comes from general revenues. This program is administered by a separate Accident Compensation Commission (ACC). Medical services needed for work injuries are simply provided in the general health program,

but for all other injuries special payments are made to providers by the ACC. Even injuries due to medical malpractice have been brought under the jurisdiction of this "no fault" compensation program. The costs of this program have been increasing gradually, to 2.6 percent of national health expenditures in 1985.

One final aspect of New Zealand health services deserves mention. Some 10 percent of the population are the original inhabitants: the Maori. For many reasons they remain an impoverished and disadvantaged section of the population, with the greatest health problems. In contrast with the policy of other countries toward native peoples, however, New Zealand has not segregated them on reservations or in any other way; they are now mostly urbanized, and their health care has been integrated with that of the rest of the population. While their health status is still poorer than the average, it has shown clear improvement with this policy of integration.

OTHER SCANDINAVIAN COUNTRIES

The health system of Norway has been examined in some detail, but other industrialized Scandinavian countries with health systems have "comprehensive" attributes: Sweden, Denmark, Finland, and Iceland. In all of these countries, the entire population is entitled to health services as a social right, but the exact organizational structures, methods of financing, and patterns of delivery differ. Some of the highlights of these differences follow.

Sweden

Sweden is the largest of the Scandinavian countries in both territory and population. With 8.4 million people, a GNP per capita of $11,890 in 1985, and an extremely good health record, it has often been regarded as the "model" of Scandinavian culture. After World War II, when nations became sharply divided between capitalist and socialist camps, Sweden was often heralded as the ideal "welfare state" demonstrating "the middle way" in politics.

Sweden's favorable economic position in the postwar decades may have been related to its neutrality during the war.

Until 1955, the health insurance program of Sweden was voluntary but heavily subsidized by the central government. Under this arrangement, about 70 percent of the population were insured, although much hospital care was given to noninsured persons by local governments at public expense. In 1955, health insurance protection was made compulsory for virtually everyone, and in 1962 legislation ensured entitlement to health care and sickness cash benefits for every resident. Since 1970, patients have been required to make a small copayment (perhaps amounting to 20 to 30 percent of the full cost) for each ambulatory visit. In the late 1970s, however, social insurance contributions from workers were ended, and the "insurance" funding was derived 75 percent from employers and 25 percent from government.

The Swedish health system has long put great stress on hospitals, and the simple functional design of hospital architecture has attracted worldwide attention. In 1985 there were 16 hospital beds per 1,000 population, of which 5 were for general short-term care, 5 for long-term care, and 6 for mental disorders. In addition, there were 7 beds per 1,000 in homes for the elderly. Of the total hospital beds, 94 percent were in facilities controlled by some level of government.

The most important level of government operating Swedish hospitals is the *county* (as the first echlon below the top, described as the *province* in the account on Norway). Sweden has 23 counties and 3 municipalities, each with an elected council. Although ambulatory medical care is financed mainly by national insurance, hospital services—including hospital physician salaries—are financed principally by the general revenues of the county governments, derived from county income taxes. In 1984, about 64 percent of hospital costs came from this source; the national government provided another 24 percent from general revenues, to equalize resources between counties and support medical education and research. Only 8 percent came to hospitals from the

health insurance fund and 4 percent from patient fees.

Swedish health leadership has for some time been quite aware of the heavy emphasis on hospital care. To increase efficiency in the use of hospitals, a movement for regional organization of all health facilities was launched in the 1960s. The country was divided into seven regions, each containing several counties. In each region there is one major regional hospital for complex tertiary care, and each county has at least one county hospital. Below the county level are districts, with populations up to 60,000 that might be served by a small hospital. All hospitals have out-patient departments for ambulatory specialist care.

The most peripheral component of the regionalized health program is the health center, to serve about 15,000 people for primary health care. In the mid-1970s, the construction of health centers proceeded rapidly, with approximately 800 in the nation by 1985. Each health center is staffed by two to four general practitioners, along with nurses and other ancillary staff; all these personel are on salaries, financed by the health insurance scheme. Several parliamentary actions promoted this transformaton of ambulatory medical care from traditionally private to organized public control—the Primary Care Act of 1974, the Health and Medical Services Act of 1983, and the 1985 Dagmar Reform. Under these measures, nearly all community physicians became salaried employees. A few local governments contract with private physicians for service, but the impact is negligible.

Nursing homes for the elderly and chronically sick are also being expanded at the municipal level (Sweden has a total of 284 municipalities). With this increased emphasis on resources for both primary health care and long-term care, Sweden intends to reduce its supply (or ratio to population) of short-term general hospital beds.

In light of the highly organized pattern of medical staffs in hospitals and the increasingly organized arrangements for primary health care, private medical practice has become relatively scarce in Sweden. Although hospital specialists may spend a few hours a week in private practice, only about 5 percent of Swedish doctors are entirely devoted to private work.

One other unusual feature of the Swedish health system should be noted. Just as the cost of virtually all health service has been collectivized, the same principle has been applied in Sweden to malpractice by physicians. Until 1975 patients who considered that they had been harmed by medical treatment could take legal action against the doctor under conventional tort law. Such malpractice suits were actually quite uncommon, but in 1976 a law was passed on Treatment Injury Insurance. This is, in effect, no fault social insurance, under which any patient who believes he or she has suffered some ill effect from medical treatment presents the claim to a Medical Responsibility Board. There is no requirement for proving medical negligence or incompetence; if some harmful effect can be shown, the patient is automatically compensated. Under this scheme, the rate of malpractice claims has risen (although it was only 15 per 100,000 people in 1976) and the size of awards has declined slightly. The insurance premiums are paid by county governments.

Swedish health functions, not surprisingly, require expenditure of a high percentage of GDP—9.1 percent in 1986. Of this amount, 91 percent came from public sources, both tax revenues and social insurance, and only 9 percent from private sources. In the mid-1980s, a purely private sector of medical practice had begun to expand in Sweden, and provoked responses by the Social Democratic Party. The counties must set limits on the number of patient visits to private doctors compensable by the insurance program, and larger national grants were allotted to the counties with weak public services.

Finland

Finland developed universal coverage and equity in health care somewhat later than the other Scandinavian countries, but since 1972 it has moved ahead rapidly. In that year, the Primary Health Care Act was passed, fundamentally changing the pattern of delivery of ambulatory health services. National health in-

surance had been enacted in 1964, with financial support shared by compulsory contributions from workers and employers. The benefits were limited, however, to reimbursement of 50 percent of official fees, for out-of-hospital care, and the physician was free to charge amounts higher than those on the official fee schedule. Hospitalization had long been financed predominantly (about 85 percent) by local general revenues, and insurance covered only the balance. Finland's population in 1984 was 4.9 million, with a per capita GNP of $11,300.

With the 1972 act, a policy of high priority for primary health care and greatly decentralized management was instituted. Unlike policy in Norway and Sweden, the basic administrative level became not the counties or provinces (12 of these), but the communes and municipalities. These local authorities in Finland number 445, averaging about 10,000 people each. For support of health services, they receive about 50 percent national subsidy (varying between 70 percent to the poorest units and 39 percent to the most affluent), conditional on their meeting national government health care standards.

The provision of primary health care in the communes or municipalities is under the direction of a local board of health, selected by a general municipal (or commune) council; the latter is elected by the general population every 4 years. The principal strategy for delivering these services is through a nationwide network of health centers, which numbered 217 in 1982. Each health center serves about 20,000 people (in one or more communes), with four to six physicians and numerous other personnel. These health workers are not all stationed in one health center building, but may be located at health posts around the area. A small hospital for chronically ill patients may also be included in the health center organization, as well as quarters for maternal-and-child health clinics and laboratories.

Physicians in the health centers are paid by salary, with supplements for overtime work; they are not permitted to engage in private practice. Hospital physicians, who must be specialists, are also salaried (for a short 37-hour work week), and are free to conduct private practice after official hours, which most of them do.

Since 1972, Finland has concentrated on health promotion and disease prevention. Great stress has been put on encouraging healthful ways of living including sound nutrition, nonsmoking, moderate use of alcohol, proper exercise, balanced interpersonal relationships, and adequate rest and recreation. The death rate among middle-aged males, which had been exceptionally high from cardiovascular disease, soon began to decline. Finland's infant mortality—5.9 per 1,000 live births—was the lowest in the world in 1985. At health centers, all preventive services are free, but small charges are imposed for all treatment services, including a nominal copayment for each day of hospital care.

Since the 1972 legislation, the major source of economic support (about 80 percent) for the Finnish health system is the general tax revenue collected by the local and the national governments. Social insurance still continues but is used mainly for cash benefits and for only selected aspects of health services, such as out-of-hospital drugs, travel costs, and partial reimbursement of fees paid to private practitioners. Altogether, Finland spent 7.5 percent of GDP on its health system in 1986, of which 77 percent came from public sources and 23 percent from private. The proportion of expenditures coming from public sources has been gradually rising.

Denmark

Because Denmark, with a population in 1984 of 5.1 million people, occupies a relatively small land area, it has the highest population density of the Scandinavian countries. Its GNP per capita in 1984 was $11,450. Denmark is also the most urbanized Scandinavian country; having 13 percent of its population in Copenhagen affects its health insurance operations.

With its southern border touching the Federal Republic of Germany, it is not surprising that, since the early nineteenth century, Denmark has financed medical care for workers and their families, as in Germany, through hundreds of small sickness insurance funds. In

1885 there were 700 such funds; however, their protection reached only a minority of the population. Coverage gradually expanded, the funds were subsidized by the government, and though insurance was technically still voluntary, some 90 percent of the population were insured by 1935. In 1961 health insurance coverage was made universal for every resident of Denmark. In 1973, administration was greatly simplified by abolition of the hundreds of sickness insurance funds, and assigning health insurance payment responsibilities to the 280 municipalities.

Denmark is unique among the Scandinavian countries in distinguishing between the affluent minority of the population and the vast majority, in their health insurance arrangements. Persons with an annual income below a specified level—constituting about 92 percent of all—are "class 1 protected." All persons of higher income are "class 2 protected." For class 1 patients, the reimbursement by the insurance must be accepted by the doctor as payment-in-full. For class 2 patients, the doctor receives the official fee payment, but may make additional charges to the patient. This was the legal stipulation in 1973, but as of 1976 anyone could decide which of the two classes he wished to be in, regardless of actual income.

The exact method of remunerating the doctor, moreover, is different for class 1 patients in Copenhagen from those in the rest of the country. In the large capital city, doctors are appointed by the Health Security Service to official panels of general practitioners, designated by district. Insured persons of class 1 select a doctor, for one year, and the GP is paid by a flat per capita amount. (A maximum of 220 persons is allowed on each doctor's list.) Outside of Copenhagen, a similar capitation mechanism is applied, but it is calculated to provide about half of the doctor's payment. For the other half, he charges fees on a fee-for-service basis, which are also paid by the insurance. For class 2 patients, both inside and outside Copenhagen, insurance payments are entirely by fee-for-service, with extra charges payable by the patient personally.

Hospitals in Denmark, as in Sweden, are financially supported mainly by the 14 county (province) governments, with a 35 percent subsidy from the national government. The staffs of medical and surgical specialists are on full-time salary; only the chiefs of various clinical services are allowed to spend up to 4 hours per week in private practice outside the hospitals.

Within the counties or provinces of Denmark, the 280 municipalities carry financial responsibilities principally for social welfare for the poor and handicapped. As noted, the municipalities also serve to administer payments under the health insurance program. They give direct health services at home to school children, mothers and infants, and the chronically sick. To advise municipal authorities on public health matters, including environmental sanitation, there are some 50 or 60 nationally appointed medical officers. On the whole, the Danish health system seems to be more complex than that of the other Scandinavian countries, in response to various political and professional pressures. The system's total cost in 1986 was 6.1 percent of GDP, of which 84 percent came from public sources.

SOUTHERN EUROPEAN COUNTRIES

In the 1970s, later than in northern Europe, Italy, Greece, and Spain in southern Europe undertook bold actions to extend health services to their entire populations. The most sweeping action was taken in Italy in 1978, establishing a National Health Service to begin in January 1979.

Italy

As in other European countries, voluntary mutual aid societies for medical care had grown up in Italy since the nineteenth century. After World War II, with the fall of fascism, coverage was made mandatory for most industrial workers, and the numberous mutual societies were converted into local branches of a national health insurance program. By the 1970s, coverage reached over 90 percent of the population, although the range of benefits differed among local societies. Then, in 1977 Italty's several left-wing political parties gained substantial strength in the parliament. By then, 96 percent of the population were estimated to have health insurance protection. In 1978, a National Health Service was legislated, under which 100 percent of the population would be covered and financial support would be gradually shifted to general revenues. Physicians would be free to remain in private practice or to be employed in hospitals and health centers. The whole system would be administered by a greatly strengthened Ministry of Health, which would manage all health resources and programs through assignment of responsibilities to Italy's 20 political regions.

It was not expected that the Italian National Health Service (NHS) would be achieved overnight. The 20 regional health authorities could be established rapidly, but the transfer of financing from the sickness insurance funds to national government revenues, administered by the Ministry of Health, would take time. Also, it would require some years before approximately 650 local health units (*unidad sanitaria locale,* or USL) could be staffed and equipped to provide the population primary health care. Hospitals would be placed under the direction of the regional authorities (similar to provinces elsewhere), directly if they were public institutions, and by contract if they were religious or private. As of 1979, about 86 percent of hospital beds in Italy were in public institutions, and 14 percent in private ones (nonprofit or proprietary). Hospital physicians have by tradition been on regular salaries, but they are also free to engage in private practice outside.

The central Ministry of Health establishes technical standards, including proper ratios of population to all health personnel, but the regions may modify these somewhat to fit local conditions. The regional authority divides its territory into local health units (USLs), in consultation with local municipalities or communes. Each USL serves a population of 50,000 to 200,000, and these may be subdivided further into *basic health districts.* The USL is responsible not only for general ambulatory medical care, but also for environmental sanitation, disease prevention, rehabilitation, pharmaceutical control, and hospital administration. Directing each USL is a management committee, chosen by municipal councils to represent all the relevant political parties.

Public hospitals in Italy had actually been transferred to regional authority administration in 1974, before the NHS legislation was passed. They were experiencing serious economic difficulties, because of the financial weaknesses of many of the sickness insurance funds. Since 1974, therefore, hospitals have been paid on the basis of an approved annual budget. The same applies to other health facilities, such as clinics, laboratories, and pharmacies, many of which are nongovernment in ownership. The day-to-day management of all health facilities, within their allocated budgets, is the responsibility of the USL.

Planning of the administrative procedures of the Italian NHS was strongly influenced by British experience. Largely for this reason, general practitioners and pediatricians, working in USLs, are paid on a capitation basis—that is, a fixed amount per year for each person registered with them. The capitation amount is not uniform, but varies with the seniority, training, and experience of each doctor. An optimal GP list is regarded as having 1,000 persons (1,400 for pediatricians), with 1,500 being the maximum allowed.

Specialists in virtually all hospitals, as noted, are paid by annual salaries. In out-patient clinics under public control, they are paid by the hour. In clinics under private auspices, specialists are paid on a fee-for-service basis. As a cost control measure, in the 1980s copayment of 15 percent was required for consultation with an out-of-hospital specialist. Nurses and other health personnel are paid by salaries set at the regional level.

Under the old sickness funds, the range of health benefits varied in accordance with the financial position of the fund. The NHS entitles everyone to the same services, which are general and specialist medical care, hospitalization, nursing care, and prescribed drugs. The patient may be treated at an ambulatory care clinic (public or private) or at home. He or she has free choice of doctor and, although payment is made by capitation for one year, another doctor may be chosen at any time. Prescribed medications can be obtained at any pharmacy; no charge is made for those on a list of "essential drugs" (numbering 800 in 1979),

but for other drugs copayments are required. Dental service was not encompassed in the NHS at the outset. Long-term care may be provided under NHS financing, if it is medically oriented, but not if it is purely custodial.

As noted, neither general nor specialized physicians are compelled to be employed by the Italian NHS, or even contract with it. In the initial years, many physicians chose to stay independent. If the physicians in a local health unit are too few and the service is perfunctory, patients can consult private doctors, and higher-income families do so frequently. Private commercial insurance coverage is available to pay for such care.

Disease prevention and health promotion are major responsibilities of USLs; much of this work is done by nurses and sanitation personnel. Occupational safety and health have traditionally received great attention in Italy, and personnel skilled in this field (formerly in the Ministry of Labor and Social Security) are assigned to the USLs. Participation of workers in the enforcement of health and safety regulations is a special feature of this preventive program.

As of 1988, the Italian NHS was not yet in smooth operation, and various administrative problems had not been solved. According to one observer, by 1988 the intended NHS policies had been properly implemented in only 8 of the 20 health regions. At the regional level, training courses in management were offered for communal USL personnel. The share of national wealth going into the Italian health system had risen from 3.9 percent of GDP in 1960 to 6.7 percent in 1986. The proportion from public sources in 1986 was 79 percent. The Italian economy has suffered from severe inflation and other difficulties in the 1980s. These economic problems and the associated political instability have undoubtedly retarded the full implementation of the Italian National Health Service.

Greece

After many years of military dictatorship, a Socialist Party government was elected to power in Greece in 1981. The Party's political agenda called for modernization and social equality in all aspects of Greek society. In the health field, it called specifically for a *national health system* that would unify all public health services under the Ministry of Health and reduce the size and inequities of the private sector. (The peasant population in rural areas of Greece had long been seriously disadvantaged and largely dependent on traditional healers for medical care.) Legislation to formalize this ambitious program was enacted in 1983, when the GNP per capita of Greece was $3,932.

Before 1983, through developments over the previous century, some 95 percent of the Greek population of about 9.8 million people were economically protected with some form of health insurance. Three-quarters of these were covered by two large insurance funds—the Social Security Fund (IKA in Greek) for industrial workers, mainly urban, and the Agricultural Workers Fund (OGA in Greek), mainly rural. The remaining fourth of the insured population was enrolled in about 80 smaller funds. The patterns for delivery of medical care and the range of benefits differed widely among the funds. The smaller funds, in general, had more "privileged" arrangements, under which members could consult private physicians, who were paid fees according to negotiated fee schedules. The two large funds operated their own polyclinics, health centers, and hospitals staffed by salaried doctors. Frequently these facilities were crowded, however, and insured patients consulted private doctors at their own expense.

Unification and fiscal consolidation of all health insurance funds under the Ministry of Health, with a uniform range of comprehensive services for all persons, meant much more equitable accessibility to health care. Enlargement of health expenditures was a high priority of the new government. The central budget for 1987 showed the expenditure for health to be more than three times higher than it had been in 1981 (in real currency terms). Capital investment in health facilities construction was actually six times higher; this was mainly to expand hospitals in the severely underserved rural areas.

The health resources, with which the new government of Greece could work, were relatively large. In 1985 physicians numbered 286 per 100,000—abundant but extremely maldistributed. Greater Athens, with 31 percent of the population, had 56 percent of the physicians, while inadequate numbers were located in most of the other 53 districts (nomai) of the country. Likewise most of the 60,100 hospital beds (6.2 beds per 1,000, not counting mental health) were in the Athens area, including secondary as well as tertiary-level facilities.

The task of the new government was to mobilize the stock of health manpower for public service, as well as to equalize hospitals and also health centers for primary health care. Of the 24,500 doctors in Greece in 1983, about 13,000 were exclusively in private practice, 8,650 worked full-time in some government post, and most of the remaining 3,050 combined private practice with government functions. As more physicians came into salaried government posts, providing service to the people without charge, the market for private practice contracted.

The Socialist government of Greece set out to build health centers in all areas, rural and urban, with a sufficient population. Most of these units were staffed with general practitioners and nurses, and often also with a dentist, a pediatrician, a microbiologist, and a radiologist. The nearest hospital would provide the backup services of specialists, who were expected to visit the health center several times a week. For rural areas with too few people to warrant a health center, peripheral *medical stations* were established, offering substantially higher salaries to attract general practitioners. If these voluntary incentives did not succeed, the ministry could assign physicians to isolated stations, at 50 percent higher salaries for periods up to 6 months.

Greece formerly had an excessive number of specialists, so that graduate education in the specialities (except "specialized general practice") was greatly reduced. Specialty posts in the main cities were also curtailed. Certification of specialists was transferred from the auspices of the Panhellenic Medical Association to the Ministry of Health. In teaching hospitals, the beds assigned to each specialty were reduced. Also the specialist title in general practice was authorized for any GP with 5 years of experience, through a 6-month special course; new graduates could spend 2 years of

training for specialized general practice qualification. Salaries of the new general practitioners became the same as those for conventional specialists and, unlike the latter, they
were entitled to overtime pay for overtime
working hours.

To establish the hundreds of health centers
needed, especially in rural areas, the Ministry
of Health appropriated and renamed the various facilities of the major health insurance
funds, as well as constructing new ones. To
transfer various private facilities to government control, the Ministry of Health used several strategies. Before 1983, the 60,100 hospital
beds were about 46 percent in government
hospitals, 14 percent in voluntary nonprofit
hospitals (mostly with religious groups), and
40 percent in private "clinics" (actually small
hospitals usually owned by physicians or professional groups). With the 1983 law, the former 50 percent national subsidy to voluntary
hospitals was terminated.

The government then offered to purchase
any of the private units, and many promptly
sold out. Regulations prohibited any transfer
of private clinics to other owners, as well as
any expansion or modificiation. Even the purchase of equipment required approval of one
of the new Regional Health Councils (RHCs,
initially about 10) set up by the new government. With these strategies, both private medical practice and private health facilities gradually diminished to small proportions in
Greece. Some will doubtless remain to cater to
a relatively affluent minority, who object to
waiting or to other conditions of the National
Health System.

Under the NHS, both the primary care doctors in health centers and the specialists in hospitals are paid salaries, adjusted according to
their experience, training, and responsibilities.
General practitioners have lists of people they
served (from 1,800 to 2,500), but they are not
paid on a capitation basis; a flat salary pays for
the first 1,800 enrolled, with increments for
others beyond this up to 2,500. For pediatricians the comparable enrollment figures are
1,200 to 2,000. All primary care doctors are
barred from any outside private practice (although, as noted, they may get overtime pay
for official work).

Management of the entire Greek National
Health System will be a difficult task, requiring
the training of new administrative personnel.
At the top, a Central Health Council, representing mainly consumers (industrial workers,
farmers, etc.) along with a minority of professional providers, will have great authority
within the Ministry of Health. The health
functions of other ministries were also transferred to the Ministry of Health—environmental health (from the Ministry of Environment and Public Works), occupational health
(from the Ministry of Labor), nutrition (from
the Ministry of Agriculture), medical education (from the Ministry of Education), and
postgraduate professional education (from the
Ministry of Social Services). There were also
plans for setting up a National Drug Industry
that might gradually replace the numerous private pharmaceutical firms.

The regional health councils will make policy and supervise all health personnel and facilities (both hospitals and health centers)
within their jurisdictions. They are expected to
carry out the policies of the Central Health
Council. These policies are directed toward
gradual minimization of the previously strong
private health sector in Greece, to achieve an
equitable National Health System. Data are
not yet available to show how successfully this
entire policy is being carried out. It may be
noted, however, that well before the NHS program was implemented, the public sector in
the Greek health system was becoming
stronger; in 1960 national health expenditures
entailed only 2.9 percent of GDP, of which
58.6 percent came from public sources. By
1986, total health expenditures had risen to 3.9
percent of GDP, of which 94.8 percent came
from public sources.

Spain

When Francisco Franco died in 1975, Spain
saw the end of a period of fascist dictatorship
that had started in 1939. The new democratic
government promptly extended the coverage
of social security and brought its health services under the control of a greatly strengthened Ministry of Health and Consumption.
The Constitution of 1978 explicitly affirms a

right to health care for everyone. After years of highly centralized authority, Spain was divided—for most administrative purposes, including health insurance—into 17 *autonomous communities* or regions.

The former social security or Compulsory Sickness Insurance program in the Ministry of Labor became the National Institute of Health (INSALUD) in the Ministry of Health and Consumption, along with other more traditional activities formerly supervised by the Ministry of Interior. The latter were preventive public health services operated by each of the 52 provinces (or districts), and also provincial and municipal medical care for the mentally ill and the indigent. Health reform legislation of 1986 called for decentralization of all these functions to the 17 regions, and as of 1989 this had been accomplished in four regions.

In 1984, an estimated 93 percent of the Spanish population were covered by the IN-SALUD program, financed 75 percent by employer and 25 percent by worker contributions. The remaining population, most of whom are indigent, may get care at the out-patient department or in the wards of public hospitals, run by the provinces or municipalities. Those with higher incomes (as well as many insured persons who want prompt and personal attention) obtain medical care privately. In the more prosperous regions, such as Catalonia, thousands of people purchase commercial insurance to facilitate their access to private medical care.

The INSALUD program operates a large network of its own hospitals and ambulatory care clinics. The doctors and other personnel working in these facilities are all salaried, although some primary care physicians are also paid by capitation fees. These formerly social security hospitals of INSALUD are generally regarded as the most technically developed institutions in Spain, but the resources for ambulatory care have frequently been criticized.

Since INSALUD has come to cover so many people, the program's own facilities are no longer adequate to serve all beneficiaries. Many services must, therefore, be obtained in public general hospitals or even in private hospitals, with which INSALUD makes contracts. In 1984, of all INSALUD health expenditures,

58 percent went for services in its own facilities, 20.5 percent for services under contract, 19 percent for private pharmacies, and 2.5 percent for other purposes.

Up to 1988, preventive public health services in Spain were provided separately. As the responsibility of the provinces and municipalities, they have been provided in small improvised quarters, inadequately equipped. Since 1984, the Ministry of Health has constructed 250 modern health centers, which are intended to promote preventive services, as well as primary medical care to populations of 5,000 to 20,000. As of 1988 about 25 percent of the population were accessible to one of these centers.

Spain has a very large stock of physicians because, until 1979, the medical schools admitted every secondary school graduate who applied. Since 1980, the enrollment has been controlled, but the country's 23 medical schools still graduate more than 10,000 new physicians a year. In 1986, Spain had 335 physicians per 100,000 population, of whom 53 percent had positions with INSALUD. Others work for different sections of the MOH, the military medical establishment, units of local government, and other organizations, but many are engaged entirely in private practice. In addition, employed doctors frequently practice privately in the afternoons.

As reflected in hospital resources, 33.0 percent of the beds are in private facilities. Altogether, Spain has 976 hospitals, with 4.7 beds per 1,000. The public hospitals, with 67 percent of the beds, are much larger than the private ones (averaging 311 and 102 beds, respectively), and generally serve the more complex medical and surgical cases. The medical staffs in both types of hospital are predominantly on full-time salaries.

A special feature of Spanish society is its large number of private charitable foundations, some originating as long ago as the thirteenth century; wealthy persons can avoid inheritance taxes by establishing such philanthropic organizations. Out of the 7,000 foundations estimated to exist in 1977, about 300 are primarily oriented to health service or medicine. Some are devoted to helping specific hospitals, some to tackling certain diseases, some to medical research, some to helping children, and so on. In 1988, some 13 of the major foundations concerned with health formed a coalition, intended to coordinate activities in Spain's 17 regions—possibly orienting their work to support research. This would include both biomedical research and studies to improve the effectiveness of the Spanish health system. Foundation leaders spoke of concern for the need to "restructure the health system in order to meet its ethical obligations."

In the late 1980s, the Spanish health system was undergoing rapid changes. The government was clearly committed to development of a national health service, in which preventive and curative services would be integrated and everyone would have access to comprehensive care. The customary pyramidal model, starting with local health centers and leading to provincial (or district) hospitals and then tertiary centers at the regional level, would be established. It was also expected that a major share of the funding would have to come from general tax revenues, rather than social insurance contributions.

In 1986, Spain's health system absorbed 6.0 percent of its GDP, somewhat less than other countries of Western Europe. Of this, 72 percent came from public and 28 percent from private sources. To reach its health service goals, a larger share of health expenditures will probably have to come from governmental sources. Even before this, however, Spain's health record was remarkably good, with an infant mortality rate in 1987 of only 9 per 1,000 live births and a life expectancy at birth of 77 years.

The development of national health services in Italy, Greece, and Spain in the 1980s was clearly the outcome of larger political forces in those countries. In all three countries, large sections of the population had long suffered under poor living conditions. Numerous political parties represented every ideology in the political spectrum, including socialism and communism. The NHS legislation in these countries was clearly the product of left-wing coalitions.

As of this writing, political movements toward NHS objectives—universal population coverage, comprehensive health services, substantial governmental control of health personnel and facilities, and financial support mainly from tax revenues—seem to be developing in Portugal also, but final actions cannot yet be reported. Data for 1982 show that Portugal was spending 5.7 percent of GDP on health, of which about 70 percent came from the public sector. Of the latter, 85 percent was attributable to the social security program, which covered essentially all employed persons and their families. Health services were provided mainly by salaried doctors and others working in polyclinics and hospitals. In all the southern European countries, the pattern of delivering health services under social insurance programs has been strikingly more organized than what is customary in northern Europe.

SUMMARY

In summary, the nine industrialized countries that have developed comprehensive health systems, covering their total populations, usually achieved these systems through a lengthy process. In Norway it took 45 years (from 1911 to 1956) and in Great Britain 37 years (from 1911 to 1948); the terrible suffering of World War II played a part in both cases. New Zealand's health system covered its relatively small total population at the outset, in 1939, but many organizational changes occurred over the years. In the other six countries, the evolutions were a fairly lengthy process.

With universal population coverage, the patterns for delivering medical care underwent various degrees of change. In countries where virtually all ambulatory medical care was customarily provided by autonomous medical practitioners, there has been a gradual extension of arrangements for organized teams of health personnel working in health centers operated by units of government. This trend has been most extensive in Finland and Sweden. In the southern European countries, where the private medical market had not previously been very strong, as in Greece or Spain, an organized pattern of health service delivery under insurance financing was used at the out-

set, but its population coverage has been gradually extended. These not-so-affluent countries
are still in the process of broadening their national health service schemes to the universal
coverage defined in their legislation.

The development of total population coverage, comprehensive services, and financing derived largely from general revenues has greatly
simplified administrative processes in these
previously pluralistic health systems. This sim-
plification is sometimes obscured by the fact
that the system management has become
clearly visible to everyone, when previously it
was out-of-sight in hundreds of small semi-independent agencies. Likewise, the broad entitlement of people to service has changed the
place of health care in national political debate. The role of the private sector and the
input of ordinary people in the management
process are sometimes contentious issues, but
the social soundness of a universal and comprehensive health service tends to be fully accepted. Once such a system is installed, its
value has not been challenged by any significant political group.

REFERENCES

Norway

Ekeid, S. E., *Health Services in Norway: Commitment to Decentralization.* Oslo: Directorate of
Health, 1984.

Evang, Karl, *Health Services in Norway.* Oslo: Norwegian Joint Committee for International Social Policy, 1970.

Fogarty International Center, *Health Care in Scandinavia.* Washington: U.S. Public Health Service, 1975.

Lembcke, Paul A., "Hospital Efficiency—A Lesson
from Sweden." *Hospitals,* 1 April 1959.

National Insurance Administration, *Social Insurance in Norway.* Oslo, December 1986.

Roemer, Milton I., and Ruth Romer, *Manpower in
the Health Care System of Norway.* Washington, D.C.: Public Health Service (DHEW Pub.
77–39), 1977.

Siem, Harold, *Choices for Health: An Introduction
to the Health Services in Norway.* Oslo: Univ-
ersitets-forlaget AS, 1986.

Tobiasson, T. K., "Insuring the Future: Costs
Threaten Welfare State." *International Herald
Tribune,* 3–4 June 1989.

Great Britain

Barnard, Keith, and Kenneth Lee (Editors), *Conflicts in the National Health Service.* London:
Croom Helm, 1977.

Beveridge, William, *Social Insurance and Allied
Services* (American Edition Reproduced Pho-
tographically from the English Edition). New
York: Macmillan Co., 1942.

Bunker, John, "Surgical Manpower: A Comparison
of Operations and Surgeons in the United
States and in England & Wales." *New England
Journal of Medicine,* 282:135–144, 15 January
1970.

Department of Health and Social Security, *Inequalities in Health: Report of a Working Group* (the
"Black Report"), 1980.

Forsyth, Gordon, "United Kingdom," in *Health
Service Prospects: An International Survey.* 1.
Douglas-Wilson and G. McLachlen, Editors.
London: The Lancet and the Nuffields Provin-
cial Hospitals Trust, 1973, pp. 1–35.

Fogarty International Center, *The British National
Health Service: Conversations with Sir George
E. Godber.* Washington, D.C.: U.S. Public
Health Service (DHEW Pub. No. 77–1205),
1976.

Godber, G. E., *The Future Place of the General Physician* (1969 Michael M. Davis Lecture). Chicago: University of Chicago, Center for Health
Administration Studies, 1969.

Hart, Nicky, "Inequalities in Health: The Individual
versus the Environment." *Journal of the Royal
Statistical Society (Series A),* 149 (3):228–246,
1986.

Kimball, Merit C., "Private Medical Care in U.K. Is
Losing Its Luster." *Health Week,* 6 September
1988, pp. 1 ff.

Kinnaird, John, "The British National Health Service: Retrospect and Prospect." *Journal of Public Health Policy,* 2(4):382–412, 1981.

Levitt, Ruth, *The Reorganized National Health Service.* London: Croom Helm. 1976.

Lindsay, Almont, *Socialized Medicine in England
and Wales: The National Health Service 1948–
1961.* Chapel Hill: University of North Caro-
lina Press, 1962.

Macmillan, Donald, et al., *NHS Reorganization: Issues and Prospects.* Leeds: Nuffield Center for
Health Services Studies, 1974.

Nelson, Harry, "Crisis Grips Health Care in Britain:
Desperate for Funds." *Los Angeles Times,* 7
March 1988, pp. 1 ff.

Orr, Douglas, W., and Jean Walker Orr, *Health Insurance With Medical Care: The British Experience.* New York: Macmillan Co., 1939.

Robb, J. Wesley, "The British Choice in Health
Care: A Report from London." *The Pharos,*
Winter 1985, pp. 33–37.

Secretaries of State for Health (Wales, Northern Ireland and Scotland), *Working for Patients,* London: Her Majesty's Stationery Office, January
1989.

Silver, George A., "The Community-Medicine Specialist—Britain Mandates Health Service Reorganization." *New England Journal of Medicine,* 287:1299–1301, 21 December 1972.

Torrens, Paul R., "Some Potential Hazards of Unplanned Expansion of Private Health Insurance in Britain." *The Lancet*, 2 January 1982, pp. 29–31.

Yates, John, *Why Are We Waiting? An Analysis of Hospital Waiting Lists*. Oxford: Oxford University Press, 1987.

New Zealand

Begg, Neil C., "New Zealand's Plunket Society: A Community-Supported Organization for the Health of Infants and Young Children." *Clinical Pediatrics*, 7(10): 614–623, October 1968.

Broughton, H. R., "A Viewpoint on Maori Health." *New Zealand Medical Journal*, 9 May 1984, pp. 290–291.

Department of Health, "A Review of Health Service Administration in New Zealand 1872–1972." Extract from the *Department of Health Annual Report*, Wellington, 1972.

Director General of Health, *Report on the Department of Health*. Wellington (New Zealand), 1984.

Emery, George M., "New Zealand Medical Care." *Medical Care*, July–September 1966, pp. 159–170.

Health Benefits Review Committee, Choices for Health Care. Wellington: Health Benefits Review Committee, 1986.

Kennedy, D. P., "School Dental Nurses in New Zealand." *New Zealand Medical Journal*, 72 (462):301–303, November 1970.

Malcolm, L. A., and J. R. Barnett, "The Availability, Distribution, and Utilization of General Practitioners in New Zealand: A Study Based on GMS Claims." *New Zealand Medical Journal*, 28 May 1980, pp. 396–399.

Malcolm, Laurence. "Progress Towards Achieving Health for All New Zealanders by the Year 2000." *Social Science & Medicine*, 25 (5):473–479, 1987.

Malcolm, Laurence A., "Towards Public Sector Goals: New Zealand's Recent Experience in Health Services Reorganization." *Journal of Public Health Policy*, 10(1):117–122, 1989.

Smith, A. G., and P. M. Tatchell, "Health Expenditures in New Zealand: Trends and Growth Patterns." *New Zealand Medical Journal*, 25 April 1979, pp. 308–311.

Other Scandinavian Countries

Andersen, Ronald, Bjorn Smedby, and Odin W. Anderson, *Medical Care Use in Sweden and the United States: A Comparative Analysis of Systems and Behavior*. Chicago: Center for Health Administration Studies (Research Series 27), 1970.

Anon., "Finnish National Health Insurance Begins in Fall." *Medical Tribune*, 18–19 July 1964.

Bjorck, Gunnar, "Trends in the Development of Medical Care in Sweden." *Medical Care*, 2(3):156–161, August–September 1964.

Bygren, Lars Olov, *Met and Unmet Needs for Medical and Social Services*. Stockholm: Scandinavian Journal of Social Medicine, Supplement 8, 1974.

Engel, Arthur G. W., *Planning and Spontaneity in the Development of the Swedish Health System* (Michael M. Davis Lecture). University of Chicago: Center for Health Administration Studies, 1968.

Fogarty International Center, *Health Care in Scandinavia*. Washington, D.C.: U.S. Public Health Service, 1975, pp. 40–52.

Gannik, Dorte, Erik Holst, and Marsden Wagner, *The National Health System of Denmark: A Descriptive Analysis*. Washington, D.C.: Fogarty International Center (DHEW Pub. No. NIH 77–673), 1976.

Haro, A. S. (Editor), *Planning Information Services for Health*. Helsinki: Nordic Medical Statistical Commission, 1981.

Holst, Erik, and Marsden Wagner, "Primary Health Care Is the Cornerstone." *Scandinavian Review*, 63 (3):30–39, September 1975.

Kalimo, Esko, "Medical Care Research in the Planning of Social Security in Finland." *Medical Care*, 9 (4):304–310, July –August 1971.

Ministry of Foreign Affairs of Denmark, *Fact Sheet/ Denmark: Health Services*. Copenhagen, 1982.

Ministries of Labor and Social Affairs, *Health Security and Daily Cash Benefits*. Copenhagen, 1974.

Ministry of Social Affairs and Health, *Primary Health Care in Finland*. Helsinki, 1978.

Ministry of Social Affairs and Health, *Health Policy Report by the Government to Parliament*. Helsinki: May 1985.

Ministry of Social Affairs and Health, *Health Care in Finland*. Helsinki, 1986.

National Board of Health and Welfare, *The Swedish Health Services in the 1990s*. Stockholm, 1985.

Rosenthal, Marilynn M. "Beyond Equity: Swedish Health Policy and the Private Sector." *Milbank Quarterly*, 64 (4):592–621, 1986.

Saltman, Richard B., "Ambulatory Care in Sweden: The Changing Legal Context." *Journal of Ambulatory Care Management*, 12(2):75–82, 1989.

Sjovall, Hjalmar, "Liability and Compensation Independent of Medical Negligence," *Forensic Science*, 6:235–239, 1975.

Sondergaard, Willy, and Allan Krasnik, "Health Services in Denmark," in Marshall W. Raffel (Editor), *Comparative Health Systems*. University Park: Pennsylvania State University Press, 1984, pp. 153–196.

Swedish Institute, *Fact Sheets on Sweden: The Health Care System in Sweden*. Stockholm, April 1986.

World Health Organization Regional Committee for Europe, *Planning & Management of Health Services in Finland—A Case Study*. Copenhagen: WHO/EUR/RC 32/Tech.Disc./BD/3, September 1982.

Southern European Countries

Bariletti, Antonio, "Background Paper on the Italian Health Services System." Rome: Instituto di Scienza delle Finanze, Univ. di Roma, 1982 (processed).

Blum, Richard, and Eva Blum, *Health and Healing in Rural Greece.* Stanford, Calif.: Stanford University Press, 1965.

Center for Medical Manpower Studies, "Regionalization of National Health Insurance in Italy." Boston: Northern University, 1978 (processed).

Kent, George D., "Socializing Health Services in Greece." *Journal of Public Health Policy,* 10(2):222–245, Summer 1989.

McArdle, Frank B., "Italy's National Health Service Plan." *Social Security Bulletin,* 42 (4):38–42, April 1979.

Minestero della Sanita, *Towards the National Health Service in Italy.* Rome (Special Report), 1979.

Paghi, Aldo, "Background Information on Primary Health Care in Italy." In *Il Medico di Base in Italia e in Gran Bretagna: Aleune Idee ed Esperienze a Confranto,* Rome 1980.

Plessas, Demetrius J., "The Greek Health Care System: Old Structures and New Prospects." Ann Arbor: University of Michigan, School of Public Health, September 1984 (processed paper).

Ramic, H., "Spain," in *Draft Report on Study on Primary Health Care Development in the European Region.* Copenhagen: World Health Organization, Regional Office for Europe, March 1988, pp. 71–85 (processed document).

Reich, Michael R., and Rose H. Goldman, "Italian Occupational Health: Concepts, Conflicts, Implications." *American Journal of Public Health,* 74 (9):1031–1041, September 1984.

Ritsatakis, Anna, "The Changing Health Services System in Greece," in Charles O. Pannenborg et al. (Editors), *Reorienting Health Services: Application of a Systems Approach.* New York: Plenum Press, 1984, pp. 347–356.

Saturno, Pedro J., "Spain," in Richard B. Saltman (Editor), *The International Handbook of Health-Care Systems.* New York: Greenwood Press, 1988, pp. 267–284.

Tsalikis, G., "Evaluation of the Socialist Health Policy in Greece." *Intenational Journal of Health Services,* 18(4):543–561, 1988.

Wood-Ritsatakis, Anna, *Unified Social Planning in the Greek Context.* Athens: Centre of Planning and Economic Research, 1986, pp. 164–226.

World Health Organization, Regional Office for Europe, "Spain," in *Evaluation of the Strategy for Health for All by the Year 2000.* Copenhagen, 1985, pp. 188–91.

CHAPTER EIGHT

Socialist Health Systems in Industrialized Countries

The national health systems analyzed in the three previous chapters have demonstrated increasing degrees of intervention in the medical market, to make health service available to the population. Actions were undertaken principally by governments to convert health care from a "commodity," traded in the market, through various transitional forms, to a service provided to everyone who needs it as a basic social right. A fourth degree of market intervention has been through social revolutions, which have virtually abolished free market economies and installed socialism, along with socialist health systems.

GENERAL FEATURES OF SOCIALIST HEALTH SYSTEMS

The first revolutionary overthrow of capitalism occurred in Russia in November (October by the Gregorian calendar) 1917. An earlier revolution in March 1917 had overthrown the autocratic Czar, and installed a provisional government of Constitutional Democrats; this government proclaimed many personal freedoms, but did little to alter control of the economy. It was the second revolution, led by Nicolai Lenin, that led to the seizure of power by the Communist Party, a complete reorganization of the economy, in which virtually all industry and land were nationalized, and establishment of the Union of Soviet Socialist Republics (USSR).

The USSR, or Soviet Union, remained alone as the world's only socialist country, adapting a Marxian philosophy, between the end of World War I in 1918 and the end of World War II in 1945. In those years, it devel-

oped a health system that differed from any other in the world. After World War II, communist parties gained power in a number of other countries of Eastern Europe and, in their health care organization as in other social sectors, they emulated the Soviet Union. These countries included Albania, Bulgaria, Czechoslovakia, German Democratic Republic (East Germany), Hungary, Poland, Romania, and Yugoslavia. A few years later China (People's Republic of China) and several other less economically developed countries also established Marxian socialist governments following revolutions; the health systems of these countries are discussed later.

The health systems of these Eastern European, and essentially industrialized, countries have much in common, although no two are identical. Just as there are differences in every national culture, the historical backgrounds and the economic and political conditions of countries create several variations in their national health systems. Nevertheless, all of the systems have certain general features that can be broadly defined:

1. Health services of almost all types are a social entitlement of everyone, without any, or with only minor, personal charges.
2. The provision of all health services is a responsibility of government, at various levels.
3. The delivery of preventive and therapeutic health services is essentially integrated, with emphasis on prevention.
4. Health resources and services are centrally planned, as part of the general planning of the entire social and economic order.

5. While local groups of citizens contribute to health policy formation, final decisions on major features of the national health system are made by central health and political authorities.
6. Insofar as resources are limited, priorities in the health system are accorded to industrial workers and children.
7. All component parts of the health system are directed or integrated under one major authority—the Ministry of Health—and its subdivisions.
8. Private medical practice (and related activity) is not prohibited, but it is subject to strict regulation.
9. All health work is to be based on scientific principles, so that nonscientific or cultist practices are theoretically not permitted.

The implementation of these basic principles, of course, is seldom perfect and, as noted, the precise methods by which they are applied differ among the socialist countries. Variations also occur at different times and in different regions of the same country. The common notion that socialist or communist countries are monolithic, with deadly uniformity in all matters, may be useful in political rhetoric, but it is far from an accurate description of the realities.

Except for the Soviet Union's health system, those of the other socialist countries of Eastern Europe are all relatively young—barely 40 years old, as of this writing. Their physical and human resources all suffered massive destruction from World War II, and great political and economic turbulence has impeded their development. Most of the countries were under fascist domination for years before their revolutions, so their transformation into socialist societies was obviously stormy. As predominantly agricultural economies, their national wealth, as measured by GNP per capita, was much lower than that of the Western European countries. They lacked the long tradition of parliamentary democracy that characterized France, Germany, and Great Britain. All of these circumstances influenced the extent to which any of the Eastern European countries could implement the principles of a socialist health system, articulated in Marxian theory and often inscribed in their constitutions.

Because the Soviet Union was the socialist pioneer and because its health system has served as the model for so many other countries, we examine that system in some detail.

THE SOVIET UNION

Before considering the five major components of the Soviet health system, some of the highlights of its background should be reviewed.

Russian Health Services Before 1917

The vast majority of the Russian population, under the czars, were rural people—impoverished peasant families. In 1861, Czar Alexander II had abolished serfdom, in response to great unrest among the peasants following Russia's defeat in the Crimean War. One of the most important social reforms was launched in 1864, when a network of local district assemblies, elected by the people, was authorized to operate many local services, including health care. These local government bodies, called *zemstvos,* brought great improvement to the health services of Russian peasants.

Election of members to the assemblies, however, was far from democratic. Large landowners and the bourgeoisie had two-thirds of the seats, while the far more numerous peasants had one-third, and yet most of the revenues to finance zemstvo activities were paid by the peasants. Nevertheless, the basic concept of zemstvo health services was sound and certainly a great advance over the past. Hundreds of medical stations were established, each staffed by a physician and several auxiliary personnel. Since salaries and other costs were supported by tax funds, the service was free. If the patient needed hospitalization, he or she was sent to the nearest zemstvo hospital, where the care was also free.

By 1890, after 25 years of zemstvo health care, 34 Russian provinces had been organized with health facilities. These were divided into 359 districts (zemstvo territories), containing 1,422 medical stations (essentially for primary care), 414 dispensaries for special health services, and 1,068 small hospitals with an average of 25 beds each. An indication of the program's expansion was the increase of physicians in these units from 756 in 1870 to 1,805 in 1890. Various auxiliary personnel—*feldshers* (see later), midwives, and pharmacists—increased from 2,794 in 1870 to 6,778 in 1890. Of all the physicians in Russia at the time, about 16 percent worked in the zemstvo program, and many of these were young and idealistic recent medical graduates.

By 1913, shortly before the Revolution, the zemstvo health care program had expanded to 4,367 rural medical stations (staffed by doctors and others), 4,539 feldsher posts (staffed only by health auxiliaries), and hospitals containing 49,087 beds. Although this was a vast improvement over the days of feudalism and serfdom, the network of health facilities had to serve more than 80 million rural people. This meant an average of about 18,500 people per medical station and 0.60 hospital beds per 1,000 population. Of course, the distribution of medical stations and feldsher posts was not exactly even; some districts had only one physician for 40,000 people. But, with all its weaknesses, the zemstvo program established certain formulations, on which the Revolutionary government later built. It demonstrated the feasibility of providing medical care as a public service, given by salaried doctors and auxiliaries, all financed (not by personal fees but) by tax revenues.

In the cities, arrangements for the medical care of industrial workers were quite different. In 1866, under Czar Alexander II, a law was passed requiring factory owners to provide one hospital bed per 100 workers—presumably along with the necessary staff; this law was often disregarded, however. Then in 1912, Russia under Czar Nicholas II took action similar to that of several other European countries at the time, enacting social insurance for medical and sickness benefits. Employees in only the larger companies were covered, however—about one-fifth of all industrial wage earners. In the typical European manner, the insurance fund came 50 percent from the employers and 50 percent from the workers. Private doctors and others were paid on a fee basis.

Thus, after the 1860s the Czarist regimes took certain actions to respond to the great health needs of the rural peasants and urban workers. The programs, however, were far from adequate for the needs. In 1913, all the territory of the Russian Empire had 23,143 physicians for a population of 159,200,000. This meant one doctor to about 6,900 people, or 14.5 doctors per 100,000 population. Russia made extensive use of auxiliary health personnel, such as other European countries used only in their overseas colonies in Asia and Africa. Most important was the *feldsher,* a type of "assistant doctor," of whom there were 29,000 in 1913. There were also 10,000 nurses and 15,000 midwives. Hospital beds numbered 207,300, or 1.3 beds per 1,000 population. Hospital distributions was so uneven that 35 percent of all towns had no hospital at all, and only 21 percent of the hospitals had more than 20 beds.

Transition to Socialism

When the majority *(Bolshevik)* wing of the Russian Socialist Party seized power from the Provisional Government (under the control of the Constitutional Democratic Party since March 1917) in October (Gregorian calendar) 1917, Russian society was in shambles. The physical and human destruction of World War I had been enormous; everything—factories, public utilities, transportation, schools, homes—was in a state of disaster. Hundreds of hospitals and medical stations, meager as they were, were destroyed. Worst of all, the population was being decimated with epidemic diseases, the worst of which was typhus fever, spread by rats and the insects they harbored. It was estimated that, soon after the Revolution, 20 million to 30 million cases of typhus fever occurred, with some 3,000,000 deaths.

The first organized health activity to take shape was a Medical–Sanitary Committee, consisting of Bolshevik physicians; it was formed on 26 October 1917, to organize medical services for the workers and soldiers of the Petrograd (later Leningrad) area. Lenin, the Bolshevik leader, was in no hurry to establish a central Commissariat (Ministry) of Health, regarding it best for social functions such as health care, to arise from the actions of local people ("the masses") rather than from central government initiatives. Therefore, sections or committees on medicine and public health were organized in many of the local councils *(Soviets)* of workers' and peasants' deputies. To promote epidemic control, the small hygienic units (later developed as *sanitary–epidemiological stations*), sometimes set up under the zemstvo health programs, were expanded. In January 1918, a central *council of medical boards* was established, to supervise and coordinate these peripheral activities.

In June 1918, a national conference was held for all the committees on medicine and public health that had been set up under local soviets throughout the country. The conference was chaired by Dr. N. A. Semashko, a physician who had previously been exiled with Lenin. This conference passed a resolution that free medical care for the entire population must be part of the health program of the USSR and a central Commissariat of Health Protection should be established to bring this about. The next month, on 11 July 1918, such a Ministry of Health Protection was established.

As so often happens when health services are reorganized, a major problem confronting the new ministry was its relationship with the medical profession. Although many of the younger physicians supported the Revolution, the older leadership of the profession was not willing to accept subordination to nonmedical political groups. In response, the government leadership accused these physicians of "medical sabotage" and "counterrevolutionary" activities. The attitude of the ruling party was that the previously dominant physicians were hopelessly "bourgeois." Egalitarian goals could be achieved only by changing the attitude of the medical profession to that of "medical workers."

A major strategy for achieving this change was to organize a new association: the All-Russian Federated Union of Medical Workers. Unlike several societies of physicians that had lingered from the pre-1917 period, this federated union was open to all categories of health personnel. At first, mainly junior health workers joined and very few physicians. By the end

of 1919, however, pharmacists and veterinarians joined, and in 1920—with special arrangements for a nonpartisan role—physicians joined the union.

The first years after the Revolution, 1918–1921, were extremely difficult; there was vast economic disruption internally and military assaults from capitalist powers externally. With famines and epidemics, the top priority was prevention, by doing everything possible for safer environmental sanitation. Pharmacies and other medical installations were nationalized, and all health personnel were made subject to "work draft" (although the latter could not be achieved immediately). Hygienic centers for communal feeding were set up. Tuberculosis and venereal disease were treated at dispensaries. Medical services for the Red Army, fighting both White Russians internally and foreign forces externally, were directed by the Commissariat of Health, and these services were available to civilians as well.

The period of Lenin's New Economic Policy (NEP), 1921–1928, saw a strategic retreat in socialization generally, reflected also in the health services. Some restrictions on private medical practice were removed, although the general movement to public medical employment continued. Many nationalized pharmacies were returned to private ownership. By 1923–1924, the major epidemics had been conquered, and greater attention could be given to the organization of health services for workers in major industries and also for the poorest peasants. In 1924, a meeting of the All-Russian Congress of Health Departments stressed the unity of sanitary (preventive) and medical (therapeutic) work, previously recognized in tuberculosis and venereal disease control, as essential in tackling all health problems.

The years 1928 to 1941 were a period of intense efforts toward industrialization and collectivization of agriculture. Forced urbanization and the reshaping of agriculture led to much violence. The Ministry of Health was evidently moving more cautiously, and was criticized by the Central Committee of the Communist Party for being too slow in collectivizing the health services. Improvement in the training of health personnel according to socialist concepts was called for, and a better geographic distribution of graduates was also said to be essential.

The first of the now-famous Five-Year Plans was launched in 1928. Under instructions from the Party leadership, the Ministry of Health set out to accelerate the organization of medical services for industrial workers (through polyclinics) and for the socialist sector of agriculture. Far more doctors and other personnel were needed, but the top priority for basic industry impeded the creation of medical school facilities and equipment. With women being drawn into industrial employment, thousands of kindergartens and creches had to be developed, mostly under Ministry of Health supervision.

In 1936, the authorities of the former Commissariat (Ministry) of Health Protection, established in 1918, were greatly broadened. As the People's Commissariat of Health for the USSR, it encompassed several previously separate administrative bodies. One was the Institute of Experimental Medicine (started in Leningrad by Nobel Laureate Ivan Pavlov), which was to become the Academy of Medical Sciences. Another was the All-Union States Sanitary Inspectorate, which supervised a nationwide network of sanitary–epidemiological stations for epidemic control (including the education of the people about hygienic behavior).

Most important, and unique in the world, was the transfer of almost all the medical faculties from the universities to the direction of the strengthened Ministry of Health. This took several years in the 1930s, and it was applied to the training programs for all health personnel. Since the graduates were to staff the programs of the health system, it was considered most reasonable for their training to be fitted to Ministry of Health policies. This crucial move affected both the quantity of medical personnel turned out and the content of their educational preparation. (The Ministry of Education, of course, continued to be responsible for all elementary school education and for university education in the humanities, sciences, and the various general nonprofessional fields.)

Still another transfer of responsibilities in this period applied to the field of pharmaceutical products and medical supplies. These items were produced by various ministries such as the Ministry of Light Industry (later a new Ministry of Medical Industry), and this arrangement continued. Decisions on which drugs should be produced, however, and standardization of drug composition, dosages, and so on were assigned to the Ministry of Health. A special Scientific Council was established to advise on these pharmaceutical questions.

Finally, a crucial action for unification of health functions under the Ministry of Health was taken in 1937 in the economic sphere. Until then, financial support for health services in the USSR essentially came from two large sources with correspondingly separate administrative authorities. The large social insurance program for industrial workers and their dependents had been administered by the Ministry of Labor, but in 1922 it was transferred to the trade unions. Soon after the Revolution, all health insurance contributions were collected from the enterprise and none from the workers. The medical establishments supported by these funds had always been under the Ministry of Health, but in 1937 the health insurance moneys were also transferred to the general government budget.

The second source of economic support for health services was that used for the rural population. From the outset, the peasants and others were not enrolled in the social insurance scheme, and their health care was financed directly from general government revenues. With the transfer of social insurance moneys to general government funds in 1937, the economic foundations of the health system became essentially unified under the Ministry of Health.

By 1941, when the Soviet Union became deeply involved in World War II, its health system had become quite well developed. Its human and physical resources, as we shall see, were greatly expanded. All the major organized entities concerned with health were under the unified control of the Ministry of Health. Most important, a comprehensive range of health services was available to virtually the entire population, without any significant charges. Then the massive destruction of

World War II substantially assaulted the operation of the whole system. The system's overall organizational framework, however, had been firmly established, and the transition to the first socialist health model in the world had essentially been accomplished.

Current Organizational Structure

The reconstruction of the Soviet Union, after the devastation of World War I, and the early development of a new socialist society were hardly complete when World War II demolished a major part of what had been achieved. Then the stresses of the Cold War in the 1950s, and 1960s, and the huge military expenditure it engendered, further handicapped the Soviet health system. By 1969, it was deemed important for the Supreme Soviet (parliament) to issue a comprehensive legislative statement on the national organization of the health services.

This legislation stated that "Citizens of the USSR shall be entitled to free and professional medical care available to all. It shall be provided by public health establishments administered by the government." Detailed responsibilities of the Ministry of Health were spelled out on medical services, pharmaceuticals, environmental controls, maternal and child health, hospitals, and all related matters. For historical reasons, special health care programs were authorized in the Ministries of Transport, Internal Affairs (police), and military defense, but these services had to be coordinated by the Ministry of Health.

The basic organizational structure of the Soviet health system is now parallel with that of the general structure of government. In the council of Ministers (the cabinet) of the central government, one member is the minister of health. The USSR Ministry of Health (MOH) headquarters in Moscow is not a very large organization, since its responsibilities have been largely delegated to several lower echelons. Central functions are largely standard-setting, consultation, and general supervision. For these functions, the MOH has technical units on medical care (including both therapeutic and personal preventive services), environ-

mental sanitation, pharmaceuticals (both technological policies and drug distribution), health professional training, planning and financial matters, and foreign relations in health. The Academy of Medical Sciences, supervising hundreds of research institutes, also comes under the central ministry.

The USSR is a union of 15 republics, with a combined population in 1984 of 276,257,000; its territory occupies 22,402,000 square kilometers, which is the largest area of any country on earth. Much the largest population is in the Russian Soviet Federated Socialist Republic (RSFSR), which has about half of the national population, and also more than half the territory (including Siberia). Of the other 14 republics, all but one have populations of less than 16 million and mostly less than 8 million. One can therefore appreciate why the Russian Federated Republic dominates most political and economic affairs. The overall GNP per capita of the Soviet Union was $7,095 in 1984, but the economic level in the western, European republics has long been higher than that in the eastern, Asiatic republics.

Each republic also has a ministry of health, whose structure and functions are largely equivalent to those of the central ministry. Certain republics might have special additional subdivisions, such as for maternal and child health or for sanitaria and rehabilitation. The republic governments carry a great deal of responsibility for managing all health services, so their power is considerable.

Below the level of the republic is the province (in Russian, *oblast*), which usually has a population of 1,000,000 to 5,000,000 people; there are a total of about 150 provinces in the entire country. The Provincial Health Department is probably the crucial organizational and administrative unit in the entire Soviet health system. This department includes special supervisors for virtually all categories of health activity. There are chief consultants in medicine and in surgery, also in obstetrics and gynecology for maternal health and in pediatrics for child health. A Provincial Sanitary Inspector supervises the network of sanitary–epidemiological stations that look after environmental sanitation. Another specialist oversees pharmaceutical matters. There are offices for planning, for personnel, and for financial accounts.

Each province is further subdivided into districts (*rayons* in Russian), which number 10 to 50 per province, with populations ranging between 40,000 and 150,000 people. The entire Soviet Union contains about 3,100 districts. Their structures vary between urban municipalities and rural areas. A small municipality may constitute one district, while a large city may contain several districts or *rayons*. At this level, the administrative organization merges with the facilities for providing health care, since the district health director (especially in rural areas) often serves as the medical director of the district hospital. In this role, he has responsibility for the operation of all health services in the jurisdiction (ambulatory, environmental, pharmacies, etc.), as well as the running of the hospital. The district health director typically has deputies to supervise the hospital, the polyclinics and other ambulatory services, and the *sanepid* station, and also to perform general administration (finances procurement, personnel, etc.).

Districts are the lowest level having a responsible administrative unit, but for purposes of health work districts are subdivided even further into sectors (or in Russian, *uchastoks*). A sector's population may vary between 1,000 and 10,000, with the average about 4,000. These people in a rural area are regarded as the "catchment" population of a local health facility for primary care. In a city, several sector populations may be served by several teams of health personnel (doctor, nurse, feldsher, etc.) in a larger health facility (usually a polyclinic).

This account of the hierarchical structure in the Soviet Ministry of Health gives the barest outline of the framework. The content of health functions differs among the republics, especially between the large and small ones; the organization charts of different provinces (oblasts) in the same or different republics also differ. Variations are most likely at the district (rayon) level, insofar as the range of health facilities varies. In some districts there may be numerous polyclinics specifically for children, in others for industrial workers, in others for women. Specialized dispensaries for cancer, tuberculosis, mental illness, university students, rehabilitation of the disabled, or venereal diseases are located in certain districts and not others. Likewise, sanitary–epidemiological stations may be much more highly developed in some areas than others. The size and functions of hospitals are also very diversified.

These several echelons of the Ministry of Health encompass the great bulk of activities in the total Soviet health system—probably 90 percent, as measured by either expenditures or volume of health services. Certain other comparatively small programs must be noted.

The special health programs of the transportation utilities, the police, and the military forces have been mentioned. These are all coordinated by the Ministry of Health, but they function independently. In time of war on home soil, the military and civilian health services are fully integrated. Moreover, personnel policies, standards of technical quality, procedures for prevention and therapy, record and reporting schemes are all essentially the same as in the general programs of the Ministry of Health (MOH).

Industrial enterprises, especially the larger ones (with 500 or more workers), play a crucial role in the Soviet health system. The staffing and operation of special polyclinics and hospitals for workers are responsibilities of the MOH, but the physical facilities and equipment are usually provided by the enterprise. Certain administrative personnel to manage these health programs may also be furnished and financed by the enterprise. If the supply of certain drugs, furnished ordinarily by the MOH, is low, it may be restocked at the expense of the enterprise. The managment of any enterprise, it must be realized, is motivated to keep its workers healthy and satisfied, if only to meet or surpass its production quota. The same general policies apply to enterprises in agriculture, both state farms and cooperatives.

Voluntary health agencies in the Soviet Union (and also in other socialist countries) are quite different from those in free-market countries. The Red Cross—or in Moslem parts of the USSR, the Red Crescent— is probably the most important agency devoted mainly to health. Its focus is on health and welfare services in emergencies or natural disasters. Collection and distribution of human blood is another function, as in many countries. Much of the work done by Red Cross personnel is voluntary, without compensation, but the MOH provides substantial funds necessary for certain full-time workers, such as nurses, doctors, and ambulance drivers. Although its management and membership are private, the Red Cross Society and its hundreds of chapters are closely integrated with the overall government health program. The Soviet Red Cross is affiliated with the International League of Red Cross Societies and participates in international Red Cross meetings.

Other nongovernment health activities in the Soviet Union are carried out by mass organizations of women, youth, workers, farmers, and others as part of their general social programs. These organizations have millions of members; subgroups participate in voluntary activities for improving environmental sanitation, getting children immunized, providing health education on special problems (such as contraception), and so on. The trade unions assume more concrete responsibilities. They develop and operate rest homes and spas for meritorious workers. These are medically staffed by the MOH, but the selection of workers, typically for 28-day stays, and the general management policies are the responsibility of the unions.

Finally, the Soviet health system has a small private sector. Private medical and dental practice by individuals is not prohibited, but it is discouraged through very high taxation on earnings. More significant are the officially sanctioned *paying polyclinics,* developed in several large cities. Specialists may spend 1 or 2 hours a day in these clinics—somewhat like private "group practices" in other countries—at which the patients pay fees personally. An administrator is assigned by the MOH to manage the polyclinic, to ensure the setting of proper fees, and to distribute proper shares of the earnings to the physicians, with additional allocations for rent, supplies, and the payment of ancillary personnel. These clinics are attended, of course, only by higher-income persons, who are able to pay personally for faster and perhaps better quality service. They are estimated to account for only about 1 percent of the ambulatory services nationally.

Production of Health Resources

The most spectacular achievements of the Soviet health system, and the essential foundation for all aspects of its system operation, have been the education of vast numbers of health personnel and the construction of a huge nationwide network of health facilities. The highest priority has gone to preparing physicians, perhaps on the ideological ground that the Revolution should ensure "the best" quality of personnel to serve all workers and peasants. Large numbers of "middle medical workers" (nurses, feldshers, etc.) are also trained, but still Soviet physicians are expected to perform many functions that are done by more briefly trained personnel in other countries.

Health Manpower. It will be recalled that, before the Revolution, in 1913 Czarist Russia had one doctor to 6,900 people, or 14.5 per 100,000, and these were concentrated in the large cities. Almost immediately after the Revolution, new medical faculties were established in the major universities. In the 1930s, nearly all of these faculties were withdrawn as separate *medical institutes* under the MOH. With MOH control, it was reasoned that medical education would be oriented more appropriately to the health needs of the population (compared to the academic interests of professors). Moreover, the ministry's concern for acquiring large numbers of doctors would govern policy, even if this meant enrolling very large classes. The priority was for quantity of manpower; quality "would come later." (The concept of linking education to social needs was not unique to the health field. Colleges of agriculture were brought under the Ministry of Agriculture, and engineering colleges were tied to various ministries of industrial production.)

By 1980, the Soviet Union had 83 medical institutes plus 9 medical departments still attached to universities. With tens of thousands of medical graduates turned out each year, by 1986 there were more than 1,200,000 physicians in the country, or 430 per 100,000 population. Their distribution was not entirely even, of course, with greater supplies and ratios being in the western republics and fewer in the eastern republics.

Specialization in the Soviet Union, as in all industrialized countries, became highly developed, and has gradually become more so. The specialist receives a higher salary and has greater prestige. There are primary and secondary grades of specialists, requiring different periods of postgraduate training. With the increasing movement to specialize, by the 1980s more than 80 percent of Soviet doctors were specialists in about 50 different fields. Since the mid-1970s, this has included a "specialty in general practice."

In a sense, a specialty orientation begins even in medical school. The first two years of the 6-year curriculum are the same for all students, but then a path must be selected toward general medicine, pediatrics, or hygiene. About 60 percent of students choose the general path, 35 percent choose pediatrics, and 5 percent choose hygiene. (The new graduate in pediatrics, for example, is not a specialist, but rather a generalist for children.) On completing medical education, nearly all graduates are required to spend 3 years in a rural area, chosen from a list of locations prepared by the Ministry of Health of the republic in which the school is located. Some exceptionally talented students are excused from this obligation, to permit immediate specialty training in a hospital, and others escape it with one or another excuse; the great majority of medical graduates, however, perform this rural service.

From the early days of the USSR, women entered medical training in great numbers for several reasons; there was no gender discrimination, the frequently short work-day (6 or 7 hours) was attractive to women with family duties, and women were regarded as particularly suitable for the high-priority field of pediatrics. With thousands of male doctors killed in the war, and with higher salaries in engineering attracting the more scientifically talented men, around 1950 some 75 percent of Soviet physicians were women. Since then the female:male ratio has been declining, and is moving toward a goal of half-and-half. Women are also beginning to hold top administrative health posts, which had been almost exclusively held by men.

Medical education, like higher education in other professional fields, is supported almost entirely by government; there are no tuitions to pay, and about 85 percent of students receive stipends for living expenses. Applicants for medical school are abundant, and one is accepted for every two or three who apply.

Continuing education, to acquaint practitioners with new developments in medical science, is required of all physicians in the Soviet health system. The periodicity seems to vary among the republics and in different specialty disciplines. Supplementary training in a hospital may be undertaken for 2 weeks each year, for 1 month every second year, or perhaps for 3 months every 5 years. It is not clear how rigorously the requirement for continuing education is enforced. In general, physicians in rural posts are provided with continuing education more often (e.g., every 2 years) and in urban posts less often (e.g., every 5 years).

In 1968, there were 13 special Institutes for Advanced Training of Physicians, plus another 14 advanced training faculties in the basic medical institutes (medical schools). These training centers are mainly for the preparation of medical and surgical specialists. In addition, almost all the larger provincial and district hospitals offer frequent courses of 2 weeks to several months. Some continuing education is even through correspondence courses, while the doctor remains at his regular post.

Dentistry, or care of the teeth and mouth, is defined differently in the Soviet Union than in other countries. The top responsibility in this field is assigned to stomatologists, as they are called, whose training is for 5 years—just 1 year less than that for a physician. Stomatology is regarded as one of the subdivisions of medicine, and statistics on Soviet physicians usually include stomatologists (about 10 percent of the total). Most of the common restorative dental work, however, is done by *dentistas* or "dental doctors" (regarded as middle medical personnel), who are trained for 3 years and work under the supervision of a stomatologist.

Almost all other types of health manpower in the Soviet Union are regarded as *middle medical personnel*. The most numerous of these health workers are nurses, who are trained for 2 years (if they have completed secondary school, a total of 10 years of basic education) or for 3 years (if they have completed 8 years of basic schooling). Much of the time is devoted to practical exercises in hospitals and polyclinics. In contrast to the multiple levels of nurses (registered, assistant, practical, etc.) in other countries, the Soviet health system trains simply one category of nurse. All nursing graduates must pass a nationally uniform examination, prepared by the Ministry of Health.

The second most numerous category of middle medical worker is the *feldsher,* a type of "assistant doctor" who, it will be recalled, dates back to the nineteenth century. In contrast to the Czarist's feldshers, who were trained mostly by apprenticeship, the Soviet feldsher receives formal and relatively rigorous training. For candidates with 10 years of basic school, the course requires 2½ years, and for those with 8 years of schooling the training is 3½ years. The extent of feldsher training is somewhat similar to that of nurses, but more time (involving greater depth) is required in both the classroom and field practice aspects. Moreover, feldsher training in the modern period is usually specialized, varying with the goal as noted later.

The policy of the Soviet government toward feldshers has changed over the years since the Revolution. Soon after the Bolsheviks took power, the feldsher came to be regarded as the very symbol of "second-class medicine" for the masses under czarism. A quotation from prerevolutionary Russia, attributed to the gentry and nobility, states that "The peasant is not accustomed and does not need scientific medical assistance; his diseases are 'simple' and for this a feldsher is enough—a physician treats the masters, and a peasant is treated by a feldsher." With such a perception of feldshers, the new revolutionary government decided to terminate their training. Then, as the enormity of the task of preparing enough doctors for this huge country became clear, feldsher training was reinstated but made more rigorous, and comprehensive. Feldshers proved to be very useful in the military medical services during World War II, as well as elsewhere.

By the 1970s, vast numbers of physicians had been trained and the role of the feldsher was again changed. Criticism frequently appeared in the medical press that feldshers were taking too much medical responsibility and not working under a physician's direction. Why should feldshers be used when physicians were available? The solution seems to have been to assign to feldshers various specialized roles—in factories, on ambulances, in sanitation work, in laboratories, and so on. The emphasis would be on supportive service, including health education. In general, the feldsher in cities works in settings where the medical supervision is close at hand. In rural areas, the feldsher–midwife, at an isolated health station, tends to have a more independent role. Nevertheless, Ministry of Health officials stress that at all places the feldsher functions as an assistant to the physician. In time, it is hoped that the rural feldsher–midwife stations will be replaced by small health centers, staffed with at least one physician.

The training of feldshers, nurses, and other middle medical personnel is conducted at *secondary medical schools* operated by the Ministry of Health, but separate from the medical institutes training physicians. Pharmacists, dental technicians, physiotherapists, and other middle medical health workers are also trained at these schools. It is noteworthy that, in contrast to practice in most other countries, the education of all these ancillary health personnel is largely integrated in multidisciplinary institutions. Instruction in many basic scientific subjects can therefore be offered in the same classroom to students working toward several different health occupations.

Regarding all health personnel, a notable feature of Soviet education is the occupational mobility that is possible. Middle medical personnel may advance to become physicians, with academic credit allotted for their previous experience. In the 1970s, some 15 percent of physicians had risen from the ranks of feldshers or nurses. The curricular content of education for all the health professions includes a strong emphasis on hygiene and the social aspects of disease.

Health Facilities. As in most countries, general hospitals play a large part in the Soviet health system. With the vast destruction of World War II, thousands of hospitals had to be rebuilt, and in 1986 there were 23,500 in-patient care facilities with some 3,660,000 beds. This amounted to 13.0 beds per 1,000 population, of which more than half were general beds for short-term care. Although the bed supply varies among the republics, in all of them the hospitals are functionally regionalized. At every jurisdictional level, all Soviet health facilities are government-sponsored; despite the small private sector in ambulatory care, there is none in hospital care.

At the most local level are small sector (uchastak) hospitals of 35 to 50 beds, serving a population of under 10,000 people for relatively simple conditions; these are each staffed by only a few full-time specialists, usually including one surgeon. As roads and transportation resources have improved, people have gained access to larger facilities (serving larger populations) and the smallest rural hospitals have been closed or converted to ambulatory care stations.

At the next level, for more difficult cases, are district (rayon) hospitals with 100 to 300 beds, to serve 40,000 to 150,000 people; in these there are 14 to 16 specialists in various fields. More technically developed is the provincial (oblast) hospital of 600 to 1,200 beds, to serve a population of 1,000,000 to 5,000,000. This type of hospital is staffed with a full range of specialists, and may serve as the teaching unit for a medical school. The x-ray and laboratory equipment in all of these hospitals is relatively modest, compared with facilities in other industrialized countries.

Besides these regional networks of adult general hospitals throughout the Soviet Union, there are also separate specialized hospitals at large industrial enterprises, hospitals for children, maternity and gynecological conditions, cancer, mental illness, tuberculosis, for acute infectious diseases, and trauma cases. Large tertiary hospitals for heart disease, cancer, eye disorders, and so on are associated with research institutes in those fields.

The rest homes or sanataria operated by trade unions have already been noted. In 1980, more than 13,000 of these existed, with over 2,100,000 beds. These should not, however, be considered institutions for long-term care: the usual patient stay is not more than a month. These facilities furnish care for convalescence or general rest-and-recreation after a period of stress. They are usually located in attractive environments with pleasant climates. Natural mineral waters may be emphasized, as at spas for rest cures in the European tradition.

Institutions for the elderly and chronically ill—known in Western Europe or North America as nursing homes or homes for the aged—do not seem to be part of the Soviet health system resources. Chronically ill patients requiring medical care are attended predominantly in general hospitals or remain in personal homes. Some senile patients are kept in special sections of mental hospitals. Under the Ministry of Social Affairs, there are custodial "homes for the elderly" to accommodate persons who lack a family; they do not provide medical service, however, except for acute episodes that may arise.

Outside of hospitals, which have out-patient departments for ambulatory patients, the key Soviet facility for ambulatory care is the polyclinic. In the early plans, each population group of 20,000 to 40,000 was intended to be served by a polyclinic staffed with several teams of physicians and allied personnel. For a population of about 4,000 (in a health sector), the medical team consisted of a general practitioner or an internist (called a *therapeutist*), a pediatrician, an obstetrician–gynecologist, and a stomatologist; in addition were nurses and clerks.

As the Soviet health system has become more specialized, this teamwork model has been modified. Now, the cities generally have polyclinics for adults, others for women with obstetrical or gynecological problems, and some 13,000 others exclusively for children up to age 15. At large industrial plants are polyclinics in which the doctors are oriented strongly to disorders of work. At universities are polyclinics with doctors oriented to the health problems of young men and women. Altogether, in 1986 there were about 40,100 polyclinics of various types throughout the USSR, which meant that the average one served about 7,000 people. (Any calculation is complicated, however, by the fact that one person might attend several different polyclinics during one year.)

In rural areas, the point of entry to the health system is the feldsher–midwife post or the medical station with a single physician and nurse. Difficult cases may be sent to a more fully staffed polyclinic in the nearest town or to a sector or district (rayon) general hospital.

Another important resource in the large cities and some rural regions of the Soviet Union is the Emergency Medical Service (EMS). By use of a simple telephone number, anyone can call a central switchboard for help. The call is received by one of a bank of feldshers or nurses, who must respond in some positive way. If the case is not urgent, an empty ambulance may be sent simply to transport the patient to the nearest health facility. If it is urgent in any degree, an ambulance carrying a doctor and a feldsher or nurse is dispatched. (More details are given later.) In a sense, the EMS programs in the Soviet Union furnish a type of primary health care that would not otherwise be rapidly available at any hour of the day or night. Altogether, there were about 5,100 EMS ambulance stations throughout the country in 1986. There are also airplane ambulances to transport patients from remote areas to a city hospital.

Sanitary–epidemiological stations (sanepids) are the final facilities established throughout the Soviet health system. Their function is not only to survey environmental sanitation, including vector control, but also to provide general health education. Their staffs must be on the alert to problems of environmental pollution, food contamination, or outbreaks of communicable disease. They are also responsible for the safety of working conditions. There is at least one sanepid per district (rayon) and a total of about 5,000 in the whole country. The typical unit includes a laboratory for bacteriological and chemical analyses, and departments for communicable disease control and disinfection. Sanepid stations come under the immediate supervision of the District Health Department, usually based at the district hospital. Overall policies and standards, however, are governed in each republic by a sanepid chief, who in turn comes under a national chief sanitary–epidemiological inspector in the central Ministry of Health.

Drugs and Commodities. As indicated earlier, most of the drugs required in the Soviet health system are manufactured in the country by one or another state enterprise. Some drugs, however, are imported. The Ministry of Health's decisions on drugs to be produced are based on investigations and clinical trials made in its research institutes. Then the Ministry of Medical Industry is responsible for shipping and distributing the products throughout the country, both to the network of hospitals and other facilities for health care and to some 24,000 retail pharmacies. The fierce competition and advertising that generate such high pharmaceutical costs and induce such complex regulatory procedures in Western capitalist countries are absent in the Soviet pharmaceutical industry. On the other hand, fixed prices and the lack of any profit motive have discouraged innovation and permitted various inefficiencies—especially long delays between the development of a new drug and its availability in hospitals and pharmacies.

Soviet health leadership seems to be well aware of bureaucratic problems in its method of development, production, and distribution of drugs. It is seeking ways of improving coordination between the Ministry of Health (including its research institutes) and the various subdivisions of the Ministry of Medical Industry. Pharmacists are also being encouraged to play a greater role in promoting new and effective products to physicians, so that they are put to use as promptly as possible.

Regarding other health commodities, most of the types of elaborate diagnostic and therapeutic equipment manufactured and used in other industrialized countries are also made in the Soviet Union. The quantitative output of such equipment, however, is much less than the need, and the quality is not highly sophisticated. Improvement in these technological matters is anticipated in future planning of the health system.

Knowledge and Technology. Research to produce new health knowledge, and its application through technology, is carried out in several ways in the Soviet health system. At every medical institute (school) for training doctors and its affiliated teaching hospital some research in clinical medicine is conducted. Medical faculty members, however, unlike their counterparts in most other countries, are not expected to devote a great deal of time to research; their main duties are to teach medical students (also physicians taking postgraduate and continuing education), to provide patient care, and to give consultations to peripheral institutions. Some research may also be conducted at nonteaching hospitals, polyclinics, and laboratories.

By far the most important centers for medical and related research are a large array of *scientific research institutes* that have been established throughout the Soviet Union over the years, for specialized purposes. A compilation of these as far back as 1958 listed more than 700 such research institutes, each of which typically included several subdivisions. The purpose of a particular institute might be as broad as biochemistry or dermatology or industrial medicine and toxicology. It might be as specific as the study of rheumatology or tuberculosis. The objective of many of the research institutes corresponds to various specialties of medicine, such as internal diseases, ophthalmology, or surgery.

The vast majority of medical research institutes come under the Ministry of Health, but the exact sponsorship varies. Those dealing with issues in the basic sciences (e.g., biochemistry or physiology) are usually under the general direction of the central Academy of Sciences of the USSR. Under the central Ministry of Health, the national Academy of *Medical* Sciences is the major sponsoring body; while this academy falls within the Ministry of Health, and is expected to focus on research problems of social significance, it functions with considerable autonomy. Another type of research institute comes under the Ministries of Health of the 15 republics; these are usually oriented specifically to problems faced by the republic ministries, such as the improvement of maternal and child health or communicable disease control.

Still another type of research institute is linked to provincial or municipal health authorities. These units tend to carry out assignments made by the public health body, and often must offer advice on the organization or local health service. A few research institutes are exceptional in being sponsored by an entity considered outside the official health system. Thus, an institute for prosthetic appliances functions under the Ministry of Social Welfare and some institutes for the study of physical education and sports function under the Ministry of Higher Education.

As new problems arise, or former problems decline in importance, changes are readily made in the functions of research institutes; some old institutes may be abolished and new ones established. The Leningrad Institute of Sanitation and Hygiene, for example, in response to problems of radioactive fallout, became the Leningrad Institute of Radiation Hygiene. Sponsorship may also be changed, such as the transfer of the Institute of Biophysics from the USSR Academy of Medical Sciences to the USSR Academy of Sciences in 1954. New departments may be added to well-established institutes, such as the addition of a Department of Preventive Cardiology to a Research Institute of Cardiology and Vascular Disorders when new epidemiological knowledge pointed to the preventability of much heart disease. The directors of research institutes, or even of the departments within them, are usually physicians of great prestige, who command the highest salaries in the health system.

Most of the findings from work done at the numerous research institutes are published in Soviet journals, which of course use the Russian language. Since 1937, there has been a central State Publishing House of Medical Literature, under the Ministry of Health. Other official medical publishers of books and journals have also developed over the years. Under the Ministry of Health is an Institute of Medical and Technical Information, which works to improve methods of dissemination of important new knowledge. To enhance communication with the rest of the world, many Soviet medical books are also published in Western languages (mainly English and French). In Russian-language journals, it is customary to include summaries of the articles in several foreign languages. Important new Soviet medical books are often published in enormous quantities, in hundreds of thousands, and their prices are much lower than equivalent books in other countries.

Health System Management

From all that has been discussed so far, it is evident that the general administrative character of the Soviet health system is highly centralized. To expect the world's first sweeping revolution to transform a semifeudal and capitalist economic system into a socialist or even quasi-socialist economy and social order without strong centralized power would hardly be realistic. Whatever one may think of socialist economic and political policies, it must be agreed that, in spite of worldwide opposition, they have survived in the USSR. With relatively little flexibility, the basic principles of a centrally planned and controlled economy, dominated by a highly structured Communist Party, have endured. This meant great repression of individual freedom in the health system, as in virtually all social sectors, to attain certain health goals.

Planning. The management process in any complex social system such as health must begin with planning. In market-dominated economies, the planning is done by each of hundreds of independent productive entities, with the phenomena of supply and demand, price and competition, theoretically resulting in an allocation of resources that is optimally responsive to needs. The market, in other words, is expected to do the planning. In a socialist system, with the market largely eliminated, planning requires some sort of objective determination of needs, with a deliberate allocation of resources based on that determination, in the light of various constraints on the supply and distribution of resources.

In health systems, determining need requires estimates of the volume of sickness in a population, adjusted by various other needs (e.g., unrecognized illnesses and the requirements of prevention), and this is exactly what Soviet health planning has attempted to accomplish. When the first overall 5-year plan was launched in 1928, it was obvious that more health resources of virtually every type—more doctors, more nurses, more hospitals, more clinics, more everything for health service— were needed everywhere. As the output of these resources was increased, the value of more refined quantification was appreciated.

In contrast to techniques for measuring health needs in other countries, no household surveys of morbidity or even disability were conducted by the Soviet health leaders. *Perception* of need was regarded as the crucial element. The significant rate of morbidity was defined as the rate of "first consultations" sought by a given population during a certain time period, such as 1 month. It was assumed that— given the occurrence of illness, the personal feeling and behavior of individuals, the transportation available, family health care resources, and so on—the patients coming to a facility for health service constitute a measure of health needs. The various environmental conditions that determine whether a given symptom will lead one to seek health care naturally differ among large cities, small towns, and rural areas, and they differ in various regions of the country and during various seasons of the year. Therefore studies of "first consultations" were conducted under these diverse circumstances, at different times and places. In all sites, an adequate supply of health care resources had to be available, so that there was no constraint on the supply side, just as the lack of any charges eliminated economic constraint on the demand side.

Soviet health planners are aware, of course, that much serious illness may be present without any symptoms to stimulate the seeking of care. They are also sensitive to the need for preventive services in children and adults who may be perfectly well. Therefore, adjustments in the "need" for health care are made for unrecognized disease and preventive services. Unrecognized disease is determined by careful medical examination of a subsample of the population; preventive service needs are based on the judgment of experts at each time and place.

To translate the findings on health needs into estimates of the necessary resources requires the judgment of medical experts, along with observations in clinics and hospitals on the average number of patients that can be served properly per hour. This, of course, varies with different specialties from perhaps two to five or even more patients per hour. Based on a work week of 40 hours, one can calculate the numbers of physicians for ambulatory care required per 1,000 population in a specified type of city or rural area. Equivalent calculations are made for hospital beds and the various specialists required to staff them. Likewise the resources required for laboratory examinations, pharmaceuticals, nursing services, and so on can be estimated.

These varied and relatively complex calculations become the *technical* foundation for various standards or norms that the Ministry of Health of the USSR uses in planning. The technically desirable quantities, however, must be adjusted for economic realities. To meet the technical requirements for physicians, for example, might require an overall national supply of 300 doctors per 100,000 population, while the national stock was only 200 per 100,000; corresponding ratios must be applied for each specialty. The same matching of technical needs with the realistic availability of resources must be carried out for nurses and other types of health personnel. Similarly, the planning process yields estimates of the number of hospital beds of various specialties that should be established, in relation to the technical needs. This adjustment of technical need to practical feasibility must also take account of the time required to train additional health personnel or to construct additional health facilities. There are obvious constraints in the availability of teachers, building materials, equipment, and so on. All of these calculations constitute *economic* adjustments to the technical needs, leading ultimately to the establishment of norms.

Both the technical and economic phases of health planning are carried out by the central Ministry of Health, which calls on republic and provincial (oblast) bodies for collaboration. Various research institutes usually conduct the empirical studies required in the technical determination of health needs. The information is collected and analyzed in the Department of Planning Expertise and Estimates of the central MOH. At this level, forecasts must also be made on changes in needs that may be expected due to changes in (a) the demography of the population (e.g., the age composition), (b) the spectrum of morbidity (e.g., infectious versus cardiovascular disease), and (c) the patterns of delivery of health care with technological advances.

Even these adjusted estimates do not yield the final determination of standards. A third essential step is *political.* The health system is only one among many sectors in Soviet society. Limited resources must serve education, construction, manufacturing, and all other sectors, as well as health. To make the ultimate decisions on how much of the nation's resources should be allotted to the health system at a given time, the plans of the MOH must be submitted to the central State Planning Commission (GOSPLAN). This agency is essentially a technical arm of the cabinet or Council of Ministers of the USSR. Usually each ministry wants a larger piece of the national economic pie, and GOSPLAN must recommend to the cabinet its judgment on a reasonable distribution. The final decisions are made by the Council of Ministers. The relative allocations to different ministries obviously vary in times of peace and war, and under varying circumstances in the flow of international trade. Only after these final political decisions are made can the Ministry of Health finalize its standards in all elements of the health system.

This complex process of health planning has been carried out every 5 years since 1928. As the Soviet Union has developed, however, the process has become less mechanistic, more flexible and decentralized. As more was learned about health problems, resources, and the methods of providing service, more responsibility for planning decisions has been delegated to local levels of government. The norms ultimately formulated centrally by the MOH serve as general guidelines, for various types of urban or rural settings, for districts, provinces, and republics to prepare their budgets each year. The human and physical resources required are based on the norms defined in the current 5-year plan, but adjusted to meet the special conditions of each local area.

This description of the Soviet health planning process is perhaps oversimplified. In the complex social and political affairs of any country, administrative procedures are seldom as clear and tidy as they are intended to be. Human judgment is often faulty, and decisions made at one time and place may yield difficulties at another time. Many events cannot be accurately anticipated, such as the influence of the weather on agriculture or the impact of the previously unknown AIDS virus on the health system. Such problems are encountered by all health systems, whether driven mainly by market forces or by central planning. In fact, health planning, insofar as its targets change every year or even more often, incorporates certain information derived from health market dynamics (such as the changing demand for certain health services) in its formulations.

Administration. Principles of administration in the Soviet health system may be generally inferred from the analysis of its organizational structure. Chapter 3 analyzed the meaning and content of *administration* in any health system as including eight elements, about each of which a few words can be said.

Regarding organization, the broad scope of responsibilities brought together under a unified Ministry of Health is perhaps the outstanding feature. The Soviet health system has departed from many long traditions, such as the autonomy of universities (providing the education of health personnel), to achieve an integrated system. As a corollary, the pyramidal hierarchy of administrative authorities, from the top through the republics, provinces, and districts, is organizationally efficient. Health-related skills are concentrated in MOH organs at all levels and not dispersed among administrative bodies with diverse objectives.

The overwhelming emphasis in staffing and budgeting appears to be given to the training and development of physicians. This policy is so dominant that many functions, assigned to physicians, could probably be done by other less extensively trained personnel. Physicians have high prestige and yet their salaries are rel-

atively low. With their short work day (6 or 7 hours), the weekly productivity of the average physician is probably below that found in other industrialized countries.

Supervision in the Soviet health system is strong. The authority of the head of each organizational unit is clear and seldom questioned. The prevention of deviant performance may have its merits, but rigid supervision can discourage innovation and originality. Health personnel at the lower echelons of a hospital or polyclinic or a district health department can stagnate and lack incentives to work hard. On the other hand, clinical physicians, who hold virtually every supervisory position, may not be competent in a supervisory role.

Regarding consultation, there are many channels through which it may be sought. On questions of clinical medicine, the faculties of medical institutes may be freely consulted without economic deterrents. On administrative matters, bureaucratic superiors in the hierarchy are available. One might suspect that some personnel would feel inhibited about soliciting advice, for fear of disclosing ignorance, but this presents a problem in every country.

The functions of procurement and logistics have special importance in a health system as unified as that of the Soviet Union, where all the parts are interdependent. (In more pluralistic systems, one agency can fail while the others continue to function.) A disorder in one part of the structure may obstruct movement in many other parts. Bureaucratic difficulties of this sort have caused shortages of drugs and supplies in many Soviet regions. Of course, pharmaceutical production also depends on international trade, in which the Soviet economy may suffer handicaps for political reasons.

Regarding records and reporting, the unified health system structure has many advantages. Contrary to conventional wisdom, bureaucracy need not breed paperwork but can reduce it. The complexity of fee payments in entrepreneurial or even welfare-oriented countries, with multiple payers and varying entitlements for different patients, is far greater than in the unified Soviet system. Payment of health personnel by salary is much simpler than by any other method, and it reduces administrative costs. Few periodic reports on health program operations are required, because general policies are assumed to be widely understood by everyone. It is mainly the unusual or difficult problem that generates a report.

Coordination is a major administrative function in pluralistic health systems, but the Soviet system has little need for it. Within the integrated structure there might, nevertheless, be poor working relationships between polyclinics and hospitals or between sanitary–epidemiological stations and polyclinics. Proper liaison is promoted through a policy of hospital doctors visiting polyclinics periodically and vice versa. The sharp separation between preventive and therapeutic health work that characterizes many countries does not complicate the Soviet health system; both types of services are given to patients in the same polyclinic or health center.

The quality of health service has not often been evaluated deliberately in the Soviet health system (note recent changes described later). Where medical practitioners in hospitals are largely autonomous, as in the United States or Canada, special *peer review* committees may be necessary to monitor performance. In the Soviet system, however, where teamwork is the general rule, self-discipline is more likely to be built into day-to-day work; evaluation is an ongoing process. On the other hand, one must recognize that the entire medical staff of a hospital or polyclinic may perform inadequately under poor leadership. As we note later, a crisis in the late 1980s led to extensive evaluation of all Soviet physicians.

Regulation. In almost all countries, the regulatory aspects of management involve principally governmental controls over the private sector. To maintain standards, prevent abuses, and protect people from incompetent service, many rules are established and enforced. In the Soviet system, however, medical graduates are registered automatically because the institutes that train them are supervised by the MOH. Continuing education is mandatory. Hospitals and other health facilities are inspected only if there is a special problem. Pharmaceutical products do not require the degree of regula-

tion that multiple competing private companies provoke in capitalist countries. As noted earlier, the Ministry of Medical Industry produces almost all the domestic drugs under simple generic names. When a new product is turned out, a special Pharmacology Committee in the Ministry of Health tests it for safety and efficacy before it can be distributed.

It has been noted that private medical practice is permitted in the Soviet health system by individual doctors and, more often, by medical groups. In spite of the limited extent of this private sector, it comes under MOH regulation. The administrator assigned to the *paying polyclinics* oversees general operations, the fees charged, and the distribution of earnings. Individual practitioners may also be visited occasionally, to ensure that they pay taxes on their earnings.

In a sense, the most pervasive regulatory influence in the Soviet health system is the nationwide network of Communist party branches, essentially parallel to government authorities. If a patient or a provider of health care has a grievance, or if there is some general evidence of unsatisfactory health service, the initial action is to seek help from the head of the relevant local unit; if this does not yield a satisfactory response, the matter is brought to the attention of local Party authorities. If they choose to investigate the matter and find evidence of culpable behavior, some corrective action is usually stimulated. A physician or health workers may be reprimanded, moved to another post, or even fined. Not all party branches are equally vigilant, but it must be recalled that this one-party nation has elections *within* that party; members who want to be elected naturally seek the good will of the general population.

Legislation. Compared with parliamentary countries, legislation plays a relatively modest part in managing the Soviet health system. The Five-Year Plans may be regarded as a form of legislation, insofar as they explicitly state policies and goals, and often outline steps to be taken to reach those goals. Nevertheless, on selected problems for which planning has been incomplete or the activities of the responsible bodies are deemed inadequate, the Supreme

Soviet of the USSR may enact laws. These seem to serve as a type of instruction to the authorities to strengthen or modify strategies for dealing with certain problems. Similar legislative actions may be taken by the Supreme Soviets of the constituent republics.

In 1936, the Supreme Soviet enacted a Constitution that states numerous principles and the designated "rights" of citizens. Article 120 affirms the following:

> Citizens of the USSR have the right to material security in old age and also in case of sickness or loss of capacity to work. This right is ensured by the wide development of social insurance of workers and other employees at state expense, free medical service for the working people, and the provision of a wide network of health resorts at the disposal of the working people.

Recall that in the 1950s and 1960s, the international Cold War led to very large military expenditures by the Soviet Union, resulting in reduced allocations for domestic purposes. This led to a broad legislative reaffirmation in 1969 of "professional medical care (being) available to all," which was noted previously. Laws on much more specific matters have been passed over the years. Citation of the titles of a sample of these statutes from different periods may reflect the role of the Soviet legislation in shaping health policies:

1924: On the professional work and rights of medical employees.

1927: On measures for struggle with venereal diseases.

1935: On cadres of blood donors.

1936: On collective farm maternity homes.

1940: On the sanitary protection of the Moscow–Volga Canal as the source of water supply for the city of Moscow.

1941: On measures for the reduction of disease in children.

1942: On the organization in collective farms of children's playgrounds and nurseries of the simplest type.

1952: On the unsatisfactory conduct of measures for the reduction of the incidence of tuberculosis in the population.

1953: On measures for improving the culture and living services for the blind.

1954: On measures for the sharp reduction of infectious diseases and the liquidation of food poisoning.

1962: On measures for the eradication of hoof-and-mouth disease in cattle.

1965: On the reorganization of agencies for the sale, installation, and repair of medical technology and the rendering of technical aid to health care institutions serving the rural population.

1972: On the system for the work of employees on jobs with vibration dangers.

1972: On measures for strengthening the struggle against drunkenness and alcoholism.

1976: On measures for providing the people with contact lenses to correct vision.

1976: On measures for the further improvement of oncological aid to the population.

1980: On measures for strengthening the struggle against smoking.

1983: On the procedure for approval of the list of diseases for which victims are given the right to priority housing space.

1983: On the free distribution of medications to individual categories of patients who are in out-patient treatment.

1983: On approval of the statute on the Department of Health Care of the Executive Committee of Province and Region (rayon) Soviets of People's Deputies.

This sample of 21 health-related laws enacted over a 60-year period by the USSR Supreme Soviet should illustrate how legislation is used in the Soviet Union to manage the health system. Most of the statutes, in fact, are intended specifically to influence the activities of the Ministry of Health, to modify its priorities, or to set up new programs. They serve as strategies for interventions by the population, as represented in the Supreme Soviet, in the performance of the national bureaucracy.

Economic Support

The sources of economic support for the Soviet Union's health system—both its operating and its capital costs—are less complicated than those in most other countries. Exact data on current economic accounts are not readily available, but the general principles are fairly clear.

Recall that around 1937, the two major sources of financing—social insurance for industrial workers and their dependents and general government revenues for the rest of the population, especially rural—were consolidated. Hence, today the overwhelming bulk of financial support for the many aspects of the health system reviewed here is derived from the revenues of the central government. In this socialist economy, those come mainly from the earnings of all state enterprises (industrial, agricultural, and other) and individual income taxes.

Yet general revenues are not the only source of funding. Although the available data are old (from 1968), there is no reason to suspect any major changes in the proportions since then. From various official Soviet sources, the English economist Michael Kaser has compiled information, published in 1976, which shows the percentage distribution reported in Table 8–1. Certain comments about these figures are in order. The large share (77.1 percent) of health costs, met by general government revenues in 1968, constituted 9.1 percent of the

Table 8.1. Sources of Health System Financing in the USSR, 1968

Source	Percent
General governmental revenues	77.1
Social insurance	5.5
Enterprises (industrial & agricultural)	13.7
Personal household payments	3.7
All sources	100.0

overall Unified State Budget of the USSR. Of these moneys, the Ministry of Health reports that more than 95 percent is spent locally, that is, within the republics at the various lower levels (see later). The amounts allocated to the different republics depend on the budgets each has submitted (hence, more developed regions receive higher allotments), but some attempt is made to give relatively larger amounts to the poorer republics. A very small share of the 77.1 percent is dispersed by ministries concerned with police or public transport, but nearly all is for the Ministry of Health.

The 5.5 percent share of funds derived from social insurance has no relation to the former large contributions made for the general medical care of workers by industrial enterprises. It is simply for the support of rest-care facilities for workers, prosthetic appliances, and special dietetic products which are entitlement of workers, administered mainly by trade unions. The 13.7 percent of total health expenditures derived from enterprises includes both capital and operating costs. Both large industrial enterprises and large collective or state farms may construct polyclinics and even hospitals at their own expense. The major staffing and financing of these facilities are then responsibilities of the Ministry of Health, but certain administrative personnel as well as drugs and supplies may be financed by the enterprise subsequently.

The small personal share of total health expenditures (3.7 percent) is an especially interesting reflection of the economic dynamics of a socialist health system. About three-quarters of these expenditures are payments for pharmaceuticals in pharmacies; these include any nonprescribed or over-the-counter drugs plus nonessential palliative drugs that have been prescribed. (Life-saving drugs, such as insulin, digitalis, or antibiotics, and any drugs for military veterans or elderly pensioners are without charge.) The other one-fourth of the 3.7 percent (or about 0.9 percent of total health expenditures) constitutes expenditures at *paying polyclinics*. Data on expenditures for medical care by individual doctors are not available; since the outlay for private polyclinics, staffed by highly qualified specialists from the official institutions, is under 1.0 percent, however, one can infer that expenditures on purely private care from solo practitioners are probably very low.

In financial accounts on Soviet health expenditures, it has been customary to combine physical culture activities with those in the health system. This may seem to complicate comparisons with health expenditures of other countries, but the problem is not significant. Thus, in 1973, all physical culture expenditures absorbed only 0.53 percent of the central government budget for health and physical culture.

The large share of total health system expenditures (77.1 percent) made by the central government from general revenues has been noted. Based on the 1968 fiscal reports, listed previously, these funds are predominantly distributed through regular allocations to the republics, from which various amounts are allotted to the lower levels to operate all the health programs. The distribution has been approximately as follows:

Administrative Level	Percentage
Central headquarters	3.0
Republic ministeries of health	10.1
Provincial (oblast) health authorities	14.7
City health authorities	41.4
District (rayon) health authorities	25.3
Local soviets	5.5
All administrative levels	100.0

A breakdown of Soviet financial data by type of health activity was published in 1987. It applied to health expenditures in 1985 and showed the following distribution:

Purpose	Percentage
Personal health care (hospitals, polyclinics, etc.)	86.4
Sanitary–epidemiological activities	3.8
Physical culture	0.7
Capital allocations (construction)	5.8
Other current expenditures	3.4
All purposes	100.0

Judging from patterns in other countries, most of the 86.4 percent for personal health care is probably devoted to the operation of hospitals.

A crucial feature of the economic support of every national health system is the percentage of the country's gross national product (GNP) spent on it each year. This figure frequently cited for the Soviet Union is quite low—4.1 percent. Consultation of Soviet sources, however, indicates that this percentage applies, not to GNP but to the Soviet national income—that is, the sum of the incomes of all households. The probable reason for use of this denominator is that, in Marxian economic theory, *products* refer to physical or material commodities; they do not include services. (GNP includes the value, at current prices, of all goods *and services* produced during a year in the country.) Hence the Soviet GNP is not comparable with that of other countries. To avoid this difficulty, and report a figure that is internationally comparable, Soviet economists evidently calculate health system expenditures in relation to "national income."

The national income of most industrialized countries, however, is lower than the GNP. In the United States, for example, between 1970 and 1986 the national income each year was 80 to 82 percent of the GNP. If we adjust the Soviet figure of 4.1 percent of national income, to be roughly comparable to the percentage of GNP spent for health in a large capitalist country like the United States, it would become even lower, or 3.3 percent. Judging by other Soviet reports, the percentage of national wealth devoted to the health system has risen slowly over the years, but between 1970 and 1980 it hovered around 4 percent of national income.

Of course, the absolute sums devoted to health have risen, but only at about the same pace as national income. Whether or not the figure is adjusted to apply to GNP (as defined by capitalist countries)—that is, whether 4.1 or 3.3 percent—the share of economic stock (to use a neutral term) used to support the health system is relatively low. Even if we add 10 percent (frequently estimated) for purely private health expenditures, not identified in national accounts, the 3.3 percent of national income would rise to only 3.6 percent devoted to health purposes. In any event, health expenditures are much lower than those found to apply to all the other industrialized countries reviewed in previous chapters. Even the extremely frugal British National Health Service, as we noted in Chapter 7, spends about 6 percent of its GNP.

One may suspect several reasons for this. Most important, the salaries of health workers are relatively low. Although physicians are the most highly paid personnel, their salaries are modest, similar to those of elementary school teachers. Not that salaries are uniform, since their level depends on the doctor's background of training, experience, and the responsibility carried. Medical salaries (except for the directors of institutes or professors), however, are only moderately higher than those of feldshers or nurses. (Perhaps the differential is greater than it seems, because of the frequent payment of "bonuses" to doctors at the end of the year. Also, male physicians often increase their earnings by taking part-time jobs.)

One must appreciate that since 1928 the highest priority of Soviet society has been industrialization; thus, the greatest financial rewards have gone to engineers, managers, and skilled workers. Analysis of the health budget of several republics in 1970 found salaries to account for only 54 percent of the total; in other industrialized countries this share would be closer to 80 percent. (One must also appreciate that rentals and many other costs of living in the USSR are very low.)

Another possible factor in the low Soviet health expenditures is the relatively modest investment in modern medical equipment. Compared with Western European countries, Soviet hospitals are rather weak in their radiological, laboratory, and other diagnostic or therapeutic technology. As noted earlier, there have also been shortages in pharmaceuticals and in some medical supplies.

On the other hand, the relatively low percentage of Soviet national income spent on the health system doubtless reflects many efficiencies. The pervasive payment of salaries, rather than fee-for-service, is economically sound and it avoids perverse incentives. Extensive use of feldshers and other ancillary personnel yields economies. The governmental production of drugs and elimination of profits from patented brand-name products, with extensive advertising, saves money. Hospitals are financed with prospective global budgets, which have been found to be economically prudent in many countries. The basic simplicity of management, under a highly unified system, reduces administrative and clerical costs. The whole process of health planning achieves a distribution of resources, which is calculated to meet needs reasonably and yet avoid duplication, excesses, or waste. Finally, one must not overlook the huge military expenditures, which the Soviet government has considered necessary, in the light of international relationships.

Delivery of Services

From all that has been said about resources, organization, management, and financing of the Soviet Union's health system, much can be inferred about the patterns of delivering health services.

Ambulatory Health Care. In a territory as large as the USSR, much of the population still lives in rural areas—35 percent (97,000,000 people), compared with much smaller shares in Western Europe. The delivery of health services differs substantially between cities and rural regions. The problem of distance and transportation is still significant in rural areas.

In the cities, virtually everyone has access to a physician in a polyclinic serving the area in which he or she lives. As noted earlier, the roughly 40,000 Soviet polyclinics average a catchment population of about 7,000, but the variations among cities and neighborhoods is very wide. The area served by a polyclinic is divided into sectors or *uchastoks,* sometimes called microdistricts, of about 3,000 to 4,000 people. The earlier concept of a team of generalist, pediatrician, and gynecologist seems to have been eroded by the great movement to specialization. Polyclinic physicians still provide basic primary care, but they are predominantly generalists or *therapeutists,* each of whom is expected to serve about 2,000 adults.

Children are seen by pediatricians, who are mainly located at separate children's polyclinics, which serve about 1,000 children per pediatrician. Women also often have separate polyclinics for obstetrical and gynecological conditions (although for other conditions women use the regular adult facilities). In large cities, polyclinics may be adjacent to general hospitals.

Since individual patients, adult or child, go to the doctor responsible for the area in which they live, there is no "free choice of doctor" in the sense that this prevails in the private medical sector of other countries. Still, if a patient is dissatisfied with the designated doctor, he or she may change to another, with the authorization of the polyclinic director. Few instances of patients desiring such changes are reported. The same general policy of linking patients to particular doctors applies in the polyclinics for children, women, and other groups.

The principal other groups for which special polyclinics render health care in cities are industrial workers. The priority for workers is based not only on political considerations (since workers spearheaded the Revolution), but also on the economic objective of maintaining a healthy work force for maximum productivity. The physicians in an industrial polyclinic try to become acquainted with the working conditions of each employee, and sensitive to special hazards of accidents or occupational intoxication. A large plant of several thousand workers normally has a polyclinic of its own, and even a hospital. In a city or town with several small plants near each other, one industrial polyclinic may serve them all. Each worker is free to attend either the industrial unit or the neighborhood polyclinic near his or her home, or both facilities at different times. Somewhat similar specialized polyclinics are located at universities and large technical schools, to serve both students and faculty members.

In rural areas, where enough people are physically near one location, typically in a small town, the general polyclinic is also the basic facility for primary health care. Where the population is thinly settled, as is true of vast territories in the USSR, the point of first contact in the health system is the feldsher–midwife station. Here the feldsher naturally does a broader scope of work than his or her urban counterpart. In the city polyclinic or hospital, the feldsher is a true assistant to the doctor or plays special technical roles (sanitarian, ambulance attendant, etc.), which were noted earlier. The rural feldsher is authorized to give first-aid and simple treatment of minor ailments. Any serious condition must be referred to the nearest polyclinic or perhaps to the out-patient department of a district hospital, if this happens to be closer.

Despite the several strategies for attracting physicians to settle permanently in rural areas (after their 3 years of mandatory duty), there are still rural shortages. The rural doctor supply has shown some improvement, however, and it is hoped eventually to replace feldsher–midwife stations with health centers staffed with at least one physician.

The principle of integrating preventive and therapeutic service is implemented at polyclinics in several ways. Where children are served, preventive check-ups and immunizations are done by the same pediatricians who treat the sick child. Perhaps to increase efficiency, immunizations and well-baby examinations may be scheduled for certain days each week. Health educational posters are displayed everywhere, and sometimes there are films and small-group discussions. For health maintenance in adults, policy calls for systematic follow-up of any person with a chronic disease. The Russian term for these regular periodic examinations is *dispensarization,* and the quality of a doctor's work is judged by the thoroughness with which his adult patients are *dispensarized.* Written notices are sent periodically to the patients and if they do not show up, their home is visited. At these examinations, patients are supposed to be advised about healthful diets, avoidance of smoking or excessive alcohol, exercise, and other features of hygienic living.

The environmental sanitation aspects of prevention are the responsibility of the sanitary–epidemiological stations. Headed by a physician, who has specialized in environmental hygiene, the staff members monitor all aspects of the local environment—water supplies, sewage disposal, solid-waste disposal, health aspects of housing, vector control, food-processing plants, restaurants, and even workplaces. Laboratories to examine food or other possibly toxic substances are maintained. The sanepid station also produces graphic materials for health education on disease prevention. In case of an epidemic, the sanepid director has great authority to take corrective actions.

The specialization of polyclinics for different demographic groups has occurred, to a lesser extent, for certain diseases. In larger cities, *dispensaries* are devoted to the ambulatory care of certain serious disorders. In 1971, the Ministry of Health reported more than 3,700 dispensaries for the treatment and follow-up of patients with tuberculosis and venereal disease (these were most numerous), and also for cancer, accident cases, and mental problems.

Soviet doctors at all facilities providing ambulatory care make visits to the patient's home much more frequently than is done in Western Europe or America. The home call has almost disappeared from medical practice in many countries, but in Soviet polyclinics it is normal for three or four afternoons a week to be spent on visits to patient homes. In this way, it is claimed, the doctor gets to know his patients better, and can appreciate their living conditions.

Another noteworthy type of out-of-hospital care in the Soviet health system is the *emergency medical service* (EMS), operated in large cities. The first systematic organization of such a program was in Leningrad in the 1950s, and since then it has been set up in all major cities. A person with any sort of health problem—not only accidents, but acute symptoms of any type—can gain access to the EMS program through a simple telephone number. All calls come to a central exchange, where a feldsher or nurse takes the message: the nature of the problem and the address or location. An ambulance is then dispatched from the nearest of several stations set up around the city.

If an accident has occurred, the ambulance dispatched is specially equipped for trauma care (blood transfusion, bandages, etc.). If a heart attack is suspected, cardiological equipment is sent along. The feldshers staffing the ambulance (occasionally a doctor) are correspondingly trained. Policies generally require response to every "call for help," even if it seems trivial. Only after the patient is seen may the attendant decide whether or not he should be transported promptly to a hospital or polyclinic.

With these several categories of ambulatory health service in the USSR, and with no economic deterrents, it should not be surprising that rates of utilization are high and increasing. Soviet Ministry of Health reports indicate that in 1974 the rate of ambulatory contacts with a doctor were 11.1 per person per year in the urban population. This was an increase from 8.5 contacts per person in 1960. The rates of contact with doctors in rural areas is much lower—4.0 per person in 1974. It must be realized, of course, that in rural areas many more health contacts occur with feldshers. A weighted average for urban and rural rates in 1974 gives a figure of 8.7 ambulatory patient–doctor contacts per person per year. About one-third of these medical services are for preventive purposes. (Equivalent national rates are not available in many other countries, but in the United States and Great Britain, doctor–patient encounters fall between 4 and 5 per person per year.)

This diversity of ways of providing ambulatory care in the Soviet Union may imply a fragmented health system. Actually all the resources come under the direction of the health departments in the province and district. The use of several different facilities by various members of one family does not seem to be an issue in the Soviet system. Specialization in medical care is, of course, a worldwide phenomenon.

Hospital Care. Hospital resources have been described, and here we consider their manner of operation. As in most of the world, Soviet hospitals are staffed by salaried full-time specialists, who are organized through various departments in a medical staff hierarchy. Norms call for a certain number of doctors per 100 beds, varying with the specialty. In 1960, for example, the internal medicine beds were supposed to have about 5 full-time physicians per 100 beds, and in obstetrics–gynecology 7 physicians per 100 beds. As standards have improved, the overall average in 1980 was about 10 physicians per 100 hospital beds.

The overall staffing of Soviet hospitals, however, is relatively modest. There are fewer nurses, technicians, dieticians, and others than found in comparably sized hospitals of West European countries. This doubtless contributes to the long average patient stays, about 18 days, and the high occupancy levels, usually exceeding 90 percent. In some regions this leads to waiting periods for admission of several weeks or months, for nonemergency conditions. With limited diagnostic equipment and staffs, it takes many days to process a patient who elsewhere might be "worked up" in a day or two. On the other hand, hospitalization in the Soviet culture is regarded as a sort of rest-period after steady work (there is very little unemployment in the USSR) and is not to be rushed.

Patients are admitted to hospitals, of course, only by the decision of a hospital doctor; the physician at a polyclinic or industrial unit refers the patient to the hospital OPD, but the examining physician there decides if admission to a bed is necessary. The annual rate of admission to general hospitals was about 156 per 1,000 persons in 1980 (similar to that in many other industrialized countries), but with the long average stays, the rate of use of hospital care is very high—2,800 days per 1,000 persons per year. As we will see, efforts are being made to achieve shorter patient stays, so that the same hospital bed supply could accommodate more cases.

Administration of Soviet hospitals is clearly in the hands of physicians, rather than nonmedical managerial personnel. The top director is almost invariably a physician, even in small hospitals, where he or she must also do clinical work. In very large hospitals, the physician-director may spend only limited time giving clinical service, but the Soviet concept is that a good administrator must be in close touch with the service he is directing. (Even the national Minister of Health is expected to spend a little time each week seeing patients, in whatever his field of specialization may be.)

The medical director is, of course, typically assisted by an administrative manager of some type. He is also often assisted by an advisory committee of various hospital employees. It must be recalled, however, that the heavy paperwork required for the fiscal operations of hospitals in other countries is not necessary in the Soviet Union, and personnel matters are also less complex. On the other hand, as noted earlier, in many district (rayon) hospitals, the medical director is administratively responsible for all health services (polyclinics, sanepids, dispensaries) in the district.

The physical amenities for patient care in Soviet hospitals are much less elaborate than those found in some other affluent countries (such as the United States or Sweden); yet they are not very different from standards in countries like Italy or Greece. A typical room has four to six beds, and private one-bed rooms are rare. Plumbing in the Soviet Union is generally not very well developed. Yet the sensitivity of nurses to patient needs is reported by foreign observers to be as tender as characterizes hospitals in richer countries. Questions of this sort, of course, are always subject to debate.

Patterns of health care delivery in specialized hospitals are naturally different from those in general short-term hospitals. Mental facilities, for example, as everywhere in industrialized countries, are usually very large, with more than 1,000 beds. Some years ago, there were smaller units for patients considered curable and responsive to therapy, while large "mental colonies" were maintained for those deemed to be chronically disordered or incurable. This dichotomy no longer prevails. Virtually all mental patients are regarded as subject to improvement, through active use of medication and energetic environmental therapy. Programs of work and occupational involvement are emphasized. The average length of stay has steadily declined.

Special Issues. The Soviet health system, as the first and most highly developed in a thoroughly socialist society, has attracted exceptionally great worldwide attention. Practices in the Soviet Union on many health matters that draw scant attention in other countires are probed deeply and broadcast widely. Just four of these aspects of health care delivery are examined here.

Superior quality health service for the top political leaders is one such matter. Indeed, special polyclinics and hospitals in the large cities provide health care for leading political figures and their families. These facilities have priority in acquiring the latest equipment, drugs, and supplies, and their medical and allied personnel are of outstanding quality. The same sort of favored and even extravagant medical care is provided, of course, for political leaders in virtually all countries. Indeed, in most nonsocialist countries this type of care is available to almost anyone of great wealth, whether the person is politically significant or not. In low-income developing countries and especially in resource-rich (but not industrialized) countries, it is customary for high political figures to be sent abroad to Europe and America for the treatment of illness of even moderate severity, at government expense. In Soviet jargon, this special service is sometimes called the *Fourth Department* of the Ministry of Health.

A second issue concerns the Soviet attitudes toward traditional healing or folk medicine. The official Marxist attitude is to base all services on scientific principles and reject unscientific doctrines of all sorts. Nevertheless, some cultist or magical form of healing persists in rural areas, especially in the Asiatic republics. Homeopathy (which arose as a reaction to excesses in regular medicine in nineteenth-century Germany) is practiced privately in many cities to a small extent; in Moscow seven homeopathic pharmacies and two large clinics exist. This medical cult is not part of the official system, but it is available to anyone willing to pay private fees.

Private medical practice, already noted, is a third issue. Though not encouraged, it has never been banned. In the 1960s and 1970s as demands for prompt medical service of good quality increased more rapidly than the official system could meet them, waiting lists lengthened and the services of polyclinic physicians became perfunctory. As a result, the demand for private service individuals would be willing to pay for increased. Aside from the service of individual doctors in the patient's home,

which had long been used, the Ministry of Health institutionalized the *paying polyclinic,* staffed by the most competent specialists after their official duties were completed. About 130 of these private clinics exist in the country (compared with the 40,000 Ministry of Health polyclinics). Although the fees are controlled, they are affordable only by relatively high-income families, so a small degree of inequity is tolerated. Since virtually all physicians in these facilities spend their full allotted time in the official service, however, this private sector—unlike the situation in many other countries—does not reduce the volume of health manpower available to the vast majority of the population.

Probably more serious is the problem of bribery or the practice of patients offering gifts or money to doctors and other personnel in hospitals; this is done to accelerate admission or attract favored attention. Giving small gifts in appreciation of medical care is a worldwide practice, but it is widely reported that it has become excessive in Soviet cities, allegedly to the point that service can hardly be expected without them. The true extent of this problem is really not known.

A final issue in Soviet health care delivery is the policy and practice on abortion. The official policy has varied with changing conditions and experience. Immediately after the Russian Revolution, abortion—which had previously been illegal but widely done under clandestine and unsafe conditions—was legalized; it had to be performed, however, by a physician in a hospital. Contraception was not widely understood or available at the time, and the rate of abortions rose rapidly—so much so that excessive uterine trauma became injurious to the health of women. In 1936, therefore, the law was changed, and abortions in hospitals were restricted to cases in which the life or health of the mother was endangered or there was a high risk of a congenitally defective baby. (Hostile foreign observers interpreted this to mean a strategy to increase the Soviet population for military purposes.)

As might be expected, the 1936 law led to a resumption of many illegal abortions, with infections and maternal deaths. As a result, in 1955 the law was changed again, to legalize abortions within the first 3 months of pregnancy simply at the request of the mother, and at later times under special circumstances. Meanwhile, various special benefits had been provided for maternity, along with creches and kindergartens for small children of working women (the vast majority of women). The 1955 law is still in effect, and abortions are freely available in hospitals. Because contraceptive use is apparently not widespread in the USSR, the rate of abortions has become extremely high. In the 1980s, it was claimed that two out of every three pregnancies end in abortions.

The problem of illegal abortions, outside hospitals or abortion clinics *(abortorias)*, has still not been solved. This is evidently explained by long waiting periods for hospital admission in some localities, the disclosure of "abortion" on the medical certificate (denying the woman cash benefits for work absence), and sometimes the shortage of anesthetics in hospitals. The vast majority of abortions, however, are being done safely in hospitals, and great efforts are being made to extend the use of contraceptive techniques (family planning).

Restructuring *(Perestroika)*

In 1985, after the death of previous top officials, the government of the Soviet Union acquired new leadership—men with attitudes very different from any that had been in control since the 1917 Revolution. The newly chosen Chairman of the Council of Ministers (equivalent to the prime minister in other countries) was a relatively young man, Mikhail Gorbachev, who spearheaded a movement for openness *(glasnost)* and restructuring *(perestroika)* of the entire socialist society. Gorbachev's election to this leading post by the Council of Ministers clearly meant that a desire for basic changes in both the economic and political structure of the USSR was widely felt throughout the country.

In the Soviet health system, early signs of difficulties were reflected in a report, published in the United States in 1980, claiming that the national infant mortality rate (IMR) had reversed its 50-year downward trend and begun to rise. Since the IMR has long been regarded

as a sensitive indicator of both living conditions and health services, this report had ominous significance. The officially reported IMR had been reduced from 273 infant deaths per 1,000 live births in 1913 to a low of 22.9 per 1,000 live births in 1971. Then, the rate rose slowly to 27.9 per 1,000 in 1974, when the Soviet MOH suddenly stopped reporting. Not until 1986 was official reporting resumed, and the IMR had declined again slightly to 25.9 in 1984. Since Soviet policy excludes from its statistics very low birthweight infants who die within 7 days (regarding these as "miscarriages"), the figure comparable with those of other industrialized countries would be slightly higher.

These adverse statistical data provoked a great deal of discussion outside the USSR. One interpretation suggested that earlier IMR figures had been underreported. Another emphasized handicaps in the less developed Asiatic regions. Other interpretations spoke of the overcrowded nursery schools (creches), with much crossinfection, since women were working more than ever and could not care for their infants at home. High alcohol consumption, even by pregnant women, was blamed. The excessive rate of abortions was said to lead to less robust babies. Then, of course, there was the Cold War and its concomitantly huge military expenditures, which resulted in much lower allocations to the Ministry of Health than were needed. Within the health services, shortages of incubators to care for premature infants were generally recognized. Basic medications were often lacking. In light of their very low salaries, nurses were leaving the hospitals for other better-paid jobs.

Whatever may have been the true cause or causes of the rise in Soviet infant mortality in the 1970s, the resumption of official reporting in 1986 was undoubtedly related to the spirit of *glasnost* (openness), brought about by Chairman Gorbachev. Reflecting this spirit, and the plan for restructuring *(perestroika)* the entire social order, was the appointment in 1987 of a new Minister of Health. Dr. Y. I. Chazov, who with an American physician (Dr. Bernard Lown) had been co-president of the International Physicians for the Prevention of Nuclear War (IPPNW), which won the Nobel

Peace Prize in 1985. Chazov was a cardiologist, with no background in public health work, but his IPPNW role made him a clear symbol of courage, initiative, and energetic behavior.

In 1987, the USSR Council of Ministers and the Central Committee of the Communist Party approved a basic plan for "reorganization of the health care system of the USSR"—a plan obviously prepared under the direction of the new minister of health. The full text of the plan was reported openly in the Soviet medical press, and its candor was impressive. After recounting the many achievements of the Soviet health system, the plan stated the following:

> In the 1970s and in the beginning of the 1980s negative tendencies began to appear and grow in the realm of health care. . . . [There was] a decrease in the share of funds devoted to health care in the governmental budget. . . . Deficiencies in organization and planning and a decrease in precision and quality control became the cause of serious errors. . . . Such phenomena as callousness, inhumanity, rudeness, lack of accountability for fulfilling professional duty, bribery, and bureaucratism have become widespread. . . . Attention has weakened toward preventive work. . . . In a number of regions the people are not provided with high-quality drinking water. . . . For many years, work toward creating a healthy basis for living has not been given necessary consideration. . . . Drinking and alcoholism are widespread. . . . The level and quality of medical care does not fully respond to the growing needs of the Soviet people. . . .

The scathing criticisms also referred to delayed admission to hospitals of patients needing urgent care, poor quality of maternal and child health service and inadequate care of premature newborns, outdated and deteriorating medical equipment, a low level of medical research and failure to apply new scientific knowledge, and so on.

As a result of these deficiencies, the plan stated frankly that infant mortality was high, life expectancy of men had stagnated or actu-

ally declined, and the levels of heart disease and cancer had not changed. Absenteeism from work due to sickness was excessive. Therefore, the Council of Ministers called for fundamental restructuring of the entire health system. This was intended to (a) strengthen preventive services, (b) develop a "dispensary scheme" (periodic examinations) to better serve everyone, (c) improve professional expertise, and (d) raise the quality of work of preventive and pharmaceutical facilities. Also greater attention should be paid to the environment, improved conditions in the workplace and the home, better personal life-styles, and stronger "moral and ideological training" for all health personnel. The plan also called for a "Soviet Fund for Health and Mercy," to be financed by voluntary contributions.

The methods of implementation of these policy objectives were spelled out in numerous sections of the twelfth 5-year plan of the USSR, for the period 1986–1990 inclusive. Major environmental protection measures were to be incorporated in all industrial enterprises, as well as in agriculture (use of pesticides, fertilizers, etc.). The State Board of Sanitation had to enforce regulations to cut environmental pollution. Absenteeism due to sickness of workers had to be reduced 15 to 20 percent. Sanitary regulations in food processing and transportation had to be enforced. The people's diets had to be improved through the production of nutritious foods and education of the population on sound dietary habits. Active health education on sound living habits had to be started in elementary school and continue throughout life; this would include sex education and physical culture. The greatest emphasis had to be put on "a resolute war against drinking and alcoholism, drug abuse, and smoking."

For preventive objectives, every citizen had an annual medical examination. From 1987 to 1991, priority goes to the chronically ill, children and teenagers, young students, pregnant women, war veterans, and workers in various types of industry and agriculture. By 1995, the entire population must be covered.

To improve the quality of all medical services, a new type of diagnostic faciltiy was planned. There would be a network of diagnostic centers, where sophisticated medical technology is available; these would strengthen the capabilities of both polyclinics and hospitals. They would eventually shorten the average length of stay of hospital patients. Polyclinics have to be reorganized to increase the numbers of people they serve. The "role and prestige" of the local polyclinic doctor had to be enhanced; he or she would be relieved of work not requiring a physician. Multipurpose or general hospitals had to be provided with better equipment and organized for handling different stages of case severity, including intensive care and (at the other end of the spectrum) rehabilitation. Specialized sanatoria for convalescence (not rest-homes or spas) had to be developed. Better home care of the chronically sick had to be organized.

Improvements also had to be made in the emergency-and-ambulance medical service and in all maternal and child health care. This would include better equipped services for premature births and also improved day care centers for small children. For workers in small enterprises, regional polyclinics had to be strengthened.

The plan called for strengthening of both district hospitals and the better-developed provincial hospitals. District hospitals also had to develop social programs for the elderly. Highly sophisticated hospitals, specialized in such fields as microsurgery, organ transplantation, and renal dialysis, were proposed. Cardiology departments were also required in all polyclinics and hospitals. More cancer treatment centers had to be developed and strengthened. Similar plans were laid out to improve general surgical care, prevention of blindness, dental health, and care of psychoneurological disorders and to treat alcoholism and drug addiction. The general approach seemed to call for numerous specialized dispensaries and hospitals for the management of all these conditions.

To carry out the various new plans, a broad program of strengthened training was required for all personnel—training along both technical and humanistic lines. "The Soviet doctor," it was stated, "must have high ideological conviction, a feeling of debt to socialist society, and be conscious of the social significance of his profession." Selection of all candidates for training in the health professions would put greater stress on previous experience. Physician training would be more oriented toward general practice; social sciences had to be included. Medical and pharmacy education would have to put greater stress on practical experience in hospitals. Preventive concepts had to be incorporated more firmly in all education. Basic medical education may be lengthened from 6 to 7 years. Examinations had to be rigorous, and medical students who failed would be allowed to enter a middle medical field (e.g., nursing or feldsher).

The training of nurses, feldshers, midwives, pharmacists, sanitarians, and other middle medical personnel had to emphasize compassion as well as technical competence. To ensure good quality performance, *probationary periods* of employment would be introduced everywhere. All educational institutions were to be reviewed and new textbooks prepared, including new *medical encyclopedias.* Salaries had to correspond more closely to competence, and specialists would require recertification periodically.

Abuses of position had to be closely monitored and penalized. The maldistribtuion of personnel in different regions had to be eliminated. To improve the conditions of rural health service, better living quarters had to be provided for health workers. Innovation was encouraged in all health work. All local Soviets of People's Deputies would review the "capital expenditures" set aside for the construction of needed facilities.

The twelfth 5-year plan (1986–1990) called for still more changes to restructure the Soviet health system. Improvements in the work of medical research institutes were planned. The construction of new polyclinics, hospitals, and other health facilities was proposed in detail. Management procedures were criticized and methods to reduce bureaucratic delays were proposed.

These health system objectives in the twelfth 5-year plan were obviously not only ambitious but also would be very costly. To accomplish them, the government budget for the health system required great enlargement—an estimated tripling by the year 2000. For the 1989 budget year, it was reported that the allocation to the Ministry of Health was nearly doubled through the transfer of funds from Soviet military expenditures.

The time had arrived, according to the new minister of health, to slow down on the quantitative output of human and physical resources and to concentrate on the quality of health care. This required a vast infusion of modern diagnostic equipment, as in the new *diagnostic centers* proposed by the 5-year plan, and also the complete replacement of about 25 percent of the country's large supply of hospital beds. Every hospital would have to be better equipped with modern technology, absorbing 20 to 30 percent of capital costs instead of the previous 10 to 12 percent. In 1988, the Ministry of Health started to require all physicians to take examinations on their basic medical knowledge. In fact, when the first 350,000 (about one-third) of the nation's doctors were tested, 30,000 got only "provisional certification" (requiring another test soon) and 1,000 were stripped of their licenses entirely.

To combat the impersonal and even "arrogant and rude" attitudes of polyclinic doctors (according to a letter published in a Moscow newspaper in 1988), patients would have free choice of doctors. Then physicians who attracted more patients would receive salary increases, of up to 30 percent. Lower rates of industrial absenteeism would warrant bonuses to industrial physicians, as long as investigations showed that disability certifications were not being unfairly withheld. To retain nurses in their profession, their salaries would also be increased. The private paying polyclinics would be slightly expanded, to increase competition with the official services. The minister emphasized, however, that enhanced private medical care would only be slight, and the massive efforts would go into improving the official system.

Psychiatric care in the Soviet Union, as in most countries, has many problems, relating to the stigma of mental illness and the inadequacies of psychiatric knowledge. In addition, Soviet psychiatry seems to suffer from the people's mistrust of the entire field, because of widely recognized abuses. Since the law has long required only three physicians to certify that a patient is "socially dangerous" to commit someone to a mental hospital, it has been misused to isolate political dissidents and even "uncooperative" industrial workers. On the other hand, genuine criminals have been kept out of prison by being certified as "mentally ill." Part of the *perestroika* movement called for a complete modification of the law on mental hospital commitment.

Most of all, the fresh Soviet policy of openness and restructuring signified the flexibility of this socialist society, and the health system within it, in spite of the common perception in Western Europe and America that it is cast in concrete. One might well criticize the long period that problems were evident before corrective action was taken, but the same must be said of almost any large national society. In the case of the Soviet Union, with the extreme hostility of Western powers who epitomized it as "an evil empire," one can understand a policy of massive investments in military defense. The entire level of living of the civilian population inevitably suffered from these huge military expenditures. The irritations in ordinary family life, with long queues for food and long delays for housing or repairs in household utilities, are bound to affect general morale.

Yet the Soviet health system has managed to make basic health care, preventive and curative, available to a huge and diverse national population essentially free of charge. It has established health facilities within easy reach of virtually all of its approximately 280 million people. A highly developed emergency medical service provides backup support for primary health care at any hour of the day or night, in every urban center. It has completely decommercialized health care as a market commodity, and made it a service to be routinely expected in modern society. Whatever aversion Marxian socialism may have to classical capitalism, the health leaders have tried to "learn from the West," and adopt many forms of medical technology, concepts of preventing chronic disease, even principles of competition with financial rewards for better performance. Because of the simple logic of its planning process and the basic rationality of its organizational structure, the Soviet health system has come to serve as a model for many newly independent and developing countries in Africa and Asia. The system will doubtless continue to change, in response to worldwide influence and domestic experience.

POLAND

With the defeat of the fascist countries in World War II, socialist political power in Eastern Europe was great. Soon after the Nazi surrender in 1945, several nations that had been under fascist control for several years were transformed into socialist states, with varying degrees of influence from the Soviet Union. These countries included Poland, East Germany (the German Democratic Republic), Czechoslovakia, Hungary, Romania, Bulgaria, Yugoslavia, and Albania. The last two countries, for many historical and military reasons, were least influenced by the Soviets. Poland, also for many historical, military, political, and economic reasons, was perhaps the most influenced by the Soviet Union.

In the general design of its health system, the People's Republic of Poland emulated the Soviet model very closely. Poland suffered enormous destruction and loss of human life during the war, making reconstruction of the society extremely difficult. Yet, during the first 30 years of the new socialist government, from 1947 to 1977, advances in the health system and in the Polish people's health were enormous. Then numerous difficulties developed, leading to major reforms. Rather than review this entire process comprehensively, we will examine certain selected features of the Polish health system experience, which were somewhat different from the Soviet model, and might be regarded as uniquely Polish. But first certain general features of Poland must be considered.

General Features

In 1984, the People's Republic of Poland had a national population of approximately 37 million people, of whom 60 percent were urban. Education had always had a high pri-

ority in urban Poland, and now it was extended everywhere, resulting in nearly 100 percent literacy. For many centuries, the Catholic religion was a major cultural influence; some 98 percent of the people are of Catholic origin. Despite Marxian antireligious ideology, churches are still numerous and Catholic priests play a significant role in daily life. National wealth is somewhat lower than that of most other Eastern European countries, with a GNP per capita in 1984 of $4,634.

The socialization of the Polish economy was never complete. Basic industry, including mining (coal, iron, etc.), was the major object of nationalization, and came to employ some 90 percent of industrial workers. Almost all agriculture, however, has remained under private ownership. There are some agricultural cooperatives, but as of 1978 70 percent of the available land was in the hands of small independent farmers. Finally, a small but significant private sector exists in various service enterprises—restaurants, transportation, various trade shops, and so on. Private medical practice also seems to be somewhat more extensive than in the Soviet Union.

Poland is divided administratively into 49 provinces (*voivodships* in Polish), which also provide an organizational framework for the health system. Each province has a Provincial Health Department, to which authority is delegated for the management of the wide range of programs directed nationally by the Ministry of Health and Social Welfare. To establish a network of centers for tertiary health care, the provinces are grouped into 10 health regions, containing about five provinces each. At the center of each region is a medical school (known as *medical academies,* since their transfer from the universities in 1952 to the Ministry of Health) and a large teaching hospital. These constitute centers not only for tertiary-level patient care, but also for consultation and continuing education to health personnel throughout the region. As in the USSR, the medical academy faculty members are expected to spend a great deal of time in services to patients, as well as to teaching, but not as much time to research. Medical research is the task of some 15 to 20 research institutes, also under Ministry of Health supervision.

Local Health Care Organization (the ZOZ)

A notable aspect of the Polish framework of health care organization has been the development, within each province, of local areas of "integrated health service" (*zespol opieki zdrowotne,* or ZOZ in Polish). Implementation of this approach began around 1974, to link the ambulatory services more closely to the hospitals, which were regarded as the centers for ensuring a high scientific quality of service.

Each ZOZ was expected to contain at least one hospital, several ambulatory care health facilities, and often other specialized ambulatory services such as emergency units, elementary school health services, and industrial dispensaries. This scheme of integration between hospital and ambulatory services was a departure from earlier patterns, under which hospitals functioned in a network from periphery to center, independent of the ambulatory services both primary and specialized. Some ZOZ responsibilities are specialized, in such fields as occupational health or mental health, if hospitals in those fields are located in the particular area. For large cities, with highly developed emergency medical services, ZOZs may also focus entirely on EMS. Certain services, such as sanitary–epidemiological activities or the supervision of pharmacies, nearly always remain under the general direction of the provincial health departments. There are actually numerous variations among provinces in the distribution of responsibilities between the provincial and local ZOZ levels.

In spite of the many variations among the provinces in the adminstration of various specialized services at the provincial level, the greatest share of day-to-day personal health service is rendered by the generalized ZOZ structures. Their essential feature is the technical integration between the hospital and the ambulatory care units—both those offering primary care and those concentrating on specialist care. Primary care in Poland is considered to include adult internal medicine, pedi-

atrics, obstetrics–gynecology, and dentistry. Throughout Poland, there were 412 ZOZ units in 1976, including both generalized and specialized types.

As early as 1967 Poland explored the local generalized ZOZ concept on a pilot basis and emphasized in certain parts of the country, but with the restructuring of the provinces from 17 to 49 in 1973 the policy became nationwide. The territory encompassed in a typical ZOZ area is roughly equivalent to that of the former *powiat* (district), but the functions are different and, outside the health services, the boundaries have no meaning as political jurisdictions. The key feature is the technical integration of each specialty of health service, whether rendered to a hospital bed patient or an ambulatory patient. Thus, the chief of pediatrics in the ZOZ hospital is technically responsible for all child health services in the ambulatory care centers of the area, and likewise for internal medicine, gynecology, and so on.

The medical director of the ZOZ ordinarily serves also as director of the main hospital. He may be a full-time administrator and practice no clinical medicine, or he may do both. He may be aided by deputies for specialist care (largely in-hospital services), for primary care (largely services in the ambulatory care units), for diagnostic services (laboratory, x-ray, electrocardiograms, etc.), for social welfare, for nursing (both in and out of the hospital), for economic and administrative affairs, and for "methodological and organizational" functions. The last type of deputy has an interesting range of responsibilities; he handles all statistical data on health problems and health services used in planning. He also promotes and conducts health education programs, supervising the continuing education of doctors and all other health personnel in the ZOZ.

The point of a patient's entry into the ZOZ health scheme is ordinarily through one of the ambulatory care facilities. In the rural sections, this unit is typically staffed by one general practitioner (who gives primary care to men, women, and children), aided by a nurse. A dentist is aided by a chair-side auxiliary. A second nurse spends part of her time making home visits to patients. A small drug depot is managed by one of the nurses. A clerk and maintenance personnel complete the *rural health center* staff. In the towns, ambulatory care centers (which would be called *polyclinics* in the USSR) usually serve a larger population and are more fully staffed with a generalist, pediatrician, obstetrician–gynecologist, and dentist, along with allied personnel.

A patient need not always enter the ZOZ scheme through an ambulatory care center; however, he is free to go directly to the hospital outpatient department without the conventional referral. If the hospital specialist considers the case within the competence of the primary care unit, he simply refers the patient back to it. Thus, as in so much of Polish society, there is a theoretically preferable procedure, but official attitudes are permissive and flexibility is readily accepted.

A uniform and essential feature of all ZOZ programs is the comprehensive range of authority delegated to the director. This is implemented largely by the system of financing, in which the Provincial Health Department allots a global sum to the ZOZ headquarters. Thus, the ZOZ director may decide how to divide the funds among the several facilities and programs under his jurisdiction; in this way he can alter the priorities from time to time. He is influenced, of course, by the standards for staffing and program emphasis issued by the Provincial Health Department, which in turn are guided by national standards from the Ministry of Health and Social Welfare. At the provincial level, a reserve fund is usually kept to assist ZOZ areas that face a deficit; likewise, any area with a surplus of funds at the end of the fiscal year is required to return them to the Provincial Health Department.

It should also be noted that each ZOZ, like each province, is funded by the next higher level of government for all the services it is expected to render, regardless of the patient's place of origin. Thus, unlike the policy of organized health care programs in many countries, when a patient from one locality is hospitalized in another the hospital serving him or her does not have to be reimbursed by the agency at his place of residence. Each facility, each ZOZ, and each province in Poland is simply funded for all services it must render; the

financial base is nationwide and not linked to local place of residence.

The broad authorities of the ZOZ director, as noted, include freedom to transfer personnel within the area, as needs change. Exchange of doctors periodically between hospitals and ambulatory care centers is a regular policy in some ZOZ programs and not in others. Geographically the ZOZ area is small enough to permit such transfers without any need for the doctor to change his residence. The benefits of such exchanges are in their educational impact; it helps the hospital specialist appreciate the problems of primary care, while enriching the community doctor's background. On the other hand, exchanges may disrupt the continuity of care for patients served in a local health center, and for this reason they are not carried out in all ZOZ programs.

Some Polish health administrators believe that ZOZ integration can be carried too far. Programs can become unwieldy, if too much responsibility is lodged in one specialist at a hospital or in a matron (director of hospital nursing). Hospital doctors, who theoretically are supposed to supervise all services in their specialty in the ZOZ area, are often unable to find the time to meet these expectations. This is aggravated when a ZOZ population is very large; ideally this should not exceed 100,000 people, but many ZOZ units have much larger populations. Naturally the current organization must be built on the framework of existing facilities, and these are often not in the ideal location or of the appropriate size. With the vertical links from ambulatory care centers to hospitals based on technical specialties, the community health center may lack cohesiveness. Each such ambulatory care unit has one physician in charge administratively, but it is sometimes difficult to distinguish an administrative from a technical matter. Clearly, the attitudes of hospital specialists dominate the ZOZ model, and this may yield policies contrary to the philosophy of primary health care.

Social Insurance and Economic Support

Nearly 100 percent of the Polish population have economic protection against the costs of health service, and physical access to medical care, but this was not achieved overnight. On the attainment of power by revolutionary groups (United Workers Party and the left wing of the Socialist Party) in 1945, the social insurance coverage of the population for health care was estimated to by only 15 percent. Then, as industrial development occurred under government control, the coverage of workers and their families was gradually extended, and insurance contributions came entirely from the enterprise (i.e., no wage deductions were made from the worker's paycheck). Administration of the health care insurance program, however, remained under a separate Central Social Insurance Board. Only in 1951 was this function transferred to the Ministry of Health.

By the mid-1950s, economic access to medical care became extensive in the cities, but it was still far from universal. Beneficiaries were required to be "insured" by virtue of employment in a public enterprise, even though earmarked contributions from "employers" were no longer used for financing health services. (Such contributions continued, for the support of monetary insurance benefits, such as old-age or invalidity pensions.) Thus, persons who were self-employed (along with their dependents) and not part of the socialized economy were not covered by the health insurance system. These were mainly farm families and independent tradespersons, an estimated 27 percent of the population in 1975. Even among these families, infants and children through the primary school years were entitled to free government health care, as were maternity cases, patients with infectious disease, and certain others. The charges made for health services rendered in public institutions, moreover, were very low (varying with family income) and much below true costs. These uninsured persons, however, obtained a great deal of their out-of-hospital care from private medical and dental practitioners. In rural areas there were also numerous agricultural producer and consumer cooperatives, some of which financed medical care.

Health insurance protection was extended to independent farmers only in January 1972. Since then, more than 99 percent of the Polish population have become entitled to comprehensive health care of all types, with only minor restrictions. (The fraction of 1 percent of the population not covered are purely private tradespersons or the owners of small private enterprises.) The principal benefit limitation is a charge to the patient of 30 percent of the cost of out-of-hospital drugs purchased in a pharmacy, but even these charges are reduced or waived for pensioners and persons with certain serious diseases. Extra charges may also be levied for use of a private room in a hospital (when not medically necessary), decorative eyeglasses, and other such nonessential items. To adjust to the heightened demand for services after 1972, hundreds of addtional health centers and hospitals were constructed in rural areas.

Production of Health Resources

Regarding health personnel and facility development in Poland certain features are noteworthy. Among personnel, pharmacists in Poland seem to have a somewhat higher status than in the USSR. They are not regarded as "middle medical personnel," although *assistanct pharmacists* are trained less thoroughly. The full-fledged pharmacist receives 5 years of higher education in one of the medical academies (most of which have a faculty in pharmacy).

The development of nursing in Poland reflects certain interesting characteristics of female employment in a socialist country. In most industrialized countries there are two or more levels of nurses. In general, the number of assistant or auxiliary nurses exceeds the number of fully qualified or professional nurses. Thus, in Great Britain for 1979, the World Health Organization reported 128,481 professional nurses and a total of 148,811 "assistant nurses" and "nursing auxiliaries." In the Netherlands, the assistant and auxiliary categories of nurses in 1978 amounted to 72,868, compared to 34,500 professional nurses. In Poland, however, the total number of assistant nurses in 1979 amounted to only 11,879, while fully qualified nurses (not counting *feldshers* or midwives) numbered 137,526.

The explanation is that, once secondary school education as well as full professional nursing education became free, applications for admission to the assistant nurse programs (only 1 year after elementary school) declined greatly. Applications were so few that, in 1967, assistant nurse training was terminated entirely.

The decline of these applications doubtless reflects an employment setting or labor market in Poland very different from that in most free-enterprise and industrialized countries. The labor market in the latter countries includes many women of limited skills seeking employment of some type. With few other job opportunities, these women—often from poorly educated ethnic minority groups—throng to low-level nursing jobs, even for very meager wages. In Poland, however, even when general economic conditions were poor, unemployment has been minimal. There is hardly any reservoir of unemployed and undereducated women. Therefore, any woman interested in nursing has been able to undertake full professional training without personal cost.

Another aspect of Polish nursing is noteworthy. In 1969, Poland was the first European country to offer university-level education in the nursing field. The Polish Nurses Association had pressed for this training, to raise the qualifications of nursing teachers and administrators. Graduate nurses were previously free to undertake university studies in sociology or other fields, but the Polish initiative established a master's degree in nursing. After 1969, 4-year university-level educational programs in nursing were established at five of the medical academies. Two years of professional nursing experience are required for entry.

In Poland, as in other European socialist countries, a majority of physicians are women. In the 1980s, a move was made against the "feminization" of medicine. Overt preference was given to male applicants for medical education; in 1982, for example, of the large number of applicants 37 percent were young men, but these were 50 percent of those accepted. As in other socialist countries, medical salaries are quite low, but the prestige of the medical profession remains exceptionally high.

Private Medical Practice

Private practice by physicians is apparently much more common in Poland than in the USSR. After working their official 7 hours a day (often 8 A.M. to 3 P.M., with no time out for lunch), some 30 percent of doctors are estimated to spend a few hours in seeing private patients at their own homes. This is only for ambulatory care, since there are no private beds in any of Poland's hospitals. A study in 1972 found 8 percent of an urban population visited individual private doctors regularly. After retirement, physicians are free to engage in private practice up to half-time.

The equivalents of paying polyclinics in the USSR are called *medical cooperatives* in Poland. Such medical cooperatives are located in almost all Polish cities. It is estimated that 20 or 25 percent of Polish doctors work in them part-time, and accordingly are subject to much more regulation, for the public good, than they would be in purely private practice. Thus, after the 7 hours of public service, a physician or dentist may work in a cooperative up to 2 hours per day. The fees chargeable to patients are fixed by the Ministry of Health, and tend to be lower than fees for corresponding service in private quarters. The usual policy allows about 50 percent of each fee to go to the doctor and the other 50 percent to be retained by the cooperative to support the cost of nurses and other associated staff, supplies, rental, taxes (about 20 percent of collections), and so on. Most important, the Provincial Health Department appoints a cooperative manager, who handles the accounts and ensures that regulations are being followed. Periodic inspections are made by officials from the Provincial Health Department and also from the local sanepid station.

Patients evidently come to medical cooperatives in substantial numbers, judging by the growth of the pattern. They are attracted by the unrestricted freedom of choice of doctors and the impression that only the best qualified specialists are allowed on the cooperative staffs. Since 1975, drug prescriptions issued by a medical co-op doctor may be filled in a regular public pharmacy, with only the usual 30 percent copayment; previously such prescriptions required 100 percent payment by the patient. Laboratory and x-ray services are provided in the co-op, for additional fees. The extent of utilization of medical co-ops by the population is not known, but a common estimate is 7 percent, or between 5 and 10 percent. A national survey in 1967 (when medical co-ops were fewer than now) found only 2.0 percent of people using them; the rate varied with educational level, however, being under 1.0 percent among persons with only primary schooling and rising gradually to about 5 percent among university graduates. At the same time, 11 percent of persons surveyed said they would like to use co-ops, and 21 percent said they would like to use private doctors if they could afford the costs.

The "Solidarity" Movement and Health Reforms

In spite of the reputation of Poland as having a form of "flexible socialism," many people have reacted to the rigidities of the entire society. In August 1980, issues came to a crisis, with the organization at Gdansk of an independent and governmentally disapproved trade union named *Solidarity*. This grew into a nationwide movement, extremely critical of the Communist Party leadership of the country. Health care issues were included among the movement's criticisms, and a dynamic industrial nurse served as chief of Solidarity's health section.

Under pressure from Solidarity, government leaders from the ministry of health began to speak and write articles about deficiencies in the health system that had evidently been long recognized but not discussed openly. In November 1981, the government's official public health journal published a sweeping criticism of the operations of the entire system, referring to such faults as long waiting periods for service, "stiff or even bureaucratic attitudes to patients," "low quality of medical care—perfunctory and inexact examinations," and so on. The official spokesmen called for "thorough and complete organizational changes." Much more emphasis, they said, should be put on preventive and primary health care, and on improvements in the quality of all services.

To achieve these objectives, the MOH leaders advocated much greater decentralization of responsibility to both the regional and provincial levels. Diversified patterns of organization, they wrote, should be encouraged in response to local conditions. The community people should have a say in local policy decisions. "The professional domination stereotype," it was said, "should be replaced by an approach in which those receiving health services are co-partners in the process or organization and control." Decisions on capital investments in facilities should be made at the regional level, in cooperation with the 10 medical academies. Provincial health directors should have much greater independence. At the local level also, the primary health care unit (with generalist, pediatrician, gynecologist, and dentist) should have greater freedom, which seemed like a departure from the ZOZ integration principles.

Professional education, it was advocated, should provide greater experience in practical service, with less emphasis on specialization. Salaries should be made more dependent on work output (for motivational reasons) and less on academic credentials. Under pressure from Solidarity, the budget for the Ministry of Health was reported to be increased in October 1981 from about 2.5 to 6 percent of national income (not GNP). A new minister of health was also appointed.

In December 1981, the Polish government declared martial law, and the Solidarity union was officially banned. Nevertheless, even under military control, the demands of Solidarity were largely adopted as official policy, within the constraints of the poor overall economic situation. In late 1980, the government had agreed "immediately to increase investments in the sphere of health protection, to improve the supply of drugs through imports of raw materials, to raise the salaries and wages of all health personnel, and to urgently prepare a governmental and ministerial program, with a view to improving health standards in the country." (This became known as *Demand 16* in a long list of Solidarity demands.) In 1987, a former critical Polish analyst of the system could report with approval about ". . . the openness [of government], and above all the desperate struggle to maintain the material base of the health system, the standards of health care, and [efforts] to prevent or at least to slow down the process of its decline. Some battles have been quite successful and have resulted in improvement in the supply of drugs, in rather better conditions of pay for some categories of health personnel, and in the slightly increased share for health in the capital investments for construction."

Primary health care (PHC) was emphasized, through various local experiments with free choice of doctor and a loosening of selected ZOZ programs, to test the liberation of PHC units from domination by hospital specialists.

Thus, it appears that the Solidarity movement in Poland stimulated changes in the health system—greater decentralization, emphasis on primary health care, participation of the people in policy decisions, and even a higher economic priority for health in national affairs—quite similar to those associated with the *glasnost* and *perestroika* political reforms, launched in the USSR 3 or 4 years later. In socialist nations, confrontation and even violence, in one setting, can evidently encourage the peaceful transformation of social structures in another. Perhaps such dynamics apply to all types of sociopolitical order.

In 1989, free elections in Poland resulted in the actual attainment of government power by the Solidarity movement. For the first time since 1945, Communist Party control was ended in an Eastern European country. The new government leaders pledged continuation of the publicly financed health system, with further development of the decentralized policies long promoted by Solidarity.

YUGOSLAVIA

Among the socialist countries of Eastern Europe, Yugoslavia is unique for its high degree of decentralized responsibility in all sectors of society, including health. Even within a socialist political framework, much of the economy follows competitive free-market principles;

thus, both scholars and politicians have regarded the country with exceptional interest.

General Features

Yugoslavia took shape as a country, carved out mostly from the Austro-Hungarian Empire, after World War I. It became an uneasy assemblage of various ethnic groups under a Kingdom of Jugoslavia in 1929. During World War II, the territory was again divided among several fascist states, and only in 1945 was it reunited as Yugoslavia, under Communist Party control. The leader of the successful Partisan antifascist movement, and the first Premier, was Josip Broz Tito.

For 3 years Yugoslavia collaborated with the USSR and other Eastern European socialist countries, and began to develop a health system on to the model of the Soviet Union. Then in 1948, Tito's sharp disagreements with Josef Stalin in Moscow led to a breakaway from the Cominform alliance of socialist countries. Asserting its independence from Soviet dominance in economic and political policies, Yugoslavia has built a society, including a health system, unique in the world.

In 1984, Yugoslavia had 23,000,000 population, divided among six semiautonomous republics and two autonomous (and relatively poor) provinces. The several republics differ largely (though not entirely) along ethnic lines. These jurisdictions, with their significant peripheral responsibilities, were designated in the Constitution of 1946. The overall economy is still largely agricultural, with 54 percent of the people living in rural areas. The GNP per capita in 1984 was $2,990, which was significantly lower than that of the other European socialist nations. With a supply of 160 physicians per 100,000 and 5.6 hospital beds per 1,000, its health system resources were also somewhat weaker than those of the other socialist countries.

In 1953, after the break with the Soviet Union was complete, the Yugoslavian government abandoned the attempt to collectivize agriculture. It also launched its ambitious program to decentralize the entire economy. Ownership of industry remained in the hands of the government, but its control and general management would be turned over to councils elected by the workers of each enterprise. Central planning would be replaced by local decision-making, competition, and profit-sharing among the groups of workers in each establishment. Political controls were also decentralized to the communes—118 in the entire country, with populations of about 50,000 to 100,000 each. The communes, and sometimes groups of adjacent communes, play a significant role in the operation of the health system.

Yugoslavia has been reported to spend about 6.1 percent of its GNP on health activities, from all sources. Social insurance is the major source, accounting for about 75 percent of health expenditures, with the remainder coming from government revenues (at different levels) and enterprises, and about 6 percent from private fees. Public revenues come principally from the republics, with very little spent at the federal level.

Social insurance for financing health care had long been independent of government in Yugoslavia, insofar as funds were handled by local workers' organizations. Before 1969, the mandatory insurance laws applied essentially to industrial workers and their families. Farmers and agricultural workers, constituting 36 percent of the population, could insure themselves voluntarily at relatively high costs. In 1969, farmers and their families were brought under the mandatory insurance scheme; they made contributions based on a percentage of net income.

All insurance funds were handled by local associations of the people in one or more communes, to aggregate at least 150,000 persons, for assurance of actuarial stability. In 1978, close to 100 percent of the Yugoslavian population were protected by general insurance for medical care. In the Republic of Croatia, for example, industrial workers and their families constituted 87 percent of the insured (a lesser percentage nationally), farm families were 12 percent (a greater percentage nationally), and the remaining 1 percent were self-employed professionals or craftsmen. Although the management of health insurance is left up to each republic, the federal government stipulates the required range of health services. If the contributions from farmers are not sufficient to finance the required benefits, funds can be transferred from the workers' insurance to help farm families, under the principle of *social solidarity*.

Health Workers' Self-Management

When the principle of local self-management of all enterprises by their workers was generally established in 1953, it was also applied to the organizations for providing health services. Just as industrial workers, through their elected representatives, managed each industrial enterprise, health workers became responsible for policy and practice in each hospital, health center, and academic health institution. These facilities, of course, still had directors and various department heads, but these executives were chosen, not by a Ministry of Health, but by all the health personnel of the local establishment; all basic policy decisions required the agreement of the *workers' self-management council.* These principles were all embodied in the new Constitution of 1963.

As experience was gained with this highly democratic and decentralized model of management, the need was recognized for some type of coordination between institutions and a rational scheme to allocate resources among institutions. In each commune, as well as in each republic, therefore, there were established "quasi-parliaments" of elected workers in every social sector. Thus, there were parliaments in the health sector, known as *Self-Managing Communities of Interest in Health,* at both the commune and republic levels.

The Self-Managing Communities of Interest (SMCIs) for health, however, differed from these bodies in other fields by including a strong voice for the consumers of health care. Thus, the SMCI for health had two houses— one representing health workers and the other composed of elected consumers from the local area. The SMCIs were responsible for coordinating individual facilities (e.g., between health centers and hospitals of different sizes and functions), planning new construction, and allocating money from the insurance funds and the government. To a limited extent, the federal government subsidized health services in the poorer republics, and republic governments subsidized the less prosperous communes.

By the late 1960s, certain undesirable consequences of many years of decentralization became apparent. Large differentials in earnings developed between workers in various enterprises, and even between workers of different levels in individual enterprises. Around 1970, demands arose for even more local autonomy and the complete rejection of socialist principles—to the point that subdivisions of one enterprise earned a profit (with higher wages), while other subdivisions of the same enterprise suffered a loss (with lower wages). Under Tito's leadership, a third Yugoslavian Constitution was enacted in 1974. This established a voice for Communist Party officers in each local commune; they would henceforth serve as a third house in the communal SMCI. The same would apply at the republic level. Republic laws required that in any enterprise (or any health institution), the highest-paid worker could not earn more than five times as much as the lowest paid worker.

The SMCI at the communal level was intended to reconcile the demands of each health facility for a larger budget every year, to respond to social needs, and in view of the constraints of social insurance funds available. Conflicts were unavoidable. Since the workers and consumers were naturally the most emphatic about social needs, the achievement of some negotiated agreement often meant suppression of their voices and increased domination by managers and technocrats. Obviously there were discrepancies between the ideal conception of workers' self-management in all forms of production, including services, and the realities of daily management practice.

Many observers, both inside Yugoslavia and outside, have gone so far as to claim that progress in the health system has depended largely on *deviations* from the principles of decentralized worker control and the application of greater centralized planning. The distribution of physicians, for example, illustrates the issue. With its permissive ideology, Yugoslavia has no mandatory rural service for new medical graduates (as do other socialist and many non-

socialist developing countries). Yet legal requirements at both federal and republic levels that minimum health services must be provided for everyone have had a crucial impact on the allocation of both social insurance and general revenue funds. Thus, areas of doctor shortage receive greater funding and have more medical positions to offer. As a result, the distribution of doctors has become more equitable.

In effect, self-managing workers' councils, in the sector of industrial production, may well be effective in providing incentives for hard work and in stimulating competitive energies. In health systems, on the other hand, where competition can create serious inequities rather than optimal social interests, marketplace competition can be harmful. The same applies to other service sectors, such as education. The Yugoslavian authorities have learned, through experience, that *market socialism* has its strengths and its weaknesses, the latter largely in sectors for socially needed services.

One other aspect of the Yugoslavian health system should be noted. Because physician salaries in the official health system are relatively low, private practice after official hours is perfectly acceptable. Nevertheless, it is rare outside the large cities, where there is a market of relatively affluent patients. In both cities and rural areas, it is also common for doctors (both from hospitals and health centers) to hold second part-time jobs. The government-supervised private group clinics found in the Soviet Union and Poland, however, do not operate. The output of physicians by Yugoslavia's 11 medical schools has contributed to a steadily increasing ratio of physicians to population, although the worldwide expansion of specialization, at the expense of general practice, is also found. The attraction of specialization is its linkage to hospitals and its high prestige; salaries are little different from those of general practitioners.

OTHER EUROPEAN SOCIALIST HEALTH SYSTEMS

Aside from the health system of the Soviet Union, we have examined those of Poland, a country closely modeled after the USSR, and Yugoslavia, the country whose social policies are most widely divergent from the Soviet model. The health systems of the other Eastern European countries all conform closely to the Soviet model, but in one respect or another each has some special characteristics. In the order of their GNPs per capita in 1984, these are the health systems of Romania, Bulgaria, Hungary, Czechoslovakia, and the German Democratic Republic.

Romania

With a per capita GNP in 1984 of $3,571, Romania had long been one of the poorest countries in Europe. With socialist transformation after World War II, the health resources were enormously expanded, but the ratios of both personnel and facilities are still appreciably lower than those of the other socialist countries. In medicine, Romania has departed from Soviet policies by deliberately minimizing trends toward specialization. In the 1970s the specialties for which qualifications could be earned were reduced from 57 to 27. Greater stress was put on broad medical knowledge and its use in general practice. Around 1980, some 60 percent of all Romanian doctors were GPs. Still, in 1979 the 2-year mandatory rural service for new medical graduates was suspended. Instead, physicians were provided with cars, which permitted them to live in cities and drive regularly to health posts in rural areas.

Until 1978, private medical practice had been authorized for government physicians up to 12 hours per week. Since then, it has been greatly restricted. Total health expenditures have been quite low. When Soviet health expenditures were estimated in 1976 as 2.7 percent of GNP, they were 1.9 percent in Romania. Social insurance remains the mechanism of economic support for personal health services, but independent farmers and self-employed tradespersons are still not covered. (They may obtain care in the public system, but they must pay for it.) Romania's Superior Health Council has 200 members, representing all population groups, in overseeing the performance of the Ministry of Health, as a generally democratic strategy.

Bulgaria

With GNP per capita of $5,014 in 1984, Bulgaria is somewhat more economically developed than Romania. Back in 1966, its total health expenditures were 2.5 percent of national income (not GNP). Because their government salaries were low, rural doctors were free to supplement them regularly with payments from rural agricultural cooperatives. Full-time private medical practice is authorized only for retired physicians, but any public physician may engage in part-time private practice after official hours.

The close linkage of health center or other ambulatory care doctors to hospitals, found in the Polish ZOZ, is implemented in Bulgaria in another form. Hospital specialists supervise the work of health center doctors by a policy that considers the latter to be extramural members of the hospital staff. The large tertiary hospitals are also expected to supervise the work of small peripheral hospitals, through regular field visits by their medical staffs. The best-qualified specialists offer continuing education courses of about 10 days in the surrounding small community hospitals.

Hungary

The health system developed by Hungary after World War II was a faithful replication of the Soviet model. At the national level, virtually all health responsibilities were vested in the Ministry of Health. Below the top, the country was divided into 19 counties (equivalent to provinces), plus the national capital, Budapest. Within each county are municipalities, and many municipalities have villages with their own adminstrative structures.

At each level is a health authority, which is adminstratively responsible horizontally to the general government council—that is, at the level of the county, the municipality, or the village. For technical policy questions, the health authority is responsible vertically to the next higher echelon, leading up to the central Ministry of Health. General health policies and standards are established by the central government. Broadly speaking, the administration of hospitals is principally at the county level, and primary health care programs are managed principally at the municipal and village levels.

Hungary's human physical resources for health service were enormously expanded after the devastation of World War II. In 1950 there had been 110 physicians per 100,000 population, and by 1987 this was increased to 320 per 100,000, nearly all trained in the nation's four medical schools. Virtually all doctors are employed in the public service, and 76 percent were specialists in 1985. Hospital construction has been emphasized, and in 1988 there was an overall supply of 9.8 hospital beds per 1,000 population.

Ambulatory care for the general population is provided mainly through a network of district physicians—general practitioners and pediatricians—located in health centers or small medical stations in the villages and municipalities. Ambulatory specialist services are provided at the out-patient department of a hospital, usually regarded as a hospital-linked polyclinic. Even if a polyclinic is distant from the hospital, since 1976 it has been considered a satellite of the hospital.

Industrially based health services have had exceptionally high priority in Hungary. In 1985 nearly 8,000 physicians were giving primary care, and of these nearly one-third were attached to industrial enterprises full-time or part-time. Although industrial units and even large polyclinics are part of the general MOH system, bonuses may be given to these personnel by the enterprise, and extra equipment may also be provided. A National Institute of Labor and Industrial Hygiene is one of the strongest of 18 research institutes operated by the MOH.

Generous tipping for medical (as well as other) services has long been customary in Hungary, even before the advent of socialism. With low medical salaries, this has come to play a significant part in professional incomes, even though it is officially frowned on. Tips are reported to augment incomes by 30 or 40 percent—even more for prestigious specialists. Unfortunately, many patients seem to believe that good service cannot be expected without a good tip. Purely private practice has never been forbidden, and it is offered in the home of the doctor or the patient in evening hours.

In spite of rising demands for private service, paid for privately, the demands on the official health system remain high. In 1987, the average general practitioner had 2,471 patients on his list (that is, to whom he gave regular care for his salary). Typically the GP sees patients 2 to 4 hours a day in his office and spends another 3 to 4 hours on home calls. He or she usually refers only about 5 percent of cases for a specialist consultation at a hospital polyclinic.

Nevertheless, Hungarians have free choice of doctors, and the demands for direct services from specialists in the hospital out-patient department and polyclinic have grown. With severe economic constraints, the MOH could not afford the resources for greater delivery of specialist care. In the 1980s, therefore, special efforts were made to strengthen both human and technological resources at the primary care level. Much of the out-patient specialist care, previously given at hospitals, was being transferred to health centers in the villages and municipalities. Hospitals will provide only highly advanced specialty service.

Furthermore, Hungary has been opening up its health system to competition from private institutions, developed with both domestic and foreign capital. Services may be purchased in these facilities with private insurance or purely private funds. It remains to be seen whether the competitive incentives lead to greater efficiencies in the public sector.

A rather poor health record in Hungary's mortality rates from heart disease, cancer, accidents, suicide, alcoholism, and cardiovascular disease since about 1960 has alerted health leaders to the need for much greater attention to health promotion and prevention. It is intended to put greater emphasis on health education, early case detection, national dietary policy, work-site health promotion, environmental controls, and general primary care.

Research on morbidity and on the operations of the national health system appears to be quite well developed in Hungary. In the 1960s, studies of the demand for medical care, as indicative of morbidity, were made at 130 consultation points. It was found, for example, that although health services were equally available to everyone, the rate of demand for medical care rose with educational level. Clinical examinations of a population sample confirmed that there was a higher rate of "unrecognized illness" among persons of lower educational levels.

An impressive demonstration of health services research in Hungary was published in 1986. (Perhaps this was related to the onset of *glasnost* in the USSR at this time.) In this year, a new Center for Regional Studies was established in the Hungarian Academy of Sciences, and the first report of this body was on regional disparities in the health system. It was shown that, although all health resources had improved (doctors, hospital beds, etc.) throughout the entire country, the differentials between the best supplied counties (or provinces) and the least well supplied had actually widened over the years 1960 to 1982. The share of government budgets devoted to health in all of the 20 provinces had declined, and the proportion of national income allocated to the health system had been virtually stationery—changing from 3.52 percent in 1965 to only 3.87 percent in 1980. This candid report also explicitly demonstrated that, in the first 25 years of the socialist state, 1945–1970, the major emphasis had been on health manpower development and primary health care (PHC). Since 1970, it was evident that PHC had become subordinated to the demands of high technology. This, in turn, contributed to the increased regional disparities in health service. With the reforms of the late 1980s, these relationships may change once again.

The difficulties in Hungary's health system in the late 1980s were obviously a reflection of the national problems of a socialist economy. With a GNP per capita of $5,915 in 1984, Hungary was one of the more affluent of the Eastern European countries, but its foreign debt was (on a per capita basis) enormous. More than most socialist states, Hungary had long allowed and even encouraged private enterprise in the marketing of many consumer goods and services. In the late 1980s, for the first time unemployment appeared, and unemployment benefits had to be added to the social security scheme.

Identifiable health expenditures in the late 1980s were estimated at between 3 and 4 percent of the overall national expenditures in Hungary, although this did not include the value of gifts, nor of private fees or official co-payments for pharmacy drugs. Official copayments for medical and hospital service had been considered and rejected. If the new reforms succeed in reducing hospital costs, while only slightly increasing primary care costs, net savings may be achieved. The government is, in any case, determined to continue the operation of its health system as essentially accessible to everyone.

Czechoslovakia

With a longer history of industrial and cultural development, even before socialist transformation, Czechoslovakia could develop its new health system relatively fast. The GNP per capita was $6,267 in 1984. The country's 11 regions (or provinces), with about 10 districts in each, yielded a total of 118 districts, with populations of about 120,000 to 150,000. Each district was placed under the supervision of an *Institute of National Health,* responsible for all health activities in the area. This included not only hospitals, polyclinics, sanatoria, dispensaries, and so on, but also sanitary–epidemiological stations, pharmacies, and schools of allied health personnel. Although ambulatory care units were supervised by hospitals, as in the other socialist countries, the overall direction of all health activities was clearly in the hands of the district institutes.

A tabulation of the distribution of all Czechoslovakian physicians, engaged in various types of ambulatory service in 1967, may shed some light on practices in many socialist countries.

Types of Ambulatory Care Physician	Percent
Community health generalists for	
adults	30.6
Industrial physicians	14.1
Pediatricians	15.5
Gynecologists	5.3
Other specialists in polyclinics	34.5
All ambulatory care	
physicians	100.0

In 1967, each community health center for primary care was expected to serve a population of only about 3,800 people—fewer than such units in the Soviet Union. The customary team of generalist, pediatrician, gynecologist, and dentist was evidently provided in small local community health centers quite regularly.

In higher-education policy, Czechoslovakia differs from the other socialist countries. There are ten faculties training physicians, dentists, and pharmacists. Although their curricula are designed largely by the Ministry of Health, these faculties remain functionally within the universities; they have not been withdrawn as separate academies or institutes under direct MOH control, as in the USSR and other socialist states. The education of nurses, technicians, physical therapists, and other middle medical personnel comes under direct MOH administration.

German Democratic Republic (GDR)

With a GNP per capita in 1984 of $7,995, the GDR is the only European socialist country with greater overall wealth than the USSR. As part of the former German Republic, where industrialization was already well developed in the nineteenth century, the background of resources and activities in the GDR health system was much richer than in any of the now-socialist countries to the East. Even 12 years of fascism, with all its bigotry and antisocial policies, did not completely destroy the ability of the East German people to function efficiently and reconstruct a viable society.

A field survey group, sponsored by the World Health Organization in 1980, reported that the GDR health system had made health services available to 100 percent of its 16,700,000 people. In spite of the massive destruction from World War II, by 1970 nearly all essential health facilities had been rebuilt, and thousands more medical and associated personnel had been trained. In 1969, private medical practice after official hours, permitted only for high-level medical directors, was still extensive, since the official system was not yet developed sufficiently. By 1984, there were 222 physicians per 100,000 population, of whom 55 percent worked in hospitals and 45 percent in out-of-hospital care (including polyclinics, enterprises, etc.). Unlike other socialist countries, the GDR had several religiously sponsored hospitals that were allowed to continue under their old management; this applied to 89 hospitals out of 584, or 15 percent. The proportion of private hospital beds was lower, and these hospitals survived only with donations from abroad to supplement the GDR financing.

Medical education in the GDR appears to be more rigorous than in any other socialist country. Basic medical training, as almost everywhere in the world (except in the United States and Canada), is 6 years following secondary school. Then, after this, 4 or 5 years of further training are *mandatory.* This lengthly educational sequence is required for all physicians, whether they are undertaking a conventional specialty or going into general medicine.

Nineteenth-century Germany, it will be recalled, was the birthplace of social security programs, which used hundreds of local sickness funds as intermediary bodies. The old system was very complicated, with diverse sets of benefits for various occupational groups. Now there is a flat 10 percent insurance tax on all wages, shared by the workers and the enterprises, up to a maximum of $24 per month. This is used to finance all benefits (old-age pensions, disability compensation, etc.), including health care. There is also a substantial subsidy from general government revenues. Trade unions perform some of the administrative functions. Every GDR resident is entitled to the same service, through the network of polyclinics and hospitals.

Since East Germany lost a great deal of its people in World War II, as well as through postwar emigration, there is a general policy of encouraging population growth. Children's allowances through social insurance are quite generous, and there is a large network of creches for children under 3 years of age; in 1981, 612 children out of each 1,000 under 3 were enrolled in a creche, supervised by a specially trained nurse. There is also an especially well-developed network of well-baby stations. Nevertheless, abortion is freely available within the first 12 weeks of pregnancy, and contraceptive measures are likewise free. The net outcome of all these policies has been a modest increase in the birth rate.

The juxtaposition of the two Germanies—one with the welfare-oriented and free-market model of a health system, and the other with a socialist model—invites comparison. West Germany (the Federated Republic) and East Germany (the GDR) are quite different in their per capita wealth. In 1984 the Federated Republic had a GNP per capita of $10,985; this was 37 percent higher than the $7,995 figure for the GDR. The infant mortality rates of the two countries in 1985, however, were identical, at 10 infant deaths per 1,000 live births.

SOCIALIST HEALTH SYSTEMS—COMMENTS

The experience of industrialized and socialist countries in the development and operation of socialist health systems has much to teach about the dynamics of centralized planning. Incentives associated with the profit motive and competition may stimulate maximum productivity in the output of steel or the manufacture of shoes. In health services, however, the same incentives may have perverse effects—a severe maldistribution of health resources and the provision of superfluous services to some people while others, in greater need, are deprived. Centralized planning, therefore, can potentially promote the distribution of resources in appropriate relation to the health needs of people at various times and places.

Yet the process of centralized planning, and the pyramidal administrative structure that usually goes with it, may cause other problems. The hierarchical organization, the relatively rigid rules and regulations, the firmly established procedures for reaching policy decisions may have adverse effects on individual creativity and personal motivations. These issues have, of course, been the subject of political debate for many decades, even centuries.

This somewhat detailed review of the health system of the Soviet Union, and of special aspects of the systems of seven other socialist and industrialized countries, leads to certain general observations. Centralized health system planning, the nearly complete elimination of market dynamics in the provision of health service, and the sponsorship and control of almost all health resources by government have been shown to be feasible strategies for making comprehensive health care available to all persons in a country. Some organized resource for primary health care has been brought within convenient reach of virtually everyone, whether through a rural health station, a polyclinic, a hospital out-patient department, or an emergency ambulance call. The application of these strategies in European and largely industrialized countries has depended on socialist revolutions. Survival of these revolutionary reforms, in the face of inevitable and strong opposition, has entailed great repression of personal freedoms and the firm leadership of a single political organization.

This is not to say, as some have argued, that significant social change in health systems to achieve universal coverage and comprehensive health services for everyone in a country can be achieved *only* with violent social revolutions. We have seen in Chapter 7 how such goals have been attained in parliamentary democracies through legislative enactments, following many years of experience with programs of national health insurance. In those countries, however, many of the resources of the health system remain under private sponsorship and control. Important aspects, such as the manufacture of pharmaceuticals, much education of health personnel, the operation of many voluntary health agencies, the provision of health services to most industrial workers, and several other health system features remain outside the sphere of government. For better or worse, the socialist health systems have established virtually complete and integrated control of all resources and services, under a unified public authority.

With such developments, at least as they have occurred in Europe since the Russian Revolution of 1917, access to essential health services has been accorded to total national populations, through a hierarchical structure of authority from a national center to provinces, districts, and small urban and rural communities. This has been done at relatively low costs to the nation—much lower than those in capitalist or free-enterprise countries. Overall expenditures for health care have been kept low, probably much too low, by greatly reducing the historical independence of the medical profession, and converting of nearly all physicians, like other health personnel, into civil servants working on modest salaries. (Physicians remain dominant decision-makers in the technical aspects of patient care, but not in the overall economics and operation of the system.)

Central planning has also governed the investment of national wealth in medical technology, so that much of this has been very frugal, much below the potential of modern scientific knowledge. Other forms of investment in national economic development and the attainment of military strength have taken precedence.

Centralized authority, planning, and power have enabled socialist health systems to achieve many efficiencies. Hospitals are established in regionalized networks, with small facilities handling simple cases and larger facilities, with more advanced staffs and equipment, serving more complex cases. Health personnel work in teams, so that labor is divided and each task is theoretically done by the person with the least elaborate training who can still perform the task properly. Because population health needs are deemed more important than the personal wishes of individual medical practitioners, periods of mandatory service must be spent in "unattractive" rural areas.

Pharmaceuticals and other products are not subject to the monopoly of patent laws, and they are manufactured at the lowest possible costs. Preventive and therapeutic personal health services are integrated, without separation based on the economic interests of the private practitioner. Duplication and even deception, associated with market competition and advertising, are eliminated. Relatively simple fiscal mechanisms greatly reduce the administrative costs of paying for services. The effort to abide by scientific principles in all health service has lessened much personal choice but has eliminated the waste or potential harm of most cultist or sectarian healing practices.

These are the major factors contributing to the effectiveness and efficiency of the Eastern European health systems, in accordance with their theoretical socialist principles. In practice, however, many of the theories have not always been successfully applied, and some of them have seriously overlooked certain realities of human behavior. Centralized planning has by no means been infallible. In previously impoverished countries, health planning has understandably emphasized the production of large quantities of health personnel and facilities, even at the sacrifice of quality. In time, however, a poor-quality product—whether it is a piece of medical equipment, a hospital ward, or a clinical physician—may be accepted as the norm. Many socialist health personnel are much less well educated than their capitalist counterparts. The schedule of drug production has often resulted in shortages of certain products, while surpluses accumulate in others.

Conversion of all health personnel to civil servants, with little independence, has had a major impact on individual motivations. The role of each health worker is explicit and clear, but there may be serious loss of flexibility and innovativeness. The adoption of new ideas may be inhibited by fear that some rule will be broken, with resultant penalties. Job security and virtually guaranteed employment, of course, have their social merits; there has been virtually no unemployment in the European socialist countries. Yet this policy does not encourage diligence and hard work; absenteeism has been high and the productivity per worker, relative to that in capitalist countries, has been low. Relatively generous cash benefits for sickness absenteeism have contributed to crowded polyclinics for certification of disability; in spite of abundant physicians, the demands on their time are great, and patient service is often rushed. Medical work pressures can lead to perfunctory care and to abrupt, even arrogant attitudes toward patients. Crowded hospitals, in spite of a large bed supply, may generate corrupt practices, such as bribery, for gaining access to a hospital bed.

It is to the credit of socialist societies that these deficiencies, in the application of their basic theories, have come to be recognized.

One may think that such insights took a long time to be grasped. In any event, the recognition of problems has generated important reforms. In practice, the rules have not always been rigidly followed everywhere. Individuals with courage and initiative have applied new ideas, so that health centers, polyclinics, hospitals, and medical schools do, indeed, show many variations. More important, a mass movement, such as Solidarity in Poland, could arise; although it was legally repressed its impact on the health system was substantial. In several socialist countries the demand for private medical services was recognized in the early 1970s, resulting in the institutionalization of paying polyclinics or medical cooperatives. In Yugoslavia, on the other hand, an extreme swing of the pendulum toward decentralized self-management by workers in the 1950s led to a return to greater central controls in the 1970s. In the USSR the massive social reform, epitomized by *perestroika* (restructuring) in the 1980s, indicates a remarkable admission of failures in classical socialist doctrine, with a basic need for changes in policy to modify human attitudes and performance.

One must not overlook the handicaps of Eastern European socialist countries, because of well-organized and often covert hostility from the industrialized capitalist countries. The so-called iron curtain, isolating the socialist states from Western Europe, was fashioned by the North Atlantic Treaty Organization (NATO) powers as much as by the Warsaw Pact countries. Attempts of United Nations organs to encourage East–West trade were only minimally successful. The Cold War period from about 1947 through 1970 created far more difficulties for the socialist states than for other nations.

The influence of Western ideas on socialist health systems has not always been beneficial. The movement in the 1970s to improve the quality of medical care was equated with the Western emphasis on specialization. Almost every population group and every major type of disease gave rise to specialized dispensaries, polyclinics, and hospitals. Much of the patient-centered integration of health services in neighborhoods of socialist lands was eroded.

The subordination of polyclinics and health centers to hospitals (in the interest of quality maintenance) surely weakened the position of primary health care. Physicians may have been deprived of their excessive dominance, through unified professional associations, but in virtually every subdivison of the health system the top authority is vested in doctors, even if other types of personnel might be better qualified. Typically Western dietary habits— excessive consumption of dairy products and high-fat meats—were adopted by socialist countries, just as epidemiological studies were leading to their reduction in the West. Excessive tobacco smoking is another custom learned from abroad.

The decades of the 1970s and 1980s have, in any case, shown that socialism and socialist health systems are much less rigid than they had been reputed to be in the parliamentary democracies. Firm control by highly disciplined communist parties was their strategy for survival against opposition, from both within their borders and outside. But the negative consequences of these policies, as in most free-market societies in the opposite direction, have come to be recognized. Problems that become widely apparent eventually generate reforms in all societies. One may expect socialist health systems, in the year 2050, to have a very different configuration from what they had in 1950.

REFERENCES

Soviet Union

Anon., "Homeopaths Flourish Behind Iron Curtain." *Medical World News,* 3 June 1966, p. 110.

Anon., "Soviet Health Law." *Soviet Statutes and Decisions,* 20:(1)(2)(3)(4), Fall 1983–Summary 1984 (M. E. Sharpe, Armonk, New York).

Becker, Carl L., *Modern History: The Rise of a Democratic, Scientific, and Industrialized Civilization.* New York: Silver, Burdett & Co., 1935.

Butrov, V. N., "Note on the System of Post-Graduate Training of Doctors in the USSR." Geneva: World Health Organization (Travelling Seminar on the Organization of Refresher Courses for Medical Staff), 1968.

Chazov, Yevgeni, *Restructuring Affects the Whole Health Service.* Moscow: Novosti Press Agency Publishing House, 1988.

Davis, Christopher, and Murray Feshbeck, *Rising Infant Mortality in the USSR in the 1970s.* Washington, D.C.: U.S. Bureau of the Census (Series P-95, No. 74), September 1980.

Field, Mark G., *Soviet Socialized Medicine—An Introduction.* New York: The Free Press, 1967.

Field, Mark G., "Taming a Profession: Early Phases of Soviet Socialized Medicine." *Bulletin of the New York Academy of Medicine.* 48(1):83–92, January 1972.

Field, Mark G., "Soviet Infant Mortality: A Mystery Story," in D. B. Jelliffe and E. F. P. Jelliffe, *Advances in International Maternal and Child Health,* Oxford: Clarendon Press, 1986, pp. 25–65.

Fry, John, *Medicine in Three Societies.* New York: American Elsevier Pub. Co., 1970.

Fry, John, and L. Crome, "Medical Care in USSR," in John Fry and W. A. J. Farndale (Editors), *International Medical Care,* Oxford: Medical and Technical Publishing Co., 1972, pp. 177–203.

Galin, Liza, "'Glasnost' Boosts Health Care: Soviet MDs." *Medical Tribune,* 11 November 1987, p. 10.

Gorbachev, Mikhail, *Perestroika: New Thinking for Our Country and the World.* New York: Harper & Row, 1987.

Hyde, Gordon, *The Soviet Health Service: A Historical and Comparative Study.* London: Lawrence and Wighort, 1974.

Kaser, Michael, *Health Care in the Soviet Union and Eastern Europe.* Boulder, Colo.: Westview Press, 1976.

Knaus, William A., *Inside Russian Medicine: An American Doctor's First-Hand Report.* New York: Everest House, 1981.

Ministry of Health of the USSR, *The System of Public Health Services in the USSR.* Moscow: the Ministry, 1967.

Nelson, Harry, "Massive Reforms—Soviet Goal: Resuscitate Health Care." *Los Angeles Times,* 15 May 1988, pp. 1, 16, ff.

Popov, G. A., *Principles of Health Planning in the USSR.* Geneva: World Health Organization (Public Health Papers No. 43), 1971.

Pustovoy, Igor V., *Health Care Planning in the USSR.* Chicago: University of Chicago, Center for Health Administration Studies (Michael M. Davis Lecture), 1975.

Raffel, Norma K., "Health Services in the Union of Soviet Socialist Republics," in Marshall W. Raffel (Editor), *Comparative Health Systems.* University Park: Pennsylvania State University Press, 1984, pp. 488–519.

Roemer, Milton I., "Highlights of Health Services in the Soviet Union." *Milbank Memorial Fund Quarterly,* 15:373–406, October 1962.

Rosenfeld, I. I., *Planning and Allocation of Medical Personnel in Public Health Services* (translated from Russian). Washington, D.C.: National Science Foundation, 1963.

Ryan, Michael, *The Organization of Soviet Medical Care.* Oxford: Basil Blackwill, 1978.

Ryan, Michael, "Funding for the Soviet Health Service." *British Medical Journal,* 295: 652–653, 12 September 1987.

Sidel, Victor W., and Ruth Sidel, *A Healthy State: An International Perspective on the Crisis in United States Medical Care.* New York: Pantheon Books, 1977, pp. 158–186.

Sidel, Victor W., "Feldshers and Feldsherism: The Role and Training of the Feldsher in the USSR." *New England Journal of Medicine,* 278 (17): 934–939, 25 April, 1968.

Sigerist, Henry E. *Medicine and Health in the Soviet Union.* New York: Citadel Press, 1947.

Sigerist, Henry E., *Socialized Medicine in the Soviet Union.* New York: W. W. Norton & Co., 1937.

U.S. Department of Health, Education, and Welfare, *A Directory of Medical and Biological Research Institutes of the USSR.* Washington, D.C.: National Institutes of Health, 1958.

U.S. Delegation on Health Care Services and Planning, *Medical Care in the USSR.* Washington, D.C.: Fogarty International Center (DHEW Pub. No. NIH 72-60), 1970.

USSR Ministry of Health, "The Basic Plan for the Development of Health Care and for Reorganization of the Healthcare System of the USSR in the Twelfth Five-Year Plan and for the Period until the Year 2000." *Meditsinskaya Gazeta,* 96: 4749, 27 November 1987 (translated from the Russian by Clifford Kaylin).

Venediktov, D., "Union of Soviet Socialist Republics," in I. Douglas-Wilson and Gordon McLachlan (Editors), *Health Service Prospects: An International Survey,* London: The Lancet and Nuffield Provincial Hospitals Trust, 1973, pp. 231–254.

Wallace, Helen M., "Primary Health Care of Mothers and Children in the Soviet Union—1979." *Clinical Pediatrics,* 19(6):420–423, June 1980.

World Health Organization, *Health Education in the USSR.* Geneva: WHO (Public Health Papers No. 19), 1963.

World Health Organization, *Health Services in the USSR.* Geneva: WHO (Public Health Papers No. 3), 1960.

Zhuk, A. P., *Public Health Planning in the USSR.* Washington, D.C.: Fogarty International Center (DHEW Pub. No. NIH 76-999), 1976.

Poland

Anon., "Health and Health Protection of the Polish Population: Experience and the Future." *International Journal of Health Services,* 13(3):487–513, 1983.

Central Statistical Office, *Concise Statistical Yearbook of Poland.* Warsaw, 1975.

Indulski, J., and J. Kaminski, "The Role of the State in the Development of the Citizens' Health Protection." *La Santé Publique* (Bucharest), 18(4):389–402, 1975.

Indulski, J. et al., "Health Care in Polish People's Republic: Attempts of Evaluation and Trends of Rationalization" (English Abstract). *Ochrona Zdrowia W. PRL* (Polish Public Health), 11 November 1981, pp. 784–787.

Kurlowicz, W., "The Role of the State Institute of Hygiene in the Protection of the Health of the Population." *Zdrowie Publiczne* (Public Health), 87:1–9, January 1976.

Leowski, Jerzy (Editor), *Health Service in Poland.* Warsaw: Polish Medical Publishers, 1974.

Ministry of Health and Soviet Welfare, *Health Care in the Polish People's Republic.* Warsaw, 1978.

Roemer, Milton I., "National Health Policy Formulation in Socialist Poland." *Journal of Health Politics and Law,* 3(2):155–162, 1978.

Roemer, M. I., and Ruth Roemer, *Health Manpower in the Socialist Health Care System of Poland.* Washington, D.C.: U.S. Health Resources Administration (NO1-MI-34090 P), 1978.

Rytel, Alexander, "Public Health and Welfare in Poland." *Polish Medical Science and History,* 14:182–192, October 1971.

Sokolowska, Magdalena, and Bozena Moskalewicz, "Health Sector Structures: The Case of Poland." *Social Science and Medicine,* 24(9):763–775, 1987.

Spivak, Jonathan, "Medical Muddle: Polish Health-Care System Is Beset by Shortages; Crisis Is Major Social Problem Facing Solidarity," *The Wall Street Journal,* 16 October 1981, p. 48.

Webster, Thomas G., "Health Policy and Solidarity in Poland." *New England Journal of Medicine,* 4 February 1982.

Yugoslavia

Association of Self-Managed Communities of Interest for Workers Health Insurance and Health Service of the City of Zagreb, *Economic Aspects of the Health Service and the Health Care in Zagreb* (English Summary), Zagreb, Yugoslavia, 1983.

Berg, Robert L., M. R. Brooks, and M. Savicevic, *Health Care in Yugoslavia and the United States.* Washington, D.C.: Fogarty International Center (DHEW Pub. No. NIH 75-911), 1976.

Federal Institute of Public Health, *The Public Health Service in Yugoslavia.* Belgrade, 1975.

Himmelstein, David U., S. Lang, and S. Woolhandler, "The Yugoslav Health System: Public Ownership and Local Control." *Journal of Public Health Policy,* 5:423–431, September 1984.

Institute for Social Medicine, Statistics and Research, Medical Faculty of Belgrade and Institute of Public Health of S.R. Serbia, *Regional Organization of Health Services and Health In-*

surance in Serbia Proper. Belgrade, December 1973.

Kunitz, Stephen J., "Health Care and Workers' Self-Management in Yugoslavia." *International Journal of Health Services,* 9 (3):521–537, 1979.

Parmelee, Donna E., G. Henderson, and M. S. Cohen, "Medicine under Socialism: Some Observations on Yugoslavia and China." *Social Science and Medicine,* 16:1389–1396, 1982.

Shain, Max, "Health Services in Yugoslavia." *Medical Care,* 7(6):481–486, November–December 1969.

Shain, Max, and T. Gjurgjevic, "Principles of Health Insurance: Decisions in Croatia and Proposals in the United States." *Medical Care,* 11(3):254–258, May–June 1973.

Yugoslavia Federal Committee of Labor, Health and Social Welfare, *The System of Health Development Planning in Yugoslavia.* Belgrade, September 1979.

Other Socialist Health Systems

Battistella, Roger M., *Role of Health Services in National Social and Economic Development Planning in the Socialist Republic of Romania.* Ithaca, N.Y.: Cornell University, Spring 1980 (processed report).

Csepanyi, Attila, *The Hospital–Polyclinic Complex in the Hungarian People's Republic.* Budapest, July 1983. Processed report.

Flahault, Daniel, et al. "Travelling Seminar on Primary Health Care in the GDR." Geneva: World Health Organization, 1980, unpublished field report.

Forgacs, Ivan, and Mihaly Kokeny, *Health, Health Care, Social Services.* Budapest: Ministry of Social Affairs and Health, 1989.

Fulop, Tamas, "Integrated Epidemiological Surveys: Rural Population of Hungary." *Milbank Memorial Fund Quarterly,* 49(1):59–92, January 1971.

Gebhard, Bruno, "Public Health in East Germany." *American Journal of Public Health,* 54(6):928–931, 1964.

Institute for Social Hygiene and Health Care Organization, *Health Care in the German Democratic Republic.* Dresden: Ministry of Health, 1981.

Lehfeldt, Hans, "Medicine in East Germany Almost Wholly Nationalized." *Medical Tribune,* 10 March 1969, p. 8.

Light, Donald W., and Alexander Schuller (Editors), *Political Values and Health Care: The German Experience.* Cambridge, Mass.: The MIT Press, 1986.

Ministry of Health of the Hungarian People's Republic, *Health Care in Hungary.* Budapest, 1978.

Orosz, Eva, *Critical Issues in the Development of Hungarian Public Health with Special Regard to Spatial Differences.* Pecs, Hungary: Center for Regional Studies of Hungarian Academy of Sciences, 1986.

Palec, Rudolf, "The Regional System and Postgraduate Medical Training in Czechoslovakia." *Milbank Memorial Fund Quarterly,* 44(4):414–425, October 1966.

Postgraduate Medical School of the German Democratic Republic, *Public Health in the German Democratic Republic.* Dresden: Ministry of Health, 1972.

Raffel, Norma K., and Marshall W. Raffel, "The Medical Care System of Hungary." *Journal of Medical Practice Management,* 4(2):142–149, 1988.

Skrbkova, Emilie, and Milos Vacek, "Some Problems of Health Care Organization in Czechoslovakia." *Medical Care,* 9(5):405–414, September–October 1971.

Stritesky, Jan, "Some Observations on the Czechoslovak Health Services." *Medical Care,* 5(2):78–84, March–April, 1967.

Vacek, Milos, and Skrbkova, Emilie, "Methods of Planning Health Services in Czachoslavvakia." *Milbank Memorial Fund Quarterly,* 44(3):307–317, July 1966.

Whitney, Craig R., "Health Care in the East German Way." *New York Times,* 8 April 1976, p. 4c.

PART THREE

TRANSITIONAL COUNTRIES

CHAPTER NINE

Entrepreneurial Health Systems in Transitional Countries

All countries that are not affluent and industrialized are sometimes described as *developing,* but here we subdivide this large array of countries into two sets: those that are very poor and *underdeveloped,* and those that are more energetically involved in the process of development, or *transitional.* The transitional countries and their health systems are moving relatively rapidly toward economic and social development. In terms of national wealth, they have an annual gross national product (GNP) of less than $5,000 but more than $500 per capita. (The figures change, of course, from year to year, and these numbers apply to the data reported for 1983 or 1984.) The great majority of these countries, in fact, have GNPs per capita between $1,000 and $3,000 per year, with a global median of about $1,500. Of course, they also demonstrate a range of political ideologies in their health systems.

GENERAL FEATURES

Aside from their economic level, the transitional countries, with entrepreneurial-type health system policies, have certain distinguishing features. Long dependent for their income on agriculture, mining, and the export of raw materials, they have developed an increasing amount of industrialization. In certain of these countries, the industrial development has been extremely rapid, commodities are mass-produced for export, and their GNPs have leaped sharply upward. This applies to South Korea and Taiwan, where free private enterprise is a central tenent of the national economic policies. In other of these countries, such as Thailand or the Philippines, industri-

alization has been largely oriented to the manufacture of consumer goods for domestic consumption.

Urbanization is increasing rapidly. In each of these countries one great metropolis, usually serving as the national capital, dominates the nation politically and culturally. A middle class of government and commercial employees, tradespersons, and professional personnel has been expanding. There are many new buildings, often with striking architectural design. The downtown sections of these large cities are like prosperous European and American metropolises. Yet a short distance away are usually thousands of marginal families in miserable peri-urban slums. The rural areas are another world, where massive poverty is the norm.

The maldistribution of family incomes associated with these conditions is extreme. Data are not available for all of these countries, but household surveys in a few have shown disparities in household incomes, such as the following:

Country (year)	Percentage of National Income		Ratio (1):(2)
	Lowest 5th (1)	Highest 5th (2)	
Thailand (1976)	5.6	49.8	1:9
Philippines (1985)	5.2	52.5	1:10
South Korea (1976)	5.7	45.3	1:8

Source: World Bank, *World Development Report* 1987, pp. 252–253.

Another common feature of all the entrepreneurial health systems in these transitional countries is the very large role played by the private sector. Well over half of all health-related expenditures are derived from personal sources. Even public facilities for health service typically require private payments for their use. Moreover, when collectivized methods of financing health service have been organized by governments, through social insurance, the moneys are spent mainly to purchase services from private providers of medical care.

Data on private spending, as a percentage of total national health expenditures, are not available for many transitional/entrepreneurial countries for the same year. Reports by World Bank economists, however, although applicable to different years, show the following:

Country (year)	Percentage of National Health Expenditures from Private Sources
Thailand (1979)	70
Philippines (1970)	75
Republic of Korea (1975)	87

In other words, funds for the health system contributed by government (for the years indicated) amounted to only 30, 25, and 13 percent of the total expenditures, respectively. As we will see, in welfare-oriented countries of the same general economic level, government health expenditures are usually a much higher proportion of the total. With time and political changes, of course, these private/public relationships in health spending may change substantially.

Because of the strength and independence of the medical profession in these entrepreneurial systems, another common feature is an exaggerated maldistribution of physicians, not only between urban and rural locations generally, but between the large capital metropolis and the rest of the country. Along with this goes an extremely high concentration of hospital beds in the capital city, and a clustering of medical schools and their teaching hospitals.

To exemplify this type of national health system, we analyze the situation in Thailand in some detail. Then we consider selected characteristics of the health systems of the Philippine Republic, the Republic of Korea (South), and South Africa.

THAILAND

Thailand is one of the few nations of Southeast Asia that has never been a colony. (*Thai* means "free," which is more meaningful than the formerly European designation, *Siam*.)

Social Setting

From its origins in the seventh century until 1932, Thailand was an absolute monarchy. In 1932, the king accepted a constitutional and representative form of government. In 1957, however, power was seized by the military forces. Since then, except for short periods in 1974 and again in 1976, the ruling government has been essentially in military hands. The king has been retained as a symbol of national authority.

The population of Thailand in 1984 was about 51,000,000. Nearly all are ethnically Thai people, with small minorities of Malays and Chinese. Buddhism is almost the universal religion, and Buddhist concepts permeate the entire culture. Urbanization has grown, but only to 20 percent, while 80 percent of the population remains rural. Literacy is reported to be 91 percent among adults, but in rural areas and among women it appears to be much lower than this. The GNP per capita in 1984 was $814.

Jurisdictionally, Thailand has 71 provinces, plus the Bangkok Metropolitan Area (BMA); if the BMA is counted as a province there are 72, with subdivisions as shown in Table 9.1. At the lower levels of communes and villages, the chief officials are elected by the people, but the provincial governors and the district officers are all appointed by the central government (Ministry of the Interior). The organizational structure of the Ministry of Health is estab-

Table 9.1. Number and Typical Populations of Government Jurisdictions in Thailand, 1985

Jurisdiction	Number	Typical Population
Province	72	600,000
District	703	60,000
Commune	5,608	8,000
Village	53,102	600

Source: Thailand Ministry of Interior, Department of Local Administration, *Annual Report,* 1985.

lished in strict accordance with these general government jurisdictions.

The Bangkok Metropolitan Area is a large, crowded, and dynamic city. It is a center of commerce and tourism, not only for Thailand but for all of Southeast Asia. The 53,000 villages, however, where 80 percent of the people live, are dull and impoverished places, though their agricultural produce—rice, corn, tapioca, and rubber—provides the foundation of the national economy.

Organizational Structure of the Health System

Several government agencies play roles in the Thai health system, the principal one being the Ministry of Public Health. There is also a small nongovernmental but organized private sector (voluntary) and a very large commercial private sector.

Ministry of Public Health. In 1918, a Division of Public Health was set up in the Ministry of Interior, to bring together various public functions related to health. This unit produced smallpox vaccine, appointed "commune doctors" (usually traditional healers), and built and operated a few provincial hospitals. Not until 1942 was this unit removed from the Ministry of Interior (largely exercising police powers) and established as a cabinet-level Ministry of Public Health.

The Ministry of Public Health (MOPH) at the central level in Bangkok has six principal departments: (1) Office of Under-Secretary of State for Health, (2) Department of Medical Services, (3) Department of Health, (4) Department of Communicable Disease Control, (5) Department of Medical Sciences, and (6) Office of Food and Drug Committees. The Under-Secretary's Office has very wide scope. In addition to coordinating the other five departments, it supervises all rural health services and trains health personnel. In 1985, this office absorbed 75 percent of the MOPH budget.

The Department of Medical Services controls the major general and special hospitals throughout Thailand. The Department of Health plans and supervises the major health promotion and disease prevention activities in the country—maternal and child health, nutrition, environmental sanitation, and others. The Department of Communicable Disease Control facilitates immunizations and other infectious disease control strategies within the general MOPH infrastructure. The Department of Medical Sciences supervises the analytical laboratories in all MOPH facilities. The Office of Food and Drug Committees is expected to monitor all such products, to protect consumers against hazards, but its activities in 1984 depended on only 0.36 percent of the general MOPH budget.

Peripherally, each of the 71 provinces has a provincial public health office, the director of which is appointed by the central MOPH. The provincial chief medical officer (PCMO) is technically responsible to the Under-Secretary of State for Public Health and administratively reponsible to the governor of the province. The PCMO's technical scope encompasses all MOPH activities in the province, both preventive and curative. Thus, he oversees the provincial general hospital (sometimes two) and typically several district hospitals, as well as the preventively oriented programs. On the staff of the PCMO is usually a medical officer, specifically devoted to health promotion programs and the distribution of vaccines and medications. The PCMO must obviously exercise great discretion in reporting to the governor on administrative matters (e.g., fiscal and personnel questions) and to the MOPH on technical matters.

With approximately 10 districts in a province, each district is headed by a district health officer (DHO). The DHO is not ordinarily a physician, but typically a senior sanitarian with brief extra training in public health administration. A few of the 703 districts are headed by senior nurses. Since the DHOs are seldom medical, they have no responsibility for the district hospitals (recently termed *community hospitals*), but they supervise small health centers for primary care in the communes. The DHO must also distinguish his technical responsibility to the PCMO and his administrative responsibility to the centrally appointed district officer.

Commune health centers are the most peripheral facilities of the MOPH, and they are staffed entirely by nurses and auxiliary health personnel. Each commune typically contains 10 or more villages. Hundreds of villages (but only a fraction of the total) have a small station (often a personal home) with a government-trained midwife. Since 1978, there have been even more peripheral health workers—volunteer and part-time personnel, regarded as employees of the village, but not MOPH. These workers are *village health volunteers* (VHVs), trained at the commune health center for 20 days, and *village health communicators* (VHCs), trained for only 5 days. The work of these village personnel was originally confined to family planning (birth control education and distribution of contraceptive materials), but it has been extended to several aspects of general primary health care, with education of villagers about use of the commune health center.

It is evident that the MOPH of Thailand has a program of quite broad scope. There are, however, many other activities within the organizational structure of the Thai health system.

Office of the Prime Minister. The Office of the Prime Minister contains several very important agencies that affect the health system. First is the Bureau of the Budget, which determines the central government funding of the entire MOPH. Second is the Civil Service Commission, which controls the numbers, categories, and salaries of all government health personnel. Third is the National Economic and Social Development Board, which is responsible for overall planning and must approve the health planning proposed by the MOPH. Fourth is the Department of Technical and Economic Cooperation, which supervises all foreign aid programs, including those related to health. Fifth is the National Statistical Office, which conducts household surveys relevant to health needs and services. Sixth is the National Environmental Board for coordinating all environmental activities. Seventh is the National Research Council for coordination and support of all research, including medical and health-related work.

Ministry of Interior. This large ministry, where the Division of Public Health was orig-

inally lodged, still carries many responsibilities relevant to health. Most important is the MOI Department of Local Administration, which was established around 1911. This department was responsibile for designing the whole structure of provinces, districts, and communes outlined earlier. Among other things, the basic law entrusted each commune, or cluster of villages, to elect a local *commune doctor.* Nearly always, this was a traditional healer; he was expected to oversee environmental sanitation, encourage vaccinations, and help out in emergencies. Although the usefulness of these local health officials has gradually declined, some still function under the supervision of district health officers and are paid small monthly fees by the MOI.

More important is the Department of Local Administration responsibility for municipalities. Within the 703 districts, about 125 urban concentrations qualify as "municipalities." They have some independence from the authority of district officers and their district health officers. In most of them, a registered physician, designated as *municipal doctor,* is paid a monthly part-time salary by the MOI. For this, he is expected to supervise environmental sanitation, control communicable diseases, hold occasional first-aid clinics, and act as coroner to investigate suspicious deaths. Occasionally he is assisted by a sanitarian or a nurse. Administratively he is responsible to the elected mayor of the municipality, and technically he may seek advice from the provincial chief medical officer.

Overshadowing all of the nation's municipalities is the Bangkok Metropolitan Area (BMA), which operates a substantial health program under the MOI. Although BMA includes no hospitals, it supervises a network of health centers, offering preventively oriented primary health care. These units are not financed or controlled by the MOPH.

Other departments of the MOI also have diverse health responsibilities. The Department of Public Welfare operates various custodial institutions. In 1978 there were 21 facilities for orphaned or abandoned children, six homes for the aged, four homes for the destitute, and three institutions for the rehabilitation of "socially handicapped women" (prostitutes). All of these facilities require medical services that the MOI provides. A Department of Public Works in the MOI furnishes standardized architectural plans for the construction of health centers and hospitals. It also constructs piped water systems in municipalities, and participates in drilling deep wells in rural villages. Finally, there is a Department of Labor, which inspects factories for work hazards; this department also administers an Industrial Injury Compensation Act, which has been gradually extending coverage since 1972.

State University Office. Since 1976, the State University Office (SUO) has been a separate authority (formerly in the Office of the Prime Minister), with substantial health system responsibilities. Thailand has eight medical schools, of which seven are in universities under the control of this office. The only separate school is under the Medical Department of the Army. Each university-based school has a large teaching hospital, the financial support of which requires a major SUO expenditure, outside the budget of the MOPH.

Two of the oldest Thai medical schools were developed with the advice and assistance of the Rockefeller Foundation in the 1920s and 1930s. In the light of later events and policies, it is significant that as early as 1923 a Thai Prince proposed that a second-class "school of lower standing" be developed, to train large numbers of "practical" doctors to serve the rural population. This proposal was rejected by the foundation, on the grounds that it would lower the standards of the modern scientific schools and lead to various abuses. The Thai leadership was pursuaded, and not until 1935 was a small school for "second-class practitioners" started. Far greater investments, however, went into the first-class medical schools, favored by the Rockefeller Foundation, and not until the 1970s was this policy radically revised.

Other Ministries. Several other government ministries perform functions relevant to the health system. The Ministry of Education operates the primary and secondary schools which, among other things, teach the pupils about personal hygiene. The schools also cooperate with the MOPH in providing immunizations and other personal health services to school children. The Ministry of Agriculture and Cooperatives is concerned with control of zoonoses (animal diseases transmissible to humans) and regulation of the use of hazardous pesticides. The Ministry of Industry is expected to prevent factories from polluting their immediate environment. The Ministry of Defense has its own medical service organizations for the several armed forces, including a network of 18 military hospitals; these institutions also serve military dependents to a limited extent. One hospital is reserved for the care of military veterans with service-connected disabilities.

Under the supervision of the Ministry of Finance there are some 72 quasi-governmental "state enterprises," such as the Bank of Thailand, the national Tobacco Monopoly, and the State Railway. Most of these enterprises operate special medical care programs for their employees. Especially important is the Government Pharmaceutical Organization (GPO), which, though a state enterprise, is technically supervised by the MOPH. The GPO was started in 1939 and has gradually expanded. In addition to manufacture of certain common products, the GPO maintains several drug depots, and distributes imported or domestically manufactured drugs to all public hospitals and other health facilities.

Voluntary Health Organizations. Outside of government, Thailand has numerous private nonprofit agencies concerned with health or health services. In 1984 a survey found about 150 such agencies. All voluntary organizations must register with the Department of Religious Affairs in the Ministry of Education.

The largest voluntary agency with health functions is the Red Cross Society. It founded and nominally runs the largest hospital in Thailand—the Chulalongkorn University Hospital, which serves as the teaching facility for this university medical school. In fact, the government meets the operating costs of the hospital through the State University Office. Similarly a few smaller hospitals outside Bangkok, financed by the MOPH, are sponsored by the Red Cross. The Red Cross operates a central blood bank in Bangkok and branch banks in most of the provinces. In the 1980s the Red Cross, in cooperation with international agencies, sponsored camps for refugees from Laos and Cambodia in the east border region. Maintenance of eye banks and the production of antiserum for treating snakebites are still other Red Cross functions. For all this work the Red Cross Society is subsidized by the MOPH.

Family planning services are provided principally through voluntary agencies. These include the Planned Parenthood Association of Thailand, the Population Development Association, the Thai Assocation for Voluntary Sterilization, and the Association for Sterilization in Private Clinics. These groups carry out general education, provide direct services, and train auxiliary health workers. Almost all their funding comes from grants by international agencies, with a little supplementation from the MOPH. This strategy, of course, protects the government from any political controversy over birth control, while still getting the work done.

The Anti-Tuberculosis Association of Thailand conducts BCG immunizations, does case-finding through chest x-rays, and offers general health education. It also operates a small tuberculosis sanatarium in Bangkok, where patients must pay most of the operating costs. Since these are relatively high, the patients are mainly government employees, whose agencies pay the necessary charges. Some funds are raised through an annual Buddhist equivalent of Christmas seal sales.

Still other voluntary bodies are a Diabetes Association, Kidney Disease Foundation, Heart Disease Foundation, and Children's Foundation; the work of these groups is largely confined to Bangkok. Professional societies, such as the Medical Association of Thailand, hold conferences contributing to continuing education. There are also charitable foundations that sponsor maternity homes and other facilities for certain ethnic groups—Chinese, Japanese, and Moslems.

Finally, religious groups contribute to the health system through fundraising and direct services. Buddhist monks raise money from ordinary families for the construction of health centers and hospitals. In rural areas, the monks offer healing services through both religious rites and traditional herbal remedies; unlike the customary traditional healer, they collect no fees. One group of monks is reported to

have an effective regime for the rehabilitation of drug addicts.

Other religious bodies from abroad have long provided certain health services in Thailand. In fact, the country's first hospital was built by a Christian missionary group in 1886. There are now about 25 general clinics and small hospitals, sponsored by religious missions, mainly in rural areas. Some poor patients are treated without charge, but most patients must pay for the service; even though missionary doctors and nurses usually work without salaries, money is needed to pay domestic personnel and buy food, drugs, and medical supplies.

Commercial Enterprises. The thousands of small industrial shops in Thailand provide no health services for employees, but legislation requires that enterprises with 500 employees or more must have the regular services of a physician. Around 1980, an estimated 450 such firms existed in the country, and the medical services were provided by a doctor who was part-time or "on call." The Department of Labor in the Ministry of Interior is supposed to monitor these practices.

Some large companies go beyond the requirements of law and, out of paternalism or the desire to maintain productive workers, finance insurance to pay for private medical care (in whole or in part) for their workers. One commercial carrier (U.S. owned), for example, insured 120 industrial groups in 1974. The insurance typically indemnifies the worker with a fixed amount, based on a schedule of fees, and any balance must be paid to the doctor or hospital by the patient.

In 1980, there was also at least one private group practice clinic in Bangkok that catered mainly to industrial workers. It sold contracts for service on a prepaid capitation basis, along the lines of American health maintenance organizations (HMOs). The clinic manager, in fact, was a former employee of a large HMO from the United States.

The Private Market. The last part of the organizational structure of Thailand's health system is the largest. In spite of its amorphous configuration, it absorbs the largest share of health expenditures in the country, as we will see later. With respect to ambulatory health care, it doubtless also accounts for the largest proportion of services. This is the private health service market. The several distinct sections of this market include (a) traditional healers, (b) drugstores and drug-sellers, (c) private physicians and dentists, and (d) private hospitals.

For centuries before "Western medicine" was brought to Thailand in the nineteenth century, Buddhist priests and a variety of nonreligious healers rendered healing services. The latter employed various treatment methods, including both magic, to invoke supernatural forces, and physical procedures such as massage and herbal remedies. Thousands of these traditional practitioners, usually part-time, still render services in rural villages and, to some extent, in the towns.

As more effective scientific services have become available in Thailand, traditional healing has declined. It has by no means disappeared, however, and as the healers have discovered the value of certain modern drugs, such as antibiotics, they have acquired and given them to patients, along with their magical procedures. Because of the widespread belief that any drug given by injection is more effective, some healers, known as *injection doctors,* specialize in this technique. (Vitamin B complex, which is generally harmless and sometimes beneficial is commonly given this way.) Occasionally a village shopkeeper or teacher also performs injections for a fee. In recognition of the continuing viability of traditional healers, the MOPH has offered short courses to orient them on some elements of modern primary health care.

Another ancient practitioner important in rural areas is the traditional birth attendant (TBA). Although the MOPH trains young women in modern midwifery, it also recognizes the popularity of TBAs in the rural areas. Therefore, every year the ministry offers hundreds of rural TBAs brief courses (one week) on hygienic childbirth practices.

The modern drugstore, selling a vast variety of medications, is perhaps the major source of personal health care for most of Thailand's population. It is clearly the principal resource for the lowest income groups in large cities and small towns, where government health facilities are either unsatisfactory or overcrowded, and is used for the care of many ailments by people who cannot afford private medical attention.

Thai drugstores are of several types: (a) shops with a registered pharmacist present during all services hours, which sell modern compounds (including some considered "dangerous"); (b) shops without a pharmacist that sell only prepackaged modern drugs; and (c) traditional drugstores, attended by a registered traditional pharmacist, that sell only traditional medicine products. In 1981, these drugstores numbered 2,390, 5,420, and 6,740, respectively.

In addition, "common household drugs" are sold in ordinary groceries and other trade shops in the towns and villages. These, and sometimes more potent drugs, are also sold by itinerant drugsellers at public crossroads, especially in rural districts.

A major part of the private health care market, of course, is Thailand's supply of modern medical and dental practitioners. Only about 10 percent of the nation's physicians and dentists are engaged entirely in private practice, and the balance serve in the MOPH or other public agencies. The vast majority of the public physicians and dentists, however, also engage in private practice, after their official hours. Since earnings from private fees are much higher than government salaries, physicians have an incentive to minimize their time in the official post and maximize their time in a private office or clinic.

Finally, Thailand has private hospitals, especially in Bangkok and some provincial capitals. Altogether, these units, as of 1981, had about 11 percent of the total hospital beds. About one-third of these were in religiously sponsored nonprofit institutions, and two-thirds were in proprietary (for-profit) units, typically owned by doctors; in both types, patients must pay privately for care. In addition, many government hospitals, especially the larger ones, maintain a small number of beds (usually in single-bed rooms) for private patients.

Thailand has a few private providers of other types of health care, such as private-duty nurses, sellers of eyeglasses, hearing aids, or other prosthetic devices, and an occasional physical therapist. Considering all types of private health care, traditional and modern, it constitutes the major share of all personal health services rendered in Thailand. As we will see, this is true whether the services are quantified by their volume or by the expenditures made for them.

Production of Health Resources

As a transitional developing country, Thailand has far fewer health resources—both human and physical—than the industrialized countries reviewed in previous chapters. It also has much fewer than necessary to meet the recognized needs of the population.

Health Manpower. Physicians have been prepared by Thailand's medical schools at a gradually increasing rate. In 1984, about 8,700 fully trained modern physicians were registered in the MOPH, but not all were in Thailand and in active medical practice. Well-informed Thai health leaders estimate that about 2,000 of these had left the country or were not engaged in active practice. The balance of 6,700, therefore, meant a ratio of 13.1 active physicians per 100,000 population, which can be compared with ratios of some 150 to 300 per 100,000 in most highly developed countries.

Virtually all doctors in Thailand have been trained in one of the nation's eight medical schools—all government supported and university-based, except one that is under the Ministry of Defense. Students pay no tuition for their medical education, but they must buy their own books and pay fees for supplies; about 20 percent receive fellowships for living expenses. Until 1984, the medical curriculum had the typical 6-year sequence, followed by 1 year of hospital internship. In 1984, to increase the output of physicians, medical studies were reduced to 5 years, and the internship was no longer required. Altogether, about 700 medical graduates are turned out by the schools each year.

Probably the most serious problem in Thailand's medical manpower situation is the severe maldistribution of physicians. Urban concentrations of doctors is a worldwide phenomenon, but in Thailand it is extreme. Bangkok, with 9.2 percent of the national population, is estimated to have 75 percent of the country's doctors. The other 91 percent of the population are served by 25 percent of the doctors, and most of these are in the provincial capitals. In Bangkok, furthermore, the doctors devote an especially high proportion of their time to private practice, and thus are less accessible to the thousands of periurban slumdwellers. For some time, the geographic disparity of physician distribution seemed to be growing worse. In 1964 the density of physicians in Bangkok was 17 times greater than that in the rest of the country; by 1970 it had become 20 times greater, and by 1978 it was 28 times greater.

In reaction to this trend and in an attempt to improve physician distribution, in 1976 the government required new medical graduates, after a 1-year internship, to spend 2 years in public service—one at a district hospital and one at a health center (at district or commune level). This action has resulted in increased district hospital staffing from 300 doctors in 1975 to 1,000 in 1985. Primary health care in rural areas, however, is still overwhelmingly dependent on nonmedical auxiliary personnel.

Specialization in medicine has been increasing in Thailand, as elsewhere. Residences in numerous fields, which were formerly undertaken abroad, are now available in the several teaching hospitals in Bangkok. Official specialty recognition comes from the Medical Council of Thailand, a semi-independent professional body housed at the MOPH. (The Medical Council is also responsible for the general registration of all physicians and for overseeing medical ethics.) About half the physicians in Bangkok have specialty status, but only a handful elsewhere.

The vast majority of Thai physicians have a salaried appointment, in addition to their private practice. In 1977, when about 5,000 doctors were estimated to be in the country and actively occupied, they were distributed approximately as follows:

Ministry of Public Health	1,800
Universities and Ministry of Defense	2,200

Municipalities and State Enterprises	600
Exclusively Private Practice	400
All physicians	5,000

Dentists in Thailand are trained by five schools of dentistry, supported by the State University Office. The 6-year curriculum, after secondary school, is the same length as that for medicine (until the shortening in 1984), but it does not involve internships. With about 200 dental graduates each year, in the mid-1980s there were around 2,000 dentists in the country, the great majority in Bangkok. In addition, Thailand recognizes *second-class dentists* (who may have dropped out or failed dental school), who are authorized to do extractions and prepare full dentures. (In some countries, these are known as *denturists.*) In 1975 there were 500 of these people, and just under 1,000 qualified dentists. The second-class dentists charge relatively low fees, and are more evenly distributed in the provincial towns, where they serve low-income patients.

Dental hygienists, who perform dental prophylaxes and health education, are trained by two schools under the MOPH. Their curriculum requires 2 years after secondary school. There are fewer than 1,000 of these personnel, and most of them work in the schools. Back in 1948, the MOPH organized a school for *dental auxiliaries,* who would be prepared for a much broader scope of dental work among school children, along the lines of the New Zealand dental nurse. Strong opposition from the private dentists, however, led to the termination of this program.

Pharmacists are trained at six university-based schools of pharmacy under the State University Office. The curriculum requires 5 years after secondary school, and about 300 graduates are turned out each year. Altogether, Thailand had around 2,500 to 3,000 pharmacists in 1985, the great majority of whom owned or worked full-time in private pharmacies. Most of the pharmacies in hospitals and health centers are staffed by assistant pharmacists, who are trained in three schools run by the MOPH. These programs last 2 years after secondary school. In a move toward equity, in 1984 newly qualified pharmacists were required to work 3 years in government service.

Nursing personnel, in Thailand as in most countries, are the most numerous type of health workers who receive formal training. There are two basic professional nursing curricula—one lasting 2 years after secondary school and the other 4 years. (A third auxiliary nurse program is discussed later.) Both programs entitle the graduate to R.N. (registered nurse) designation, but the 4-year program also earns a B.Sc. degree. The 2-year R.N. is known as a *technical nurse* and the 4-year trainee is considered a *graduate nurse.*

There are 17 hospital-based schools, under the MOPH, that train technical nurses. To train the graduate baccalaureate nurse there are four schools, based in university teaching hospitals. The number of active professional nurses in Thailand is not certain. According to the World Bank, Thailand had about 47 "nursing persons" per 100,000 in 1981, which comes to about 23,800 nurses of all grades. The great majority of these are doubtless technical or even auxiliary nurses, although some may do further studies to upgrade to graduate nurse. Also, graduate nurses can do advanced work to become a *nurse practitioner* (entitled to provide general primary care) or nurse anesthetist, or to earn a master's degree in nursing or public health.

Besides the two types of registered nurse, Thailand also trains auxiliary or practical nurses. The curriculum lasts 12 to 18 months, after 10 years of basic schooling. Sixteen hospital-based schools under the MOPH offer this training. There were 16,000 such nurses in 1975, nearly all of whom served in small district hospitals or commune health centers. Since these women come predominantly from poor families, their earnings are important, and relatively few become inactive.

Midwives constitute still another personnel category trained by the MOPH. Some have had training equivalent to that of a registered nurse and become nurse-midwives, but most go through a shorter course of training. They are trained in a hospital for 18 to 24 months, following 10 years of basic schooling. Six schools for this training are operated by the MOPH. Nearly all these young women work in the rural areas, out of a commune health center or frequently from their own small houses in the villages. Since the 1970s, most of these rural midwives have been given supplementary training to provide family planning services.

Traditional healers, noted ealier as part of the private market, were estimated in 1977 to number about 35,000 in Thailand. This is much more than the number of trained physicians, but nearly all of these practitioners have other occupations and engage in healing only occasionally. Their techniques combine occult or magical procedures with the use of medicinal herbs, the latter based principally on the Indian doctrines of Ayurvedic medicine.

The estimate of 35,000 applies only to healers "registered" with the MOPH, a status theoretically required for anyone selling drugs. Still others are practicing without being registered. In recent years, the MOPH has given an annual examination, which must be passed. The healers who took this examination in 1974 were investigated, and the occupations they reported were merchants (28 percent), farmers (21 percent), government officers (21 percent), and nonspecified (30 percent). Of the total, 94 percent were men. The very limited time devoted to healing practices is reflected by the finding that only 6 percent said they could "make a living" from this work.

Finally, since the late 1970s, the Thailand MOPH has undertaken a massive program to prepare and deploy very briefly trained volunteer health workers at the village level. Since the 1960s, young volunteers had been trained briefly for specialized programs, such as family planning or malaria control, and their functions had gradually been broadened. By 1982 an estimated 33,300 *village health volunteers* (VHVs) had received 20 days of instruction on the simplest elements of primary health care; special emphasis is still put on education on family planning. In addition, about 325,000 *village-health communicators* (VHCs), trained for only 5 days, were expected to promote health consciousness among 8 to 15 households each. The training is usually given at commune health centers.

Continuing and graduate education is also fairly well developed in Thailand. Public health personnel are provided a number of short courses. District health officers and assistant DHOs are offered courses of 10 and 5 weeks, respectively (these men, it will be recalled, are mainly sanitarians). Health administrators, who work in large hospitals or Provincial Health Offices, take a 1-month course. Provincial chief medical officers often attend 2-week workshops on selected subjects. Short workshops are also held for specialized personnel, such as hospital pharmacists or provincial-level dentists. The National Economic and Social Development Board (in the Office of the Prime Minister) offers seminars on the health planning process.

A notable type of graduate training is provided by the Faculty of Public Health at Mahidol University. This special school prepares doctors, nurses, and others for the master's degree in public health, and also offers master's degree programs in nutrition, health education, family health, and other fields. Students from many Asian countries, beyond Thailand, attend this school.

Health Facilities. In spite of Thailand's general entrepreneurial character, the hospital resources in its health system are predominantly governmental. The great majority of beds are in general hospitals—at district, provincial, or central levels. Counting all types of beds, there were about 72,000 in 1980. This amounted to 1.52 beds per 1,000 population, of which 89.1 percent were under government control. Of the remaining 11 percent, about one-third were religious and nonprofit, mainly in rural regions. The two-thirds of these beds that were proprietary were located mainly in Bangkok and owned by doctors.

Of the overall hospital beds, about 24 percent are for specialized types of care, such as 7,400 beds for mental disease, 2,300 for leprosy, and 580 for tuberculosis. (Nearly all these beds are in government institutions.) Since the latter conditions require very long patient stays, the number of persons served per year is relatively small. In the general hospitals the opposite is true. In provincial general hospitals, the average length of stay is only about 6 days, so that the bed turnover rate, or number of patients served per bed per year, is high.

The early 1980s saw quite a large expansion of private for-profit hospitals in Thailand; these were typically small units (under 30 beds), owned by four or five doctors, mainly in Bangkok. Even though few people could afford to use these hospitals, government actually encouraged their construction. They were exempted from taxes on the importation of equipment and supplies for the first 5 years.

It is noteworthy that, even in the public hospitals of Thailand, care is not free. For drugs, laboratory tests, x-ray examinations, and various supplies, the vast majority of patients must pay. The very poor are theoretically exempted, but in practice relatively few qualify for completely free care.

Facilities for ambulatory care have been gradually expanded by the MOPH. Before 1975, there were two grades of health centers—Class I medical and health centers, containing 10 to 30 beds, and Class II health centers, without beds. When 288 Class I centers were converted into district hospitals, all health centers became exclusively for ambulatory care. In 1981, there were 4,167 health centers to serve the 5,608 communes, or 74 percent coverage. (Planning called for coverage of all communes by 1986.)

Another form of ambulatory care under the MOPH is the small midwife station, noted earlier. In 1981 there were 1,674 of these in the villages, in most cases providing some infant health care, family planning advice, and other preventive service outside of childbirth deliveries. Only a small percentage of the 53,000 villages were covered, however. A small number of selected districts also have special *village health posts,* usually financed by foreign aid for "demonstration projects." These are discussed later.

Finally, the purely private facilities for care of ambulatory patients must be recognized; they play a very large part in Thailand's health system. In 1981, there were 14,550 drugstores of the three types described earlier. Of these, 46 percent sold mainly traditional drugs and 54 percent sold modern drugs. Nearly all are heavily patronized.

Private clinics in Thailand provide mainly the services of physicians or dentists, but some offer the services of other health personnel. In 1983, the Division of Medical Licensure of the MOPH reported the following licensed private clinics:

Physicians	4,255
Dentists	944
Second-class dentists	525
Nurses	86
Nurse-midwives	514
Midwives	172
Traditional healers	698
Traditional midwives	6

It is generally assumed that the provinces have many more clinics of allied health personnel, which are not licensed. The 4,255 physician clinics include those of doctors in full-time private practice, plus many that are shared by several government physicians for different hours of the week.

Commodities. The major commodities in the Thailand health system, of course, are drugs. These include both modern and traditional compounds. Both types are either manufactured in the country (usually from imported raw materials) or imported in final packaged form.

Thus, in 1981 there were 187 drug factories, preparing modern products (pills, capsules, ampoules, etc.) almost entirely from imported materials. A somewhat larger number of firms simply imported various finished modern drug products. For traditional drugs, the number of firms is even greater. Although their average size is typically quite small, in 1981 there were 834 firms manufacturing traditional drugs from both domestic and imported materials. A much smaller number (about 90) were devoted entirely to importing finished traditional drug products.

In 1983, roughly 26,000 official brands of drugs were sold in Thailand (nearly all modern drugs, since most traditional preparations are never registered). To control government expenditures on this large variety of drugs, a National Drug List Committee was appointed in the MOPH in 1980. The next year, it issued a National Drug List of only a few hundred compounds, which became the basis for drug orders by the Government Pharmaceutical Organization (GPO). The GPO, as noted earlier, is responsible for distributing most of the drugs to all government health facilities.

Practically all equipment for the diagnosis or treatment of disease in Thailand must be imported. The use of highly sophisticated technology is illustrated by computerized tomography (CT) scanners, which became available in the 1980s. More than 20 of these expensive machines were in operation in Thailand in 1985, but most were in small private hospitals. To amortize their high cost, hospitals charge high fees for a CT scanning. Competition among private hospitals, in turn, has led many of them to return 10 percent of the CT scanning fee to physicians by sending them suitable and affluent patients. This has led inevitably to excessive use of and expenditures for CT scanning, beyond the objective needs of the case.

Knowledge and Its Dissemination. The final resource in the Thai health system, scientific knowledge, is derived from a moderate amount of domestic medical research and a great deal of disseminated literature from abroad.

Scientists are researching many health problems in several medical schools and teaching hospitals in Bangkok and Chang Mai. The budgets of all the schools include small amounts for research, but the chief source of support is the National Research Council, which has a branch on medical science. Priority subjects have included infectious diseases, malnutrition, environmental pollution, family planning, medical demography, mental health, and health services research.

Some research grants to Thai investigators may come from foreign sources. In hematology, for example, internationally recognized work has been done on thalassemia (formerly called Mediterranean anemia), with the financial support of the U.S. National Institutes of Health. A Thai university faculty serves as the Central Coordinating Board of the Tropical Medicine Program of SEAMEO (South-East Asian Ministries of Education Organization). Universities also sponsor special research institutes, such as one on population studies and another on nutrition.

The Ministry of Public Health is likewise engaged in health research. Its Department of

Medical Sciences has research laboratories in virology and entomology. This department is also testing the pharmaceutical effects of various traditional herbs. The MOPH is doing field studies in family planning, environmental sanitation, nutrition, and dental health. The Department of Communicable Disease Control is studying malaria and tuberculosis. The Thai Army has an Institute of Pathology, which conducts both laboratory and clinical studies.

Despite this exceptionally broad range of medical research in the country, most of Thailand's health science knowledge and technology is drawn from the rest of the world. Since the early nineteenth century, Thailand has eagerly sought lessons from Western medicine, particularly from Great Britain and the United States. Perhaps some of the "high-technology lessons" have not been the most appropriate for Thailand's health needs. The books in Thai medical libraries are mainly from the United States, and since 1945 most foreign postgraduate studies by Thai doctors are undertaken in North America.

New health knowledge is disseminated in Thailand through journals sent to provincial hospitals and through frequent conferences. As in many developing countries, however, dynamic exchanges of new ideas are largely concentrated in Bangkok. One sees little evidence of public health or medical literature in the district hospitals or anywhere peripheral to the provincial capitals. The skewed distribution of physicians, noted earlier, seems to mirror the distribution of new scientific knowledge in Thailand.

Management of the Health System

Even before the Ministry of Public Health was established in 1942, planning and certain aspects of management of the health system were carried out in the Ministry of Interior. The old commune doctors contributed a little to the development of sanitation and to vaccination against smallpox. The current era of health system management, however, began after World War II.

Planning. Although many steps were taken to establish a provincial infrastructure of public health service in the 1950s, the first formal 5-year plan for national development was launched in 1962. The National Economic and Social Development Board (NESDB) formulated the first general 5-year plan for 1962–1966, to emphasize the development of an economic infrastructure, such as roads, power, and irrigation, but also including health facilities. The first and second plans apparently resulted in a widened gap in income distribution among various population groups and regions, so that the third plan for 1972–1976 gave greater attention to income, health, and social services.

Parallel with the general NESDB planning has been the national health planning in the MOPH, also beginning in 1962. The plans for 1962–1966 and 1967–1971 stressed the physical infrastructure (hospitals and health centers) of the MOPH and also communicable disease control. The third health plan (1972–1976) also stressed maternal and child health and family planning services. The fourth health plan (1977–1981) adopted the WHO goal of primary health care as the main strategy to achieve "health for all." With this plan, greater attention was given to the decentralization of certain health planning procedures to the provinces.

The Division of Health Planning achieved formal status in the MOPH in 1972, and is now within the strong Office of the Under-Secretary of State for Public Health. The fifth health plan, for 1982–1986, became the responsibility of a National Health Planning Committee, including top executives of the MOPH, the NESDB, the Bureau of the Budget, the Civil Service Commission, and several universities. Each year the MOPH Health Planning Division solicits proposals from the provinces and submits an annual plan to the NESDB and the Bureau of the Budget.

In the fifth 5-year health plan (1982–1986), the primary health care strategy was reinforced with major efforts to stimulate community participation and intersectoral collaboration at the most peripheral level. In its health planning methodology, Thailand has been greatly influenced by the World Health Organization. In 1976, WHO began to stress a simplified approach to planning called *Country Health Programming.* Instead of relying on complex computations, when data were often lacking or extremely unreliable, the method called for the identification of problems by well-informed observers, brainstorming sessions, and arrival at group consensus on specific health targets. These targets largely concerned (a) the achievement of population coverage with designated services and (b) the reduction of specific health problems. Several different working groups would be appointed to tackle various questions.

In 1976, for example, 19 discrete working groups were established, one of which coped with the problem of health manpower shortages in the rural areas. It was this group that came up with the plans to train hundreds of village health volunteers (VHVs) and village health communicators (VHCs), to recommend the 2 years of mandatory rural service for new medical graduates and train nurse-practitioners at one university.

Nevertheless, some basic limitations in the Thai health planning process should be recognized. Most important, the whole planning effort has been confined to activities in government. The private sector of health care—which is, in fact, much larger in aggregate than the entire public sector—is ignored. Moreover, even within government, planning concerns essentially the programs of the MOPH. Yet the output of physicians and other professional personnel is under a separate body, the State University Office. There may be some interchange between these two agencies, but we know that the education of physicians is oriented largely to specialized technology rather than to primary health care. In response to these criticisms, planners point out that, if public services are strengthened, people will not make as great use of private services.

In Thailand, as in many countries, there are serious discrepancies between theory and practice. Thai national health policy calls for "better medical care for the rural population by improving the efficiency and effectiveness of medical care services rendered by hospitals and health centers." Yet, in practice, tax exemptions are allowed to encourage the construction of high-cost private hospitals in the main cities. Such policies are sometimes rationalized as "reducing the burden on public hospitals," while in reality the opposite occurs.

Scarce personnel are withdrawn from the public hospitals, serving the great majority, and are attracted to private hospitals, serving a small affluent minority. Publicly employed physicians and other health workers are, of course, paid to serve the general population. Yet, their salaries are so low that almost all of them cut corners on their official duties to maximize the time they can devote to private practice.

Policy calls for "effective control and eradication of communicable disease through the development of effective surveillance networks." Accordingly, prostitution is legally prohibited. Yet in Bangkok, thousands of young women serve every day and night in "massage parlours" as prostitutes in everything but name—with open advertising and complete tolerance by official authorities. Meanwhile, the Public Welfare Department of the Ministry of Interior operates rehabilitation centers for some of these "socially handicapped women," while thousands more are exploited.

Administration. With the military domination and the monarchistic history of the Thai government, it is not surprising that authority generally has been highly centralized. Provincial governors and their chief medical officers are not elected but appointed by the central government. The same applies to district officers and district health officers. Any of these officials can be removed if they do something that displeases the central government.

Nevertheless, since the late 1970s, efforts have been made to decentralize greater authority and responsibility to the provinces. This has been noted for the health planning process, and it also applies to the appointment of field health personnel, the procurement of certain supplies, and the management of budgets. As long as a total budgetary maximum is not exceeded, provincial and district health officials may transfer funds between budget lines. This permits the occasional development of wholly innovative programs.

The responsiblity of health officials, technically to the MOPH and administratively to the provincial governor or district officer, creates an obvious administrative challenge in the daily work of these health executives. In effect, they must keep their superior from the Ministry of Interior informed on almost everything they do, to be certain that they are not breaking some administrative rule.

Coordination, as an aspect of administration, may be illustrated by certain initiatives in the 1980s. To promote health manpower development—specifically, the training of physicians—more suitable to population needs, the national cabinet set up a Center for Medical and Health Coordination. Its operation was entrusted to a committee composed of representatives of both the MOPH and the universities. Similar coordinated action is seen in the Training Center for Primary Health Care Development, established in 1983. This center is operated jointly by the MOPH and one major university.

Evaluation, as an aspect of administration, is built into the functions of many adminstrative units in the Thai health system. The MOPH is most important, since several of its divisons are expected to monitor regularly the performance of their programs. Thus, the Health Planning Division has a Monitoring and Evaluation Section. The Epidemiology Division issues Mortality and Morbidity Weekly Reports to keep everyone informed on health status changes, especially for communicable diseases. The Health Statistics Division reports data on use of health facilities, and sometimes, in conjunction with university personnel, conducts household surveys on special health questions.

Outside the MOPH, the National Economic and Social Development Board monitors progress on basic aspects of health resource development. The National Statistical Office conducts a regular population census and several types of household surveys that are relevant to evaluation of the health system. Some of the crucial findings of this office, on the personal expenditures of families for health service, are discussed later.

Universities, through various social science departments and institutes, have conducted many studies that contribute to health system evaluation. Research grants from international sources have supported several household surveys on knowledge, attitudes, and practices with respect to family planning. The findings have provided guidance in the organization of family-planning programs, and have permitted evaluation of the effectiveness of various strategies.

Regulation and Legislation. Regulation within the MOPH and other organized health programs of government is virtually synonymous with managment, but regulatory controls on the private sector have been the subject of much legislation in Thailand. Legislation in five categories of health system regulation, enacted between 1922 and 1979, is shown here. Almost all of the 26 statutes provide a legal basis for various regulations and actions by government agencies.

Legislation on health professions has included the following:

1. Act for control of the practice of the healing art 1936
2. Medical premises act 1961
3. Medical profession act 1968

Communicable disease control legislation has included the following:

4. Infectious disease act 1934
5. Malaria control act 1942
6. Leprosy control act 1943
7. Act for protection against rabies 1955

Food and drug control has been the subject of many laws:

8. Narcotic act 1922/1979
9. Act for control of disease agents and toxins from animals 1932
10. Indian hemp act 1934
11. Kratom act 1943
12. Food quality control act 1964/1979
13. Drug act 1967
14. Poisonous substance act 1967
15. Cosmetic act 1974
16. Psychotropic substance act 1975

Environmental health legislation has included the following:

17. Act for control of cemeteries and crematories 1938

18. The public health act 1941
19. Act for control of the use of human excreta as fertilizer 1943
20. Act for the cleanliness and orderliness of the country 1960

Legislation indirectly concerning health has involved the following:

21. Civil service act 1975
22. Act for the suppression of prostitution 1960
23. Building construction act 1936
24. Mineral act 1967
25. Factory act 1969
26. Labor act 1972

It may be noted that most of these laws establish constraints on certain forms of human behavior—on what persons are permitted to do—in the interests of protecting health. The preceding list is doubtless incomplete. It does not include, for example, the Industrial Injury Compensation Act, noted earlier, under which workers injured on the job are entitled to coverage of medical care costs. The 1936 Act to Control the Practice of the Healing Art has very broad implications for modern as well as traditional healers.

Unfortunately, wide gaps may exist between the provisions of laws and their enforcement. The disparity between the 1960 law on "suppression of prostitution" and the thriving massage parlors has been noted. Not only is the law essentially ignored, but government physicians, in their private practices, examine the young women from massage parlors and issue them "health certificates" to reassure their clients. The same sort of sham applies to abortion, which is illegal unless the pregancy results from rape or the woman's health is endangered. Most physicians refuse to do abortions, largely on grounds of Buddhist prohibition, but many illegal abortions are performed by various nonmedical personnel—nurses, midwives, injectionists, and others. Thus, abortion is commonly practiced and its complications are a frequent cause for hospital admission and maternal death.

The Factory Act of 1969 and the Labor Act of 1972 are likewise only meagerly enforced.

Regulations require, for example, minimum levels of light and maximum levels of noise, as well as various types of protective equipment. In practice, the Department of Labor has so small a staff that proper enforcement is virtually impossible. Regulations requiring industrial establishments with 500 workers or more to have a doctor in attendance are also rarely enforced.

Perhaps the most widely flaunted regulations relate to the sale of drugs. Legislation requiring medical prescriptions for all but the simplest drugs (such as aspirin or vitamins) are on the books, but the numbers of drugstores and drug sellers are so great that little is done to enforce them. Except for addictive narcotics (and the extent of their distribution is not clear), virtually any drug can be purchased "over the counter" for the asking. Also all sorts of untested dyes are added to foods to brighten their color, without any effective restriction.

Under the Medical Profession Act of 1968, the Medical Council of Thailand was established. Although this body is housed within the Ministry of Public Health, it has a semi-independent status. The council's 25 members consist of 10 who are elected by the doctors and 15 appointed by the Minister of Public Health. In addition to its registration of physicians, the council must approve the curriculum of every medical school in Thailand, although this is little more than a formality. Final examinations are given only by the schools.

The Medical Council is also responsible for monitoring the ethical performance of all doctors. A Code of Ethics has been issued to specify standards. Among these are general integrity in the care of patients, confidentiality regarding a patient's condition, prohibition of advertising and so on. Only about 10 to 20 offenses involving the Code of Ethics are reported to be brought to the council's attention in a year, most commonly for advertising or fraudulent reports by a doctor (e.g., under the Workmen's Compensation Program). Likewise, charges of medical malpractice are rare, although there is no specific law on this subject. If a doctor is charged with unethical behavior, the case is investigated by a committee of the Medical Council. A guilty finding may result in (a) simply a warning, (b) temporary withdrawal of medical registration, or (c) permanent withdrawal of registration; in event of the third decision, however, the doctor may reapply for registration after 2 years.

Other health professions have no bodies equivalent to the Medical Council, but registration is required directly in the Ministry of Public Health. Recall that such registration applies not only to dentists, nurses, pharmacists, and other modern health personnel, but also to various categories of traditional healers. Both modern and traditional practitioners ordinarily register only once. Although a change of status, such as retirement, change of location, or even death, is supposed to require notification of the ministry, this is often not done. As a result, the listing of Registered Nurses, for example, does not reflect how many are active.

Outside of legal regulation, there are, of course, policies and procedures prescribed in provincial and district health offices and in all hospitals and health centers. As an overwhelmingly Buddhist country, much of the behavior of Thai people is influenced by the education and leadership of Buddhist monks. With the incentive of accumulating "credit" for meritorious acts, individuals can make special efforts to maintain sanitary homes and keep their bodies clean.

Considering the large part played by the private medical practitioner in the health system in Thailand, one must conclude that overall regulation is relatively weak. Within the public services for health care or protection, the dynamics of organized programs are the principal regulatory influences. In the substantial sphere of drug consumption, and the services of private physicians, dentists, nurses, traditional healers, and others, regulation in Thailand contributes little to health system management.

Economic Support

With the many programs functioning in the organizational structure of Thailand's health system, along with a substantial private market, it is clear that the sources of economic support for the system must be numerous. The figures on Thai health expenditures for the most recent year that data are available can be reviewed under the following headings: (a) Ministry of Public Health, (b) other government agencies, (c) enterprises and voluntary bodies, (d) private households, and (e) foreign aid. Then we can determine the relative importance of each source and the share of total national wealth that is spent on the health system.

Ministry of Public Health. As the principal governmental body concerned with the health system, one would expect MOPH expenditures to be substantial. The total MOPH budget in 1985 (at all jurisdictional levels) amounted to a sum equivalent to U.S. $368,000,000. This was 4.4 percent of the overall national government budget—a proportion that fluctuated only slightly between 4.0 to 5.0 percent during the previous decade.

A breakdown of these MOPH expenditures is available for 1974, when it was as follows:

Purpose	Percentage
Personal health services	67.0
Environmental health services	6.2
Communicable disease control	14.6
Health education	0.2
Health personnel training	3.6
Laboratories and research	1.1
Health planning and administration	7.3
All purposes	100.0

The lion's share of expenditures for personal health services applies, of course, to the operation (and construction) of the large MOPH network of hospitals and health centers. An estimate for 1985 suggested that about three-fourths of the 67 percent, or 50 percent of the total outlay, went for the support of curative services in hospitals. On this assumption, one can infer that 17 percent of the total went for the services of health centers that are mainly preventively oriented. Along with the other items listed here, this means that MOPH activities are divided among (a) preventive services (38 percent), (b) curative services (50 percent), and (c) other functions (12 percent).

The allocation of 38 percent of MOPH funds for preventive purposes constitutes a trend upward, in accordance with the government's policy emphasis on primary health care. This is also reflected in a shift of health expenditures in the rural areas from 43 percent of the total MOPH budget in 1981 to 56 percent in 1985.

Other Government Agencies. It is dificult to be certain about the health-related expenditures of various public agencies, outside the MOPH; the subdivisions of the large Ministry of Interior budget, relevant to health services, are not explicitly reported, and there is obvious confidentiality about the health expenditures of the Ministry of Defense. To adjust to these problems, the estimate by an official of the Health Planning Division of the MOPH may be acceptable. In the mid-1980s, all non-MOPH health expenditures amounted to between 7 and 8 percent of total national health expenditures in Thailand. Rounding off this figure, these expenditures came to about U.S. $131,000,000.

The largest proportion of this figure in the 1976–1983 period went to support the nation's medical schools and their associated teaching hospitals—about 80 percent of it. Most of the balance went to support Ministry of Interior activities, especially for the substantial government health activities in the Bangkok Metropolitan Area. All other ministries, while performing a great variety of functions, accounted for only 2 to 3 percent of non-MOPH public expenditures.

Enterprises and Voluntary Bodies. Although a large number of nongovernment organizations make health expenditures, a 1978 estimate found the aggregate to constitute only 0.7 percent of total health expenditures. Because of the expansion of private industry and the associated health services for workers since then, an estimate for 1983 may be an even 1.0 percent, or U.S. $17,400,000. This relatively low figure corresponds to the proportions found in even the economically advanced countries.

Private Households. Expenditures for health from purely private sources are difficult to determine in any country, but Thailand is fortunately among the few developing countries where regular household surveys are conducted. These were started by one of the universities, but are now a regular function of the National Economic and Social Development Board (NESDB). The survey is based on a carefully chosen nationwide sample, and questions solicit information on expenditures for doctors, drugs, traditional healers, and other elements of medical care.

As a proportion of family income, health expenditures have generally turned out to be surprisingly high. They are higher in the urban areas, where health care resources are greater, than in the rural areas. In terms of family incomes, the absolute amounts spent in the poorest families are low, but as a proportion of family income they are greater than health expenditures by higher income families.

The crucial finding of these NESDB household surveys emerges when they are compared with the health expenditures by the MOPH and other public and private agencies. Before doing this, we should break down the purposes for which private health expenditures are made. Such a breakdown is available for 1981, for households in Thailand (about 75 percent of the total) that reported sickness and some personal health expenditures. The distribution was as follows:

Health Care Purpose	Percent
Government facility private charges	40.8
Private health practitioners (modern and traditional)	55.3
Private drugstores	5.1

It is noteworthy that even the government hospitals and health centers in Thailand absorb more than 40 percent of private expenditures, since they make significant charges for their services.

The 5.1 percent figure for private drugstores is undoubtedly misleading. In fact, high proportions of the expenditures for the other two purposes are actually for drugs, dispersed both by private physicians and drug sellers and by public hospitals and health centers.

A more detailed analysis of private household health expenditures is available for an

Table 9.2. Health Expenditures by Private Households, by Type of Service, in Thailand (Percent Distribution), 1970

Type of Service	Bangkok	Provinces	Nation
Private physicians	54.8	37.6	39.3
Drugstores and drug sellers	16.6	23.9	23.2
Traditional healers	0.3	12.0	10.8
Government hospitals	27.9	22.4	23.0
Government health centers	0.4	3.8	3.5
Other	0	0.3	0.2
All services	100.0	100.0	100.0

Source: Thai Ministry of Public Health, *Report on the Result of Survey of Health Manpower and Expenses Incurred in Medical Treatment of the People.* Bangkok, 1970.

earlier period from a survey made in 1970. At that time, private expenditures, reported by all households (not limited to those with sickness), were distributed in the way shown in Table 9.2. If these distributions are still valid (and one can speculate about various changes), several conclusions seem evident. Private expenditures on personal physician's care (including also physician-owned private hospitals) are the greatest cause for spending both in the provinces and in Bangkok, but in Bangkok the proportion is much higher. The purchase of drugs accounts for nearly one-fourth of the total health expenditures; it is probably higher than 23.2 percent, since a large share of the charges made by doctors and hospitals is actually for drugs. Expenditures for traditional healers are extremely low in Bangkok, but in the provinces they were also relatively low even in 1970; their share of the total is doubtless lower today. Payments of private fees to government health facilities, accounting for 26.5 percent of household expenditures, were surprisingly high even in 1970, although they were still higher in 1981. Taken as a whole, one may conclude that urban people (of higher average incomes) make greater use of private medical practitioners, while the lower-income rural people depend much more on drugs (usually self-prescribed) and traditional healers.

Foreign Aid. One more source of health funding must be recognized, although it overlaps with data already discussed. Several foreign agencies support the Thai health system, usually through financing of specific projects. These may involve specific health services (such as immunizations or family planning), training personnel, supplies and equipment, construction, consultation on planning or administration, and so on. The sources may be international agencies (often called multilateral) or individual countries (bilateral). Although predominantly governmental, the sources are sometimes private (e.g., religious bodies or foundations). In the main, this financial support is included within the budget of the Ministry of Public Health or other public agencies, and so has been included in the figures given here.

Calculating the aggregate financial support from foreign sources of all types, the amount is not very great. Such a calculation done in 1978 gave an estimate of 0.9 percent of total health expenditures. A more recent estimate suggests an aggregate total of from 1 to 3 percent. The effect of international collaboration, in stimulating new ideas may, of course, be much greater than is suggested by monetary measurements.

Total Expenditures. In 1983, the NESDB calculated that total health system expenditures of Thailand, expressed in U.S. dollars, was $1,740,000,000. This amounted to 4.6 percent of the GNP that year. In U.S. dollars, this was $35 per person per year. Though low by the standards of industrialized countries, this constituted an increase from $26 per capita and 3.5 percent of GNP in 1979. As we noted earlier, this rise in health spending has come largely from the private sector, as one would expect in a country with predominantly entrepreneurial health policies.

Table 9.3 summarizes the health expenditures from all sources in Thailand, as of 1983. The expenditures by private households (families and individuals) were derived from the household surveys, analyzed by the NESDB. An equivalent survey in 1979 found that private spending accounted for 66.5 percent of the total. Therefore, even though government spending has increased, the 70.3 percent from

Table 9.3. National Health Expenditures, by Source: Amounts and Percentages of Distribution in Thailand, 1983

Source	Amount (U.S. $)	Percentage
Ministry of Public Health	341,900,000	19.6
Other government agencies	131,000,000	7.5
Voluntary agencies and enterprises	17,400,000	1.0
Foreign aid[a]	26,100,000	1.5
Private households	1,223,600,000	70.3
All sources	1,740,000,000	100.0

[a]This is an estimate, which assumes that all foreign aid is expended through the Ministry of Public Health.
Source: National Economic and Social Development Board, Bangkok, Thailand (unpublished data), 1985.

private sources in 1983 suggests that private expenditures have risen at a greater rate.

Delivery of Health Services

The patterns by which health services are delivered to the people of Thailand obviously vary between the cities and the rural areas and between the high- and the low-income groups. There is also much exploration of new methods of delivery, in the interest of improving the efficiency and effectiveness of the whole health system.

Ambulatory Care. From a review of the economic data, it is evident that the services of a scientifically trained private physician are the most common form of ambulatory medical care in the cities. Even though medical fees are relatively high (so that dollars cannot be simply equated with services), the relationship of 54.8 percent of expenditures for private physicians to 0.4 percent for the use of government health centers is overwhelming, and must reflect a far greater use of private doctors for ambulatory care in Bangkok. The contrast between private and public ambulatory care in the provinces is not as great, but still substantial.

The heavy concentration of physicians in Bangkok results in a certain stratification of medical practices, such that certain doctor's offices (or private medical clinics) are located in low-income neighborhoods, where poor patients are served. Other doctors, usually specialists associated with the leading hospitals, are located in elegant or commercial sections of the city, convenient for service to the middle- and upper-income groups. Grouping of doctors in private clinics is rare in Thailand; almost all private medical service is provided by individual practitioners.

In the provinces, medical services from private physicians is also predominant in the provincial capitals and larger towns, though not to the same extent as in Bangkok. Greater use is made of government health centers in very isolated areas, although even here village drugstores or itinerant drug sellers are more frequent sourses of care. Health centers or midwife posts are more often used for preventive services to pregnant women and newborn infants, including immunizations.

In Thailand, as in many other developing countries, the rate of use of health centers is much below their capacity. As rural people become better educated, they become less satisfied with the services of auxiliary health personnel, or sometimes even of general medical practitioners. Therefore, they bypass both the village health post and the local health center to seek care at the outpatient department (OPD) of a district or preferably a provincial hospital, where specialists may be available. If a private physician is within reach, if the illness seems serious, and if they can afford it, they consult him. The hospital OPD is usually overcrowded, with long waits; to avoid uncomfortable delays, patients must resort to more costly private doctors both in the rural regions and the main cities.

A survey by the MOPH and a university in 1981 asked a sample of the population what actions they took in response to their last illness. Of those who had experienced some illness or disorder in the previous month, 6 percent had not sought any help outside the household. Of the 94 percent who sought care, the most frequent action was to purchase something in a drugstore. (Two-thirds of the drugs purchased in Thailand are nonprescription.) The proportions, however, differed for urban and rural populations, as is shown in

Table 9.4. Utilization of Ambulatory Care in Urban and Rural Areas, by Type of Facility: Percentage Distribution in Thailand, 1981

Type of Facility	Urban	Rural	Total
Government unit	24.8	35.4	33.0
Private practitioner[a]	36.4	21.0	24.5
Private drugstore[b]	38.8	43.6	42.5
All facilities	100.0	100.0	100.0

[a]Includes traditional healers.
[b]Includes private drug sellers.
Source: Ministry of Public Health and Mahidol University, *Community Household Survey.* Bangkok, 1981.

Table 9.4. In rural areas drugstores are more important, and in the cities private medical practitioners are much more important. It is significant that only 33 percent of the population used any public resources (health center, hospital OPD, or any other), while 67 percent resorted to the private sector.

For more refined data on ambulatory care utilization in Thailand, we must refer to the findings of a 1970 household survey. At this time a nationwide sample of 24,000 persons were asked about illnesses occurring during the previous month, and any actions taken. Table 9.5 shows the distribution of the responses. It is noteworthy that, compared with the 1981 situation, the preponderance of self-medication was even greater, and the use of private physicians was slightly less nationally. The

Table 9.5. Utilization of Ambulatory Care, by Type of Service: Percentage Distribution in Thailand, 1970

Type of Service	Bangkok	Provinces	Total
Drug purchase for self-care	37.1	56.2	51.4
Private physician	43.3	15.5	22.7
Government hospital OPD	13.0	9.6	10.5
Government health center	1.3	5.4	4.4
Traditional healer or midwife	1.3	4.8	3.9
Injectionist	0.3	5.1	3.8
Specialized public clinic	——	0.8	0.6
No treatment or no response	3.7	2.6	2.7
All services	100.0	100.0	100.0

Source: Ministry of Public Health. *Report on the Result of Survey of the Utilization of Health Manpower and Expenses Incurred in Medical Treatment of the People.* Bangkok, 1970.

much greater use of government facilities in 1981—counting both health centers and hospital OPDs—than in 1970 is also noteworthy, probably reflecting the substantial development and staffing of these facilities throughout the 1970s. Traditional healers and injectionists were used only to a small extent in 1970, even in the provinces outside Bangkok.

Another study in 1985 showed the trend toward greater use of government health resources, as they were developed in Thailand. Although the categories differ in the various studies, a household survey in 1985 reported that the services for illness (defined as absence from work for at least one day) in the past month were distributed as follows:

Service	Percentage
Self-treatment (or no care)	28.6
Government hospitals (as outpatients)	32.5
Government health centers	14.7
Private practitioners	21.8
Traditional healers	2.4

The use of traditional healers, it should also be noted, continued to decline.

In light of the extensive anthropological research done on traditional medicine, these findings might suggest underreporting by families. Another study of a smaller sample (120 families), however, included weekly interviews for 1 year in 1971; nonreporting under such circumstances would be very unlikely. The percentage of family contacts with traditional healers in this study was almost identical: 3.7 percent of the total. It seems likely that as people became educated and modern drugs became available in Thailand, traditional healers were replaced by drugstores and drug sellers.

The popularity of the drugstore or drug seller (in both the 1970 and 1981 studies), so much outranking the government health center, is not difficult to understand. As noted earlier, Thailand has nearly 15,000 drugstores (14,550 in 1981)—far more than the commune health centers, which would number 5,600 if every commune were covered. Thus, drugstores are more conveniently accessible to people. There is virtually no waiting time. The patient describes his or her symptoms or asks

for a particular compound and a package is quickly selected from the shelf. The service is inexpensive, and no discomfort or embarrassment is involved, as might come from a medical examination.

Most drugstores in Bangkok or the provincial capitals are attractive places. The walls are covered with shelves holding many-colored packages. The very abundance and variety of medications give the patient confidence. The experienced drug seller has learned to be sympathetic with his clients; as he takes their money, he gives them reassurance. Whatever the price, it is less than a physician would charge, and only slightly more than the patient would be expected to pay at a government health center or hospital OPD, where the drugs usually come in duller packages and are regarded as inferior in quality.

The mode of delivery of ambulatory care by physicians depends very much on the setting. In health centers, even when the patients are few, very little time is spent with each case—perhaps 5 to 10 minutes. This has usually been preceded by a long wait on a hard bench, or even on the floor. In hospital OPDs, which are usually crowded, the pressure is greater, and 10 to 12 patients are seen per hour. The doctor's typical workday starts at 8 in the morning and theoretically goes until 3 or 4 in the afternoon. It is widely recognized, however, that, when all the patients are seen (usually by midday), the doctor leaves for his much more lucrative private practice.

In his private quarters, the doctor does everything he can to win the good will of the patient. He asks carefully about the symptoms, tries to develop a warm personal relationship, and finally dispenses from his own drug supply the prescribed medication, usually two or three items. Because the supply of each drug is usually enough for only a few days, however, the patient must return soon. The fee, based mostly on the pharmaceutical costs, varies with the doctor's estimate of the patient's income level—the time-honored "sliding scale."

With the doctor's split loyalties between his government position and his private practice, abuses are almost inevitable. Patients seen hastily in a health center, if they appear affluent enough, are advised that "for really good quality care" they might come later to the doctor's private clinic. Government drugs are even pilfered from the health center and hospital pharmacy for use in a private practice. (Small wonder that health center drug supplies are usually depleted rapidly.) Even nurses and sanitation personnel see patients privately after their official working hours. Such abuses, of course, are not unique to Thailand. MOPH officials recognize the abuses, but they feel helpless to cope with them.

Village Primary Health Care. Peripheral to the commune health center and private medical clinic are the elementary health services available in an increasing number of Thai villages. Longest established, though still serving only a small fraction of the 53,000 villages, are the midwifery stations. As noted, their functions have steadily broadened to include family planning service and various elements of primary health care (PHC), including first-aid and referral of patients to health centers or hospitals, when necessary.

The major "competition" to use of the MOPH midwifery station is the traditional birth attendant (TBA), who has served rural families in Thailand for centuries. As recently as 1977, the MOPH reported that 64 percent of all rural childbirths were delivered by TBAs in the mother's home. In that year, only 30 percent of rural expectant women had received any prenatal examinations. More detailed data on childbirths are available for 1974, when the percentage distribution for the rural population was as follows:

Attendance at Last Childbirth	Percentage
Traditional birth attendant	62.9
Official MOPH midwife	14.2
Family members	11.5
Self-delivery	6.4
Friends or neighbors	1.8
Traditional healers	0.6
Others	2.6
All attendants	100.0

Another study by the NESDB in 1976 compared TBA attendance in two districts; in the high-income district, TBAs handled 54.7 percent of the childbirths, and 72.1 percent in the low-income district.

The preference of village women for TBAs is understandable. Not only are they usually personally known to the family but, compared with the trained MOPH midwife, they are typically older women with long experience. The TBA's charges, furthermore, are not a deterrent, since government midwives, despite their salaries and the official policy of free service, often charge fees the same as or higher than those of the TBA.

The newest aspect of village PHC is the service of village health volunteers (VHVs) and village health communicators (VHCs), whose brief training was described earlier. As of 1982, nearly two-thirds of the villages were served by these volunteers, and full coverage was expected by 1986 or 1987. The individuals selected for training had been chosen by the village people, but their contacts with families turned out to be quite limited.

To heighten their effectiveness in the villages, the VHVs were entrusted with an important new responsibility in the early 1980s. The MOPH furnished them with a small supply of medications, which they were free to sell. Then, with the earnings, they could purchase a new drug supply from the nearest health center or hospital. Supervision of this "revolving drug fund," however, was meager and the program often terminated after a few months.

To fortify the idea, the MOPH promoted the organization of *village drug cooperatives* (VDCs). Each village family was invited to contribute the equivalent of U.S. $1 into the cooperative fund, which would then be used to purchase drugs. To encourage joining, the MOPH gave $30 worth of free drugs to any VDC that enrolled at least 70 percent of village families. The drugs were then sold by the VHV at a 25 percent profit. The profits were distributed to the cooperative members or used for loans to support health promotion activities, such as constructing latrines.

By 1984, there were reported to be 18,400 VDCs in Thailand, and the number was continuing to grow. Some had extended their functions to establish funds for nutrition or sanitation. The whole VDC idea was, in effect, the MOPH strategy to reduce the great dependence of rural people on commercial drugstores and drug sellers.

Around 1985, still another innovation was launched in Thailand, designed to increase the use of health centers and other public facilities. Building on the success of the VDCs, the ministry sponsored a voluntary insurance program to finance access to government health facilities. It should be recalled that personal fees are now charged for attendance at MOPH health centers and hospitals. For the *Health Card Fund* (HCF) the MOPH, with the aid of VHVs and VHCs, sells health cards to families for U.S. $12 per year. This card entitles any four members of the family to free care at a health center or hospital, up to six times a year. Drugs can also be purchased from the local village drug cooperative at a 10 percent discount. If the local health center refers the patient to a hospital, the cardholder gets priority attention, without the usual wait and without an OPD charge. Later the HCF pays the facilities for the services used by cardholders. If funds are left over at the end of the year, they are distributed as "dividends" to all members of the HCF.

The effects of these various cooperative financing programs on rural health services in Thailand are not yet clear. The various strategies for strengthening primary health care, however, reflect the entrepreneurial ideology of Thailand. They all require people to help themselves, with personal expenditures, rather than enlarge the contributions of government. The village-level PHC workers are expected to be volunteers, not public employees. The village drug cooperative, though it is a collective action, is financed by the villagers themselves and not a burden on the public treasury. The health card fund is another self-help strategy, even for the support of government facilities. Altogether the approach is oriented to enhancing private support for health services—already predominant in Thailand—and does nothing to strengthen the public support of the national health system.

Aside from these general PHC strategies, Thailand has been a country highly favored for international health projects. Both multilateral and bilateral agencies have launched several special projects for extending PHC in selected

areas, according to various designs. With 71 provinces and 700 districts, Thailand offers many locations to test different designs for PHC organizations, and in a dozen or more places this was done. The objective seems to have been to improve PHC at the local level at low cost, with the training and use of auxiliary personnel.

Best known, perhaps, was the Lampong Health Development Project, financed largely by the U.S. Agency for International Development (USAID) in the northern province of Lampong. In 1974, when the project started, the province's 600,000 people, divided among 11 districts, was typical of Thailand's rural areas. There were relatively few government midwives, sanitarians, nurses, and other personnel in each district. The total province had 17 physicians, less than 0.3 per 100,000 population. After 5 years, in 1979, local training had produced significant numbers of four new types of health personnel:

Village health volunteers (VHV)	918
Village health communicators (VHC)	5,359
Trained traditional birth attendants	352
Paraphysicians *(wechakorn)*	92

As we have already seen, the VHV and VHC village health workers were soon adopted as a nationwide type of PHC personnel. The paraphysician, or *wechakorn,* was the Thai version of the U.S. nurse-practitioner—that is, a nurse taught about prevention and the treatment of common ailments in a 1-year course. These advanced nurses have not been as widely deployed in rural areas.

In addition, the Lampong project enlarged the ratios of other health personnel available per 100,000, by 38 percent for government midwives, 500 percent for assistant nurses, 300 percent for graduate nurses, and 233 percent for physicians. Health centers, village child nutrition stations, and beds in district hospitals were also substantially expanded.

To evaluate the effects of the project, comparisons were made with conditions in an adjacent province on which equivalent data were collected. It was found, for example, that the project area had (a) broader coverage of children with disease prevention and health promotion services, (b) a much higher percentage of childbirths delivered by trained personnel, (c) an increased use of contraception, (d) a slightly increased use of government health facilities, and (e) a slightly decreased use of private drugstores and drug sellers.

Nevertheless, the impact of 6 years of effort on the health status of the Lampong Province population was disappointing. With surprising candor, the Thai MOPH made the following conclusion in its final report in 1981:

> Despite the increased rates of utilization of health services and general improvements in household environmental conditions (particularly in improved water supply and waste water disposal), little change was observed in the health or nutritional status of the target populations or of the general population. The slight effects observed cannot be clearly attributed to project interventions.

In the light of health status improvements achieved from health service interventions in other, less market-oriented countries (as we will see in later chapters), perhaps the major lesson of these findings is the great importance of social and economic conditions (which were untouched) in determining the health of rural people in certain developing countries.

Organized Prevention. Primary health care, of course, includes organized preventive services, but in developing countries, like Thailand, they can have such large impacts that they warrant special attention.

Urban and rural water supply systems in Thailand are the responsibilities of separate agencies. For the cities, the Bangkok Metropolitan Authority operates its own piped water network, and the Provincial Water Supply Division of the Department of Public Works in the Ministry of Interior handles piped water in the provincial capitals. Piped water in cities brings water into only those homes or buildings for which the owner can afford to pay for the connections with the main line. This was estimated to be about 55 percent of the population in 1978.

Rural water supplies are the responsibility of

seven different agencies, located in various departments of the MOPH and the Ministry of Interior; a National Rural Water Supply Committee attempts to coordinate the work of these agencies. The usual technique is to drill wells in the village square, from which families can pump water, carried in large jugs to their homes. The percentage of rural families served by such clean water is believed to be much lower than that in the cities.

Government responsibilities are not as fragmented for excreta disposal, except that the Ministry of Interior is responsible for cities and the Ministry of Public Health for rural areas. The standard rural modality is the outdoor pit latrine. In rural villages in 1976, only 24 percent of households had even such humble facilities. Judging by the limited supply of sanitation personnel trained for rural work, the priority for such environmental resources in rural Thailand is not high.

Communicable disease control, it should be recalled, is the function of one of the major departments of the MOPH. Separate divisons are responsible for the control of malaria, filariasis, tuberculosis, leprosy, venereal disease, and other infectious diseases. For many years, campaigns against these diseases were launched and directed by the central ministry; only in the early 1970s was some decentralization started. For venereal disease control, for example, in 1972 the nation had 98 VD control units, of which only 16 were under the direction of provincial or municipal health authorities. VD test specimens are examined by the centrally directed network of provincial laboratories. Tuberculosis control, by BCG vaccination, case detection, and treatment, has become much more decentralized through district health authorities.

Maternal and child health (MCH) preventive services are probably more decentralized in Thailand than any other type of prevention. MCH activities are the major preoccupation of most commune health centers and village midwifery stations. They are also provided by outpatient departments of the district hospitals. Family planning services are usually linked closely to MCH services, even though they may be sponsored by nongovernment agencies. (In addition, these agencies attempt to spread the word about family planning through other resources—small shops, drugstores, private doctors, and of course the village health workers. Contraceptive pills are distributed free by the agencies but, as an incentive, the village health worker may make small charges for them.) Yet we know that the majority of rural childbirths are still delivered by untrained TBAs. One may hope that the efforts of thousands of new VHVs and VHCs will educate women to make greater use of trained personnel.

Preventive health services for school children were started by the Ministry of Education in 1925, and transferred to the MOPH in 1942. Elementary school children are examined by teams of a doctor, a nurse, and a dental hygienist, occasionally in Bangkok and a few other cities, but seldom in the rural schools. Children's health and hygiene education is a responsibility of the teachers.

Malnutrition has not been reported as a very extensive problem in Thailand, which is a food-exporting country. Taken as a whole, the population in 1984 had more than enough food to meet calorie requirements, but the distribution has not been entirely equitable, and there are shortages of certain nutrients, such as protein, iron, and vitamin A. Therefore, the Division of Nutrition in the MOPH has organized 250 *child nutrition centers* in 46 provinces. Here mothers can go for supplementary foods for newly weaned infants. Iodized salt may also be distributed to certain remote regions, where goiter is epidemic.

Preventive services in workplaces are principally the responsibility of the Department of Labor in the Ministry of Interior. An occupational Health Division in the MOPH also surveys working conditions, and can formulate standards on occupational safety and health. Thailand's industries, however, are believed by knowledgeable observers to have generally very poor and unsafe working conditions.

The objective of Thailand's commune health centers is to provide integrated ambulatory services—both preventive and therapeutic. There is much evidence to show that both rural and urban populations seek personal preventive services more regularly if a health center or similar facility acquires the reputation

for giving effective treatment. The frequent resort to drugstores and private physicians to treat sickness is, therefore, a major obstacle to preventive strategies in Thailand. It is hoped that health educational efforts of VHVs and VHCs will increase the rate of use of the national network of commune health centers.

Hospital Services. The great majority of Thailand's hospital beds, as noted earlier, are in facilities under governmental auspices. The director of these hospitals is invariably a physician, appointed by the central Ministry of Public Health. This applies to both provincial and district hospitals; for the university teaching hospitals, appointments are made by the central head of the State University Office. Other supervisory personnel in public hospitals are also appointed by the central authority on the recommendations of the hospital director. All such appointments require approval of the Civil Service Commission. The hospital director is often assisted by deputies for nursing, business, and so on. All physicians on the medical staff report straight to the hospital director, without going through any intermediary.

The medical staffs of all public hospitals in Thailand are "closed," that is, composed of selected physicians on salaries. Patients are admitted to a bed only by a hospital physician, whether the case is referred by an outside doctor or the patient comes on his or her own. The majority of patients are self-referred to the hospital OPD.

Nearly all physicians in large hospitals are specialists and also engage in private practice outside the hospital for several hours a day. Private practice generates referral to the hospital of private patients, who may occupy one of the relatively few private or semiprivate rooms in a public facility. The private patient then pays the hospital for drugs and procedures, as do public patients, but he also pays a room charge and a physician's fee. Medical earnings from private patients in public hospitals are much greater than the official salaries. One can speculate on the incentives for admission of private patients.

The Ministry of Public Health attempts to apply standards for staffing hospitals of various levels. Provincial general hospitals are expected to have one physician for 15 beds, but this standard is not always met. In a district hospital, although the bed patients are not as severely sick, the doctor must also serve a large volume of out-patient cases; the standard therefore calls for one physician for 10 beds. In small district hospitals, the doctor also carries administrative responsiblities. Corresponding standards apply for nurses (graduate and auxiliaries), for technicians, maintenance personnel, and others as well.

Most beds in public hospitals are in six- to eight-bed wards. If the hospital is large, the wards are divided among departments—medicine, surgery, pediatrics, obstetrics–gynecology, and so on—but in small hospitals they may be separated only for men and women. Rooms for private patients usually hold about 10 percent of the hospital beds.

The occupancy levels of district hospitals in Thailand have typically been quite low, under 50 percent, since most patients bypass them to get more specialized medical service at provincial hospitals. The latter institutions are, therefore, usually occupied at a high level—near 100 percent and sometimes more, with beds in the corridors. Occasionally 10 beds are jammed into a 6-bed room, and one may see two patients in one bed. Because of this great pressure for beds, the average length of stay in provincial hospitals has been exceptionally short—only about 6 days.

Hospital secretaries, working as administrative assistants to the director, are found in large hospitals. They supervise the kitchen, laundry, housekeeping, and other functions, and handle financing and personnel matters. Their training usually consists of only a 2-week orientation course at the MOPH. The master's degree course in hospital administration, offered at the Faculty of Public Health in Bangkok, is open only to physicians, nurses, and other health professionals.

The charges to patients for drugs and various procedures in all public hospitals of Thailand has been noted. Even though low-income patients are not forced to pay, nearly everyone pays something. People have been led to believe that, unless they make some payment, they will not receive proper care. It is possible that very low income patients, who may need

hospitalization, do not seek it because they cannot afford the charges and are too proud to seek complete charity care. Data published in 1978 indicate that all general hospitals of the MOPH in Thailand were utilized at the rate of only 64 days per 1,000 persons per year. Even if this figure is doubled or tripled, to take account of non-MOPH hospitals, and an overall national rate of 190 days per 1,000 persons per year is estimated, the rate is still very low. It may be compared with a rate of about 500 days of hospital care per 1,000 persons per year in neighboring Malaysia or rates of more than 1,000 days per 1,000 persons per year in the industrialized countries.

The causes of hospital admission reflect something about the major health problems of a country. Although the data are somewhat old, the following were the 10 leading causes of admission to Thai provincial hospitals in 1967:

1. Fractures and injuries
2. Diarrheal diseases
3. Respiratory diseases
4. Childbirth—uncomplicated
5. Complications of pregnancy
6. Malaria
7. Abortion
8. Peptic ulcer
9. Appendicitis
10. Gynecological disorders

These 10 causes accounted for 59 percent of all admissions.

The amenities for patients in public hospital wards are extremely frugal. The beds are simply flat cots, with well-worn and thin mattresses. At the bedside is a small utility table, but seldom a lamp or walllight for illumination or any other device for patient comfort. The meals are extremely simple, served on a metal or plastic tray, with indentations for the food; platters are not used. Sanitary facilities are limited, so that one toilet must serve 6 to 12 patients or more.

Private hospitals in Thailand are quite different. In Bangkok, there are several large private institutions—both nonprofit and proprietary. Their staffing with nurses and other personnel is much better, their beds are of comfortable modern design, their meals are served with hotel-style elegance, and television sets are generally available. It is reported that patients are kept as long as possible, since each day yields additional earnings; some of the surgical operations are said to be of questionable necessity.

Management of the relatively few private hospitals that are nonprofit is by a board of directors, chosen by the sponsoring body, usually a religious group. Under the board, a medical director is in charge, usually full-time. The hospital physicians are on salary, as in public hospitals, but this is typically for only part of the day. The rates paid per hour are much higher than in public service. Patients pay separate amounts for the hospital and the physician's service, but all the funds go to the hospital, which then pays per-hour salaries to the doctors.

The for-profit private hospitals in Thailand are typically small and owned by one or more physicians. An administrator is appointed to work under the direction of the owners. Most of the physicians come from the staffs of public hospitals, and devote 3 or 4 hours to the private unit in the late afternoons. They are also paid on a part-time salary basis, even though the patients pay separate medical fees. Thus, these are also "closed staff" facilities, and the patient of an outside doctor must be referred to a staff physician if he wishes to use the private hospital.

Services for Special Populations. Outside the general framework of programs and services discussed so far, Thailand provides special services for selected populations.

Most highly developed is the network of 18 hospitals to serve military personnel (Army, Navy, and Air Force). To some extent, the families of men on active military duty may be served in these hospitals, as well as in ambulatory care clinics at military posts. High officials from all ministries may also be served without charge at military facilities. Private citizens regarded as "important" may likewise be treated at military hospitals for payments.

The police in Thailand are national, rather than local, under the Ministry of Interior. A few special hospitals serve the national police,

but they are also cared for in regular provincial hospitals, where they receive favored attention. Both the police and the armed forces are provided all necessary immunizations, carefully balanced diets, and other forms of health promotion. The robust health of these men is quite evident, as one sees them throughout the country.

Veterans disabled in the line of military duty are entitled to continuing care for these disorders. This care may be given at any military hospital, but there is also a special Veterans Hospital for severely disabled cases. After retirement, all veterans have certain entitlements to use military hospitals if a bed is available. For conditions not connected with military service, the veteran must pay part of the costs.

All government employees and their families also have certain benefits, if they use public hospitals; they are not obligated to pay for drugs and procedures, as are other people. If a private doctor or private hospital is used, the civil servant is reimbursed for part of the costs.

Employees of state enterprises are not considered civil servants, but many of these organizations operate their own health facilities. There are 72 state enterprises, including the railways, the port authority, and the Bangkok electrical utility; if one does not operate its own polyclinic, it may contract with a private hospital or clinic for service to its employees.

Finally, in northern Thailand, there is a small population (about 500,000) of mountain tribes that do not speak the Thai language or observe Buddhism. They live under very primitive conditions, and the Department of Social Welfare of the Ministry of Interior has encouraged their settlement in agricultural projects. About 55 such settlements have been established, and many of these are served by auxiliary health personnel.

This completes the account of Thailand—a transitional developing country, with basically entrepreneurial policies in its national health system. In spite of great efforts by government authorities, particularly in the Ministry of Health, to build a nationwide network for primary health care and hospital services, the use of those services is much less than adequate to meet the health needs. The vast majority of day-to-day health problems generate demands for care from private sector providers—drugstores, drug sellers, and private physicians. Private medical care is quite widely available in the cities and small towns, since the very low government salaries lead nearly all public physicians to supplement their earnings through private practice.

When illness becomes severe and requires hospitalization, it is usually obtained in a public hospital. The weakly staffed small district hospitals are usually bypassed for the larger provincial hospitals with specialists, even though services are frugal and conditions crowded, and patients must pay for drugs and technical services. As a result, the overall rate of hospital utilization is very low. Even health centers for primary health care charge fees and are used at rates far below capacity.

The strategy of the government to heighten the use of health centers and village stations with trained midwives is based largely on the training and use of thousands of village-level volunteers. Small village cooperatives (privately financed), for the purchase of drugs or the payment of fees at public facilities, are being encouraged, but government economic support is notably absent. The people of Thailand are spending a relatively large fraction of GNP on health (4.6 percent in 1983), but 70 percent of this is spent through private channels that are least likely to yield efficiency and equity in use of the nation's scarce health resources.

THE REPUBLIC OF THE PHILIPPINES

As a nation of more than 7,000 islands off the coast of Southeast Asia, the Republic of the Philippines has been independent since 1946. From 1899 to 1946, the country was a territory of the United States, as an outcome of the Spanish-American War of 1898–1899. Before that, going back to 1564, the Philippines were essentially a colony of Spain, whose Catholic Church greatly influenced the life of the people. Thus, the combined impacts of domestic tradition, Spanish colonialism, Catholicism, and American imperialism are clearly discern-

ible in today's general culture of the Philippine people, and specifically in their national health system. Even after full liberation in 1946, following World War II, the entrepreneurial free-market ideology of U.S. society continued to permeate health system strategies.

General Features

The Republic of the Philippines had a population of 56,700,000 in 1984. Its GNP that year was $568 per capita—much lower than one would expect from a visit to its dynamic capital city, Manila, on the principal island of Luzon. After impressive economic growth at the rate of 6.4 percent annually in the 1950s, rapid population growth in the subsequent decades contributed to virtual economic stagnation and major problems of underemployment and poverty. The vast disparity between the incomes of the highest and lowest social classes was noted earlier. Yet the transitional/developing status of the Philippines is reflected in the urbanization of 40 percent of the population and the engagement of 73 percent of the people in occupations outside of agriculture.

The entrepreneurial nature of the Philippine health system was dramatically shown in the survey finding that 75 percent of all health-related expenditures came from private sources. Although this study was made in 1980, and public spending may have become stronger since then, we will see that the recent or current health situation still has a highly entrepreneurial character. Adult literacy, in the indigenous language, Tagalog, or in English, was reported to be 86 percent in 1984, but only 54 percent of school-age children were enrolled in schools.

For administrative purposes, the scattered Philippine islands are divided into 12 regions—54 percent of the people live on Luzon and other northern islands, 23 percent in a central cluster (the Visayas), and 23 percent in the southern cluster (Mindanao). Each of the 12 regions includes several provinces, amounting to 76 in all. The provinces, in turn, are subdivided into a total of 228 districts, which play a significant role in the health system, reflected in a network of district hospitals. Within the districts are 1,700 municipalities (or subdistricts) and 43,000 villages or *barangays.*

The 76 provinces have elected governors, but the central ministries also have their own representatives in the provinces, who can bypass the governor and make policy decisions directly. This applies to the Ministry of Health (MOH), among others. Municipalities also have elected mayors, and villages have elected captains. The dominant tradition in Philippine government has been one of great centralization; this has long been very clear in the health system, in which numerous specialized MOH programs were operated vertically, with power starting in Manila and extending outwardly to the provinces and down to the community level.

In 1982, under a Presidential Executive Order, major steps were taken toward decentralization, with responsibilities for the vertical health programs delegated to the provinces. The former central authorities were transformed into consultative offices, to assist provincial operating officials on request. Also, the hospitals and rural health services in each province were brought together under unified direction.

Organizational Structure

Since the 1982 reorganization, the Ministry of Health (MOH) functions through five operational levels. At the top, the Office of the Minister has responsibility for health planning, financial management, manpower development, and other overall functions. There are 12 staff bureaus, including preventive health services, medical services (hospitals), food and drug control, family planning, malaria eradication, nutrition, and other such fields. These bureaus all serve to advise offices at lower levels throughout the country.

The second MOH level consists of 12 Regional Health Offices, which have considerable freedom in managing the health budgets allocated to them from the top. The RHO also conducts public health training, operates a regional laboratory, and supervises medical centers and regional hospitals outside metropolitan Manila. Each of the 76 provinces has a provincial health officer (PHO), who is respon-

sible for all preventive health services, as well as supervision of the main provincial hospital. The PHO also carries the ultimate responsibility for district hospitals.

At the level of the 228 districts, there are usually small primary/emergency care hospitals, the heads of which serve as district health officers. The DHO may or may not be a physician. He or she is also responsible for *rural health units* in the municipalities and the *barangays,* or villages. The village health station is staffed entirely by briefly trained auxiliary health workers. Many international agencies, both multilateral and bilateral, as well as nongovernmental, sponsor special demonstration projects on primary health care in selected districts and villages.

Other government agencies, besides the MOH, contribute to the Philippine health system. The Ministry of Social Services and Development provides nutritional services. The Bureau of Agricultural Extension offers health education to farm families. The Ministry of Labor and Employment monitors health services at the workplace. The National Commission on Population integrates an extensive nationwide program to promote family planning, in which numerous voluntary and public agencies play roles. The reduction of the high Philippine rate of population growth (around 3 percent per year) is regarded as a crucial factor in economic development.

Perhaps the most important government agency concerned with health, outside the MOH, is the Philippine Medical Care Commission, established in 1969 to administer a social insurance program for hospital services and associated physician's care. The Medicare program, as it is called, applies to two major population groups: (a) government employees and their dependents and (b) employees of private industries and their dependents. However, the employee (as of 1985) had to earn 150 pesos or *more* per month, to be eligible; if eligible, the employer was required to contribute 50 percent of the premium. The collection and disbursement of funds for the hospital and related services are handled by two separate agencies: the Social Security System (SSS) for private employees, and the Government Service Insurance System (GSIS) for government employees. In 1979, some 4,000,000 persons in all were eligible for Medicare support, as primary beneficiaries. Assuming about 3 dependents per worker would mean a total of 16,000,000 persons, or about 28 percent of the population.

Several features of the Philippine medical care insurance program reflect the basically entrepreneurial character of this health system. The limitation of eligibiilty to employed persons is not unusual; virtually all social insurance or social security programs start this way. The Philippine policy, however, is to cover only the *higher* paid employees, excluding those who earned less than 150 pesos per month in 1985. Thus, the lowest paid workers, whose health needs are usually greater, are not protected. (Traditionally, social insurance was designed to protect the lowest income families.)

Second, unlike policies in nearly all other developing countries, the Philippine social insurance program does not take advantage of the economies achieved by the "direct" pattern of medical care organization—that is, engaging its own doctors and other health personnel on salaries and operating its own facilities. Instead, the insurance funds are used for making fee-for-service payments to independent doctors and hospitals, private or public. Around 1980, this involved agreements with some 14,000 practicing physicians and 1,648 hospitals. Only in certain isolated places—81 in the whole country—did Medicare find it necessary to establish its own health facility for primary care, because none was otherwise available.

Third, as medical and hospital costs have risen, the administrative response was not to apply regulatory cost controls, nor to increase insurance contributions from employers or employees. Instead, increasing proportions of cost-sharing were imposed on the workers. By 1979, the hospitalized worker had to pay out-of-pocket 34 percent of the total costs. For hospitalization, of course, this can mean a heavy financial burden.

The entire Medicare program is undoubtedly helpful to millions of Philippine working people. Yet its administrative design clearly suggests that it is also meant to give substantial financial support to the private market within the national health system—both private doctors and private hospitals.

Another part of the organizational structure of the Philippine health system incudes numerous voluntary health agencies. These have been developed mainly in the fields of child care, nutrition, and family planning. Much of their financial support comes from international agencies, both multilateral and bilateral, public and private. Religious organizations, educational institutions, and private foundations support local community health projects in some 65 locations throughout the country. The U.S. Agency for International Development (USAID) has played an especially large role in supporting both government and voluntary health projects in the Philippines.

Finally, the purely private market for medical care is very highly developed. As in most developing countries, there are substantial numbers of traditional leaders, but modern medical practitioners and modern drugstores play larger parts. Even hospitals—which in other entrepreneurial countries, such as Thailand or South Korea, are predominantly public—are predominantly private in the Philippines. The great strength of the private sector in the Philippine health system, of course, reflects the overwhelmingly free-market ideology in the total national economy.

Resource Production

The development of health manpower, facilities, and commodities in the Philippines strikingly reflects the entrepreneurial character of the national health system.

Health Manpower. The output of physicians, nurses, and other health personnel in the Philippines is exceptionally high, but a large proportion of the new graduates leave the country. One study in the mid-1980s reported that 68 percent of all Philippine doctors were living in other lands. The domestic national supplies, therefore, are not as great.

In 1984, there were 14.3 physicians per 100,000 people. This meant about 8,100 physicians in the whole country, of whom more than half were concentrated in metropolitan Manila and the central Luzon region, with 22 percent of the national population. An exceptionally large number of medical schools are approved for training physicians—23 schools, graduating 1,300 new doctors a year. Only 3 of the schools are government-sponsored, although these have the largest enrollments; no fewer than 20 are small private schools, typically established by private physicians as profit-making enterprises.

The output and training of nurses is similar. There are 132 schools preparing graduate-level (R.N.) nurses, and 87 percent of these are privately owned. During the period 1977–1980, more than 12,000 nurses passed the official examinations each year. Since this was many more nurses than the health system could absorb, a large share of them emigrated—mainly to the United States, where their training was found acceptable as well as their ability to speak English. A World Health Organization study in the 1970s found that 37 percent of Philippine nursing students intended to emigrate on completion of their training. A later study reported that 80 percent of Philippine-born nurses were living abroad, not only in the United States, but also in Saudi Arabia, Hong Kong, and elsewhere.

The predominantly private character of professional education seems to apply to virtually all the health disciplines. There are 97 schools for preparing midwives, 14 schools for pharmacists, and 26 for medical technologists—all predominatly private. Only sanitary inspectors and village-level community health workers are trained by the Ministry of Health. Volunteer *barangay health workers* (BHWs) get 3-week courses in family planning and certain other services.

The work settings of health personnel parallel their educational preparation; they are predominantly private. A MOH report in 1981 stated that 59 percent of physicians in the Philippines were engaged entirely in private practice. Among the 41 percent in government employment (mainly the MOH), nearly all did some private practice part of the time. Among dentists, private practice was even greater, applying to 84 percent, in relation to 16 percent in public service. Among nurses, 58 percent

worked in private facilities and 42 percent in government.

With the massive emigration of so many nurses, physicians, and others, the Philippine people are forced to rely increasingly on the briefly trained volunteer local village health workers. By 1983, some 150,000 village health workers had been trained by the MOH, but not all of these are in active service. About 20 percent of those trained discontinue their work each year; a study showed that this was due to their frustration with the lack of supplies, the absence of refresher training, and the irregularity in their supervision.

Health Facilities. Hospitals are relatively abundant in the Philippines, with 1.8 beds (of all types) per 1,000 population in 1981. Of the 1,607 hospitals in operation that year, 1,194, or 74 percent, were private. Since private hospitals are generally smaller than government ones, the proportion of private beds was not so high, but still constituted a majority. Based on data for general hospital beds (excluding mental, tuberculosis, etc.), private facilities had 55 percent of the beds in 1980.

Philippine hospitals are classified as primary, secondary, and tertiary, according to their size and complexity. In 1981, 48 percent of the hospitals were small primary facilities (averaging 15 beds each), with 14 percent of the total beds; many of these are essentially general practitioner clinics with a few beds. The secondary hositals averaged about 40 beds in capacity, and were 36 percent of the hospitals with 28 percent of the total beds. The 16 percent of hospitals in the tertiary class were the dominant institutions. They had an average capacity of 185 beds and held 58 percent of all hospital beds. This hierarchy includes both public and private institutions.

Patients using private hospitals must pay the full cost of care, although, as noted, some may be financially protected by the Medicare insurance program. A small share of patients may be insured through private commercial companies. Even public hospitals, however, are not entirely free. Charges are made on a sliding scale, in proportion to family income. Indigent patients, who are the majority, are theoretically not required to pay fees, although they are encouraged to make voluntary contributions. The charges made on a sliding scale are especially for drugs and diagnostic procedures. As a share of total MOH expenditures in hospital services, patient fees contributed only 8 percent in 1982, but for low-income patients even these small charges may be very burdensome.

Public hospital wards, meals, and amenities provided vary with the patient's income level. Patients with insurance, or who are otherwise affluent, have private or semiprivate rooms. The indigent are kept in large overcrowded wards. Two patients in one bed is not unusual, nor are beds placed in dark corridors.

For ambulatory care, the Philippine health system in 1982 had nearly 2,000 health centers in the 1,700 subdistricts or municipalities. These *rural health units* are theoretically staffed by a municipal health officer (a general medical practitioner), along with a public health nurse, a sanitary inspector, and several midwives. Some 70 percent of these structures have been established by the MOH, and the remainder by local government. Each is expected to serve about 20,000 to 30,000 people, but numerous vacancies in the medical posts result in low utilization. While these health units theoretically offer general primary health care, in practice their services are almost entirely preventive. Except for first-aid in emergencies, patients coming for medical treatment are usually sent to a private physician or a hospital out-patient department for care.

Most peripheral are the village *barangay* health stations. These have been established in 8,000 of the 43,000 villages. They are staffed by a trained midwife and several volunteer health workers. Each station is expected to serve about 3,000 people with first-aid, family-planning services, and advice on environmental sanitation. An international review published in 1984, however, reported 53 percent of the accommodations for rural health units and village health stations "are in need of considerable repair or are badly dilapidated."

Drugs. The manufacture of drugs in the Philippines—except for certain vaccines and oral rehydration salts (furnished by UNICEF)—is carried out entirely by private firms. All basic drugs or raw materials are imported and then processed into dosage form. About 15,000 brand-name drugs are on the market, the majority of which are sold over-the-counter directly to consumers.

As in Thailand, drug consumption is the major response to primary health care needs in the Philippines. More than 80 percent of all drugs are purchased in some 7,750 private drugstores or small village *boticas.* Counting these private expenditures and the 20 percent coming from government agencies, drug spending in 1982 was much more than double the total budget of the MOH that year.

Economic Support and Health Care Delivery

With these strong private-sector attributes of health resources in the Philippines, one may naturally expect the utilization of services and health expenditures to be correspondingly private in character.

In 1982, overall health expenditures were estimated to absorb 3.0 percent of the gross national product. Judging from household survey data of 1980, this money came about 25 percent from government and 75 percent from private sources.

Of the government expenditures on health, more than 70 percent went for the support of MOH activities. These were, however, only 3.8 percent of total central government spending—a figure that has fluctuated between 3 and 4 percent since 1975. The breakdown of MOH expenditures in 1982 was as follows:

Purpose	Percentage
Hospital services	53.4
Field health units and stations	28.9
Special disease-control projects	4.6
Administration and planning	3.4
Other	9.7
All purposes	100.0

The purposes of private health expenditures were analyzed in a household survey made in the Philippines in 1975. These were estimated to be as follows:

Purpose	Percentage
Drugs and medical supplies	45
Hospital and similar fees	30
Physicians and other providers	25
All purposes	100.0

An overview of health service utilization in the Philippines was given in a national MOH household survey conducted in 1978. Of the total sample, most had some illness during the survey period (previous month), and the actions taken in response were distributed as follows:

Response to Illness Problem	Percentage
No action taken	59.6
Self-prescribed drugs taken	21.1
Government health center or station	6.9
Private hospital consulted	3.6
Government hospital consulted	2.3
Private health care provider	1.9
Response unknown	4.6
All responses	100.0

Another study in 1976 did not tabulate the large percentage of cases on which no response to illness was reported, but found that, among persons who took some action, 28 percent consulted private health care practitioners and another 8 percent saw traditional healers. Regarding childbirths, traditional practitioners have been of much greater importance. In 1978, of all rural births, 65 percent took place at home, handled by a traditional birth attendant; 27 percent were also at home but attended by trained midwives. Only 8 percent of births took place in a public or private clinic. MOH reports in 1982 estimate that 70 percent of the population had access to general primary health care, but this may be an exaggeration.

These conditions in the Philippines are a legacy of more than two decades of corrupt dictatorship, ending only in 1986 with the election to the presidency of Mrs. Corazon Aquino. Soon after she came to power, Mrs. Aquino replaced the minister of health with a professionally competent physician. She also ordered an immediate increase in the MOH budget. Whether a stronger government health program will reduce the great dependence on the private sector and increases health equity in the Philippines remains to be seen.

OTHER ENTREPRENEURIAL HEALTH SYSTEMS IN TRANSITIONAL COUNTRIES

Two other countries with very distinctive characteristics are of a transitional economic level and have health systems that show highly entrepreneurial policies. In spite of their quite different backgrounds, they fit together here in a review of the world's national health systems: the Republic of Korea (South) and South Africa.

Republic of Korea (South)

The Republic of Korea was established after World War II, with the termination of colonial control by Japan. The entire Korean peninsula in the northeast part of Asia had been under Japanese domination from 1910 to 1945. In 1948, however, two separate governments were established, north and south of the 38th parallel. The northern part, dominated by the Soviet Union, became the People's Democratic Republic of Korea, with a clearly socialist orientation. The southern part was dominated by the United States, and became the Republic of Korea, with an equally clear capitalist orientation. In 1950, armed conflict broke out between the two Koreas, each side supported by thousands of troops from its respective political sponsor. After massive loss of life and physical destruction on both sides, an armistice was reached in 1954, resulting only in greater determination by North Korea to develop socialism and by South Korea to build a land of free private enterprise.

The Entrepreneurial Korean Health System. The development of the Republic of Korea

Table 9.6. National Health Expenditures, by Source: Percentage Distribution in the Republic of Korea, 1975

Source	Percentage
Central government	6.2
Local governments	7.2
All public	(13.4)
Personal consumption	84.0
Industry	1.6
Voluntary health agencies	1.0
All private	(86.6)
All sources	100.0

Source: Park, Chong Kee, *Financing Health Care Services in Korea.* Seoul: Korea Development Institute, 1977.

from an agricultural economy to a largely industrial and urbanized society, between 1960 and 1985, has been remarkable. In spite of underlying capitalistic principles, the government launched an initial 5-year plan in 1962, stressing industrialization. The rate of growth of the gross national product (GNP) since then has been close to 10 percent per year—one of the highest rates in modern economic history. Even with a rapid population growth of 2.3 percent annually, the net growth of GNP has been impressive. The per capita GNP rose from $87 in 1962 to $2,126 in 1984. Most observers would agree that national economic planning, combined with capitalist incentives, extensive foreign investment, and a highly industrious population all contributed to South Korea's achievements. The Korean health system has many, though not all, of the attributes of the larger society. Changes occurring after 1977 might warrant classifying South Korea's health system as "welfare oriented," but as we shall see, its philosophical assumptions are still highly entrepreneurial.

In 1975, the Korean Development Institute conducted a national survey of all health expenditures in South Korea, with the support and advice of the U.S. Agency for International Development. Data on expenditures by government and other organized agencies were solicited from those sources, and private expenditures were determined from a nationwide household survey. The findings were astonishing. Nearly 87 percent of all health-related expenditures came from private sources, and overwhelmingly from indivduals and families.

Only 13.4 percent came from government at all levels. The details are given in Table 9.6.

Further analysis of the breakdown of personal household expenditures in 1975 in several cities produced the following findings:

Purpose	Percentage
Drugs (modern and traditional)	57.3
Physician's services	33.5
Hospital care	8.4
X-rays	0.7
All purposes	100.0

As in Thailand, the major personal expenditures of South Korean people in 1975 in response to illness, was the purchase of drugs, typically without medical advice. At this time, total national health expenditures amounted to 2.7 percent of GNP.

In 1984, the population of the Republic of Korea was 40,513,000. With rapid industrialization, the country changed from 26 percent urban in 1955 to 65 percent urban in 1984, facilitating the provision of both personal and environmental health services. Urban settings were also conducive to the expansion of higher education for health professions and the construction of hospitals.

In 1986, South Korea had 85.8 physicians per 100,000 population, an increase from 64.4 per 100,000 in 1979. (A small portion of these were registered herb doctors.) In the decade from 1976 to 1986, medical schools doubled, from 14 to 28. Many of these schools are sponsored by voluntary nonprofit organizations, but several are entirely proprietary. The expansion of other health personnel between 1979 and 1986 has been equally impressive. Pharmacists increased from 62.2 to 77.0 per 100,000, dentists from 8.8 to 14.4 per 100,000, and nurses from 98.3 to 154.6 per 100,000.

Hospitals and hospital beds increased even more rapidly. Between 1975 and 1987, the bed supply increased from 21,000 to 80,000—by nearly four times; this meant a rise from 1.3 to 2.6 beds per 1,000 population. Especially significant is the overwhelmingly private sponsorship and control of the new hospitals. In 1975, they were already mainly under private control; 53.7 percent of the beds were in private facilities. By 1987, private beds constituted

81.4 percent of the total, and public beds only 18.6 percent.

As an overall indicator of this expansion of health resources, the share of GNP devoted to health purposes rose from 2.7 percent in 1975, noted earlier, to 4.0 percent in 1984. A substantial influence on this growth of health expenditures was the development and gradual expansion of a major program of social insurance for medical care, which warrants special consideration.

Korean National Health Insurance. As far back as 1963, South Korea had enacted a law to encourage, through public subsidies, the organization of voluntary health insurance schemes. Eleven programs were started, but their growth was very slow, and they got into financial difficulties by attracting exceptionally high-risk members. In 1976, therefore, the law was amended to require all employers of 500 workers or more to establish health insurance societies. The premium costs had to be shared equally between employers and employees. Gradually the threshold of 500 workers was reduced to 16 workers in 1983; even firms with fewer than 16 workers could be insured on a voluntary basis. This became known as the Class I scheme, and it was administered by 149 separate and autonomous insurance societies.

In 1978, government employees, private school teachers, and some others were required to be enrolled in a Korean Medical Insurance Corporation, through one of its 14 regional offices. This became known as the Class III scheme.

The Class II scheme, for self-employed persons, farmers, and fishermen was launched in 1981. Being difficult to reach administratively, these people were approached gradually on a county or community basis, and were enrolled through the 14 regional offices set up under the Class III scheme. Special occupational groups, such as taxi drivers, were permitted to enroll in separate schemes on a voluntary basis. In all three classes of health insurance, dependents in the immediate family were covered.

Through this variety of mechanisms, the numbers and percentage of the South Korean population, protected economically for medical care costs, have steadily expanded. The largest share is in Class I, but altogether the enrollment has risen from 8.8 percent of the population in 1977 to 49.9 percent (nearly 21 million people) in 1987.

The pattern of service delivery under all three classes of health insurance scheme reflects the entrepreneurial character of the South Korean health system. Essentially delivery is through private (or sometimes public) physicians, hospitals, and other health care providers, who are paid on a fee-for-service basis. Benefits include a broad range of medical, hospital, drug, ambulance, and related services, but both in-patient and out-patient care are limited to 180 days per year. Details on benefits vary slightly among insurance societies, and generally the self-employed (Class II scheme) have greater benefits.

As might be expected, the rate of utilization of medical and hospital services rose rapidly as soon as the social insurance took effect. The response, in expansion of both human and physical resources, was noted earlier. But high utilization also created financial pressures on the insurance agencies. Two adjustments were generally applied: (a) reduction of the fees payable and (b) the introduction and elevation of copayments by the patient. Professional fees and hospital payments were reduced to slightly over half of customary charges. Required copayments fluctuated over time and among the several schemes. Copayments for Class III scheme members in 1980, for example, were 30 percent for ambulatory care and 20 percent for in-patient hospital care. Generally copayment obligations are higher for dependents.

The perverse economic incentives of fee-for-service methods of remuneration are well understood by health insurance administrators in South Korea, as elsewhere. The rates of provision of both ambulatory and hospital services have climbed every year—mainly, of course, because doctors spend little time with each patient and ask him or her to return soon. Thus, in the Class I scheme, ambulatory visits rose from 1.3 per person per year in 1977 to 6.9 in 1985. In the Class II scheme, the rise was from 0.5 visits per person per year in 1981 to 3.8 in 1985. Great increases also occurred in the rates of hospitalization. Nevertheless, the reduction of medical fees and the cost-sharing obligations of patients have caused widespread dissatisfaction, among both providers and consumers in the whole health insurance program.

Aside from reducing the fees paid and increasing the copayments required, economies have been sought in administrative procedures. Through coalescence of many small insurance societies, their total number has been reduced from 513 in 1977 to 144 in 1985. Proposals to unify the three basic schemes administratively and financially, in a spirit of "social solidarity," however, have been rejected by the government.

The great extension of mandatory health insurance coverage in Korea has, of course, modified the sources of health expenditures reported in the 1975 survey. Spending for health services by government and the several health insurance programs raised the share derived through public sources from 13.4 percent in 1975 to 36.0 percent a decade later. Still, the result of large copayments required with insurance and the noncoverage of many people was 64 percent of health expenditures in 1985 still being derived from private sources.

Of the three classes of health insurance coverage in South Korea, the weakest is that of the self-employed in both rural areas and cities (Class II scheme). These include small farmers, artisans, casual workers, and service employees, who are often out of work. The government plans to provide general medical care for many of these people through a different strategy. Instead of attempting to enroll them in the Class II scheme, it hopes to upgrade the network of health centers and subcenters that has been developed throughout the country since the 1950s. Thus, the low-income and marginal self-employed people and their families would be served through these public facilities.

As in most other developing countries, South Korea's Ministry of Health and Social Affairs, by 1982, had gradually established 202 health centers—one in each of the 140 counties, one in each small city, and one in each ward of the five largest cities. These were intended to provide preventive services and simple primary medical treatment. Each health center was theoretically staffed by one general doctor and several allied health personnel, but

typically the medical post was not filled. In addition, in 1982 there were about 1,000 subcenters, staffed only with auxiliary health personnel, in the townships (clusters of villages). Most of these units for ambulatory care were only meagerly utilized, because people had little confidence in them.

The plan in the mid-1980s was to improve both the staffing and the equipment of these health centers and subcenters, and to put greater emphasis on treatment of the sick. Patients needing specialty services would be referred to a public hospital for out-patient or in-patient care. Also in 39 rural counties without any hospital, public or private hospitals were planned to be built with government subsidy.

This arrangement for Class II eligibles seems, except for the financial aspects, the same as that used in Korea's separate Medical Assistance Program for the poor, implemented in 1977. This categorical scheme, for persons certified by the Ministry of Health and Social Affairs (MHSA) as impoverished, covered 5.7 percent of the population in 1977 and grew to 11.0 percent, or 4,629,000 people, in 1987. Of this number, however, hardly 20 percent—the aged, the disabled, and children without any means of support—are entitled to out-patient and in-patient care in public hospitals without charge. All other certified poor persons may obtain free care only at one of the MHSA health centers or subcenters. For hospitalization, however, they are charged up to 50 percent of the cost in a public hospital, which must be repaid within 5 years.

If the currently noninsured persons in the Class II category (self-employed) are to become insured (through premiums paid to one of the 14 regional offices), and to receive services under a pattern similar to the very poor, the quality of those services will have to be improved. This will put greater demands on the budget and resources of the MHSA. Such changes may modify the South Korean health system from an entrepreneurial to a more welfare-oriented pattern. (By 1989, in fact, unofficial reports indicated that expansion of enrollment in all three schemes—Classes I, II, and III—had achieved insurance coverage of nearly 100 percent of the South Korean population.)

South Africa

Another country at a transitional level of economic development with a health system of basically entrepreneurial character is South Africa. Unique in the world, with its rigid and explicit separation of health resources and services for different racial groups, it must be analyzed as two or more subsystems. Yet its gross national product of $2,611 per capita in 1984 is the net outcome of the work of a population of 32,000,000, divided between a small minority of affluent families and the majority of people who live at a bare subsistence level.

Basic Social Features. The influence of race and racial background on social policy in South Africa is so crucial and pervasive that we must outline the basic features of the society before the health system can be understood. The vast majority of South Africa's population consists of black Africans, but the country is ruled and completely dominated by a small minority of white Europeans—about 60 percent with Dutch backgrounds and 40 percent of largely British origin. Racial backgrounds are regarded as so overwhelmingly important, however, that government policies are formulated according to four racial groups. In the 1980 census these were subdivided as follows:

Racial Group	*Percentage*
Africans *(Bantus)*	71.5
Mixed races (colored)	9.4
Asians (mostly from India)	2.9
Whites (mostly European)	16.2
All races	100.0

Domination of the Europeans over the native Africans was evident in some degree from the first settlement of the Dutch East India Company in 1652, and it became increasingly prominent over the centuries. The Boer War between the South Africans and the British (1899–1902) resulted in a British victory, and the Union of South Africa became a British colony with dominion status. Only after World War I, through legislative actions in 1926 and 1931, did South Africa gain full independence, but these political events promoted the formation of distinctive political parties that sharply influenced policies toward the Africans. After World War II, the South African Nationalist Party won the election of 1948, and became increasingly the party to implement a policy of *apartheid* or rigid separation of the races in all aspects of life and work. In 1961, South Africa left the British Commonwealth completely, and the voice of the Afrikaaners (Dutch background) became clearly dominant in the Nationalist Party.

South Africa is divided into four provinces and about 800 local authorities. At the national level, the central government is located in three cities: for administration, the capital is Pretoria; for legislation it is Cape Town; and the judicial capital is Bloemfontein. Since the 1950s, government policy has set aside about 15 percent of the land, in several scattered small areas, as *homelands,* or *bantustans,* reserved for various tribal groups of black Africans. By the mid-1980s, 11 of these had been established and were self-governing in domestic affairs, including health service. Approximately 40 percent of the African population had "chosen," or more often been forced, to live in one of the so-called homelands—more accurately described as ghettoes. The bantustans are predominantly congested settlements on arid, unattractive land.

In 1984, a new Constitution carried South African apartheid policy one step further. In a strategy, manifestly designed to separate the "colored" and the Asian population groups further from the black Africans, the government established three parliaments—white, colored, and Asian. There was no parliament for the black Africans, and the voting ratios in the three official parliaments were designed to ensure that the whites would outnumber the other two combined on any decision. Thus, actions of the central government administration—on allocation of resources or any other matter affecting the lives of people—were determined essentially by the white parliament.

The injustices and cruelties of apartheid policies cannot be properly elaborated here. The housing, nutrition, schools, transportation—all aspects of life—are grossly inferior for the Africans compared with the whites. People must carry passes at all times, although these are monitored solely for blacks, and there are curfews for them in the cities. Male workers who do the mining, on which the economy is based, are separated from their families; they are housed in crude "hostels" near the mines, while their families—wives, children, and elderly parents—live in some distant homeland.

Health System Infrastructure. Since the Health Act of 1977, South Africa has had a central public health authority, known now as the Department of National Health and Population Development. This is responsible for general coordination of public health (preventive) services, health planning, promotion of contraception, communicable disease control, operation of a national laboratory service, and provision of long-term psychiatric care. Other responsibilities are left to the provinces and local authorities.

The four provincial health administrations (Cape, Transvaal, Natal, and Orange Free State) provide and operate facilities for personal health care, both in public hospitals and in ambulatory service units. The 800 local authorities are responsible for environmental sanitation, for local communicable disease control, and for general health promotion in their areas. However, the homelands or bantustans, also called Black National States, are responsible for all health services within their borders. Of decisive importance is the method of public funding for all these provincial, local, and bantustan health services; it is wholly dependent on allocations from the central government. These are based fundamentally on the races of people served by the hospitals and other resources, as we will see later.

In spite of the bigotry in apartheid policies, or perhaps to ensure their enforcement, the construction and operation of hospitals in South Africa are principally governmental. In 1985, of the 720 hospitals in the country, 495 or 68 percent were governmental. (This included a small number of hospitals founded by religious or other nonprofit groups, but now financed almost entirely with public funds.) The rest were private, but even these facilities receive significant government subsidy. The overall hospital bed supply in South Africa amounts to 3.2 beds per 1,000 population, and 87.5 percent of the beds are in public institutions.

The racial designation of *public* hospital beds is 25 percent for whites (16 percent of the population), 49 percent for Africans (72 percent of the population), 3 percent for the colored (9.4 percent of population), 1.5 percent for Asians (2.9 percent of population), and 21.5 percent unclassified. It must be further recognized that the private hospitals are almost entirely for white people, with perhaps some beds for colored and Asians. If both private and public hospital beds are counted, there are vastly more beds per 1,000 population for whites than for African blacks.

The several hundred government health centers intended for black Africans are poorly equipped and badly deteriorated. They are staffed mainly with auxiliary health workers, since physicians will not accept appointments in them. Africans usually prefer medical care in hospital out-patient departments. Environmental sanitation facilities—both for water supply and excreta disposal—are extremely deficient in the rural areas. Although exact data are not available, we know the African population is overwhelmingly rural while the white minority lives in the cities, where environmental resources are good.

Outside the government, a few voluntary health agencies, such as associations for combatting tuberculosis, are organized within the separate racial communities. A few hospitals and clinics, sponsored by overseas religious missions, still operate in rural areas, but they are financed almost entirely by the government. Large enterprises—mining gold, diamonds, and other minerals—also operate medical care programs, including hospitals, for their workers (but not serving dependents).

Of growing importance in South Africa is the private medical market and its supporting structure. As we have noted, with the country's early colonial history, hospital care has been provided mainly by government, even though its extent and quality vary greatly among the racial groups. Ambulatory care by private general practitioners and specialists, however, is readily available in the cities for persons who can afford to pay the private fees. Of about 18,000 doctors in South Africa, approximately half are in government positions and half are in private practice. Of the latter a handful work for private commercial enterprises, but the vast majority maintain private quarters. The earnings of private practitioners exceed those from public sector work by two to four times.

To support the costs of private medical care, various groups in South Africa have developed voluntary health insurance, known generally as medical aid schemes. (A few such insurance schemes had been developed for European miners and railroad workers back in the 1930s.) About 300 of these schemes have now been developed, predominantly through employment groups, with employers and employees sharing premiums; some schemes, however, also enroll individuals (with certain restrictions). Altogether the medical aid schemes by 1983 had enrolled some 16 percent of the total South African population, but this consisted of 75 percent of the whites and 5.8 percent of all the other racial groups. The rate of growth of enrollment has been quite rapid, at about 5 percent, per year.

These are the essential features of the South African health system structure, and it is quite obvious that the entire system, in both its public and private sectors, is sharply divided along racial lines. Hospitals, clinics, health centers, pharmacies, and most private medical and dental quarters are all separated for the different racial groups. (A movement for well-staffed comprehensive community health centers for black Africans, financed wholly by government funds, was launched by a small group of progressive physicians in the 1940s. Starting at Pholela in 1942, the network grew to 44, but with reduced government funding, the facilities eventually deteriorated or closed down.)

Economic Support. Overall expenditures on health in South Africa are somewhat higher than in most developing countries, mainly be-cause of the relatively high expenditures by or on behalf of the relatively affluent 20 to 25 percent of the population of nonblack racial background. In 1984, health expenditures were estimated to absorb 5.2 percent of GNP (excluding the sales of over-the-counter medication; see later). This was an increase from 4.5 percent of GNP in 1976. The composition of these expenditures in 1982 was approximately as follows:

Source	Percentage
Government (all levels)	52.1
Voluntary medical insurance schemes	25.1
Enterprise health programs	1.4
Private payment for public or private services	21.4
All sources	100.0

The expenditures by government came almost entirely from the central level, for operation of health facilities in the provinces, but some came from local authority spending for environmental sanitation. Money spent through medical insurance schemes goes almost wholly to pay for the services of private physicians and dentists and private hospitals. The private payment for care at public or private facilities is out-of-pocket expenditure, made for user charges at public hospitals or for fees paid to private practitioners. (A portion is for copayments required even under the medical insurance schemes.) Public hospitals usually make moderate personal charges, varying with the patient's estimated household income and family size.

The exclusion of personal spending on self-medication from this analysis calls for an important adjustment in these health expenditure data. Judging from the findings on this matter in other developing countries, low-income people typically spend a great deal of their personal earnings on self-prescribed drugs. In Thailand, the Philippines, and South Korea, such spending exceeded all other personal health expenditures. Therefore, if we were to adjust the preceding tabulation to take account of private drug purchases, by increasing the "private payment for health services" by a conservative 20 percent, the resulting distribution of expenditure sources would be as follows:

Source	Adjusted Percentage
Government (all levels)	49.0
Voluntary insurance schemes	24.0
Enterprise programs	1.3
Private payment for services	25.7
All sources (adjusted)	100.0

With this adjusted calculation, we see that health expenditures in South Africa in 1982 came 49 percent from government and 51 percent from private sources.

Nevertheless, to reduce its public obligations, the South African government has actively encouraged further privatization. The medical insurance schemes are provided certain tax benefits, and user charges imposed at public facilities are being increased. (Of the total central government budget in 1984, the allocation reported for health purposes was 13.2 percent, which seems paradoxically high and questionable.)

The drive for greater privatization is propelled by the government's realization that most white people pay for their own medical care through the voluntary insurance schemes or out of pocket. One objective, therefore, is to enroll more black and other nonwhite people in these schemes, so that they are paying their own way. This strategy has been somewhat successful, in that between 1979 and 1983, most increased voluntary insurance coverage came from the black population. Theoretically this might reduce the pressure on the congested black public hospitals.

Part of the governmental health expenditures goes for the support of health professional education. There are seven medical schools in South Africa, all heavily subsidized by the central government, even though they still charge relatively high tuitions. Five of these schools are exclusively for whites; one admits some black, colored, and Asian students; and one school is intended specifically for nonwhite students. In 1985 the schools

graduated about 900 young doctors—80 percent white.

The education of nurses is also supported mainly by government. The white dominance in nursing is not as overwhelming as in medicine. In 1980, of the 55,000 registered nurses (of whom 40 percent, mainly white, were inactive), 53 percent were white, 38 percent were Africans, 7 percent were colored, and 2 percent were Asian. The less thoroughly educated "enrolled nurses" consisted of only 7 percent white, 50 percent African, 35 percent colored, and 8 percent Asian. In nursing service, because the hospitals have been forced to overlook segregation policies, some white patients are served by black nurses, and vice versa.

Interracial Comparisons. This account of the South African health system gives only a sketchy picture of the results of apartheid policies. They permeate every aspect of the country's social resources and services. Beyond the obvious social conditions, apartheid dictates enormous disparities in the wages paid and incomes earned by the several racial groups, with impacts, of course, on every aspect of life. A few indicators of these differentials are shown in Table 9.7.

The profound interracial health inequities are reflected in the division of health expenditures between public and private sectors. We have noted that of all health expenditures, 49.0 percent come from public sources, but these are the main support of the nonwhite population, constituting 83.8 percent of the total. (They also support services for a significant fraction of the whites.) The European whites, constituting 16.2 percent of the people, are benefited mainly by the private sector, which accounts for some 51.0 percent of the total health expenditures.

Regarding hospitals, the availability of beds is extremely uneven. In 1975, the disparity in overall (both public and private) bed supplies was 16.3 beds per 1,000 whites and 3.0 beds per 1,000 blacks. (This ignores the far greater need for hospitalization among blacks.) Since 1975, the disparity has become greater, especially because of the construction of many private hospitals exclusively for whites. The public hospitals used by the Africans, furthermore,

Table 9.7. Some Social Indicators of Interracial Differences in South Africa, about 1980

Indicator	White	Colored	Asian	African
Average annual income per wage earner (rands)	9,207	3,042	4,032	2,267
Education: per capita annual expenditure (rands)	1,021	580	286	176
Old-age pensions—average per year (rands)	1,010	534	532	269
Life expectancy at birth (years)	68.7	50.9	58.8	46.2

Source: Champak, C. J., H. M. Coovadia, and S. S. Abdool Karim, "Socio-Medical Indicators of Health in South Africa," *International Journal of Health Services,* 16(1):163–176, 1986.

are typically deteriorated, overcrowded, and provided with much lower operating funds per bed than those used by whites. The latter are well financed and have low occupancy levels.

The availability of qualified physicians also differs enormously for the races. In 1975, of all registered doctors in South Africa, 66 percent practiced in metropolitan cities, where white people are concentrated. Forty percent of the doctors are settled in the two largest cities (Johannesburg and Cape Town) which contain 11 percent of the population. Only 6 percent of doctors are located in the villages and rural areas where 50 percent of the population, almost all black Africans, lives. The homeland areas, with about 40 percent of the black population, have about 500 doctors in all; this means one physician to 21,000 people or 4.7 doctors per 100,000. The equipment and facilities for medical practice, furthermore, are extremely deficient.

These differentials, of course, follow from many causes, including the admission policies of the medical schools. In 1979, the racial composition of medical students was almost the exact converse of that in the general population. In that year the proportions were as follows:

	Percent of	
Racial Group	*Population*	*Medical Students*
White	17.3	84.8
Colored	9.4	1.8
Asian	2.9	8.3
Black	70.4	5.1
All groups	100.0	100.0

Perhaps it is remarkable that, with their miserable primary and secondary schooling, even 5.1 percent of medical students are Africans.

The salaries of black health workers at all levels are much lower than those of their white counterparts. Overall expenditures for the health care of blacks, compared with whites, is not easy to calculate from the figures officially released by the South African government. One can compare per capita expenditures for health in the homelands, settled entirely by blacks, however, with such expenditures in the entire neighboring provinces, which contain both white and black populations. As of 1981, the comparative expenditures in three regions were as follows:

	Annual Health Expenditures Per Capita (Rands)	
Region	*Province*	*Homeland*
Natal	73.63	19.02
Cape	99.34	25.39
Transvaal	57.23	25.26

In light of all the racism and associated oppression in South Africa, one must admire the struggles of some courageous people to achieve greater equality. Thus, in Cape Town, the leadership of university medical professors has led to a policy of almost completely integrated patient care in the main teaching hospital. A National Medical and Dental Association (NAMDA) has been formed, with the deliberate objective of bringing together health professionals of all racial backgrounds, to extend their strongest efforts to achieve social justice in the South African health system.

In the larger political arena, the struggles of the African National Congress and other movements inside the country, and countless supporters of democracy in South Africa working in other countries, are well known. The effects of social and economic pressures from outside may be subject to debate, but there is much evidence that they have succeeded in forcing the South African government to reduce some of its most extreme forms of oppression.

With the large role played by government in the health system of South Africa, some may question the placement of this system in an "entrepreneurial" category. In a purely legalistic and econometric sense, all of the people are theoretically entitled to governmentally financed health services, and almost half of total health expenditures come from public sources. The atrociously poor services provided to nonwhite people, however, for the 49 percent of health expenditures (in 1982) derived from public sources (much of this money, in fact, channeled to services for whites) must be recognized. This is not to mention the candidly inhumane attitudes of government and private enterprise toward the great majority of the population who are black. These antisocial realities permit no other conceptual decision. Within the one-sixth of the population of European background, who rule the country, the objective is clearly to maximize private entrepreneurial health service, and to orient all public policy toward that end.

SUMMARY COMMENT

Regarding all four countries discussed in this chapter—Thailand, the Philippines, Republic of Korea, and South Africa—certain general features stand out. The disparities between high-income and low-income people are enormous; an extreme maldistribution of material wealth causes corresponding inequalities in housing, nutrition, education, and general standards of living. Associated with these inequalities are extreme disparities in the resources and all conditions of life between the main cities and the rural areas. Yet many rural people, seeking a better life, migrate to periurban slums. Public policy in all four countries favors the maximum development of private enterprise, even with deliberate planning, as the path to economic development. Public policy is also violently opposed to communism and socialism, applying strongly repressive measures to any social activity

deemed to be even faintly suggestive of such orientations.

In the health systems of these countries, the quantity and quality of health services, both personal and environmental, show gross disparities between population groups, equivalent to their income levels. Expenditures for health, in spite of the massive poverty of most of the people, are drawn largely from private sources, which constitute the majority of health expenditures and far more than the percentage of affluent families in the populations of each of the countries. In spite of governmental efforts to develop organized health service for the poor, most of the available time of physicians and pharmacists is spent on selling their services to patients for private fees. The delivery of health care from private medical and pharmaceutical quarters is the predominant pattern. This is true even when the financial support for medical care has been collectivized through either social or voluntary insurance. In all these systems, the provision of primary health care by auxiliary personnel in local health units has been generally unsatisfactory; this has led people to travel greater distances to hospital outpatient departments, to purchase self-selected drugs in commercial drugstores, or to consult private physicians or private traditional healers, when they could afford the price.

It is especially noteworthy that in all of these entrepreneurial health systems of transitional countries, even governmental health facilities typically require payment of some private fee, if the patient can possibly afford it. Personal health expenditures, therefore, are made for services from both private and public providers. In the rather extensive medical care insurance programs of the Philippines and South Korea, furthermore, fees are paid for the services of private physicians and private hospitals—a departure from the health insurance delivery patterns in nearly all other developing countries. When faced with the inevitable abuses of overservicing under this private fee pattern, these systems have simply reduced the insurance benefits through large increases in the personal copayments imposed on the patient. The entrepreneurial interests of the private sector are evidently regarded as outweighing the health care interests of the population.

REFERENCES

Thailand

Bureau of the Budget, *Thailand's Budget in Brief: Fiscal Year 1978*. Bangkok, 1978.

Cook, Michael J., and Boonlert Leoprapai, *Some Observations on Abortion in Thailand*. Bangkok: Mahidol University, Institute for Population and Social Research, November 1974.

Day, Frederick A., and Boonlert Leoprapai, *Patterns of Health Utilization in Upcountry Thailand*. Bangkok: Mahidol University, Institute for Population and Social Research, December 1977.

de Ferranti, David, "Strategies for Paying for Health Services in Developing Countries." *World Health Statistics (Health Costs and Financing),* 37(4):428–450, 1984.

Donaldson, Peter J., "Foreign Intervention in Medical Education: A Case Study of the Rockefeller Foundation's Involvement in a Thai Medical School." *International Journal of Health Services,* 6(2):251–270, 1976.

Government of Thailand, *Fourth National Economic and Social Development Plan 1977–1981*. Bangkok: National Economic and Social Development Board, 1976.

Komol Keemthong Foundation, *Monks and Community Development*. Bangkok, 1977.

Kunstadter, Peter, "Do Cultural Differences Make Any Difference? Choice Points in Medical Systems Available in Northwestern Thailand," in Arthur Kleinman et al. (Editors), *Culture and Healing in Asian Societies,* Cambridge, Mass.: Schenkman Pub. Co., 1978, pp. 185–217.

Mahidol University, Institute for Population and Social Research, *The Morbidity and Mortality Differentials, ASEAN Population Programme, Phase III Thailand,* May 1987.

Ministry of Interior, Department of Public Welfare, *Facts and Figures as of January 1978*. Bangkok, 1978.

Ministry of Public Health, *The Lampong Health Development Project: A Case Study in Integrated Rural Health Care*. Bangkok, November 1978.

Ministry of Public Health, *Primary Health Care in Thailand*. Bangkok, 1978.

Ministry of Public Health, *Public Health Statistics 1977–1981*. Bangkok, Thailand, 1983.

Ministry of Public Health, *Report on the Result of Survey of the Utilization of Health Manpower and Expenses Incurred in Medical Treatment of the People*. Bangkok (processed), 1970.

Ministry of Public Health, *The Role of Provincial Hospitals and Community Health Departments in Integrated Health Services*. Chiang Mai, Thailand, November 1978.

Ministry of Public Health—*Summary Final Report of the Lampong Health Development Project, Vol. 1*. Bangkok, 1981.

Ministry of Public Health, *Thailand Health Profile*. Bangkok, 1980.

Ministry of Public Health, *Village Health Communicators and Village Health Volunteer Scheme 1977–1981*. Bangkok, 1977.

Ministry of Public Health and Mahidol University, *Community Household Survey*. Bangkok, 1981.

Muangman, Debhanom, *New Approach to Rural Health Care in Thailand and Its Possible Application to Other Developing Countries*. New Delhi: World Health Organization, South East Asia Regional Conference on Schools of Public Health, November 1978.

Muangman, Debhanom, *The Role of Drugstores in the People's Health*. Bangkok: Mahidol University, Faculty of Public Health, 1974.

Myers, Charles N., Dow Mongkolsmai, and Nancyanne Causino, *Financing Health Services and Medical Care in Thailand*. Bangkok: U.S. Agency for International Development, April 1985.

National Statistical Office (Office of the Prime Minister), *Preliminary Report of National Census Survey 1980*. Bangkok, 1980.

Nondasuta, Amorn, and Prapont Piyaratn, "Basic Minimum Needs." *World Health Forum,* June 1987, pp. 14–15.

Pisamai, Chantavimol, *Public Health in Thailand*. Bangkok: Ministry of Public Health, Health Planning Division, 1981.

Porapakkham, Yawarat, *Songkhla—Integrated Rural Development Model*. Bangkok: Mahidol University, Faculty of Public Health, December 1977.

Riley, James Nelson, and Santhat Sermsri, *The Variegated Thai Medical System as a Context for Birth Control Services*. Bangkok: Mahidol University, Institute for Population and Social Research, June 1974.

Roemer, Milton I., *The Health Care System of Thailand: A Case Study*. New Delhi: World Health Organization, Regional Office for South-East Asia (South-East Asia Series No. 11), 1981.

Secter, Bob, "Teen 'Pharmacists': In Thailand, Drugstore A Risky Place." *Los Angeles Times,* 16 November 1982, pp. 1, 12.

Snoh, Unakol, *National Development Strategy of Thailand*. Bangkok: National Economic and Social Development Board, 1982.

Southeast Asian Medical Information Center, *SEAMIC Health Statistics 1978*. Tokyo, 1978.

Tongpan, Saowaros, "Health Planning Process: Thailand," in *Consultative Meeting on Health Planning Process in ASEAN Countries,* Jakarta, Indonesia: U.N. Asian Development Institute, March 1977, pp. 179–189.

Umphol, Chindawatana, *Analysis of Health Manpower in Thailand*. Bangkok: Ministry of Public Health, Health Planning Division, 1983.

United Nations Fund for Population Studies, *Thai-*

land: Report of Second Mission on Needs Assessment for Population Assistance. New York: UNFPA Report No. 55, May 1983.

Varakamin, Somsak, and Debhanom Muangman, *Health Problems in Thailand.* Honolulu: University of Hawaii, March 1976.

Wasi, Prawase, "Thailand," in John Z. Bowers and Elizabeth F. Purcell (Editors), *The Impact of Health Services on Medical Education: A Global View.* New York: Josiah Macy Jr. Foundation, 1979, pp. 279–304.

Wongpanich, Malinee, *Statistical Survey of Industrial Premises in the Bangkok Metropolitan Area on the Health Protection of Workers.* Bangkok: Mahidol University, Faculty of Public Health, December 1977.

Woolley, Paulo, *Syncrisis: The Dynamics of Health—Thailand.* Washington, D.C.: U.S. Office of International Health, June 1974.

Yoddumnern, Benja, *The Role of Thai Traditional Doctors.* Bangkok: Mahidol University, Institute for Population and Social Research, 1974.

World Bank, *Thailand: Appraisal of a Population Project.* Washington, D.C.: Bank Report No. 1663-TH, January 1978.

Republic of the Philippines

Akin, John S., et al., "The Demand for Adult Outpatient Services in the Bicol Region of the Philippines." *Social Science and Medicine,* 22(3):321–328, 1986.

Anon., "Philippine Health Care: Good MDs Work in Poor, Overextended Facilities." *American Medical News,* 14 March 1986, pp. 3 ff.

Denoga, José C., "The Philippines," in International Social Security Association, *Medical Care under Social Security in Developing Countries.* Geneva, 1981, pp. 83–89.

Fineman, Mark, "Neglected for Years—Health Care: Philippines Crisis Looms." *Los Angeles Times,* 6 March 1987, pp. 1 ff.

Roemer, Milton I., "Political Ideology and Health Care: Hospital Patterns in the Philippines and Cuba." *International Journal of Health Services,* 3(3):487–492, 1973.

Sen, Pedro, "Financing of Medical Care Insurance in the Philippines." *International Social Security Association Bulletin,* 1975, No. 2, pp. 139–150.

Tadiar, Alfredo F., "Legitimating Change: The Expanded Role of the Filipino Professional Paramedical in the Delivery of Family Planning Services." *Philippine Law Journal,* 51:428–439, 1976.

United Nations Fund for Population Activities, *Report of Mission on Needs Assessment for Population Activities: Philippines.* New York: UNFPA (Report No. 19), August 1979.

U.S. Office of International Health, *Syncrisis: The Dynamics of Health—The Philippines.* Washington, D.C.: U.S. Department of Health, Education, and Welfare, July 1972.

World Bank, *Population, Health and Nutrition in the Philippines: A Sector Review.* (Volume II: Main Report with Tables and Technical Annexes). Washington, D.C., January 1984.

Republic of Korea

Dunlop, David W., et al., *Korean Health Demonstration Project.* Washington, D.C.: U.S. Agency for International Development (Project Impact Evaluation No. 36), July 1982.

Kwon, S. W., *Trends in National Health Expenditures and Policy Issues of Cost Containment in Korea.* Seoul: Korean Development Institute (Working Paper No. 8809), 1988.

Ministry of Health and Social Affairs, *Major Policies and Programmes in Health and Social Welfare Services.* Seoul, 1981 (processed document).

Moon, Ok-Ryun, *The National Health Insurance Policy in Korea.* Seoul: Seoul National University, School of Public Health, 1987.

Moon, Ok-Ryun, "Towards Equity in Health Care." *World Health,* May 1986, pp. 20–21.

Park, Chong Kee, *Financing Health Care Services in Korea.* Seoul: Korea Development Institute, July 1977.

Park, Chong Kee, *Planning and Coordination of Social Security Medical Systems with Public Health Programs.* Seoul: Korea Development Institute (Monograph 8102), July 1981.

United Nations Fund for Population Activities, *Report of Mission on Needs Assessment for Population Assistance: Republic of Korea.* New York: UNFPA Report No. 47, April 1982.

Yu, Seung-Hum, and Timothy Baker, *Health Insurance and Utilization of Hospital Services in Korea.* Seoul: Yonsei University, 1982 (processed document).

South Africa

Benatar, S. R., "Medicine and Health Care in South Africa." *New England Journal of Medicine,* 315(8):527–532, 21 August 1986.

Botha, J. L., et al., "The Distribution of Health Needs and Services in South Africa." *Social Science and Medicine,* 26(8):845–851, 1988.

de Beer, Cedric, *The South African Disease: Apartheid, Health and Health Services.* Trenton, N.J.: Africa World Press, 1984.

Jinabhai, C. C., H. M. Coovadia, and S. S. Abdool-Karim, "Socio-Medical Indicators of Health in South Africa." *International Journal of Health Services,* 16(1):163–176, 1986.

Price, Max, "Health Care as an Instrument of Apartheid Policy in South Africa." *Health Policy and Planning,* 1(2):158–170, 1986.

Price, Max, "The Consequences of Health Service Privatization for Equality and Equity in Health

Care in South Africa." *Social Sciences and Medicine,* c. 1988, (publication pending).

Sigerist, Henry E., "A Physician's Impression of South Africa," in M. I. Roemer (Editor), *Henry E. Sigerist on the Sociology of Medicine.* New York: MD Publications, 1960, pp. 267–272.

Susser, Mervyn W., "Apartheid and the Causes of Death: Disentangling Ideology and Laws from Class and Race." *American Journal of Public Health,* 73:581–583, 1983.

World Health Organization, *Apartheid and Health.* Geneva: WHO (Report of an International Conference held at Brazzaville, People's Republic of the Congo, November 1981), 1983.

Yach, Derek, "The Impact of Political Violence on Health and Health Services in Cape Town, South Africa, 1986: Methodological Problems and Preliminary Results." *American Journal of Public Health,* 78(7):772–776, July 1988.

CHAPTER TEN

Welfare-Oriented Health Systems in Transitional Countries of Latin America

In contrast to the countries discussed in Chapter 9, many other countries at a similar economic level have taken substantial actions to make modern health services available to their populations. We describe their health systems as welfare-oriented, since they place a higher priority on human welfare than on purely entrepreneurial considerations in a marketplace.

Most of these welfare-oriented health systems are in Latin America, where national independence from European colonial control was won in the early nineteenth century, more than 160 years ago. Others are in Asia and the Middle East, where freedom from foreign domination was achieved more recently. Because of the diversity and complexity of these numerous health systems, we need two chapters to analyze them—those in Latin America here and those elsewhere in Chapter 11. Illustrative of the welfare-oriented systems in Latin America is that in the region's largest country, Brazil.

BRAZIL

Brazil is the largest country in Latin America, in both territory and population. Its population in 1984 was 136,300,000, of whom 73 percent lived in cities and 27 percent in rural areas. In 1985 Brazil's GNP was $1,640 per capita—a figure that does not reflect the enormous differentials between wealthy families in the south and impoverished ones in the north. Data on income distribution are not available for a recent year, but in 1972 (after rapid industrial development was already well under

way) the highest 20 percent of households earned 66.6 percent of the national income, while the lowest 20 percent of households earned a total of 2 percent.

Social Background

The land that is now Brazil was visited by both Spanish and Portuguese explorers in the fifteenth century, but in 1494 it was conceded to belong in Portugal's sphere of influence. The first permanent urban settlement of Europeans was in 1532 where Sao Paulo is now located. Over the next two centuries, other countries tried to stake out claims in this large land until, in 1822, Brazil's independence was declared. A monarch of Portuguese descent ruled until 1889, however, when a republican form of government was achieved. In the mid-nineteenth century, extensive migration from several European countries contributed to the economic development of southeast Brazil, and a further economic boom came with World War II. Industrialization, mining, and general socioeconomic development, however, were heavily concentrated in the region around Sao Paulo and nearby Rio de Janeiro, while the north and especially northeastern regions remained very poor.

In 1964, following a period of economic recession and inflation, a military coup occurred, and the country came under the control of various military groups for more than 20 years. The years 1966 through 1976 were a time of rapid economic growth, described by some as the "Brazilian economic miracle." The GNP per capita grew rapidly, along with heavy urbanization. Between 1960 and 1980, Brazil changed from a nation with 65 percent rural people and 35 percent urban to the very converse, even though many of the new city-dwellers were people living in periurban slums, or *favelas.*

The period of economic boom (1966–1976) gave rise to actions that led to economic and social problems in the years ahead. Enormous investments were made in various enterprises, based on loans from foreign banks. The buoyant economic attitude led to construction of hundreds of private hospitals, among other things. Then around 1974 the international oil crisis began, with a world monopoly launched by the Organization of Petroleum Exporting Countries (OPEC). The impact on Brazil became serious around 1976, and a period of economic decline set in. The large foreign debt accumulated could not be repaid, and vast efforts were needed simply to pay the interest on the loans. Unemployment rose steadily, and inflation became more serious week by week. The worldwide recession, beginning in the United States around 1980–1981, made matters worse. In 1984, unemployment was reported to be 12 percent, but many people said it was really higher, and was compounded by great underemployment and partial employment. The maldistribution of wealth was aggravated further. Mounting discontent led to elections in 1985, and civilian parliamentary government was resumed in Brazil that year.

All of these developments, in both the period of boom and the ensuing decline, had a major impact on the health system. In the boom period, government policy was to encourage more and more private investment. The construction of private hospitals and the increased output of health personnel were integral parts of the general expansionary movement. When the decline set in, there were inevitable repercussions on living conditions influencing health, on the collection of revenues and social insurance contributions supporting medical care programs, and on the employment of health personnel, along with others. When hospitals are half empty and doctors have few private patients, abuses of various sorts are generated, as we shall see later.

This is only the sketchiest review of social and political events affecting the health system of Brazil. The numerous other social forces, inside the country and from abroad, will be evident as we analyze first the various features of the organizational structure of the system.

Organizational Structure

The structural configuration of Brazil's health system is especially complex. As in all Latin American settings, the cultural and political influences on the system have been so diverse, each with its distinctive characteristics, that our analysis departs somewhat from the model applied in the chapters on other countries. We start with a brief note about traditional healing, because it is the oldest element in the structure that still exists. Then we examine the first impact on Brazil of "modern civilization," mediated through the religious accompanists of Europen colonialism. Finally, we examine the several impacts of sociolpolitical forces maturing in the twentieth century and operating prominently today.

Traditional Healing. Before European colonists set foot on Latin America, the thousands of native Indian people depended on many types of healers for treating their ills. They used magic to invoke spiritual powers for exorcising disease from the body, but some healers also used herbs and other physical measures. In isolated areas of Brazil, such as the Amazon river valley and the Andean mountains, where unmixed Indian tribes are still found, magical healers or "witch doctors" still function. But, considering the Brazilian population as a whole, as modern medical services have become available, including countless drugs available in pharmacies and other places, the role of the ancient healer has declined.

The traditional healers, in current times, invoke the spirit not only of ancient Indian gods, but also of Catholic saints. Their decline, however, has been due to several factors. One is the decline in rurality of the population. A second factor is the increase in general literacy. Third is the greater availability of modern medical care resources, for which no charges are made. Fourth, in Brazil, as in most Latin American countries, magical healing has been banned by law. Unlike policies in many Asian and African nations, the healer, or *curandero,* is not registered with the government and is, in fact, considered illegal.

The number of healers, and the extent of their use in Brazil are not known, but a survey made in the mid-1960s in a neighboring country, Colombia, had findings that are probably relevant. A nationwide sample of the population was interviewed and asked to report any services for illness in the previous 2 weeks. The sample was large (nearly 60,000 persons), and thousands of health care encounters were analyzed. Of all encounters, it was found that in the urban population the contacts with traditional healers were 3.4 percent of all health care contacts, and in the rural population it was 17 percent; the overall national rate was 11 percent of health care contacts. This was about 1965, and the rate is doubtless lower now.

Attitudes of the people, and also of governments, toward traditional birth attendants (TBAs) are quite different. In most developing countries on all continents, TBAs are accepted and even trained by ministries of health. In Brazil, nevertheless, except in the northeast region, even the TBA has declined in importance. The proportion of childbirths occurring in hospitals has steadily increased. By 1981, for all Brazil this proportion had reached nearly 80 percent. Many of these infants are delivered by midwives, but these women are trained and working in hospitals under supervision. The nonhospitalized childbirths are heavily concentrated in the northeast region. Of this 20 percent of births in the nation, 84 percent is still delivered by TBAs, or 17 percent of the national total. This is, of course, a much smaller share than prevailed in previous years.

Charitable and Voluntary Health Services. As in most of Latin America, the earliest systematic organization of medical care in Brazil was undertaken by priests of the Catholic Church. Seeking help from wealthy laypeople, they formed welfare societies that came to be known as *Santas casas da misericordia,* or holy houses of mercy. (In Spanish-speaking countries they were *beneficencias publicas.*) The original *Santas casas* in Brazil typically operated homes for the elderly, orphanages, and cemeteries, as well as hospitals. Before 1960, santa casa hospitals were the most numerous type in Brazil, in both number of facilities and aggregate beds.

The typical santa casa hospital in 1950 was a dull and sordid building, or group of small buildings, with large wards (20 to 30 beds), very limited sanitation and medical equipment, relatively few nurses (directed usually by nuns), and medical services given by a handful of doctors, making periodic visits for small annual honoraria. They were often located near cathedrals in the large cities, and their patients were the urban poor, who were the great majority of the city populations.

As standards of medical care rose generally, and as the earnings of these charitable societies declined, they had to become subsidized by government, usually the Ministry of Health, to continue in operation. In several Latin American countries, these hospitals were taken over completely by the ministries, even though they retained their saintly names and sometimes even kept the church-dominated boards of directors for certain limited functions. In Brazil, the santa casa facilities still exist to a large extent, but their character, financing, and mode of operation have become very different. Ownership, in general, still remains with the boards of local citizens, but the hospital services are no longer oriented to the poor, nor are they financed mainly from charitable sources. Santa casa hospitals now serve principally persons insured by the social security program (see following), and they are financed almost entirely by payments from this source. Usually a small proportion of beds, under 10 percent, is reserved for patients who are not insured and indigent.

Many santa casa hospitals have been essentially turned over to private physicians for their entire management. These facilities have generally been remodeled and are much better staffed and equipped than previously. Although they remain theoretically nonprofit, they have the appearance of private for-profit (proprietary) hospitals. The modernization of many santa casa hospitals has been financed by loans from the Ministry of Health. The lotteries, formerly operated by the santas casas, are now run by the government; the lottery proceeds go to a national *Fund for Social Development* (FAS), from which grants or loans are made for hospital construction. A National Federation of Santas Casas has been formed, and it is attempting to revive a greater role for the local boards through community participation in health policy matters.

Aside from the initially charitable santa casa hospitals, other voluntary nonprofit organizations in Brazil play small parts in the health system. The Brazilian Red Cross gives health services in natural disasters, and it is partially subsidized by the Ministry of Health. There are also a few voluntary health agencies in the larger cities, concerned with special problems, such as cancer or crippled children.

In some isolated rural areas, such as the Amazon jungle, religious missions from other countries operate small hospitals and clinics. Patients may be asked to pay small fees for the services, but the missionary personnel receive no compensation beyond their living requirements.

Beneficencias privadas are cooperative societies of families who typically have immigrated to Brazil from certain parts of Portugal or from other countries. They charge a relatively large membership fee to join, and they require annual dues. Some of these societies own and operate hospitals for their own members, and occasionally give free care to an indigent person from the same ethnic group.

Ministry of Health. Brazil is, today, a federation of 22 states, plus a federal district (Brasilia). In the central government, under law, the major health authority is the Ministry of Health (MOH), although its command of funds is much less than that of the Social Security program, as we shall see. The MOH originated in 1904 as the Public Health Directorate under the Ministry of Justice, and was later transferred to the Ministry of Education as the National Public Health Department. Only in 1953, did it become the cabinet-level MOH, with corresponding Secretariats of Health in each of the states. With the enormous growth of funding, as well as functions, in the social security system, the MOH has actually declined in importance in recent years,

and its health responsibilities are essentially more supportive than operational. Between 1978 and 1982, the MOH share of total health-related expenditures, from all branches of government in Brazil, declined from 13.9 to 10.4 percent of the total.

Ministry of Health functions in Brazil can now be classified under three main groups: (a) sanitary vigilance, such as control of food and drugs; (b) basic health services, including communicable disease control, health education, and surveillance of environmental sanitation; and (c) organization of health services, including health planning, human resources, and administrative modernization. In many fields, such as communicable disease control or public health laboratory services, the ministry sets standards that the state health secretariats are expected to follow. Most of the ministry's responsibilities, however, are dispatched by making grants to the states, which involve 60 percent of its budget. The ministry has therefore been called simply a "big bank," which passes federal money on to the states.

To a limited extent, the federal Ministry of Health operates special hospitals, such as those for mental disorder or leprosy. These constitute only 2.0 percent of the beds nationally. More important is the ministry's close integration with the Foundation for Special Public Health Services (SESP in the Portuguese acronym), which was initially set up with funding from the U.S. Institute of Inter-American Affairs in 1942, during World War II. The SESP Foundation, within the framework of the MOH, operates several hundred health centers in isolated and difficult areas, such as the Amazon region. With its quasi-independent status and external financial support, SESP is able to pay higher than regular MOH salaries and attract exceptionally well-qualified full-time personnel. The health centers offer comprehensive primary health care, but they emphasize preventive services for mothers and children. The SESP program was estimated in 1984 to be giving services to 8 percent of the national population.

Relatively independent of the Ministry of Health are the Secretariats of Health in each of the 23 states. As noted, they follow certain technical standards laid down by the national ministry, and they receive financial grants (much larger grants per capita going to the poorer states), but their general programs and policies are determined autonomously. The state secretary of health is appointed by the governor of each state, who is elected. Likewise other state health employees are appointed locally. Certain national functions (e.g., the registration of health personnel or food sanitation) are delegated to the states from the national ministry, but most are undertaken at the state's own initiative. Activities in maternal and child health, mental disease control, adult health (detection of diabetes, hypertension, etc.), occupational health, dental fluoridation, and so on are carried out directly by the state secretariats of health.

The state secretariats are also responsible for the delivery of medical care in their own hospitals, health centers, and health stations. They control hospitals, both general and special, with 9.1 percent of the country's total beds. They operate hundreds of health centers which, in the past, concentrated on preventive service, but now increasingly offer medical treatment to ambulatory patients. It is noteworthy that in the state of Sao Paulo, Brazil's most populous and wealthiest state, the top priority for 1985 was emphasizing primary medical care as a function of its 850 health centers. Emergency units, staffed by doctors 24 hours a day, are also operated by the state secretariats of health.

The lowest level of government under MOH surveillance, through the state secretariats of health, is the municipality (equivalent to a county). Brazil has about 4,000 municipalities altogether; most of these are quite small and poor, but the larger ones, especially major cities, have municipal secretariats of health, which have public health responsibilities and may operate hospitals and health centers. Hospitals under municipal control are general or special (such as for maternity or the care of children), and in 1983 they contained 4.3 percent of the hospital beds in Brazil.

In past years, the Brazilian MOH, like many other Latin American health ministries, competed with the usually more affluent social security program. It is noteworthy, therefore, that many of the health facilities of both the

state and municipal secretaries of health are now significantly subsidized by the social security program.

Social Security Program. After the pioneering social security law of Chile in 1924, legislation of the same sort, to finance medical care of workers, was enacted in Brazil in 1934. A very limited public medical care program for railroad workers has operated since 1923, but in 1934 legislation authorized mandatory insurance contributions by employees and employers to build up a large fund for financing medical care and other social benefits. The insurance mechanism was to be applied separately for various occupational groups.

The first occupational group for which a social insurance institute *(instituto de previdencia social)* was established in 1934 was commercial workers. Soon after, a second *instituto* was established for industrial workers, and then came autonomous institutes for transport workers, utility workers, maritime workers, bank workers, and federal civil servants. By 1960, there were seven separate social insurance institutes for these several occupational groups. Altogether, they enrolled 4,060,000 workers who, with their dependents, consisted of about 15,000,000 people. This covered around 25 percent of the national population of Brazil at the time. Noticeably absent from insurance coverage, however, were Brazil's agricultural workers, who were the largest occupational category of all.

The manner in which medical care was provided for covered persons varied among the several institutes, but on the whole it was substantially different from the national health insurance pattern that had grown up in Europe. Instead of using insurance money to pay private doctors and local (private or public) hospitals for their services, the institutes established and staffed their own polyclinics (and a little later, hospitals), staffed by doctors and other personnel on salaries. The doctors were often part-time, being paid for 3 or 4 hours of service a day. Likewise, drugs were dispensed by the institute's own pharmacies. Persons covered by each institute used that institute's facilities. This method of direct provision of health service by the social insurance program was much more economical and fiscally predictable than the "indirect" method of contracting with independent providers, paid by fee-for-service, as in Europe.

This direct pattern of medical care could be implemented in Brazil and elsewhere in Latin America for several reasons. The medical profession, in contrast to that in Western Europe, was relatively weak, and could not insist on maintaining independent private practices; doctors were happy to get regular salaries. The workers, in turn, were accustomed to care in organized clinics; they did not demand private settings. Third, the whole level of insurance contributions in Latin America was relatively low, so that the most prudent and economical use of insurance funds was essential.

These factors explain the predominance of the direct pattern of medical care in Brazil, but it was not the only pattern; polyclinic buildings, and especially hospitals, could not be constructed and all the necessary administrative procedures organized as rapidly as enrollment was expanding. Therefore, it was necessary in later years to pay private physicians and hospitals, under contract, for the care of some insured people. Development of hospitals was especially expensive, and it was some years before enough of them could be built.

With seven separate social insurance institutes serving different occupational groups, diversities in financing, services, and administration were inevitable. Demands therefore arose for greater coordination, in the interests of administrative efficiency, economies of scale (e.g., in purchasing drugs and supplies), and also equity. In 1960, therefore, a new "organic social security law" was passed, requiring greater uniformity in policies and cooperation among the several insurance institutes.

In 1967, 3 years after the origin of military government, a law was passed to amalgamate the seven institutes. It took a few years to implement, but the policy changed, to permit a person belonging to any one of the institutes to be served by a hospital or ambulatory care facility of any of the other institutes. Initially the unified program was known as the *Instituto Nacional da Previdencia Social* (INPS); however, autonomy was maintained by the program for government employees, IPASE. It

must be recalled that the entire social security program provided not only medical services, but also monetary benefits for pensions (retirement) and disability.

In 1975, with Brazil still in a period of great economic prosperity, an important new law was passed. The government decided that the time had come to greatly extend the coverage of the social security program, in both its medical and its monetary aspects. Law Number 6229, of 17 July 1975, provided for the organization of a National Health System. Several ministries would be involved in developing policies and administrative practices in the program: (a) the Ministry of Health for general policy, with special reference to prevention and health promotion, (b) the Ministry of Social Security and Assistance (Ministerio da Previdencia e Assistencia Social) for direct personal medical care, (c) the Ministry of Education and Culture for training of health personnel, (d) the Ministry of Interior for environmental sanitation, (e) the Ministry of Labor for the health protection of workers, and (f) the states, territories, and municipalities.

Funds to support the program would come from several sources. The principal source was a tax shared by workers and employers. Self-employed persons were required to contribute the entire tax. In addition, funds were contributed by a special tax on agricultural products (2.0 percent) collected at the point of marketing, initiated in 1971—the FUNRURAL. (Agricultural workers were not taxed directly, but large agricultural employers were.) Certain funds also came from smaller sources, such as the National Foundation of Child Welfare (FUNABEM) and the Brazilian Assistance League (LBA).

For administrative purposes the overall program, or National System of Social Security and Welfare (SINPAS), was lodged principally in the Ministry of Social Security and Welfare (MPAS). To distinguish the medical aspects from the fiscal benefits, the medical side was administered by a National Institute of Medical Care in Social Security, or Instituto Nacional de Assistencia Medica da Previdencia Social (INAMPS). The fiscal benefits (pensions, etc.) were administered by another government agency. Thus, in the health system of

Brazil, it is INAMPS that has come to contribute the largest proportion of financial support to the cost of health services rendered by its own resources, as well as by those of many other sponsorships.

The 1975 law on a National Health System established entitlement or "insured status" to millions of people beyond those covered by the various specialized institutes in 1960. Virtually all employed persons and their dependents were covered, including the self-employed. Agricultural workers were covered, even though they made no direct contributions, and the FUNRURAL of 1971 raised much less money than the costs of their care. It is usually estimated that, altogether, between 80 and 90 percent (commonly stated as 83 percent) of the Brazilian population are currently entitled to medical and hospital care through the financial protection of INAMPS, to the extent feasible.

"The extent feasible," however, indicates an important limitation. The INAMPS program, and the institutes for medical care on which it was built, owned or controlled only a small fraction of the hospitals and ambulatory care facilities necessary to provide health services to 83 percent of the Brazilian population of more than 136,000,000 people. The solution reached was to make agreements and contracts for the use of other physical and human resources throughout the nation. The health care resources could be either public or private, and government policy since military control in 1964 had, indeed, been to encourage maximum development of the private sector in every field. In effect, the strategy designed in Brazil was to abandon the long-established Latin American pattern of direct provision of medical care in a social security body's own resources, and to adopt the European and North American pattern of using government funds largely to purchase health services provided indirectly by private and independent health care providers. (These could be private nonprofit or private for-profit resources, and they could also include units of state and local government.) As it turned out, the largest share of medical and hospital services to insured persons (and some others) was given by private entities—both nonprofit and for-profit. As we

Table 10.1. National Institute of Medical Care in Social Security (INAMPS): Budget Breakdown by Percentage Distribution in Brazil, 1984

Purpose	Percentage
Services in INAMPS own facilities	20.7
Services contracted with private entitles	49.9
Services by agreements with state or local governments	5.0
Help to university hospitals	3.2
Maintenance of drug supplies	1.8
Helping philanthropic entities	3.1
Helping syndicates provide care	1.5
Helping business enterprises	1.7
Helping to modernize installations	3.0
Support for retired INAMPS personnel	4.4
Contributions to government pension fund	0.5
General administration	5.2
Other	0.1
All purposes	100.0

Source: Brazil Ministry of Social Security and Social Assistance. Brasilia, 1984 (processed report).

will see later, many problems have arisen from these arrangements.

To give a better idea of the diverse mechanisms by which INAMPS provides medical and related services to its beneficiaries, we examine the INAMPS budget that was drawn up for 1984. This is presented in Table 10.1, based on data from the Ministry of Social Security and Social Assistance.

It is evident that about half of INAMPS expenditures goes to financing health services rendered under contract by private entities, one-fifth for services in its own hospitals, ambulatory care units, and other resources, and 5 percent for services rendered through agreements with secretariats of health in state and local governments. It should be noted that many of the latter are preventive services to mothers and children, and services for the control of tuberculosis and other communicable diseases. (In other words, social security supports public health activities.)

As we will see, the theoretical entitlement of 83 percent of the population to services, as insured persons, does not mean that these services are equally available to everyone. Inevitably the availability of medical care depends on the health resources accessible at different times and places in this large country. Means of transportation are obviously important.

Maintenance of insurance status is also crucial, and difficulties in Brazil's economic situation have meant that many persons have lost this protection in recent years.

Other Government Agenices. Several other federal ministries contribute to the national health system of Brazil. The Ministry of Interior, with its general responsibility for cities and towns, promotes and assists in the construction of public water supplies and sewage disposal systems. Surveillance of the proper maintenance of these resources is a task of the state public health authorities.

The Ministry of Education and Culture is responsible for the general supervision and a large part of the financing of the nation's universities. Less than half of Brazil's 76 medical schools are in public universities, but they have the largest enrollments, and many of the university-level nursing schools are public. Private universities also receive limited supervision from the Ministry of Education and Culture. Part of the costs of operating university teaching hospitals is also borne by this ministry.

Other federal government agencies with some concern for health include the Secretariat of Planning in the Presidency of the Republic, the Ministry of Justice (prison health), and the Ministry of Agriculture (diseases of animals and their control). Finally, like almost all countries, Brazil has a well-developed health program for its military forces.

Business Enterprises. In earlier years, before social security became highly developed in Brazil, large enterprises operated comprehensive medical care programs for their workers and often families. In 1960, there were dozens of such programs at mines, sugar refineries, automobile assembly plants, and other companies, sometimes operating hospitals and maintaining medical and nursing staffs with relatively high qualifications (usually paid salaries much higher than the average). Companies that provided these services were exempted from paying the share of social security contributions required for medical care.

In recent years, INAMPS has discouraged this type of special service for industrial workers as "elitist." Now the programs may continue to provide services, but they are simply financed by INAMPS on a contract basis, like other private hospitals and clinics. The same applies to medical care programs that were formerly operated by associations of private companies, such as the Servico Social da Industria (SESI).

Related to industrial medical services are ambulatory care centers operated by certain labor unions or syndicates, especially in agricultural areas. As indicated in Table 10.1, these are now subsidized through the INAMPS budget.

The Private Medical Market. The final part of the organizational structure of Brazil's health system, of course, is the private market of health care—modern and traditional. Quite aside from the extensive services of doctors, pharmacies, and other providers, financed by social security, most practitioners spend some time each week in conventional private practice. Some older physicians work exclusively as private practitioners. In recent years, many private doctors have formed medical groups or private clinics. Younger doctors may join such clinics as employees, to provide ambulatory care, and later become partners, sharing in the profits. The same applies in for-profit (proprietary) private hospitals, usually owned and operated by groups of private doctors. Private dental practice is also highly developed.

Private pharmacies are an important section of the private medical care market. As is shown later, among low-income families the largest share of personal spending for health services goes for purchasing drugs.

Finally, it must be realized that the provision of traditional healing, discussed earlier, is part of the private market. Even though the fees charged tend to be lower than those of modern practitioners, they must ordinarily be paid by patients in cash or barter. Aside from any beneficial effects of the service of tradiional practitioners that may or may not be demonstrable, the closeness of these healers to village people and their low prices are factors that help explain the survival of this form of health service.

Health Resources

Since about 1960, all types of human and physical resources in the health system of Brazil have greatly expanded. The period of rapid economic expansion, combined with the broader support for medical care by social security, has created economic support for more health personnel and facilities.

Health Manpower. Most impressive has been the increase in the national supply of physicians. In 1959 Brazil had 27,100 physicians or a ratio of about 40 per 100,000 population. By 1984, the number had increased to 122,800 or a ratio of 90.1 per 100,000.

The geographic distribution of these doctors, however, remains extremely uneven. In 1982, the prosperous southeast region of Brazil, had 175 doctors per 100,000, compared with 66 per 100,000 in the northern region. The northeast region also had a ratio of only 69 doctors per 100,000. Likewise for dentists in 1982, there were 79 per 100,000 in the southeast and 28 per 100,000 in the northeast.

The greatly enlarged supply of Brazilian doctors has come partly from an expansion in medical school enrollments, but principally from the rapid multiplication of medical schools. In 1960 there were 31 medical schools, almost entirely governmental and attached to public universities, with 1,600 graduates a year. By 1985, Brazil had 76 medical schools with 8,000 graduates a year. Some of the new schools are governmental (federal or state), but most are private. The basic curriculum in both types of school requires 6 years (5 academic years plus an internship before the degree is earned), but the private schools are commonly regarded as technically inferior and somewhat commercialized. Most of the professors are part-time and engaged principally in private practice. Yet the private tuition costs are high, while the public medical schools are almost free of charge (a nominal annual fee is payable). Altogether there are 43 private medical schools and 33 public schools, the public ones being larger.

With so many doctors in Brazil, competition among them has naturally been mounting. The great majority of doctors seek and obtain some type of salaried employment, with either a public or a private organization, or both. In addition, almost all employed doctors spend part of every day or every week in private practice. Holding three or four different positions is not unusual. The possible combinations of private and public posts is bewildering. A study in Sao Paulo in 1982 found 27 combinations of purely private activity carried out by the sample of doctors studied, and 36 combinations of private and public activity. In the total sample, 1.1 percent of doctors were unemployed or did only volunteer work.

This pattern of multiple types of employment creates obvious inefficiencies and abuses. Moving about a city every day to different clinics and hospitals is time-consuming; the doctor seldom becomes closely attached to any one team of health colleagues. More important is the abuse that occurs when the doctor, working in a public clinic (a public hospital out-patient department or an ambulatory care center), also works in a private clinic. It is well known that such doctors frequently advise public patients to visit them later at the private clinic for "better quality and more personal care." At both places the cost is paid by INAMPS—at the public place through a medical salary and in the private practice through a fee. The entire fee-for-service method of remuneration inevitably generates superfluous services that command payments, most extravagantly for hospitalization. Thus, in 1981 government-sponsored facilities provided 43 percent of ambulatory services, but these led to 86 percent of hospital admissions, predominantly in private institutions. Of course, the difficulties caused by multiple medical positions ultimately result in the low salary levels in organized health programs of all types. In effect, private practice and private fees are indirectly encouraged by government, to enable it to recruit doctors at low cost. In the end, Brazilian medical incomes become relatively high—nine times the per capita GDP (gross domestic product), a higher ratio than that in most developed countries.

To represent physicians in negotiations on salaries and related matters, there is a *Syndicato dos Medicos* in each state and also a national Federation of Medical Syndicates. In addition, the Brazilian Medical Association, with branches in each state, is intended to be a scientific body, which also oversees qualifications for the specialties. (Residencies for training in the specialties are all tied to medical schools.) A third body, the Conseillo da Medicina, is concerned with medical ethics, and every new graduate is legally required to join it.

The great emphasis in Brazil, and in Latin America generally, on training physicians has been due in part to a traditionally negative attitude toward the use of auxiliary personnel. South America was the last of the developing regions to respond to the World Health Organization's (WHO) call for briefly trained *community health workers* to provide primary health care in rural areas. Limited training projects for such personnel were started in the 1980s, but the major rural health strategy in Brazil (and neighboring countries) was to depend on auxiliary nurses, theoretically serving under medical supervision.

As in most Latin American countries, the Brazilian supply of professional nurses—that is, nurses fully trained after high school—is less than that of physicians. The proportion of young women who complete high school (secondary school) is relatively small, they tend to be from the upper social classes, and most who have gone this far academically prefer to go on to the university to study a field with greater social status than nursing. As a result, Brazil, like many other countries, must depend largely on nonprofessional (or less than fully trained) nursing personnel, to meet most of its needs.

In 1983, the Federal Council of Nurses estimated that Brazil had a total of about 160,000 nursing personnel of all types. A breakdown for 1982 (when the number was smaller) showed the following:

Fully registered nurses (college level)	22,452
High school–level nurses	71,739
Auxiliary nurses	44,673
Total	138,864

It should be noted that fully registered nurses are regarded as college level because, to attract greater numbers, they have been granted university credentials and are trained (after high school) for 4 or 5 years. There are 80 such college-level schools in Brazil, graduating 3,000 nurses a year. The high school–level graduates, sometimes known as *technical-level* nurses, receive 3 years of training (after 6 or 8 years of schooling) entirely in a hospital, without any university linkage. The auxiliary nurses are undoubtedly more numerous than the preceding figure indicates, because most of them are not listed with the Federal Council of Nurses. They are trained for 1 or 2 years after elementary school (6 years), usually in a hospital, but sometimes part of the time in a health center.

In response to the worldwide movement for putting greater emphasis on primary health care in the 1980s, Brazil developed a "Plan for Integrated Action for Health and Sanitation" (PIASS), in which the key personnel are a new type of briefly trained multipurpose community health worker. Usually a young woman, chosen by the community, she is called an *attendente* and receives training for 4 to 6 months, following only 4 years of elementary school. Hundreds of health posts have been set up for these community health workers in the depressed northeast region, under the management of the SESP Foundation. Also in a project of the World Bank in the state of Sao Paulo, these attendentes are being trained for the rural areas. At the state level, the integrating committees for interministerial activities (CIPLAN, also known as CIS), are attempting to link the attendente primary health care posts with the health centers and the general structure of the state public health program.

Midwives in Brazil are less important in community work than they are in most developing countries. Since 80 percent of all childbirths were delivered in hospitals in 1981 (undoubtedly more now), the training midwife works mainly within hospitals of all types, handling most of the normal deliveries; physicians are called only if there is an obstetrical complication. The 20 percent of nonhospital births, as of 1981, were concentrated in the northeast and northern regions, and the great majority of these were, indeed, handled by untrained traditional birth attendants. Some of these older women have received brief training in hygienic practices by the state health secretariats.

Health Facilities. The numbers and sponsorships of physical resources for health in Brazil—hospitals, health centers, and health posts—have changed markedly in recent decades. This has been due in large part to the expanding impact of the social security program, in financing services for both hospital and ambulatory care.

The overall ratio to population of hospital beds in Brazil has risen only moderately, since much new construction was required only to keep up with the growth of population. In 1959, Brazil had 2,622 hospitals in all, with a ratio of 3.4 beds per 1,000. In 1981, it had 5,272 hospitals with a bed ratio of 4.0 per 1,000 people. These included hospitals of all types, and the share of beds in specialized institutions for leprosy, tuberculosis, mental illness, and other disorders has declined, while general hospital beds have increased.

More important are the changes that occurred in the ownership and management of hospitals. In 1960, the largest share of hospital beds was in the charitable *santa casa* facilities. Their standards were very modest, their wards were large and impersonal, but they provided a great deal of free hospital care, much of it subsidized by the Ministry of Health. Today the santa casa hospitals still exist, and their legal ownership usually remains with the charitable societies, but their management is quite different, as noted earlier. Considering all types of sponsorship, the hospital bed distribution nationally in 1981 was as follows:

Sponsorship	*Percentage of Beds*
Private	(74.7)
Nonprofit	36.5
For-profit	38.2
Public	(25.3)
Federal	14.7
State	6.3
Municipal	4.3
Total	100.0

In this tabulation, the federal beds include those built and operated by the original social

Table 10.2. Hospital Beds in Brazil by Sponsorship, 1950 and 1979

Sponsorship	1950		1950	
	Number	Percent	Number	Percent
Public	74,976	46.1	124,806	26.1
Private	87,539	53.9	352,785	73.9
Total	162,515	100.0	477,591	100.0

Source: De Azevedo, Antonio Carlos, *Seminar on National Health Administration: Country Report—Brazil.* Tokyo, Japan, 1984.

security institutes (only about 2 percent of the total beds), plus the beds of other federal agencies—principally the Ministry of Health and the Armed Forces. Another formulation of the great privatization of hospital beds that has occurred in Brazil is shown in Table 10.2. It is evident that between 1950 and 1978, the total hospital beds in Brazil increased nearly three times. This, however, consisted of an increase of public beds by 1.66 times and an increase of private beds by 4.02 times. It is not surprising that the occupancy level of most private for-profit hospitals is quite low. The explosion of private hospital bed construction in Brazil was consistent with the economic ideology of private enterprise that dominated the nation during the period of military control.

The staff, equipment, and general amenities of the variously sponsored hospitals differ considerably. Hospitals of the original social security institutes are still exceptionally generous in their staffing. The Ipanema Hospital, for example, built by the former Institute for Commercial Workers in Rio de Janeiro, has a staff of 1,730 health personnel (including doctors) for 241 beds or a ratio of 7.2 personnel per bed. By contrast, the very old Santa Casa de Misericordia Do Rio has a total staff of 1,450 for 600 beds (exceptionally large, since this is a university teaching hospital), or a ratio of 2.4 personnel per bed. The private for-profit hospitals are said to manage with relatively frugal staffs (to enhance their earnings), while the state and municipal hospitals hire large numbers of workers, in the interests of providing employment to local residents.

Regarding facilities for ambulatory care, expansion has also been substantial. In the state of Sao Paulo, for example, there were 550 units for ambulatory care in 1962 and more than

1,000 in 1985. A nationwide tabulation for 1982 showed the following:

Type of Ambulatory Care Facility	Number
Health centers	5,237
Health posts	4,824
Polyclinics (multispecialty)	7,011
Emergency stations	181
Mixed units (health centers with beds)	450
Hospital out-patient departments	5,075
Total	22,778

Unlike hospitals, the majority of these ambulatory care facilities are under public auspices; they are about 60 percent public and 40 percent private. Many of the polyclinics, the emergency (first-aid) stations, and hospital out-patient departments are private. Polyclinics under public auspices—known as medical care posts (PAMs)—are typically well organized.

The functions of these several types of facility differ. Health centers, operated predominantly by state secretariats of health, emphasize preventive services—largely for mothers and children—but they also offer general primary medical care to anyone who comes. Health posts are small units, usually rural, for primary care (preventive and therapeutic) rendered by an auxiliary health worker; there is no doctor in attendance. Polyclinics are mostly large establishments, usually urban, staffed by many different types of medical and surgical specialists. As private facilities, they are equivalent to group practice clinics. As public facilities or PAMs, they are typically operated directly by INAMPS and were constructed by one of the original *Previdencia* institutes. They are usually highly developed, with every patient seen by a specialist in a separate consulting room. Several also include emergency rooms with 24-hour service. Independent emergency stations are small units whose special feature is their coverage by a physician 24 hours a day. Mixed units are simply health centers, typically operated by state governments, with a few beds to take care of patients (accident cases, maternity, etc.) for a day or two, pending transfer to hospital. Hospital out-patient departments are typically staffed by specialists from the regular medical staff. In public hospitals the OPDs are usually large and congested; in private hospitals of nonprofit sponsorship (santas casas) they are also frequently large, but in private for-profit hospitals, they are usually quite limited in size and hours of operation.

Beyond all these formally organized facilities for ambulatory care, there are hundreds of small *clinicas privadas* in Brazil, where groups of doctors, often in the same specialty, practice medicine privately; often only one or two of these doctors are full-time in the private setting, while most are part-time, coming after their hours of service in a public medical position.

Technology. Many factors determine an institution's technological development. Taking account of these, a knowledgeable observer in Sao Paulo rated the levels of technological development of different types of hospitals in Brazil in the following order:

1. University hospitals (public or private)
2. INAMPS' own original *Previdencia* hospitals
3. Private for-profit hospitals
4. State and municipal government hospitals
5. Santa casa hospitals under original charity management

The large staffs of many public hospitals, as noted, may simply reflect public policy to provide maximum employment, rather than technological development. Small staffs in private hospitals may be associated with the use of automated laboratory and x-ray equipment. Staffing, in other words, should not necessarily be regarded as a reflection of technological development. In fact, the excessive number of rather poorly trained personnel in some public hospitals is believed to contribute to a rising problem of crossinfection in hospital patients. The maintenance of x-ray and other equipment in hospitals, outside the large cities, is difficult, as is generally true in developing countries.

It is commonly believed in Brazil that private for-profit hospitals give a higher quality of care than any public institution. This view is probably based on the fact that most private facilities are smaller, newer, and have patients in single or semiprivate rooms. They may well give more personally sensitive patient care than is possible on a large 12- to 30-bed ward, but this really tells nothing about the technical quality of the diagnostic and treatment services provided.

For reasons of both quality and economy, the public hospitals obtain drugs from a central depot operated by INAMPS—the *Centro da Medicamentos* (CEME). This program undoubtedly contributes to the more discriminating use of sound "essential drugs" in INAMPS-supported facilities.

Economic Support

The great extension of organized social financing for health care in Brazil has made both curative and preventive services available to a very large proportion of the population. Even though many serious inequities remain, economic support has been mobilized for a greater volume of health care than was available in previous decades.

In 1960, medical care was not accessible to the great majority of the Brazilian population, and it was estimated that not more than about 1.0 percent of the GNP was spent for health purposes, counting money from all sources, public and private. By 1984, about 4.0 percent of GNP was devoted to the health system. Thus, even adjusting for inflation, four times the share of national wealth were devoted to health purposes, compared with earlier years.

This vast increase in health spending has been due mainly to an expanded mobilization of financial support through social mechanisms—most important, through social insurance, and second, through state, federal, and local taxation. At the same time, there has been a large increase in purely private spending, even though as a share of the total, private health spending has probably grown less rapidly. Brazil demonstrates very well a basic principle of health economics: if social support for health service is increased, private spending will be relatively less.

Sources of Funds. In Table 10.3, the proportions of total health expenditures in Brazil, from all sources, are reported, as calculated by a multiagency investigation (including the Ministries of Education, Health, and Social Security, and the Pan American Health Organization). The simplicity of this table conceals the several techniques necessary to calculate these data for 1982.

Most important, the health expenditures derived from government sources were 71.5 percent of the total. In fact, if we recognize that several of the "private" sources are, indeed, social (e.g., enterprises and voluntary insurance) rather than purely individual, only 16.5 percent of the total health expenditures in Brazil comes from individual out-of-pocket sources, and 83.5 percent could be regarded as social in origin. Of the public expenditures, roughly two-thirds are from social insurance contributions of employers and workers, and one-third from general taxation—half from the state level and the balance from federal and municipal levels. An unpublished study in 1989 showed that overall health spending in Brazil had risen to more than 5.0 percent of GDP, but that the mix of funds derived from public and private sources was still approximately 70 to 30 percent.

A tabulation of this sort may remind one that social security is basically a special form

Table 10.3. Health Expenditures, Percentage Distribution According to Source, in Brazil, 1982

Source	Percentage	
Public		
General taxation	(24.6)	
Federal	6.8	
State	12.4	
Municipal	5.4	
Social Security (for health care)	46.9	
Total public		(71.5)
Private		
Enterprises	6.3	
Voluntary health insurance	2.9	
Trade unions	2.1	
Philanthropy	0.7	
Persons and families	16.5	
Total private		(28.5)
All sources	100.0	(100.0)

Source: Ministry of Education and Culture, Ministry of Health, Ministry of Social Security, Pan American Sanitary Bureau—Principal Evaluation Group, *Program of Research in Health Services (PRSS).* Brasilia, 1982.

of taxation. The money is channeled to government from workers and employers, but its ultimate source is still the general population, who purchase the products that each enterprise or business is selling. The social insurance contributions were about 8 percent of wages, up to a certain ceiling, from workers plus another 8 percent from employers (up to a maximum), and the full 16 percent from self-employed. It must be realized that these social security taxes are used for the support of many benefits beyond health care—old age pensions, maternity leave, disability compensation, survivor payments, and so on. In 1982, the total of these monetary benefits amounted to 78.7 percent, and the costs of health care (INAMPS) accounted for 21.3 percent of the total; only the latter expenditures are included in Table 10.3.

The revenues from both taxation and social security vary, of course, with the economic development level of the different regions of Brazil. Money derived from state and municipal taxation naturally varies in the same way, but that from federal taxation, and especially social security (INAMPS), is to some extent redistributed to the different regions according to their use of services rather than the amounts they have contributed. The limitation on this redistributive effect is the availability of health resources for providing care in the different regions.

Unfortunately, the financial position of the entire social security (MPAS) program was in serious jeopardy in the mid-1980s. In 1984, the economically active population in Brazil was estimated to be 50,502,000 workers, of whom 70 percent were urban and 30 percent rural. Rural workers (as noted earlier) make no contributions, beyond what is collected from the FUNRURAL and from a relatively small proportion of rural employers. Altogether contributions were received from various groups as follows:

Urban workers	19,476,000
Employers	2,280,000
Self-employed	1,653,000
Domestic servants	668,000
Other	737,840
Total	24,814,840

Thus, in relation to the economically active population (50,502,000), only about half were making the required contributions. The other half were unemployed, underemployed, students, women who had left the labor force, and large numbers of small employers and their employees, who simply failed to make the contribution legally mandated. Collecting social contributions in all developing countries is inherently difficult.

The social security law specifies that the first claim on all funds collected must be the pensions and other monetary benefits. Because of inflation, these have risen and absorbed 83 percent of the total collections, leaving only about 17 percent for all health services, compared to 21 percent noted for 1982.

Complicating matters further is the rising cost of medical care. A major portion of the care is purchased from private hospitals and doctors, among whom financial incentives encourage excessive service. A new source of taxation in 1982 was a value-added tax of 0.5 percent on all economic production, called FINSOCIAL. How Brazil will cope with the rising total costs of its health system remains to be seen.

Purposes of Health Expenditures. No breakdown of the purposes of total Brazilian health expenditures is available, but insight comes from examining the percentage distribution of expenditures by INAMPS (47 percent of the total) in 1981, shown in Table 10.4. It is evident that the mix of expenditures for ambulatory care, hospital care, and special services is quite different among the different types of agency that INAMPS (social security) supports. Perhaps most striking is the very large share of total INAMPS health expenditures that goes to payment for services in private hospitals—44.4 percent of the total and 69.2 percent of all hospitalization expenditures.

It is noteworthy that INAMPS supports "government units" and "rural care," which include health centers and health posts providing primary care (including prevention). Yet both of these categories account for only 8 percent of the total expenditures. The great bulk of Brazilian health expenditures is for curative medical and hospital service. In 1982, a per-

Table 10.4. Health Care Expenditures by INAMPS: Percentage Distribution for Different Services in Brazil, 1981

Expenditure Outlet	Ambulatory Care	Special Services	Hospitalization	Total
INAMPS' own units	28.3	16.3	1.6	20.6
Government units	13.9	20.7	4.3	5.2
Rural care (health posts, etc.)	13.5	6.4	18.1	2.8
Enterprises	10.1	9.3	4.2	4.1
Private hospital contracts	—	—	69.2	44.4
Private medical contracts	31.7	45.8	—	17.7
Teaching hospitals	2.0	1.5	1.4	2.5
Work accidents	0.5	—	0.7	2.7
Total	100.0	100.0	100.0	100.0

Source: CONASP, "Plan for Reorientation of Health Care under Social Security." Brasilia, August 1982.

centage breakdown of Ministry of Health expenditures showed the following:

Purpose	Percentage
Medical and hospital care	84.2
Food and nutrition	4.8
Basic health services	3.1
Control of infectious diseases	2.2
Prophylactic and therapeutic substances	2.6
Other purposes	3.1
All purposes	100.0

Another way of learning the purpose of health expenditures in Brazil comes from a household expenditure survey made in 1975. Families were classified into five income levels and their personal outlays for four different types of health service were analyzed. The overall money spent by families, not surprisingly, tended to increase along with total family income. The proportions of health expenditures for different purposes varied greatly, however, in families of different income levels.

These percentages are shown in Table 10.5. Especially conspicuous is the very high proportion of their limited health expenditures that low-income families use for purchasing drugs (both prescribed and nonprescribed, doubtless more of the latter). Higher-income families, on the other hand, spend relatively much more on physicians and dentists. Of course, in Brazil, there are far more families in the three lowest-income groups than in the two highest.

The expenditures for all health services in Brazil vary greatly by geographic region; they are highest in the very urbanized and industrialized southeast region and lowest in the rural and depressed northeast region. The social security program and the federal Ministry of Health both attempt to adjust allocations to achieve a better balance of expenditures among the regions, but the great differentials in human and physical resources—not to mention in the levels of education and demand—seriously impair the balance achievable. Thus, the impoverished northeast region contributed

Table 10.5. Personal Family Expenditures for Health Care: Percentage Distribution of Spending for Various Types of Health Care by Families of Different Income in Brazil, 1975

Family Income[a]	Physicians & Dentists	Drugs	Hospitals & Surgery	Other	All Services
Poorest	14.1	64.5	12.5	8.9	100.0
Second	18.7	53.7	16.7	10.9	100.0
Third	26.7	42.0	18.3	13.0	100.0
Fourth	40.5	21.6	24.6	13.3	100.0
Richest	50.5	10.5	28.0	11.0	100.0
All levels	28.3	40.4	19.5	11.8	100.0

[a]Family income is classified according to the relationship of each level to the Brazilian "minimum wage" (legally defined) in 1974, ranging from under 2 minimum wage standards for the poorest to 30 or more such standards for the richest.
Source: Rodriguez, R., et al., *The Role of Information Processing in the Reorganization of the Social Security System of Brazil.* Sao Paulo, Universidad de Sao Paulo, Centro de Informacao e Analise, January 1984.

9 percent of social security (SINPAS) revenues in 1981 and received 17.2 percent of INAMPS health expenditures. The rich southeast region contributed 62.6 percent of SINPAS revenues that year and received 52.6 percent of INAMPS health expenditures.

In spite of this approach to "redistributive justice," Brazil makes great use of patterns of medical care delivery that are relatively expensive and provide incentives for abuse. A rough calculation of the expenditures per consultation in a large public polyclinic (PAM) in Rio yielded an estimated cost of Crs 7000, which compares with charges of Crs 25,000 or 30,000 per private consultation. To help cope with these private charges, commercial health insurance is being sold to enable upper-income and some middle-income families obtain private medical care. Large banks sell this insurance, the best known of which is called Golden Cross. Several hundred corporations have purchased such private health insurance for their employees.

This analysis of the sources and the purposes of health expenditures in Brazil is not as integrated and comprehensive as one would like. The great predominance of collectivized financing is clear, however, and it underscores the welfare-oriented policies of the Brazilian health system.

Health System Management

Health planning has come to play an explicit role in managing the Brazilian health system, even though its effectiveness has been reduced by market dynamics. In the federal government, the Secretariat of Planning in the Presidency of the Republic has been noted, and within the Ministry of Health there is also a unit in the Division of Organization of Health Services devoted to planning. These offices propose standards or norms that are applied in the operation of disease control programs or the staffing of hospitals throughout the nation. Budgets are then prepared on the basis of these norms. A good deal of the planning at the national level is intended to demonstrate the inequalities in resources among different geographic regions, which requires various adjustments.

The larger states, such as Sao Paulo, also have planning units in the Secretariat of Health. On the basis of demographic and epidemiological information, these units recommend where new health centers and health stations are needed. It must be regretfully pointed out, however, that neither the states nor the federal government in Brazil has taken action (as have many other Latin American countries) to require new medical graduates to devote a period of time to public service in a rural area, before being officially registered.

In fact, the production of both physicians and hospitals in Brazil reflects a lack of planning. The free-market ideology has been so strong since the early 1960s that numerous private medical schools have been organized and scores of private hospitals established entirely for private monetary motives. Brazil is now faced with the problems of underemployed physicians and half-empty private hospitals, along with the resultant abuses of unjustified medical and hospital services generated by these unplanned excesses.

Regarding the organizational relationships within the entire health system, Brazil seems to have a reasonable balance between responsibilities carried at the central and the state levels. Major standards and policies are issued at the top, but their implementation is the responsibility of the states; at the same time the states have a great deal of autonomy and can initiate programs by themselves. Since the state secretary of health is appointed by each state's elected governor, he is not responsible to the central minister of health (as in most other Latin American countries). This freedom of state governments has little meaning in the many poor states that require federal money to carry out most of their work. In the richer states, however, some programs can be carried out entirely with state funds. The states also get funds from INAMPS, special foundations (like SESP), or foreign aid as well as from the Ministry of Health.

Administrative competence is frequently criticized in Brazil, at both the "macro" level of state or municipal administration and the "micro" level of individual institutions (especially hospitals). Many top administrative positions are held by physicians, specialized in clinical fields, without any training in public health or health care administration. Brazil actually has several schools of public health, to which physicians and others may go for administrative training, and the Foundation for Public Administration (FUNDAP) in Sao Paulo gives short courses to orient personnel in basic principles of management.

A flow of reliable information is essential to good management, and INAMPS gives special attention to this process, with a large computerized information program, known as DATAPREV. Data reported in this chapter on resources, services, and expenditures in Brazil were derived largely from this program. The heavy use of the private sector in INAMPS, and the information on expenditures by hospitals and doctors, shed valuable light on the nature of private market health services.

The regulation of food and drugs is a responsibility of the national Ministry of Health, but implementation of these duties has been handicapped by inadequate budgets. Likewise, the inspection of hospitals by the state secretariats of health has had to be superficial, because of the lack of staff. Probably the most significant surveillance of facilities occurs as a by-product of the arrangement for contracts between INAMPS and private hospitals or local public institutions. Another form of regulation is the registration of doctors, pharmacists, professional nurses, and other personnel by the Ministry of Health. This is essentially routine, without any systematic monitoring of performance.

In response to various abuses, or suspected abuses, in the INAMPS program, certain new forms of regulation are gradually being imposed in Brazil. One is the requirement for *prior authorization* by an INAMPS doctor, before a patient can be admitted to a private hospital (either nonprofit or for-profit) when the condition is not an emergency. This is intended to reduce admissions of questionable necessity. The policy is being implemented on a state-by-state basis, although it is impeded by the frequent claim of doctors that their cases are "emergencies."

The other regulatory response to abuses has been to change the method of payment to private hospitals from fee-for-service (i.e., fees for each procedure or each day of care) to a flat

amount for each diagnosis. This amount is based on the national average computed from INAMPS experience in the previous year. Because the initial trial of this mechanism took place in one town of Sao Paulo state in 1982, it is known as the *Curitiba Plan.* As expected, hospitals argue that the amounts paid for various diagnoses are too low, but the procedure is a cautious response to abuses by private sector hospitals.

Because of the several organizations concerned with health care in Brazil at the national and state levels, various actions have been taken to promote their coordination. The most important such action was the organization in 1980 of the National Council for Administration of Health and Social Security (CONASP). This council was placed directly in the Office of the President and includes representatives of several key ministries—Health, Education, Interior, Social Security, and others. Later, representatives of the Brazilian Medical Association, labor syndicates, and the Federation of Santas Casas were added. In 1981–1982, CONASP made a critical analysis of the whole health system. It concluded that there were many abuses from excessive use of private providers. Many people had inadequate access to care, especially in the rural areas. Far too much emphasis was placed on hospitalization, and inadequate primary and ambulatory care was provided. The whole system was fragmented and seriously in need of greater coordination.

In reaction to these problems, CONASP recommended careful regionalization of all services in each state. To give greater emphasis to primary health care, every patient should first be examined in an ambulatory care unit, before being given access to a hospital. First preference for hospitalization should go to INAMPS' own hospitals, then to state and local government hospitals, and to private hospitals only as a last resort. The scheme of payment to all private hospitals should be a flat rate based on diagnosis, as described earlier. In each state a Commission for Inter-Ministry Planning and Coordination (CIPLAN), including the state Secretariats of health, social security, and education, would implement the whole coordination plan.

Because both private doctors and private

hospitals objected to the CONASP plan, it was implemented only in the state of Santa Catarina. Yet other special projects have been launched. A major undertaking, the *Cotia Project,* substantially supported by the World Bank, has functioned in Sao Paulo state since 1975. This project links numerous health centers as satellites to a hospital (together forming a *module*). Several modules make up a *health region,* with a high-level hospital at the center. The medical staffs of the hospitals also serve in the health centers. The whole program is supported by funds from INAMPS. Private medical and hospital providers may also function in the region, but they receive no support from INAMPS—only from private individuals. It is evident that the CONASP plan would take much time and effort to implement nationally. Not many states have the administrative strength and political will to carry it out. From several sources, it has been suggested that progress would be hastened if INAMPS were transferred from the Ministry of Social Security to the Ministry of Health.

Delivery of Health Services

All of the components of the Brazilian health system discussed so far culminate in delivery of services to people. The crucial question is: What proportion of the people receive the services they need, or what is the system's coverage? Also, what are the characteristics of the services provided?

Coverage. A health system's coverage has two dimensions, people and services. Coverage may be one percentage for immunizations and quite another for emergency care or hospitalization. Broadly speaking, an impressive extension of health care coverage has occurred in Brazil over recent decades. Regarding the most readily quantifiable component of the system—the social security program—coverage has been extended from about 25 percent of the population in 1962 to some 83 percent in 1984. The latter figure includes 30 percent of the people who are insured workers plus 53 percent who are eligible as dependents. For serious emergency care, however, virtually 100 percent population coverage has been achieved, since it is a policy of the several programs supported by social security (INAMPS) to furnish needed service to any acutely sick person coming to a facility, whether or not he or she is officially insured.

On the other hand, certain basic services, even primary health care, show serious deficiencies in coverage, although the trend has been toward improvement. With respect to potable water, for example, accessibility for the national population improved from 24.3 percent in 1960 to 53.2 percent in 1980; with respect to waste disposal, coverage was adequate in 1960 for only 23.8 percent of the population but for 41.5 percent in 1980. In both environmental services, improvement has been much greater for the urban population; in rural areas, in fact, access to water has shown no real improvement, and the overall change is a result essentially of the general urbanization.

Coverage should also be considered in terms of the numbers and ratios of health personnel and physical facilities available in a geographic area. Resources are much more abundant, and therefore coverage is greater, in the more affluent urbanized regions. Within any region, furthermore, the availability of all types of medical care is much greater for the higher- than for the lower-income groups. In Brazil the most complete medical care utilization data apply to the population covered by social security.

Utilization Rates. In 1982 the INAMPS population had 1.65 consultations with a physician per person per year. This was an increase from 1.25 such services in 1978. (Both figures are understatements, since they do not count privately purchased medical care.) In 1982, this amounted to 206,000,000 consultations, obtained at various places as follows:

Place	Percentage
State, municipal, and university health units	31.7
Private hospitals and private medical clinics	31.2
INAMPS polyclinics and medical posts	26.8
Santa casa and small rural units	10.2
All places	100.0

This rate of use of ambulatory care in 1982, however, varied between 1.02 consultations in the northern region and 2.10 in the southeast region. Furthermore, if we examine the urban population separately, the national rate in 1982 was 2.13 consultations per person per year, and the rural rate was only 0.56 consultations per person. In the northern region the rural rate was as low as 0.19 consultations per person per year. We know that rural people in Brazil are not healthier than urban; the differentials therefore obviously reflect differences in the availability of medical services. As one might expect, dental services are less available than medical services. In 1981, the average person in Brazil as a whole had 0.31 dental consultation a year, with the usual differences among regions. Still, this was an improvement over the rate of 0.13 such services in 1975.

In many highly developed countries, hospitalization rates paradoxically are relatively higher among the poor than among the affluent. This is usually interpreted to mean that illnesses in poor families are frequently neglected until they are so far advanced that hospital admission is necessary. To some extent a similar phenomenon may be occurring in Brazil. Examining the urban population, the rate of hospital admissions in the affluent southeast region in 1982 was 119.1 per 1,000 per year, and in the depressed northern region it was almost the same, 114.4 per 1,000 per year. (For ambulatory care, the southeast region had double the rate of consultations reported in the northern region.)

As suggested by the predominantly private ownership of hospitals in the 1980s, hospital utilization rates are much greater in private settings than the rates of ambulatory services. In 1982, INAMPS financed 7,416,000 hospital admissions to facilities distributed as follows:

Type of Hospital	Percentage
Private hospitals (nonprofit and for-profit)	66.1
Government hospitals (federal, state, and municipal)	10.0
Social Security hospitals	1.0
Other facilities	22.9
All hospitals	100.0

Characteristics of Service. In spite of the great expansion of health services in Brazil, supported mainly by stronger social security financing, serious disparities remain among regions and different income groups. Even when resources are theoretically available in a state, problems of transportation, personal education, attitudes, and patient–doctor relationships may obstruct their use. In any geographic region, public facilities are likely to be overcrowded, with long periods of waiting. This is aggravated by the widely recognized fact that physicians, who are customarily paid for a certain number of hours of work (2, 4, or 6 hours per day), seldom actually spend the designated time on the job. They often leave sooner to go to another job or to their private medical practices. Low-income patients must simply wait or return another day. Somewhat higher-income patients—able and willing to pay a private fee—seek care from a private doctor or private clinic.

Whether this is the course of events or the patient is deliberately referred to a private hospital with which INAMPS has a contract, the medical care received in a private setting is typically different from that in government settings. The doctor is more often a specialist, and likely to be less rushed and more personally sensitive. Greater use is made of laboratory, x-ray, and other special procedures. Because each of these procedures yields a special fee from the individual or from INAMPS, its medical justification is often questionable. Perhaps excessive procedures do no harm, but they waste money. Sometimes, especially with elective surgery and Cesarian sections, actual harm is done. Private hospitals have the reputation for accepting only simple cases, while complex and difficult cases must be sent to teaching hospitals or government institutions.

On the positive side, one must recognize that financial abuses sometimes help the patient medically. The INAMPS policy of never rejecting an emergency case, even if the patient is not currently insured, leads many uninsured patients to be falsely labeled "emergencies." For the 15 or 20 percent of patients who are not currently insured in Brazil, one must recall that several resources are available in the states where the majority of the people live: (a) municipal hospitals, (b) state hospitals, (c) the 10 percent of beds in santa casa hospitals reserved for charity cases, as well as (d) designation as an "emergency case" in any hospital.

The use of both the direct and indirect patterns for health care delivery by INAMPS, of course, permits great diversity in the arrangements for care. Thus, ambulatory services under the Brazilian health system may be obtained (a) at one of the INAMPS medical posts of PAMs, (b) at an out-patient department of an INAMPS hospital, (c) at an out-patient clinic under contract with INAMPS in a non-profit or a for-profit hospital, (d) at a state or federal university hospital out-patient department, (e) at a state or municipal government health center, (f) at a trade union or syndicate clinic, predominantly in rural areas, or even (g) at the private practice of an individual doctor, who may be paid by fees up to a maximum number of patients per day.

The delivery of drugs is generally regarded as beset with problems. The pharmacies attached to INAMPS and government facilities (health centers or medical posts) use formularies and dispense reasonable prescriptions. At ordinary private pharmacies, the patient can generally obtain any drugs, with or without a prescription, or perhaps on the advice of a clerk.

With respect to Brazilian health services as a whole, it is evident that the lion's share goes to pay for hospital care, as in nearly all countries, both industrialized and developing. Yet there is great awareness in Brazil of the need to put more emphasis on ambulatory care. The construction of health centers by the states and municipalities has been active. In the Northeast the PIASS program, operated by the SESP Foundation, is bringing primary health care to the interior rural areas through newly trained community health workers. It is also worth noting that, though basic health services accounted for only 3.1 percent of expenditures in 1982, this was an increase from 0.9 percent in 1978.

The multiplicity of agencies with health responsibilities in Brazil has generated widely recognized bureaucratic problems. Leaders of both the Ministry of Health and the many-faceted social security program have sought to improve coordination. The CONASP coordi-

nating council, organized in 1980, had only limited success, but plans for decentralized delegation of authority for *all* health programs to a *single* health office in each state continue to be advocated at national meetings. Effective leadership at the highest level is obviously necessary to implement such plans.

Insofar as health status is affected by health services, the record of Brazil over the past decades has been good. Life expectancy at birth for men increased from 33.4 years in 1910 to 61.3 years in 1975–1980. For women, the increase was from 34.6 years to 65.5 years over the same period. There are, of course, vast differences between the affluent and the depressed economic regions, and between high- and low-income families everywhere. Still one cannot say that conditions in the depressed northern regions are getting worse or that they are failing to improve. The fact is that in the poorest regions health conditions are improving, though less than in the affluent industrialized regions.

PERU

As a country of 19,200,000 people (1984) with an annual GNP per capita of $1,066, Peru is closer than Brazil to the average of the 21 Latin American countries. Its long Pacific Ocean coastline constitutes its western border, and more than half of its inland territory consists of the high and rugged Andean mountains. Ironically, Peru's political history in recent years, marked by a military government from 1968 to 1980, is also typical of Latin American countries. The several health service subsystems reviewed for Brazil have also functioned, in different proportions, in Peru. The changing character of national health systems in Latin America over recent decades is also well illustrated by conditions in Peru, for which much data are available on the period around 1960 and a quarter-century later, around 1985.

Conditions in 1960

Traditional healing was highly prevalent in Peru in 1960. About 64 percent of its population was rural, and among these people the local healer—empirical, magical, or both—was the most readily available source of medical care. Some 50 percent of the national population of 10,300,000 were pure-blooded Indians, whose confidence in the traditional healer was especially great. By far the largest source of hospital care was the network of *beneficencia* or charitable hospitals, with 42 percent of the total beds. The out-patient departments of these facilities gave a great deal of ambulatory care to the sick, although their quarters were typically small, poorly equipped, and overcrowded. All of these institutions received significant subsidies from the Ministry of Health, which, supplemented by proceeds from lotteries and special taxes, supported more than 50 percent of their costs.

In 1960 the Peruvian Ministry of Health had only 71 health centers, with teams of health personnel, including physicians. There were 142 medical posts with doctors in part-time attendance, but vacancies were common. The most technically developed health services were those of the social security program, which started in 1936, limited initially to manual workers. Peru has the distinction of having built the first social security hospital exclusively for insured workers (opened in 1941)—a pattern that was soon emulated by social security programs throughout Latin America. Then, in 1948, a second and separate insurance program was started for white-collar employees. Together, these two social security programs provided fairly modern medical care for between 6 and 7 percent of the population. Many hospitals and polyclinics were constructed and operated for eligible persons. In the *obrero* program (manual laborers), dependents were not covered, and in the *empleado* program wives were covered only for maternity care. The empleado health facilities were relatively luxurious, and the insured white-collar workers were also free to seek care from private doctors if they paid part of the fee (the balance payable by the insurance fund).

Industrial enterprises often developed their own medical and hospital services, where the quality of care was well above average. Special facilities and services were also provided for members of the armed forces and the national police.

In 1960 Peru had about 4,000 physicians, or a ratio of 38.5 per 100,000 population. Most were graduates of San Marcos University, but three additional medical schools had recently been established. Maldistribution of doctors was extreme; 72 percent were located in the Lima metropolitan area, with 15 percent of the national population. More than 80 percent of physicians had salaried positions of some type, but most of these also engaged in private practice. The supply of fully trained nurses (2,200) was only slightly more than half that of doctors, so great reliance had to be placed on briefly trained nursing auxiliaries. Hospital beds of all types amounted to 24,000, or 2.15 per 1,000 population.

In some of the small towns, there was coordinated use of hospitals by the Ministry of Health and the social security program. Thus, a Ministry of Health hospital provided care to insured persons who were reimbursed by the social security fund, or vice versa. On the whole, however, the several subsystems operated entirely independently. Various committees were set up to discuss integrated administration on a regional basis, but as of 1960 little had been accomplished.

Transition, 1960 to 1985

In 1960, Peru was among the poorest third of Latin American countries, and in 1985 it remained in about the same position. The population grew from 10,300,000 in 1960 to 19,200,000 in 1984, but the later population was much more urbanized; it changed from 36 percent urban in 1960 to 67 percent urban in 1984. In the late 1980s, the vast differences in living conditions between the well-to-do (perhaps 10 percent of the population) and the very poor (at least 60 percent) remained as serious as ever.

In the mid-1960s, economic conditions were deteriorating in Peru, and in 1968 the government was seized by a military coup. This was an unusual military government, however, because instead of reflecting the ideology of the upper social classes, it put through sweeping agrarian reforms, and many wealthy families left the country. It also nationalized oil mining, fish meal and other industries, and took over the banks. Food subsidies and price controls were introduced. Much of this populist reform was done in haste, however. Because agricultural cooperatives, for example, were not organized to handle modern agriculture technology, food production actually declined, and the nation's foreign debt increased.

As a result, another military coup seized power in 1976, and the social reform programs were slowed down or reversed. Conditions did not improve, and a successful general strike was called in 1977. In 1980, general elections were held and a civilian government was reinstated under President Fernando Belaunde Terry (who had been president in 1967). The new government attempted to encourage the return of private enterprise and free-market principles. Nevertheless, inflation continued and even worsened, and the foreign debt mounted. Guerilla movements (identified as the *Sendero Luminoso,* or Shining Path) arose in the Andes mountain areas. The worldwide economic recession, starting in the United States in 1980, aggravated conditions further. Border quarrels with Ecuador, Brazil, and Chile were used to justify exceptionally large military expenditures.

All of these political and economic developments have naturally had their impact on the Peruvian health system. Much progress can probably be traced to the populist military period of 1968 to 1976, despite certain deficiencies. The more conservative military government, and the current civilian government of the Accion Popular Party (usually described as center–right), are associated with a strengthened private market for health services.

The Health System Structure

The several subsystems providing health services in Peru in 1960 were still identifiable in 1985, but their characteristics and proportions had changed.

Traditional Healing. The decline of the rural population from 64 percent in 1960 to 33 percent in 1984 inevitably meant a decline in the importance of the traditional *curandero.* In the isolated Indian population of Andean villages, traditional healers—using both ritualistic and empirical methods of treatment—undoubtedly still play a significant role. But the increased literacy of the population and the greater availability of modern health facilities have reduced the dependence of Peruvian people on the traditional practitioner.

Many healers in Peru specialize in certain conditions, such as bone-setting, treatment of snake bites, and the use of massage for various bodily pains. Most healers farm or do other work, and practice healing only part of the time. A research institute in San Marcos University has been studying traditional herbal remedies, to discover which can be scientifically shown to have therapeutic value.

Charity Services. In 1960, it may be recalled, the *beneficencia* hospitals were heavily subsidized by government. Even with these subsidies, their resources (both equipment and personnel) were very modest. By 1985, almost all of these once-charitable institutions had been transferred entirely to the control of the Ministry of Health. Some were closed down completely. The beneficencia societies may still exist for other purposes, but they no longer manage the hospitals. One exception is a mental hospital in Cuzco, still under the original control.

Physical conditions and equipment in these hospitals were somewhat improved. The staffing was also increased, with personnel becoming employees of the Ministry of Health (usually meaning a higher salary scale). As in the past, the patients served by former beneficencia hospitals are mainly the poor, who pay nothing for the service. A few private pay beds, however, are still maintained in most of these facilities. In isolated parts of Peru, some foreign religious missions still operate clinics with 10 to 20 beds.

A new activity of the beneficencia societies is the operation of a drug-producing enterprise. Known by the acronym LUSA, it manufactures products that are widely used, such as oral rehydration solution. These products are sold to all Ministry of Health facilities.

Ministry of Health. Compared with 1960, the Ministry of Health in 1985 was a much stronger agency. Because of the transfer of beneficencia facilities, it controlled hospitals with 16,190 beds, or 54 percent of the total hospital bed supply in Peru, compared with 16.0 percent in 1960. The 71 health centers and 142 medical posts of 1960 had expanded to 612 such centers and 1,700 such posts in 1985; their medical staffing became much more complete. This augmentation of physical facilities obviously reflects substantial increases in ministry personnel. In 1985, the ministry had nearly 35,000 full-time personnel, plus another 18,000 under temporary contractual employment.

The functions of the Ministry of Health have become much broader. In addition to the usual ministry functions for personal health services, disease control programs, and so on, there are units for health planning and rationalization that did not exist in the past. The latter unit is devoted to development of more coordinated and efficiently organized preventive and therapeutic health services.

Reporting directly to the vice-minister of health are the directors of Peru's 17 health regions (in 1960 staffs had been established in 14 health regions). Theoretically the regional director is responsible for all health activities in his region within the Ministry of Health, including the hospitals. Actually, the hospitals operate quite autonomously. The regions were divided into health areas, which included the health centers and several health posts surrounding them; there are 57 health areas in all. The posts are supposed to be supervised by medical officers at the health centers, but in reality little such supervision is given. All of these facilities emphasize maternal and child health services and prevention, but they definitely provide curative services at the same time. Each unit maintains a small pharmacy or a supply of drugs for treatment of the sick.

In 1969, under the military government, greater importance was attached to hospitals, and they were expected to supervise the health centers in each health area. The hospital directors, however, were heavily occupied with their clinical responsibilities and gave little attention to the health centers, just as the latter gave little supervision to the health posts. In the 1970s, relationships changed again, with regional directors placed firmly in charge of the regions. Under the prevailing military ideology, however, policy making and power were still highly centralized, and the regions essentially carried out directives from the headquarters in Lima. With respect to certain formerly vertical campaigns for immunizations and the control of malaria and yellow fever, responsibilities were delegated to the regions.

Community participation in the operation of health centers and health posts was not encouraged by the military government. Occasionally a citizen advisory council was established, but it was seldom very active. School health services were another theoretical responsibility of the health center staff that, in fact, had a low priority. With some international assistance, selected health areas put special emphasis on the delivery of primary health care provided by new types of primary health workers, trained in 3-month courses.

Social Security Program. The population covered by the social security program for medical care in Peru has expanded greatly. In 1960, about 400,000 obreros and 220,000 empleados were covered, together amounting to 6.1 percent of the population (this excluded dependents who had only maternity coverage). In 1985, 2,787,000 persons (again excluding dependents) were covered, which amounted to 14.1 percent of the population. Coverage, furthermore, was expanded to include maternity care for the dependents of *all* insured persons (both manual and white-collar workers) and care of infants during their first year of life. Counting dependents, 18.6 percent of the Peruvian population was covered.

Of special importance was the action in 1975 to unify the two separate social insurance programs for obreros and empleados, as the Instituto Peruano de Seguridad Social or IPSS. Even though the fiscal contributions of the empleados were higher, everyone became legally entitled to use the hospitals and polyclinics of either program. (In reality, some stratification in the use of different facilities by the white-collar and blue-collar workers understandably persisted for several years.) To accommodate the greatly increased population covered by the unified and enlarged social security program, several actions were taken.

The hospital and ambulatory care facilities of the IPSS program itself were increased. In

1960 both programs included 14 hospitals with 3,414 beds. In 1985 the unified program had 21 hospitals with 4,730 beds. Second, there was a great expansion of IPSS contracts with the Ministry of Health to use beds in its hospitals; contracts in some localities were also made with private hospitals. Third, the right of empleados to choose private doctors and use private hospitals, with personal copayments, was extended to everyone. Thus, in 1983, out of 156,000 IPSS hospital admissions, 77.1 percent occurred in the program's own hospitals, 16.8 percent in hospitals under contract, and 6.1 percent in *libre eleccion* (free choice) private hospitals.

For ambulatory care, the strategy was similar, although relatively greater emphasis was given to expansion of the IPSS program's own facilities. By 1984 there were 29 relatively large polyclinics (with multiple specialties), 109 medical posts (with one or two doctors plus other personnel), and 117 first-aid health stations. In addition, 12.3 percent of ambulatory consultations were at facilities under contract and 7.9 percent were through free choice of doctor (with copayment). In Lima, where more than half of all insured persons live, 10 new IPSS polyclinics were constructed; the use of private doctors was becoming increasingly expensive. Contrary to common opinion, the health services of the social security program are not limited to curative care. A special administrative unit promotes immunizations, prenatal care, health education of workers, and other preventive services.

The Private Market. The supply of physicians in Peru has greatly increased, from 4,000 in 1960 to over 17,000 in 1985, and with this the availability of private medical care. Nearly 30 percent of all doctors are not employed by government, and many are engaged entirely in private practice. Of the 70 percent in some type of public employment, the great majority also have part-time private medical practices. When conditions are crowded in a public clinic or hospital out-patient department, one of the unfortunate realities in Peru is the tendency of doctors to refer some patients to their own private offices "for more careful attention."

The supply of dentists is much smaller than that of physicians, but only 28 percent are in public employment; 72 percent are entirely engaged in private practice. Among pharmacists, 87 percent are entirely engaged in private pharmacies or other private pharmaceutical work.

In hospital care, growth of the private market has been conspicuous. In 1960, there were 25 private hospitals with 1,113 beds; by 1985 there were more than 100 private for-profit hospitals, with 5,384 beds. This represented an increase from 6 to 18 percent of the total national supply of beds, not counting the private beds in public hospitals for either period. An Association of Private Hospitals promotes the economic and political interests of these institutions.

Pharmaceuticals are another part of the private market. A household expenditure survey in metropolitan Lima in 1984 found that 2.64 percent of family expenditures were devoted to medical and related services. Of this, nearly half went for the personal purchase of drugs.

Other Subsystems of Health Care. Note should be taken of the well-developed programs for the armed forces, the national police, the other public employees. In 1985 they were served by hospitals with 3,687 beds, or 12 percent of the national total.

Some large private enterprises may also operate special medical care programs for their employees. In 1960 41 hospitals were under such auspices, with 1,539 beds. In 1982 there were 43 such hospitals, but the beds had declined to 996. This also represented a decline in the proportion of beds of this sponsorship from 8.1 to 3.4 percent. This possibly reflects the greater reliance of industrial and other companies on the beds available in private, as well as public, hospitals. Some cooperatives, organized in the period of the first military government (1968–1976), developed special health care programs for their members.

Health Resources

Parallel with the many changes in the organized structure of Peru's health system, the expansion of human and physical resources for health care has been great. The growth is documented most clearly for physicians and health facilities.

Physicians. As noted, Peru's 4,000 doctors in 1960 meant a ratio of 38.5 per 100,000 population. Almost all were graduates of one medical school at the venerable San Marcos University, but three more schools had recently been established. In 1985 Peru had 17,565 doctors, coming from seven medical schools, plus two more in process; all but one of the schools are public. The 1985 doctor-to-population ratio was 91.5 per 100,000.

In 1985 the maldistribution of doctors was still great, but the increased urbanization of the population has reduced its severity. Nearly half the doctors are specialists, although specialty qualifications are not as rigorous as elsewhere. Residencies to train for specialty status are all connected with a university, and universities are supposed to certify doctors in a specialty. After this, the specialist is registered as such with the *Colegio Medico.* Many specialists, who have not come through a university-based residency, however, may be registered as specialists by the college on the basis of experience. Still other doctors practice as specialists without being registered at all.

The maldistribution of physicians—especially between the national capital, Lima, and the rest of the country—is extreme in all types of health program. Lima had 16.1 percent of the national population in 1985, but a study that year showed that 70 percent of all doctors in the Ministry of Health were located in Lima, as were 59 percent of all social security doctors and 65 percent of all doctors in private practice.

As noted earlier, some 70 percent of Peruvian doctors work on salaries, full-time or part-time, for public agencies, even though most have some private practice. In 1981, the percentage distribution of physicians according to their major type of work was as follows:

Type of Work	Percentage
Ministry of Health and its subdivisions	28.0
Social security program	22.2
Armed forces and national police	13.7
Other public agencies	6.6
Private practice or private employment	29.5
Total	100.0

Even among the 29.5 percent of doctors not employed by government agencies, there are many in salaried employment, working for industrial enterprises, religious missions, voluntary health agencies (such as the Red Cross), or other bodies. Some, of course, are entirely in private practice, especially the older practitioners. Among the 72.5 percent of dentists not employed in government, there is little doubt that the great majority are fully engaged in private practice.

The earnings of physicians vary greatly in different types of program. Most vexing for interagency relationships is the differential between work for the Ministry of Health and for social security. Theoretically, all monthly salaries in government are the same, but the social security program pays its physicians for 14 or 15 months in one year. Physicians serving the military forces receive various fringe benefits, through subsidized food and housing. In private practice, the earnings per hour are usually much higher than in any government employment.

To equalize the geographic distribution of doctors in Peru, in 1975 (under the military government) a law was passed requiring all medical graduates to perform one year of rural service. With the resumption of civilian government, however, the policy was changed. Since 1981, after medical licensure, one year of rural service is required only as a condition for appointment to a government post. Most new medical graduates have wanted to do this rural service, but ironically Ministry of Health funds have been inadequate to support the necessary rural posts.

The Colegio Medico has a general regulatory role in medical ethics. In addition, a medical Federation of Peru is concerned with protecting the personal economic interests of the doctor. This is the body that engages in negotiations with the Ministry of Health, the IPSS, or other bodies on the salaries paid to physicians. Only about half the doctors join the federation; yet they all feel represented by it in economic affairs. In the 1980s, for example, doctors working for government agencies went on strike three times to gain their demands. (During strikes, emergency cases are typically served as necessary.) In many countries the medical association, representing the eco-

Table 10.6. Hospitals, Hospital Beds, and Percentage Distribution of Beds, by Sponsorship, in Peru, 1982

Sponsorship	Hospitals	Hospital Beds	Percentage of Beds
Ministry of Health	118	16,190	55.2
Public beneficencias	3	168	0.6
Social security	18	4,554	15.5
Armed forces & police	13	2,093	7.1
State enterprises	10	394	1.3
Other public entities	2	160	0.5
Total public	159	23,559	(80.3)
Private for-profit	115	3,773	12.9
Private enterprises	43	996	3.4
Philanthropic	5	421	1.4
Cooperatives	13	581	2.0
Agricultural society	1	15	0.05
Total private	177	5,786	(19.7)
All sponsorships	341	29,345	100.0

Source: Ministerio de Salud, *Informacion Basica Sobre Infrastructura Sanitaria, Peru 1982.* Lima, 1983.

nomic interests of doctors, is totally unrelated to the body concerned with medical ethics. In Peru, however, the Colegio Medico is closely allied with the Medical Federation, supports its general positions, and looks upon it as the economic arm of the Colegio. Both the college and the federation have been trying to equalize compensation between the Ministry of Health and the social security program, but so far without success.

Health Facilities. Physical facilities for health service have expanded during the quarter-century from 1960 to 1985, but the impressive growth has been in structures for ambulatory care. As a hospital bed-to-population ratio, the supply has actually declined. In 1985, there were 338 hospitals of all types in Peru, with 29,984 beds. This was a ratio of 1.56 beds to 1,000 people. In 1960 there were 24,000 beds, with a ratio of 2.15 beds per 1,000; many of the latter, however, were for mental disease, tuberculosis, and leprosy. If we consider only general hospital beds in 1960, there were 18,833, or a ratio of 1.83 per 1,000—still more than in 1985. Over the last two decades, most of the beds for mental disease, leprosy, and tuberculosis have been closed down, with the current supply of 1.56 beds per 1,000 almost entirely in general hospitals.

Probably more important than simple ratios is the rate of utilization of the hospital beds available. With improved hospital staffing, the average length of stay of hospital patients has shortened steadily, allowing more patients to

be accommodated in each hospital bed during the year. The average length of stay in the beneficencia hospitals in 1960 was 23 days, and these were the most numerous hospitals at the time. In the 1980s, analysis of Ministry of Health data indicates that the average patient-stay in all hospitals of Peru is only about 10.0 days. This means that the current supply of 1.56 hospital beds per 1,000 is accommodating twice the number of patients as the hospital beds were in 1960. In other words, the current stock of beds is equivalent to 3.6 beds per 1,000 in the 1960 patterns of hospital utilization and length of stay.

Because of the transfer of beneficencia hospitals to the Ministry of Health and the expansion of IPSS and other government facilities, Peru's hospital installations in 1982 were 80.3 percent government and only 19.7 percent private. In 1960, of all hospital beds only 44 percent were public and 56 percent were under private auspices. Table 10.6 shows the 1982 distribution of hospitals and hospital beds in Peru, by sponsorship.

The staffing and other characteristics of hospitals, of course, vary under different sponsorships. Ministry of Health hospitals with 55.2 percent of the total beds in 1982 were better staffed than 25 years ago, but still had fewer personnel per bed than social security (IPSS) hospitals. The hospitals of the armed forces and police have still larger personnel-to-bed ratios. Physicians in all the public hospitals are on regular salaries, usually for 6 hours per day (private practice being permitted after this).

The private hospitals are typically much smaller, but they tend to be very well staffed and equipped, particularly those operated for profit. The latter have an average capacity of only 33 beds, compared with an average of 148 beds for all public hospitals. The proprietary (for-profit) hospitals typically have a small medical staff of only two or three full-time doctors who own the hospital, and a large "open staff" of almost any physician who wishes to admit a private patient. These hospitals, as well as those of private enterprises, are usually well staffed with nurses, professional and auxiliary.

The trend in ambulatory care facilities from 1960 to 1985 has been clearly upward. In 1960, the Ministry of Health reported a total of 71 health centers (of all sponsorships), 142 medical posts (staffed usually by one general doctor), and 177 health stations (staffed only by auxiliary personnel). In 1985, the number of health centers expanded to 785; of these 612 were under the Ministry of Health and 173 under other sponsorships. The expansion of smaller primary care posts was as great. Medical posts and health stations were no longer distinguished, but these units together had increased from 259 in 1960 to 1,925 in 1985. Peru has clearly given high priority to the establishment of facilities for primary health care. At present, moreover, the primary care provided by the health centers and health stations includes treatment of minor ailments (with referral of difficult cases to the nearest hospital); in 1960, these units limited their services essentially to prevention, except for the treatment of communicable diseases such as malaria and tuberculosis.

The figures on ambulatory care facilities in 1985, given earlier, include those operated by the IPSS, 67 in all. Among these are 29 large polyclinics, where patients are seen by a wide spectrum of specialists. These facilities, therefore, provide more than primary health care. The distribution of health centers and health stations among the 17 regions (or the 24 departments) is fairly equitable. Hospitals and hospital beds, on the other hand, are heavily concentrated in Lima. The national capital, with 16 percent of the population, has hospitals with 55 percent of the total supply of beds.

A somewhat greater proportion of beds should be expected in the national metropolis, to which patients from everywhere are referred, but this disparity is surely excessive.

Economic Support

In Peru, as in so many countries, the mixture of sources for the health system's economic support tells us a great deal about the entire system's dynamics. As of 1984, Peruvian health system expenditures amounted to 4.5 percent of GDP (gross domestic product). In U.S. dollars this was about $40 per capita, 66.5 percent of which came from public sources and 33.5 percent from private sources. Greater details are shown in Table 10.7.

From Table 10.7, it is evident that, with some two-thirds of its health expenditures derived from public collectivized sources, Peru's health system is much more welfare-oriented than the systems analyzed in Chapter 9. (Within the percentage of expenditures linked to the Ministry of Health, about 2 percent is derived from foreign aid.) Yet, as we shall see, health services are by no means accessible to the total population. In the early 1980s, moreover (between 1980 and 1984), the share of central government expenditures devoted to both the Ministry of Health and the social security program declined significantly. This probably meant less availability of health services from social sources and relatively greater dependence on the private health care market.

Information on the various health activities

Table 10.7. Health System Expenditures, by Source: Percentage Distribution in Peru, 1984

Source	Percentage
Ministry of Health	27.3
Social security	32.9
Other governmental agencies	6.3
Total public	(66.5)
Private households (urban)	2.7
Private households (rural)	2.7
Organized private programs	8.2
Private pharmaceuticals	19.8
Total private	(33.5)
Total health system	100.0

Source: Zschock, D. K. (Editor), *Health Care in Peru: Resources and Policy.* Boulder, Colo. Westview Press, 1988, p. 14.

for which expenditures are made is not explicitly available in Peru. One expert health economist estimates, however, that three-fourths of all health expenditures supports hospital services and only one-fourth supports primary health care and other functions. Numerical breakdowns are available only for expenditures by separate agencies. Thus, a report of the social security program (IPSS) in 1984 showed the following distribution of expenditures:

Service	Percentage
Medical consultations	51.9
Hospitalization	45.4
Dental care	2.6
Vaccinations	0.1
All services	100.0

These hospital costs are probably understated, insofar as medical consultations doubtless include services rendered within hospitals.

Analysis of Ministry of Health expenditures shows a breakdown of services along different lines. Of the total, 17 percent is spent at the central level and 73 percent in the regions. Although figures are not reported, it is almost certain that the great bulk of regional-level expenditures goes for the operation of hospitals.

Regarding personal family expenditures in Peru, repeated community household surveys provide useful information. Thus, in May 1984, a household survey conducted in metropolitan Lima found that 2.64 percent of total household expenditures were devoted to health. A breakdown of these private expenditures showed the following percentage distribution of purposes:

Service	Percentage
Drugs	48.5
Medical equipment	6.4
Physician services	28.0
Hospitalization	14.8
Health insurance	2.3
All purposes	100.00

As so many studies in developing countries have found, the largest share of private expenditures goes to purchasing drugs, prescribed and nonprescribed. Another household study in 1984, based on a nationwide sample, fails to analyze expenditures by types of health service, but does identify those for drugs. Nationally (in contrast to Lima), private drug expenditures accounted for 59.2 percent of the total. It is noteworthy also that in Lima, although the proportion is small (only 2.3 percent), some expenditures are made for private commercial health insurance; this is usually purchased to enable families of modest income (not covered by social security) to use private hospitals.

The very high proportion of private health expenditures going to drugs explains why so much of the overall pharmaceutical market of Peru is in the private sector. Of all drugs sold in the country, only about 20 percent are distributed through government programs (IPSS being the largest). Eighty percent are sold to private buyers. The pharmaceutical companies producing and selling these products are predominantly foreign, such firms accounting for 75 percent of the sales. Their raw materials for drug manufacture are almost entirely imported, and even in the domestic firms with 25 percent of the market, most raw materials must still be imported from abroad. Peruvian inflation, with devaluation of its currency, has caused obvious difficulties in the purchase of these foreign materials.

Delivery of Services

Estimates of the proportion of the Peruvian population reached by the various organized programs of health service and through the private market are difficult to make. With substantial expansion of the resources of both the Ministry of Health and the social security program over the quarter-century from 1960 to 1985, there is reason to expect an expansion of population coverage. With increased urbanization of the population and the known concentration of both human and physical resources in the cities, one would expect greater use of health services.

Calculations have been made of services provided by the Ministry of Health in 1979. Consultations at health centers numbered

4,326,000 that year, and at hospital out-patient departments they numbered 5,401,000. One can only guess at the population denominator of these 9,727,000 patient services. In 1979, however, the rate of encounters in the social security program was 2.5 per eligible person per year. Other data indicate that in the ministry's health centers 52 percent of consultations were for largely preventive maternal and child health services and 48 percent for the general health problems of adults. Based on data of this sort, in 1984 an international health research group drew certain rough conclusions on the accessibility of people in Peru to various types of health service. They estimated as follows:

Program (Source)	Population Served	Percentage Covered
Social Security	3,700,000	18.6
Ministry of Health	5,000,000	26.0
Private market	4,300,000	22.4
Voluntary agencies	2,000,000	10.4
None	4,200,000	22.6
All sources	19,200,000	100.0

There must, of course, be various overlaps among these categories; a single individual may seek Ministry of Health services at one time, voluntary agency services at another, and the private market at another time. The 22.6 percent of people who presumably have no access to any organized health program doubtless purchase some self-prescribed drugs, consult traditional healers, or even use an organized program on some occasions. Still, the preceding proportions may give a rough idea of the operations of the health system in Peru. A possible confirmation of these estimates was made by a former Minister of Health of Peru, who said in 1984 that "about 50 percent of the Peruvian population have regular access to health services, 25 percent have access sometimes but not always, and 25 percent are without any real access to modern health services."

Of course, the nature and quality of services delivered in the several major programs vary. In-patient care in ministry hospitals is of poor quality; many of the hospitals that were former charitable beneficencia facilities have patients still crowded into large poorly equipped wards. In heavily used and overcrowded out-patient departments of Ministry of Health hospitals patients get quite perfunctory care. The ministry's health centers and health stations, on the other hand, are only meagerly used; people seem to lack confidence in the quality of their service, and drugs are often in short supply.

To stimulate greater use of rural health stations and health centers, Peru's Ministry of Health, like those in several other Latin American countries, has trained hundreds of village youth (usually young women) to be *promotores de salud,* or health promoters. These young people visit homes to encourage families to obtain preventive services at the nearest health unit, and to seek medical care if necessary. The promoters are not paid, but they acquire a certain prestige from their functions. Later they may be favored for training as nurses or sanitary inspectors. Efforts to increase the use of rural health services began in Peru and other countries around 1960, shortly after the Cuban Revolution.

Social security program resources are generally much better. They are more fully staffed and equipped and they give much higher rates of service to their insured beneficiaries. In 1979, social security hospitals admitted 65 per 1,000 injured workers per year, for a total of 827 days per 1,000. In that year, the nationwide rate of admissions to all hospitals was only 25 per 1,000 population, and a total of 255 days per 1,000.

The type of health service given in private medical clinics (offices) is inevitably more gracious. Since the physician wants to attract the good will of the paying patient, he tries to be attentive and thorough. Because private hospitals are expensive, relatively few people can afford them, and their occupancy levels are low. Since they are well-staffed with nurses, however, the personal patient care is very agreeable.

In spite of the various deficiencies in Peru's national health system, the available data suggest an improvement in health status between 1960 and 1985. Infant mortality declined from 142 to 94 per 1,000 live births between those years. Although the 1985 rate is higher than that of most other Latin American countries, the improvement is still clear. The deaths of children under age 5 declined from 233 per 1,000 to 133 between 1960 and 1985. Overall life expectancy at birth improved from 47 years in 1960 to 60 years in 1985.

Data on tuberculosis shed light on the influence of Peru's health system on health status. The Ministry of Health reported morbidity of 225 cases per 100,000 population in 1962, with a decline to about 100 cases per 100,000 in 1977. Then the morbidity rose again to 150 cases per 100,000 in 1983. Meanwhile the tuberculosis mortality rates were reported to be 37.8 per 100,000 in 1970, declining to 22.8 per 100,000 in 1980, and down further to 17.6 per 100,000 in 1984. One can infer that between 1977 and 1983 socioeconomic conditions in Peru led to an increase in tuberculosis infections but medical care prevented a greater proportion of deaths. In spite of the poor economic conditions in Peru throughout the 1980s, as of this writing, no impact on national mortality rates has been evident.

MEXICO

Another welfare-oriented country in Latin America at a transitional economic level is Mexico. With a 1984 population of 78,000,000 and a GNP per capita of $3,027, Mexico has a powerful influence in all Latin American society. Its history is especially notable because, even after its independence from Spain in 1821, the country was involved in two major periods of hostility with other foreign powers: war with the United States in 1846–1847 (resulting in the formation of California and other U.S. states) and a period of domination by France, from 1864 to 1867.

History and Health Developments

Survival and recovery from these conflicts has made Mexico a proud nation, whose people make strong demands for social reforms. The most direct consequence of these demands was the Revolution of 1910, which led to the redis-

tribution of much land from large estates (latifundias) to poor peasants. Later many ejidos, or rural land-holding communities, were formed, which eventually played a part in the rural health program.

The 1910 Revolution also led to the Constitution of 1917, which required separation of church from state. In the health system, this brought an end to the beneficencia hospitals (occurring much later in other Latin American countries), and the transfer of these facilities to government. The Mexican Constitution of 1917, which is still in effect, also established health as a federal responsibility.

With the worldwide economic depression of the 1930s Mexico elected Lazaro Cardenas to the 6-year presidency in 1934. During the years 1934 to 1940, the government took control of the petroleum industry, railroads, and other enterprises under foreign ownership. Special medical services were developed for workers in these industries. Further government health services, requiring hospitals and health centers for ambulatory care, were developed by both federal and state authorities. Many hospitals were designated as "coordinated," that is, managed jointly by the federal and state governments. Other hospitals were purely state or purely municipal in their management.

In 1942, a law establishing the Mexican Institute of Social Security (IMSS in the Spanish acronym) was enacted. IMSS covered workers in almost all private industry, along with their families, but initially excluded domestic and part-time workers. The largest portion of social security income was spent on health services, and a nationwide network of modern hospitals, polyclinics, and health centers was constructed. The innovative architecture in IMSS facilities soon became a model for all Latin American countries. To arrange services for all its beneficiaries, IMSS also contracted with government and some private hospitals and clinics.

To provide similar health services to government employees and their families, in 1960 an Institute for Security and Social Services to State Employees (ISSSTE, in Spanish) was established by law. Quite separately from IMSS, this new social security program constructed exceptionally impressive health facilities with the most sophisticated staffing and equipment.

Meanwhile the population of Mexico was growing rapidly, and the economy—through major new discoveries of oil and substantial industrialization—was expanding. The national population of 35,000,000 in 1960 had more than doubled in 1984, and the supply of health resources—physicians, hospitals, health centers, and others—had greatly increased. The population coverage of both IMSS and ISSSTE steadily expanded. The benefits of social security in Mexico were also extended well beyond health services to include old-age pensions, operation of family centers for recreation and training, day care centers for the children of insured working mothers, and so on. In 1979, the federal government appropriated tax funds for providing modern health services specifically to the noninsured and marginal rural population, assigning the responsibility to IMSS, as the IMSS–COPLAMAR program.

At the federal level, the Secretariat of Health and Welfare (SSA) was also expanding its programs. More and more of the state and municipal health facilities were being converted into the "coordinated" type, with joint state–federal management. Hundreds of small health centers were established and staffed by the SSA in rural areas. The medical staffing was often by *pasantes,* or new young medical graduates, required to spend one year in government social service (under a law of 1936, when Cardenas was president). Despite the expansion of health resources and services in Mexico, however, it was difficult to keep pace with the growth in population, especially in rural areas, and millions of people remained without access to modern health services. Mexico, like so many other Latin American countries, had developed a highly pluralistic national health system, with services of very uneven quantity and quality for different population groups.

Pluralism and the Drive to Integration

In the 1970s, there arose a political sensitivity to the need for coordination or integration among Mexico's several separate and autonomous health programs. The two major social security programs, IMSS and ISSSTE, covered nearly 50 percent of the population, but the other 50 percent had to depend on public or private services that were often of limited quality or not at all accessible.

In 1980, the president appointed a commission to study all aspects of the Mexican health system and recommend improvements. The study was completed in 1982 and published under the title *Toward a National Health System.* Based on the study's findings, with updating of the numbers to Mexico's estimated population of 80,500,000 in 1986, the several major health programs served various sections of the population as shown in Table 10.8.

Closer coordination among the programs listed in Table 10.8 was advocated for years, and in 1984 Mexico enacted a General Health Law. The objectives of the new law were formulated under five headings, for the attainment of which major responsibility was assigned to the secretary (minister) of health. The objectives were as follows:

1. Decentralization of responsibilities
2. Modernized administration
3. Integration within the health sector

Table 10.8. Major Health Programs of Mexico: Estimated Population Coverage in 1986

Health Program	Population Covered (millions)	Percentage
Mexican Institute of Social Security (IMSS)	31.5	39.1
Institute for Governmental Workers (ISSSTE)	6.8	8.4
Health programs of other federal agencies	1.5	1.7
Secretariat of Health & Welfare (SSA)	16.7	20.7
Marginal families program (IMSS–COPLAMAR)	10.9	13.5
Private medical care	3.7	4.6
Unprotected population	9.5	11.8
Total	80.5	100.0

4. Intersectoral coordination
5. Community participation

Just as the reorganization program was getting under way, Mexico City was struck by a severe earthquake. In addition to the deaths of thousands of people, thousands of buildings were partly or entirely destroyed. Among these were several major hospitals of the IMSS and the SSA programs, with some 4,000 beds, in the center of the city. After the earthquake, the authorities decided not to reconstruct large tertiary-level hospitals in a central place, but rather to build 10 smaller general hospitals in the peripheral regions around Mexico City. This meant, in a sense, a step toward physical decentralization, which would contribute to the overall objective of the SSA.

The content and quality of services provided by the programs listed in Table 10.8 vary greatly. The programs' economic support and the resources, both human and physical, were extremely unequal. For the 39.1 percent of the national population served by the IMSS, for example, in 1984 health expenditures amounted to 62 percent of the total health spending of government. Yet for the 32.5 percent (20.7 served by SSA plus 11.8 unprotected) of people not covered by social security, the national health expenditures constituted only 22 percent of the total. These disparities translated into enormously greater health resources and services for the socially insured population than for others dependent on the SSA facilities, whether people were accessible to them or not.

Decentralization. Mexico is divided into 31 states plus the Federal District of Mexico City. A minor degree of decentralization developed in the late 1930s when Coordinated Services, linking the federal and state governments, were started. Under these coordinated federal–state health schemes, hundreds of hospitals and health centers were built and operated, predominantly at the expense of the federal government. The health officers responsible for directing these facilities in the states were appointed by the federal SSA and responsible to the federal authorities. Thus, although the governors of each state are elected, the "coor-

dinated" services did not really come under the control of their offices nor of their official health appointees.

The decentralization program launched in 1984 was much more far-reaching. Up to 1986, it involved 12 of the 31 states, containing about 40 percent of the national population. These states were selected for no single reason. Some are quite poor, others affluent. Some are geographically close to the national capital and others are far away. Some have large populations, others small. Their only common feature is that the state authorities were willing to carry the increased responsibilities required and to contribute a greater share of health service funding than in the past. The decentralization objective, however, applied only to the SSA programs, and not to the health services of IMSS, ISSSTE, the oil workers (PEMEX), or other specially insured populations.

Each Mexican state is divided into jurisdictions—246 in all. Although the average is 8 jurisdictions per state, the range is very wide, from 19 jurisdictions to only 3. Each jurisdiction is supposed to be headed by a physician with public health graduate training, but at present master's degrees in public health (MPH) are held by only 47 percent of the 246 jurisdiction directors.

The jurisdictions are usually divided into municipalities or sometimes simply into local health areas served by a health center. The health center is typically staffed by a young physician, doing mandatory social service as a *pasante,* along with one or more auxiliary nurses and other personnel. There is typically a small pharmacy, but for any drugs dispensed the patients must pay a share of the costs. A health center usually serves between 2,000 and 5,000 people.

Peripheral to the health centers are *casas de salud,* or health houses, which may also be staffed by a medical *pasante* but more likely only by an auxiliary nurse. Both health houses and health centers predominantly offer preventive services for mothers and small children; services in health houses are almost entirely of this type.

For a population of 100,000 or more a small SSA general hospital is expected. The medical staffs of these facilities include specialists in the four basic specialties (internal medicine, surgery, obstetrics–gynecology, and pediatrics) plus some general practitioners. Nationally the SSA hospital bed occupancy is only about 50 percent.

The decentralization policy means that the management of all these facilities is being entrusted to state health personnel. Periodic visits are made by officials of the central SSA, but day-to-day policies are made and carried out by the state, with considerable autonomy. Decentralization also means that greater shares of financial support are contributed by the state governments. In 1986, for the 12 decentralized states, this amounted to 21 percent. Of the 79 percent of expenditures derived from the federal government, 68 percent came from SSA and 11 percent from the IMSS–COPLAMAR scheme. (The 21 percent of costs met by state sources is nevertheless much higher than in the past.)

Much of the funding for the construction of new health centers, health houses, and hospitals is provided by the Inter-American Development Bank (BID) through grants and loans. In the general BID program for supporting development in the rural areas of Mexico, priority is given to the 12 decentralized states.

Another aspect of decentralization, originating before the current period, should be noted. For training public health personnel in Mexico, a school of public health has been attached to the central SSA since 1922. In recent years five other peripheral schools of public health have been established throughout the nation. Their faculties are modest, but they provide a great deal of training to doctors directing the health jurisdictions in all the states.

Responsibilities for the well-established and traditionally vertical programs of categorical disease control have also been delegated to the 12 decentralized states. In malaria control, for example, this was done since 1983. General guidelines and supplies of the new pesticides are furnished from the central headquarters, and training courses are still conducted by federal SSA staff at regional centers throughout Mexico. But the campaigns of house-spraying and other control measures are conducted by the states. Programs for immunization, diar-

rhea control (with oral rehydration salts), tuberculosis case-finding, and Pap smears for detection of cervical cancer (the second most common cancer in Mexican women) have also been decentralized. The success of this strategy has actually been somewhat uneven.

Because of the general economic crisis in Mexico, and all of Latin America in the 1980s, the ability of the states to contribute to funding of the decentralized programs has sometimes been less than expected. Nevertheless, the states have undoubtedly made greater contributions to the health programs than previously. It is relevant that the decentralization movement has been an overall policy for the entire government, but priority efforts have gone to health and education. State governors have explicitly agreed to put greater funds into the health services.

Modernized Administration. The objective of modernizing administration has paralleled that of decentralization. The numbers of personnel and administrative tasks were reduced at the central headquarters of the SSA, while they increased in the decentralized states.

One statistical problem on human resources should be noted. The number of physicians employed in all organized health programs of Mexico in 1984 was reported as 54,440. (The vast majority of these also engage in private medical practice part of the time.) A survey of 16 cities by the Center for Public Health Research in 1986 estimated the existence of 97,000 doctors—a figure that, when corrected for underreporting, comes to 102,000. If we assume an approximate number of 100,000 physicians in the country, this would mean that about 46,000 are not in organized employment and are either in private practice or not working as physicians. Yet the central government reports that in 1986 there were 14,000 physicians living in the largest cities who were "unemployed or underemployed." One cannot easily reconcile the difference between 14,000 and 46,000, because neither the national government nor the states seem to maintain a regular or current registry of active physicians.

In spite of these inadequacies of health program information, one must note one positive reflection of administrative style—the apparently high level of morale in virtually all personnel, at both the central and state levels of the SSA. Health personnel of all types appear dedicated to their work and show an attitude of confidence toward the future.

An aspect of financial management is relevant. Hospitals in the decentralized states are supported by budgetary allotments from the state level. The initial preparation of the budget is done by each hospital's administration, based on the last year's experience. After funds are allotted, the hospital still has reasonable freedom to transfer expenditures between budget lines.

Integration within the Health Sector. Judging from the 1982 report *Towards a National Health System,* integration of the organized entities within Mexico's health sector seems to warrant the greatest emphasis in the reorganization movement. The initial action taken to promote integration was to enact a constitutional amendment, which authorizes the secretary of health and welfare (SSA) to promote and coordinate all activities in the health sector. The constitutional language is very broad, and it seems to empower the minister of health to harmonize the component entities of the health sector at a rate and in a manner that he considers prudent.

To implement this policy, the SSA has become "the intelligence center for the national health system," responsible for overall health planning, development of standards, and promotion of research oriented to improving the health system. The secretary of health now participates in the governing bodies of the two major social security agencies, which includes preparation of their overall plans and budgets. Through his influence, for example, the IMSS program has put greater emphasis on the provision of primary health care. Yet the various strategies of decentralization, modernized administration, community participation, and so on have been directed predominantly to the SSA program and have had only modest influence on the entire health arena of social security.

An Inter-Institutional Commission for Education and Health has been established, to co-ordinate the training of physicians and other health manpower with the requirements of the health services. Because of this joint planning, the output of Mexico's 52 medical schools has been reduced, in recognition of an apparent "surplus" of doctors, who could not find employment.

Another coordinating mechanism operates for the standardization of drugs and medical technology, purchased and used by the organizations that provide health care. A unified mechanism was developed for purchasing the large quantities of drugs dispensed in the different programs.

Perhaps the most concrete type of integration has applied to the IMSS–COPLAMAR program launched in 1979 for health services to marginal rural families. Although this was developed and entirely operated by the IMSS organization (with funds alloted from general revenues), in 1985 it was transferred in the 12 decentralized states to the jurisdiction of SSA. This meant the strengthening of SSA resources by hundreds of health centers and hospitals.

At the state level also, Councils for Health Coordination have been established, on which the social security bodies, university medical schools, and other agencies sit along with the state SSA director. In all states, the polyclinics of IMSS and ISSSTE will now serve any emergency patient who may be uninsured. In some states, these polyclinics have agreed to accept for treatment certain uninsured patients, even outside of an emergency situation.

Any socially insured person is free to make use of SSA resources, in spite of his or her entitlement to social security services. This is especially relevant to the general programs of malaria and tuberculosis control and to the provision of immunizations to children. In recognition of this, the SSA has solicited funds from both IMSS and ISSSTE. As of March 1987, ISSSTE had responded favorably. While the funds involved were small—less than 1 percent of the social security annual budgets—the principle is important, and it may lead to larger grants in the future.

In several large cities of Mexico the municipal governments have operated ambulance services and emergency clinics. Gradually most of these services have been transferred to the control of the SSA. Such health facilities were especially well developed in Mexico City, where 29 hospitals (12 for children) were operated, plus numerous first-aid stations and mobile clinics. These resources will eventually be absorbed into the SSA program. In one aspect of health, there are no signs of integration. A major responsibility for environmental sanitation in the cities is vested in the Ministry of Urban Ecological Development. This program continues to operate quite autonomously.

Intersectoral Coordination. Perhaps the best illustration of intersectoral coordination has been the development of policies on drug production, involving relationships of the Ministry of Commerce and Industry with the SSA. Pharmaceutical manufacture is predominantly private in Mexico, but research and development are government-sponsored. Mexican patents are recognized for 10 years, after which less expensive generic drugs may be produced. The SSA drug-purchasing program gives priority to generic products. For the control of narcotic addiction, a program has been launched with the cooperation of about 20 public and private agencies.

Though not brought under SSA, the previously separate health programs for railroad workers and for workers in public utilities (under parastatal organizations) have been coalesced into the IMSS. Only the health services for military personnel and for petroleum workers (PEMEX) remain independent.

We referred earlier to the separate responsibilities of the Ministry of Urban Ecological Development for environmental sanitation in the cities. However, the SSA issues basic sanitary regulations. Responsibilities are divided along functional lines. The Ecology Ministry handles macrowaste disposal, while the sanitary aspects of water supply come under SSA. Restaurant and food inspections are also SSA responsibilities.

In some of the states, interagency health councils may be chaired by the governor, with the SSA health director serving as secretary. These councils may include representatives of agencies for education, agriculture, labor, and other sectors. The control of mosquito breeding will doubtless require the cooperation of agriculture and other sectors. In all countries, intersectoral coordination is one of the most difficult policies to implement in developing improved health systems.

Community Participation. An important feature of the decentralization program is the involvement of community representatives—farmers, women, religious leaders, teachers, and others—in policy development at the state and also the municipal levels. SSA policy calls for the formation of Committees for Social Mobilization at every hospital and health center. Effective campaigns for immunization depend largely on the efforts of such committees.

In one important respect, the involvement of community people in the SSA health program appears to be inadequate. The people, in general, do not make a great deal of use of the SSA health centers or health houses. The Department of Evaluation at the SSA headquarters, on the basis of data from all decentralized states, estimates that doctors in these facilities see only about 8 patients per day. They should see 16 to 24 patients a day, but the people do not come. Likewise the hospitals of SSA and the IMSS–COPLAMAR program report an average occupancy level nationally of only 47 percent. The reaons for these low utilization rates require investigation, if corrective actions are to be taken.

Toward a Unified Mexican Health System

The several strategies outlined in Mexico's General Health Law of 1984 were all directed toward an overriding objective of welding several separate programs of health service, for distinct population groups, into a unified national health system. The approach was not revolutionary, but very cautious, by increasing the authority of the secretary (minister) of health to oversee and even approve the budgets and activities of the other autonomous programs. The spectacular growth of the social security programs, both in population covered and in technological development, made the need for coordination all the more conspicuous. Nevertheless, the decentralization strategy—doubtless, the most important of all—applied essentially to the SSA programs and hardly to the social security health services at all.

After 1982, when a new federal administration came to power in Mexico, economic conditions took a sharp turn for the worse. Following several decades of sustained economic growth, the country was faced with a sudden drop in the world price of oil, its major export, a huge foreign debt, and steep devaluation of the peso. As a response, austerity in public spending was necessary. The share of the overall government budget allotted to public health (SSA activities) at both federal and state levels began to decline. (Social security spending meanwhile continued to increase.)

In this environment, administrative unification of programs seemed to be a strategy for achieving economies as well as greater equity among the several population groups served by the diverse programs. We have noted strategies for coordination in health manpower development, the use of technology, the purchase of drugs, and the allocation of general revenues to IMSS for serving marginal rural families—a function later transferred to SSA. Attempts were also made to equalize salaries across programs and to offer training in health system management, to strengthen decentralization.

The disproportionate share of public spending made for the insured beneficiaries of IMSS and ISSSTE has been noted. Yet the ultimate source of social security contributions, in Mexico as elsewhere, is the purchase of products sold by the industries with covered workers. Serious questions of social ethics therefore arise concerning the expenditure of social security funds. The various forms of coordinating authority vested in the secretary of health, reviewed earlier, may be only the first step in unifying the resources and economic support of the diverse programs in the interests of equity.

The issues faced by Mexico's pluralistic health system have been faced in most Latin American countries over the decades since about 1950. The growth of social security in

economic strength, coinciding with the maturation of ministries of health, in their scope of service and general role in society, were bound to generate political tensions and conflicts. Each country has resolved these conflicts in its own way, according to its special political circumstances. The course of events in Chile provides many insights.

CHILE

More than in most Latin American countries, events in Chile dramatize the influence of larger political events on the configuration and operation of the national health system. Since 1886, when local beneficencia societies came under national regulation, the health system has gone through organizational stages that illustrate major health strategies applied throughout the world at different times and places.

In 1985, Chile had a population of 12,100,000, about 85 percent urbanized, with an annual GNP per capita of $1,891. Its educational development was much higher than that of other nations of this economic level, with a literacy rate of 94 percent. This long thin nation in the southern cone of South America gained independence from Spain in 1810—earlier than other Latin American countries—and its population is composed of more persons of European background. Some Indian ancestry, however, is still extensive among the people.

The Chilean national health system can be reasonably analyzed within four major historical periods, although of course some overlapping occurs between them.

Period of Local Health Services, 1886–1914

Throughout the seventeenth and eighteenth centuries, health services in Chile, as in Europe, were largely a local responsibility. Smallpox vaccinations were given by local authorities in the late eighteenth century, and in the nineteenth century general hospitals for the poor were developed in the main cities by local boards of welfare *(juntas de beneficencia)*, linked to the Catholic Church.

Unlike policies in other Latin American countries, however, central government regulations strongly influenced the structure and operation of the beneficencia hospitals. In 1886, a major body of national hospital regulations was enacted, and enforced by the Ministry of Interior. A national congress of all the beneficencia societies was held in 1917; here these local bodies were given a quasi-governmental status, with clear responsibility for social assistance, rather than being simply voluntary charities. In 1927, a Central Board of Welfare was established to coordinate all the local boards, and in 1932 its authority was greatly extended. There were uniform medical standards, joint purchasing of supplies, fixed salary scales, and other features of coordinated management.

These latter administrative steps were substantially influenced by another crucial legislative action in 1924. In that year, Chile became the first developing country in the world to establish a program of social security for workers—initially along the lines of the Western European nations. This was shortly after World War I, when many countries responded to the new international slogan: "Peace through social justice." To be sure, the Chilean social insurance program was not built on a network of local workers' insurance funds, as in Europe, but it established a single national fund in the Ministry of Labor. For hospitalization, insured workers were admitted to the beneficencia hospitals, and for ambulatory care they went to hospital out-patient clinics or saw private physicians who were paid by fees; this delivery pattern corresponded to European policies. Only workers were covered, not dependents.

Another feature of the Chilean health system had its origins in this period. The first national public health law had been enacted in 1886, establishing certain minimum standards of environmental sanitation in the cities. Responsibility was vested in the Ministry of the Interior, and in 1918 a General Directorate of Health *(Direccion General de Sanidad)* was formed within this ministry. In 1924, the same year social security was enacted, a new Ministry of Hygiene, Assistance, and Social Welfare was organized.

Period of Health System Maturation, 1914–1952

As experience was gained with the medical care program under social insurance, deficiencies in the ambulatory services became conspicuous. The insured population was growing, and their rate of demand for services was rising. After 1932, therefore, the national Social Security Fund *(Caja de Seguro Obligatorio)* constructed several large *consultorios* in the main cities. They offered services in several specialties, dispensed prescribed drugs, and were equipped to perform many diagnostic laboratory tests. The fund also established medical posts in the small towns. These facilities were all staffed by physicians on salary, usually part-time.

The compulsory social security program applied to low-income manual workers, but after 1925 small groups of white-collar workers began to organize voluntary insurance funds for medical care. Typically these funds financed free choice of private doctors, on a fee basis, and hospital care in private beds. A government innovation in 1938 promoted coordination of several of these voluntary funds.

In that year, Chile enacted the Preventive Medicine Law, in response to the criticism that insured workers were being treated for diseases that could be prevented. The initial intention was to provide preventively oriented annual medical examinations, but the focus was soon shifted to tuberculosis, syphilis, heart disease, and later cancer—prevalent conditions that were detectable through relatively simple diagnostic procedures. The 1938 law, moreover, was not limited to the mandatorily insured workers, but applied also to voluntarily insured white-collar employees. To facilitate the screening examinations of the latter employees an amalgamated Servicio Medico Nacional de Empleados (SERMENA) was organized. The SERMENA program played a broader part in later health developments.

The years from 1924 to 1952 also brought

development of the public health program of the Chilean Ministry of Health. There were improvements in environmental sanitation, communicable disease control, and maternal and child health (MCH) services. A nationwide network of health centers was constructed, especially for MCH services, immunizations, and simple first-aid. During and after World War II, Chile received assistance from the Inter-American Cooperative Health Service financed by the United States.

During and after the years of World War II (1940 to 1950), Chile experienced economic difficulties. There were worker and peasant uprisings and great social unrest. In that atmosphere, the great health reform of the United Kingdom—introduction of the British National Health Service in 1948—appeared very attractive to the many Europe-oriented leaders in Chile. In the Chilean Senate, a Socialist Party member and physician, Salvadore Allende, introduced landmark legislation establishing a Chilean Servicio Nacional de Salud (National Health Service), or SNS, in 1952.

Chilean National Health Service, 1952–1973

The objective of the Chilean National Health Service (SNS) was to ensure complete health care to all working people, their families, and all poor people in the country. Middle-class families, who could obtain medical care privately or through voluntary insurance, were not included. The financial support to attain this objective had to come mainly from general revenues (as in Great Britain), but some support would still come from the social security fund for manual workers (not dependents).

This basic strategy was to build on the organized health programs already in operation in Chile, but to weld them into a unified system. Thus, the SNS brought together under the Ministry of Health all the following resources:

- The beneficencia hospitals, already coordinated nationally under the General Board of Public Welfare.

- The social security program, with its numerous ambulatory care centers and medical posts.

- The Ministry of Health resources, including scores of health centers and other units; these were under two major departments: a Servicio Nacional de Salubridad and a Direccion General de Proteccion a la Infancia y Adolescencia.

- Several other special programs, such as a Bacteriological Institute (producing vaccines), the Ministry of Labor factory inspection unit, and some municipal facilities for emergency care and sanitation.

Along with this transfer of programs went all the associated personnel, so that no one lost his job, and additional personnel were appointed. Notably absent from the new conglomerate of programs were those for industrial injury compensation and treatment and the voluntary *empleado* health insurance groups for white-collar employees. Intermingling middle-class and working-class patients was not considered politically appropriate at the time. Two further laws were also passed—one to establish a Colegio Medico for licensure and ethical discipline of the medical profession (controlled by the physicians themselves), and the other to establish salary rates and working conditions for all professional health personnel.

The director-general of the SNS was appointed by the president of Chile, although he was legally under the minister of health. He was advised by a National Health Council, representing workers, employers, physicians, the universities, the social security body, and others. At headquarters, the SNS had two main departments, administrative and technical. Actual management of the health service program was delegated to 13 "health zones" into which Chile was geographically divided. Since Chile had 25 provinces, this meant a distribution of one, two or three provinces per zone.

Each health zone was headed by a health officer who, by law, must have had graduate training in public health. This officer was assisted by specialists in MCH, sanitation, nutrition, and other fields. The most local units of administration were *hospital areas,* with a base hospital at the center and all less developed hospitals plus ambulatory care units and health posts functioning as satellites. It was emphasized that all of these facilities provided both treatment and preventive services, regardless of their former functions. The three largest cities of Chile also had large polyclinics for highly specialized ambulatory care. Whatever program may have previously governed a hospital, health center, or other resource, in the new health zones all the resources came under the supervision of the SNS zone health officer. Integration was the essential theme.

The SNS soon became a model for integrated health services throughout Latin America. Almost all the other countries had developed multiple autonomous programs, and most ministries of health were calling for closer coordination, especially between social security funds and the Ministries, in various ways. Chile was demonstrating that full integration was possible and effective.

In 1962, 10 years after the SNS began operation, it was estimated that about 70 percent of the Chilean population were being served. Studies showed, however, that the proportion actually using the public service was lower than this, since many people preferred to consult private physicians. Of the 70 percent, or 5,391,000 Chilean people, estimated to be covered by the SNS in 1962, 23.4 percent were insured workers, 60.6 percent were their dependents, 14.0 percent were indigent persons, and 2.0 percent were others. Indigence is supposed to be determined by social workers, but there was frequent contention with doctors over the criteria. White-collar employees, of course, were not included, being regarded as the major market for private medical practice.

The cost of operating the SNS in 1962 was 67 percent covered by general revenues, 16 percent by social security, 8 percent by the income of enterprises of the beneficencia societies, and the balance by other sources; only 4 percent came from special fees charged to patients (such as for private hospital rooms).

The financing of health services for Chile's salaried employees, public and private, was relatively complicated. One large public fund—the Caja de Empleados Publicos—covered the majority of civil servants, plus other funds for military personnel, police, and railroad workers. Also a large fund covered salaried private employees, supplemented by special funds for bank employees and others. Some of these groups organized special clinics for their medical care, but most saw private doctors, paid by the voluntary insurance on a fee basis.

The SERMENA program, growing out of the Preventive Medicine Law of 1938, has been noted. All salaried employees, private and public, could obtain preventive screening examinations through this program. If one of the four statutory diseases was found (tuberculosis, syphilis, heart disease, or cancer), a public employee could be treated, but a private employee had to consult a private physician. Neither type of employee, however, was entitled to hospital care at SERMENA expense, except for tuberculosis and heart disease in public employees. The great majority of SERMENA services were provided to employees in Chile's two largest cities, Santiago and Valparaiso. Because of the limitation to the four statutory diseases and the emphasis on preventive case-finding, most of the medical care of white-collar employees had to be obtained through private medical practitioners. The entire arrangement for health care of white-collar employees was obviously complicated and unsatisfactory, and thus its modification in 1968 with the Curative Medicine Law was in response to long-felt needs.

The Curative Medicine Law of 1968 did not bring salaried middle-class employees and their dependents into the SNS, but it provided them the protection of social insurance (that is, mandatory) for virtually complete health service. The services were obtained through private doctors and private beds (in private or public hospitals), paid for by the insurance on a fee basis. Almost all services required personal copayments by the patient. It is noteworthy that the Curative Medicine Law was passed under a politically moderate government, concerned to retain the good will of the private medical profession. Shortly thereafter, in 1970, the Popular Unity government—a coalition of left-wing political parties—was elected to power, under the leadership of Dr. Salvador Allende, the same physician who sponsored the SNS law in the Chilean Senate in 1952.

In the new Allende government the health system was not a major issue, but regarding health there were several clear objectives: (1) the integration of all branches of the health system (except the military), especially the SERMENA program, into the SNS; (2) democratization of all health programs in their operations; and (3) a shift of priorities from hospitals to prevention and ambulatory services.

The first objective of integrating almost all health service programs under the SNS was potentially most explosive; it might have forced the middle classes to lose their free choice of private doctor (with fee payments) and receive care in organized clinics, along with the manual workers. Strong opposition came from both the white-collar SERMENA employees and private doctors. Implementation was therefore delayed, opposition mounted, and in the end the idea was never implemented.

The second objective, to democratize the SNS, was more nearly achieved, though not completely. The previous government of Eduardo Frei, a moderate liberal, had established *community health councils* at several levels, to encourage citizens to participate in the operation of the health program; they were only advisory, however. The Allende administration went further, with executive councils,—representing consumers, health workers, and government, at the head of each institution; these were policy-making bodies, and they injected far more democracy in the entire SNS operation.

The third objective was most concretely achieved. The strong priority for hospitals and local hospital areas, under the original SNS design, was appreciably modified. Greater financial support was given to health centers and ambulatory care generally. Every physician working 6 hours per day in the SNS had to spend 2 hours in a health center. Child health

services and immunizations were freshly emphasized. Half a liter of milk per day was provided to all children up to 15 years old (previously the age limit was 5 years). The hospitals, in turn, were more frugally financed.

These adjustments of the health system were unfortunately only a small element in the 3 years of power of the Allende government. In spite of the constitutional electoral process by which the Popular Unity government came to power, its policies engendered severe opposition both internally and externally. The Chilean mining industry, dominated by foreign corporations, was nationalized and government took control of banking and most foreign commerce. This led to a sudden reduction of credits from international lending bodies, by more than 90 percent in one year. The United States and other countries reduced their trade with Chile precipitously, causing serious shortages of food. Internally, the owners of trucks, essential for the internal transport of food and other goods, went on "strike." (It was not the working truck drivers, but the trucking companies that shut down.) Middle-class housewives, banging pots and pans, held demonstrations in the streets of the national capital. A decline of 28 percent in the world price of copper, Chile's major export, compounded the difficulties.

The first year of the Allende government had brought remarkable progress. Unemployment declined from 6.0 to 3.8 percent. Workers received a 20 to 30 percent increase in real wages. Inflation was slowed from 26.5 to 22 percent per year. But as pressures mounted from the external boycotts and internal middle-class opposition, including condemnations by the Chilean Medical Association, living conditions grew worse. For the middle classes, accustomed to a fairly comfortable standard of living, the situation appeared desperate. (The faculty and students of the Santiago School of Public Health were almost alone in supporting the government.) Finally, after long preparation, starting 6 months after the Popular Unity government was elected, in September 1973 the military leaders of Chile launched a violent coup. Dr. Allende was assassinated and a strictly military government was installed.

The Military Government, 1973–1988

The military government, headed by General Augusto Pinochet, immediately pursued a policy of reversing the social reforms of Allende. All government spending was severely cut; this allowed taxes to be reduced. Almost all nationalized enterprises were returned to private ownership. Tariffs were greatly reduced and massive foreign capital investment flowed into Chile again.

Military strategies in the health system reflected the general economic and political policies. Basically, financial support for the SNS was significantly reduced. The SNS was not dismantled, but it was weakened. The military leaders recognized that millions of low-income workers and indigent people would still depend on SNS facilities for their medical care. The method of operation of the SNS, moreover, was changed, so that funds were no longer allocated to 13 health zones, according to their budgetary needs; instead they were distributed to 27 districts on a flat capitation basis (not adjusted for local health conditions). The SNS program, now renamed the National Health Service System, or SNSS, was estimated to serve the 50 percent of Chilean people with lowest incomes.

The most important strategy of the military dictatorship was to shift the financial support of health services, as much as possible, to the private sector. This applied, of course, mainly to the middle class. Financial support was still mobilized through insurance contributions, but the services were delivered by private medical practitioners. These arrangements were intended to serve the 50 percent of Chilean people regarded as being above the poverty level.

For the latter 50 percent of nonpoor people, the fiscal arrangements and delivery patterns were complex. The SERMENA program was terminated and replaced by a National Health Fund (FONASA), which derived its money from mandatory deductions from all salaries of people above the poverty level. A majority of these were white-collar employees or skilled workers, constituting abut 35 percent of the national population. On receipt of ambulatory or hospital care, these presons had to copay at

least 50 percent of charges personally. There was free choice of private doctors, but charges were made according to a fee schedule.

For the remaining highest-income groups—about 15 percent of the Chilean population—there was a complex system of medical care vouchers. Individuals could purchase vouchers of three values (worth approximately $3, $6, and $9). Higher-income persons, of course, tended to purchase the more expensive vouchers, which entitled them to see more highly qualified physicians. The patient's copayment was also higher with the use of the costlier vouchers, so that the wealthiest patients might copay as much as 100 percent of the official fee. A study showed that in 1983 the lowest-valued vouchers were used by 48.6 percent of patients attended, the second-level vouchers by 41.5 percent of patients, and the most expensive vouchers by 10.1 percent of patients.

The military government has also encouraged the organization of *provisional health institutes* (known as ISAPREs), which are quite similar to health maintenance organizations in the United States. Any contributor to FONASA may choose to have his contributions go to one of some 17 ISAPREs that have been organized. This strategy for limiting health expenditures, however, has been much less successful than expected.

The overall strategy of the military government in Chile has modified the economics of the health system as intended. The proportion of total health expenditures derived from public sources in 1970 was 51 percent (an increase from 43 percent in 1968). Then under military leadership, the public proportion of health spending declined quite steadily to 42 percent in 1975, 37 percent in 1978, and 34 percent in 1980. This trend, of course, reflected people's gradually increasing dependence on private health expenditures, probably aggravated by the aging of the population and the return to priority of sophisticated technology under the elitist military policies. Private health expenditures have probably continued to expand through the 1980s.

Judging by health status outcomes, one cannot find evidence of any general deterioration of health under the military government in Chile. The infant mortality declined from 114 per 1,000 live births in 1960 to 22 per 1,000 in 1985. Life expectancy at birth increased from 64 years in 1973 to 70 years in 1985. Both of these measures, of course, reflect overall levels of living and not only the health system. Yet they may well mean that the shift of health costs from the public to the private sector, affecting largely the more affluent half of the population, did not significantly reduce health services to the poorer half, among whom avoidable infant deaths are heavily concentrated.

Insofar as general opinion can evaluate a society, a plebescite was held in Chile in 1988, to solicit popular attitudes toward the Pinochet military government. The outcome was clearly negative, and general elections for a new government were being planned.

GUATEMALA

The small Central American country of Guatemala, with 8,000,000 people in 1984, may be taken to illustrate those nations of Latin America with very poorly developed health systems. It barely belongs in the welfare-oriented category of country, and borders on the entrepreneurial type, judging by the weakness of its public sector for health services. Yet, for its limited GNP per capita of $1,157 a year (1984), it has made modest attempts at improving services for the people. Unlike the other Latin American countries considered so far, only 39 percent of its people live in cities; the 61 percent living in rural areas have serious deficiencies in access to even rudimentary health care.

Income levels, land ownership, employment, and all aspects of living are extremely unevenly distributed in Guatemala. In 1980, of all landowners 3 percent controlled 66 percent of the farmland. The poorest 20 percent of the population had an average per capita income only one-tenth that of the richest 20 percent. Unemployment and serious underemployment in 1984 was estimated at 40 percent of the economically active population. One-half are pure-blood Indians, living mostly in some 18,000 villages of fewer than 1,000 inhabitants each and working at subsistence farming; some Indians provide itinerant labor for the production of export crops. The rest of the population are mainly of mixed Spanish–Indian ancestry. In 1982, only 45 percent of adults were functionally literate in any language.

Guatemala was liberated from Spain in 1821, but became part of the Mexican Empire and then of the Central American Federation until 1839, when it acquired its current status as a nation. In the twentieth century, after years of political turbulence and economic difficulties, a liberal government, led by Jacobo Arbenz, was elected to power in 1951. A law was passed expropriating large foreign agricultural estates, particularly those owned by the United Fruit Company. In 1954, with unconcealed support from the United States, military forces seized power and held it intermittently for 30 years. In 1985 a civilian government was reelected and a constituent assembly drew up a new constitution. It was generally suspected, however, that military power lurked in the background.

Health System Structure

In microcosm, Guatemala has a health system with subdivisions similar to those in Mexico. Its main component parts are as follows:

1. Ministry of Public Health and Social Assistance (MOH)
2. Guatemalan Institute of Social Security (IGSS)
3. Other government health programs
4. Organized private or voluntary health organizations (PVO)
5. Enterprises—industrial or agricultural
6. Private health care sector—traditional and modern

Like Mexico, but unlike Brazil or Peru, the church-linked or beneficencia hospitals play no part, although foreign religious missions give a little service under the fourth category.

Ministry of Public Health and Social Assistance (MOH). Since its establishment in 1944, this ministry has gradually expanded its resources and programs throughout Guatemala.

Its strongest parts have been in the national capital, Guatemala City, and the *departamento* in which it is located, but since about 1970 increasing attention has been given to building up services in the rural areas. The services provided, both preventive and therapeutic, are furnished through a network of ambulatory care facilities and hospitals.

Administrative direction of the Ministry of Health (MOH) program is highly centralized in the national headquarters. Some years ago, the nation was divided into 8 health regions, each of which contains 2 to 4 local departamentos, but now the regional offices have been abandoned. Instead, the country's 22 political departamentos constitute 24 *areas de salud* or health areas, which report directly to the national headquarters. Each health area has a medical health chief, only a few of whom have had public health training. He or she is theoretically responsible for all MOH activities in the area, both preventive and curative, except for certain vertical programs directed from the top. Currently the major vertical programs are tuberculosis and malaria control, although the intention is to decentralize these also.

In 1984, there were 690 health posts, theoretically serving 4,800,000 rural people, or an average of 7,000 people each. More than 100 posts, however, were not operational for lack of staff or supplies, and those that were functional were very unevenly distributed. At the next higher level in 1984 were 209 health centers, but these were accessible to no more than half of the target population.

MOH hospital beds in 1985 numbered 7,420 in 28 general short-term hospitals, or a ratio of 1.2 beds per 1,000 target population (excluding persons covered by the social security program). One-third of these hospital beds are in two large tertiary hospitals in the capital city, and the balance are handicapped with inadequate staff and equipment. The staffing of the nation's most sophisticated institution (the Roosevelt Hospital with 830 beds) was at an overall ratio of 1.6 personnel per bed in 1977, and that of a typical rural hospital of 70 beds was staffed with 0.4 personnel per bed. Yet hospital costs are estimated to absorb three-quarters of the entire MOH budget, leaving only one-quarter for primary health care and all the rest.

Because of the weak resources and also difficulties in transportation, the rate of utilization of the hospitals, as well as the health posts and health centers, is quite low. Of the 28 general hospitals, 22 are occupied at a level of only about 50 percent. The ambulatory care facilities are likewise used at levels much below their capacity. The health centers, theoretically staffed by physicians and others, have many vacancies. The health posts, supposedly staffed by *rural health technicians* (a special type of Guatemalan auxiliary since 1972, who are trained for 2 years) lack these RHTs in 50 percent of the units. In 1982, the MOH provided a national average of only 0.3 consultation per person per year, mainly in urban centers. Yet large percentages of all trained health personnel are not employed because the MOH lacks the funds. More than one-half of Guatemala's 4,000 physicians in 1984 were underemployed, mainly in Guatemala City; yet they are seldom willing to go to rural areas where they could be usefully engaged.

Social Security Institute (IGSS). Since 1946, Guatemala, like virtually all other Latin American countries, has developed a special program of health service for steadily employed workers, both public and private, and to a limited extent their dependents. In several respects, however, the population coverage and medical benefits provided by the Guatemalan Institute of Social Security (IGSS) are more restricted than in most other Latin American countries.

As of the early 1980s, the IGSS program covered only 8 percent of the Guatemalan population for general medical care. This included workers employed in firms with five or more employees in the capital city (Guatemala City) plus eight other departamentos out of the 22 in the country. (Establishments with five or more employees include agricultural as well as industrial establishments.) It also included the care of children up to 5 years of age. Beyond these beneficiaries, IGSS provided medical care and cash benefits for employed workers in the rest of the country only for accidents—not only accidents in the workplace but those occurring anywhere. If the latter workers, with limited accident benefits, are included, the percentage of people covered by IGSS rises to 13 percent. Administratively IGSS comes under the Ministry of Labor.

The IGSS-covered workers and some of their dependents are clearly a favored population in Guatemala. They are served by 35 hospitals with 1,800 beds, exclusively for social security beneficiaries, and 20 ambulatory care units. Expenditures for health services to this relatively small eligible population are almost as much as those for the total national population served by the Ministry of Health. The rate of consultations of fully insured workers is about 1.0 per person per year—three times the rate in the MOH program. This has engendered a sense of rivalry between those two government agencies, as occurs in several Latin American countries. Yet studies have shown that social security expenditures do not have a negative impact on MOH budgets; rather, they seem to simply enhance funds going into the overall health system and probably reduce expenditures in the purely private medical market.

Other Government Health Programs. Certain other government agencies provide health services or are related to health care in some manner:

1. The military forces, in Guatemala as in almost all countries, have a well-developed health program, with their own personnel and facilities. The national police likewise have a special health program.
2. In the Office of the President (under the direction of the president's wife) a separate social welfare (Bienestar Social) program is devoted mainly to nutritional and related health services for impoverished children.
3. Below the level of the departamentos, there are 327 local municipios in Guatemala; many of them, especially the larger ones, take responsibility for water supply, refuse disposal, and other aspects of environmental sanitation. It is also common for municipalities to construct health posts, which are then staffed and operated by the MOH.
4. The University of San Carlos is a semi-autonomous entity, linked to the Ministry of Education and financed almost entirely by the central government. It is a large institution with a long tradition and great prestige. Guatemala's only school of medicine as well as its schools of dentistry and pharmacy are in this university. These professional schools have an open admission policy, allowing any secondary school graduate to be admitted, although the great majority fail and only a small fraction are graduated. Guatemalan law requires that, before earning the academic degree, every medical student must work for 6 months at a rural health post.

Private Voluntary Organizations (PVO). A great variety of voluntary organizations, largely although not entirely under religious auspices, offer health services throughout Guatemala. A 1977 study estimated that 150 of these were health-related, including nutritional programs. While the ultimate objective of most of these organizations may be religious, they provide at the same time a certain amount of health service.

Enterprises. Private enterprises—industrial or agricultural—provide limited health services in Guatemala. A few large factories in the metropolitan area have in-plant health services, related largely to industrial injuries or occupational diseases.

In Guatemalan agriculture, a great share of the output is by large *fincas,* or plantations, with hundreds of workers. Living conditions for the great majority of these farmworkers are extremely poor, and they are most deleterious to health for those who are migratory (an estimated 80 percent, or about 500,000). Nevertheless, two Associations of Guatemalan Coffee Growers have taken the initiative to provide limited ambulatory medical services to these workers. These are provided through two clinics, staffed by physicians, each of which serves several thousand workers and their families. Although the main support comes from the finca owners, the patient must also pay a small fee for each service.

The Private Health Care Market. Finally, the private health care market in Guatemala is a large part of the health system structure. From various sources, one may draw certain inferences on its extent.

Most ubiquitous is undoubtedly the health service provided by *curanderos,* or traditional healers in Guatelama's several thousand small villages, especially in the central highlands inhabited almost wholly by pure-blood Indians. Along with the traditional healer, usually male, is the *comadrona* or the village midwife who attends the great majority of Guatemalan childbirths.

The number of traditional healers in Guatemala may only be guessed. Of the 1984 national population of 8,000,000, those living outside the metropolitan center were about 6,000,000. Assuming about one curandero for each 1,000 people would yield an estimate of 6,000. Most of these are, of course, not full-time in healing activities, but they make their living principally in agriculture or other pursuits. The same applies to village birth attendants, on whom there are more definite data. The law requires registration of midwives in their municipality, and a 1975 survey of these registers yielded a count of about 16,000. Considering that village midwives probably work more episodically and less regularly than general traditional healers, the estimate of 6,000 for the latter seems plausible.

The Colegio Medico registers all physicians qualified to practice medicine in Guatemala. The register, however, is not corrected regularly for physicians who die, leave the country, discontinue medical practice, or otherwise are not medically active. A 1982 report of 5,000 physicians registered in Guatemala, therefore, might be adjusted to about 4,000 in active practice. Of these, approximately 2,500 are employed by the two major public agencies, the MOH and the IGSS, and by the military forces, by the medical school, and by organized voluntary bodies. This leaves about 1,500 who must rely entirely (or nearly so) on private medical practice. In addition, almost all the salaried physicians employed in organized settings spend part of their time in private practice.

Another component of the private market is the private hospital. In 1977 there were 60 of these with about 1,200 beds (an average of 20 beds each), numbers that were doubtless greater in the 1980s. Of the approximately 500 dentists, the great majority are in full-time private practice, since organized programs in this field are quite weak.

Local community pharmacies are still another component of the private health care market, in fact, a very important one. In Guatemala, as throughout Latin America, a great proportion of the population go directly to a pharmacy for medication to cope with their symptoms; since a doctor's prescription is seldom demanded, the patient thereby saves the doctor's bill. In addition, of course, thousands of drugs are prescribed by doctors. In 1977, there were 224 pharmacists in Guatemala, but fewer than 20 were employed by the two major public programs. Thus, the great majority are probably engaged in retail pharmaceutical practice. In addition, drugs are frequently dispensed at general stores in the smaller towns, without a pharmacist on the premises.

Finally there are a few other providers of private health service in Guatemala—opticians, prosthetic shops, and others. Altogether, even though most of the health personnel data offered here are approximations, it is clear that the private health care market in Guatemala must be substantial.

Health System Expenditures

To gain a sense of proportion on the several component parts of the Guatemalan health system structure, information on the annual expenditures for each part can be helpful. Recent data on these expenditures were not available, but in 1977, the author undertook a modest study of the costs of the Guatemalan health system. The expenditures, per se, were not the objective so much as their serving to reflect the relative importance of various programs and activities in the system. The results of this exercise are given in Table 10.9.

The 10 items in the table are numbered (four public and six private) to permit explanation of how each expenditure figure has been estimated. This was as follows:

1. The 1976 MOH expenditures were reported as $39,900,000. Of this

Table 10.9. Estimated Expenditures for Health Services in Guatemala, by Agency Responsible and by Component of the Private Health Care Market, 1975 or 1976

Agency or Health Care Component	Expenditure	Percentage
1. Ministry of Health (adjusted)	$34,980,000	
2. Social Security–IGSS (adjusted)	31,677,000	
3. Presidency *(Bienestar)*	4,305,000	
4. Municipality health expenditures	1,000,000	
Total public		(47.5)
5. Private voluntary organizations	4,500,000	
6. Private drug purchases	40,000,000	
7. Private physician's care	24,000,000	
8. Private hospitals	5,400,000	
9. Private dental care	4,500,000	
10. Private enterprises + miscellaneous	1,000,000	
Total private		(52.5)
Grand total	$151,362,000	(100.0)

amount, however, 12.3 percent were for transfer payments on behalf of all government employees to the social security system. (The ministry acts as a "conduit" through which to pay the IGSS contributions of all central government agencies as employers of government employees.) This segment of MOH expenditures was subtracted to avoid double counting, leaving $34,980,000.

2. The IGSS expenditures for 1976 were reported as $42,637,000. Of this amount, however, 25.7 percent was referrable to cash benefits. Subtracting this proportion leaves adjusted expenditures for medical purposes of $31,677,000.

3. This expenditure by the *Bienestar* program for maternal and child health services was given in a government report.

4. This estimate of $1,000,000 spent by the municipalities was somewhat arbitrary, but one can be confident that the amount is relatively small.

5. The figure of $4,500,000 for health-related purposes was estimated by USAID (U.S. Agency for International Development) in its 1977 study of these 150 private organizations.

6. The $40,000,000 estimate for private drug purchases was derived from a marketing study in 100 community pharmacies, conducted by several foreign pharmaceutical companies.

7. The estimated expenditure of $24,000,000 for private physician's

care was derived from a blend between two different methods of tackling this problem. One method was based on combined estimates of two knowledgeable physicians about the average monthly income of sets of Guatemalan doctors in four brackets of earnings. This method yielded a total figure of $25,200,000. The second method was based on the earlier estimate that private physicians give 6,000,000 ambulatory consultations a year, and at an average of $3 each (to be conservative) this would yield $18,000,000 for ambulatory service. In addition, the supply of about 1,200 private hospital beds—assuming an occupancy of each bed for 300 days a year (about 82 percent) and a short average stay of 6 days—would yield roughly 60,000 private in-patient cases (360,000 hospital days) per year; at a conservative average of $100 per case, this would yield gross medical income of $6,000,000. Added to the estimated earnings for ambulatory care, the sum is $24,000,000—remarkably close to the estimate of $25,200,000 by the first method. The lower figure of $24,000,000 was used simply in the interests of conservatism.

8. The figure of $5,400,000 for private hospital care was derived from the previous estimate of 360,000 hospital days of care in the 1,208 private hospital beds at an overall charge of $15 per day. In the larger metropolitan

private hospitals, daily charges were well over $20, but in the many smaller maternity-focused hospitals the charges were less, leading to the estimated average of $15 per patient-day.

9. Private dental costs were based on the official registry of 376 dentists in Guatemala and an estimate from two observers that their average private earnings were about $1,000 per month, yielding an annual figure of $4,500,000.

10. Finally, the estimate of $1,000,000 spent by private enterprises for medical care and for miscellaneous other purposes (eyeglasses, prosthetic appliances) was somewhat arbitrary, but conservative, in the light of deficient information.

Altogether we may note that this analytical exercise yielded an estimated expenditure for health purposes in Guatemala of about $151,362,000 in 1976. No allowance was made in the private sector for traditional healing which, while fees are low, would doubtless increase this figure significantly. Nor have the appreciable health expenditures for the military forces or police been considered in the public sector. The expenses of constructing water and sewerage systems have also been omitted, as only indirectly related to health, and the university training of health personnel was not counted because it is commonly attributable to the education sector.

Of the total expenditures, over half are in the private sector—a much higher proportion than are found in Brazil, Mexico, or Peru. It is important to recognize, furthermore, that the Ministry of Public Health's expenditures account for only 23.1 percent of the total. Thus, if a substantial improvement is to be made in the efficiency and effectiveness of the Guatemalan health system, actions must be taken on a much broader scale than the Ministry of Health program.

Guatemala illustrates well the economic impact on a national health system of the somewhat inconspicuous private sector. Another Central American country with similar dynamics is Panama.

PANAMA

In contrast to other Central American countries, Panama took shape as a nation only in 1903, breaking away from Colombia, on the northern edge of South America. The Panama Canal, connecting the Pacific and the Atlantic Oceans, was built by the United States during 1904 to 1914, and the U.S. Canal Zone inevitably had a great influence on the economics and politics of this small nation. Sovereignty over the zone was held by the United States until, after lengthy disputes, it was ceded to Panama in 1978. The canal provided employment to thousands of Panamanians, and the income from ship traffic contributed enormously to Panama's economy. As a result, this small country of 2,133,000 people in 1984 had a relatively high per capita GNP that year of $1,965.

The customary Latin American conflicts between the Ministry of Health and the social security program in Panama have been resolved by a policy that is unique in the Americas. An Integrated Health System, as it is called, has been achieved in most of the country, through administrative agreements between the ministry and *Caja Seguro Social* (CSS), even though financial support is predominantly from the CSS. (In the 1970s, the Ministry of Health had compensated for the weaknesses of its program in rural areas by promoting the organization of hundreds of community health committees to help themselves, especially in sanitation and food production. With the integrated program in the 1980s most of these committees died out.) Since statistical data on the population coverage, resources, and expenditures are available for 1982, the analysis of Panama's health system applies to that year.

Health System Structure: Organized Programs

The 1982 population of Panama was 2,043,653, divided politically among nine provinces. The largest province, containing the capital city of Panama, had a population of 945,678 people, or 46.3 percent of the total. Directly covered for health care by the CSS program were 1,132,127 persons (counting workers and dependents), most of whom live in Panama City. Since 1973, however, virtually the entire population in the eight provinces outside of the national capital, whether insured or not, have been brought under the umbrella of the Integrated Health System; this amounted to another 714,909 people for a total of 1,847,076, or 90.4 percent of the national population.

With this large a proportion of the national population entitled to general health care, there is naturally a great deal of pressure on the available resources. Compared with many other Latin American countries, Panama has a good supply of resources, but not necessarily enough of them under public auspices to meet the demands. In 1982, there were 98 physicians per 100,000 population and 91 nurses. There were 44 hospitals with a bed supply of 3.2 per 1,000 population—exceptionally high. There were 157 health centers for ambulatory care, 131 subcenters of health, and 301 health posts. Of the relatively large supply of physicians, 66.5 percent were located in the capital province with 46.3 percent of the population. The maldistribution of nurses and dentists was similar. Of the 44 hospitals, 14 were privately owned and they contained 13 percent of the beds. Moreover, most of the Ministry of Health hospitals reserve about 10 percent of their beds for private patients. The health centers are medically staffed only with one or two general practitioners, while the subcenters and health posts are staffed only with nurses and auxiliary personnel.

These realities suggest the reasons for existence of a substantial sector of private medical care in Panama. The literacy rate is high (86 percent), and there is a substantial demand for medical service. Only in a few Atlantic Coast provinces, with significant Indian populations, is there any appreciable use of inexpensive *curanderos.* Thousands of people, in both the cities and the rural areas, seek specialist care and are not satisfied with the general practitioner service available in health centers or with the nonmedical personnel in the subcenters or health posts; as a result, they often seek care (which may require some difficult travel) at a hospital out-patient department (OPD). The OPDs are usually crowded, with long waiting periods and hasty attention by the doctor. A natural alternative is to seek care from a private doctor.

To a small extent, private resources are officially used by the public medical care system of Panama. Because of inadequacies in its own hospital bed supply, the CSS has contracted with six private hospitals, to provide some care to insured patients at negotiated per diem rates. Similarly, CSS payments are occasionally made to private physicians. Drugs and supplies are issued by the CSS from its own pharmacies for the care of insured patients.

One aspect of administration of the Integrated Health System in Panama requires clarification. Each of the nine provinces has a provincial health director, appointed by the minister of health; he is responsible in the eight integrated provinces for all health activities— those controlled by the Ministry of Health and those controlled by the CSS. The CSS personnel and all other resources, however, remain economically dependent on the CSS. In other words, the integration applies to the entitlements of patients to health care, but does not mean administrative unification. The provincial director, in effect, reports to both the minister of health and the director of the CSS.

Finally, small charges are made to patients using public medical resources. In the integrated areas, however, these charges are made only to the uninsured patients. The collection policy is said to be lenient, and no one is turned away for lack of money. (Perhaps personal pride may discourage some people from seeking health care.) These payments go into an Administrative Fund, which may be used at the discretion of the local community. In 1982, the fund amounted to only about 3 percent of the costs of operating the government health facilities.

The Private Medical Market

Of the approximately 2,000 physicians in the nation, the vast majority are employed with the Ministry of Health, the Social Security Fund, or both; some may be employed with special programs of industry or the armed forces. Perhaps 10 percent (usually older physicians) are entirely in private practice, but much more important is the fact that almost all employed physicians spend part of their time in private practice.

The customary arrangement for medical employment is for physicians to be salaried by the month for a stated number of hours of work each day. A full-time doctor is paid for 8 hours per day, but many doctors have contracts for 6 hours, 4 hours, or even 2 hours per day. In the remaining hours of each day, the physician is free to engage in private practice. Moreover, and this must be emphasized, it is generally acknowledged that publicly salaried physicians seldom serve in their official positions for the allotted hours for which they are paid. An 8-hour physician often works less than 4 hours, a 6-hour doctor less than 3 hours, and so on.

The financial attractions of maximizing the time spent in private medical practice in Panama are easy to appreciate. Salaries paid in government employment are modest, varying with qualification and seniority. Even the highest level of these salaries would not support a comfortable standard of living in Panama. (To make these salaries more attractive, although regulations prohibit special increments, there seems to be no objection to payment of physicians for 13, 14 or 15 "months" in a year.) By contrast, earnings from much less time spent in private practice are much greater.

An especially important aspect of the private medical market in Panama, as in most developing countries, is the private pharmacy. Thousands of low-income people go to pharmacies or drugstores to buy some medication, as their first response to the symptoms of an illness. They may request a specific drug or simply explain their symptoms, and ask the pharmacist or pharmacy clerk to dispense something. This practice is facilitated by the extremely weak enforcement of drug control legislation in Panama. Almost any medication can be purchased for the asking, with or without a prescription.

Private hospitals (14 out of 44) and private beds in public hospitals are a final component of the private medical market, used by those who can afford to pay the relatively high charges. To increase the size of this population, commercial health insurance has recently been offered for sale in Panama. Eight companies are now selling such insurance, the largest being Mutual of Omaha.

Every national health system, no matter how extensively organized, may expect a certain proportion of private financial transactions to take place. Even in highly collectivized systems, some individuals, with the money to spend, are willing to pay for service, which they could get free in a public facility at somewhat less convenience. The crucial question is: *How much* of a private sector operates within a health care system? Is it large enough to compromise the effectiveness of the public services?

To attempt quantification of private health spending in Panama, three approaches were used: (a) a survey of household expenditures, (b) determination or estimation of the gross earnings of health care providers, and (c) inductive reasoning based on data from several sources.

A household survey in Panama showed that in 1972 expenditures for health services amounted to 2.3 percent of household income. Several trends suggest a rise to at least 3.0 percent by 1982. The purposes of these personal health expenditures were distributed as follows:

Expenditures For	Percentage
Drugs and other supplies	33.0
Physician's care	28.4
Hospitalization	22.6
Dental care	12.2
Optical care	3.8
All services	100.0

On the assumption of 3 percent of household income being spent for health services, expenditures, by this method, would have been $116,491,000.

The gross earnings of health care providers were determined or estimated in various ways. The Income Tax Division of the Ministry of Treasury was cooperative enough to provide statistical averages for the principal types of provider in private practice (physicians, pharmacists, etc.). For some types of practitioner, the "declared income" figures were manifestly unreliable, but for pharmacies (where sales are recorded in cash registers) the declared amounts appeared reasonable. By suitable adjustments, this method found overall personal health expenditures to be $183,000,000.

The third method estimated the gross earnings of physicians on the basis of the average volume of private patients seen per year and average charges per consultation. Expenditures for other types of health care were estimated in various proportions to these. This method resulted in an overall estimate of $178,827,000 for personal health spending.

The average of these three methods of estimation of private health expenditures was $159,439,300. The total expenditures of the Ministry of Health and the social security program in 1982 were $235,923,000. Grand total health expenditures (omitting the military in the public sector and various charities and traditional healing in the private sector) amounted to roughly $395,362,000. Thus, the private health sector accounted for 40.3 percent and the public sector to 59.7 percent of health expenditures in Panama.

What does this finding mean? The central goal and slogan of the Panamanian Ministry of Health for years has been *Salud Igual para Todos*—Equal Health for All. The integrated health system has made headway toward this goal, but there is still a long way to go. The substantial private sector, insofar as it includes medical and dental fees, means that the government is not getting its money's worth from the professional salaries paid. If a doctor is paid for 8 hours of service and he gives 4 hours, the population is being cheated. This may be a sensitive issue, but it should not be ignored or concealed. A vicious circle is created. Hasty medical care in public clinics means poor quality care. Poor quality public care drives many patients to consult private physicians or simply to seek help at a pharmacy without medical advice. As more patients obtain private care, private practice becomes more lucrative. The doctor naturally tries to maximize the time spent in his private clinic and minimize the time in public service. And so the vicious circle continues.

This problem, of course, is not unique to Panama. It is found to some extent in almost all developing countries and many that are industrialized. To the extent that health service is personally purchased, it goes most frequently to those who can afford to pay. The fee payment system, furthermore, may generate unnecessary or excessive services. In either instance, economy, equity, or both are sacrificed.

ARGENTINA

Argentina is, in many ways, different from all other countries in Latin America. Its 30,000,000 people were 86 percent urban in 1984, and came largely from Western Europe ethnic backgrounds. The economy has been relatively strong, with a GNP per capita in 1984 of $1,907. Mining, industry, livestock, and other forms of production are quite well developed, so that for consumer goods the country is largely self-sufficient. The literacy level is 96 percent. The 24 provinces vary greatly in their affluence, but each is largely self-governing, with its own elected governor and other officials.

In the 1970s, there was a period of military dictatorship, which led to economic stagnation and accumulation of a large foreign debt. The 1980s brought enormous inflation, reaching 600 percent per year in 1984. In 1983, however, military rule was ended and a democratically elected government assumed power. The return to democracy brought a gradual improvement in the economic situation, and more rapid development of the health system, especially with respect to the availability of medical care.

Health Resources

Argentina has an especially great supply of physicians, with a ratio of 270 per 100,000 population in 1984—the highest of any country in Latin America. All but one of the nine medical schools are operated by national or provincial governments, and they observe a policy of open admissions. Although many students admitted fail, there are still more than 8,000 graduates each year; the enrollments in all schools are large.

Hospitals and hospital beds are also abundant. There were a total of 5.4 beds per 1,000 population in 1983 (second only to Cuba in Latin America). The ownership of beds was distributed approximately as follows:

Ownership	Percentage
Government (all levels)	63.2
Social security	5.4
Voluntary nonprofit	11.4
Proprietary	20.0
All sponsorships	100.0

The government beds were in institutions controlled by national, provincial, or municipal ministries of health or their equivalent. In addition to public hospitals, the provinces also operate (as do some municipalities) more than 2,600 health centers and dispensaries for general ambulatory care.

Drug consumption in Argentina is especially high. In 1980, it was reported to involve expenditure of $69 per capita, which was by far the highest of any country reporting in Latin America. The great bulk of these drugs were imported, although the country also exports some drug products made domestically.

Public health activities, oriented mainly to prevention, are carried out principally at the provincial and municipal levels. In the central government budget, Argentina's expenditures for health were only 1.09 percent in 1982, a decline from 2.24 percent in 1978. In each of the provinces, public health services tend to vary with provincial wealth, although the central government gives some financial aid to the poorer provinces.

Health Insurance and Medical Care

The conspicuous feature of Argentina's health system is its large network of autonomous health insurance organizations that finance medical care for the great majority of the population. Unlike most Latin American countries, Argentina does not have one or two large government insurance funds that provide services to most beneficiaries through their own facilities and personnel. Much more like the Western European pattern, it has hundreds of relatively small insurance funds that pay for medical care rendered predominantly by private practitioners and hospitalization furnished in either private or public hospitals.

As early as 1910, Argentine labor unions organized small insurance funds to pay for medical care of their members and dependents. These programs were called *obras sociales,* and they were allowed great freedom by the government. Their numbers grew to more than 320 by the 1980s, although the 12 largest ones enrolled more than 50 percent of the total membership. In 1970, membership in a *social work,* or O.S., was legally made compulsory, and by 1984 the funds were estimated to cover 74 percent of the population. Because of some overlap or double counting of O.S. enrollment, however, an adjusted estimate puts their coverage at 63 percent of the population.

In 1970, along with the mandatory legislation, the O.S. programs were coordinated under a National Institute of Obras Sociales (INOS), within the Ministry of Social Welfare. The objective was to establish standards for financial and medical management, even though the government hesitated to strictly regulate these offshoots of the powerful labor unions. In 1984, however, the INOS was transferred to the Ministry of Health, which has been more rigorous in its regulatory activities. Since the financing of O.S. programs depends on the wages of the members, there are inevitably differences in the scope of services offered by each.

Government policy over the years has discouraged the O.S. programs from building and operating their own facilities. The vast bulk of services, therefore, are purchased from private or public providers, and paid for on a fee basis. Nevertheless, some 30 O.S. programs have established their own facilities, with salaried medical and other personnel. These amount to some 114 hospitals and 260 ambulatory care clinics; they account, however, only for 15 percent of consultations and 5 percent of total hospital admissions.

The balance of the Argentine population, not protected by O.S. programs, has other arrangements for obtaining medical care. Several million people (the number is not clear) have organized voluntary mutual funds *(mutuali-*

dades), often along lines of their ethnic or religious backgrounds. These are usually self-employed persons and families, which would not be affected by the O.S. law of 1970 on mandatory enrollment. Their medical care is typically purchased from private providers. In the 1980s the mutual funds declined in importance and have been replaced by medical care insurance sold by commercial insurance companies. Some of these are organized along lines similar to U.S. health maintenance organizations.

Finally, there are people not insured by an O.S. or any of the voluntary insurance mechanisms. These people may obtain medical services at the out-patient department of a public hospital, if they are poor, and otherwise from a private physician. If hospitalization is required, the affluent patient would go to a private hospital and the indigent patient to a public hospital.

The proportions of these several sources of financing medical care have been calculated for medical consultations in 1980, when they were as follows:

Financial Source	Percentage
Obras sociales	45.6
Voluntary insurance	8.5
Public facility	14.4
Personal payment	31.5
All sources	100.0

It is evident that Argentina's national health system is highly organized in its financial aspects. Regarding the delivery of services, the system has intervened very little in the private world. The great bulk of ambulatory medical care is furnished by physicians in their private offices, even when the financing has been collectivized by mandatory or private insurance. Hospitalization is provided mainly in public hospitals (with 68.6 percent of all hospital beds), but the attending physicians are predominantly engaged in private practice every day.

In 1987, the Chamber of Deputies of the Argentine Congress enacted a far-reaching law, which would ensure financial protection for health services to everyone in the country. The structure of obras sociales, hospitals, private medical practice, and so on would not be altered. Through one mechanism or another, however, everyone would be assured of needed health services. As of this writing, final action on this legislation had not been taken.

BARBADOS

Barbados is a small island of 294,000 people (1984) that, until 1966, was a British colony. Unlike the other countries analyzed in this chapter, it is not Latin American, but with a GNP per capita of $3,850 in 1984 it is at a transitional economic level and its health system is clearly welfare-oriented. Though it is not served by a large social security program for medical care, like the larger Latin American countries, other strategies have been effective in making the great majority of its people accessible to needed health services.

With its high production of sugar cane, and a setting and climate very attractive for tourism (from both Europe and America), Barbados was favorably treated by the colonial government. This included development of an infrastructure for the health services that was already quite well developed by the time of independence. In 1976, the Barbados Labor Party was elected to power. The Minister of Health attended the WHO/UNICEF Conference on Primary Health Care at Alma Ata in 1978, returning with enthusiasm for developing a health system built on a firm foundation of primary health care for everyone. Eventually it developed into a comprehensive National Health Service.

Primary health care, on which this account concentrates, has been available in Barbados from several sources, not efficiently integrated. In 1984 there were 77 doctors per 100,000 population, about half of whom were in private general practice. Their fees were relatively low and, since the entire island is only 166 square miles, distances are short, so that most of the population have easy access to care. Based on studies made in 1977, nearly 60 percent of all primary care encounters in Barbados have been with these general practitioners.

Other resources for aspects of primary

health care (PHC) are provided by the Ministry of Health (MOH). Shortly before independence, the colonial government constructed a large 530-bed general hospital. Service in this facility was entirely without charge, except for use of one of the few private rooms. There is a large out-patient department, staffed by specialists and residents-in-training. Most of the OPD is regarded as a "casualty service," to which patients may come at any time for any complaint. It is estimated that two-thirds of the cases are not true emergencies but conditions within the proper sphere of PHC. Patients come because it is convenient, it is free, and it requires no appointment, as does a private doctor.

Another MOH service is given at 11 district clinics held weekly throughout the island for indigent persons, but especially elderly patients with chronic disease. These are staffed by local general practitioners, paid on a per-session basis. The clinics are located adjacent to 11 small government facilities for long-term care, constructed many years ago.

Still another component of PHC is provided through a small network of MOH health centers and polyclinics offering preventive services for mothers and children, immunizations, treatment of venereal disease cases, health education, and other preventive services. These units also serve as an official base for public health nurses and sanitarians. In 1980 there were six of these, but more were being developed. Through the services of these health units, Barbados children have had a high record of immunization, and the incidence of preventable infectious diseases is very low.

A final source of PHC is not intended for such services, but must be recognized. Many of the salaried specialists on the large government hospital staff are free to engage in private practice when their hospital duties are finished. Typically this is in the late afternoons, when patients are also at the end of their working day. Hence, many visits to these specialists are for simple conditions that fall properly within the domain of PHC.

Of the five types of PHC available in Barbados, the two providing the greatest volume of services—general practitioners and hospital specialists off-duty—are paid for privately; they account for about two-thirds of the services. Organized clinics or health centers under the MOH provide the remaining third of PHC services.

A plan was considered to organize general practitioners, with nurses and clerks, into small teams that would provide PHC to groups of people selecting them. Capitation payments, as in the British National Health Service, would be made to each team from a social insurance fund, to which all employees and employers would contribute. The foundation for such a fund already existed in an old-age pension program operating since 1966.

Calculations demonstrated that a very small increment, added to the old-age insurance contributions (less than 2.0 percent of wages, shared by employees and employers), plus the expenditures already being made by the Ministry of Health (for health centers and district clinics) would cover the costs of this universal PHC program. Most of the funding would simply constitute a shift of money from private to public sectors—that is, from fees paid by private patients to social insurance contributions. Barbados government leaders were initially enthusiastic about the plan. Then, objections from hospital specialists (who would lose fees from many of their private patients) led to political controversies that obstructed implementation.

Even without a public program of primary health care, financed largely by social insurance, expenditure data show the health system of Barbados to be welfare-oriented. Of all central government expenditures, 16 percent are devoted to the health system; less than 1.0 percent goes for military purposes. As a share of GNP, the health system as a whole absorbs 7.3 percent—an exceptionally high figure for a transitional developing country. Approximately 65 percent of this comes from the public sector, and much of this money is doubtless used for the support of public hospitals (a 700-bed mental institution supplements the 530-bed general hospital), with 10.2 beds per 1,000 population. This unbalanced spending, however, may eventually rekindle political interest in the development of a sronger integrated program of primary health care.

Barbados is only one of several Caribbean islands that were formerly colonies of European powers. The pattern of providing free medical care through large hospitals, with salaried medical staffs, was commonplace. In the 1970s and 1980s, steps were taken to modify this approach and give higher priority to primary health care. Mandatory insurance was frequently regarded as the most feasible method of financing. Fundraising by insurance, outside the general government budget, and the feasibility of using insurance funds to pay private sector providers, were considered great advantages. In 1988, these strategies were being actively studied by Trinidad and Tobago, the most affluent of the Caribbean island-states.

OTHER WELFARE-ORIENTED HEALTH SYSTEMS IN LATIN AMERICA

Several other countries at a transitional level of economic development have welfare-oriented health systems. We now consider highlights of three more such national health systems in Latin America.

Colombia

The health system of Colombia, in both its strengths and weaknesses, is quite typical of the Latin American scene. The 1984 population of 28,811,000 had an annual per capita GNP of $1,582. The population was 67 percent urbanized, but most of the national wealth came from the export of agricultural products, especially coffee. The literacy level for adults in 1984 was 88 percent.

The Ministry of Health is the major organized Colombian health agency, theoretically in charge of the development of a broad National Integration Plan, legislated in 1975. This plan was intended to ensure that every Colombian resident would have access to needed health services, through one program or another, by 1990. Implementation of the plan called for cooperation between the MOH and the social security sytem, voluntary provident funds, and the private sector. Below the national level are 23 departamentos and 8 territories; the governor of each departamento appoints the health director, although the governor himself is not elected but is designated by the central government. Each depart-

mental health director is also theoretically expected to coordinate the several organized programs within his jurisdiction, but this has seldom been achievable.

The Ministry of Health services are provided through a national network of 617 hospitals and some 2,000 health centers and small health posts. The latter are staffed only by auxiliary health personnel (mainly assistant nurses and sanitarians), but health centers each have at least one physician, and hospitals have several full-time doctors. *Promotores de salud,* or health promoters, with 3 weeks of training, are attached to the health centers and health posts, to visit village households and encourage the use of preventive and treatment services. Initially in the 1970s, health promoters were customarily young volunteers. Paying them minimum salaries in the 1980s, however, resulted in much improved performance.

Since 1938, Colombia has had a national system of social security, under the Instituto de Seguro Social (ISS), which covers industrial and commercial employees as well as the self-employed, for comprehensive medical services. Government employees are also covered, through a special subdivision, which also provides services for military personnel and police. Dependent spouses are covered only for maternity care, along with infants in their first year of life. Although the population covered has gradually expanded, by 1982 only about 15 percent of all Colombians were eligible.

Health services are provided to ISS beneficiaries through a network of well-staffed ISS hospitals and "basic care centers" in the main cities, where most covered persons live. Services are also provided in selected MOH and also private facilities, under contract. With periodic contributions from both employees and employers, the ISS beneficiaries receive a much higher quality and quantity of health services than the rest of the population.

Based on ethnic or religious backgrounds, a number of small "provident funds" or welfare funds support medical care costs in Colombia. These funds ordinarily pay for services rendered by private providers, and their expenditures are included within the private sector.

Finally, there is the population that must depend on the purely private market for medical care. A small percentage consult traditional healers, especially in the rural areas. A major household survey in 1967 found that, of all ambulatory care encounters, only 3 percent in the cities and 17 percent in rural areas (11 percent nationally) were with curanderos. The rate of such contacts has undoubtedly declined since then.

Also in the private market are affluent people who customarily seek medical care from private physicians and private hospitals. Even low-income people, without easy access to Ministry of Health resources (or not satisfied with them), may consult private practitioners, although they more often purchase drugs directly in a pharmacy. Then, of course, there are impoverished and many physically isolated people—often in the Andean mountains of Colombia—who have no access to any type of modern health service.

Taking these sources of health service together, the population of Colombia obtained care in 1978, according to the following percentage distribution:

Source of Care	Percentage
Ministry of Health	52.3
Social security	15.0
Private services (provident funds and individuals)	10.0
None (population without access)	22.7
All sources	100.0

The proportion of persons without any access to health care in the late 1980s may well have been reduced. Regarding the content of these services, if the expenditures of the Ministry of Health and the ISS are related to the populations they serve, one finds that for each person served by the MOH the cost was $28 per year in 1978, and for each ISS beneficiary it was $108.

In 1978, the total health system of Colombia absorbed 5.4 percent of GDP (gross domestic product). This money was divided approximately in thirds among the major sources of health care as follows: Ministry of Health, 31.5 percent; social security, 35.2 percent; and private market, 33.3 percent. One can appreciate the concern of the government of Colombia to

integrate these major entities within its health system.

To analyze Colombia's health system in its public/private proportions, the preceding data mean that the public sector accounts for 66.7 percent of health expenditures and the private sector for 33.3 percent. In terms of the ownership of hospital beds, public bodies control 85 percent and private bodies control 15 percent. In spite of its many difficulties, Colombia's health system is clearly welfare-oriented.

Ecuador

Another Andean country, Ecuador, has similar proportions of public and private sectors in the health system. Much smaller than Colombia, Ecuador's population in 1984 was 9,137,000, of whom 51 percent were urban. The GNP per capita was $1,455 in 1984 and the literacy level for adults was 82 percent.

As almost everywhere, the Ministry of Public Health is the major public agency. Its resources provide health services to most of the population, it employs most of the country's doctors, and it controls more than half of the national supply of hospital beds. Ecuador has 19 provinces, each of which is directed by a provincial health officer, appointed by the central ministry of public health (MOPH).

After the MOPH, the most important public agency in the health system structure is the social security program, or the IESS. The major part of the IESS-insured population are industrial, commercial, and government employees, whose coverage began in 1935. The numbers have gradually increased to some 8.5 percent of the 1983 population. Since 1968, coverage has been extended, although for a less comprehensive scope of services, to rural agricultural workers in selected provinces; these constitute 4.5 percent of the population. Altogether, therefore, the two branches of the IESS cover 13.0 percent of the national population. Services to both these groups are provided by dispensaries and hospitals owned and staffed by the IESS itself. Some of the agricultural beneficiaries may use facilities of the MOPH, with reimbursement by the IESS.

Still other organized health programs operate under the government. These include the

National Institute of the Child and Family (INNFA), the Ministry of Social Welfare, with creches for children and homes for the aged, the Ministry of the Interior, and the Armed Forces Health Service (FFAA).

The private sector in Ecuador includes a beneficencia, or welfare board, in one city, Guayaquil, and several voluntary health agencies—the National Red Cross, the Cancer Association, the Child Protection Society, and others. Finally, a for-profit market includes privately practicing physicians and private hospitals in the main cities, pharmacies, and the health programs of industrial enterprises (sometimes financed by commercial insurance). In rural areas, traditional healers are believed to play a significant role, estimated by some anthropologists to account for 50 percent of first encounters during an illness.

The most numerous health facilities in Ecuador are the health centers and health subcenters established by the MOPH, along with the urban and rural dispensaries of the IESS. Altogether these came to 1,230 facilities for ambulatory care in 1983. Hospitals numbered 362, and their bed distribution according to agency sponsorship gives a good picture of the array of organized health programs in the country. As of 1983, the hospital beds were distributed as follows:

Sponsorship	Percentage of Beds
Ministry of Public Health	52.5
Social security	10.0
Welfare Board of Guayaquil	14.7
Military forces	4.7
Other government agencies	0.5
Private market	17.6

The 82.4 percent of hospital beds under public sponsorship is certainly larger than the percentage of health expenditures in the public sector. Health spending in private pharmacies, and for the services of private physicians or *curanderos,* are not reflected by these figures. The great majority of graduates from Ecuador's five medical schools are employed by the MOPH, the IESS, or some other agency, but most of them also engage in private prac-

tice. While the economic private sector is therefore doubtless more than 17.6 percent, the public sector of Ecuador's health system probably includes well over 60 or 70 percent of the total.

Venezuela

Much more affluent than the two preceding countries, Venezuela had a per capita GNP in 1984 of $3,756. Its population of 16,863,000 was also more urbanized at 76 percent; the literacy level was 87 percent among adults.

Venezuela's exceptionally high GNP is due mainly to its supplies of petroleum, even though the initial exploitation of this natural resource was by foreign corporations; in the 1930s and 1940s, Venezuela acquired a larger share of the oil revenues. This income permitted a great deal of industrial development and urbanization. In 1976, the oil industry was completely nationalized, with compensation to the foreign owners. After this, an expanding program of social security came to provide medical services, by the late 1980s, to more than half of the national population.

The Venezuelan Ministry of Public Health has put its major emphasis on primary health care in the rural areas, especially because of the extensive services of social security in the cities. In 1983, there were 2,443 rural dispensaries, medically staffed, and 426 rural health posts, staffed by auxiliaries. Somewhat larger urban ambulatory care centers, operated by the MOPH, numbered 548.

In the 1960s, Venezuela was one of the pioneers in Latin America to prepare and deploy briefly trained community health workers to serve rural populations. Although the idea was strongly opposed by the Medical Federation, a courageous public health leader developed courses of about 4 months in *medicina simplificada* for young men, many of whom were former border guards or sanitary inspectors. Private physicians opposed the idea as constituting a degradation of medicine, even though physicians would not settle in rural areas. Eventually, the concept prevailed, and in the 1970s community health workers became widely accepted throughout Latin America and elsewhere.

In 1976, by legislation a National Coordinated Health Service was established in Venezuela. Theoretically, the funds of social security and the MOPH were to be consolidated in each of the 20 states and two territories, to provide general health services. The extent to which this consolidation has been implemented is not clear, but Venezuela's long life expectancy of 70 years in 1985 and its low infant mortality of 36 per 1,000 live births in 1986 suggest progress in its national health system. A slight decline in the ratio of hospital beds to population from 2.9 per 1,000 in 1978 to 2.7 per 1,000 in 1983 reflects the emphasis on primary health care.

The distribution of the overall Venezuelan hospital bed supply is a reflection of the welfare orientation of the country. In 1983, the MOPH controlled 59.8 percent of all hospital beds, the social security program 16.4 percent, and the private sector 23.8 percent. Before 1960, Venezuelan political power was in the hands of several military dictators, but since then the dominant ideology has yielded significant social reforms in several societal sectors, including the health system.

SUMMARY COMMENT

Each of the 11 transitional-level countries with welfare-oriented health systems examined in this chapter obviously has unique characteristics, and yet some common traits are evident. Leaving aside Barbados—a small non-Latin island state—all 10 of the Latin American countries have taken substantial steps to organize health services for important sections of their population. By economic criteria, the greatest attention has been paid to employed workers and their families, even though these constitute minorities of the national population. The population coverage, as a percentage of national totals, however, has gradually increased, especially in the large countries (Brazil, Mexico, and Argentina), but also in Costa Rica. The old European strategy of social insurance or social security has been employed to raise the funds but, unlike the customary European model, the pattern of delivery of service has

usually been through salaried teams of medical and allied personnel working in special polyclinics and hospitals. The major exception is Argentina, where private physicians, paid by fees, predominate.

At the same time, ministries of health (MOH) in all the Latin American national health systems have organized services for the relatively large rural populations, in pyramidal frameworks that generally correspond with the country's provinces and other subdivisions. Regional hospitals have been built in urban trade centers serving rural districts, and the old church-supported beneficencia hospitals have been largely transferred to MOH control. Health centers for ambulatory patients now offer general medical care to anyone, after their initial focus on preventive services for mothers and children. These centers are typically surrounded by small health posts, staffed by auxiliary health workers, but consultation of these posts by the people has often been disappointingly low. The quantity and quality of services, provided by MOH resources, are usually quite below the standards in social security programs serving mainly urban families. Many poor people, dissatisfied with public services, purchase self-prescribed drugs in private pharmacies.

Since the end of World War II, a movement has grown in Latin America to coordinate or integrate the health programs of ministries of health with those of social security organizations. A model of such integration was demonstrated in Chile, in 1952, with the combination of MOH and social security resources, along with the network of beneficencia facilities, into a new Chilean National Health Service, financed mainly from general revenues. Except for revolutionary changes launched in Cuba and Nicaragua (discussed later), however, no other country followed Chile's lead. Several Latin American health systems did undertake elements of integration, such as the unification of initially separate social security programs in Brazil and Peru or the sweeping coordination of hundreds of obras sociales in Argentina.

Local traditional healers are still functioning in the rural areas of these countries, but their role has been declining. A slightly growing percentage of the overall GNP is being devoted to the national health systems. Various forms of decentralization of authority are also being explored by the ministries of health in several of the systems, partly as a gesture of democratization and partly as a strategy for inducing local units of government to assume some of the burden of health system costs.

REFERENCES

Brazil

Anon., "Social Security for Rural Workers in Brazil." *Social Security Bulletin,* June 1970, pp. 18–20.

CONASP, *Plan for Reorientation of Health Care Under Social Security.* Brasilia, August 1982.

De Azevedo, Antonio Carlos, *Seminar on National Health Administration: Country Report—Brazil.* Tokyo, Japan, 1984 (processed report).

Del Nero, Carlos Roberto, *Structuring Inequality: The Development of Health Services in Brazil.* London: University of London, School of Economics and Political Science (Ph.D. dissertation), 1984.

Donnangelo, Maria Cecilia, *Condicoes de Exercicio Profissional da Medicina na Area Metropolitana de Sao Paulo.* Sao Paulo: Universidade de Sao Paulo, 1982.

Goncalves, Ernesto Lima, *Administracao de Saude no Brasil.* Sao Paulo: Livraria Pioneira Editoria, 1982.

Knight, Peter T., "Brazilian Socio-economic Development: Issues for the Eighties." *World Development,* 9:1063–1082, 1981.

McGreevey, William Paul, "The High Costs of Health Care in Brazil," *PAHO Bulletin,* 22(2):145–166, 1988.

McGreevy, William, *Brazilian Health Care Financing and Health Policy: An International Perspective.* Washington, D.C.: World Bank, November 1982.

Ministerio da Previdencia e Assistencia Social (MPAS), *INAMPS em Dados 1982.* Brasilia, 1983.

Ministerio da Saude, Centro de Documentacoa, *Cadastro de Estabetecimentos de Saude: Brasil 1981 (Vol. II).* Brasilia, 1982.

Ministry of Education and Culture, Ministry of Health, Ministry of Social Security, Pan American Sanitary Bureau—Principal Evaluation Group, Program of Research in Health Services (PISS). Brasilia, 1982.

OPS/OMS, Grupo de Trabajo Sobre Characteristicas de Organizacion de Atencion Medica, *Informe Final.* Washington, D.C., 9–13 April 1984.

OPS/OMS Representacao no Brasil, *Primeira Approximacao ao Perfil e Analise de Pais.* Brasilia, 1984.

Pinto, Victor Gomes, *Saude Para Poucos on Para Muitos: O Dilema de Zona Rural e das Pequenas Localidades.* Brasilia: Instituto de Planejamento Econmico e Social, February 1983.

Rodriguez, R., et al., *The Role of Information Processing in the Reorganization of the Social Security Health Care System of Brazil.* Sao Paulo: Centro de Informacao e Analise (Hospital das Clinicas, Universidad de Sao Paulo), January 1984.

Roemer, Milton I., "The Changeability of Health Care Systems: Latin American Experience." *Medical Care,* 24(1):24–29, January 1986.

Roemer, Milton, I., *Medical Care in Latin America.* Washington, D.C.: Organization of American States (Studies and Monographs III), 1963.

Roemer, Milton, I., *The Organization of Medical Care under Social Security.* Geneva: International Labour Office (Studies and Reports, New Series No. 73), 1969.

Peru

Bravo, A. L., "Development of Medical Care Services in Latin America." *American Journal of Public Health,* 48:434–447, April 1958.

Bustios Romani, Carlos, *Atencion Medica y Su Contexto: Peru 1963–1983.* Lima: Escuela de Salud Publica del Peru, 1985.

Hall, Thomas L., *Health Manpower in Peru.* Baltimore: Johns Hopkins Press, 1969.

Institute Nacional de Estadistica, *Cuentas Nacionales del Peru 1950–1982.* Lima, August 1983.

Instituto Peruano de Seguridad Social, "Informacion Basica de IPSS." Lima, 1984.

Keaty, Charles, and Geraldine Keaty, *A Study of Private Voluntary Organizations in Peru.* Boston: Management Sciences for Health, 1983.

Mesa-Lago, Carmelo, *Social Security in Latin America: Pressure Groups, Stratification and Inequality.* Pittsburgh: University of Pittsburgh Press, 1979.

Ministerio de Salud, *Informe Estadistica: Produccion de Actividades de Salud.* Lima, 1979.

Ministerio de Salud, *Informacion Basica Sobre Infrastructura Sanitaria Peru 1982.* Lima, 1983.

Ministerio de Salud, *Recursos Humanos en Salud Periodo 1970–1985.* Lima, 1982.

Pan American Health Organization, *Health Conditions in the Americas, 1981–1984,* Vols. I and II. Washington, D.C.: PAHO, 1986.

Sotelo, Juan Manuel, "La Salud: Reto y Accion para Nuestra Partido." Lima, 1984.

Suarez-Berenguela, Ruben M., *Financing the Health Sector in Peru,* Washington, D.C.: World Bank (LSMS Working Paper No. 31), 1987.

Zschock, Dieter K. (Editor), *Health Care in Peru: Resources and Policy.* Boulder, Colo.: Westview Press, 1988.

Zschock, Dieter K., "Health Sector Disparities in Peru." *Bulletin of the Pan American Health Organization,* 23(3):323–336, 1989.

Mexico

Crarioto Menses, Adalberto, "Recent Progress in the Program for Extending Health Service Coverage to Rural Mexico." *Bulletin of the Pan American Health Organization,* 13(3):244–248, 1979.

Davis Tsu, Vivien, "Underutilization of Health Centers in Rural Mexico: A Qualitative Approach to Evaluation and Planning." *Studies in Family Planning,* 11(4):145–154, 1980.

Estados Unidos Mexicanos, Poder Ejecutivo Federal, *Programa Nacional de Salud 1984–1988.* 1984.

Federacion de Sindicatos de Trabajadores al Servicio del Estato, *Seguridad y Servicios Sociales para los Trabajadores del Estado.* Mexico, 1961.

Frenk, Julio, J. L. Bobadilla, J. Sepulveda, J. Rosenthal, E. Ruelas, M. A. Gonzales-Block, and J. Urrusti, "An Innovative Approach to Public Health Research: The Case of a New Center in Mexico." *Journal Health Administration Education,* 4(3):467–481, Summer 1986.

Instituto Mexicano del Seguro Social, *Servicios Medicos Proporcionados durante el Amo de 1961,* Mexico, 1962.

Lopez-Acuna, Daniel, "Health Services in Mexico." *Journal of Public Health Policy,* 1(1):83–95, 1980.

Ministry of Health, Mexican Government, *Mexico's Report 1982–1986.* Washington, D.C.: Pan American Health Conference, July 1986.

Secretaria de Salud, Subsecretaria de Planeacion, *Programa de Fortalecimiento y Descentralizacion Municipal en Materia de Salud.* 1986.

Secretaria de Salud, Subsecretaria de Planeacion, *Evaluacion del Proceso de Descentralizacion.* Marzo de, 1987.

Secretaria de Salud, *Programa de Descentralizacion de los Servicios de Salud.* Mexico, 1985.

Secretaria de Salubridad y Asistencia, *Direccion de Servicios Coordinados: Direction General.* Mexico, 1962.

Soberon, Guillermo, Julio Frenk, and Jaime Sepulveda, "The Health Care Reform in Mexico: Before and After the 1985 Earthquakes." *American Journal of Public Health,* 76(6):673–680, 1986.

Young, James Clay, *Medical Choice in a Mexican Village.* New Brunswick, N.J.: Rutgers University Press, 1981.

Chile

Belmar, R., "Evaluation of Chile's Health Care System, 1973–1976: A Communique from Health Workers in Chile." *International Journal of Health Services,* 7(3):531–540, 1977.

Chanfreau, D., "Professional Ideology and the Health Care System in Chile." *International Journal of Health Services,* 9(1):87–105, 1979.

Debray, R., *The Chilean Revolution: Conversations with Allende.* New York: Vintage Books, 1971.

Duran, Hernan, "Sintesis de la Historia de las Acciones de Salubridad en Chile." Santiago: Escuelade Salubridad, 1954.

Feinberg, R. E., *The Triumph of Allende: Chile's Legal Revolution.* New York: Mentor Books, 1972.

Haignere C. S., "The Application of the Free Market Economic Model in Chile and the Effects on the Population's Health Status." *International Journal of Health Services,* 13(3):389–405, 1983.

Hall, T. L., and S. Diaz P., "Social Security and Health Care Patterns in Chile." *International Journal of Health Services,* 1(4):362–377, 1971.

Hall, Thomas L., W. A. Reinke, and D. Lawrence, "Measurement and Projection of Demand for Health Care: The Chilean Experience." *Medical Care,* 13(6):511–522, June 1975.

Kritzer, Barbara E., "Chile Changes Its Health Care System." *Social Security Bulletin,* December 1983.

Medina, Ernesto, and A. M. Kaempffer, "An Analysis of Health Progress in Chile." *Bulletin of the Pan American Health Organization,* 17(3):221–232, 1983.

Navarro, Vicente, "What Does Chile Mean: An Analysis of Events in the Health Sector Before, During, and After Allende's Administration." *Milbank Memorial Fund Quarterly,* 52(2):93–130, Spring 1974.

Roemer, Milton I., "Medical Care in Chile," in *Medical Care in Latin America.* Washington, D.C.: Pan American Union, 1963, pp. 193–245.

Scarpaci, Joseph L., *Primary Medical Care in Chile: Accessibility under Military Rule.* Pittsburgh: University of Pittsburgh Press, 1988.

Valdivieso, Ramon, and B. Juricic, "The National Health System in Chile." *Boletin de la Oficina Sanitaria Panamericana,* Selections from 1970.

Viel, Benjamin, *La Medicinos Socializada y su aplicacion en Gran Bretana, Union Sovietica y Chile.* Santiago: Universidad de Chile, 1964.

Waitzkin, H., "Medicine, Socialism, and Totalitarianism: Lessons from Chile." *New England Journal of Medicine,* 291(4), 1974.

Guatemala

Consejo Nacional de Planificacion Economica, *El Sector Salud.* Guatemala, 1975.

Direccion General de Servicios de Salud, *Memoria Anual de Actividades de Areas de Salud 1975.* Guatemala, 1976.

Keaty, C. A., and G. A. Keaty, *A Study of Private Voluntary Organizations in Guatemala.* Washington, D.C.: U.S. Agency for International Development, May 1977, processed document.

Ministerio de Salud Publica y Asistencia Social, *Republica de Guatemala Recursos Humanos y Distribucion de Camas en Instituciones de Salud Publica, 1975.*

Nelson, Harry, "Guatemala's Health Problems Unsolved: Most Doctors in Capital, Most Need in Rural Areas." *Los Angeles Times,* 1 September 1983.

Robertson, Robert L., et al., *Financing the Health Sector of Guatemala.* Washington, D.C.: U.S. Agency for International Development, June 1977, processed document.

Roemer, Milton I., and Anthony Ormasa, *Health Service Coordination in Guatemala.* Washington, D.C.: American Public Health Association, 1975, processed document.

United Nations Fund for Population Activities, *Guatemala: Report of Mission on Needs Assessment for Population Assistance.* New York (Report No. 31), 1979.

World Bank, *Guatemala: Population, Nutrition, and Health Sector Review.* Washington, D.C. (Report No. 6183 GU), July 1986.

Panama

Caja de Seguro Social, *Memoria 1982–1983.* Panama, October 1983.

La Forgia, Gerard M., *Local Organizations for Rural Health in Panama: Community Participation, Bureaucratic Reorientation, and Political Will.* Ithaca, N.Y.: Cornell University Center for International Studies, 1985.

Panama, Direccion de Estadistica y Censo, *Panama En Cifros Anos 1978 a 1982.* Panama, November 1983.

Roemer, Milton, I. and Joseph Kessler, *Integration of Social Security and Ministry of Health Programs for Improved Delivery of Health and Family Planning Services in Panama.* Washington, D.C.: American Public Health Association, 1973, processed document.

Woolley, P. O., C. A. Perry, and R. N. Eccles, *Syncrisis: The Dynamics of Health, I. Panama.* Washington, D.C.: Office of International Health, U.S. Public Health Service, revised May 1972.

Argentina

Brett, Mary T., "Primary Care and the Pattern of Disease in a Rural Area of the Argentine Chaco." *Bulletin of the Pan American Health Organization.* 18(2):115–126, 1984.

Mera, Jorge Alberto, *Politica de Salud en la Argentina: La Construccion del Seguro Nacional de Salud.* Buenos Aires: Libreria Hachette, 1988.

Mera, Jorge, "Politica sobre Obras Sociales." *Medicina y Sociedad,* 7(4):119–125, 1984.

Ministerio de Salud y Accion Social, *Institute Nacional de Obras Sociales.* Buenos Aires, 1983, processed document.

World Bank, *Argentina: Population, Health and Nutrition Review.* Washington, D.C.: Report No. 6555 AR, October 1987.

Barbados

Carr, Peter R., "Health Systems Development in the English-Speaking Caribbean: Toward the Twenty-first Century." *Bulletin of the Pan American Health Organization,* 19(4):368–383, 1985.

Hoyes, M. D., et al., "Family Practice in Barbados." *Bulletin of the Pan American Health Organization,* 15(1):3–10, 1981.

Hoyos, M. D., et al., *Morbidity Survey in General Practice in Barbados, 1977–1978.* Bridgetown, 1979, processed document.

Kaiser Foundation International, *Study Findings and Recommendations for the Establishment of the National Health Service for Barbados.* Oakland, Calif., November 1979.

Ministry of Health and National Insurance, Barbados, *Annual Report of Chief Medical Officer for the Year 1977.* Bridgetown, 1978.

Ministry of Health and National Insurance, Barbados, *Development Plan 1977–82.* Bridgetown, December 1977.

Ministry of Health and National Insurance, Barbados, *Health Care: Polyclinic Project.* Bridgetown: September 1978.

Ministry of Health and National Insurance, Barbados, *National Health Service Steering Committee Interim Report.* Bridgetown, December 1977.

Ministry of Health and Welfare, *Health Services in Barbados.* Bridgetown, 1973.

Other Welfare-Oriented Health Systems in Latin America

American Public Health Association, *Ecuador: A Health and Population Brief.* Washington, D.C., 1979, processed document.

Liisberg, E., et al., *Venezuela.* World Health Organization (WHO/UNICEF Joint Study on Alternative Approaches to Meeting Basic Health Needs of Populations in Developing Countries), Geneva, 1974.

Pan American Health Organization, "Venezuela," in *Health Conditions in the Americas 1981–84, Vol. II.* (Scientific Pub. No. 500), Washington, D.C., 1986, pp. 242–250.

Roemer, Milton, I., "Colombian Health Services in

the Perspective of Latin American Patterns." *Milbank Memorial Fund Quarterly,* 46(2), Part 2: 203–212, April 1968.

United Nations Fund for Population Activities, *Ecuador: Report of Mission on Needs Assessment for Population Assistance.* New York, Report No. 46, September 1981.

World Bank, *Colombia Health Sector Review.* Washington, D.C.: Report No. 4141-CO, December 1982.

World Bank, *Ecuador: Population, Health, and Nutrition Sector Review.* Washington, D.C.: Report No. 6078-EC, February 1986.

Yates, Ann S., "The Venezuelan *Medicina Simplificada* Program." *Public Health Reports,* 90(3):247–253, 1975.

Zschock, Dieter K., "Medical Care under Social Insurance in Latin America." New York: State University of New York at Stony Brook, 1985, processed document.

CHAPTER ELEVEN

Welfare-Oriented Health Systems in Transitional Countries: Middle East and Asia

Outside of Latin America, there are several countries at a transitional economic level with welfare-oriented health systems. Most are in the Middle East and some in southern Asia. A prototype of these countries is Egypt, whose health system we examine in some detail. More focused analyses are made of Iraq, Turkey, and Malaysia.

In one basic cultural respect, all of these countries differ from the countries of Latin America. The dominant religious faith in all of them is Islam, in contrast to Roman Catholicism in Latin America. The forms the Moslem religion takes, and its influence on the health systems, differ in different nations. Despite many political and cultural differences, all of these governments have undertaken initiatives to make modern health services available to their people, through various forms of collectivized financing and organization of services.

EGYPT

The Arab Republic of Egypt, as it is officially named, traces its history to a remarkable civilization that developed along the Nile River more than 3,000 years before Christ. Much later, when Europe was in the Dark Ages (roughly A.D. 700–1400), Arabic culture in North Africa kept alive the knowledge of ancient Greece and Rome for eventual transmission back to Europe during the Renaissance.

In modern times, Egypt was adopted as a protectorate of Great Britain during World War I. In 1923, a Constitution was proclaimed, establishing Egypt as a kingdom, with a Parliament that had only limited powers. This status continued until 1952, when a military coup ended the monarchy and established a republic. In 1954, a new Constitution was proclaimed, and many features of Egypt's current health system are traceable to the revolution of 1952 and the Constitution that followed it.

Modern Egypt is a country of 47,765,000 people, whose per capita income in 1984 was $718. Although its territory in North Africa exceeds 365,000 square miles, 99 percent of the population are settled in 3.5 percent of this area, along the banks of the Nile River. While much industrialization has developed, the population is still 54 percent rural and 46 percent urban. Land ownership in the rural areas is extremely uneven; 1.0 percent of the landowners own 27 percent of the cultivated land, 4.0 percent own 21 percent of the land, and 95 percent of the owners (peasants with holdings under 5 feddan) depend on some 52 percent of the land. The adult literacy rate is only 44 percent, and is appreciably lower in women.

Since the 1952 revolution, when Egypt changed from a kingdom to an Arab republic, a constitutional principle proclaims that everyone is entitled to free health service, provided by the government. At the same time, as Egypt states in a report to the World Health Organization, "fee-for-service private practice [is available] for those who desire it." Those who use private medical care providers, of course, must have the money to pay for it.

Health System Structure

To the casual observer, Egypt's government health programs are prominent, but the private market is much stronger than is readily apparent.

Ministry of Health. In the government sector, the Ministry of Health is clearly the dominant agency, although other ministries also play a part. The organization of the Ministry of Health (MOH) corresponds to the general framework of the government as a whole. At the central level, the MOH has eight major subdivisions. High priority was given in the 1980s to primary health care, spearheaded by an undersecretary for the overall supervision of basic health care and family health. This includes general directorates of urban health services, rural health services, maternity and child welfare, family planning, school health, and endemic disease control. These directorates are expected to maintain continuous relationships with MOH services throughout the country.

Egypt is divided into 24 governorates (provinces), the heads of which are appointed by the president. Each governorate has a health director (or undersecretary) responsible for all MOH activities. He is aided ordinarily by a deputy director for public health and another for hospitals. The governorates are divided into districts, headed by a general district officer appointed by the governor. Each district has a district health director, aided by a chief nurse, chief sanitarian, and others. Altogether, the governorates of Egypt contain 131 districts.

Closest to the people are local health areas within the district, each consisting of one to three villages. The basic resource for providing health services is a health facility staffed with several personnel. Most numerous are rural health units, or RHUs—simple structures with examining rooms, a drug dispensary, a small laboratory, and other features. If the local population is larger, it may be served by a rural health center (RHC), similar in basic conception to an RHU but also containing 10 to 15 beds. All of these health facilities are staffed with one or more physicians—quite remarkable for a developing country.

Other Government Agencies. Officially under the minister of health but virtually autonomous in their operation are three other major health care programs. The *Health Insurance Organization* provides social insurance protection for comprehensive health services to some 2,700,000 Egyptians (in 1985) employed by government and also by other large enterprises. This amounts to 5.7 percent of the national population. About 70 percent of its members are government employees, for whom government contributes 3 percent of wages and the employee 1 percent. Another 25 percent are employees of quasi-public enterprises, such as the railroads or the Arab contractors. The remaining 5 percent are employees of purely private enterprises with 500 or more workers. (In 1982 enrollment was made mandatory for employees of smaller firms.) This population of workers is entitled to a remarkably comprehensive range of health services, including not only complete medical (general and specialist) care and hospitalization, but also dental care, drugs, and prosthetic appliances. Dependents of employees, however, are not covered.

As in Latin America, these services are provided mainly in polyclinics and hospitals owned and operated by the Health Insurance Organization. There are 54 polyclinics and 23 hospitals; most facilities are in Cairo and Alexandria, but some are located in almost all of the governorates. These facilities are staffed by general practitioners and specialists who are salaried full-time or part-time. Salaries are much higher than those in the general MOH program, and the level of supplies and equipment is better. Only where there are too few workers to warrant establishment of a physical structure, does the organization contract with private medical practitioners, who are paid on a capitation basis, according to the number of beneficiaries they serve.

The second major semiautonomous operation coming under the minister of health consists of two groups of hospitals, known as the *Curative Organizations* of Cairo and of Alexandria. The first operates 11 hospitals and the second 5 hospitals. These hospitals have more amenities than those of the MOH generally, and they require payment by the patient for both the hospital care and the physician's care. The Curative Organizations were established to meet the demands of middle-class families who were not satisfied with the regular MOH facilities and yet could not afford the high charges of purely private physicians and hospitals. The MOH controls the charges made by Curative Organization hospitals, which are to be kept moderate, and 20 percent of the beds must be reserved for indigent patients. It is estimated that about 5 percent of the Egyptian population make regular use of the 16 health facilities of the Curative Organizations.

A third semiautonomous activity, supervised indirectly by the minister of health, is a constellation of functions involving the *production and distribution of drugs.* There are numerous pharmaceutical companies in Egypt, 11 of which have been put under the control of the government. Some 85 percent of drug production in the country comes from these quasi-public companies, and the activities of all drug companies are regulated by the MOH. In spite of this large government role, drug costs are high, and 30 percent of all national health expenditures (public and private) are estimated to be for drugs and vaccines.

Other government agencies are entirely independent of the Ministry of Health but clearly relevant to the health system. Important among these is the *Ministry of Education,* which control's Egypt's nine university-based faculties of medicine training doctors. Attached to each is a relatively large teaching hospital, financed and controlled by this ministry and providing tertiary-level specialty services. These hospitals contain 8,844 beds, or 11 percent of the nation's total of 81,905 beds under all auspices. Ambulatory care is also provided in the out-patient departments of these hospitals. And through its control of the entire national public school system (primary, secondary, and prepatory levels), of course, the Ministry of Education is responsible for instructing students in personal hygiene and health education generally.

Several other ministries have major responsibilities for environmental sanitation, which has special importance in the light of the large burden of water-borne infectious disease in Egypt. Several organizations are concerned with public water supply and sewage disposal systems in the towns and cities (although the water is examined periodically by the MOH sanitarians and laboratories). Concerned especially with rural water supply and sanitation is the *Ministry of Housing,* particularly its governorate authorities. Various irrigation canals breed the snails that are vectors of Egypt's major endemic disease, schistosomiasis (also called bilharziasis). Under the *Ministry of Defense,* of course, there is a substantial health care organization for the military forces. Even the ministry responsible for prisons operates its own hospitals, with 900 beds.

Finally, associated with government are numerous *quasi-public enterprises,* which operate general health care programs for their employees. Several of these concern transportation, like the railroads and airlines. Public utilities providing electricity and telephone service are also among these, as is a large construction enterprise, known as the Arab Contractors. (In Egypt, these are described as "public sector" activities, to be distinguished from the government sector as well as the private sector.)

Organized Nongovernment Programs. There are estimated to be as many as 9,000 voluntary organizations in Egypt, a large number of which provide health services. Many of these concentrate on services to mothers and children, and they are often associated with religious mosques. Many agencies provide family planning; the Egyptian Family Planning Association operates 500 family planning clinics throughout the country, under the auspices of the Ministry of Social Affairs. Other voluntary health agencies provide services for the blind, crippled children, cancer patients, and others. The Red Crescent (equivalent to the Red Cross elsewhere) helps during national disasters and emergencies.

Private industrial firms also provide limited in-plant occupational health services to their workers, as required under law. If a firm employs 500 workers or more, it is obligated to have a full-time or part-time physician available for work-related accidents or diseases.

The Private Health Care Market. Whether or not people are entitled to "free" services in an organized health program, the majority of Egyptians seek private medical care for some or all of their ailments. Broadly speaking, this care is obtained either from formally trained personnel or from untrained traditional healers. In general, trained or modern personnel are used by higher-income families and traditional personnel by lower-income families. Modern care tends to be used more extensively in the cities and traditional care more in the rural areas, but the two types of care play a definite role in both urban and rural sections.

Privately purchased care of *physicians,* both general practitioners and specialists, is extensive. Only about 10 percent of Egypt's total supply of physicians are exclusively in private practice, and these are mainly in Cairo and Alexandria. The great majority of physicians in the Ministry of Health, however, as well as in other organized programs, engage in private practice after their official work is done. Since normal working hours in government are from 8 A.M. to 2 P.M., there is ample time for private medical practice in the afternoons and evenings. The usual estimate in the Ministry of Health is that 80 percent of MOH physicians engage in private practice, the number of hours per day, of course, varying. This service is paid for on a fee basis, the amount being typically higher in the cities than in rural areas and higher for specialists than for general practitioners.

The supply of *dentists* in Egypt is quite small, in comparison with physicians, but a higher proportion (perhaps 25 to 50 percent) are entirely in private practice. The great majority of government dentists are women, whose household responsibilities probably discourage their doing private dental work after official hours.

The vast majority of *pharmacists* are in the private health market, as owners or employees of some 4,400 private pharmacies. As noted, some 30 percent of all Egyptian health expenditures are for drugs, and a large portion of these are purchased in private pharmacies. Regulations requiring medical prescriptions for drugs are weakly enforced, so most are sold over-the-counter, directly to the patient. In addition, many drugs may be purchased in food shops or general markets. Appliances, such as eyeglasses and crutches, are also sold privately in the main cities.

The market for *traditional healers* is more difficult to analyze, but it is undoubtedly large, particularly in rural areas. Most ubiquitous is the *daya,* or traditional birth attendant. Usually an older woman who has had several children herself and has learned by apprenticeship, she is found in every Egyptian village, as well as in the cities and towns. Official policies on the daya have changed over the years. In the 1940s, a formal training program was launched, and by 1950 more than 5,000 dayas had taken the course and been granted government permits. Then in 1969, no further permits were issued and daya activities were made illegal. In spite of this, it is estimated that 80 percent of childbirths among both rural and urban poor are done by dayas in the mother's home. Even when trained nurses are available to handle deliveries without charge, most village families prefer the friendly and emotionally supportive service of the daya.

For general medical care, the major traditional healer in Egypt is the barber, descendant of the medieval barber-surgeon. While cutting hair and shaving beards, village barbers do minor surgery, give injections, perform circumcisions on boys, extract teeth, incise abscesses, and so on. They also often give nonsurgical treatment by advising patients or prescribing drugs to be purchased in a pharmacy. Until 1969 barbers, like dayas, were issued permits by the Ministry of Health and were often officially responsible for the registration of births and deaths, reporting them to the district health office.

Less common, but found in many Egyptian villages, are still other types of traditional healer. There are bone setters, who bandage injuries (even if there is no fracture). Herb vendors, not as frequent as in Asian countries, sell both herbal and modern medications. The *daka,* a form of healer who is disappearing, uses music, dancing, and various rites to treat illnesses believed to be emotional in origin.

In spite of the high regard of many Egyptians for traditional healing, it is still part of the private health care market, and must usually be paid for. The fees are typically low and sometimes are payable by barter. Occasionally a healer with a good reputation charges the same fees as a physician. Current Egyptian policy opposes the use of healers (except for the daya, about whom local policies vary), insofar as physicians, nurses, and other trained personnel are now widely available. People's continued confidence in traditional healers, nevertheless, reflects deficiencies in the official health services, as they are perceived by low-income families.

Health Resources

Egypt has relatively strong resources for its health system, particulary medical manpower. An outgrowth of the revolution of 1952 was free university education for everyone, and the notion developed that any young person wishing to study medicine should have the opportunity. As a result, the university medical schools have an "open admission" policy and, although many of those admitted fail, thousands of medical students graduate each year.

Health Manpower. Special emphasis has been put on the training of physicians, and their supply in Egypt has been expanding rapidly. In 1945 (before the revolution), 4,300 physicians were registered with the Ministry of Health, and this grew to 23,725 by 1973 and to 43,550 by 1980. About 9,500 of the doctors registered, however, were retired, outside the country, or inactive, leaving about 34,000 active physicians. Including new graduates and attrition, by 1981 there were 38,000 active physicians. For a population of 41,500,000, this meant a ratio of 91.7 physicians per 100,000 persons in Egypt—an exceptionally high ratio for a developing country.

The national distribution of the 34,000 active physicians in 1980 was estimated in a major study, conducted by the Ministry of Health in collaboration with the U.S. National Center of Health Statistics. This showed the following:

Agency	Percentage
Ministry of Health	45.6
Other government agencies and quasi-public bodies	11.8
Exclusively private practice	8.8
Military services (estimated)	13.2
In-hospital trainees	11.8
Immigrant physicians	8.8
Total	100.0

Since the great majority of physicians in the Ministry of Health and other agencies also have private practices after their official hours, the effective medical manpower is probably greater than suggested here. This unusually large supply of physicians in modern Egypt undoubtedly explains the government's decision against embarking on the training of the new types of community health workers for primary health care, being trained in so many other developing countries.

In 1980, two major changes were launched in Egyptian medical education, in response to problems that had long existed. It was decided to strengthen instruction in community medicine by including courses on various aspects of the field throughout the 6 years of the medical curriculum. Second, specialty status was granted to general practice (a worldwide trend), incorporating instruction in this "holistic" field into the medical school program.

Because of Moslem customs, it is important to have an adequate supply of female physicians in a country like Egypt. Most women do not wish to be examined by a male physician, especially for any gynecological condition. It is relevant, therefore, that the proportion of female medical students has been increasing significantly—from 9.7 percent in 1952 to 29.4 percent in 1979. The proportion of dentists who are women is even higher.

The categories and training programs for nurses in Egypt have changed over recent years, with a general tendency toward upgrading qualifications. Formerly there were large numbers of assistant nurses and assistant midwives, who were trained for 18 months after 9 years of basic schooling. There were also health visitors, trained for health work in the schools, without being nurses; their 3-year curriculum was taken in a regular secondary school (not a hospital). Then there were *hakima,* or nurse-midwives, who started with the 3-year diploma course in a hospital after 9 years of basic schooling; after a year of hospital practice, a fifth year was spent in midwifery training.

In 1972, this was all changed, and the great majority of nurses were trained in 3-year courses in secondary technical schools, located in or near a hospital. Entrance to one of the 138 schools requires 9 years of basic education. A relatively small number of nurses are also trained in one of two health institutes, in a 2-year program of study; these institutes also train sanitarians, laboratory technicians, and other health personnel. Finally, there are two university-based high institutes of nursing, which require 12 years of basic education for entrance, and a 4-year baccalaureate course, followed by one year of internship. After this, the graduate can continue to a master's or doctoral degree in nursing or a related field.

The present supply of nurses in Egypt, therefore, is a mixture of persons with diverse types of training. As of 1977, there were about 41,000 nurses, the majority of whom were graduates of the 3-year course in secondary technical schools but many were assistant nurses or midwives graduated before 1972. The overall nurse–population ratio in 1977 was 105 per 100,000, at a time when there were 91 physicians per 100,000.

In other health science fields, the supply of trained personnel is relatively weaker than that of physicians and nurses. In 1978 there were 13,367 pharmacists, or 32 per 100,000 population. Dentists numbered 5,133, only 13 per 100,000 population; about 550 dentists are graduated annually from the five dental schools.

The numbers of various types of traditional practitioner in Egypt are not known, even though numerous field studies in selected villages always identify several of them. Based on data from 1969, however, when dayas and barbers were trained and registered, estimates can be made. In the 1980s about 10,000 active

dayas and a total of about 20,000 traditional healers of all types existed. Most healers are also engaged in other work, as farmers or shopkeepers, for example, and provide their healing services part-time when requested.

Until the 1980s, the output of trained health personnel in Egypt was based simply on a policy of steady expansion. In 1973, counting enrollment in the faculties of medicine, dentistry, and pharmacy, the number of students in the nation was 39,434; in 1978 this had grown to 52,740. With an output of so many more young doctors than the Egyptian health care system could economically absorb, many hundreds of physicians and other professionals left the country each year to work, typically for much higher salaries, in other countries—principally the oil-rich Arab countries in the Arabian Gulf region.

In 1982, for the first time, a national decision was made to reduce the admission of students to medical school by 10 percent. This decision was made by a Joint Board on Medical Education, which included representatives of the universities, the Ministry of Education, the Ministry of Health, and the Egyptian Medical Syndicate (or medical society).

In 1955, the High Institute of Public Health was established in Alexandria, with the support of WHO, UNICEF, and the U.S. foreign aid program. It was sponsored jointly by the Ministry of Health and the University of Alexandria, but in 1963 was transferred fully to the university. This institute is unique in the Arab world in offering intensive 1-year study leading to a Diploma of Public Health (DPH), equivalent to that of graduate schools of public health in other parts of the world.

The institute has a remarkably large faculty, with 160 members full-time and some 200 part-time. All specialties within public health seem to be covered, including statistics, epidemiology, vector control, environmental engineering, occupational medicine, nutrition, hospital administration, dental public health, maternal and child health, geriatrics, and more. The student can major in one of 20 fields.

Health Facilities. The health programs in the structure of Egypt's health system each constructed hospitals and operate them for various sections of the population. In 1982, the Egyptian Ministry of Health reported an overall hospital bed supply of 2 per 1,000 population. Considering hospitals under all sponsorship in 1982, the total quantity of beds was nearly 82,000, the great majority being in governmental institutions. Reports in the 1980s referred to a trend of expanding private hospitals, but, as of 1982, the distribution of beds in the nation was as follows:

Sponsorship	Hospital Beds	Percentage
Ministry of Health	49,600	60.6
Health Insurance Organization	3,000	3.7
Curative organizations	3,200*	3.9
Other ministries	2,147	2.6
Universities	11,391	13.9
Quasi-public agencies	7,454	9.1
Private (proprietary)	5,113	6.2
All sponsorships	81,905	100.0

The capital construction costs for all of these facilities were derived from government revenues, social insurance income, and (for the private ones) mainly from bank loans made by private physicans. Depending on how one considers the beds controlled by quasi-public agencies, Egypt's hospital beds are between 84.7 and 93.8 percent within the government sector.

To implement its constitutional pledge on health care, Egypt is supplied with hundreds of health centers and rural health units. The health centers number about 600, each containing 10 or 15 beds for maternity care, trauma cases, or acutely ill patients pending referral to a hospital. Rural health units are somewhat smaller and have no beds; they number about 1,700. All 2,300 of these health facilities are staffed with physicians, most of whom are recent medical graduates, serving their periods of mandatory rural service.

The health centers operated by the MOH in both urban and rural areas provide primary health care, both preventive and therapeutic. In 1981 59 urban health centers and 39 addi-

*Estimated on the basis of 16 hospitals, averaging 200 beds each.

tional rural health centers were upgraded to *rural hospitals.* In all of these facilities, maternal and child preventive health services are offered, along with immunizations. In some, health education is offered on nutrition, personal hygiene, or family planning. Sanitarians doing environmental work are stationed at nearly all of them. Every health center also offers general ambulatory medical care to patients who come with complaints. In addition 236 small urban clinics provide maternal and child health services exclusively.

Rural health units (RHUs) are closest to the people for the provision of primary health care. They are simple structures, with rooms for examining patients, storing drugs, conducting laboratory tests, and housing personnel. The basic RHU staff consists of a physician (general practitioner), two or more nurses, a sanitarian, a laboratory technician, and clerical and maintenance workers. The levels of training of the nurses, sanitarians, and technicians may vary, but all the physicians are qualified (usually young) medical graduates. Housing is usually provided for the physician, sometimes for two physicians. Unlike the situation in many developing countries, there are few if any vacancies in the RHU medical posts.

In both hospitals and health centers, most drugs are provided free of charge. They are produced mainly by the quasi-public pharmaceutical companies in Egypt. There is a theoretical policy of referring patients, as necessary, from rural health units, to rural health centers, to district hospitals, and finally to urban general hospitals.

Under the Ministry of Health, there are a total of 171 district and general hospitals, with an average capacity of 124 beds. In addition, the MOH operates 156 specialized hospitals for infectious diseases, chest disorders, leprosy, endemic diseases, children, and other special purposes. All of these hospitals provide out-patient as well as in-patient service. Because hospitals are staffed by specialists, their out-patient departments are heavily utilized; patients frequently bypass nearby ambulatory care units to get specialist service at a hospital OPD. In 1980, the OPDs of the 171 general and district hospitals served 14,803,000 ambulatory patients. The vast majority of hospital OPD patients come on their own initiative, rather than by referral for specialist care.

Economic Support

Only minimal data are available on expenditures in Egypt for support of the health system. Within government, the Ministry of Health, at both central and local levels, absorbed 9.1 percent of the total government budget in 1966. With some irregularities, this declined to 5.6 percent in 1976. Over the same years, expenditures for the Health Insurance Organization and the Curative Organizations, though much lower in absolute amounts, remained about constant at 3.8 percent of government expenditures.

In 1978, the Egyptian government, in cooperation with the U.S. Agency for International Development, undertook a national study of overall health expenditures. The government share was calculated from the official records of the Ministry of Health and other authorities. Private expenditures were estimated on the basis of income tax returns of private physicians, pharmacies, hospitals, and so on. It was concluded that 46 percent of health expenditures were government and 54 percent private. There is much reason to believe, however, that the private sector proportion is substantially larger. It is widely agreed that income tax returns underreport incomes. The private earnings of rural government doctors, moreover, are officially *not* reportable (i.e., they are tax-free). Private payments to all traditional healers and birth attendants were not included in the study at all. In the light of these and other considerations, it would seem reasonable to estimate the government health sector at no more than 40 percent of the total, and the private sector at 60 percent.

Health System Management

It is evident from relationships between health services in the governorates (including the central appointment of all governors) and the central Ministry of Health, that the general management of Egypt's health system is highly centralized. The health director of each governorate is expected to carry out the policies of the ministry headquarters, and on specialized questions, such as endemic disease control, MCH, nutrition, and environmental sanitation, he must turn for guidance to the national supervisors in these fields. Governorate health directors have no responsibilities for local activities of the Health Insurance Organization or any other national agency.

Recognition of the value of greater decentralization in the Egyptian health systems arose with respect to efforts in health planning. In the 1970s the MOH established a Division of Health Planning at headquarters. The first steps, however, were taken at the local level. Plans were to be submitted to the governorate level, where they might be modified and then transmitted to the central Division of Health Planning. From these submissions, an overall national health planning document would be prepared.

Some promotion of decentralized work has also occurred with respect to intersectoral cooperation. MOH personnel have been encouraged to join councils, including various other sectors—education, agriculture, social service—at the governorate and the village levels. Some local areas have combined structures, which house officials from these several social sectors. Less cooperation has been evident at the national level.

Problems of coordination within the health system seem more conspicuous. In family planning services, for example, volunteer women workers have been recruited by various public and private agencies, with no planning to avoid overlap. Some of these volunteers relate to official health personnel, while others do not.

With foreign aid programs involving the health system, problems of coordination have been severe. Egypt receives considerable technical cooperation in health matters from both multilateral and bilateral agencies. Within the MOH, certain relationships have been maintained by the Directorate for International Health, others by the Directorate for Planning and Health Investment, and still others by various specific program offices. Furthermore, among the international agencies working in Egypt, coordination of efforts occurs only on a very informal level; overlap and even friction is avoided by selection of geographically separate governorates, in which agencies conduct their projects. Comparative evaluations of the effectiveness of various health strategies have not been carried out.

Much health legislation has been enacted by Egypt's Parliament. Decrees of the minister of health also have the force of law. For example, in the years from 1973 to 1977, laws were enacted on such subjects as the following:

- At least 2 years of compulsory government service for new professional graduates—physicians, dentists, pharmacists, nurses, sanitarians, technicians, and other health professions—with priority for service in rural and remote areas.
- Regulation of medical practice of physicians, midwives, nurses, and dentists.
- Regulations for nursing education.
- Compulsory immunization against measles.
- Regulation of the importing of pharmaceutical and medical equipment.
- Compulsory registration of births and deaths.

Egypt's perception of itself as a "socialist" society is reflected in a decree by the minister of health in 1974, on the Rule of Ethics and Charter of Honour for the Profession of Medicine. Among other things, the decree states that "The doctor has to study and solve the health problems in society, and to participate in the Syndicate's (i.e., medical association's) share in directing health policy according to socialist rules. . . . The doctor has to be a good example in his society in order to strengthen the thoughts and socialist values."

Egypt has also put a good deal of effort into evaluating health services in both rural areas and cities. Major projects have been conducted, with international assistance, on the effectiveness of family planning, primary health care, and services for mothers and children.

Delivery of Health Services

In spite of the extensive network of medically staffed health centers and rural health units that Egypt has developed, the use of these MOH primary health care resources has not been high. Counting all patient visits, for both prevention and treatment, in 1980 all RHUs reported 12,452,500 visits. For 1,700 RHUs, this would mean 7,325 visits to each unit per year. Assuming 250 working days (allowing for weekends and holidays) in a year, this amounts to 29 patients per day. It is widely reported that physicians spend only 1 or 2 minutes on each case, but even if we assume 5 minutes, this volume of ambulatory service would require less than 3 hours—hardly half of the doctor's 6-hour official working day. In rural health centers, a similar analysis of utilization yields an average of 50.3 patient-visits per day, but these facilities are usually staffed with two or more physicians (as well as larger staffs of nurses and others).

Estimating the rate of ambulatory services provided by both RHUs and RHCs, one may relate the services to the rural population of Egypt. In 1980, this consisted of about 23,500,000 people. The aggregate of rural health facility (both RHUs and RHCs) ambulatory services was 20,343,400, or 0.87 services per rural person per year. Almost everywhere, health care utilization is lower among rural than among urban people, but it may be noted that under the Egyptian statutory health insurance program, in 1979 ambulatory care encounters occurred at a much higher rate (see later).

By comparison, the program of Egypt's Health Insurance Organization demonstrates a rate of service delivery that is possible in the same country. The organization's 54 polyclinics offer both primary and secondary medical services to ambulatory patients, and its 23 hospitals operate out-patient departments that do likewise. In 1979, out-patient visits numbered 7,193,000, 75.1 percent of which were the services of general medical practitioners. For the total of 1,390,000 members at that time, this meant 5.17 medical services or 3.89 services of general practitioners per person per year. This rate was between four and six times the annual rate of services provided to Egypt's rural population (0.87 services) by the MOH health centers and RHUs combined.

Among the 34,000 active physicians in Egypt (in 1980), 3,000 were exclusively in private practice. Another 3,000 physicians were classified as immigrants, and presumably they were also mainly in private practice. (The 4,500 physicians in military service cannot engage in private practice, and this is also true of the 4,000 in-hospital trainees.) Of the 15,500 MOH doctors, the common estimate of 80 percent engaging in private practice means about 12,400 part-time private practitioners. Similarly, 80 percent of the 4,000 physicians employed in other programs suggests another 3,200 part-time private doctors. Thus, there are 6,000 full-time private physicians 15,600 part-time. Assuming the latter to be providing about 50 percent of full-time service, in full-time doctor-equivalents, therefore, they would amount to 7,800 practitioners. Adding these to the full-time private doctors, the total comes to 13,800 doctors. At a conservative estimate, the average private medical practitioner would see in his office or private clinic about 20 patients a day. (In the large cities, they doubtless see many more than this.) For a year of 250 working days, this would mean 5,000 patient encounters per doctor. The total of 13,800 doctors (in full-time equivalents) would therefore give medical services of 69,000,000 patient visits. Most of these patients are doubtless from middle- or upper-class families, but some are from poor families who are desperate for help and not satisfied with public services.

This analytical exercise may be crude, but the magnitude of private medical consultations in Egypt is obviously large. The total of patient visits in all rural health facilities (20,343,000), in all MOH hospital out-patient departments (14,803,000), and in the resources of the Health Insurance Organization (7,193,000) is 42,339,000 services—appreciably less than the estimate of ambulatory services obtained from private doctors.

The 2 years of MOH service, required of all new medical graduates in Egypt, has been noted. This provides a steady flow of young physicians to staff the MOH's rural health units and rural health centers, as well as their urban equivalent. Exceptions to this mandatory service are granted to the highest-ranking medical graduates, who may go directly into specialty training in a university hospital. (About 30 percent of graduates achieve this privilege, which unfortunately leaves the impression that a rural post signifies poor academic performance.) Many of these young rural doctors, furthermore, are free to leave after one year, to make room for the new crop of graduates.

Before the 2-year period of rural service begins, the young doctor is required to take a 2-month orientation course in rural health service. This has been necessary because of the weak preparation of medical graduates in public health and the problems of general family medicine. The course is given at the governorate level, by doctors and others on the staff of the Governorate Health Directorate.

The low rate of use of rural health facilities is easy to understand. Typically these small structures are not very cheerful or sanitary, and they are not well equipped. The waiting areas may even lack benches, forcing patients to stand or sit on the floor. The hastiness of medical consultations has been noted, and the young physician may offer to visit the patient's home later for a fee. (Regulations even encourage this practice, since medical fees collected for "home calls" are officially tax-free.) It is reported that doctors remaining at a rural post for several years do so because of the relatively high earnings from private practice. Near the facility, the rural doctor is also usually provided a suitable dwelling rent-free. Nevertheless, after their rural assignment, most young doctors depart for specialty training, urban practice, or employment outside Egypt at a higher salary.

A household survey, made in Egypt in 1979, provides information on the sources of health service given to preschool children. Five possible sources were identified, and their percentage distribution in urban and rural areas was found to be as follows:

Source	City (Percent)	Rural Area (Percent)
Private doctor	33.6	10.1
Hospital out-patient department	22.3	2.5
Health center or unit	23.2	24.3
Other source	5.0	0.3
No care received	15.9	62.8
All sources	100.0	100.0

Considering the high priority for children in official health programs, the large percentage of rural children receiving no care in the study period is noteworthy, as is the high proportion of urban children consulting private doctors.

Regarding environmental health services, limited data on Egypt are available for 1980. For water supply, the urban situation appeared good, with 88 percent of homes having indoor water connections, and 9 percent having access to public standposts. For the rural population, however, 56 percent of households had "reasonable access" to a public water source, and 44 percent did not. Sewage disposal problems were more serious. Public sewage lines were available in 19 cities, with a combined population of 13 million people (about 28 percent of the population). The majority of the Egyptian population had to depend on individual sewage disposal (septic tanks, latrines, etc.), and many of the public systems did not function well. There were extensive plans, however, to undertake major projects for both water supply and sewage disposal.

In 1982 a personal interview study was done on a sample of 2,100 patients visiting various health facilities in Cairo, the national capital. A central finding was that the great majority of patients used multiple sources for their health care—hospital OPDs, private physicians, pharmacies, health centers, or simply self-care at home. Three-quarters of the patients seen at a facility had taken some other action before visiting the place where they were interviewed. Clients were also interviewed in their homes, and expressed significant dissatisfaction with government health facilities in Cairo.

In their order of frequency, the reasons for dissatisfaction were that (1) government health facilities were too crowded; (2) services offered were regarded as ineffective; (3) doctors and other personnel treated patients rudely, and they expected to be tipped to give good care; (4) since the service was free, it was felt to be degrading; (5) doctors and other personnel seemed careless in their work. Because of these and other complaints, many persons interviewed said they preferred to see private physicians and purchase prescribed drugs, in spite of the personal costs.

In summary, Egypt's health system reflects a national policy of investing major efforts to provide health service to the people. For a country with a per capita GNP of only $718, it has developed an exceptionally large supply of health personnel (especially physicians) and health facilities. Major priority is assigned to primary health care, and resources, both human and physical, are remarkably well distributed to serve the rural population. A study in 1979 estimated that 95 percent of rural people lived within 5 kilometers of a health facility that provides primary health care. A beginning has also been made in developing higher-quality services under a social insurance program. The performance of most personnel in government programs, however, is apparently poor; they do not seem to win the approval of most patients. As a result, many people avoid using public services and turn to the private sector. Physicians and pharmacists in private practice are abundant. Most Egyptian health expenditures are therefore made in the private market.

TURKEY

The Republic of Turkey lies in the eastern part of Europe, between the Black Sea and the Mediterranean, with its great land mass (Anatolia) serving as a bridge to western Asia. The Turkish population in 1984 was 49,518,000, of whom about 46 percent were urban and 54 percent rural. Nearly 100 percent of the people are of the Moslem faith, although the government is secular. Unlike other Moslem populations in the region, the language and culture are not Arabic, but Turkish.

Since Turkey's change from an empire to a republic in 1923, under the leadership of Kemal Ataturk, the country has undergone great economic and social development. In 1985, its gross national product was derived 35 percent from industry, 19 percent from agriculture, and 46 percent from services. The GNP per capita in 1984 was $1,420.

General political power in Turkey is highly centralized, with the national seat of government in Ankara, near the nation's geographic center. Istanbul, the largest city, is located in the western part of the country, as is Izmir, the third largest city. The nation is divided into 67 provinces, the governors of which are appointed by the central government. Each province is, in turn, divided into districts—572 in all. The director of each district is also appointed by the central authorities. Only below this level are political leaders elected by the people—that is, the heads of municipalities, towns, and villages. A military takeover in 1980 ended with a transfer of power to an elected parliament in 1983.

Literacy has been gradually improving in Turkey, although it remains low in the eastern provinces. In 1984, the literacy level of adults was 69 percent, although it was much lower in women. Generally speaking, social and economic development is weakest in the eastern provinces, growing stronger as one moves toward the west. The capital, Ankara, marks a general border between the more developed western and less developed eastern regions. Periurban belts around the larger cities of the west, however, have extensive slums, holding thousands of depressed rural families who have come in search of employment. Because of the generally high unemployment, more than 2 million Turkish citizens are employed as "guest workers" in other countries.

The structure of the Turkish health system is as pluralistic as that of other welfare-oriented countries at a transitional economic level. Special efforts have been made, however, to achieve at least partial integration of programs. Several health service functions of other ministries, state enterprises, and local governments have been transferred to the Ministry of Health. The full array of health programs can therefore be analyzed under four main headings: (1) Ministry of Health, (2) Social Security, (3) other organized public programs, and (4) private health care market.

Ministry of Health

The full title of Turkey's major governmental health agency is the Ministry of Health and Social Assistance. Its central framework has changed frequently in recent years, in response to changing priorities in national health policy. The ministry was created in 1920, with a small range of infectious disease control functions, but its responsibilities have gradually been broadened. In 1983, there were six general directorates, reflecting the major importance of these fields: (1) primary health care, (2) hospital services, (3) family planning and maternal and child health, (4) education of health personnel, (5) social affairs, and (6) MOHSA personnel management. Other directorates (not general) included (7) malaria eradication, (8) tuberculosis control, (9) "socialized" health services, (10) cancer control, and (11) sport.

The General Directorate of Primary Health Care had several subdivisions, including (1) environmental health, (2) communicable disease control, (3) food control and nutrition, (4) public health laboratories, (5) trachoma control, (6) leprosy control, (7) venereal disease control, and (8) the provincial health directorates.

Each of Turkey's 67 provinces has a provincial health director, under the administrative control of the appointed provincial governor and the technical control of the MOHSA in Ankara. Below this level are two major types of health service organization, which were differentiated in 1961. In that year a military government enacted a law on the nationalization of health services. This law set in motion, on a province-by-province basis, a program to provide integrated preventive and treatment services, through health center teams serving 5,000 to 10,000 people. As satellites to each health center, there would be midwife stations or "health houses" to serve the maternal and child health needs of about 2,500 people. Every resident was theoretically entitled to services without charge, except for small payments for drugs. Private medical practice was not banned from the area, but the free health center services were expected to meet nearly all the needs.

The "nationalization" or "socialization" process, as it was later called, was started in the eastern province of Mus in 1963. The plan called for gradual extension westward. By 1970, 25 provinces had been socialized, and a total of 47 provinces by 1983. These provinces included 26,000,000 people, or about 54 percent of the national population.

The second type of health service organization applied to the 20 provinces that were not yet socialized. In these provinces, under the provincial health director, were simply health districts corresponding to the political districts. In each district, with some 50,000 or more people, there was typically a single medical officer. There might also be maternal and child health centers for purely preventive services to mothers and children.

The theoretical plan for the socialized provinces—to cover the entire population with accessible primary health care—did not prove to be feasible in practice. By 1980, hundreds of health centers had been constructed, but there were serious deficiencies in their staffing. The ideal staff included a physician (as head of the health center team), a nurse, a male nurse (who would sometimes give treatment), a sanitarian, two or three midwives, a record clerk, a maintenance worker, and a driver. Seldom was this complete team available, but most serious was the shortage of doctors. Only about 30 percent of the health centers had physicians, so treatment services were not available. Moreover, small charges were levied for all treatment services, except to the very poor.

In 1981, another fundamental policy change was launched, also under a military government. All new medical school graduates were required to give 2 years of service in a MOHSA health facility. With about 1,500 graduates each year, this meant that by late 1982 about 3,000 new young doctors had been stationed throughout the country. The selection of posts was based on a lottery.

Before starting his or her medical assignment (about half the graduates were women), the young doctor received a 2- to 4-week period of field training at one of the better staffed health centers in the province. Under the socialization scheme, political district lines were no longer followed, and there was no district medical officer. Instead, the cluster of five or six health centers, serving about 50,000 people, was regarded as a *health center group,* and the most experienced physician served as the chief of group. If a small hospital served the same population, the chief of group might also be the hospital director.

The 47 socialized provinces in 1983 contained 1,995 health centers. All were staffed to some degree, but only about 75 percent had a complete staffing complement. The *health*

houses, staffed by midwives, numbered 7,119. One must realize that the midwife is trained to do much more than midwifery. She examines the newborn babies and gives immunizations. She advises the mother on infant feeding and other matters. She gives injections or other medications that have been ordered by the doctor. She provides first-aid to accident cases, when necessary, and refers patients to the health center or to a hospital. Being close to the village people, the midwife is really the crucial primary health care worker.

Beyond the various provisions for primary health care, the MOHSA maintains a large network of hospitals. In 1984, there were 451 hospitals with 60,500 beds. These institutions are staffed by full-time specialists, employed by the ministry, along with nurses and other auxiliary personnel. MOHSA beds, however, constitute only about half of the national total, as we will see later.

The nonsocialized provinces, are much less well provided with health care, but they do not lack MOHSA services completely. In addition to the medical officer in charge of each district (about 50,000 population), there is a network of 185 *maternal and child health centers,* which offer preventive services including family planning. Peripheral to these are also 415 *MCH stations,* staffed by trained midwives.

Social Security

Social insurance protection for medical care goes back to the nineteenth century in Turkey, but numerous autonomous programs were consolidated into a national scheme in 1945. Since then coverage, initially for industrial workers, has been gradually widened to include government employees, agricultural workers, and the self-employed. The benefits vary, however, for different population groups. The broad umbrella concept of "social security" actually covers several separate programs.

The largest is the Social Insurance Organization (SIO), started in 1964. Originally it covered all industrial and commercial workers, but not government employees. In 1973, "permanently employed" agricultural workers were included. As of 1984, the total primary workers covered by the SIO came to

2,400,000, and with dependents it was 12,800,000. Premiums are paid by both employers and employees; for health benefits alone (not pensions, etc.) the rate is 6 percent of salaries from employers and 5 percent from employees.

Health services for SIO beneficiaries are provided through the organization's own network of hospitals and clinics, with salaried health personnel. Its 77 hospitals are better equipped than those of the MOHSA, and at least one hospital is located in 44 of the 67 provinces. The SIO also operates 141 health stations, all staffed by general practitioners. At the next higher level are 85 dispensaries, staffed by numerous specialists. There are also some specialized hospitals for geriatrics, tuberculosis, and mental disorders. And the SIO has a factory to prepare many of its frequently used drugs. In areas with no SIO facility, contracts are made for services from other public or private resources.

Self-employed persons and their dependents are covered by the Social Insurance Agency of Merchants, Artisans, and Self-Employed (BAG-KUR), established in 1972. Benefits for these people were limited at first to long-term care but in 1986 were expected to be broadened to general medical care. This program covered 2,325,500 people, but it did not operate its own facilities; services were purchased from existing health resources.

For certain population groups, still other insurance bodies operate. Employees of banks and certain other commercial firms are covered by 26 small autonomous funds, enrolling 273,000 people. Finally, there is a small Mutual Assistance Fund for primary school teachers and also a long-established (since 1921) Coal Mine Workers Assistance Fund. The numbers enrolled are not reported, but are probably not more than 100,000.

Turkish government employees at both central and local levels are covered by still other separate social security programs. The costs are fully met by the public agency, without employee contributions. Dependents are also covered, including the civil servant's parents. Medical and related services are purchased through fees paid to public or private providers, since no special facilities are operated by these programs. With some overlap in statistics for different social insurance benefits, an exact count of persons covered is difficult to make, but in 1984 it seemed to be about 2,040,000.

Altogether, social security protection for health services covers about 17,540,000 people in Turkey, or around 35 percent of the national population. Utilization data suggest that many of these people also sometimes use the services of the MOHSA, although the latter are really intended for people without insurance protection.

Other Organized Public Programs

Most important among other ministries with health functions is the *Ministry of Defense*. As in all countries, the Turkish military services maintain a large medical establishment providing comprehensive curative and preventive services. The dependents of military personnel are also covered. The magnitude of this program is reflected in its complement of 15,100 hospital beds—almost as many as under the SIO, with its 13,000,000 covered persons. The medical staffing of this program is ensured by a law mandating 2 years of compulsory military service for every Turkish male, including medical graduates; this is over and above the 2 years of required government health service for medical graduates, instituted in 1981.

Other health functions are the responsibility of the *Ministry of Labor*. Periodic inspections of workplaces are made, to identify health or safety hazards and to require their correction. Workers injured at work are entitled to cash compensation from the employer and to free medical care from the SIO system. An Occupational Health Institute for research and training in this field is also operated by the Ministry of Labor.

The development of water supplies and sanitation in Turkey is an important responsibility involving other branches of government. Sanitarians of the MOHSA test and monitor water supplies, but the actual construction of these resources is done by different agencies. In the larger cities, both water supply and sewage systems are developed by the *State Hydraulic Works* (DSI), along with municipal governments. Rural water supply systems are promoted by the *Ministry of Rural Affairs,* through its Department of Roads, Water, and Electricity. (It was estimated in 1981 that 63 percent of Turkey's rural population were provided with satisfactory water, and another 23 percent with possibly safe water, leaving 14 percent with a definite deficiency.)

The training of health science professions has been gradually expanding in Turkey, both in the universities, controlled and financed by the *Ministry of Education,* and within the resources of the Ministry of Health and Social Assistance. Of great importance are the 22 universities with medical faculties, which turn out hundreds of new physicians every year. Pharmacists, dentists, and high-level nurses are also trained in university settings.

To provide proper training in all these fields, it is necessary to have good access to patients. Accordingly, each of these universities operates its own hospital, with financial support from the Ministry of Education. Altogether, the 13,800 beds in university hospitals are a significant share of the national total. Turkey also has a *State Planning Organization,* which oversees the programs of all Turkish ministries. One unit within the SPO is responsible for reviewing and approving the budget of the Ministry of Health and Social Assistance.

Several enterprises in Turkey, such as electrical power, railroads, coal mining, and the airlines, are operated by special government corporations. The employees of these "parastatal" organizations, and usually their dependents, are entitled to medical care offered directly by the enterprise. A total of 2,072 hospital beds were in the health facilities under these programs in 1986.

Municipalities. There are 36 cities in Turkey with more than 100,000 population. In these and certain other municipalities, the local government takes much responsibility for local water supplies and sewerage. A municipal medical officer is typically appointed by the Ministry of Health and Social Assistance, although his salary is paid by the municipality.

In addition to overseeing environmental sanitation, and supervising trained sanitarians, the medical officer does medicolegal work that

may be ordered by a court of law. He examines applicants for any type of municipal employment. Sometimes he is called on to examine disabled and poor persons, who are seeking charitable support from the city. In the largest cities, municipal hospitals are maintained for special purposes, such as maternity or infectious disease; these facilities contained 928 beds in 1984.

Private Health Care Market

Permeating the entire Turkish health system, with its several organized programs, is the operation of a private health market, both traditional and modern.

In 1984, about 34,195 physicians were actively practicing in Turkey. Of these, 14,244, or 41.6 percent, were in full-time private practice. The remaining 58.4 percent of physicians worked for the MOHSA and the several other organized public programs reviewed earlier (19,951). A substantial share of these government physicians, however, also engaged in private practice when their official duties were completed. This applies mostly to the great majority of the government doctors who were trained as specialists. In effect, well over half of the time of Turkish doctors is devoted to private medical practice.

Regarding dentistry and pharmacy, private practice is of even greater importance. In 1981, of the 6,790 dentists, 5,269 or 78 percent were wholly in private practice. Of the 11,423 pharmacists, 8,741 or 77 percent worked entirely in private pharmacies. This private market for health service is heavily concentrated in the large cities, where more affluent people live. The nation's three largest cities—Istanbul, Ankara, and Izmir—have 18 percent of the national population and more than 60 percent of the national supply of health professionals.

Finally, in Turkey's private health care sector, one must count a variety of traditional healers that people consult for their ailments, particularly in rural areas. Most numerous are traditional birth attendants, who still deliver about one-fourth of the babies in rural Turkey. In addition, there are thousands of needlemen, bone setters, mystics, and a variety of other healers.

One category of health personnel, the male nurse or *saglik memeru,* perhaps occupies a borderline position between modern and traditional health practice. Starting in 1910, these multipurpose health workers were trained in government schools, which eventually grew to 14 in 1965. Today there are only two schools, and the functions of these personnel have become focused on sanitation and laboratory technology. In 1982, there were 11,956 of these male nurses, and 33 percent of these were reported to be illegally in private practice; this was mainly in rural areas, without proper medical personnel.

The general proportions of the private market for health services in Turkey can be inferred from two surveys of household expenditures made in the 1970s. As is shown later, in terms of expenditures they even exceed the aggregate of all public programs.

Health System Overview

The proportions of the several parts of the Turkish health system structure may be gathered in two general ways—by the distribution of resources and by analysis of health expenditures.

The output of physicians has increased rapidly in Turkey in recent decades. In 1964 there were four medical schools with an enrollment of 900 students, which expanded to 22 medical schools in 1984 with 5,500 students. The 34,195 active physicians in 1985 were distributed, based on their principal activity, among the major health programs as follows:

Program	Percentage
Ministry of Health and Social Assistance	27.5
Social Insurance Organization	10.6
Other public organizations	6.2
Universities	14.0
Private market	41.7
All programs	100.0

The breakdown of sponsorship for hospitals is available in slightly more detailed categories. In 1984, Turkey had 730 hospitals with

115,600 beds—a ratio of 2.4 beds per 1,000 population. The sponsorhsips of these hospital bed supplies were distributed as follows:

Sponsorship	Percentage of Beds
Ministry of Health and Social Assistance	52.3
Social Insurance Organization	15.3
Ministry of Defense	13.2
Universities (Ministry of Education)	11.9
Parastatal economic enterprises	1.8
Other ministries	0.7
Municipalities	0.8
Voluntary nonprofit agencies	1.7
Private proprietary owners	2.4
All sponsorships	100.0

Examining the overall Turkish health system in terms of its economic support, the frequency distribution suggests a different picture. Of Turkey's national GNP in 1983, approximately 3.5 percent was spent on the health system as a whole—a figure quite close to that of other countries at the transitional economic level with welfare-oriented policies. The distribution of these health expenditures in 1983, by source, was as follows:

Source	Percentage
Ministry of Health and Social Assistance	17.2
Social Insurance Organization	11.5
Government Employees Insurance	1.1
Other government agencies	2.8
University hospitals	8.3
Parastatal enterprises	1.1
Personal households	58.0
All sources	100.0

Figures for 1982 cast some light on the relatively small share (17.2 percent) of national health expenditures attributable to the MOHSA. Out of the total budget of the central government, the share allocated for health has varied from year to year; in 1970 it was 3.48

percent of the total, but in 1982 it was 2.94 percent. The Ministry of Defense in 1982 absorbed 17.4 percent of the national budget.

Considering these several sets of data together, it seems that the resources of the Turkish health system are predominantly public. Of all hospital beds, almost 96 percent are sponsored by government bodies, and of all physicians, 58.3 percent work principally in government programs. The money to support health services, on the other hand, comes mainly (58 percent) from personal households. Even though there may be some inaccuracies in these data, the government of Turkey seems to have done a great deal to develop a health system infrastructure, without making equivalent expenditures to finance the system outputs or services.

Indirect support of this inference can be drawn from data on ambulatory services applicable to 1981. Based on a report of the MOHSA for the 47 socialized provinces, in 1981 the overall visits to all Ministry health centers were estimated at about 6,000,000. Visits to MOHSA hospital out-patient departments were far greater, numbering 14,700,000. (People obviously prefer seeing specialists at an OPD, even if it means more travel.) Relating these 20,700,000 ambulatory services to the noninsured population of about 28,000,000 people that year, an average of 0.74 visits were made per person each year. A similar calculation for ambulatory services to the socially insured population in 1981 yields an average figure of 1.23 visits per insured person per year.

Both of these rates of ambulatory consultations are quite low. Yet we know that more than half of the available physician time in Turkey is spent in private practice, and it is generally recognized that private medical earnings are much higher than salaries in any government post. The ambulatory services provided by physicians through private practice, therefore, are undoubtedly equal to or greater than those provided by the various government programs in health centers, hospitals, and OPDs. In effect, the private medical personnel of Turkey are compensating for the inadequacies of a large public infrastructure, at the expense of personal households.

IRAQ

Another Middle East country at a transitional/developing economic level with a welfare-oriented health system is Iraq. Its population in 1986 was 16,190,000, of which 68 percent were urban. Like other countries in the region, it has significant reserves of petroleum, but not large enough to raise its per capita GNP (in 1984) above $1,837.

Information on the Iraqi health system is not readily available, especially since the turmoil of the war with Iran, which lasted from 1980 to 1988. The history of the land that is now Iraq can be traced back to ancient Mesopotamia, along with its capital city, Baghdad. In the sixteenth century, the land was dominated by the Ottoman Turkish Empire, but after World War I it came under British control. A British Mandate, established by the League of Nations, lasted until 1932. Oil was then discovered, greatly strengthening the national economy. In 1936, the first of several military coups occurred. The military group seizing power in 1958 was oriented toward a socialist ideology, which was reinforced by still another coup in 1968. Large land holdings were broken up, and most industry was nationalized. In 1972 the internationally developed oil explorations were nationalized and a 15-year friendship pact was signed with the Soviet Union.

A provisional Constitution, promulgated in 1970, espoused socialist principles. For a period the Communist Party was legalized, but this ended in 1978, when Iraq attempted to attain a neutral posture between East and West superpowers. The adult literacy level in 1984 was only 58 percent overall, and much lower among women. Food consumption in 1984 was reported as 18 percent above the average daily requirements. Iraq's president in 1989 was Saddam Hussein, a military leader described as seeking a balance between Western technology and socialist ideology.

Health System Organization

Serious development of resources for health care of the population in Iraq began in the

1930s, with the discovery of oil. Under the British Mandate (1921–1932), the country had been divided into governorates for general public administration. These numbered 15, plus 3 autonomous regions. The governorate is divided into 15 to 20 smaller administrative units. A chief officer of health, appointed by the national minister of health, is in charge of governmental health services in each governorate.

At the national level, six major departments under the Ministry of Health carry out a wide range of responsibilities: (1) preventive medicine (epidemiology), (2) medical supplies (including pharmaceuticals), (3) rural health services (both preventive and curative), (4) health services (largely nationwide disease control programs), (5) medical services (management of hospitals), and (6) health inspection (mainly environmental sanitation). Each of these departments provides technical backup to the governorate officers of health, and for certain functions, such as hospital operation and vector-control campaigns, services are managed directly from the top.

Each governorate has a network of general regional and district hospitals, main health centers, branch health centers (or subcenters), and specialized dispensaries. These are all governmental and, until recently, their services were given entirely without charge. In 1987, due to the economic derangements from the war, small fees were imposed for each visit to a health facility and for each drug prescription.

Separate from the MOH framework of health activities is a program of mandatory insurance for nonagricultural workers and their dependents. All government employees are covered, along with industrial workers in private firms with five employees or more. Petroleum workers are covered, insofar as this industry has been nationalized. To support the program, contributions are made principally by employers, with a lesser fraction of wages from workers.

The program is administered by the Iraqi Directorate of Social Security for Workers, which is supervised by the Ministry of Labour and Social Affairs. In 1987, this agency reported that 234,670 primary workers were covered. If we assume, for this Arab country, three dependents per worker, 938,700 persons would be covered by medical care insurance, or about 5.8 percent of the national population.

Covered persons are entitled to virtually complete medical care without charge. Unlike that of Egypt, however, the Iraqi social security program has not established health facilities of its own. Instead, for both ambulatory and hospital service, beneficiaries use designated resources of the Ministry of Health. The social security organization reimburses the MOH for these services.

Voluntary health agencies in Iraq include the Red Crescent, which is subsidized by the government. There are also the customary societies for children, against tuberculosis, and so on. Moslem religious groups operate some shelters for the aged.

In the private market, fewer than 10 percent of all medical practitioners in Iraq work exclusively in private practice. The great majority of government physicians, however, including the governorate officers of health, spend part of each day seeing private patients. Services in private practice are subject to some supervision by the MOH.

Health Resources

The supply of physicians has increased rapidly in Iraq since 1950, when there were 15 per 100,000 population. At that time there was one medical school in the country (founded in 1927) at the University of Baghdad. Since then five additional medical schools have been established, four of them outside the national capital. By 1981, Iraq had 7,630 physicians or a ratio of 56 per 100,000. All new graduates are required to spend 6 years (an exceptionally long period of mandatory service) in a position assigned by the MOH. Licensure is granted, not by a government agency, but by the Iraqi Medical Association.

The ratio for professional-level nurses and midwives in Iraq was 58 per 100,000 population in 1982. That for dentists was only 10 per 100,000.

Hospitals are relatively numerous in Iraq. In 1986, there were 234 hospitals with 31,700 beds, or a ratio of nearly 2.0 beds per 1,000 population. Practically all of these beds were controlled by the Ministry of Health or other public agencies. Fewer than 2 percent of the beds were in small private facilities.

Health centers for primary health care are distributed throughout the country. In 1986, there were 177 main health centers and 587 subcenters. Each main center is expected to be staffed by at least one doctor and allied personnel; the subcenters have only auxiliary-level personnel. The main health centers are theoretically meant to serve about 20,000 people and the subcenters about 5,000; many more structures would be needed, however, to reach these standards. There were also 231 dispensaries in 1986 for tuberculosis, venereal diseases, and maternal and child health services. The MCH clinics also provide family planning services. Specialist services are available to ambulatory patients at all hospital out-patient departments, numbering 132 in 1979. More than 100 mobile clinic units serve the most thinly settled rural population, and some of these travel by river.

Drugs are relatively abundant in Iraq, constituting a major responsibility of the MOH. About half are produced in the country and half are imported.

Health Service Delivery and Expenditures

Health centers and hospital OPDs are rather heavily used, and the recent imposition of small user fees was intended, in part, to reduce their rate of use. A study in 1982–1983 found a rural utilization rate of 4.3 ambulatory consultations per person per year, the great majority at government health facilities; aside from sickness, distance from the facility was the main factor determining the utilization rates of various households. On the other hand hospital occupancies, outside the national capital, are relatively low—45 percent for the national average. Hospital admissions occur at the rate of 68 per 1,000 persons per year, for an average patient-stay of only 5 days.

As in many other countries, the physicians of Iraq are heavily concentrated in the national capital. In spite of the 6 years of mandatory public service, a great share of the doctors go

to Baghdad when this service is completed. In 1976, when the capital contained 27 percent of the population, it had 49 percent of the doctors, and the disproportion has grown worse since then.

The effectiveness of the network of health centers and subcenters is reflected in Iraq's high rate of immunizations. In 1987 the MOH had immunized 91 percent of the children for diphtheria, pertussis, and tetanus. The record on poliomyelitis was also 91 percent. The MOH reported in 1987 that 100 percent of the urban population and 80 percent of the rural population had access to basic health services. Childbirths were handled by trained health personnel at a rate of 70 percent in urban areas and 40 percent in rural areas, although only 35 percent of all deliveries in the nation were performed in health institutions. Infant mortality was reduced from 139 per 1,000 live births in 1960 to 70 in 1987. Life expectancy in 1987 was 64 years.

Urban environmental sanitation in Iraq has been remarkably good, with 100 percent of the city population reported to be served by safe water and sewage disposal in 1987. In rural areas, however, 54 percent of the population had access to safe drinking water in 1987 and only 11 percent to sewage disposal.

The expenditures (public and private) for the Iraqi health system as a whole amounted to 4.5 percent of GNP in 1983. Of the overall government budget, 5.5 percent was allocated to the Ministry of Health. The share of total health expenditures absorbed by the private sector is not reported but, judging by the extensive national coverage with government health resources and the very small charges made for public services, it is very likely a small fraction. Even though the socialist character of the total Iraqi economy may be debatable, the national health system is clearly welfare-oriented.

MALAYSIA

Malaysia is a nation of 15,080,000 people (1984) in Southeast Asia that won its independence from Great Britain in 1957. The ethnic composition of its population is strikingly varied, with Malays constituting 47 percent, Chinese 33 percent, Indians (and some Pakistani) 9 percent, and indigenous people plus a few others 11 percent. The national health system embodies so many features from the country's past that the historical background warrants more than cursory review.

Historical Background

Five hundred years ago the Malay Peninsula was peopled by rural tribes, whose healing arts were believed to be influenced by the ancient medical lore of the great Asian continent. Malay traditional medicine was a blend of local folklore, Hindu mythology, Moslem orthodoxy, and Arabic pharmacopeia. This stream of development, despite the enormous influences of the West, is still very much alive in the work of *bomohs* and other traditional healers in the several thousand villages or *kampongs* of modern Malaysia.

The impact of the West started with the Portuguese settlement in what is now Malacca in 1511. In 1641 the Portuguese were succeeded by the Dutch in Malacca and in 1786 the British came to the island of Penang and, in 1795, replaced the Dutch in Malacca. A generation later, in 1819, the British acquired control of the island of Singapore by purchasing it from a local ruler. In all three of these early trading stations, the Dutch and then the British established small garrison hospitals or infirmaries for the care of European officials and their families. Perhaps local persons were occasionally treated at these infirmaries, but there was no significant spread of Western medicine inland until about 1873, when the British intervened with the warring Malay State Sultanates. The civil administration of the three coastal cities—Malacca, Penang, and Singapore—was strengthened by the formation of the Straits Settlements authority under the British Colonial Office in 1867, including limited responsiblity for health protection.

In the early nineteenth century, tin was discovered in Malaya, and Chinese settlers came to extract it. They brought Chinese traditional medicine, and in 1880 they built a small hospital of 28 beds for their countrymen in Kuala Lumpur. In 1883, the British Resident established a "general hospital," also in Kuala Lumpur—the first of what now constitutes a network of general hospitals in each of the state capitals of the 11 states of West Malaysia. As the Chinese continued to come to Malaya in the later nineteenth century, Chinese herbalists, with hundreds of remedies from plants and animal organs, settled in the slowly growing towns.

In 1896, the Federation of Malay States was formed by agreement between the British and the Sultans of four states. In these federated states, the advice of the British Resident was followed on all matters (including health), except religious and Malay customs. A few years later, five other states passed from Thai (Siam) to British "protection" in foreign relations. These came to be known as the "nonfederated states," with greater autonomy in the management of their internal affairs. Thus, by about 1910 an administrative structure, under different forms of authority, had been established in the three Straits Settlements, the four federated states, and the five nonfederated states of the Malay Peninsula.

With this extension of European influence, between 1883 and 1910, general hospitals were established in the capital cities of each state. The emphasis of this period was obviously on curative medicine and the hospital treatment of the desperately sick. There was, however, a dawn of sensitivity to preventive health needs in the main cities. Kuala Lumpur, in fact, set up among the British governmental personnel a Sanitary Board that was concerned with cleaning the streets, maintaining public markets, and so on.

The challenge of research into the causes and control of infectious tropical diseases was met by the establishment by the British of the Institute for Medical Research in 1900. This important center in Kuala Lumpur, tied originally to universities in London and Liverpool, now plays a key role in the health services of all Malaysia. The Singapore Medical College was founded in 1905, evolving later into the Faculty of Medicine of the University of Malaya.

In 1910 an organized Health Department was established on a permanent basis in Kuala Lumpur. It was staffed by colonial government medical officers, and its functions were chiefly related to environmental sanitation in Kuala Lumpur and the surrounding areas. By 1920, the staff had expanded to 31 medical officers and 8 sanitary inspectors.

Meanwhile in the early twentieth century, rubber estates had begun to take form (after the introduction of the trees in Singapore in 1877). By 1920 there were 1,200 such estates, and a Labour Code, including provisions for health and sanitation, was enacted. Outside the main cities, it was on the rubber estates (rather than in rural areas generally) that public health efforts were concentrated. Swamp drainage and application of mosquito larvacides to control malaria in these locations, along with smallpox vaccination and some quarantine, were the chief activities.

In the decades between 1910 and 1930, medical officers of health were appointed in the capital cities of each of the Malay states. In some, their functions were confined to the interior of those cities and in others they extended to enforcement of sanitary conditions at the rubber estates and tin mines. In a few cities, maternal and child health clinics were established and some school children were examined. Each of the federated, as well as the unfederated states, had a public health adviser assigned by the Colonial Medical Service.

Quite separate from the public health work, general hospitals were also expanded in the state capitals during this period, and some small district hospitals were built in other towns. As satellites of some of the hospitals, small *town dispensaries* were established in a few cities, staffed mainly by hospital assistants. These were male dressers or medical auxiliaries who learned their skills by apprenticeship in the hospitals.

Thus, two sides were taking shape in the health services: a "public health" side and a "hospital" side. After 1948, both were transferred to the control of the state governments. At the federal level in Kuala Lumpur, health authority was limited to enforcement of quarantine and control of epidemics, the allocation of personnel, the operation of certain federal hospitals (mental, military, etc.), and general advisory services. Not until 1958 did the national government of the then independent

federation again take over control of both public health and hospital functions in the states.

From 1930 to 1942, the colonial public health and medical services were faced by the setbacks of the worldwide economic depression. Outside the estates and mines, the only services for rural areas were a few traveling dispensaries emanating from the hospitals. In 1942, war spread in Asia and the country was conquered and occupied by the Japanese army until 1945.

With the end of the war and the formation of the Malayan Federation in 1948, civil government became more systematized throughout the states. Among other things, this meant the establishment of 70 admininstrative districts as smaller units of political jurisdiction. Health districts, however, were somewhat fewer.

The postwar period also saw a large expansion of district hospitals to 50, in addition to 10 general hospitals, by 1956. Emanating from most of the general and district hospitals, usually located in the headquarters town of an administrative district, were various static dispensaries in the towns. Some additional traveling dispensaries to rural locations were also organized. Maternal and child health clinics were established in scores of cities and towns.

After the departure of the Japanese, the British turned over authority to the sultanates. This led to an antigovernment guerilla movement, starting in 1948—a civil war that became known as the Emergency. Since the Communist guerrillas derived much of their sustenance from Chinese settlers, wresting a living at the edge of the Malayan jungles, a major counterinsurgency program consisted in resettlement of about a half million of these people into *New Villages*—some 500 throughout the country. This was done between 1950 and 1953. Although curfews were imposed and movements restricted, the inhabitants of the New Villages were often provided with midwife clinics or small first-aid facilities.

The Emergency, therefore, not only contributed to the belated recognition of rural needs, it also highlighted the special deficiencies in the hundreds of kampongs peopled by Malays who had taken no part in the guerilla movement. With all the attention given to the Chinese in New Villages, it was argued in Parliament, what about the social needs of the greater number of rural Malays? Thus, a series of national programs were started, focusing on improving conditions in rural areas; these led eventually to a very active Ministry of National and Rural Development. It was part of this swelling tide of concern for rural welfare that led to the formulation of the Rural Health Services Scheme, starting in 1953.

This historic background of sultanic states, British colonial government, and wartime experience helps explain the current contours of the Malaysian health system, with its separate management of preventive and hospital services, its emphasis on rural health programs, and its orderly general division of responsibilities between national and state governments. Malaysia in 1984 was still predominantly rural, with only 32 percent of its population living in cities. National productivity had been gradually rising, to a per capita GNP of $2,112. The adult literacy rate was 73 percent, and lower among the Malay ethnic population.

Organizational Structure of the Health System

The major government body responsible for protecting the health of the Malaysian population is the Ministry of Health, but several other entities play a part both inside and outside government.

Ministry of Health. The range of the responsibilities of the Ministry of Health (MOH) is very wide. The minister is a member of the national cabinet and participates in all major political policy decisions. The ministry's programs encompass the entire range of preventive and curative health services, which are provided through a pyramidal administrative framework through the entire country.

The preventive services include family health (maternal and child health promotion), environmental sanitation, occupational health protection, food safety, control of vector-borne diseases (e.g., malaria), tuberculosis and leprosy control, prevention and control of acute communicable diseases (immunizations, etc.), health education, and preventive dental care.

The curative services included both ambulatory and bed care of the sick through a large network of hospitals, health centers, health clinics or posts, and other facilities staffed with trained personnel. Treatment is furnished to both acute and chronic diseases and to both physical and mental disorders. Personal dental care is also provided for certain sections of the population.

Many other services are necessary to support these programs, particularly the diagnostic and therapeutic aspects of the curative work. These include the operation of laboratory and x-ray services. The maintenance of pharmacies and drug supplies is an essential supportive service. Other supportive services are biomedical research, some health services research, engineering, and general health planning and development.

To manage the operation of all these programs, of course, the central government must perform functions of finance, personnel, procurement of equipment and supplies, and others. Peripherally, each of Malaysia's 13 states (11 in peninsular Malaysia, plus Sabah and Sarawak in Borneo), has an Office of Medical and Health Services representing the MOH. The state director of this office is responsible for the operation of almost all MOH programs, especially the hospital, health centers, and other health facilities. (The control of vector-borne diseases, however, is largely a "vertical" program, managed at the federal level.)

Below the state level are health districts, about 50 in all. The district medical officer of health, however, is responsible only for public health (essentially preventive) activities in the district, while the district hospital comes under the direction if its medical officer-in-charge, who reports directly to the state health office. Dental services in the district come under the direction of a senior dental officer. (Only in the state of Sarawak are these three types of health services administered by a single district medical officer of health.)

Within the rural districts there are subdistricts, with a network of health centers, health subcenters, and rural or midwife clinics, staffed to provide primary health care to Malaysia's large rural population. The conception of the Rural Health Services Scheme, starting in 1953, was to cover rural populations of 50,000 people with a main health center, four health subcenters (serving 10,000 people each), and 25 midwife clinics—5 around each health center and subcenter, serving 2,000 people each. Initially only one physician would be posted at the main health center, and the rest of the staffing consisted mainly of hospital assistants (for general medical care), nurses, assistant nurses, assistant midwives, sanitation personnel, clerks, and others.

Over the years, great progress was made in the Rural Health Services Scheme (RHSS). Many more doctors were appointed, and numerous subcenters were upgraded to main health centers. Hundreds of additional facilities were established, and many of the small midwife clinics were upgraded to general primary health care posts, through supplemental training of the assistant midwives. In 1985 it was estimated that some 93 percent of the rural population of Malaysia had convenient access to an RHSS facility.

Other Government Agencies with Health Functions. Several other government agencies do work relevant to the Malaysian health system.

The Ministry of Education is responsible for the operation of the nation's universities, three of which have medical schools. Dentists are trained in one university and pharmacists likewise. The institutions of higher learning also maintain general medical service programs for all their enrolled students. One of the universities also operates its own teaching hospital (although the other two make use of general state-level hospitals of the MOH). The Ministry of Education also runs a supplementary feeding program for certain undernourished school children.

The Ministry of Labor inspects factories to enforce regulations designed to protect the safety and health of workers. Also in this ministry is the administrative body operating a program of industrial injury compensation, known by the acronym SOCSO. In 1982, SOCSO covered 2,181,000 workers, defined by their employment in firms with five or more

employees, whose income was less than $1,000 per month. The compensation includes partial replacement of wages lost due to occupational injury or disease and, within stated limits, the cost of medical care. Initially this care is usually given by a private physician, but any necessary hospitalization is in a public hospital, since the SOCSO award is seldom large enough to cover private hospital charges. This social insurance program on work-connected problems is financed by regular contributions from both employer and worker, rather than solely from employers, as in other countries.

The Ministry of Land and Mines operates a relatively large hospital for aborigines, along with a network of radio-linked health posts in jungle areas. This special facility functions quite independently from the MOH network of hospitals.

Programs for rehabilitation of drug addicts are conducted by the Ministry of Home Affairs and the Ministry of Social Welfare. The latter ministry also operates institutions for the mentally retarded and custodial homes for the aged. These facilities provide their guests a certain amount of medical care.

The Ministry of Culture, Youth, and Sports provides certain health services in connection with its management of sports facilities. The Ministry of Science, Technology, and Environment is concerned with standards for protection against air pollution. Along with local authorities, it enforces regulations of this problem. The Veterinary Department in the Ministry of Agriculture is concerned with measures for the prevention of zoonotic diseases.

The armed forces, as in all countries, have a well-organized health service program for military personnel. In Malaysia, the families of these personnel are also eligible for care.

Aside from the local health activities of the Ministry of Health, municipal authorities participate in the regulation of environmental sanitation, especially regarding food safety, vector control, housing, and solid waste disposal. In some larger cities, maternal and child health services are provided for the whole population, and general primary care clinics are operated for city employees.

About 75 large enterprises in Malaysia are operated essentially as government corporations. These statutory or quasi-public bodies include the Malaysian Airlines, the national railways, the national petroleum corporation, and the Management Board for Pilgrims. Many of these organizations operate special clinics for their employees. The agency for pilgrims even operates its own hospital.

Finally among government agencies is an independent body (i.e., not under any ministry) that has great potential importance for the health system—the Employees Provident Fund (EPF). This is essentially a scheme of compulsory saving, launched in 1951, which requires all employed persons (but not the self-employed) to make regular contributions to a national fund. By statute in 1983, the employee had to pay 9 percent of his wages into the fund, and the employer must contribute 11 percent of payroll. The money is invested (mainly in government securities) and draws interest, so that it grows over the years. The main objective is to provide funds for pensions on retirement, which normally occurs at 55 years of age in Malaysia. The individual may, however, make withdrawals before retirement for such purposes as purchasing a home, education of children, or to meet the costs of private medical care within certain constraints.

It should be noted that the EPF is not the same as social insurance, in that there is no pooling of funds to meet the risks of any contributor. Rather, each person has claim only to the contributions made by himself and his employer. In 1984, more than 4,300,000 persons contributed to the fund. If we assume, conservatively, 1.5 dependents per employee, the EPF involved about 10.8 million people, or 72 percent of the national population of 15 million. In 1985 it was proposed that the SOCSO program for industrial injury compensation be integrated with the EPF, to achieve a national social security organization. This might gradually widen its scope to include sickness and disablement benefits.

Voluntary Health Agencies. Outside of government, a number of voluntary agencies in Malaysia perform health functions. Important among these are the Red Crescent Society, St.

John's Ambulance Service, National Cancer Society, the Society for Prevention of Tuberculosis, Association for Mentally Retarded Children, Association for the Blind, and the Family Planning Association.

Some of these agencies, like the Association for the Blind, operate small facilities, and all of them do educational and general welfare work. Most of them are subsidized by the national government—usually, though not always, through the MOH—on the grounds that their functions complement those of the government.

Among voluntary health agencies one must also count the several associations of professional personnel in the health field. The Malaysian Medical Association, for example, sponsors a certain amount of continuing education for physicians. It also sometimes arbitrates questions of medical ethics. The MMA plays a part in designating what training standards are proper for attainment of specialty status in various fields.

Enterprises with Health Functions. Quasi-public enterprises that provide health services to their employees have been noted. In addition, hundreds of private enterprises in Malaysia provide employees a wide range of medical and hospital services. The national Employment Security Act requires firms with more than 500 employees to provide a comprehensive scope of medical services for workers and, if the enterprise is in an isolated location, their families as well. Large rubber estates and tin mines often operate hospitals under the requirements of this legislation. Smaller firms are required by law to provide only for emergency medical care. Altogether in 1985 the estates and mines maintained 65 small "hospitals" or sickbays with 2,056 beds. They employed 68 doctors, but almost all were part-time.

The Private Health Care Market. Beyond all the organized health programs, there is a substantial private market for medical care in Malaysia. Probably most important are the private medical practices of 2,200 physicians functioning in 1983. The great majority of these are individual practitioners, but some form small medical groups. These constituted 52 percent of all doctors in the nation at that time, although before 1982 the majority were in public service. In Malaysia (unlike so many other countries), publicly employed physicians may not engage in private practice after official hours; thus, all of these private practices are full-time pursuits.

Of the 858 registered dentists in Malaysia, a lesser proportion (42 percent) were engaged in private practice in 1983. In addition, there were 315 Division II dentists in private practice; these are less than fully trained practitioners, who are authorized mainly to do extractions and fit full upper or lower dentures.

In recent years, the number of privately owned hospitals has grown rapidly in Malaysia. In 1983 there were 119 of them, owned and operated mostly by doctors. With a total of 3,521 beds, they tend to be small, with an average capacity of 30 beds.

In the private health care market, one must also count 327 private pharmacies or drugstores, which sell both prescribed and over-the-counter drugs. The larger cities also have shops that sell corrective eyeglasses, hearing aids, and prosthetic appliances.

Finally, the entire field of traditional healing must be counted in the private health care market. Almost all observers agree that there are large numbers of *bomohs* in the rural areas, as well as *bidans* (traditional birth attendants). In 1976, it was estimated that there were 20,000 bomohs in peninsular Malaysia—that is, not counting the two less developed states in north Borneo. The vast majority of these practitioners, however, are not full-time but are engaged mainly in farming or some other rural occupation. As illiteracy declines in Malaysia and the availability of modern health services increases, the use of traditional healing lessens. The Chinese herbalist, who sells "natural" products for any and every ailment, is still another part of the health care market in the small and large towns of Malaysia. In the cities there are also some Ayurvedic practitioners, although in lesser numbers, who cater to people of Indian background.

Production of Resources

As economic development has proceeded in Malaysia, the number and diversity of health resources have increased.

Health Manpower. At independence in 1957, Malaysia's only medical school was the one established by the British in Singapore in 1905. When Singapore broke away in 1963, Malaysia was left with no medical school. Then at the University of Malaya in Kuala Lumpur, a medical faculty was established, and the first class of Malaysian medical graduates was turned out in 1969. Soon a second medical school was established at the National University in Kuala Lumpur, and a third one was started in 1980 at the University of Science in Penang.

The great majority of graduates of these medical schools remain in Malaysia, and they are also supplemented by many doctors immigrating from other countries. For some years, Malaysia found it necessary to invite into the country physicians from South Korea, the Philippines, India, and elsewhere to staff rural health centers and other rural posts. Then in 1970, a law was enacted requiring that all new graduates of a Malaysian medical school devote 3 years to work in the public service. The effect of this was to greatly improve the medical staffing of district and (state) general hospitals. Better medical staffing of the health centers by Malaysian doctors was slight, however, and it has still been necessary to import doctors from abroad; now they come mainly from Indonesia and Bangladesh.

In 1983 the annual output of the Malaysian medical schools was 352 graduates, and there were 4,324 doctors in the nation—a ratio of 29 doctors per 100,000 population. As everywhere in the world, there is an imbalance between the cities and the rural areas, and the urban concentration is aggravated by the high proportion of doctors (52 percent) in private practice.

Specialization is not highly developed in the Malaysian medical profession. Of the 2,034 doctors in public service in 1983, about 13 percent were registered specialists. In private practice there were also some specialists, but the proportion was less. Until the 1980s specialty training was available only abroad—principally in Great Britain—but since 1985 such training has been offered at the domestic medical school teaching hospitals.

There were 858 dentists in Malaysia, or about 6 per 100,000 population. As noted earlier, the majority of dentists work in the public service, but the 363 who are in private practice are supplemented by the services of Division II dental personnel, who are not trained to give full dental care. Perhaps more important are the 647 *dental nurses* whose training is based on the New Zealand model. These young women are prepared by 2 years in a special center following high school graduation. They work exclusively with school children and give a wide range of preventive and restorative services under the general supervision of professional dentists.

Pharmacists are trained at only one university-based school in Malaysia, which graduates about 70 per year. In 1983 there were 585 pharmacists in the nation, of whom about 200 worked in the MOH.

The vast majority of other allied health personnel in Malaysia work in institutions of the Ministry of Health. The largest category is nurses staffing the hospitals—7,148 in 1983. Assistant nurses numbered 5,669, in both hospitals and health centers. Staffing mainly the midwife clinics of the Rural Health Services Scheme are midwives II, numbering 3,065. For the training of nurses, there are 8 schools in Malaysia, all connected with hospitals. Assistant nurses are trained at 17 schools, mostly connected with health centers in the rural areas. Likewise, the Division II midwives are trained mostly in rural settings at 13 schools.

A very important type of allied paramedical health worker in Malaysia is the hospital assistant, whose functions were originally formulated under the British colonial government. Initially, these personnel, always males, learned about medical care simply by serving apprenticeships in hospitals, under the tutelage of doctors. Now they receive 3 years of formal training, mainly at centers connected with hospitals, after high school graduation. Some work in hospitals, but most are posted at rural

health centers and subcenters, where they do almost all of the curative work, including minor surgery and the prescribing of drugs. Three schools for training hospital assistants turn out about 200 per year. A less comprehensive training regime also produces *junior hospital assistants.* Altogether, in 1983 Malaysia had, 1,749 hospital assistants and 302 junior hospital assistants.

A very new category of personnel for primary health care is the *rural nurse,* who is an upgraded version of the rural midwife II personnel serving in the RHSS. Supplemental training of 6 months is given at two schools linked to rural health centers, and by 1985 about 380 rural nurses had been trained.

Environmental sanitation work in Malaysia is done by senior personnel, known as *public health inspectors,* and junior personnel, known as *public health overseers.* The inspectors are trained at a special Public Health Institute, located in Kuala Lumpur, where they take a 3-year course; there were 527 inspectors in the nation in 1985. The overseers receive only a 1-year course at schools located at two rural health centers.

Still other types of health personnel are produced in Malaysia to staff hospitals and, to some extent, other health facilities. These include laboratory and x-ray technicians, physiotherapists, dental technicians, dental assistants, and pharmacy assistants. Training of each of these personnel categories is done at only one or two schools under the Ministry of Health.

Beyond the basic education of all of these types of health manpower, postbasic or postgraduate training is available in several fields. A registered nurse, for example, can be trained to qualify as a *public health nurse.* Nurses are trained in hospitals for special qualifications in ward management, psychiatric nursing, or intensive care. Laboratory technicians get specialized training in advanced medical microbiology or parasitology. Continuing education, however, is not provided on a systematic basis, although clinical conferences are held from time to time at the state general hospitals.

Health Facilities. The origins of state general hospitals and smaller district hospitals in the

British colonial period have been reviewed. In 1984, the Ministry of Health operated 12 general hospitals and 48 district hospitals in peninsular Malaysia. There are two large mental hospitals under the Ministry of Health, and certain beds are also set aside for mental patients in some of the general hospitals. As noted earlier, other government agencies besides the MOH operate hospitals for selected populations. Counting beds in all of these types of institution, as well as hospital beds in Sabah and Sarawak, the distribution in 1984 was as follows:

Sponsorship	Beds	Percentage
Ministry of Health	25,797	81.59
Other government agencies	2,301	7.28
Private owners	3,521	11.14
All sponsorships	31,619	100.00

The ratio of hospital beds overall in 1984 was 2.1 per 1,000 population. Counting only beds for short-term general illness, the ratio is 1.6 beds per 1,000. These figures do not include the 2,056 beds in the health facilities of 65 estates and mines, since those are usually too modest to qualify as proper hospitals.

Hospital operating costs absorb some 61 percent of Ministry of Health annual expenditures. Small charges are made to patients admitted to MOH hospitals, although collections of these are quite weak. In the district hospitals, all the beds are classified as class III (large open wards), for which the charge in 1986 was $3 per day. In the larger general hospitals, class III beds constitute about 60 percent of the total; about 25 percent of beds are in much smaller class II rooms (for which $20 per day was charged), and 15 percent are in class I rooms (for which charges of $30 to $80 per day were made). For some 75 percent of patients obviously of very low income, no serious attempt is made to collect these charges. All these collections are estimated to amount to hardly 2 percent of the ministry's total health budget.

The types of patients and occupancy rates in the different hospitals vary significantly. The small private hospitals in general serve principally maternity cases, simple elective surgery, and other uncomplicated diagnoses. The large state general hospitals (500 to 1,000 beds) are staffed with well-trained specialists and have relatively sophisticated equipment. They serve patients from all socioeconomic levels, with serious and complex diagnoses. Rates of occupancy of the general hospitals tend to be high, particularly in the class III wards; there are often waiting lists for admission of nonemergency cases. The district hospitals, whose medical staffs include only general practitioners, have much lower rates of occupancy—often below 25 percent (see later).

The other important health facilities in Malaysia are those providing primary health care in the Rural Health Services Scheme. The main features of this program have been described, and the impressive growth of its resources are as follows:

Facility	1960	1968	1982
Main health centers	8	39	82
Health subcenters	8	139	249
Midwife clinics	26	703	878
Primary care clinics	—	—	640

The main health centers are staffed with physicians (general practitioners) plus nurses, assistant nurses, midwives, sanitary inspectors, clerks, and others. The other three types of facility are staffed entirely with auxiliary health personnel. The primary care clinics, developed only after 1975, are staffed with the new type of rural nurse, who was upgraded from an assistant midwife.

Before the RHSS was launched in 1953, there were numerous special clinics for maternal and child health services, dental care, tuberculosis control, and other services, which were absorbed into the RHSS program. In the cities, however, many of these specialized facilities remain, and are known as *static dispensaries* or *traveling dispensaries.* Administratively, they function usually as satellites of hospitals, which furnish their medical staffs.

Commodities. Almost all drugs and equipment required in the health care system of Malaysia must be imported, although certain foreign companies maintain packaging plants in the country. Modern pharmaceuticals are relatively expensive. One can understand why many people purchase medications directly from Chinese herbalists, at low prices.

Drugs dispensed in MOH hospitals, health centers, and clinics are obtained from a central supply depot maintained by the ministry. The central Pharmaceutical Division of the MOH purchases large quantities of drugs overseas and stores them under proper conditions. Periodically supplies of drugs and other materials are distributed to each of the state medical and health offices, which in turn distribute them to all MOH hospitals and health centers in the state. Emphasis is on the selection of generic, rather than brand-name compounds, and use of a carefully composed drug formulary achieves quality and cost controls for the MOH.

For the ambulatory patient, modern drugs can be obtained either at a governmental health center or clinic or from the private market. In the latter case, the patient can purchase drugs with or without a prescription. Prescribed drugs, however, are more frequently dispensed by medical practitioners directly. The physician typically buys a supply of drugs from a pharmacy at a reduced wholesale rate. He then charges the patient about double the amount that the drug cost him.

The Pharmaceutical Division of the MOH, in addition to its procurement, storage, and distribution functions, has in recent years acquired the ability to manufacture certain drugs (from imported chemicals). A National Pharmaceutical Laboratory has also been established for testing and registering all drugs, whether produced domestically or imported. Improved methods of formulation and packaging are the subject of research.

Knowledge. Much the greatest proportion of knowledge, and its application in technology for the health system, is acquired from abroad. Each of the 12 general hospitals maintains a medical library, as do several of the larger district hospitals.

Within Malaysia, the principal center for production of new knowledge is the Institute for Medical Research (IMR) in Kuala Lumpur. The establishment of this institution in 1900 has been reviewed, and its scope of scientific investigation has gradually broadened. The IMR serves as a reference center for the World Health Organization, and it conducts various studies in cooperation with the University of California. The IMR also serves as a central clinical laboratory for backup of the national network of laboratories maintained in the general and district hospitals. The medical faculties, of course, also carry out research.

Management

In each of the entities in Malaysia's organizational structure management practices are somewhat different, but this analysis concentrates on the Ministry of Health.

Health Planning. In the Office of the Prime Minister of Malaysia is an Economic Planning Unit (EPU) concerned with the large questions of economic and social development. Since independence (1957), Malaysia has engaged in formal overall planning, but in 1966 a new series of 5-year Malaysia Plans was launched. The Fourth Malaysia Plan (1981–1985) called for further strengthening of rural health services, which was indeed accomplished. On the other hand, only 1.5 percent of national development expenditures (mainly capital construction) were for the health sector, compared to 7.6 percent for education, and 18.3 percent for national defense. The Fifth Malaysia Plan called for, among other things, greater private support of health system costs.

Within the Ministry of Health there is also an Office for Health Planning and Development. The jurisdiction of this office, however, is limited to the programs of the MOH. It is concerned largely with the construction and renovation of physical facilities of the ministry and with the training of personnel within its orbit. The training activities to upgrade rural assistant midwives to rural nurses for general primary care were first proposed by this office. On the other hand, the MOH Office of Planning has no influence on the training activities of the universities, which come under the Ministry of Education.

It is particularly significant that the MOH planning activities include no concern for the construction of private hospitals, neither their location nor their size. The only approval by government for such construction involves their operation as new "businesses" in a locality. Also, there are no official standards for the features of various hospital departments nor any schedule for inspection of private hospitals. Likewise there is no planning of the geographic distribution of physicians in Malaysia. During the 3-year period of mandatory public service, new medical graduates are placed in MOH facilities where they are needed, but after this they are free to engage in private practice wherever they choose.

Soon after independence, health planning and general planning called for input of ideas from the states and even the administrative districts. But by 1985, planning seemed to be confined to the central government. A rough national guideline called for 2 short-term general hospital beds per 1,000 population. Yet, the national supply of 1.6 such beds was far from fully occupied, particularly in the 48 district hospitals. Planning procedures for appropriate referral of patients from the district to the state level might correct the imbalance between district and general hospital utilization, to make more efficient use of resources.

Health Administration. Administration of the health system includes many functions, most important being the relationships between central and peripheral parts of organized health activities. In Malaysia, health authorities are strongly concentrated at the top. The medical and health officers in each of the states are appointed by the central Ministry of Health, and their duty is to carry out national policy. They have very little discretion to undertake innovative activities on their own. Their responsibilities, furthermore, are restricted to the program of the MOH, and include no concern for health activities of other ministries, nor for any aspect of the private health sector.

As noted, the medical officers of health at the district level are responsible only for preventively oriented public health activities, along with the RHSS program. They have no jurisdiction over district hospitals whose medical directors report directly to the state chief medical and health officer. In each module of the RHSS (health center, subcenters, and rural clinics), the physician at the main health center is theoretically responsible for the proper functioning of all the peripheral units. In practice, however, these physicians devote nearly all their time to clinical medicine in the main health center, and provide little health supervision.

Medical records are reasonably well designed and used within the programs of the Ministry of Health. Data are regularly produced on the use of services in the MOH hospitals, health centers, and other units. They are absent, however, on services rendered in the private sector, in either private hospitals or private medical practices.

Another aspect of administration is to attract the participation of ordinary citizens in the policy making and operations of the entire health system—the concept defined and advocated by the World Health Organization as *community participation.* At the district level in Malaysia, there are citizen committees for development and security, with equivalent committees in almost every village. Their many functions include cooperation in the local programs for primary health care.

Evaluation, as an aspect of administration, is carried out at several levels within the public sector of Malaysia's health system. Regarding inputs, the increasing supplies of personnel and facilities have been reported. Regarding utilization of services, the measurement of the health care process, the trend has also been upward (as reported later). Here we can note some evaluative highlights of the health status "outcomes" of the Malaysian health system.

Data on the infant mortality rate (IMR) for Malaysia are available for the period 1960 to 1986. Over these 26 years, the IMR fell from 73 to 27 infant deaths (under 1 year of age) per 1,000 live births. Death rates of children from ages 1 to 4 showed an even steeper decline. They fell from 10.65 per 1,000 in 1957 to only 1.83 in 1981. The maternal mortality rate also declined steeply from 3.2 per 1,000 childbriths in 1957 to only 0.50 per 1,000 in 1982. Life expectancy at birth was 57.0 years in peninsular Malaysia in 1957 (it was doubtless lower in Sabah and Sarawak). By 1985, it had extended to 68 years for all Malaysia (including the two eastern states). These improvements, of course, cannot be attributed only to the health system.

Regarding causes of death, the available data are not as clear. Unfortunately as recently as 1980, only 37.5 percent of all deaths in Malaysia were certified by a physician. The rest occurred at home or elsewhere, without medical attendance. As a result, mortality can be identified only for those deaths occurring in government hospitals. In 1983 the major causes of such in-hospital deaths were (1) heart diseases, (2) diseases of early infancy and childhood, (3) accidents, (4) cardiovascular diseases, and (5) neoplasms, in that order. In Sabah and Sarawak, where general socioeconomic development is much less, the five leading causes of in-hospital deaths did not even include cardiovascular diseases or neoplasms.

Regarding morbidity, we must also rely on data reported by government hospitals. In peninsular Malaysia for 1983, the major causes of hospital admission, in order of frequency, were (1) accidents, (2) complications of pregnancy, (3) heart and cardiovascular diseases, (4) gastroenteritis, (5) mental illness, and (6) diseases of early infancy.

Data on trends are available for certain communicable diseases that are legally reportable. By this criterion, there has been definite improvement in the rate of occurrence of childhood infectious diseases against which immunizations are widely provided; these are diphtheria, whooping cough, tetanus, and poliomyelitis. Between 1976 and 1981, the rates for all four of these diseases declined steeply in Malaysia.

For other communicable diseases, on which effective immunizations are not available, the picture is not as bright. Such diseases, associated with poor sanitation, include cholera, typhoid fever, dysentery, food poisoning, and infectious hepatitis. For all five of these diseases, between 1976 and 1981, improvements were slight or the reported cases actually increased. When an increase has appeared, one cannot be certain whether it is real or simply reflects more complete reporting.

Trends between 1977 and 1981 for vector-borne diseases, in spite of major attempts at vector control, were mixed. For filariasis, dengue, and dengue hemorrhagic fever, the trends were inconsistent, but the rates were slightly lower in 1981 than in 1977. The rate for malaria, which is much higher per 100,000 than the other three mosquito-borne diseases, was higher in 1981 than in 1977.

Regulation and Legislation. The elected Parliament of Malaysia is an active legislative body, in spite of the substantial power of the sultans in each state. There are many laws and regulations in Malaysia for environmental sanitation. These have been enacted mainly by the state governments and the larger municipalities. Also, with respect to prevention of dental caries, almost all public water supply systems in peninsular Malaysia have been fluoridated under law.

Because of the problem of diseases spread by insect vectors, especially mosquitoes, various federal regulations have been enacted to eliminate or control breeding places. To reduce sexually transmitted diseases, there have been regulations on the medical examination of prostitutes, although prostitution is now legally prohibited.

Within the jurisdiction of the Ministry of Labor, there are numerous regulations on conditions of work, designed to reduce the hazards of accidents or occupational diseases. As in many countries, however, proper enforcement of these laws and regulations is limited by the inadequate number of trained personnel to carry out workplace inspections.

In the 1960s, laws were passed on the registration of hospital assistants in the states, the control of traditional birth attendants, nursing, and dangerous drugs. In the 1970s, legislation was enacted on dental health care, private hospitals, malaria eradication, destruction of disease-bearing materials, and general medical services. In the 1980s a law was passed on mandatory use of seat belts in automobiles.

Regulation of private medical practice and of private hospitals, however, is weak. Once a physician, dentist, nurse, or hospital assistant is registered, his or her entitlement to practice is permanent. There is no requirement for reexamination to determine if the individual has kept informed on recent developments. Initial registration is based on completion of a specified course of study, without further examination. Only for expatriate physicians is licensing or registration restricted to a certain number of years, after which (when their services are no longer needed) they must leave the country. The Malaysian Medical Council is a quasi-public body, appointed from the leading members of the Malaysian Medical Association, which is responsible for the registration of physicians, and it oversees questions of medical ethics.

In private pharmacies of Malaysia, almost any drug can be purchased without a medical prescription. For all practical purposes, regulatory restrictions apply only to narcotic and addictive drugs. Drug addiction, particularly with heroin, has become a serious problem in Malaysia—to such an extent that persons selling it or bringing it into the country are subject to the death penalty.

Economic Support

Based on data collected from several sources, the health expenditures of government agencies in 1983 are presented here. (It should be emphasized that these are actual expenditures, which may be less than the financial allocations given to the several ministries and agencies.)

Agency	Expenditure ($U.S.)	Percentage
Ministry of Health	$830,726,876	66.2
Ministry of Defense	54,915,148	4.4
Ministry of Education	83,941,116	6.7
Other ministries with health functions	16,746,052	1.3
Statutory (quasi-public) bodies	189,590,801	15.1
State and local governments	79,534,333	6.3
Total public	$1,255,454,326	100.0

The Ministry of Health obviously accounts for the lion's share of government health expenditures—66.2 percent in 1983. Over the years these MOH expenditures have risen. Using figures on financial appropriations, rather than actual expenditures, they rose from $112,663,747 in 1961 to $1,034,468,227 in 1983. In relation to the GNP of Malaysia, which was also rising rapidly over these years, the increase of public funding for health was not as sharp, going from 2 percent of GNP in 1961 to 3.15 percent of GNP in 1983. The overall government budget, in fact, was expanding even more rapidly than the GNP, so the proportion allocated for health actually declined, from 7.97 percent of the public budget in 1961 to 3.60 percent in 1983.

If the health expenditures from private sources could be analyzed on a basis comparable to public expenditures, we would present data on economic support from voluntary health agencies (charity), enterprise health services, voluntary health insurance, and spending by private individuals or families. Since this is not feasible, private health expenditures are estimated on the basis of the gross earnings of various types of private health care providers. In 1983, from an analysis of questionnaire returns, these were as follows:

Private Provider	Gross Earnings	Percentage
Private hospitals	$ 75,250,462	17.3
Private physicians	264,000,000	60.9
Private dentists	40,000,000	9.3
Private pharmacies	14,913,168	3.4
Other private providers	39,633,094	9..1
Total private	$433,796,724	100.0

This is doubtless an underestimate of private sector spending, since it overlooks expenditures of families on traditional practitioners, traditional birth attendants, and traditional Chinese herbalists. It also does not consider expenditures by voluntary health agencies and by private business enterprises for the health care of employees. Judging from findings in other countries, expenditures from the latter two sources are probably quite small, but expenditures on traditional healing might be significant.

Commercial insurance companies, numbering about 60 in Malaysia, sell life and casualty insurance to groups and individuals. Some seven or eight of these companies sell insurance to meet the costs of medical care, usually for major medical expenses—that is, medical costs exceeding a high threshold (such as $5,000), after which the insurance covers 75 or 80 percent of the obligations. About 100,000 persons have purchased this insurance protection. These expenditures are included in the gross earnings of health care providers, listed earlier (except for the administrative expenses and profits of insurance companies).

One other form of private health expenditure not captured here should be noted—the payment by individuals for service in governmental health facilities, especially for class I and class II services in hospitals. This money is transmitted to the Ministry of Finance and is not available for use by the Ministry of Health. The amount, however, is said to be small—only about 2 percent of the operating expenditures of the MOH. In 1983, this would have come to about $15,000,000, and would raise the private sector expenditures by only 3.5 percent.

Considering overall health expenditures from both public and private sources, we derive the following proportions for 1983:

Source	Amount	Percentage
Public	$1,255,454,326	74.3
Private	433,796,724	25.7
Total	$1,689,251,050	100.0

Thus, about three-quarters of Malaysia's health expenditures are derived from public sources, and about one-quarter from private sources. Even if adjustments were made for the omissions in the private sector noted previously, the changes would probably not be large. Attempts of the government in the mid-1980s to maximize private health spending may have had a greater effect.

Relating these findings to Malaysia's overall wealth or GNP, the health system in 1983 was found to absorb 2.6 percent of GNP. This figure is fairly typical of developing countries, but less typical is the substantially greater share coming from public than from private sources. This predominant public responsibility for the health system has undoubtedly contributed to the exceptionally favorable health status and health trends of the Malaysian population.

Delivery of Health Services

Personal health services in Malaysia are delivered predominately in organized settings, but this applies less to primary health care than to hospitalization.

Primary Health Care. The oldest form of delivery of primary health care in Malaysia was doubtless the service, both magical and empirical, of traditional healers or *bomohs.* Such therapeutically oriented care is still given by thousands of healers in the rural areas, although its extent has undoubtedly declined, as modern services have become available and the educational level of the population has increased. In 1984 some 73 percent of the adult population was literate, and almost all children attended school. With 32 percent of the population urbanized (living in places with 10,000 or more people), the purely rural population has been proportionately declining.

The gradual extension of the organized Rural Health Services Scheme (RHSS) since 1953 has brought this network of primary health services within reach of more than 90 percent of the rural population. Most of the services are provided by paramedical personnel—assistant nurses, hospital assistants, assistant midwives, and others—working in small clinics or health centers. A physician theoretically supervises this work, but he personally sees only a small fraction of the patients, and the basic training of the auxiliary personnel is relatively brief.

A good deal of the effort of the RHSS staff goes into preventive maternal and child health services, including immunizations and family planning. Treatment is given mainly by the hospital assistants (with 3 years of training after high school), furnished with a small selection of the important drugs. Environmental sanitation is promoted by the efforts of public health inspectors and health overseers, who visit the homes and assist in the construction of latrines, safe wells, and promotion of a generally sanitary environment around the houses. Vector-control activities, to eliminate mosquitoes, are carried out by teams of health workers coming to the villages from a higher administrative level. All of these RHSS services are free to the people and financed wholly by the Ministry of Health.

Data on the use of these primary care services are not complete. In 1982, counting the ambulatory services at health centers and static or traveling dispensaries in both rural areas and cities, there were 6,147,729 attendances in all. This was an increase from 4,224,299 such attendances in 1970. In addition, a great many people with access to the health centers and health subcenters prefer to bypass them, as in so many developing countries, and go directly to the out-patient department of a hospital, where they can see a doctor. In 1982, there was an even greater number of such medical attendances—8,849,067. This was an increase over 5,487,120 of such hospital out-patient attendances in 1970. For 1982, the total attendances amounted to 14,997,000 or about 1.0 per person per year for the nation.

These utilization data take no account of the services rendered at the rural midwife clinics and rural health clinics. Before the initiation of the RHSS in 1953, the great majority of rural childbirths in peninsular Malaysia were managed in homes by traditional birth attendants. By 1982, of all the estimated pregnant mothers, 61.6 percent received some prenatal care by the trained assistant midwives and 43.2 percent received some postnatal service. Of all the childbirths in 1982, 53.1 percent were delivered in hospitals and (counting home deliveries) 76.4 percent were attended by trained government personnel.

In the cities, where private physicians are concentrated, a great deal more primary care is provided in the offices of private medical practitioners. It is generally believed that this service is more personal and sensitive than the services rendered in crowded out-patient departments. It is estimated that in Malaysia, the private physician sees an average of about 50 patients a day; for an 8-hour day this means hardly 10 minutes per patient. Assuming about 260 working days a year, the 2,200 private medical practitioners in Malaysia provide a total of 28,600,000 attendances. For the nation as a whole, this would mean 1.9 attendances per person per year, or more than the total ambulatory services in MOH facilities.

Insofar as prescribed drugs are part of primary health care, they are dispensed along with the clinical care. In government health centers or hospital out-patient departments, drugs are ordinarily dispensed on the spot. In private medical practice, the physician typically dispenses his own prescribed drugs, for which the charge is included in the medical fee. Drugs purchased at pharmacies are usually self-prescribed medication taken on the informal advice of the pharmacist. Traditional herbal drugs are usually purchased at the shop of a traditional Chinese practitioner, largely on the basis of the symptoms reported.

As part of primary health care, dental services are provided at clinics in the health centers or in separate facilities. The government services employ both professional dentists on salary and dental nurses. In 1983, there were 3,471,318 attendances for this public dental service, all of which was without charge. The volume of services provided by private dentists is not known, but it is probably greater.

Hospital and Specialized Care. With nearly 90 percent of hospital beds in Malaysia being under government sponsorship, their staffing is by full-time medical and allied personnel. In district hospitals, the doctors are typically general practitioners, often young medical graduates putting in their 3 years of mandatory service. With this requirement for public service since 1970, the district hospitals have much larger medical staffs than in previous years; yet their occupancies are very low, since patients often bypass them to seek the services of specialists at the larger state general hospitals. As noted earlier, neither the general practitioners in district hospitals nor the specialists at general hospitals are permitted to engage in private practice, even after their official work is done.

The patterns of health care delivery in private hospitals of Malaysia are quite different. These hospitals are supported entirely by the fees they charge. They tend to serve mainly simple cases, but their amenities are attractive and their charges are relatively high. Their average lengths-of-stay are shorter than those in public hospitals, and they naturally cater to well-to-do families in the cities. Their medical staffs are not salaried, but are paid by patient fees for each service. These staffs are loosely organized and open to almost any private physician who has a patient to admit. Their outpatient departments are not well developed and, except for emergencies, serve only patients who can afford to pay private fees.

The method of financing of government hospitals is based on a global budget, which is calculated for each institution every year. No public payments are made on the basis of units of service rendered or per diem charges. In 1985 the average length-of-stay in all public general and district hospitals was about 6 days. Small personal charges are made to patients, but they are seldom collected for class III services, which apply to the great majority of beds (all the beds in district hospitals). Somewhat higher charges for class II and class I accommodations in the large state general hospitals have been noted. (Government employees are, however, entitled to any class of service for very small charges.) The annual global budget is paid in quarterly installments. If there is a shortfall of funds, a supplemental allotment may be granted, but any surplus at the end of the year must be returned to the treasury.

Care of Special Population Groups. Military service personnel and also their families are served by a wholly separate subsystem of health services. The doctors and other personnel are all on full-time salaries and work together in a highly organized framework. The services are free to both military personnel and families. Environmental sanitation and personal preventive services are especially well developed in this program.

Malaysia's aboriginal population, who live in the central hill areas, are served by a special network of health posts and a unique hospital located near Kuala Lumpur and designed appropriately for their rather primitive way of life. When a patient is admitted, usually brought in by airplane, the entire family comes along to feed and take care of him.

For workers at larger rubber estates, tin mines, and certain other enterprises, special programs of health service are provided. A

general practitioner, on either part-time or full-time salary, is usually in charge, aided by various assistant nurses and other auxiliary personnel. The small infirmaries that exist provide little more than bed rest, because any patient requiring medical care is transferred to a district or state general hospital.

Patients with serious mental disease are usually admitted to one of the two large mental hospitals operated by the Ministry of Health. In some states, the general hospital maintains a special section for mental patients. Occasionally the static dispensary in the larger cities provides a part-time psychiatrist for ambulatory mental patients.

SUMMARY COMMENT

In spite of the differences, in both their historic backgrounds and their current structures, the health systems of these Middle East and Asian countries clearly demonstrate a welfare-oriented ideology. The social security mechanism does not play as crucial a role as in Latin American countries, although its place is expanding. More important have been the energetic strategies of government to address the health deficiencies of rural areas. The national supplies of physicians have been substantially enlarged, and auxiliary personnel have also been extensively trained and used. Health centers and health stations have been widely constructed, although their utilization has not been as great as the out-patient clinics of hospitals, staffed by specialists.

In all of these countries there seems to be an unsteady equilibrium between the public and the private sectors. Government salaries for physicians are relatively low, making private practice attractive either full-time or after official duties. At the same time, government may even encourage private medical practice to reduce professional pressures for higher salaries. Drugs are usually given free-of-charge in government health facilities, but their quantity and quality are not always adequate. The private pharmacy, therefore, becomes a major resource for low-income people, usually without use of any medical prescriptions.

The trend of private health expenditures in

these countries has been upward, although that for government expenditures seems to be increasing even more. The overall percentage of GNP devoted to the health systems of these countries has been growing larger. In the 1980s, all the countries in this welfare-oriented category have been emphasizing priority for primary health care, even though tertiary hospitals continue to be a great drain on public budgets. The benefits of primary health care, in extending life expectancies and reducing infant mortality rates, have generally been dramatic.

Of the four countries discussed in this chapter, all except Malaysia had tumultuous social conditions in the 1970s and 1980s, with wars, periods of military dictatorship, massive inflation, and various sorts of domestic strife. The Moslem faith is dominant in all four, but with less intensely orthodox than in other Middle East countries. Each government, in its own way, seems committed to strengthening the official health services, but at the same time it responds to demands for the support of private enterprise. The health system is obviously marginal to other issues, and its future prospects will depend on these larger events.

REFERENCES

Egypt

Arab Republic of Egypt, Ministry of Health, *Egyptian Experience in Primary Health Care.* Cairo, 1978.

Bicknell, William, and A. Fairbank, "Health Development in Egypt: A Proposal." Boston: Boston University, August 1981, processed document.

Carney, Kim, "Health in Egypt." *Journal of Public Health Policy,* 5(1):131–142, March 1984.

Dalton, James, "Private and Public Sector Health Services Delivery Systems in Egypt." *Health Sector Assessment:* Cairo: U.S. Agency for International Development, April 1982, processed document.

Egyptian Ministry of Health, *Basic Statistical Information of Health Services.* Cairo, July 1981, processed document.

Experimental Center for Training and Evaluation of Social Programs, *Urban Health Delivery System Project: Health Sector Assessment.* Cairo, October 1982.

Furnia, Arthur H., *The Arab Republic of Egypt.* Washington, D.C.: U.S. Office of International Health: Syncrisis—The Dynamics of Health, September 1975.

Hassouna, W. A., "Summary of the Three-Country Health Services Coverage Study." *The Health Services Researcher,* 2(2):7–31, 1981.

Lamb, David, "Egyptian Paradox: Medical Clinics Abound But Care Is Questionable." *Los Angeles Times,* 31 August 1984.

Ministry of Health, *Health in Egypt.* Cairo: Publication No. 15, March 1982.

Nadini, Nawal El Messiri, *Rural Health Care in Egypt.* Canada: IORC (T515e), 1980.

Nazif, Kamal M., et al., "Evaluation of Activities Performed by the G.P.s Concerning Primary Medical Care in the Outpatient Clinics." *Bulletin of the High Institute of Public Health* (Alexandria), 11(4):183–210, 1981.

United Nations, "Egypt," in *The International Drinking Water Supply and Sanitation Decade Directory,* 1st edition. New York: United Nations, June 1981, pp. 34–35.

United Nations Fund for Population Activities, *Report of Second Mission on Needs Assessment for Population Assistance: Arab Republic of Egypt.* New York: Report No. 78, October 1985.

U.S. Agency for International Development, *A Report on Health Development in the Arab Republic of Egypt: A Sector in Transition.* Cairo, 1982.

World Health Organization, "Egypt," in *Sixth Report on the World Health Situation 1973–1977, Part II.* Geneva, 1980, pp. 281–285.

Turkey

Goodman, Neville M., "Turkey's Experiment in the 'Socialisation' of Medicine." *The Lancet,* 4 January 1964, pp. 36–38.

Kapil, Iris, *Final Report on the Management of Primary Health Care in Turkey.* Ankara: UNICEF, March 1980, processed document.

Ministry of Health and Social Assistance. *Health Statistics Yearbook, 1979–1982.* Ankara, 1983, preliminary tables.

Taylor, Carl E., R. Dirican, and K. W. Deuschle, *Health Manpower Planning in Turkey: An International Research Case Study.* Baltimore: Johns Hopkins Press, 1968.

United Nations Development Program, *Turkey: Development Cooperation Report, 1981.* Ankara, 1982.

United Nations Fund for Population Activities, *Turkey: Report of Mission on Needs Assessment for Population Assistance.* Report No. 28. New York, May 1980.

Voniatis, Michael N., *A Comparative Study of Primary Health Care in Three Mediterranean Countries.* Leeds (England), August 1981, pp. 77–105, processed document.

World Bank, *Turkey: Health Sector Review.* Report No. 6089-TU. Washington, D.C., September 1986.

World Health Organization, Regional Office for Europe, "Turkey," in *Health Services in Europe, 3rd edition.* Vol. 2. Copenhagen, pp. 191–197.

Iraq

Habib, Omran S., and J. P. Vaughan, "The Determinants of Health Services Utilization in Southern Iraq: A Household Interview." *International Journal of Epidemiology,* 15(3):395–407, 1986.

Mann, George J., "Rural Health Facilities in Developing Countries." *World Hospitals,* 15(2):129–131, May 1979.

Ministry of Labour and Social Affairs, *Annual Survey of Developments and Trends 1983.* Baghdad, 1984.

Nyrop, R. F., *Iraq—A Country Study.* Washington, D.C.: American University, Foreign Area Studies, 1979.

Republic of Iraq, Ministry of Planning, *Annual Abstract of Statistics.* Baghdad, 1987.

Republic of Iraq, Ministry of Planning, *Result of Census 1977,* Vol. 31, Baghdad, 1978.

World Bank, *Financing Health Service in Developing Countries.* Washington, D.C., 1987.

World Health Organization, "Country Report: Iraq." Baghdad, 1987, processed document.

Youssef, Enaam Y. Abou, *Analysis of the Nursing Manpower Situation of the Eastern Mediterranean Region.* Alexandria: EMRO Health Services Journal No. 2, 1985.

Malaysia

Bolton, J. M., "Medical Services to the Aborigines in West Malaysia." *British Medical Journal* No. 5608, pp. 818–823, 29 June 1968.

Chee, Heng Ling, "Health Status and the Development of Health Services in a Colonial State: The Case of British Malaya." *International Journal of Health Services,* 12(3):397–417, 1982.

Chen, Paul C. Y., "Traditional and Modern Medicine in Malaysia." *Social Science and Medicine,* 15A:127–136, 1981.

Chen, Paul C. Y., et ai., *Health and Aging in Malaysia.* Kuala Lumpur: University of Malaya, 1986.

Harlan, William R., L. C. Harlan, L. O. Wee, "Policy Implications of Health Changes in Rapidly Developing Countries: The Case of Malaysia." *Journal of Public Health Policy,* 5(4):563–572, 1984.

Ho, T. M., "Family Practice in Malaysia." *Family Practice,* 1(4):197–198, 1984.

Ho, Tak Ming, "The Present Problems and Future Needs of Primary Health Care in Malaysia." *International Journal of Health Services,* 18(2):281–291, 1988.

Jayesuria, L. W., *A Review of the Rural Health Services in West Malaysia.* Kuala Lumpur: Ministry of Health, 1967.

Kanapathy, V., "Health-care Industry in Malaysia: Problems and Prospects." *UMBC Economic Review,* 20(2):7–19, 1984.

Malaysian Medical Association, *The Future of Health Services in Malaysia.* Kuala Lumpur, April 1980.

Martinez, E. J., *Statistics on Health Matters.* Report No. 1. Kuala Lumpur: Ministry of Health, October 1966.

Ministry of Health Malaysia, *Annual Report 1985.* Kuala Lumpur, 1986.

Ness, Gayl D., *Bureaucracy and Rural Development in Malaysia.* Los Angeles: University of California Press, 1967.

Office of the Prime Minister, *Fourth Malaysia Plan 1981–1985* (Health and Social Welfare). Kuala Lumpur, 1981.

Roemer, Milton I., *Rural Health Services Scheme of Malaysia.* Manila: World Health Organization, Regional Office of the Western Pacific, February 1969, processed document.

Sandosham, A. A., "The Medical and Health Services in the Context of National Development." *The Medical Journal of Malaya,* 22:259–262, June 1968.

Sorkin, Alan, *Health Economics in Developing Countries.* Boston: Lexington Books, 1976.

Sundram, Chellie J., "The Education of Dental Nurses in Malaya, Malaysia." *The Dental Delineator,* Summer 1967.

Westinghouse Overseas Service Corporation. *Health Services Financing Study: Final Report.* Kuala Lumpur: Asian Development Bank, September 1985.

Wylde, E. M. B., "Short Outline of Growth of Public Health in Kuala Lumpur and Malaya. *The Medical Journal of Malaya,* 13:316–321, June 1959.

CHAPTER TWELVE

Comprehensive Health Systems in Transitional Countries

Only a few countries at a transitional/developing economic level have developed or attempted to establish national health systems in which every resident is entitled to comprehensive health services. In Chapter 7, we discussed eight free-market countries that had implemented such a policy, all industrialized and all but one European. Though not politically socialist, each of these countries has developed, in some degree, a socialized health system. For countries of weaker economic development and much more limited health resources, implementation of such a policy is very difficult. There may be a considerable gap between theoretical health policies and the health services actually available to people.

In a few transitional countries, nevertheless, government policy has explicitly declared that everyone is entitled to complete health care as a "right"—that is, a service essentially without cost to the individual. Health care is no longer subject to trading in a market. Countless economic and environmental problems, nevertheless, at certain times obstruct the prompt availability of services. Insufficient hospital beds, for example, means a waiting period for elective surgery. The physician staffing a health center may be temporarily absent, without a replacement. Drugs may be in short supply or x-ray equipment may be out-of-order.

The health care entitlements in these countries, therefore, must be qualified by the current realities; that is, they are "rights" to the extent that resources allow. It is also understood that, if resources are inadequate at any time or place, the government must make every effort to provide them as quickly as possible.

With these provisos, there are two Latin American countries that belong in the specified category: Costa Rica and Nicaragua. A third, from the Middle East, is borderline in its level of economic development; its per capita GNP in the 1980s was above $5,000, hence at an "affluent" economic level. This is the state of Israel, whose economic growth has been very rapid, along with an exceptionally large volume of foreign assistance. The Israeli health system is described as it was in the 1970s, when its economic development was, indeed, at a transitional level.

COSTA RICA

Costs Rica had a national population of 2,587,000 in 1984, and 48 percent of the people lived in urban areas. Among the Central American countries, Costa Rica stands out as a nation with a rich tradition of democratic social reforms that have significantly shaped the structure and functions of the health system. The per capita GNP in 1984 was $1,362—surprisingly low in the light of the country's many social achievements. The adult literacy level that year was 94 percent.

After liberation from the Spanish in 1821, land ownership in Costa Rica was acquired predominantly by thousands of small peasants. Although the marketing and exporting of coffee, and then other crops, came to be controlled by a small elite class, the two groups (peasants and marketers) were dependent on each other, and no sharp class conflicts occurred. By the early twentieth century, the United Fruit Company acquired large banana plantations; this led to the organization of labor unions and in the 1930s the birth of a

Communist Party. With the worldwide economic depression and a sharp drop in coffee trade, there was a great deal of social and political strife, leading to numerous social reforms in the 1940s.

In 1941, social security legislation was passed in Costa Rica, starting the provisions for medical care insurance that were eventually to become universal. A labor law affirmed the rights of workers to organize into unions and to strike. The University of Costa Rica was established and public education was generally extended. After World War II and the rise of the Cold War, violence developed between left-wing and conservative political groups. It was settled in 1948 through seizure of power by a National Liberation Movement, led by José Figueres. Although the Communist Party and the labor unions were suppressed, the reforms in health, social security, and education were retained and even strengthened. The movement evolved into a political party, which has retained power to the present day.

The National Liberation Party nationalized the banks and electrical utilities. Agriculture was diversified and, although the United Fruit Company was left undisturbed, the share of its profits going to the Costa Rican government was raised from 10 to 30 percent. A new Constitution written in 1949 institutionalized the social reforms. Most important, it explicitly banned the maintenance of an army; only a small police force for domestic purposes was allowed. This unique and crucial policy decision has been observed faithfully over the years. Thus, in 1980 Costa Rica's expenditure on its police force amounted to $3 per person per year, in comparison with military expenditures by the other Central American countries averaging $16.25 per person per year.

In the period 1965 to 1974, Costa Rican economic growth continued at a high rate. Then in the late 1970s and the 1980s, the country entered a period of inflation and increasing foreign debt. Some unemployment developed and a great deal of underemployment. A very poor quality of housing for at least half of the population became conspicuous. In the midst of these and other problems, the Costa Rican government has stalwartly defended its special achievements in two fields: education and health. This is evident in analysis of the health system in 1985.

Health System Structure

In a legal sense, the Ministry of Health is the major health authority in Costa Rica, but in terms of power and resources the Social Security Bureau (CCSS) is much more important. Because of its earlier origin, nevertheless, we consider first the development and characteristics of the Ministry of Health.

Ministry of Health. Organized public health activities acquired importance at the national level in Costa Rica in 1922, with the creation of an Under-Secretariate of Hygiene and Public Health. Before this, there had been a Program Against Hookworm Disease, starting in 1907, followed by a Sanitation Department and Nursing School in 1916, and a Tuberculosis Sanatorium in 1918. The Under-Secretariate of Hygiene was elevated to a Ministry of Health in 1927.

During its first years Ministry of Health (MOH) activities concentrated on communicable disease control and environmental sanitation. In the 1930s, programs were broadened to include the control of drugs and foods. An antimalaria campaign became important in the 1930s, and local health agencies were established to provide village doctors to small communities throughout the country.

The Social Security Law of 1941 eventually exerted great influence on the MOH, but the 1940s were also marked by extension of public health activities, especially for malaria control. In 1950, with advice from the World Health Organization, the MOH was reorganized into two major parts: one for relationships with hospitals and the other for coordination and promotion of preventive services. New technologies against tuberculosis (streptomycin) and malaria (house-spraying with DDT insecticide) were widely applied, with spectacular results. There were also massive immunization campaigns. Nutrition centers were widely established for distributing food to mothers and preschool children, increasing from 37 centers in 1959 to 446 in 1980.

These preventive and health promotion

strategies brought rapid benefits in reduction of infant mortality and extension of life expectancy. Within the health system, coincident with an overall increase in human resources and programs, the relative supply of hospital beds was actually reduced; they declined from 5.6 per 1,000 in 1940 to 4.6 per 1,000 in 1960 and down to 3.3 per 1,000 in 1980. The benefits of prevention were dramatically demonstrated. Their strength and effectiveness probably contributed to the harmonious relationships that the MOH developed later with the social security program.

Social Security Bureau. After its statutory establishment in 1941, the Costa Rican Bureau of Social Security (CCSS) gradually extended its population coverage. Initially there were only limited medical benefits for workers with low wages in the national capital, San José, and the seven provincial capitals; dependents were not included. By 1950, coverage had reached only 8 percent of the national population. Then, in the 1950s, coverage was extended to agricultural workers outside the Central Valley, and the wage ceiling for eligibility was substantially raised; by 1961 coverage had reached 18 percent of the national population.

Along with the extension of coverage, CCSS proceeded to construct its own hospitals and ambulatory care centers in San José, with salaried physicians and nurses. In the other provinces, CCSS purchased services for its beneficiaries from local charity or municipal welfare hospitals. In 1961, the National Legislature was sufficiently confident of CCSS capabilities to enact a constitutional amendment, calling for "universal" national population coverage within 10 years. This led to rapid extension of coverage to rural areas and to all dependents of the primary worker. By 1971, however, coverage had not reached 100 percent but 45 percent of the population.

Costa Rica's political determination to achieve universal population coverage was then dramatized by the General Health Law of 1973. This called for a radical reorganization of all health services in the country, along lines that were unique in Latin America if not in the world. Basically all therapeutic health services, especially hospitals and major clinics for am-

bulatory care, were put under the control of the social security program. This meant the transfer to the CCSS of not only the hospitals of the MOH, but also numerous small charity hospitals in the municipalities (financed largely by lotteries) and even several hospitals still operated by the banana corporations. In the meantime, population coverage by CCSS was extended further, to reach 78 percent of the nation by 1982. All income thresholds were eliminated, and everyone in any type of private or public employment, with their dependents, as well as the self-employed, were enrolled.

Resources for prevention, as well as for general primary health care of the noninsured population, remained under the control of the MOH. To carry out health promotion and prevention programs, the MOH in 1978 operated 60 health centers, 16 dispensaries, and 240 rural health posts. The 22 percent of people not covered by social security could obtain primary health care at these units, and they could be hospitalized at a CCSS hospital, if necessary, at the expense of the government.

Other Government Agencies. Aside from the all-important CCSS and MOH in Costa Rica's health system, other public agencies have certain responsibilities. A National Insurance Institute gives cash disability benefits during illness and provides medical care for work-connected accidents. There is also a separate national Institute of Aqueducts and Sewers, which has developed safe water and sewage disposal throughout the country, both in cities and in rural communities. Its effectiveness is reflected in the achievement by 1980 of piped drinking water for 84 percent of the Costa Rican population and proper sewage disposal for 93 percent.

Nongovernment Agencies. Because of the remarkably broad coverage and services through government agencies in Costa Rica, voluntary health agencies have not played much of a role. The Costa Rican Red Cross operates ambulances and responds to emergencies and major natural disasters. Its women members also provide volunteer services in many hospitals. Most Red Cross expenses, in fact, are met by grants from the government. The same applies to the Costa Rican Demographic Association, which carries out extensive education on contraception and family planning.

Health services, formerly provided by the banana plantations and a few other companies, have now been absorbed within the CCSS program.

Private Market. About 90 percent of Costa Rican doctors are employed by the CCSS or the MOH, meaning that about 10 percent—predominantly specialists, retired from employment—are entirely in private practice. About one-third of the employed physicians also engage in private practice for a small part of their free time. Costa Rican government salaries are relatively higher than those in other developing countries, so both the proportion of doctors involved and the time spent in private practice is much less than elsewhere.

Costa Rica also has private pharmacies, but they are not as numerous as elsewhere because prescribed drugs are provided without charge, as part of the services in both the CCSS program and the MOH primary care units.

Production of Resources

In light of the remarkable achievements in the Costa Rican health system, it is surprising that physicians have been trained in the country only since 1961; before that, Costa Ricans had to seek medical education abroad, or foreign physicians had to be attracted. In 1961, a Faculty of Medicine was finally established in the University of Costa Rica, and the physician supply rose rapidly. A second medical school was established in 1976, under private auspices.

In 1930, Costa Rica had only 27 physicians per 100,000 population, and the ratio remained at about this level until 1960. After the medical school started in 1961, the ratio rose to 56 per 100,000 by 1970 and to 78 per 100,000 by 1980. Even this is a relatively modest supply of doctors, which apparently serves the country's needs quite well because of extensive use of auxiliary nurses (164 per 100,000 in 1980) and health assistants; these

personnel work in the rural health posts, health centers, and hospitals. The nursing auxiliaries are trained for one year after eighth or ninth grade, and the health assistant for only 4 months. Both of these types of worker, however, profit from continuing education every month and also from regular supervision. The personnel at rural health posts spend most of their time on visits to households, usually by motorcycle, rather than passively waiting for patients to come to the post.

Since the integration after 1973, virtually all Costa Rican hospitals have come under the control of the CCSS. Furthermore, the decline in the nation's ratio of hospital beds has been noted. The resources for ambulatory care, and especially primary health care, on the other hand, have steadily increased. Health centers, staffed by at least one physician, grew to 174, as of 1980; 99 of these (with somewhat larger staffs in the cities) were operated by the CCSS and 75 (mainly in small towns) by the MOH. In 1980 there were 4 MOH dispensaries for special disorders and 297 rural health posts of the MOH. The latter are key facilities for providing primary health care to the rural population. Nutrition centers for small children numbered 530 in 1984, so low-income families had ready access to one of them. The MOH also operated 28 dental clinics for school children and 9 treatment units for alcoholism. Instruction in and devices for family planning are part of the services of all health centers and health posts, and this has been effective in achieving a relatively low birth rate of 29 per 1,000 in 1986.

Drugs are nearly all imported. Great controls, however, are exercised through the massive purchasing power of the CCSS program. When serious economic constraints were felt in 1982, for example, the number of different drugs imported was reduced from 1,000 to 400.

Health-related research, to produce new knowledge in fields of special importance, is exceptionally well developed in Costa Rica. At the University of Costa Rica, there is an Institute of Investigations in Health (INISA), financed by the Ministry of Education. INISA conducts studies in infectious diseases, nutrition, genetics, aging, maternal and child health, and other fields. Other institutes supported by the Ministry of Health do research in immunology, food safety, alcoholism, and vector-transmitted diseases. Even the social security program supports research in such fields as oncology and hematology. In the National University there is an institute for research on social and demographic problems, including determinants of disease and mortality.

Economic Support

The generous investment in health resources and services in the Costa Rican health system has been possible only with a steadily increasing expenditure of funds. In 1960, before the massive integration brought by the General Health Law (1973), the national health system absorbed 3 percent of the total GNP. By 1980, this had risen to 7.4 percent of an enlarged GNP.

The integration strategy meant that increasing proportions of national health spending came from the CCSS, corresponding to the increased social security coverage of the population. In 1974, of total public expenditures for health, 44 percent came from the CCSS—about the same amount as the funds from general revenues for the MOH. By 1979, the CCSS expenditures constituted 63 percent of government health expenditures, and the MOH budget accounted for less than 25 percent. Considering central government health expenditures as a whole, according to the World Bank, they rose from 4 percent of the national budget in 1972 to an amazing 30 percent in 1981. With a general economic recession in 1980 to 1983, government spending for health inevitably declined, and by 1985 it constituted about 12 percent of overall national public expenditures, still a large share.

Data on the composition of overall government expenditures for health or health-related purposes are available for 1982. The percentage distribution includes expenditures by agencies concerned with nutrition, improvement of housing, and general support of children, as well as the more strictly defined health services. Even so, the large percentage of funds going to support of the essentially therapeutic services of social security (CCSS) is evident:

Health-related Agency	Percent (1982)
Ministry of Health (MOH)	12.8
Social Security (CCSS)	64.9
Aqueducts and Sewers (AA)	3.7
Office of Family Allowances (OCAF)	13.6
Institute of Medical-School Assistance (INAMES)	3.7
International Cooperation for Health (OCIS)	1.3
All agencies	100.0

The OCAF and INAMES are agencies whose funds are spent largely for nutrition and other forms of assistance to children in low-income families. If these agencies were not included in the tabulation, the CCSS share of public expenditures, principally supporting hospitals and clinics, would be even greater than 64.9 percent.

Regarding private sources of health expenditure in Costa Rica, data are strangely lacking. Although numerous reports have been published on the Costa Rican health system and the spending in its public problems, nothing is available on private expenditures. One may infer that the strong programs of public service probably result in lower private expenditures than in other developing countries of comparable economic level. Yet we know that in the main cities, many government employed physicians engage in private practice after their official hours. In San José, there are three large private clinics and several smaller ones. The CCSS permits covered persons to be hospitalized at social insurance expense, and yet be served by physicians whom they pay privately.

Dental care for adults is provided predominantly in private offices. More than half of Costa Rican pharmacists are employed in private pharmacies or pharmaceutical companies. Even though most microbiologists are employed by the government, some 30 private laboratories serve the patients of private physicians.

With all these available private health resources, many people with high or moderate income must be willing to pay for private medical care, to avoid the waiting time and perhaps depersonalized attention in the public facilities. After 1982, with the economic difficulties found throughout Latin America, pressures mounted to reduce public spending. The obvious alternative in the health system was to increase private spending. Political leaders in Costa Rica therefore began speaking of a pattern of "mixed medicine," which would permit greater private spending by those who could afford it. In 1983, insured persons were allowed to select and pay a private physician, while diagnostic tests and prescriptions were still financed by the CCSS.

In the perspective of other Latin American countries, nevertheless, there is no question about Costa Rica's exceptionally strong government commitment to financing health services. Taking account of the available data, one can only guess on the mix of public/private support of the health system. Until the private side is quantified, a reasonable guess would put its contribution at about 25 percent of total costs, with 75 percent coming from public sources.

Management

As a small country, geographically as well as in population, Costa Rica has highly centralized authority and policy making. The president is elected for 4 years and may not succeed himself, but he has great power; he appoints the Minister of Health and also the Director of Social Security, who are the major supervisors of the entire health system. The planning that brought about the major integration of the MOH and CCSS was done at the national level; it involved not only the two top officials, but also the president and a committee of the Parliament (unicameral) that drafted the General Health Law of 1973.

For general political purposes, Costa Rica has seven provinces, in addition to the capital city of San José. Provincial health directors are appointed by the minister of health to carry out central policy. Each province is divided

into several cantons—81 in all. The canton is the usual setting for the organization of community committees. Such community participation was especially effective from 1964 to 1980 in reducing infant mortality, through the efforts of Rural Health and Community Health Programs. In 1979, an important National Health Council was organized, to coordinate all national agencies in the health system, especially the MOH and CCSS. In the 1980s, community participation became more broadly motivated, through the organization of health and social security councils in every canton.

Intersectoral coordination also became a prominent objective in the 1980s, promoted by the newly established Ministry of National Planning and Economic Policy (MIDEPLAN). This ministry started interministerial councils in each major region and subregion of the country. (For CCSS purposes, five regional jurisdictions had been mapped out.) The typical council has representatives of (a) the municipal government, (b) the CCSS, (c) the MOH, and (d) six population groups chosen freely from the community.

The focus of intersectoral efforts is on solving the problems of "critically poor" slum populations. The scope of these efforts is illustrated by a Council of Development, set up in one subregion of Puriscal in 1981. This council included representatives of the following agencies:

- Ministry of Planning (MIDEPLAN)
- Ministry of Health (MOH)
- Social Security Bureau (CCSS)
- Ministry of Agriculture (MAG)
- Ministry of Education (MED)
- Family Allowances Program (OCAF)
- Municipality of Puriscal
- Institute of Investigations in Health (INISA)
- Branches of Banks in Puriscal
- National Institute of Alcoholism (INSA)
- National Patronage of Childhood (PANI)

- Mixed Institute of Social Aid (IMAS)
- National Directorate of Communities (DINADECO)

In 1982, the health record of Puriscal children showed remarkable improvement.

Delivery of Health Services

The exceptional development of organized health care programs, by both the CCSS and the MOH, indicates that personal health services in Costa Rica are delivered predominantly in settings where organized teamwork is the general rule. A household study of ambulatory consultations in 1978 found that 86 percent occurred at a health center, hospital OPD, or health station, and only 14 percent in the quarters of a private physician. Virtually all hospitalization is provided in government institutions. In the 1980s only three small private proprietary hospitals existed.

The rate of consultations has been gradually rising, as more persons are covered by social security and the facilities of the MOH in rural areas have increased. The national rate of consultations in 1970 was 2 per person per year, and this rose to 3 by 1978. The rate in more recent years has doubtless risen further.

The accessibility of essential health services to all Costa Ricans in the 1980s is customarily analyzed in terms of the urban and rural populations. Of urban people (48 percent of all in 1984), 80 percent make use of CCSS resources and the remaining 20 percent get service at MOH resources. Of the rural population (52 percent of all in 1984), 70 percent are served by CCSS resources and 30 percent by resources of the MOH. In the cities, a small percentage of people prefer to consult private practitioners at their own expense, and in the rural areas an even smaller percentage do so. Entitlement to free, or nearly free, publicly financed health care, however, is legally universal.

The regionalized framework of health facilities, where both urban and rural people obtain their care, includes resources operated by both the MOH and the CCSS. Each of five regions, defined by the CCSS, is furnished with facilities at four levels; if we think of the scheme as a pyramid, the MOH and CCSS resources at each level in 1980 were as follows:

Level	Resources	MOH	CCSS
Peripheral	Health posts	297	—
	Health centers	75	99
Second	Out-patient clinics	16	10
	Small hospitals	—	16
Third	Regional hospitals	—	5
Central	National	—	8

Services among the four levels are intended to be completely integrated. Patients of both insured and noninsured status enter the framework at the most peripheral level; in the rural areas this is typically a health post and in the cities a health center. Insured persons at this level use CCSS units, and others use MOH units. If the care cannot be handled here, it is referred to the second level—an out-patient clinic (perhaps polyclinic would be an appropriate term)—under either MOH or CCSS sponsorship.

Patients requiring hospitalization are referred to a small hospital or a regional hospital at the third level. This applies to both insured and noninsured. The insured are entitled to CCSS hospital care without charge. The noninsured are similarly served, but they must pay small fees. They may also buy drugs at CCSS hospitals or clinics at low cost.

Only the most difficult cases, whether insured or noninsured, are referred to one of the central-level national hospitals. Here again, service is free to the insured but requires small payments from the others. The sequence of referrals is not always this regular. A patient with manifestly serious diseases may be sent from the first or second level directly to a national hospital at the center.

The whole process, of course, may not always flow this smoothly. As Costa Rican health leaders have expressed it:

In practice, this potential access [to health care] is greatly limited by socioeconomic and cultural factors; undoubtedly a middle-class state employee or university professor living in San José has a much better opportunity of receiving appropriate care in a quick and efficient manner than a poor peasant living thirty kilometers from the nearest health center or rural post. These differences are hard to eliminate under any health system; but, at least formally, the State openly recognizes, and the people are conscious of, the right that every Costa Rican citizen has to be adequately cared for when ill, with little cost, and with the least possible delay.

Outcomes and Trends

The Costa Rican strategies have clearly been to extend greatly the population coverage of social security, simultaneously increase the general revenue support for health, unify most therapeutic services for everyone under the CCSS program, and concentrate preventive services and primary health care for the uninsured in the Ministry of Health. At the same time, general education and nutrition supplements for poor children have been emphasized. What have been the outcomes of these strategies?

According to conventional measurements of health status, the results have been phenomenal. The infant mortality rate was reduced from 131 per 1,000 live births in 1940–1944 to 18.6 in 1980–1982. Life expectancy at birth in 1940 was 46.9 years and it rose to 73.7 years in 1983. The age-standardized death rate for tuberculosis declined from 52 per 100,000 in 1950 to 3 per 100,000 in 1980. The corresponding mortality decline for malaria was from 64 in 1950 to zero in 1980. Of course, one cannot attribute these achievements entirely to the health system, but health services undoubtedly played a crucial part.

The worldwide economic recession, starting around 1980, was a blow to the prosperity of Costa Rica, as of other countries. The population living below the poverty level rose from 25 percent in 1977 to 71 percent in 1982. Children hospitalized with severe malnutrition increased from 152 cases in 1981 to 322 cases in 1982. Malaria cases (not deaths) rose from 189 in 1981 to 569 in 1984.

Yet, there were no significant changes in Costa Rica's rates of mortality. The government tried hard to maintain the gains in health achieved in the 1970s. From 1981 to 1982, there was a moderate decline in government health spending—about the same as for overall public spending—but in 1983 health expenditures rose again. One of the few deteriorations in health service was a decline in CCSS pediatric consultations from 84 per 100 children per year in 1981 to 77 in 1985.

In the 1970s, Costa Rica's great health progress was partially attributable to solid assistance from international agencies, particularly the Inter-American Development Bank and the U.S. Agency for International Development. Yet, in the 1980s, when greater assistance was sorely needed, the policies of these agencies changed toward promotion of "government austerity and maximum private-sector spending." Despite these external pressures, the Costa Rican government demonstrated its continued commitment to health by establishing 150 new rural health posts between 1982 and 1985.

Conservative forces in the country nevertheless echoed the call for privatization, leading to the policy of mixed medicine for higher-income CCSS families, as noted previously. By 1986, the debate over health care financing seemed to subside, and the Costa Rican health system, with massive government support, was effectively providing virtually complete health services to everyone in the country.

ISRAEL

The state of Israel was established in 1948, as a sequel of World War II, although with origins traceable to the fourth millennium b.c.; few nations have had a longer and more tumultuous history. Since this eastern Mediterranean country was carved out of Palestine, it has developed a health system unique in the world, and one providing virtually comprehensive health services, through a variety of organized mechanisms, to all of its citizens. Although Israel's GNP per capita in 1984 was slightly above $5,000, it was $4,150 in 1979 and $3,500 in 1978. Our analysis applies principally to the late 1970s, when the country's economic development was at the developing transitional level.

The Recent Past

Until 1917, the land that is now Israel was a remote section of the Ottoman Turkish Empire. It was part of a province occupied by Arabs, Jews, and Christians. Social conditions were miserable, infectious disease was rampant, and mortality rates were high. After World War I, Great Britain gained control of the region known as Palestine, and in 1922 the League of Nations assigned to Britain international responsibility to govern the area—the so-called British Mandate. With this authority, the substantial immigration of Jews and the development of Jewish communities was facilitated, as the British Balfour Declaration of 1917 had called for.

Jewish interest in establishing a national homeland in the Palestine region had been actively promoted since the rise of the Zionist movement in 1882. In 1912, Jewish labor groups from Central Europe began to organize a sickness insurance fund, linked to the Jewish Labor Federation. With the British Mandate, assistance in developing medical facilities in Palestine came from various foreign sources, most notably from *Hadassah,* a U.S. Zionist women's group. Hadassah and other charitable agencies helped organize maternal and child health centers for both Jewish and Arab families. Under British governance, improvements were made in environmental sanitation and in control of the major infectious diseases. Several hospitals, built by the Hadassah organization, were turned over to the local municipalities (Haifa, Tel Aviv, etc.) in the early 1930s.

When the United Nations carved out the small, oddly shaped state of Israel in 1948, therefore, several elements of a health infrastructure already existed. In the subsequent years, each of the elements was greatly developed—the hospitals, the maternal and child health clinics, the environmental sanitation, the health insurance programs. Great stress was also put on education, with attainment in Israel of a literacy rate of 88 percent by 1980 and 95 percent by 1984.

Israeli development, however, was impeded by repeated bouts of war with the surrounding Arab States. In May 1948, soon after the United Nations established the new nation, there were attacks from five surrounding Arab countries. With great loss of life and property, these attacks were repelled. In 1956, Israel took aggressive action to gain access to the Suez Canal in Egypt. In 1967, the Six-Day War resulted in Israeli occupation of the West Bank of the Jordan River, inhabited by more than a million Arabs, and also the Gaza Strip near Egypt. In 1973, Arab aggression in the Yom Kippur War had little effect, except for the later U.S. intervention, which led to the Camp David Peace Agreements between Israel and Egypt in 1979.

During all these hostilities, Israel received a great deal of financial and military assistance from the United States. With the rapid expansion of its population, mainly through immigration—from 1,370,000 in 1950 to 4,006,000 in 1984—and with the exceptional energy and determination of its people, Israel succeeded in building a health system of great effectiveness. In spite of many administrative complexities, reflecting various social and political interest groups, the system provides a remarkable scope of health services to virtually every citizen. Our account analyzes the Israeli health system as of around 1980.

Health System Organization

Within the government of Israel, nearly all health responsibilities are vested in the Ministry of Health. Although the vast majority of the population are covered by health insurance, unlike other countries whose people have such medical protection, no public agency has supervisory authority. Legally the insurance is voluntary.

Ministry of Health. The Ministry of Health (MOH) has general responsibility for planning and supervising the national health system, as well as for direct administration of many parts of it. Numerous hospitals, health centers, and other health care facilities are operated by the MOH, even though much of their cost comes from other sources.

Centrally, the MOH is organized through

three main divisions: (1) the Medical Division, (2) Planning and Budgeting, and (3) Administration. The Medical Division has very broad scope. It supervises hospitals, both those it operates directly and those managed by other bodies. In the same sense, it supervises and operates psychiatric services and also geriatric and rehabilitation services. The ministry also oversees the maintenance of standards in pharmacies.

Under the Medical Division is the national Public Health Service, which administers many laws and ordinances, some of which were enacted under the British Mandate, with later amendments. The PHS has four major subdivisions: (1) environmental health (water, sewage, air pollution, etc.), (2) food supervision, (3) epidemiology, which includes public health laboratories, and (4) personal and community health services.

To administer all these services, the MOH maintains 6 district offices and 14 subdistrict offices throughout this small country. The medical directors of these offices are trained in public health and centrally appointed. The personal health services are provided through numerous hospitals, clinics, and health stations, the numbers of which are discussed later.

Other Government Agencies. Besides the MOH, few health activities are carried out by other branches of the Israeli government. Occupational health protection is principally a responsibility of the Ministry of Labor and Social Welfare; this ministry also provides custodial care for the mentally retarded. The Ministry of Agriculture has a veterinary health program that includes the control of animal diseases transmissible to humans.

Municipal governments carry major responsibilities for local water supplies and sewage disposal. Several of them also own and operate general hospitals.

Voluntary Health Insurance. As noted, since 1912 Jewish labor unions have organized insurance programs first to finance, and then to provide, health services to their members and families. These have grown steadily, especially since statehood; today they are the major or-

ganized health program in Israel alongside the MOH.

Health insurance programs or voluntary sickness funds *(Kupat holim)* started in Israel, unlike in Europe, with cooperative coverage of agricultural workers. Eventually they spread to all workers in the General Federation of Labor *(Histadrut).* Much the largest insurance organization is the *Kupat Holim Klalit,* with 2,900,000 members (workers and dependents) in 1980. In addition, there are three smaller sickness funds that altogether cover about 650,000 people. Counting all persons with voluntary health insurance, about 92 percent of the national population in 1980 were covered for a wide range of health services. Financial support through insurance premiums is shared between employees and employers, the latter's share being greater; self-employed persons pay the full premiums.

Also unlike the European pattern, from the outset medical services in the major sickness fund, linked to the Federation of Labor, were provided by salaried teams of doctors and nurses. If hospitalization was needed, it was given in government hospitals. Several dispensaries or health centers were established wherever there were groups of workers, and in 1923 the Kupat Holim Klalit built its first hospital. The number and quality of facilities for ambulatory care, as well as hospitals, have steadily increased, so that almost all health services needed by members are provided in the sickness fund's own facilities and by its own salaried personnel. For their administration, the General Kupat Holim (as the major fund is known) has divided the country into 12 districts.

The three smaller sickness funds insure medical costs for their members, but do not usually operate their own resources. The insurance pays for medical care provided principally by private doctors and government facilities, although a few special clinics are operated. Sometimes even the General Kupat Holim has to purchase services from government facilities, if one of their own units is not accessible to the member.

Voluntary Health Agencies. Aside from the important health insurance funds, several other voluntary agencies play significant parts in the Israeli health system. Much of the economic support for these comes from overseas charities.

The Hadassah Medical Organization, started by Jewish women from the United States, has played a major part in establishing the nation's first medical school at Hebrew University. Although the current Hadassah Medical School started instruction in 1947, its beginnings can be traced to medical work done at the Rothschild Hospital, founded in Jerusalem in 1854. The Hadassah agency also started the first school of nursing in 1919. Numerous hospitals and health centers, which emphasize services for mothers and children, were established over the years of the British Mandate, and eventually turned over to the central or municipal governments to operate. As this was done, Hadassah directed its efforts to other goals, such as strengthening medical education and research.

Another important voluntary health agency is Malben, which grew as an offshoot of the American Jewish Joint Distribution Committee, formed in the 1940s to help Jewish refugees from war-torn Europe and North Africa. Malben has focused on institutional care and rehabilitation of the physically handicapped and chronically ill. It also provides protective services for the frail aged and sheltered workshops for the disabled.

Numerous other voluntary health agencies focus on antituberculosis work; ambulance and first-aid services (the Red Shield of David); cancer control, research, and education; care of handicapped children; rehabilitation of the mentally retarded; education of the deaf and the blind; and still other problems. A notable feature of voluntary health agencies in Israel is a general policy of attempting to coordinate their work with that of the Ministry of Health, as well as the sickness funds. Though each group has its pride and wants credit for its accomplishments, voluntary agency programs are usually planned in cooperation with the public health authorities, to ensure that they are addressing needs not otherwise being met.

Private Health Care Market. Although the vast majority of Israel's relatively large number of physicians and dentists (see later) are employed by one of the sickness funds, the MOH, or some voluntary agency, there are still several hundred doctors entirely in private practice. In addition, any salaried doctor may also engage in practice privately in his off-hours.

Two of the three small sickness funds apply the principle of "free choice of doctor" and maintain panels of physicians, from whom members of the fund choose their preferred practitioner. The doctor is paid on a fee-for-service basis. Furthermore, anyone who is already insured by the General Kupat Holim may consult a private physician separately at his own expense.

In 1962, a purely commercial insurance company, organized in cooperation with the Israel Medical Association, was established. This insurance pays for prescribed drugs and diagnostic tests, as well as for medical and dental services, on a fee basis. Hospitalization is also paid for separately in government hospitals.

Since a large proportion of Israeli physicians are immigrants, trained in various other countries, their competence and attitudes are not uniformly satisfactory to all patients in the organized programs. As a result, there is much demand for consultation from outside doctors or second opinions, which creates a considerable market for private medical care.

A few hospitals are privately owned and operated, mainly for psychiatric and geriatric patients. Many pharmacies are also private businesses.

Production of Health Resources

The people and the government of Israel have always put a high priority on health services. It was Jewish tradition that gave rise to the cliché "Everything will be all right as long as you have your health." Much emphasis, therefore, has been put on acquiring an abundance of health resources of all types.

Health Manpower. Until statehood was achieved, all doctors in Israel were educated in other countries. The great majority of these doctors were in the later years of life. Soon after 1948, therefore, postgraduate courses were organized to help these physicians learn about modern advances in medical science. The first initiative was taken by the Israel Medical Association (founded in 1912 largely to disseminate scientific information), next by the Medical Council of the General Kupat Holim, and then by the Hebrew Univeristy–Hadassah Medical School, in cooperation with the MOH.

The Hadassah Medical School, located in Jerusalem, turned out its first graduates in 1952. Then, between 1964 and 1974 three more medical schools were established at the three other major cities of the country (Tel Aviv, Haifa, and Beersheva). By 1980, the four medical schools were turning out 285 graduates per year, following 6 years of university study plus a 1-year internship. In addition, many young Israelis, not admitted to one of these schools, go abroad for study and return to practice medicine in Israel. Still other physicians continue to immigrate to the country from abroad.

As a result, Israel has an unusually large supply of physicians—about 8,400, or 210 per 100,000 population. As in most countries, concentration of physicians is heavy in the main cities, but the country is so small that relatively few people have no access to a doctor. Specialization is strong, particularly among the younger and better trained physicians. The newest of the medical schools, at Beersheva, is stressing general family practice as a "specialty" in its undergraduate and postgraduate studies.

The stock of other health personnel in Israel is also large. Nurses are trained to the professional (R.N.) level in 17 schools and to the practical nurse level in 15 schools. In all, there were 19,000 actively employed nurses in 1980, or a ratio of 460 per 100,000. The trend is toward more academic content in nursing education, with increasing stress on university training and gradual reduction in the proportion (45 percent in 1980) of practical nurses.

Regarding dental service, Israel has two university-based schools of dentistry and a supply of 2,450 dentists in 1980, or 77 per 100,000 population. Not all dentists work full-time, but their productivity is heightened by many dental hygienists and dental assistants. Since 1978, there has also been a school for dental technicians to prepare oral prostheses.

In 1980 pharmacists numbered 2,300 in Israel, or 57 per 100,000; there were also 600 assistant pharmacists. In a 4-year university-level course, one school of pharmacy turns out 60 pharmacists per year.

Additional health personnel include physical and occupational therapists, laboratory and x-ray technicians, dieticians, and others. All of these fields have several special schools, most of which are hospital-based. Sanitary engineers and sanitarians are trained in special technical institutes, connected with the MOH. In the 1980s, a school of public health was organized in Jerusalem, to train public health leaders from both Israel and other countries. A separate National Center for Public Health was also established, in affiliation with the country's four medical schools, to promote research in public health problems.

Because of the numerous organized health programs in Israel and the extensive financial support through insurance or government revenues, virtually all of these health personnel are employed, unless they personally wish to retire. In spite of the very large stock of physicians, nurses, and others, there does not seem to be any sense of "surplus," nor any plan to reduce the output of new graduates. The major policy issue is that, because many health personnel are not fully abreast of modern scientific developments, continuing education courses are frequently being launched.

Health Facilities. Israel's physical resources are as abundant as its human resources, and this applies to both hospitals and facilities for ambulatory care. The sponsorships of both types of facility are also diverse.

Hospitals, as noted, have been constructed by numerous public and voluntary agencies, resulting in facilities with about 25,800 beds or about 6.6 per 1,000 people in 1980. More than half of the beds were in specialized, mainly long-term care institutions, but 2.96 beds per 1,000 were in short-term general hospitals.

Although 92 percent of the population are insured through the sickness funds, these funds own only a minority of the beds; fund mem-

Table 12.1. Hospital Beds in Israel by Ownership:
Percentage Distribution, 1978

	Hospital Beds (percent)	
Ownership	General[a]	Long-Term[b]
Central government	36.8	39.4
Municipal government	11.0	2.0
General sickness fund	30.7	8.8
Voluntary nonprofit	18.3	10.7
Private proprietary	3.2	39.1
All ownerships	100.0	100.0

[a]Short-term.
[b]Principally for psychiatric and geriatric patients.
Source: Ellencweig, A. Y., "The New Israeli Health Care Reform:
An Analysis of a National Need." *Journal of Health Politics, Policy
and Law,* 8(2):366–386, Summer 1983.

bers, therefore, must mainly use beds under government and other sponsorships. The distribution of both general and special types of hospitals beds in Israel, according to their ownership, is shown in Table 12.1. It is evident that the central government (essentially the MOH) controls the largest portion of both general (short-term) and long-term beds. The second most important sponsorship for general hospital beds is the major sickness fund (Kupat Holim Klalit), and for long-term beds it is numerous proprietary individuals or groups. Some general hospital is easily accessible to everyone in Israel—not a very difficult accomplishment in such a small territory.

Facilities for ambulatory care are also highly developed. For general primary medical care, as well as much ambulatory specialty care, the sickness funds (the major one, as well as two of the three small funds) operated 1,260 clinics throughout the country in 1980. Virtually every agricultural settlement, village, and urban neighborhood is served by one or more of these. Even a noninsured person can be treated in these clinics for a small fee, although such persons are usually served by a government hospital out-patient department or a private physician. Beyond these general medical clinics, the sickness funds operate 89 mental health clinics, 12 child development units, 5 drug addiction centers, 200 dental clinics for children, 20 chest disease clinics, and 7 public health laboratories.

Prevention oriented family health stations, mainly for maternal and child health services, are operated throughout the country also. The Ministry of Health maintains 583 of these, providing prenatal care and also family planning services. Examinations, immunizations, and advice are given to babies, preschool children, and also to school-age children. Similar preventive health services are provided in an additional 203 family health stations maintained by the sickness funds, 51 operated by municipalties, and 3 by the Hadassah organization. Altogether in 1980 there were 840 family health stations providing these preventive services to the entire population of mothers and children.

A gradually increasing proportion of pharmaceuticals and medical supplies are being manufactured in the country. Some, though probably a minority of the total, pharmaceuticals, however, must still be imported from abroad. The rate of consumption of prescribed drugs in Israel is very high, but the volume is included in the data on overall expenditures of hospitals and clinics (see later). Expenditures for drugs and medical supplies in community pharmacies in 1979 was only 4 percent of total health expenditures—exceptionally low for the health system of a transitional/developing country.

Knowledge and technology are produced at an exceptionally high rate in Israel. Research institutes in almost every subdivision of the health sciences have been organized in all the universities, the Ministry of Health, and the General Kupat Holim, as well as several separate entities, such as the Weizman Institute of Science, the Institute for Biological Research, and the Hadassah Medical Organization. In 1959, the government established the National Research and Development Council, to formulate an overall research policy and coordinate the numerous research programs. In the specialties of medicine there are 28 separate national societies. Several journals are published to disseminate the results of Israeli research, as well as worldwide developments in the health sciences.

Economic Support

With such a highly developed health system, it is only to be expected that Israel devotes a relatively high percentage of its gross national product for support of the health system. In 1960, the overall health system absorbed 5.3 percent of GNP and in the fiscal year 1979–80, health expenditures rose to a little over 8 percent of GNP. These percentages put Israel in the class of a developed and industrialized country, even when its total GNP was below $5,000 per person per year.

The proportion of health expenditures derived from governmental sources has been changing rather rapidly. In 1962–63, when government was relatively weak and private charities as well as voluntary health insurance were relatively strong, the proportion of total health spending derived from government (central and local) was 32.2 percent, and nongovernmental sources supported 67.8 percent of expenditures. By 1979–80, these relationships were almost reversed. Not only was a much higher percentage of GNP devoted to the health system, but the sources in 1979–80 were approximately as follows:

Source		Percentage
Government		63
Central	(60)	
Municipal	(3)	
Private		37
Sickness funds and		
other agencies	(21)	
Private households	(16)	

Within the central government budget, the allocation for health has remained around 5 percent of the total for many years, but the overall public budget has grown steadily every year since 1949. Nongovernment health expenditures did not grow less over recent decades, but government expenditures grew much more.

From the perspective of health activities, the purposes for which these funds were spent were predominantly curative. In 1978–79, the breakdown of operating expenditures (i.e., excluding 11 percent for capital purposes) was as follows:

Health Activity	Percentage
Hospitals (including physicians	
employed)	44
Clinics for treatment and	
prevention	33

Dental clinics	15
Private physician's care	3
Privately purchased drugs and	
supplies	4
Government administration	1
All activities	100.0

The expenditures by the sickness funds are voluntary in a legal sense, but the entire Kupat Holim program is, of course, highly organized. Some observers, in fact, have called it a government within a government. If we classify the overall health expenditures as organized versus individual, in 1979–80 they would have been as much as 84 (63 plus 21) percent organized and only 16 percent individual.

Management

The most obvious feature of management in the health system of Israel is that it is highly pluralistic. In the overall health system there is no central planning body. Each of the major organizations—the Ministry of Health, the sickness funds, the Hadassah, and other charitable agencies—does its own planning. Likewise, the universities establish medical and other professional schools according to their own judgment. The municipalities develop water supply and sanitation networks and also establish many facilities for personal health care on their own initiatives.

Nevertheless, in the 1970s a commission for hospital planning and construction was established, under the chairmanship of the Ministry of Health. Its purpose was to coordinate hospital construction by the several agencies, to the extent that each agency was agreeable. Likewise a public body, funded by several ministries, was established to coordinate, as much as possible, the construction of facilities for the elderly and chronically ill.

Quality standards for all health structures are neverthless promulgated by the MOH, and each institution must be licensed to indicate compliance. Over the years, a heavier concentration of hospital beds has been established in the major cities, but regionalization concepts would find this reasonable. The ambulatory care centers, for both prevention and treatment, are remarkably well distributed throughout the country, simply because decisionmakers in each agency take account of the needs at different times and places.

Administration in the major organizations follows conventional principles, but there is virtually no integration across organizations. Within the MOH, the directors of each of the districts report to the central authority, and this also applies in the General Kupat Holim. Still, within budgetary limits a local health official is allowed freedom to explore new ideas that are consistent with general policies. Standardized record forms make possible the compilation of useful statistics on health care utilization and expenditures.

In the 1980s, a multiagency planning body was set up to coordinate and promote health personnel education by the universities and other training centers. In medicine, this body has encouraged greater emphasis on family practice. Expanded training of paramedical and paradental personnel has also been encouraged.

Regulation and legislation are extensive in Israel. The licensure of physicians and other major health personnel is handled by the MOH. If the applicant is a graduate of an Israeli school (approved by the Ministry of Education), licensure is automatic. If the person has been trained in a foreign school, licensure depends on the approval of that school by the Ministry of Health; new examinations are not required, but special postgraduate education may be recommended.

The health legislation inherited by Israel from the time of the British Mandate was extensive. A major Public Health Ordinance of 1940 contained 73 sections on almost every aspect of the health system—environmental sanitation, infectious disease control, registration of vital events, licensure of personnel and facilities, drug regulation, and much more. Amendments were made to this and several other laws up to about 1964. At the same time, new laws were passed in the 1950s and after—for example, laws on treatment of the mentally ill in 1955, on maintenance of local sewerage systems in 1962, on acquiring medical specialty qualifications in 1964, and on the use of food preservatives in 1965.

Performance in the Israeli health system is evaluated principally through comparisons of morbidity and mortality rates in different districts of the country. Studies are conducted both by the MOH and the General Kupat Holim. In Israel as a whole, the life expectancy at birth in 1986 was 75 years and the infant mortality rate was 14 infant deaths per 1,000 live births. The trends of both these indices have shown steady improvement since 1950. Thus, from 33 deaths per 1,000 lives births in 1960, the infant mortality rate declined to 15 per 1,000 in 1980, and then to 14 per 1,000 in 1986. Maternal mortality was down to nearly zero by 1980.

Although the Israeli population is composed overwhelmingly of Jews, around 12 percent of the people are non-Jews, mainly Arabs of the Moslem faith. For many historical reasons, the socioeconomic conditions of the Arabs, almost all of whom live in separate agricultural settlements, are poorer than those of the Jews. Non-Jews have access to essentially the same organized health services as the Jewish population, but their health record is inferior. In 1980, for example, when the overall infant mortality rate (IMR) was 15 per 1,000 live births, it was 12.1 per 1,000 among Jews and 24.2 among non-Jews. These differentials have caused some political tension, even though the non-Jew IMR in Israel is much lower than that in neighboring Arabs countries; in Lebanon, for example, the IMR in 1984 was 48 per 1,000 live births, and in Syria it was 53 per 1,000.

Similar controversies have arisen over the health conditions of Arabs in territories occupied by the Israeli Army since the 1967 war. Here, too, the health services and health record of the Arab population are significantly lower than those in the general Israeli population. Yet, official data for the occupied Gaza Strip show that in 1967, before the military occupation, the IMR had been 140 per 1,000 live births, and after 20 years of occupation (and services by Israeli authorities) it had declined to 30 per 1,000 in 1987. Before 1967 only 10 to 15 percent of childbirths in Gaza and the West Bank area had been in hospitals; in 1987 of all childbirths in Gaza, 79 percent were hospitalized and 63 percent in the West Bank. All health facilities and health manpower in both areas have been greatly expanded by the Israeli occupation authorities, even though they have not reached the level of Israel generally.

Delivery of Health Services

With the abundance of health resources in Israel and the size and scope of organized programs, the volume of services provided to the population is high. With the numerous and widely distributed clinics and preventive health stations, almost every Israeli resident has easy access to a physician. Counting both therapeutic and preventive services, the rate of patient–doctor contacts was found in a 1977 survey to exceed 10 per person per year. Counting dental services, the rate in 1980 has been stated to be 14 contacts per person per year. A study within Kupat Holim clinics reported 7.2 contacts with a primary care physician per person per year, and the balance would be the services of specialists.

The sickness funds, as noted, operate 1,260 treatment clinics, of which three-quarters serve fewer than 5,000 people. In the cities, each team of a family doctor and nurse serves a list of about 1,500 persons, and in rural settlements it is about 1,200 persons. Patients can change their primary care doctor at any time, but they are encouraged to stay with the one they chose originally, for continuity of care. (The doctor's salary is not affected by the number of patients on his list, as with capitation programs.) As backup for the doctor–nurse team, there are social workers, health educators, and dieticians, especially in the larger urban clinics.

The various ambulatory care units do not organize personnel in an administrative hierarchy, as do the hospitals. In units with large staffs, however, one "area physician" is designated as the person mainly responsible for harmonious work and achievement of overall clinic objectives. In many places, primary care clinics are used to teach medical and nursing students, to supplement the customary work on hospital wards. Any necessary services in the patient's home are arranged with an affiliated district home care team (including nurses, physical therapists, homemakers, etc.).

Hospitalization in Israel also occurs at a high rate. Although 92 percent of the population have health insurance protection, the sickness funds own less than one-third of the hospital beds. Most hospitalization is therefore in government hospitals, for which the sickness funds pay the MOH. Patients who are not members of sickness funds use MOH or municipal hospitals for almost all their hospital care; if they are indigent, there is no charge, and if they can afford to pay, small charges are made.

Considering Israeli general hospitals of all sponsorships, their occupancy level is high. In 1980 it was 92 percent. The average length-of-stay in general hospitals was 6.4 days—very short for any country; this meant that each bed was occupied by 52.5 patients in a year. From the vantage point of the population, 148 persons per 1,000 were admitted to a general hospital annually. Thus, each 1,000 persons experience 958 days of hospital care per year—nearly one day per person. Reflecting the priority assigned by Israel to primary health care is the trend in its ratio of general hospital beds to population. This was 3.27 beds per 1,000 in 1975, declining to 2.96 beds per 1,000 in 1980.

Hospitals are well staffed, with full-time salaried specialists, as well as nurses, technicians, and other personnel. The same applies to the many facilities for ambulatory care. Since the demands for service are high, the doctors and others must work hard and can spend only a short time on each patient. A study of the patients in one sickness fund in 1981 reported that only 48 percent evaluated the behavior of doctors toward patients as "humane."

Physicians, on the other hand, feel that they are overworked and underpaid. In 1983, feelings were so strong that all the doctors working for the General Kupat Holim, as well as for government health agencies, went on strike. The strike was settled after 118 days, during which the Israel Medical Association set up a network of private clinics, where patients were treated only for substantial fees. Similar arrangements were made in the hospitals. Even though only high- or moderate-income people could afford to pay for this medical care, there was evidently no measurable adverse effect on the population's health.

In summary, the pluralistic Israeli health

system results in convenient access to health services, therapeutic and preventive, for virtually the entire national population. For the 92 percent who are insured, there is financial protection, as well as assured resources for delivery of care. Of the remaining 8 percent, some are doubtless affluent and able to purchase care privately. Preventive services are free for noninsured people at the MOH family health stations. Ambulatory treatment can be obtained at any sickness fund clinic for a small fee. Ambulatory care is also available, without charge, at any MOH hospital out-patient department. Anyone who is clearly indigent is given necessary medical treatment, as an out-patient or an in-patient, at an MOH hospital. The same general policies apply to geriatric care or the treatment of mental illness.

The great predominance of organized settings for the delivery of health services in Israel is reflected by the financial data reviewed here. The share spent for private physician's care in 1978–79 was only 3 percent of the total, and for private medications and supplies only 4 percent. Much of the use of private physicians, furthermore, is by insured persons who want a second opinion on their case or who lack faith in the sickness fund clinic or the hospital physician.

For many years, certain health leaders in Israel have been calling for integration of the sickness fund programs with the Ministry of Health, to achieve greater effectiveness and efficiency. The goal put forward has been a program of National Health Insurance covering the entire population. The resources of all agencies, public and private, would be mobilized and administered through a regionalized scheme of 22 regions. At the hub of each region would be a major hospital, with all the ambulatory care facilities regarded as satellites. The currently separate therapeutic and preventive services would be brought together in the same clinics or health centers. Each region would be headed by a medical director, on behalf of the Ministry of Health. Financial support would continue from a combination of insurance contributions (which would become compulsory) and government revenues.

This proposal was put forward by a relatively conservative government that came to power in 1977. Paradoxically, opposition has come from the Labor Party and its allies, which controlled the government almost continuously since statehood (1948). The explanation is no mystery; the General Kupat Holim of the Jewish Federation of Labor is virtually an appendage of the Labor Party. Absorption into a unified government health system would mean loss of its independence and its strong political identity. For other nonpolitical reasons, independence was also cherished by the smaller sickness funds. With such powerful opposition to the 1977 proposal, and similar calls for integration been made long before, the two major entities of the Israeli health system and the several smaller ones have remained independent and autonomous.

In spite of its persistent pluralism, the health system of Israel has been successful in assuring comprehensive health services to its entire population. Perhaps because of the independence of its parts, it has fostered creative innovations of several types—in primary health care, community-oriented family services and intensive home care for the aged chronic sick. (In the region around Beersheva, however, an experimental integration of the MOH, Kupat Holim, and medical school programs under unified leadership has been only partially successful.) Throughout the physical and social disruptions of repeated hostilities, the complex Israeli health system has remained intact and functioned effectively. Even under pressure the health personnel, wearing different hats, have generally worked together. It is plausible to expect that, when political conditions are ripe, a unified national health system, managed through a network of health regions, will develop in Israel.

NICARAGUA

Nicaragua is a small Central American country, with a tumultuous history since its liberation from the Spanish in 1821. Its populatin in 1984 was 3,100,000, and its GNP per capita was $1,044. Because of revolutionary events in 1979, Nicaragua developed a health system that entitled everyone to basic health services, although many difficulties obstructed the implementation of this policy objective.

Historic Background

Hostilities have dominated life in Nicaragua since 1848, when U.S. business interests clashed with the British in the country's eastern region. Clashes occurred later between Liberals and Conservatives within the country, and between the governments of the United States and Nicaragua. Allegedly to protect U.S. property, U.S. military forces intervened in Nicaraguan political affairs repeatedly between 1853 and 1933. In 1927, the United States organized a Nicaraguan National Guard, to maintain peace and order. In 1932, Anastosio Somoza was appointed head of the National Guard, and in 1934 he assumed dictatorial powers.

The only Nicaraguan military leader to oppose U. S. influence was Augusto Cesar Sandino, but in 1934 he was assassinated by Somoza's forces. Anastasio Somoza and members of his family held absolute power for the next 45 years. Meanwhile in 1961, an armed opposition was organized, under the name of the Sandinista Front for National Liberation (FSLN). Slowly and cautiously, the FSLN won support from the impoverished peasants. A severe earthquake in 1972 further disrupted the society. In July 1979, the FSLN succeeded in seizing national power, and the Somoza family fled the country. That month, the Front proclaimed a new Sandinista government.

Aside from the massive destruction and deaths from the insurrection, the Sandinistas were faced with an extremely deficient and inequitable health system. Most of the country's health resources, especially the physicians and hospitals, were concentrated in the national capital, Managua, where about 25 percent of the people lived. The Ministry of Health had supervised a number of vertical disease-control programs, but there was little in the way of health infrastructure at the local level. There were 172 health centers and posts, built largely with U. S. foreign aid funds, but only 35 of these units were in rural areas. They were staffed mainly by auxiliary nurses, and their utilization rate was very low.

In 1975, Nicaragua had 63 physicians per 100,000 population—principally graduates of its single medical school. In Managua and a few other main cities, the ratio was 138 physicians per 100,000, and 41 per 100,000 in the rest of the country. Professional nurses numbered only 27 per 100,000. The rural population depended largely on the health services of *curanderos.*

Hospitals of all types had 5,017 beds in 1972, for a ratio of 2.5 beds per 1,000 people. Their distribution, however, was 5.4 beds per 1,000 in the capital city and 1.8 per 1,000 in the rest of the country. A study of the 25 short-term general hospitals, made by the U.S. Agency for International Development (USAID) in 1973, found "a combination of poor physical plant, lack of equipment, uncleanliness and poor quality of medical attention.... Fifteen hospitals lacked proper hygiene, adequate preventive medicine programs, and effective plant and equipment maintenance. Nineteen hospitals lacked any emergency facilities, a basic means of access of local patients to hospital services."

Totally unrelated to the Ministry of Health was the Nicaraguan Social Security Institute (INSS), which provided medical care for insured workers (and limited maternity services for wives) in the major cities, constituting about 9 percent of the population. A third major health agency was the National Social Assistance and Welfare Board (JNAPS), which operated central general hospitals. Local hospitals, however, were controlled by 19 largely autonomous local Social Welfare Boards (JLAS). A large relatively well-equipped military hospital was quite independent.

Another USAID study in the early 1970s estimated that only 28 percent of the population had reasonable access to medical care. It is small wonder that Nicaragua's health record before 1979 was extremely poor. Although mortality reporting was weak, the life expectancy at birth in 1979 was 52.5 years. Infant mortality (estimated by the Latin American Center for Demographic Studies) was 121 per 1,000 live births. Studies by INCAP (Institute of Nutrition for Central America and Panama) found 66 percent of children under 5 years of age to have some degree of malnutrition. Diarrhea and other preventable infectious diseases were the number one cause of death.

The Sandinista Health Approach

In spite of allegations, the new Sandinista Front policies were not based on communist ideology. The FSLN did not set out to nationalize agriculture or industry, although the government did take over the widespread assets amassed by the Somoza family. As of 1986, to which period this account largely applies, most of the land and most of the businesses were in private hands. An approach of fundamental social reform, however, was applied to the health system, to make essential services, as much as feasible, available to everyone.

Less than a month after the triumph of the Sandinista Front, the new government established the Unified National Health System (SNUS) on 8 August 1979. This brought all public hospitals (but not a handful of private ones) under the Ministry of Health (MINSA), along with all health centers. The health resources of the Social Security Institute, including hospitals and urban polyclinics, were transferred to MINSA, as well as the periodic flow of funds derived from employer/employee contributions for medical care. It established in MINSA a National System of Technical Supplies (ATM), which increased and rationalized the domestic production and distribution of drugs and supplies, although most pharmaceutical firms and pharmacies remained under private control.

The law establishing the Unified National Health System was based on six principles: (1) health is a right of every person and a responsibility of the government; (2) health services should be accessible to the total population geographically and legally, as well as economically and culturally; (3) health services should be integrated; (4) health functions should be based on teamwork; (5) health activities should be planned, with the understanding that planning is the most sensible strategy for rational-

izing resources; and (6) the community should participate in all activities of the health system.

These principles could not, of course, be implemented overnight. Human and physical resources had to be greatly expanded, which would take time. The tasks were enormously complicated by the mounting in 1983 of a counterrevolutionary movement of dissident Nicaraguans, based in Honduras and Costa Rica. Substantial military, technical, and all sorts of logistic assistance was provided by the United States, both openly and covertly. The *contras,* as these armed opponents were called, killed civilians and destroyed public utilities, bridges, housing, and specifically scores of health facilities. By May 1986, they had caused more than 4,400 deaths (which would be proportionately the equivalent of 352,000 in the United States population).

The Nicaraguan government was forced to devote the lion's share of its resources to military defense; one estimate claimed that 40 percent of the government budget was required. As a result, the health system progress, which had been substantial in the years 1979 to 1983, was seriously slowed down. Nevertheless, the basic structure of the system stayed reformed, and its characteristics as of 1986 may be presented. So much of the organized health activity was brought under the Ministry of Health that MINSA deserves separate analysis.

Ministry of Health (MINSA): The Main Pillar

The health service unification law of 1979 (SNUS) brought nearly all government health activities under the jurisdiction of the Ministry of Health (MINSA). To carry this broad range of responsibilities, MINSA had to be completely reorganized, in both its central headquarters and its framework for health administration throughout the country.

The minister of health was supported by four vice-ministers for (1) medical services (preventive and curative), (2) research and training, (3) hygiene and epidemiology, and (4) technical and medical supplies. There were also two directorates serving the entire ministry for (1) planning and (2) finance.

The Ministry of Health supervises a national network of hospitals, health centers, and health posts that provide personal health services, preventive and therapeutic, to the entire population. MINSA is also responsible for training health personnel and for planning and supervising the production of drugs and medical supplies. The Planning Office of MINSA also sets goals for the output of health personnel trained outside the ministry, such as physicians and dentists educated in universities, and it establishes technical standards for all health facilities and services. (Pregnant women, for example, were expected to receive four prenatal examinations, although in 1986, 2.3 such examinations were actually being provided.)

Under Sandinista control, the formerly vertical programs of the Ministry of Health were transferred to a regionalized framework, bringing the management of all health services closer to the people. Previously Nicaragua had been divided into 16 *departamentos,* each of which simply followed directions from the top. Now the country was divided into nine jurisdictions—six regions (in the more heavily populated Pacific side), and three zones (on the more thinly settled Atlantic side). Each of these nine regions or zones (averaging 340,000 people) is headed by a medical director-general; six of these officials have also had public health training. The staffs of the six health regions include personnel responsible for medical service, training, and the other major functions found at MINSA headquarters. In the zones, the staffing is more limited.

The directors of the health regions and zones are appointed by the minister of health, and are technically responsible to her. At the same time they come under the surveillance of the regional delegate of the presidency, an official with overall responsibility for public affairs. Nevertheless, the regional health director has great leeway in the work and is encouraged to take initiative to develop new programs in response to local needs. He has no clinical duties to detract from his administrative work. This includes responsibility for all MINSA hospitals, health centers, and health posts. Coordination and supervision of regional health work are provided through periodic visits of central MINSA officials to all the regions, and also by monthly meetings of the regional directors in Managua.

Below the regional level are 90 *health areas* of approximately 20,000 to 50,000 people. Each area has a health center, staffed with at least one physician and several auxiliary personnel. Health centers offer general primary health care, preventive and therapeutic. The physician is usually a recent medical graduate serving his 2 years of "social service," required of all new graduates. The regional health director tries to visit each of the health areas at least twice a year, and meetings of health area personnel are also held periodically at the regional headquarters. About 20 health centers also contain a few beds for emergencies, childbirths, or temporary bed care, usually pending transfers of the patient to a hospital. The local political subdivisions of Nicaragua are municipalities, numbering 140, and steps were being taken in 1986 to recast many health areas to conform to the boundaries of the municipalities.

Still closer to community life are health posts. In 1986 these numbered 379, with each intended to serve 5,000 to 10,000 people. In the larger cities, health posts were staffed by one physician and usually an auxiliary nurse, but in the rural areas the staff was usually limited to one or two auxiliary nurses. The health post is expected to furnish preventive services, including health education, to give first-aid treatment, and to encourage people to make use of the health centers. In contrast to the situation in many developing countries, the rates of utilization of health posts and health centers seem to be quite high.

In rural areas, very briefly trained *brigadistas* serve as outreach workers in the villages, under the supervision of health post auxiliary nurses. These are usually volunteers and are considered agents of the community, not MINSA (see later).

At all administrative levels of MINSA, community participation in health policy determination and program implementation is fostered by popular health councils, which include representatives of all major social groupings. Among these are the local Sandinista Defense Committees, organizations of women, youth, farmers, workers, and other groups. These councils meet regularly with MINSA personnel, to express their concerns, to give advice, and also to provide a channel for general education of the people on health programs. The councils, along with the brigadistas, are of special importance in carrying out campaigns, such as for immunizations, malaria control, and environmental cleanups. Despite the many hardships faced by the entire MINSA staff, in 1986 the espirit de corps from the center to the periphery was remarkably high.

Other Organized Health Programs

Besides MINSA, several other government and nongovernment agencies contribute to the operation of the health system in Nicaragua.

Other Public Agencies. Certain public authorities affect every branch of government, including health. Thus, the *Ministry of Planning* has a Division of Social Services and Population, which reviews the plans of the Ministry of Health, to see that they are consistent with overall national socioeconomic planning. The *Ministry of Finance* establishes a ceiling for the health expenditures of MINSA; this naturally sets limits on all MINSA activities. More specifically concerned with the provision of health services are several other ministries or autonomous government institutes.

The *Nicaraguan Institute of Social Security and Welfare* (INSSBI) was established by law in 1955. Before the Sandinista victory it covered 120,000 workers in the main cities, with limited benefits for wives and infants. In 1986 it covered 350,000 workers for numerous risks—occupational injuries and disease, old age, permanent disability, and death. Workers in firms with one or more employees (previously 10 or more employees were required) are now covered, and 30,000 agricultural workers became insured. As noted, the previous responsibilities of INSSBI for providing medical care were transferred to MINSA in 1979, along with its health facilities. However, under the concept of "welfare," INSSBI still conducts programs for infant and child care, child nu-

trition, and rehabilitation of children, and it operates orphanages, homes for the aged, and institutions for the blind and deaf.

When the Unified National Health System (SNUS) was established in 1979, two well-developed hospitals (in Managua and Léon) of INSSBI and numerous polyclinics were turned over to MINSA. Most of the polyclinics became regular MINSA health centers, but a few in larger cities remained as multispecialty polyclinics. These facilities are now open to the entire population. The former INSSBI doctors are paid the same salaries as all MINSA doctors (although they had previously been paid at higher rates).

Most important is the monthly transfer of funds from INSSBI to MINSA, for support of health services, not only to insured workers and their dependents, but also to the rest of the population. INSSBI derived its funds in 1986 from a 4 percent tax on all covered workers and 12.5 percent tax on their employers. (There is no wage ceiling for these taxes.) In a spirit of social solidarity, 60 percent of the social security money raised is transmitted to MINSA each month to support the entire SNUS program. Part of this funding must be used for payment of cash disability benefits (for loss of wages due to sickness), but most is devoted to financing health services.

In spite of their special contribution to the financial support of the nation's health services, insured workers do not have any special privileges in use of hospitals or health centers. They do, however, receive one financial benefit. Drugs for most ambulatory patients at MINSA facilities require payment of small fees; insured workers are exempted from these payments. The INSSBI also operates a small program for selling eyeglasses to anyone at very low prices.

Nicaragua is primarily an agricultural country, but there is a small industrial sector. Industry employs about 188,000 workers, and the health and safety aspects of their workplaces are monitored by the *Ministry of Labor.* Labor legislation requires that establishments with 200 workers or more must have a full-time (at least 6 hours per day) physician at the workplace. There are 120 such large firms in Nicaragua, mostly in or near Managua, and they employ 260 industrial physicians. Most of these doctors, however, are not trained in occupational health, and they provide essentially general medical care. Smaller enterprises, which are much more numerous, engage nurses at the workplace.

The enterprise must finance these workplace health services. In a firm with fewer than 200 workers, however, if the labor union demands a regular physician, one is provided at the expense of MINSA. Many industrial physicians work partly for MINSA and partly for an enterprise. A few purely private physicians may work at three or four different companies.

Still another government entity with substantial responsibility for environmental sanitation is the *National Institute for Aqueducts and Waste Disposal (INAA)*. This autonomous agency is responsible for public water supply systems everywhere, in both urban and rural areas. MINSA does no work involving water supplies, but it does promote latrine construction in rural areas, complementing INAA activities. By Nicaragua's definition of urban (places with over 2,000 people), the country is 57 percent urban and 43 percent rural. Piped water systems have been established in 200 urban communities, constituting 76 percent of the urban population (compared with 63 percent before the FSLN victory). Of the 1,350,000 rural people, 11 percent have been provided with potable water (mainly by wells), which compares to 6 percent before the revolution.

In the cities, water piped into houses or buildings is metered and paid for by the users. Even rural communities must find ways of paying for water drawn from wells. Thus, this essential public health service is self-supporting, or supported by private families and other users. The construction costs of new water supplies are borne 50 percent by the national government, 23 percent by INAA, and 27 percent by external sources (foreign aid).

Most education of nurses and other allied health personnel is provided by MINSA, but physicians, dentists, and pharmacists are prepared entirely at the universities, which come under the control of the *National Council of Higher Education*. This council is separate from the Ministry of Education but coordi-

nated with it. One university and one polytechnical institute are under private religious sponsorship.

The *Ministry of Interior (MINT)* in Nicaragua, as in many other countries, is concerned with internal national security. This includes the maintenance of a national police force and the operation of prisons, both of which functions include the provision of health services.

MINT operates one general hospital in Managua and about 11 special clinics and 20 health posts around the country. Supplies are furnished by MINSA but paid for by MINT. To staff these facilities, MINT has 130 full-time doctors who, unlike those with MINSA, are not permitted to engage in part-time private practice; they receive other perquisites. The MINT health services also cover the spouses of police and other official personnel and their children up to 6 years of age. Health care absorbs about 2 percent of the total MINT budget. The International Red Cross monitors the medical care and general conditions of all MINT prisoners.

Finally, as almost every country, Nicaragua has a *Ministry of Defense,* which includes a relatively well-developed health service for the army, the navy, and the air force. The military services operate two general hospitals. There are also health posts throughout the country, staffed by specially trained medical auxiliaries. Military physicians, (about 14 to 19), serving full-time, are all specialists. General practitioner services are furnished by residents who rotate in the Managua military hospital, and by interns (who are sixth-year medical students).

Voluntary Agencies. Several nongovernment organizations (NGOs) or voluntary agencies in Nicaragua contribute services and resources to the health system.

As most countries, Nicaragua has a *Red Cross,* which is especially well developed. It operates, under contract with MINSA, a national blood bank program, that furnishes blood to the hospitals. It also maintains a network of ambulance stations throughout the country, available at all times. It handles 90 percent of the patients transported from accidents or other places to hospitals. In 1986, 37 vehicles were functioning—largely donated by

Red Cross societies from other countries. Disaster relief is the third major Red Cross function, whether the disaster is natural or manmade. Thousands of people displaced by the contra war have been provided food and shelter by the Red Cross. In 1985, the agency started a dental service for children, with help from Scandinavia.

The principal Red Cross work is done in Managua, where there are 243 paid employees. Throughout the nation are 37 chapters, each with 10 to 15 employees and a much larger number of volunteers—5,000 nationwide. The funds necessary to maintain this program are raised mainly through voluntary efforts—recreational events, donations of businesses and individuals, and gambling. A national lottery, conducted by the Social Security Institute, contributes to the Red Cross, and government (MINSA) provides a few salaries for health personnel who maintain the blood bank services.

Religious medical missions were numerous in Nicaragua at one time, but now they are mainly limited to the *Evangelical Committee for Support and Development* (CEPAD). The health program of this body, known as PROVADENIC, is maintained by only one of the 46 Protestant denominations of CEPAD—the Baptist Convention. Funds are contributed largely from other countries.

PROVADENIC carries out health work in 22 villages, mainly providing primary health care by community health workers. Each village has at least 500 people, and about 16,000 people are served in all. The community health workers are trained for 8 weeks by the full-time staff of seven health personnel. This staff visits the villages regularly for consultation and to bring drugs and supplies. Drugs are purchased at low prices through religious groups in Europe. (In fact, PROVADENIC assists MINSA in purchasing drugs economically from European sources.) The communities selected for work by PROVADENIC are chosen carefully, to serve people not reached by the MINSA program.

Another health-related activity of the Baptist Convention is the University of Polytechnical Institute (UPOLI). This is a higher educational center for training various types of technical personnel for banking, statistics, industrial design, and so on, including professional nurses and vocational nurses. Although UPOLI is owned and operated by the Baptist Convention, it is heavily subsidized by the National Council of Higher Education. About 40 nurses graduate per year, and they are deployed to places designated by MINSA.

Nicaragua has several mass organizations, promoted by the FSLN to mobilize youth, women, farmers, and others to build a new egalitarian society. Most actively concerned with health services is the *Association of Nicaraguan Women—Luisa Amanda Espinoza (AMNLAE)*. During the period of FSLN insurrection, in 1977, AMNLAE was organized to help the Sandinista fighters; for example, they collected and stored drugs and provided first aid. After the FSLN triumph, they were organized with chapters throughout the country and acquired a full-time staff of 150 women.

AMNLAE women work with brigadistas to carry out campaigns against malaria and for immunizations. Their members are also encouraged to become brigadistas. They help establish infant development (child day care) centers, to enable mothers of small children to work, in cooperation with the Social Welfare Division of INSSBI. They educate women on family planning, nutrition, prenatal care, and so on. They promote the performance of Pap smears for detection of cervical cancer. They are calling for liberalization of Nicaragua's antiabortion law, which permits this procedure only to save the life of the woman. They provide special support for the U. S.-based *Madre* project of the Women's Hospital Bertha Calderon. Th entire AMNLAE program is subsidized by the government, along with support from voluntary national and international donors.

Finally, among voluntary agencies, one should not overlook the *Sandinista Front for National Liberation (FSLN)* itself, which is concerned with health development, as with all other aspects of society. There are seven political parties represented in the Nicaraguan National Assembly, but the FSLN has majority control. (Unlike many developing countries, Nicaragua is not a one-party nation.) While it had the support of a clear majority of the voters in 1986, formal membership in the FSLN is limited to persons who are deeply committed to FSLN goals and willing to work hard. Therefore, fewer than 1 percent of the population are formal party members, who attend monthly meetings. It should be emphasized, however, that appointment to MINSA or another government position does not require FSLN membership.

The Private Medical Care Market. Nicaragua, under FSLN leadership, has a pluralistic economy. In spite of allegations to the contrary from some foreign sources, almost every field has a substantial private sector. Most of the agricultural and industrial production is in private hands, as we noted earlier, and health services are no exception. There is no ban on private medical or dental practice, and it is extensive (see later). The great majority of pharmacies, where people may purchase prescribed or nonprescribed drugs, are privately owned and operated.

Since precolonial days, *traditional healers,* or *curanderos,* were widespread in the land that is now Nicaragua, and they still exist in the rural areas. As modern health resources have been developed and people have become educated, the volume of these healers has steadily declined, but it is widely recognized that they still provide care in isolated villages, and are consulted when patients are not satisfied with the results of conventional modern health service. They are most numerous in the East Coast zones, where government health services are least developed. Curanderos are essentially private practitioners, although their fees are usually low or paid by barter. If there were one curandero for every 1,000 rural people in Nicaragua, they would number about 1,500.

Traditional birth attendants (TBAs), or *parteras,* are much more fully recognized and, indeed, incorporated in the official health programs. They are also in private practice, but the policy of MINSA is to provide them training on hygienic methods of handling childbirths and to accept them without reservation. About 55 percent of childbirths in the nation are estimated to be handled by TBAs in the home.

Much the largest component of the private medical market is the service of modern *physicians.* This service takes two forms in Nicaragua: (1) a relatively small number of physicians work exclusively in private practice, almost entirely in the larger cities, and (2) the vast majority of doctors employed by MINSA and the universities engage in private practice 3 or 4 hours a day, after their official duties are over. Together, these two sets of physicians provide a great deal of curatively oriented medical care to persons who can afford to pay for it.

Private medical practice is not discouraged in Nicaragua, because government salaries are quite low, and few doctors with family responsibilities could maintain a decent standard of living on these salaries alone. Private earnings are much higher per day than government salaries; in a few days of private work the medical official can earn more than his monthly public salary. Without this extra source of livelihood, MINSA and other public programs might not be able to retain their medical staffs; some of these doctors might even leave the country.

Private hospitals also operate in Nicaragua—three in all. The largest is the Baptist Hospital in Managua; it has 42 beds, down from 75 beds before the 1972 earthquake. Although it is sponsored by a religious group and is nonprofit, patients must pay for care. There are 12 full-time private physicians on the staff, 52 nurses, and a total staff complement of 225, or 5.4 personnel per bed. (This is much higher than the staffing of public hospitals.) About 3 percent of the services provided are given free to qualified persons with low income. There are also small private bed units attached to six or eight private clinics in other major cities of the country.

Another large component of the private medical market are the *private pharmacies,* which are the most common drug dispensers in Nicaragua. In 1986, there were 284 private pharmacies in the country. With one or two exceptions, the drugs dispensed by government programs come from small dispensaries located in hospitals or health centers.

Most of the private pharmacy's drug supplies are purchased from the government.

Some are purchased from private distributing companies, which obtain them from overseas. About three-quarters of the drugs dispensed by pharmacies are sold over-the-counter, without a medical prescription. All drug prices are regulated by the government and are kept quite low.

Among *dentists,* a higher proportion than among physicians are devoted exclusively to private practice. Out of some 350 dentists in Nicaragua in 1985, about 220 worked for MINSA, and 130, or about 35 percent, worked entirely privately. The government dentists also engage in private practice after their official duties. Private earnings, as in medicine, are much higher than public. The special problem in dentistry is to obtain necessary supplies and equipment. There are two private dental supply depots in Nicaragua, but dentists sometimes must resort to use of a black market. Gold for fillings is purchased from the Central Bank, and a private German dental enterprise maintains a firm in Managua.

About 50 private *dental laboratories,* prepare dental prostheses. Although it is illegal, many dental laboratories also make complete dentures for patients directly, without the intervention of a professional dentist. Such service is, of course, much less expensive for the patient. Numerous private *clinical laboratories* also function in the main cities, examining specimens sent by private physicians. Government laboratories in hospitals or health centers will not examine specimens from private practitioners.

Production of Health Resources

Since the Sandinista victory in 1979, the rate of production of all health resources, especially personnel, has greatly accelerated.

Health Manpower. Expanding the output of *physicians* was a high FSLN priority. Before the revolution, there was just one medical school at Léon, which admitted about 100 students a year and turned out about 70. In 1981 a second medical faculty was established at the University of Nicaragua in Managua, and in the two schools, 500 students were admitted each year, of whom 400 graduated. About 30 percent are women. Medical education requires 6 years after secondary school, the last year being regarded as an internship. After graduation, every young doctor must spend 2 years on assignment by MINSA, as a condition for official registration. In the first years of FSLN control, hundreds of doctors from Cuba, Europe, and elsewhere were invited to Nicaragua to help staff the rural health units.

By the mid-1980s, the availability of physicians in Nicaragua had increased greatly. Considering only the medical staff of MINSA and other government agencies, the ratio rose from 52 per 100,000 population in 1977 to 69 in 1984. The Federation of Nicaraguan Medical Societies (FESOMENIC) estimated that in 1986, counting all physicians in the country, the supply was 2,400; for a population in 1986 of 3,300,000 this meant a ratio of 73 physicians per 100,000. Since the Ministry of Health and other government agencies employed 2,172 physicians (including 297 from other countries), this meant about 228 physicians outside the government and presumably in exclusive private medical practice. Thus, 90.5 percent of all physicians worked for the government and 9.5 percent were essentially in private practice. About one-third of Nicaraguan doctors are specialists and two-thirds are general practitioners; the specialists spend more time in private practice.

The output of *dentists* is much less, but has also increased since 1979. The one dental school at the University of Nicaragua in Léon was enlarged to admit 200 students for the 5-year course, graduating about 160. Altogether the 350 dentists in Nicaragua in 1985 meant a ratio of 10.6 per 100,000, which was a slight improvement over the past.

The training of *professional nurses* has been greatly expanded by opening up two additional nursing schools, beyond the four that had existed. The six schools of nursing can accommodate about five times the pre-1979 enrollment. Nevertheless, as in most Latin American countries, there are still fewer fully trained nurses than doctors—1,271, or 38 per 100,000 in 1985. Professional nurses receive 3 years of hospital-based training after secondary school, and one can appreciate why most young women who complete this basic schooling prefer to go on to university to study medicine, dentistry, or pharmacy.

Nursing needs are met by training relatively large numbers of *nursing auxiliaries,* which requires only 1 year after elementary school (six grades). There were 13 schools for training auxiliary nurses in 1986, spread throughout all nine regions/zones of the country. About 4,400 auxiliaries were working in 1985, constituting 133 per 100,000 population.

Pharmacists are trained in a 5-year university course in Léon; about 75 students enter each year and 60 graduate. Altogether Nicaragua has about 350 pharmacists, of whom 256 or 73 percent work in private pharmacies. The opportunities for employment in government pharmacies, attached to hospitals and health centers (about 80 such facilities), are relatively fewer.

Other health personnel in Nicaragua include laboratory and x-ray technicians, anaesthesia technicians, physiotherapists, and auxiliary sanitarians. These personnel are trained principally at a national Polytechnical Institute for Health (POLISAL) and at the nongovernment UPOLI school (under Baptist control) described earlier.

All this higher education is free to the students, except for the cost of textbooks. To cover living expenses, some 72 percent of health profession students receive scholarships from the national government. Clinical training for all health science students is given in the hospitals and other health facilities of MINSA.

Finally, among human resources are the *brigadistas,* young community health volunteers who were initially trained to help in certain disease control campaigns. In the fight against malaria and other mosquito-borne diseases (such as dengue fever), about 25,000 were trained. Others were prepared for immunization and sanitation campaigns. Altogether about 70,000 brigadistas had been trained by 1985, but not all of these remained active.

The initial brigadista training lasted only 1 week, but periodic refresher sessions lasted about one day each month. For qualification, a brigadista needed only to be literate and willing to work without pay. The training usually took place in a local school, and was given by nurses, professional or auxiliary. More than half the brigadistas were women, and 80 percent were under 30 years of age.

After the initial disease-specific campaigns, or *jornadas,* in 1982, brigadistas began to be trained for a wider role in general primary health care (PHC). For this, their training was extended. Their functions came to include general health education (particularly on hygiene and sanitation), cooperation in immunizations and malaria prophylaxis, first-aid and treatment of minor illnesses, and administrative recordkeeping. They were provided a small first-aid kit and they worked under the supervision of auxiliary nurses.

Health Facilities. Physical resources in the Nicaraguan health system consist principally of hospitals, health centers, and health posts. In 1986, there were 31 *hospitals* in the country; counting the small groups of beds in certain health centers, there were 5,280 beds or 1.6 beds per 1,000 population. This ratio has remained constant for several years, because Nicaragua has deliberately put priority on the construction of facilities for primary health care.

Because of the trade embargo and war launched by the contras, hospital equipment has been in short supply. At least one new hospital building (constructed with USAID funds for the Somoza regime) remained completely empty for lack of equipment. In several hospitals, whole sections were not used because no beds and equipment were available.

The major physical resources for primary health care in Nicaragua are *health centers* and *health posts.* Together these units numbered 172 in 1977, before the Sandinista triumph. In 1986, there were 487 units, consisting of 108 health centers, all medically staffed, and 379 health posts. The health posts in cities and some rural health posts also had doctors (typically recent graduates doing their social service), but most rural posts had only one or two auxiliary nurses. The health center doctor is expected to supervise the work of the health posts.

Of the 108 health centers, 19 had four to six beds for emergencies, maternity cases, and temporary patients usually pending transfer to a hospital. There are small separate rooms for maternal and child health care, immunizations, medical examination and treatment by the doctor, a modest laboratory, and the storage and dispensing of drugs.

Among health facilities in Nicaragua, one must not overlook the 284 private *pharmacies,* plus 80 "popular pharmacies" attached to hospitals or health centers. In addition, there are 18 warehouses for drugs, used as midway depots for distribution of the drugs produced domestically or imported by government.

Commodities. The procurement of drugs and supplies is relatively complex. Of all drugs consumed in Nicaragua, only 16 percent are produced domestically and 84 percent are imported. Of the *imported drugs,* about 70 percent are bought by a government trading enterprise, known as COFARMA. This body also approves the 20 percent of drug imports handled by private enterprises. The remaining 10 percent of imports are obtained through international agencies, such as UNICEF, and religious missions. Imports come principally from Europe (both East and West) and from Cuba, Peru, and Mexico. The decisions on drugs to be imported, as well as those to be produced domestically, are made by MINSA. The policy is to limit drug use to 395 essential products. Of the *domestically produced drugs,* about half are made by a relatively large enterprise, known as SOLKA, which is jointly owned by government and private investors. It comes under the control of the Ministry of Industry. The other half of domestic drugs are produced by 12 small firms, privately owned.

Another health commodity is *medical equipment.* Nicaragua has special problems in this regard, since most of its basic diagnostic and therapeutic equipment had formerly come from the United States, which has embargoed the provision of all spare parts. As a result, much equipment no longer functions. There are, for example, 89 x-ray machines in the country, for which replacement parts must be sought from firms in Europe.

Knowledge. A final health resource is knowledge, for which Nicaragua must depend mainly on the world's medical and public health literature. Foreign exchange necessary to obtain books and journals, however, is very limited. A certain amount of medical research is done by the two medical faculties and some public health research is done by the Center for Health Research and Studies (CIES).

CIES is equivalent to a school of public health and, in addition to conducting research, it trains epidemiologists and health administrators for MINSA. As an institution of higher education, CIES has links to both the University of Nicaragua (which confers degrees) and to MINSA. The full-time faculty is only six teachers, but about 80 part-time lecturers are drawn from MINSA and the University of Nicaragua.

Economic Support

The economic support of the Nicaraguan health system, as in all countries, comes from several sources. Of course, government support is substantial, but in the pluralistic economy guided by the FSLN philosophy, there is also a significant private sector. Some funds also come from charity (domestic and foreign) and from industrial enterprises.

Because of the rapid rate of inflation in Nicaragua, it is difficult to quantify correctly the funds derived from different sources, especially when data are reported for different years. Thus, between 1985 and 1986, the consumer price index in Nicaragua rose by about 700 percent. In the estimates offered here, therefore, we try to use figures applicable only to 1986.

The largest share of *government revenue financing* in Nicaragua is the general tax support that sustains the Ministry of Health. Even MINSA, however, derives funds from certain sources beyond general public revenues. Thus, as we noted earlier, a substantial share of the income of the Social Security and Welfare program (INSSBI) is transferred regularly to

MINSA. Separate funds from the National Lottery, managed by INSSBI, also contribute to the MINSA budget, as does a limited amount of foreign aid. In 1986, the total budget of MINSA amounted to U.S. $11,350,000 (at the 1986 exchange rate of 2,100 cordobas to the U.S. dollar). This absorbed 14 percent of the overall government budget. These MINSA funds were derived from five sources as follows:

Source	Percentage
General government revenues	79.9
Social security transfers	11.7
Lottery	5.9
Foreign aid	2.4
Other	0.1
All sources	100.0

MINSA expenditures in 1986 were expected to be slightly less than the budgeted amount. The purposes for which these funds were spent were as follows:

Purpose	Percentage
Hospital services	48.4
Primary health care (health centers and posts)	24.7
Vector control (malaria and dengue)	3.8
Administration	12.9
Training	2.3
Capital investment	1.9
Other	5.1
All purposes	100.0

Although hospital expenditures were still relatively high in 1986, they had been higher before 1979, and the trend has a decline in hospital expenses and more emphasis on primary health care.

The expenditures for water and waste disposal (INAA) are derived partly from government, for capital development, but mainly from charges to consumers for water. The latter must be regarded as private. Public sources in 1986 accounted for 31 percent of the total, and private sources (household payments) for 69 percent. (This does not consider MINSA work in rural sanitation.)

Health expenditure for the armed forces and Ministry of Interior can be only roughly estimated. Official estimates of the costs of supporting the university-based professional schools, and also the medical services in social welfare institutions, are presented here.

Estimates of *private health financing* for medical care in any health system are especially difficult to make. In Managua, a household survey made in 1983 found that 2.17 percent of urban family expenditures went to pay for medical care and drugs. Because of the severe inflation, changes in family income, and the special character of this urban sample, using these findings in estimating national private health expenditures would not be sound. Instead, estimates could be based on information gathered on the gross incomes of physicians and dentists in private practice, and likewise for other health care providers.

Estimates of the gross earnings of private physicians were made with advice from the Nicaraguan Federation of Medical Societies (FESOMENIC). Annual figures were calculted for 228 physicians exclusively in private practice in 1986, and for the 2,172 government-employed physicians, of whom 90 percent did some private practice. In aggregate, these expenditures (in U.S. dollars) could be estimated at $6,718,000 in 1986.

Equivalent information from the Nicaraguan Dental Association (CON) indicated the gross private earnings of dentists in 1986 to be about $833,000. It was assumed that this figure included the cost of dental laboratories for making prescribed prostheses, or it might be raised slightly for amounts paid by patients directly to these laboratories for full dentures.

Calculation of the probable gross income of 284 private pharmacies from drug sales yielded $1,623,000 in 1986. Private gross hospital income, based on information from the Baptist Hospital, was estimated at $571,400. The relatively large private expenditures for water and waste disposal, supporting the INAA program, was noted earlier; in dollars for 1986, this came to $2,533,000. The charges for drugs that MINSA collected at health centers from noninsured patients in 1986 amounted to $219,000. Private payments to clinical laboratories and to optical shops for eyeglasses in 1986 were estimated at $238,100.

To estimate private expenditures on traditional practitioners, one should note that the crude birth rate in Nicaragua was 46.1 per 1,000 persons per year in 1985. This meant about 152,000 births, about half of which (76,000) were handled by traditional birth attendants *(parteras)*. At a modest fee of $2.50 each (equivalent to the normal fee for one consultation with a general practitioner), this would mean $190,000. Traditional healers are much less common, so expenditures for their services can be assumed to amount to about one-third as much, or $65,000. Together these expenditures for traditional health service add to $255,000.

Finally, one must consider expenditures that are nongovernmental but not purely private— health expenditures from *charitable* sources or *business enterprises*. On the basis of data furnished by the Red Cross for 1985, expenditures in 1986 were estimated at $667,000. Likewise, expenditures by the religious PROVADENIC program in 1986 were $143,000. The numerous mass organizations that contribute to health activities (women, youth, farmers, workers, etc.) pay salaries to certain full-time personnel; an estimated $95,000 would be allocated to the health system in 1986 as part of these costs.

Industrial and other enterprises engage about 260 industrial physicians and 500 nurses. Since the salaries paid correspond to those of MINSA, one may calculate that the overall expenditure from this source in 1986 was about $286,000.

It is now possible to combine these various estimates of health expenditures and draw some tentative inferences on the relative proportions of the public and private sectors in the Nicaraguan health system. The results of these calculations are presented in Table 12.2. It is evident that in 1986, of all health-related expenditures in Nicaragua 49.6 percent were governmental. Among nongovernmental sources 46.2 percent came from private fami-

Table 12.2. Expenditures in the Nicaraguan Health System, Classified by Sources or Purposes, and Their Percentage Distribution, 1986

Source	Percentage	
Ministry of Health (MINSA)	40.4	
Water & Waste Disposal (INAA)—government share	4.1	
Armed Forces and Interior (MINT)	3.4	
University Health Science Training	0.8	
Social Welfare (within INSSBI)	0.8	
All government		(49.6)
Private physicians care	23.9	
Private dental care	3.1	
Water supply private payments	9.0	
Private pharmacies	5.8	
Private payment for public drugs	0.7	
Private hospital care	2.0	
Laboratory tests and eyeglasses	0.8	
Traditional health services	0.8	
All private		(46.2)
Red Cross	2.4	
PROVADENIC	0.5	
Mass organizations	0.3	
Enterprise health care	1.0	
Charity and enterprises		(4.2)
All health expenditures	100.0	(100.0)

lies and individuals and 4.2 percent from charity and business enterprises. In light of the relatively rough estimates on which many of the figures are based, it would probably be wise to conclude that about 50 percent of health system costs in Nicaragua came from public sources and 50 percent from private sources.

This key finding strongly supports the claims of the FSLN leadership that they favor pluralistic principles in the economy. (Perhaps the private sector, however, is larger than is desirable for the efficiency and effectiveness of the health system.) It also reflects the difficulties faced by the government in fulfilling its pledge that "health is a right of every person and a responsibility of the government." It means that, in large part, health services are accessible to the population only with substantial private expenditures.

Health System Management

Central planning is a prominent aspect of the Sandinista approach to the Nicaraguan health system. Even though the general economy includes a substantial private market, as do the health services, all government health activities are carefully planned.

MINSA has a well-staffed planning division, and the Ministry of Planning has a Division of Social Services and Population, which includes health. The great expansion of health personnel and facilities, of course, has followed from planning decisions. The development of a School of Health Research and Training (CIES) was a planned response to the need for public health leadership.

Administration in the Nicaraguan health system seems to show a reasonable balance between centralized policymaking and decentralized implementation. Regional directors of health have freedom to develop programs, within the limits of their budgetary allocation. Community participation is fostered by the regular functioning of People's Health Councils at the levels of the regions and health areas. Intersectoral collaboration is crucial and its impacts on the population's health have been obvious. The land distribution program of the Ministry of Agriculture has clearly improved nutrition. The literacy rate increased from 66 to 88 percent between 1980 and 1984, because of the efforts of the Ministry of Education.

Administrative practices are illustrated by budget-making policies. The budgetary process begins in the regions, which gather information on needs from the health areas under their jurisdiction. Tentative budgets are then submitted to MINSA headquarters, where adjustments are made to achieve a proper balance among regions. Negotiations with the Ministry of Finance determine the final MINSA budget, which is necessarily affected by other requirements in the total society. Based on the finalized MINSA budget, budgetary allocations are then sent back to the regions.

Regulation has been conspicuous in some parts of the Nicaraguan health system and not in others. Imports of pharmaceutical products are largely controlled, and the pricing of drugs in private pharmacies appears to be well regulated. The private practice of medicine and dentistry, on the other hand, seems to be quite unregulated.

The charges made for a private medical consultation are uncontrolled. General practitioners commonly charge around $2.50 per visit, but specialists may charge three to five times as much. Private earnings are supposed to be reported annually to the Ministry of Finance, for payment of income taxes. The surveillance of these reports from doctors, however, is lax. The attitude of this ministry toward doctors is deliberately "soft," to avoid alienation that might result in their leaving the country. A physician employed full-time by the government is ordinarily expected to work for 6 hours, but he often works only 3 or 4 hours to maximize his private practice time.

Evaluation is based essentially on health outcome data. The crude death rate in Nicaragua was 16.4 per 1,000 population per year in 1977, and it declined to 9.7 per 1,000 in 1984. Life expectancy at birth increased from 52.5 years in 1977 to 59.8 years in 1984. The infant mortality rate was estimated by the Latin American Demographic Center (in Costa Rica) to be 121 per 1,000 live births in 1977, declining to 71.5 per 1,000 in 1984. Morbidity data are available on only a few communicable diseases. The incidence of measles reported for 1977 was 36 cases per 100,000 population per year; by 1983 this had declined to 3.4 cases per 100,000. Poliomyelitis attacked 40 to 50 persons in 1978, but no case has occurred in Nicaragua since 1982. Blood smears positive for malaria parasites were found in 12 percent of persons surveyed before 1979, but in 1984 this rate had declined to 3 percent.

Since 1984, social turmoil from the contra hostilities has been so great that more recent health data are not reliable.

Delivery of Health Services

The patterns for delivery of ambulatory health care in Nicaragua obviously differ for the public and private sectors. In the MINSA and other public programs, services are provided by salaried doctors and other personnel working in organized health centers, health posts, and hospital out-patient departments; the latter are staffed by specialists. Examinations are relatively brief, because there is usually a long queue of patients. Immunizations and examinations of well babies are customarily done by auxiliary nurses, and the sick patients are usually seen by a doctor. In some rural areas, where health posts are staffed only by auxiliary nurses, they handle sick patients as well, referring difficult cases to a health center.

MINSA has made primary health care (PHC) available to almost the entire population of Nicaragua. In the cities, about 85 percent of the population actually make use of the health facilities each year, and experience shows that in any population 15 to 25 percent of people have no illness during the year that leads them to seek care. In most rural areas, the equivalent utilization of PHC is 65 to 75 percent of people during the year. All services in Nicaragua are free, except for a small charge for drugs (from which insured workers and some others are exempted).

During the few years of FSLN control of the health system, the rate of utilization of ambulatory services has gradually increased, except for a decline in 1984, when the disturbances caused by contra military activity were especially great. Thus, counting consultations at hospital out-patient departments (OPDs), health centers, and health posts, before the Sandinista government (1977), there were 1.1 ambulatory care contacts per person per year. This figure rose gradually to 2.1 such contacts in 1982. Of these, about 70 percent occurred at community PHC units and 30 percent at hospital OPDs. In 1984, however, with the severe hostilities, the rate declined to 1.9 consultations per person per year. In the rural areas, health centers seem to be heavily used, but in the cities, where hospitals are nearby, they are often bypassed by patients wishing to see a specialist in the hospital OPD.

The achievements on immunizations of infants indicate progress, though limited. National data show the following trends in percentages of infants immunized;

Disease	1977	1984
Diphtheria	25.6	33.3
Pertussis	25.6	33.3
Tetanus	25.6	33.3
Measles	—	47.1
Poliomyelitis	62.5	80.8
Tuberculosis	19.1	98.0

Dental visits rose from 80 per 1,000 persons per year in 1977 to 150 per 1,000 in 1984.

These data apply only to the MINSA program; they take no account of ambulatory services in private medical offices or clinics. As reported earlier, 228 doctors are exclusively in private practice and 1,955 in part-time practice after their government work, for a total of 2,183 practitioners. Very conservatively, one might assume that the average private doctor sees 10 patients per day (estimates of 20 patients per day are commonly given). If these physicians work privately for 260 days per year, their consultations would amount to 5,675,800. This would mean an additional 1.72 medical contacts per person per year in Nicaragua. Added to the services in MINSA, the total rate would exceed 3.6 consultations per person per year.

Private medical practitioners cannot serve private patients in public facilities, as is permitted in some developing countries. This must be done in separate private quarters. To save on overhead expenses, it is customary for several physicians—as many as 10 or 15—to have examination rooms together in a private clinic. They do not work as a "group practice"; each has his or her own patients, but there may be a common waiting room and a small laboratory serving all the doctors.

All but a few hospitals in Nicaragua are governmental, and they are moderately well staffed. A regional hospital has 1.5 to 2.0 personnel per bed. Medical care is given by salaried specialists, assisted by young doctors undertaking residency training. Outside physicians cannot admit patients.

Although the ratio of hospital beds to population in Nicaragua declined in the 1980s, the rates of occupancy increased and the average length of patient stays decreased. As a result, the rate of hospitalization rose from 49 admissions per 1,000 per year in 1977 to 69 per 1,000 in 1983; then, with the hostilities, it declined to 63 per 1,000 in 1984.

Regarding environmental sanitation, the population served with potable water rose from 34.5 percent in 1979 to 46.0 percent in 1983. The improvement in sanitary excreta disposal was less—from 17.2 percent of the population in 1979 to 20.5 in 1983. The urban situation, as everywhere, was better than the rural.

Implementation of the six principles of the health system by the Sandinista government has obviously been greatly handicapped by political and military conflict. In 1988, matters were further complicated by a very destructive hurricane. In 1988, all of Nicaraguan society suffered from severe inflation, unemployment, massive physical destruction, and demoralization.

Yet, in spite of the enormous difficulties, the Sandinista movement for social equity and its applications in the health system was very much alive. Political commitment to comprehensive health services for everyone remained strong and, in fact, was high on the nation's political agenda. Lofty objectives for human welfare can hardly be achieved, however, without first attaining peace. When vast expenditures for military defense are no longer necessary, and when the entire Nicaraguan economy can be rehabilitated, people's energies can be directed to building the national health system, defined by the principles formulated in 1979.

SUMMARY COMMENT

Far greater differences than similarities characterize the national health systems of Costa Rica, Israel, and Nicaragua, and yet they all share a strong commitment to health protection. The government of each country, in its own way, has pursued a policy of putting maximum effort into the provision of health services to all people on the basis of their needs.

Costa Rica is a nation at peace, without any standing a.my, while both Israel and Nicaragua devote major shares of their GNP to military defense. In Israel, the greatest part of all health activities is under the control of a nongovernment health insurance organization, while the bulk of health responsibilities in Costa Rica and Nicaragua is in public hands. Both Nicaragua and Israel permit their salaried medical personnel to engage extensively in private practice after official hours, and this is also

allowed in Costa Rica with lesser consequences. But everyone's entitlements to health service are perfectly clear, and the record of health status accomplishments is impressive in each country.

These three small countries illustrate very well the importance of political commitment to the development of a national health system. Historical background, economic foundations, technological developments, and the place of the country in the global political scene all determine the contours and strategies of the health system. But under very different circumstances, these countries have been able to support their health systems with a political will strong enough to serve their people more effectively than other countries of the same economic level.

REFERENCES

Costa Rica

Casas, Anatonio, and Herman Vargas, "The Health System in Costa Rica: Toward a National Health Service." *Journal of Public Health Policy,* 1:258–279, September 1980.

Gonzalez-Vega, Claudio, "Health Improvements in Costa Rica: The Socioeconomic Background," in Scott B. Halstead et al. (Editors), *Good Health at Low Cost.* New York: Rockefeller Foundation, 1985.

Harrison, Paul, "Success Story." *World Health,* March 1981.

Jaramillo A., Juan, "Changes in Health Care Strategies in Costa Rica." *Bulletin of the Pan American Health Organization,* 21(2):136–148, 1987.

Jaramillo, Juan, C. Pineda, and G. Contreras, "Primary Health Care in Marginal Urban Areas: The Costa Rican Model." *Bulletin of the Pan American Health Organization,* 18(2):107–114, 1984.

Mata, Leonardo, and Luis Rosero, *National Health and Social Development in Costa Rica: A Case Study of Intersectoral Action.* Pan American Health Organization, Technical Paper No. 13, 1988.

Morgan, Lynn M., "Health Without Wealth? Costa Rica's Health System under Economic Crisis." *Journal of Public Health Policy,* 8:86–105, Spring 1987.

Rosero-Bixby, Luis, "The Case of Costa Rica," in Jacques Vallin and Alan D. Lopez (Editors), *Health Policy, Social Policy and Mortality Prospects,* Liege, Belgium: Ordina Editions, 1985.

Vega Carballo, José L., *Costa Rica: Coyunturas Economicas, Clases Sociales y Estado en su Desarallo Reciente, 1930–1975.* San José: Universidad de Costa Rica, 1976.

Villegas, Hugo, "Extension of Health Service in Costa Rica." *Bulletin of the Pan American Health Organization.* 11(4):303–310, 1977.

Israel

Central Bureau of Statistics, *National Expenditure on Health 1978–79 and Preliminary Estimate for 1979–80.* Jerusalem (Reprint from Supplement to the Monthly Bulletin of Statistics No. 2), 1981.

Consulate General of Israel, *Response of the Government of Israel to "The Casualties of Conflict—Medical Care and Human Rights in the West Bank and Gaza"* (March 30, 1988). Boston, May 24, 1988, processed document.

Doron, Haim, "Planning Community-Oriented Primary Care in Israel." *Public Health Reports.* 99(5):450–455, September–October 1984.

Doron, H., and A. Ron, "The Kupat Holim Hospitalization Plan," *Kupat Holim Yearbook, Vol. 6 1977–78,* Tel-Aviv, 1978, pp. 7–24.

Ellencweig, A. Y., "The New Israeli Health Care Reform: An Analysis of a National Need." *Journal of Health Politics, Policy and Law,* 8(2):366–386, Summer 1983.

Evang, Karl, *Report on a General Evaluation of the Health Services in Israel, November 1959–January 1960.* Alexandria: World Health Organization, Regional Office for the Eastern Mediterranean, 1960.

Grushka, Theodor (Editor), *Health Services in Israel.* Jerusalem: Ministry of Health, 1968.

Hadassah Medical Organization, *Sixtieth Anniversary Report 1972–1973.* Jerusalem: Jerusalem Post Press, 1974.

Halevi, H. S., *The Bumpy Road to National Health Insurance: The Case of Israel.* Jerusalem: Brookdale Institute of Gerontology and Adult Human Development, 1980.

Halevi, H. S., "Health Services in Israel: Their Organisation, Utilisation and Financing." *Medical Care* (London), 2(4):231–242, October–December 1964.

Kanev, Itzhak, *Mutual Aid and Organized Medicine in Israel.* Tel-Aviv: Central Kupat Holim, 1953.

Kupat Holim, *The Health of the People Is the Wealth of Society.* Tel-Aviv: Kupat Holim Health Insurance Institution, 1983.

Lazin, Frederick A., "Comprehensive Primary Care at the Neighborhood Level: An Israeli Experiment that Failed." *Journal of Health Politics, Policy and Law,* 8(3):463–479, Fall 1983.

Margolis, Emmanuel, "Health Care in a Changing Society: The Health Services of Israel." *Medical Care,* 13(11):943–655, November 1975.

Nizan, A., *National Insurance in Israel.* Jerusalem: National Insurance Institute, April 1979.

Palley, H., et al., "Pluralist Social Constraints on the Development of a Health Care System: The Case of Israel." *Inquiry,* 20:65–75, 1983.

Pilpel, D., "Coping with Doctors' Strike in Israel." January 1985, processed document.

Shuval, Judith, *Israel Study of Socialization for Medicine.* Washington, D.C.: National Center for Health Services Research (NCHSR Research Digest Series), October 1978.

State of Israel, Ministry of Health, *The Israeli Health Services Profile: Survey on Hospitals' Services.* Jerusalem, 1981.

Tulchinsky, T. H., "Evaluation of Personal Health Services as a Basis for Health Planning: A Review with Applications for Israel." *Israel Journal of Medical Sciences,* 18:197–209, 1982.

Tulchinsky, T. H., "Israel's Health System: Structure and Content Issues." *Journal of Public Health Policy,* 6:244–254, June 1985.

Tulchinsky, T. H., "New Concepts in Primary Care: Prevention as Policy." *Israel Journal of Medical Sciences,* 19:723–726, 1983.

Tulchinsky, T. H., V. Lunenfeld, S. Haber, and M. Handelman, "Israel Health Review." *Israel Journal of Medical Sciences,* 18:345–355, March 1982.

Nicaragua

Bossert, Thomas John, "Health Policy Making in a Revolutionary Context: Nicaragua, 1979–1983." *Social Science and Medicine,* ISC:255–231, 1981.

Braveman, Paula, and David Siegel, "Nicaragua: A Health System Developing Under Conditions of War." *International Journal of Health Services,* 17:169–177, 1987.

Braveman, Paula A., and Milton I. Roemer, "Health Personnel Training in the Nicaraguan Health System." *International Journal of Health Services,* 15:699–705, 1985.

Donahue, John M., *The Nicaraguan Revolution in Health.* South Hadley, Mass.: Bergin & Garvey, 1986.

Downing, Theodore E., and Peter K. New, "The Politics of Health Care in Nicaragua Before and After the Revolution of 1979." *Human Organization,* 42:264–272, Fall 1983.

Garfield, Richard M., "Health and the War Against Nicaragua, 1981–84," *Journal of Public Health Policy,* 6:116–131, March 1985.

Garfield, R. M., T. Frieden, and S. H. Vermund, "Health-Related Outcomes of War in Nicaragua." *American Journal of Public Health,* 77(5):615–618, May 1987.

Garfield, Richard M., and Pedra F. Rodriguez, "Health and Health Services in Central America," *Journal of the American Medical Association,* 254:936–943, 16 August 1985.

Garfield, Richard M., and Eugenio Taboada, "Health Services Reforms in Revolutionary Nicaragua." *American Journal of Public Health,* 74:1138–1144, October 1984.

Halperin, David C., and Richard Garfield, "Developments in Health Care in Nicaragua." *New England Journal of Medicine,* 307:388–392, 5 August 1982.

Heiby, James R., "Low-Cost Health Delivery Systems: Lessons from Nicaragua." *American Journal of Public Health,* 71:514–519, May 1981.

Ministerio de Salud, *Condiciones de Salud y Logros Alcanzados 1982–1985* (Informe Presentado en la XXIII Conferencia Sanitaria Panamericana). Mangua, Nicaragua, September 1986.

Scholl, Edward A., "An Assessment of Community Health Workers in Nicaragua." *Social Science and Medicine,* 20:207–214, 1985.

CHAPTER THIRTEEN

Socialist Health Systems in Transitional Countries

A few countries at a transitional/developing economic level have undergone social revolutions and developed socialist health systems. These have all occurred since the end of World War II, and all the health systems have been substantially influenced by the Soviet Union model. The countries are in three different continents: Cuba in the Americas, Albania in Europe, and North Korea in Asia. Because most information is available on Cuba, its health system is examined in some detail. Only a few words can be said about the Korean Democratic People's Republic and Albania.

CUBA

Cuba is an island in the Caribbean Sea, just 90 miles south of the Florida coast of the United States. Because of this proximity to the great American superpower, its sociopolitical attitudes and actions, including its health system, have aroused worldwide interest.

In 1985, Cuba had a population of 10,100,000, of whom 71 percent were urban. Its principal economic base has been the production and export of sugar. The GNP per capita in 1984 was $1,911, putting it at about the midpoint in a ranking of the Latin American countries. Adult literacy in 1984 was 96 percent. The characteristics of the Cuban health system have been influenced overwhelmingly by its revolution of 1959, when a guerilla group, headed by Fidel Castro, gained national power. The previous government, headed by Fulgencio Batista, was essentially a military dictatorship that arose in 1933. To understand the current socialist health system, prerevolu-

tionary health circumstances should be reviewed.

Prerevolutionary Health Patterns

Cuba had been settled and colonized by Spain, like most of Latin America, after Columbus's voyage in 1492, but it did not win its independence until some 80 years after the 1820s, when most of the American nations became self-governing. Slaves were brought from Africa for agricultural labor in 1513 and were not emancipated until 1868. Important health care patterns, like the *mutualistas* (see following), were established by families from the mother country, who naturally dominated Cuban life until independence. After independence, in 1902, Cuba came under considerable influence from the United States, its giant neighbor to the north. For various reasons, the Catholic Church was not very strong, which may account for the minor role of *beneficencia* hospitals, so important in numerous other Latin American countries. The dominance of the United States, on the other hand, meant correspondingly less influence of Europe, which may account for the weak development of social security health care programs—likewise important in nearly all other countries of Latin America.

Cuban prerevolutionary health services, however, were like those of the rest of Latin America in several respects. In the main cities, there was a great deal of private medical practice for members of the middle class who could pay the charges. There were also many small private hospitals. The maldistribution of doctors was extreme, with a surplus in the national capital (one of the reasons for organizing the mutualistas) and severe deficiencies in the rural areas. A government health service was established in 1906, initially for preventive purposes but evolving into the Ministry of Health and Social Welfare after World War II. This ministry operated hospitals for the poor in the cities, it supervised environmental sanitation, conducted some research, and supervised certain other aspects of health. In addition, as in other Latin American countries, small hospitals were operated by private enterprises (like sugar mills) for their workers. Medical facilities for the military forces were well developed.

A number of important developments occurred in Cuban health service before 1940. After the Secretariat of Sanitation was established in 1906, the period from 1910 to 1925 was sometimes considered the Golden Age of Public Health in Cuba. In these years the work was done that led to eradication of smallpox, through vaccination, and of yellow fever through elimination of the *Aedes aegypti* mosquito. In 1926, the Carlos Finlay Institute was founded—named after one of the discoverers of the mode of transmission of yellow fever and the first secretary of health—to produce vaccines and offer short courses of instruction in hygiene. In 1916, the first social insurance was enacted, providing compensation for wages lost due to industrial injuries and the associated costs of medical care. In 1934, the first nonoccupational social insurance was enacted, but it was limited to maternity benefits for working women and the wives of insured workers.

In the 1930–1940 decade, in response to the worldwide economic depression, the *mutualista* health insurance plans expanded in Havana and other main cities; these nongovernment programs helped finance medical care for people with steady income and also helped keep doctors and hospitals solvent. In the three decades before 1940, many government (mostly municipal) hospitals were built and hundreds of doctors had been graduated by the University of Havana Medical School (in 1958 at the rate of about 80 graduates per year).

Thus, at the time of the revolution in 1959, Cuban health services were moderately developed in several ways. Certain organized components of the health system, as they existed around 1958, should be described.

Ministry of Health and Social Welfare. The most important unit under this ministry was the Directorate-General of Health. This department was responsible for sanitation of ports and airports, supervision of health professions, drug control, food sanitation, health statistics, venereal disease control, disinfection, and general environmental sanitation also. Below the top, were 126 municipal health districts that reported directly to headquarters, but no health offices at the level of the six provinces.

Another unit of the ministry was the Directorate-General of Welfare, which was in charge of 46 hospitals for the poor, 1 dispensary, 13 blood banks, and a small dental service. There were also some first-aid stations *(casas de socorro)* in the larger cities, aided by the Red Cross. A third unit was a separate National Council for Tuberculosis, which operated 28 dispensaries, 5 sanatoria, and 2 preventoria. A fourth unit was the Directorate-General for Prevention of Leprosy, Syphilis, and Skin Diseases, which operated 2 leprosaria and 10 dispensaries. A fifth unit was the Directorate-General for Child Guidance, which operated 8 maternal and child health centers and certain services in the schools. Three other units of the Ministry of Health and Welfare were the National Corporation for Public Welfare (operated creches and homes for the aged), the Carlos Finlay Institute (producing vaccines and offering some training), and the National Institute of Health (conducting research).

Thus, the Ministry of Health and Welfare in 1958 consisted of eight quite separately functioning national programs, with little if any coordination at the provincial or local levels. All eight directorates were staffed by 1,458 doctors (both full-time and part-time), which constituted about 23 percent of the 6,421 physicians in the country (in 1956). The other 77 percent of physicians were predominantly in private practice, and many of the ministry doctors also engaged in private practice part of the time. For dentists, the ministry engaged 90 out of 2,100 in the country, or under 5 percent. Of the approximately 28,500 hospital beds in Cuba in 1958, about 9,000 were controlled by the Ministry of Health and Social Welfare. These included beds in provincial and municipal, as well as national, government hospitals. The balance of hospital beds come under nongovernmental auspices.

Military Medical Services. Before the revolution, one hospital served the armed forces in each of Cuba's six provinces. In addition, each of the two main cities, Havana and Santiago, had a second large military hospital. A separate hospital was also maintained in Havana for the police.

Social Security. As noted, the medical benefits before the revolution were limited to compensation for industrial injuries and provision of maternity care. To provide childbirth service, four or five maternity hospitals with about 200 beds each were operated in the main cities. Agricultural workers and their families were not covered by the social security law. The industrial accident insurance was carried mainly by private insurance companies (principally foreign-owned), and injured workers were served by private doctors and hospitals on a fee-for-service basis. Some private clinics in Havana specialized in these trauma cases.

Industrial Medical Services. Some large companies operated hospitals and clinics for their own employees. The United Fruit Company had one such facility in Oriente Province. These industrial medical programs were financed half by the employer and half by employee wage deductions. Two labor unions— the transport workers and the schoolteachers—operated their own hospitals.

Religious and Voluntary Facilities. There was no typical *beneficencia* hospital program in Cuba. Two or three small hospitals and a few clinics, supported by bequests, were sponsored by religious bodies. Lotteries were used for the support of orphanages, but not for hospitals.

Doctors sometimes worked in the religious units without compensation. A few voluntary nonsectarian agencies, like the League Against Cancer, were supported by donations. The Red Cross operated ambulances and emergency services, and these were subsidized by government.

Mutualistas. Perhaps the most important programs for medical care in prerevolutional Cuba were these nongovernment insurance schemes. The *mutualistas* or mutual benefit societies had been started by Spanish immigrants and colonists for themselves and their families in the nineteenth century. Persons from certain provinces of Spain banded together for self-help, the largest groups being the Society of Asturians and the Society of Galicians. Monthly premiums were paid to finance medical care, supplemented by fees for each service, and indigent persons from the same Spanish province were sometimes helped.

In the 1930s, with the general economic depression, new mutualistas were organized by small groups of physicians, as a means of attracting financial support for their services. Membership was sold to any buyer, and the funds were used to build facilities, as well as for operating costs. Occasionally all the employees of an industrial or commercial enterprise would be enrolled in one mutual society. Through this mechanism many small hospitals, or *clinicas,* were constructed in the main cities. After World War II, the mutual societies grew rapidly to a membership, at the time of the revolution, of about 600,000 persons. Of these, about 60 percent lived in Havana, 20 percent in Santiago de Cuba, and 20 percent in the rest of the island.

The mutualistas were an important mechanism for both financing and providing medical care for families with steady income. The insurance payments sustained numerous clinic facilities that would have failed without the financial support. Yet mutual society hospitals and other private facilities were commonly half empty, while the public hospitals were overcrowded, with two patients in a bed. Moreover, many mutual and private facilities became commercialized, performing unnecessary surgery or unjustified Cesarean sections, for which fees were levied.

Thus, before the revolution, health services in Cuba, as in most Latin American countries, conformed largely with social class. The very small wealthy class was served by purely private doctors and hospitals. The middle class and some skilled workers—about 10 percent of the population—were served largely by the resources of the mutual societies. The large class of rural peasants and urban proletariat were served in crowded and understaffed government hospitals and clinics, if they received care at all. The Ministry of Health and Social Welfare was an administrative umbrella for eight separate health programs. Insofar as this ministry exercised quality controls, they applied to its own facilities, and not to the mutualista or private hospitals and clinics. A fee schedule used by doctors was established by the Medical Association and insurance companies, not by the ministry. Preventive services of limited scope were provided quite separately from the treatment services.

Transition to Socialist Health Policies

When Fidel Castro and his guerilla comrades attained power in January 1959, they did not bring with them a blueprint for the reorganization of the health services, nor any other aspect of Cuban society. The revolution had been launched to overthrow the Batista dictatorship, to gain land and a better life for the *campesinos,* and to extend the benefits of democracy to everyone. Concepts of Socialism, on the Marxist model, did not crystallize until 2 or 3 years later. The socialist ideology was shaped through a series of crucial events, including (a) the United States blockade (1959–60), (b) the Bay of Pigs invasion (April 1961), and (c) the Soviet Missile Crisis (November 1962). These historic events naturally influenced the development of health services.

First Steps: The Ministry of Public Health. For the first 6 months after the triumph of the revolution, very few changes were made in the health services. A new minister of health was,

of course, appointed—Dr. Martinez Pais. He was a young orthopedic surgeon, the first doctor to join the revolutionary guerrillas in the Sierra Maestra. It is significant that a revolutionary viewpoint, rather than technical knowledge of public health, was the main consideration. (One is reminded of Lenin's appointment of Dr. N. A. Semashko as the first People's Commissar of Health in the USSR, based not on his technical knowledge but on his revolutionary background.)

In mid-1960, with hostility mounting from the United States and from foreign-owned enterprises in Cuba (especially oil refineries), the Cuban government began to turn more resolutely toward a socialist pattern of health services. Initially the Ministry of Health and Social Welfare was reorganized at the central level. A law in 1961 established the new Ministry of Public Health (Ministerio de Salud Publica—MINSAP). The previous directorates, with their relatively autonomous structures, were blended into a new ministerial structure with five vice-ministries. These were for (1) medial training, (2) medical care (including hospitals and polyclinics), (3) medical supplies (especially drug production), (4) hygiene and epidemiology (including communicable disease control, environmental sanitation, and the operation of research laboratories), and (5) economics (including planning, financing, and external relations).

At the top, helping the minister, were a general advisory council, made up of the five vice-ministers plus other key health officials, and a scientific council, made up of the country's most qualified technical personnel. Reporting directly to the minister was a health director of each of the nation's six provinces. The functions of MINSAP were defined in terms of a series of 15 program objectives: (1) extension of preventive and curative health service to the whole population, (2) emphasis on services to mothers and children, (3) health promotion among adolescents, (4) medical guidance in physical culture and sports, (5) improved environmental rural and urban sanitation, (6) worker health protection, (7) epidemiological control of disease, (8) food and drug control, (9) health statistics, (10) health education, (11) hospital construction and surveillance, (12) application of advancing science to health services, (13) research, (14) regulation of cadaver disposal, and (15) national production of drugs.

Converting these program objectives into practical administrative operations was not easy. To reach these goals, nine principles of health administration had to be followed: (1) health planning within the general planning of the nation, (2) concentration of all health activities in the Ministry of Public Health, (3) integration of preventive and curative health work, (4) centralization of standards and decentralization of execution, (5) collective direction of all activities, (6) a "mass line," with participation of the people in health tasks, (7) a scientific basis for all work, (8) coverage of the entire territory with health services, and (9) international cooperation. A later formulation of these basic principles consolidated some of them, and added one further principle: (10) transformation of the goals of medical education to train professional and technical personnel with both scientific and humanistic attitudes appropriate to the new (socialist) society.

Aside from the reorganization of the Ministry of Health and Social Welfare, two other laws relevant to health were enacted in 1960: one required that all graduates of the medical school of the University of Havana serve for 2 years in a rural post, designated by the Ministry of Public Health; the other law reorganized the Ministry of Labor, among other things, consolidating various social insurance programs under that ministry. At the same time, the medical and hospital establishments, formerly under the Health and Maternity Insurance Scheme, were transferred to the Ministry of Public Health.

Regionalization of Authority. To build a new administrative structure for the health services of Cuba, perhaps the most important principle among those listed here was the fourth: centralization of standards and decentralization of execution. The major task was to convert an array of numerous separate health programs, "vertically" autonomous from top to bottom (that is, from central, to provincial, to local levels), into a system in which "horizontal" integration would be achieved among all health activities at the local and provincial levels, as well as at the top.

The strategy began to take shape after the attempted invasion at the Bay of Pigs was repelled in April 1961. With continued open advocacy for further invasion in the U.S. Congress, Cuba began to look seriously to the USSR and other countries of Eastern Europe for substantial advice and assistance. In the health sector, counsel was especially sought from and offered by Czechoslovakia. The process of decentralized execution of health services, then, began in 1961 with clarification and strengthening of the authority of the public health directorates in each of the provinces; the six established provinces were recast as eight *health provinces.*

At the same time, each of these health provinces was divided into *health districts* (which were later termed *health regions*). These regions varied from 60,000 to as much as 500,000 population, with an average of about 200,000. By 1962, 36 health regions were established. Each of these was placed under the direction of a health official, who reported to the provincial health director and was made responsible for all health activities in the region, both preventive and curative. Typically, the regions were designed to include one or more regional hospitals, but the directors of these hospitals were not synonymous with the regional health directors; rather, the former reported to the latter.

Within the health regions, the more difficult task was to organize a network of health areas, which would be the principal framework for delivery of preventive and therapeutic service, especially to the ambulatory person. The plan conceived of health areas with a population of 25,000 to 35,000, each of which would be served by a polyclinic for ambulatory care or by a small rural hospital. The delineation of these health areas was a gradual process, because it meant education of the population to seek health care from a specific facility serving their geographic area. It also required the construction of many new facilities or the absorption into the integrated system of old and previously independent facilities. This process began around 1965, and by 1968 there were 268 functional health areas. A final task was to subdivide each health area into *health sectors* of about 4,000 people, for the purpose of carrying out work assignments. Eventually 2,209 such sectors were defined.

Integration of Resources. The process of developing an integrated network of health facilities and services took place in two main phases. The first phase was the placement under MINSAP control of all resources for health care, which had previously been under some branch of government. More complicated was the second phase of the integration process—namely, the absorption and integration of the many health resources coming under nongovernment or private control. These included principally the resources of (a) the mutualistas, (b) industrial and agricultural enterprises, (c) religious and other voluntary bodies, and (d) purely private owners.

It is noteworthy that in Cuba, despite the revolutionary power, the socialist integration process was very gradual. The objective was clear, but MINSAP moved only step by step. The general policy was for government, if possible, to take control of a hospital or clinic only if it met proper health standards and when a specific cause made such action reasonable. One such cause might be a labor dispute developing in a hospital between employees and management; the Ministry of Labor would intervene to settle the dispute, and then turn over the facility to MINSAP. Another cause might be a serious shortage of supplies (drugs, instruments, etc.); with the embargo against Cuba, supplies from the United States dwindled and the government naturally reserved those supplies imported from the USSR and elsewhere for government facilities. Under these pressures, the private hospitals and clinics would have to close down of their own accord; if the facility met reasonable standards, MINSAP intervened and took it over.

Another cause for intervention, especially for the purely private and some mutualista facilities, was the departure of their owners. Soon after the revolution, many upper- and middle-class people, including doctors who owned private hospitals, left Cuba. The hospital property they left behind, if it met MINSAP

standards, was then taken over by the government. Still another cause, involving some mutualista facilities, was a decline in the insured memberships. As health services under MINSAP expanded, mutual society members sought care from public resources and dropped their society ties; with income from members declining, the mutual societies were willing to sell out to the government.

It should be noted that, when owners of a hospital or clinic of suitable standards remained in Cuba, their property was not seized without compensation. A deliberate policy of integration of the private and mutual society facilities began only 3 years after the revolution, in 1962. The value, for compensation purposes, was based on the previous declared value of the property for real estate tax purposes. When this had been artificially low, the owners were compensated accordingly. Finally, there were many small *clinicas,* under either mutualist or purely private ownership, which MINSAP regarded as inefficient or unsanitary. Some of these were simply converted houses and were far below minimum health standards. These units (eventually 230 of them) were simply closed down and not absorbed into the network of government health facilities.

In the initial organizational structure of MINSAP, there was a special Directorate of Mutualist Clinics under the vice-minister for medical care. Then after 1962, society memberships began to decline as the component facilities, for the causes explained earlier, were gradually eliminated or integrated into the overall regionalized health care network. In the mid-1960s, some mutualista resources finally had to be seized by the government (with compensation), to complete the regionalization scheme. Not until 1968, however, were all mutual society insurance dues terminated. And only in 1970 were the last mutualista hospitals and clinics of adequate standards drawn into the MINSAP network.

Drugs: Production and Distribution. Another significant aspect of the transition to socialism in the health system was in the pharmaceutical industry. Before the revolution, of course, drug production and distribution was entirely in private hands. In 1958, there were about 500 drug companies in Cuba, but the great majority were only distributors of imported products. The basic plan of MINSAP was to nationalize and rationalize the drug industry, for both production and distribution of pharmaceutical products, but this was done in stages.

Initially, when conflicts developed between labor and management in a pharmaceutical manufacturing company, the Ministry of Labor intervened. Some of these companies were taken over by the Ministry of Labor and then transferred to the Ministry of Industries. In 1959 and 1960 several Cuban owners of drug companies left the country, as did many of the foreign owners; these companies were taken over directly by the Ministry of Industry. Then in March 1961, this ministry drew up a general plan for government drug production. A study by the Association of Cuban Laboratories in 1959 showed that of the original 500 drug companies, 110 met minimal standards; the rest sold unethical or poor-quality products. Of these, 72 accepted control criteria, and the Ministry of Industries selected 14 that were considered reasonably efficient. Those that had not been acquired by one of the methods noted here were taken over with compensation.

These 14 drug-production firms were organized as the Enterprise of Pharmaceutical Products within the Ministry of Industries. Equipment and personnel from the other companies were transferred to the 14 main units, to the extent considered efficient. For a time about 250 other smaller companies were allowed to stay in private business, until the nationalization process was completed about 1965.

Both before the revolution and since, the raw chemicals from which most drugs are prepared have been imported. After the revolution, however, the source of these chemicals shifted from the United States to the Soviet Union, some Western European countries (Great Britain, Holland, and Switzerland), and Canada. To handle these imports, the Ministry of Foreign Trade organized a special government unit called *Medi-Cuba,* turning over the materials to the Ministry of Industries for fabrication into usable drugs. For a period, the distribution of drug products to hospitals and polyclinics was done by the Ministry of Domestic Products.

This unwieldy system was changed in 1963, by assignment to MINSAP of the task of distribution of all drugs to local health facilities. Then, in 1965, responsibility for drug production was also transferred from the Ministry of Industries to MINSAP. Finally, in 1966 the task of importing finished drugs, or the raw materials for fabrication of drugs, was also transferred from the Ministry of Foreign Trade to MINSAP. Thus, nationalization and unified administration of the production (including importation of supplies) and distribution of drugs required seven years.

Throughout this period, of course, a major change took place in the number and types of drug products (formulas) available to doctors. Before the revolution, about 30,000 to 40,000 different products (that is, drugs with different names) were used in Cuba. As in most free-market countries, a large proportion of these were duplications of the same chemical compound, with different trade names, and many were products of dubious medical value. As the drug companies were nationalized and consolidated, the list of available drugs was reduced to about 4,000, which were registered with the Colegio Medico as meeting quality standards; these were compounds formerly produced by the 72 companies noted earlier. Many of these, however, were still duplicate preparations, and a final "national formulary" was developed, with only about 1,000 different drugs specified as necessary for the practice of modern scientific medicine. (This was still much more than are on the World Health Organization list of "essential drugs," developed much later.)

The technical controls and surveillance necessary to ensure quality standards in drug production were vested in a subdivision of MINSAP. At first, foreign advisers had to be called on for this function, but Cuban personnel were gradually trained. Inevitably there were difficulties in this whole transitional process and, according to MINSAP officials, there were sometimes shortages of certain needed drugs.

By 1969, however, a satisfactory supply of all needed drugs was achieved.

The distribution of drugs to the population in Cuba, as in most countries, was traditionally through numerous private pharmacies. In most Latin American countries, the multitude of small private pharmacies, where people buy drugs directly without a doctor's prescription, reflects the inadequacies and costs of modern medical care. Before the revolution there were 2,223 such pharmacies in Cuba, whose locations were largely related to local purchasing power; thus, an excessive number were located in wealthier urban areas and very few in rural districts.

A law passed in October 1960 started the nationalization of wholesale drug distributors. This process was completed in 1962. In November 1963, the process of developing a reasonable network of local pharmacies was completed, and 1,250 out of the original 2,223 were acquired, with compensation, by MINSAP. The process of rationalized planning of local pharmacy services resulted in a great reduction of them in cities, from more than 2,100 to about 950, and an increase of rural pharmacies from about 60 to 300. In small towns and villages, where the population was not large enough to warrant a pharmacy, a neighborhood general store was allowed to dispense drugs. With centralized control, 24-hour availability of drugs was arranged in every community.

Drugs outside the hospital in Cuba, as in the Soviet Union, were not made a free benefit, as was all other health service. Patients must generally pay for prescriptions, with the exception of pregnant women, persons with tuberculosis or syphilis, and certain other categories. Aged persons and children got a 40 percent reduction on prescription prices. Soon after the revolution, moreover, in March 1959 a decree brought about a 15 percent reduction in the price of all domestically produced drugs and a 20 percent reduction in the price of imported drugs. About 85 percent of drugs were obtained through prescription, but simple remedies for minor ailments could still be obtained over-the-counter.

A similar process of gradual rationalization and integration under MINSAP applied to the optical industry. Before the revolution, there were 114 optical supply houses in the country, 62 in Havana. To make eyeglasses more generally available to people, these shops were gradually taken over by MINSAP and new units were established in rural regions. Prices were also reduced—50 percent for eyeglass frames, 40 percent for the lenses, and 60 percent for contact lenses.

Priority for the Health Service. This whole transition of the health services from the prior Latin American to the Socialist pattern was probably most intense between 1962 and 1968. After 1968 came a period of consolidation of previous gains, with an emphasis on improvement in the efficiency and quality of services. New resources, of course, also continued to be developed.

In the whole process of the Cuban Revolution, health services seemed to occupy a high priority. Even without statistical data on the percentage of GNP devoted to health purposes in Cuba, compared with other countries, it was widely judged to be relatively high. This has been noted by relatively conservative observers such as Lee Lockwood, no less than by such radical economists as Leo Huberman. In spite of serious economic difficulties in general economic development, after the U.S. embargo, heavy investment was made in education and health which, many argue, contribute only indirectly to overall development.

There were doubtless many reasons for the great importance attached to health in the Cuban Revolution. One was surely the importance of health for national strength and efficiency of production in both industry and agriculture. Another was that health services are appreciated and help win the hearts and minds of the people for the government in power. A third reason, of course, was the basic humanitarianism of the socialist ideal.

Perhaps a fourth reason was the relatively strong role of doctors in the revolution itself. Several important Cuban revolutionaries were trained as physicians. Most famous was Dr. Ernesto "Che" Guevera, who came from Argentina and worked closely with Fidel Castro both before and after the revolution, until his death in Bolivia. Less widely known are several other doctors who played leading roles outside the medical arena—the minister of interior, the director of the Institute of Hydraulic Resources, the director of the Cuban Port Authority, the rector of the university, the vice-minister of foreign trade, and even high officers in the Cuban army. Thus, one might expect a special sensitivity to health questions at many places in the structure of the Cuban government and the revolutionary movement.

As noted earlier, other socialist countries gave Cuba assistance and advice in formulating its health service patterns. Significant aid was also received from the Pan American Health Organization. As one MINSAP official said, in explaining the whole process of transition to a socialist health system: "We received helpful ideas from some capitalist and from all socialist countries. We blended these with creative initiative of our own."

Health System Organization in the Mid-1980s

It was in 1962–63, that Cuba became firmly committed to develop a socialist health system, but the first 20 years were not static. With experience and general socioeconomic development, several changes were made. The contours of the system in the mid-1980s can now be summarized.

Ministry of Health (MINSAP). The scope of responsibility of the Ministry of Health (MINSAP) gradually became even broader than it was in 1962. Several reorganizations were made at the headquarters level—first consolidating the original five vice-ministries into two, then recasting authorities around 1980 into six vice-ministries. In 1975, the medical schools and other faculties within the universities were transferred to the control of MINSAP. Special health programs for workers in selected industrial enterprises were also transferred.

The nationwide framework of MINSAP administrative offices was substantially changed. The original 8 *health provinces* were increased to 14. In 1976 a major change was made in the overall Cuban policies of governance. With the revolutionary government firmly in command, the political leadership felt sufficiently confident to arrange for popular elections of local officials. Cuba had 169 municipalities, and delegates were elected to municipal assemblies—3 for every 5,000 people. From these bodies, representatives were elected to provincial assemblies, and from the latter representatives were elected to a National Assembly. At each echelon, the assembly chose an executive council of full-time officials. These councils appoint, among others, municipal and provincial directors of public health, and they bear ultimate responsibility for the health program. With all this governance at municipal and provincial levels, the former health regions were found to be redundant, and were eliminated. (The "regional" level continues only insofar as hospitals, serving the population of several municipalities, may be regarded as having a regional function.)

Other Organized Health Activities. Aside from the functions of MINSAP, there is almost no specific health activity at the national level. For financial support, of course, the Ministry of Finance makes ultimate decisions on allocations to all ministries, including MINSAP. Likewise, the health planning done by MINSAP must be reviewed and approved by the overall national planning body, known as JUCEPLAN.

Only environmental sanitation (water supplies and sewage disposal) is not controlled by MINSAP but by the municipal authorities. MINSAP establishes general standards and advises on the design of sanitary mechanisms, but ultimate responsibility is at the local level.

Voluntary agencies for health purposes in Cuba are not significant, except for the "mass organizations." These are principally the Committees for the Defense of the Revolution, the Federation of Cuban Women, and the National Association of Small Farmers. Volunteers from these groups assist in mass campaigns, such as house-spraying with insecticides for malaria control and mobilizing families for immunization of their children. To some extent these groups may do voluntary work to construct simple health posts or facilities for water supplies and sanitation.

The private market in medical care has remained very small in Cuba since the transition to socialism. Private care by dentists has been somewhat more common than by physicians, probably because dental service has not been well-developed in MINSAP facilities. The pharmacies are now all under MINSAP control, but some nonprescribed drugs may be purchased privately from them.

Production of Health Resources

As in other socialist health systems, Cuba has put great emphasis on increasing all types of resources on which the health system depends.

Health Manpower. Educating large numbers of physicians was given the highest priority. Before the revolution, Cuba had one medical school, at the University of Havana. Nearly all the professors also had private practices, and soon after the fall of Batista 90 percent of the medical faculty left the country.

Physicians, in general, had high incomes, and a large proportion of them fled Cuba (mainly to the United States) after the revolution; the new government did not obstruct their departure. Estimates of the volume leaving vary between 33 and 50 percent. The need to replace the physicians lost and expand the number well beyond the previous total was obviously urgent. This departure of doctors with the Cuban Revolution was not unusual. After the American Revolution, thousands of well-to-do New Englanders—the United Empire Loyalists, loyal to the British king—fled to Canada. After the Russian Revolution, thousands of White Russians (supporters of the Czarist regime), including doctors, fled to Western Europe and the United States. Likewise after the Chinese Revolution, a substantial share of the scientifically trained doctors, identified with the Kuo-Mintang government, went to Taiwan, Hong Kong, or elsewhere. Perhaps in Cuba the medical exodus was more massive because the United States, only 90 miles away, extended so warm a welcome and was so easy to reach, and also because the Revolutionary Government was so permissive. In Miami, Florida, a special Postgraduate Medi-

cal Program for Cuban Physicians was established by the University of Miami, to help these doctors pass examinations for U.S. licensure.

The actual reasons for departure of the Cuban doctors can be summarized as follows: (a) political involvement of some kind with the Batista dictatorship, (b) ownership of major industrial or rural properties, which were expropriated by the revolutionary government, (c) previous earning of very high incomes from wealthy patients, which could not be expected to continue in Cuba but might be realizable elsewhere, (d) possession of unusually high qualification by some doctors (e.g., neurosurgeons), who were offered attractive positions in the United States, and perhaps most important (e) the petit bourgeois mentality of many doctors who simply opposed the Cuban Revolution as a threat to their future lives. Whatever the reasons may have been, a substantial share of all Cuban doctors departed. Since these were mainly older physicians, those remaining in Cuba were younger and more likely to adjust to the social concepts of the revolution.

To replenish the supply of physicians, a second medical school was established in 1962, a third in 1966, and a fourth in 1968. By 1983, the four medical schools were graduating more than 2,000 young doctors a year. About half the new physicians were women. Entry to medical school depended mainly on secondary school grades and also on having "the right moral characteristics and a revolutionary feeling." About 7 or 8 percent of the medical students come from other countries. Medical education requires 5 years plus a 1-year hospital internship.

The conception in back of medical education in Cuba is summarized in 11 basic principles, as follows: (1) a foundation in the teachings of Marxism–Leninism; (2) forging a body of scientific thought—avoiding dogmatism and pragmatism alike; (3) avoiding a gap between theory and practice; (4) integration of basic sciences and clinical medicine; (5) recognizing psychological factors in health and disease; (6) a humanistic and social concept of medicine; (7) inclusion of productive manual labor within medical training; (8) socialist teamwork and elimination of bourgeois individualism; (9) a broad cultural education as part of medical training; (10) emphasis on prevention; (11) orientation on the administrative structure of the nation's health services.

On graduation, the young doctor does not take the classical Hippocratic Oath, but a special Cuban oath, which declares his or her intention to serve the people, to renounce private practice, to cooperate with government policies, to emphasize prevention and human welfare, and so on. On completion of medical studies, all graduates must spend 3 years in a rural post. After rural service, the great majority of young doctors take specialty training through a hospital-based residency. Emphasis in recent years, however, has been given to general internal medicine or "family practice."

With these policies, Cuba soon trained far more physicians than were needed to replace those who left. By 1982, there were 17,000 active physicians, for a ratio of 170 per 100,000. Similar expansion of training applied to other categories of personnel, especially nurses. Nursing schools were increased to 34, turning out 500 graduates per year by 1975. In 1982 there were 20,300 fully trained nurses and 11,600 auxiliary nurses—207 and 118 per 100,000, respectively. Dentists numbered nearly 4,000 or 40 per 100,000, but professional pharmacists numbered only 700 or 7 per 100,000. Without private pharmacies, the need for pharmacists was not great. The geographic distribution of all these personnel was remarkably balanced across the long, narrow Cuban island. The simple fact that doctors, nurses, and others must go where positions in health facilities are available virtually ensures this even distribution of health manpower.

Among middle-level technical personnel, special technical schools (not the universities) trained various laboratory and x-ray technicians, dental assistants, pharmacy assistants, and others. Notably absent from Cuban health manpower, however, is the general medical assistant, typified by the *feldsher* in the Soviet Union. Cuban thinking has regarded such personnel as second-class doctors, who should have no place in a revolutionary health system. (This echoes the attitude of health leaders immediately after the Russian Revolution, except that the Soviet policy later changed.) With its

large number of doctors, nurses, and assistant nurses, Cuba has not used any "barefoot doctors" or community health workers (trained for only a few months), so widely used in other developing countries.

Also absent is the trained midwife. Traditional birth attendants had served the poor extensively before the Cuban Revolution, but they have gradually died out. Childbirths are now delivered by physicians, and in 1982 nearly 100 percent of these occurred in hospitals. Some nurses have received special training in obstetrics, since 1967, but their function is to assist doctors in maternity cases.

In the 1960s, a school of public health was organized in MINSAP for postgraduate education of physicians and others in epidemiology, health administration, environmental hygiene, nutrition, and other fields. The training program is unique, in alternating periods of academic study with periods of placement in MINSAP administrative settings, for a course of 2 years leading to a master's degree. The school faculty is well-developed, and there are many graduate students from other Latin American countries.

Another aspect of personnel training in Cuba is continuing education. Most of this occurs in hospitals and some in teaching polyclinics (see later). There are also numerous short courses, which the health professional attends on full salary. This training is not compulsory, but is encouraged in many ways; it contributes to advancements in salaries and positions.

Salaries of Cuban physicians are relatively modest. Doctors in 1983 earned from $250 a month as hospital residents to $700 a month for a full professor. This is much higher than earnings of the average Cuban worker, whose wage averaged $200 a month in 1983. The differentials between physicians and other health personnel, however, are not as great as in nonsocialist countries. The prestige of the physician is exceptionally high.

Health Facilities. Hospitals have been greatly improved in their distribution, total bed-capacity, and quality of equipment since the revolution. In 1958 there were 339 hospital structures but, as noted earlier, many were inadequate and were closed down or converted to other purposes. Altogether there were 28,200 hospital beds, many in very small units, or 4.4 beds per 1,000 people. In 1982 there were fewer hospital structures (256), but they contained 47,300 beds or 5.3 beds per 1,000 population. Of these institutions, 26 were teaching hospitals for training in numerous specialties and for continuing education. Average hospital size had risen from about 80 beds before the revolution to about 200 beds in 1983.

More significant has been the change in the geographic distribution of hospital beds over the years. Before the revolution, 62 percent of the hospital beds were in metropolitan Havana and 38 percent for the larger population in the rest of the country. By 1982 this relationshp had been reversed, and 39 percent of the hospital beds were in Havana, with 61 percent serving the rest of the country. Hospital staffing has also improved. Pre-1959 data are not available, but after the training of thousands of new personnel, in 1975 there were about 1.6 health workers per hospital bed. There were doubtless more in the 1980s.

By 1985, a suitable hospital was readily accessible to everyone. The size, staffing, and functions of each hospital depended on its place in the regionalized scheme. At the national level (Havana) there were a few large hospitals for highly complicated and difficult cases. Each of the 14 provinces had one or more provincial hospitals with a 350- to 800-bed capacity. Below the provincial level, groups of municipalities (formerly constituting regions) were served by regional hospitals with 150- to 350-bed capacity. Most of the 169 municipalities, rural and urban, had small hospitals with 50 to 100 beds. Patients were admitted first to the nearest hospital facility, and then were transferred to higher-level hospitals, as medically necessary.

The customary point of entry to the Cuban health system is not the hospital and its outpatient department, but the polyclinic. Cuban health leadership takes pains to refer to its ambulatory care facilities as *policlinicos*, rather than *centros de salud*, since each unit is staffed by teams of specialized doctors—a generalist, a pediatrician, an obstetrician–gynecologist,

and a dentist—as well as nurses, technicians, clerks, and others. The original jurisdiction at the most local level, as explained earlier, was the *health area* of 25,000 to 35,000 people, each served by a polyclinic. By the mid-1980s, for 169 municipalities there were 423 polyclinics. For Cuba's population of more than 10,000,000 in 1984, this meant a ratio of about 25,000 persons per polyclinic.

The internal organization of polyclinics has been modified over the years, and in the 1980s greater emphasis was put on community-oriented primary health care. Individuals and families were attached to a particular doctor, based on the sector in which they lived—a pattern discussed further later.

For thinly settled rural areas there are medical posts, numbering 159 in 1982. These were staffed simply by one general practitioner and a nurse; for all but the simplest conditions, patients are referred to the nearest polyclinic. There are also some small medical posts in the large cities, 66 in 1982.

Still other types of facilities have been established in the Cuban health system. In 1982 there were 142 dental clinics, 36 public health laboratories, 21 blood banks, and 8 psychiatric day centers. For in-patients, aside from hospitals, there were 81 maternity homes, 68 homes for the aged, and 18 homes for the physically handicapped. Beyond these, MINSAP listed in 1982 (without indicating functions) 177 "other units of medical care."

Commodities. With the nationalization and reorganization of the pharmaceutical industry discussed earlier, Cuba is capable of producing domestically the great majority of the drugs it needs. In 1982, there were 71 factories producing drugs and medical supplies and another 34 units for producing scientific and technical equipment. Chemicals and other raw materials are imported from Eastern Europe and also from Sweden, Spain, and several countries of Latin America. With these, Cuban enterprises produce 83 percent of the drugs used in the country, although certain preparations remain in short supply.

MINSAP distributes the drugs to all its health facilities for patient care. Drugs are also distributed to the 1,444 pharmacies (one per

7,000 people) under MINSAP control, where anyone can obtain prescribed or nonprescribed drugs. There were also 90 shops for dispensing eyeglasses and seven for orthopedic prostheses in 1982. For oral prostheses there were 19 dental laboratories.

Knowledge. MINSAP tries hard to acquire medical books and journals from all European countries and to publish review articles in its own journals, devoted to the diverse medical specialties. Abstracts of important articles are also published from some 800 periodicals reguarly received by MINSAP. Within MINSAP there is a National Center for Information in the Medical Sciences, which publishes almost all this material. This includes, of course, reports of research work done by Cuban investigators. The National Center maintains a central medical library that furnishes books and journals to teaching hospital libraries around the country. The center also responds to requests for information from individual researchers or clinicians.

Emulating the Soviet model, Cuba has established numerous special research institutes, over and above the medical research done by the faculties of the medical and related schools. On a smaller scale, there are research units in hospitals at the provincial level. In 1983, the various places where research was conducted and the projects under study were as follows:

Type of Institution	Number	Research Projects
Research institutes	12	453
Higher medical science schools	46	344
Pharmaceutical enterprises	3	47
Provincial institutions	151	539
Total	212	1383

For a country of only 10,000,000 people, this seems to be a remarkable investment in health science research. The 12 major research institutes are devoted to such special subjects as cardiology, gastroenterology, epidemiology, neurology, oncology, child development, and other areas. In all this research, efficiencies are

achieved by integrating the studies with the regular work of MINSAP hospitals and polyclinics. A study of child development in the 1970s, for example, was carried out as part of the regular MINSAP program of child health services. Visits to the children's homes to collect information on diet, family conditions, and so on were made by volunteers from the Federation of Cuban Women.

All of the research in Cuba is motivated by social objectives of tackling important health problems, rather than in pursuit of the intellectual curiosity of the scientist. It may be noted that, like the teaching program, research is tied to the system of health services. Thus, unlike the usual pattern in other countries, research is not linked closely with teaching in socialist Cuba, but rather manpower training and medical research are both tied to the overall national program of health services.

The several specialized medical journals, which are widely distributed (without charge) to all health facilities in the country, publish articles that report the results of new research as well as general educational reviews. This is illustrated by the table of contents of articles in a 1984 issue of the *Cuban Review of Health Administration* ("Revista Cubana de Administracion de Salud"):

- Marxist social hygiene as a science.
- Prevalence of coronary risk factors in a health area of a teaching polyclinic.
- Automation of hospital management.
- The services of internal medicine and general surgery as organized systems.
- The volume of water consumed, wasted, and left over in a teaching hospital.
- The randomized response technique: a method for reducing evasive behavior in population surveys.
- Epidemiological surveillance in occupational medicine.
- Some indicators of health status of children at the primary school level.
- The organization and functions of public health services in a region of Czechoslovakia.

- Supervision of the national system of vital statistics in Nicaragua.
- The woman in Cuban medicine from the sixteenth century to the first quarter of the nineteenth century.

Health System Management

Much about the management of the Cuban health system has already been discussed. As described in the early postrevolutionary transitional period, central planning played a crucial role. The vast increases in personnel, facilities, and all health resources resulted from planning decisions. With experience, administrative arrangements were modified, from the original use of health regions within the provinces to the later elimination of regions and vesting of responsibilities in municipalities, with elected councils.

Establishment of locally elected bodies to be responsible for community services was legally incorporated in a new Constitution drawn up in 1975. This action, according to one interpretation, was a response of Cuban political leadership to economic difficulties in the 1970s (such as the failure to reach official goals in the sugar harvest). It was considered important to reduce the strong linkage of the Communist Party to the government and to involve the general population more actively in governance at all levels. The popular slogan for the new role of the various elected bodies became "people's power."

In the health system, this meant that virtually all local health services became the responsibility, not of the central government, but of the locally elected councils. The general standards for hospital operation, for example, were established nationally, but their implementation in each facility was the responsibility of the local council. In the words of Fidel Castro, expressed in a speech in 1977:

> The key principle [of people's power] is that all productive and service units, which provide their goods and services to the community, have to be run and controlled by the community. . . . This decentralization does not mean, however, that every community or province is going to

fly on its own. . . . They will have to follow certain norms, so as not to allow disparities and inequities across the country. . . . A municipal hospital, for example, cannot do whatever it pleases. It will provide similar medical services with similar norms of quality, similar for the whole country. . . . Otherwise, the local People's Power will be the unit of government responsible for what happens in that hospital, how it is being run, how the staff responds to the needs expressed by the population.

Accordingly, municipal health directors, who have direct administrative responsibility for the hospitals, polyclinics, and other units in their jurisdiction, are themselves responsible to the local people's councils. On technical matters, relevant to the maintenance of standards, they must be guided by the leadership of higher levels—the province or the central government. But for day-to-day operations or for response to any local grievances, they must report to the elected municipal council. These councils, it should be added, are expected to consult with the local chapters of "mass organizations" (such as the Committees for Defense of the Revolution) in making policy decisions.

To underscore the principle of democratic control, rather than dictatorship by a political party, the National Assembly (which has been elected) enacts a great deal of legislation. Especially significant for the health system was a new Public Health Law, enacted in July 1983. This comprehensive law repealed all earlier conflicting statutes, and established the principles that should govern virtually every aspect of the system. Chapters were included on (a) general preventive and therapeutic health service, (b) maternal and child health care, (c) health care for the elderly, (d) out-patient and hospital care, (e) mental health, (f) rehabilitation, (g) sanitary and epidemiological services, (h) environmental protection, (i) nutrition, (j) occupational health, (k) school health services, (l) health manpower development, (m) pharmaceutical transactions, and (n) still other fields.

Regarding evaluation, as an aspect of health system management, Cuban health leadership has taken great pains to collect data and publish reports on both the process and outcomes of its system. In a later section, we will take note of "process measures" on the delivery of health services, and here we report some basic data on health outcomes.

Life expectancy at birth in Cuba in 1960 was 61.8 years. By 1982 it had increased to 73.5 years. Infant mortality before the revolution in 1958 was reported to be 33.0 infant deaths per 1,000 live births. It is very likely, however, that this constituted underreporting. After 10 years of the new government, in 1968 the rate was officially stated to be higher—38.3 deaths per 1,000 live births. Then, the infant mortality rate declined to 23.3 per 1,000 live births in 1976 and to 17.3 in 1982. For 1986, UNICEF reported a rate in Cuba of 15.0 infant deaths per 1,000 live births.

For disease-specific causes of death, tuberculosis in Cuba took 14.9 lives per 100,000 population in 1960 and only 1 per 100,000 in 1982. Tetanus caused 4.4 deaths per 100,000 in 1960 and 0.1 per 100,000 in 1982. Mortality from acute diarrheal disease (mostly in infants and small children) was 57.3 per 100,000 in 1962 and 4.1 per 100,000 in 1982. Maternal mortality declined from 118.2 per 100,000 live births in 1960 to 48.2 per 100,000 in 1982.

These indicators of remarkable improvements in Cuban health status cannot, of course, be attributed solely to the health system. Many other features of Cuban society are relevant to health, such as the provision for adequate nutrition, the educational services bringing about virtually 100 percent literacy, and arrangements for modest but adequate housing at very low costs. These social benefits, along with the health services, have resulted in an infant morality rate and a life expectancy in 1982, which constituted the best record of any Latin American country or perhaps of any country in the world at a transitional/developing economic level.

Economic Support

The abundant resources and services in Cuba's health system obviously require a great deal of expenditure. Nearly all of this spending now comes from government sources. The extent of health expenditures from private sources is ac-

tually not known, but it must be very small. In the official system, only the cost of drugs outside a hospital or polyclinic must be paid for privately, and there are numerous exceptions for children, the elderly, and pregnant women, and for the treatment of tuberculosis, cancer, and certain other diseases.

Expressed in millions of Cuban pesos, government health expenditures have risen from 20.5 in 1958, before the revolution, to 535 in 1976 and 875 in 1986. On a per capita basis, this was an increase from 3.02 pesos per person in 1958 to 85.9 pesos in 1986. As a share of the overall national government budget, MINSAP used more than 10 percent in 1986.

As a share of the GNP, the health system must absorb a large percentage, but no reliable figure has been reported. One estimate by a foreign observer in 1983 suggested that as much as 15 percent of the GNP was devoted to the health system, although this high a figure is hard to believe. Some economists, both inside and outside of Cuba, have questioned whether the extremely high investments in both health and education may have retarded overall industrial and agricultural development.

Substantial indirect subsidies from the Soviet Union have undoubtedly helped to strengthen the entire Cuban economy, including the health system. This support has been through the purchase of Cuban sugar at prices higher than the world market level, and the sale of Soviet oil to Cuba at prices lower than the world level. Thus, in the 1970s, the USSR purchased most of the Cuban sugar output at 36 cents per pound (when the world price was down to 10 cents), and it sold oil to Cuba for $10 per barrel (when the world price had risen to $30). Cuba, nevertheless, owes a substantial debt to the Soviet Union and other Eastern European countries.

Delivery of Health Services

The central features of Cuban health care delivery are that (with the minor exception of certain drugs), all services are available without charge to everyone, and they are provided by salaried teams of personnel in government facilities.

Ambulatory Care. Most prominent in the health care delivery pattern are the multiple preventive and therapeutic services of the 423 polyclinics that were located throughout the country in 1984. Each structure served about 25,000 people, and each medical team of four doctors (internist, pediatrician, obstetrician–gynecologist, and dentist) and allied personnel served about 5,000. Thus, each polyclinic included about five teams.

From the postrevolutionary outset of the Cuban health system, polyclinics were the point of entry to the system, the place where primary health care (PHC) was provided and from which referrals were made to hospitals or other resources. By 1975, enough personnel had been trained to provide complete health teams to most polyclinics, and to put greater emphasis on the comprehensive scope of modern PHC. As the WHO/UNICEF Conference at Alma Ata in 1978 pointed out, PHC had to stress prevention and outreach to families, not merely therapeutic responses to patient complaints.

The importance of community participation was emphasized in the 1975 Constitution, just as it was in the 1978 Declaration of Alma Ata on PHC. Efforts were made to involve the local Committees for the Defense of the Revolution in both policy making and operations of the polyclinics.

With expansion of polyclinic staffing, it was possible to "sectorize" the population served by each medical team. Thus, the approximately 5,000 people living in a geographic sector would be served by a particular team; in this way the patients became well acquainted with their doctor, for better continuity of care. (A dissatisfied patient was free to change to another team, but this was said to happen rarely.) With the relative stability of the patients living in each sector, preventive services, such as immunizations or cervical Pap smears, could be more fully performed. Many home visits could also be made in the afternoons to patients living in the nearby sector of each polyclinic team.

As communicable diseases have declined in Cuba, as well as the general mortality of infants and children, the chronic diseases of later life, such as cancer, have naturally increased in prevalence. This has heightened the importance of periodic health examinations of adults, for early case-detection and for the monitoring of patients with chronic disorders, such as heart disease or diabetes. Using the Soviet term, Cuban polyclinics in the mid-1970s began to emphasize *dispensarization.* Health examinations and diagnostic tests were performed systematically on the adults in each sector. If patients did not come to the polyclinic, as scheduled, they would be contacted by mail or by a home visit. Health education on smoking, diet, and other chronic disease risk factors has also been enhanced.

In 1983, Cuba set about exploring the concept of the *family practitioner* in selected polyclinics. With this concept, physicians trained as specialists in family medicine (through a broadly oriented residency) would serve a population of only about 130 families, or 600 to 700 people. There would still be four-doctor teams in this polyclinic to back up the generalist. If this pattern proves to be successful, it may be extended throughout the country.

Another innovation of the late 1970s was establishment of the *teaching polyclinic.* Some 32 of these had been developed by 1984 at locations convenient to the four medical schools. The objective was to provide settings where medical students and others could see and participate in model programs of PHC. Hopefully, this would increase the interest and competence of young physicians in the PHC concept.

The growth and development of Cuban polyclinics are well reflected in the rates of utilization of ambulatory care. Polyclinic consultations (both preventive and therapeutic) were reported to be made at a rate of 1.4 per person per year in 1965. They rose gradually to 3.3 per person per year in 1982. In addition, emergency services are provided at hospital out-patient departments, and these increased from 0.5 to 1.8 per person per year between 1963 and 1982. Combining these two rates of ambulatory care gives a figure of 5.1 contacts per person per year in 1982.

The services of dental clinics were provided at a rate of only 0.1 per person per year in 1963. They increased 10-fold, to 1.1 dental services per person per year in 1982.

Regarding personal preventive services, immunizations are, of course, done routinely on children at the polyclinics. The best indication of their effects is the trend in rates of the communicable diseases responsive to immunization. Morbidity rates are not available, but death rates from the six main immunizable diseases were as follows:

Disease	Deaths per 100,000	
	1960	1982
Diphtheria	0.7	0.0
Tetanus	4.4	0.1
Pertussis	1.0	0.1
Measles	1.1	0.2
Poliomyelitis	0.5	0.0
Tuberculosis (BCG)	14.9	1.0

Cervical cytology examinations, through Pap smears of adult women, have been done at the polyclinics at an increasing rate. The figure was 91.5 per 1,000 women over 19 years of age in 1969, rising to 164.6 examinations per 1,000 such women in 1982.

Cuban policy on population and birth control has been moderate. Family planning is not actively promoted, since the country does not feel any pressure of overpopulation. (Indeed, since the revolution there has been a shortage of labor, especially for agricultural harvesting.) Women or men who request contraceptive advice or materials, however, are provided these as part of the regular polyclinic services. There is no religious objection. Regarding abortion, the law remains the same as it was before the revolution—namely, that a pregnancy may be interrupted only to preserve the life or the health of the mother. In practice, there is said to be no significant opposition to induced abortions. When a woman requests an abortion, the reasons are discussed and an effort may be made to persuade her to have the baby; if she has a sound medical or social reason (e.g., being unmarried or simply not wanting another child although married) for terminating the pregnancy, the abortion is usually performed. This is considered preferable to denial and risking an illegal abortion outside of proper medical facilities. In 1977, in fact, two induced abortions in hospitals were reported for every three live births.

Hospital Services. The staffing of hospitals with full-time specialists and allied personnel is adequate but not abundant. Large teaching hospitals have about 2 health personnel per bed, but the average municipal or provincial facility has 1.0 to 1.5 personnel per bed. As medical standards have risen, Cuban health leaders have perceived a shortage of nurses, similar to that in developed countries. Also, as in affluent industrialized countries, most young physicans seem to prefer being appointed to a hospital staff rather than a polyclinic staff. The top administrative officer of every hospital is invariably a physician, who may spend part of his time doing clinical work. He is usually assisted by a nonmedical administrator for various management functions. Outside of Cuba's 26 large teaching hospitals, modern equipment for diagnostic or treatment purposes is relatively modest. Because of the U.S. embargo, most sophisticated equipment comes from Europe or Japan.

Most hospital beds are in small wards of six to eight patients per room. Although there is little privacy, at each bedside there is a comfortable chair, in which a relative may stay throughout the day and overnight; free meals are also provided to relatives. Medical examinations of patients are done in separate examining rooms. A few single-bed rooms are available for special leaders and dignitaries.

The emphasis on ambulatory care in Cuba has understandably slowed down the rate of increase in the utilization of hospitals. The rates of admission to all types of hospital bed (general, psychiatric, maternity, pediatric, etc.) were as follows:

Year	Admissions per 1,000 per Year
1963	94
1970	126
1977	125
1982	143

The average length of stay in 1963 and 1970 was about 10 days. It declined to 9.3 days in 1977 and 9.0 days in 1982.

The great reduction in both infant (especially in the neonatal period) and maternal mortality has doubtless been associated with the increased rate of childbirths occurring in hospitals. In 1963, of all childbirths 62 percent were delivered in hospitals by physicians or under their immediate supervision. By 1982, this had risen to more than 98 percent of all childbirths.

The overall accomplishments of the Cuban health system have made a worldwide impression, especially in other developing countries. Young people come from Africa and Asia, as well as Latin America, to study in Cuban medical and other technical schools. The Cuban government also feels an obligation to other developing countries, in a "spirit of international cooperation." In 1983, Cuba sent more than 3,000 health workers, including 1,743 doctors, to serve in 26 other countries; these were not only socialist nations, such as Vietnam and Angola, but also struggling nonsocialist countries, such as Tanzania or Iraq.

Cuban efforts to build a socialist society have clearly been successful in the national health system. In education, nutrition, social security, housing, and the general level of living, progress for the general population has also been substantial. The achievement of greater social equity is reflected in changes in income distribution between 1953 and 1978. Over that 25-year period, the share of total income received by the lower half of the population increased from 6.2 to 32.8 percent; the share of total income of the highest tenth of the population declined from 38.5 to 21.1 percent. (In Mexico, by contrast, over essentially the same period, the income of the lowest three-fifths of the population declined from 30.6 to 20 percent, while the share of the top tenth rose from 38.6 to 43.5 percent.)

The gains in economic productivity of Cuba have not been as great as those in health and personal well-being. Industrial development has been slight, and Cuba's earnings still depend mainly on the export of sugar. But real increases have occurred in the output of citrus fruits, fish, textiles, meat and dairy products, and other consumer goods—even refrigerators and television sets. Cuba has nearly achieved self-sufficiency in food production, but is far

from this in other sectors. The national health system has probably been the brightest feather in the socialist cap, and has been attracting increasing attention of other developing countries as a model. As stated in 1988 by a West German observer of Cuba's *internacionalismo* in health services, "Today, many Third World countries view Cuba not as Moscow's representative but as its successor." Officials of the World Health Organization have repeatedly pointed to Cuba as proof that the goal of "Health for All" is achievable.

ALBANIA

Couched between Yugoslavia and Greece on the east and the Adriatic Sea on the west, Albania is a small country of 3,000,000 people (1986) in Eastern Europe. Although not religious in the usual sense, its population is predominantly of Moslem background. Albania became an independent nation in 1912. Italian fascism controlled the country from 1939 to 1944, when a communist guerilla movement gained power.

Since 1944, political and economic policies have become clearly socialist, although relationships have grown increasingly strained with other socialist nations. After periods of close ties with the Soviet Union and then with China, Albania's fiercely independent interpretatin of Marxist–Leninist principles led to its consideration of these powers as "revisionist." In spite of isolation from almost all other nations, Albania has been able to develop a health system that provides greatly improved services to its population. Also by 1984 the adult literacy level was raised to 75 percent, although the GNP per capita, $1,655, was still very low for a European country.

Health System Organization

Soon after its liberation from fascist occupation in 1944, the People's Socialist Republic of Albania established a Ministry of Health to which virtually all responsibilities for health services, education, research, and regulation were assigned. At the national capital, Tirana, there were directorates for (1) curative and prophylactic institutions, (2) hygiene and epidemiology, (3) maternal and child health, (4) health personnel training, (5) planning and finance, (6) pharmaceuticals (production and distribution), (7) health statistics, (8) scientific research, and (9) administration.

Under MOH supervision several other major entities perform research and also provide certain services. These are (1) the Institute of Research in Hygiene and Epidemiology, (2) the Institute of Tuberculosis, (3) the Institute of Folk Medicine, (4) the Directorate of Health Education, (5) the Pharmaceutical Industry, (6) the Central Laboratory for Control of Drugs, and (7) the Institute of Military Medicine.

Albania is much less urbanized than other European countries—only 34 percent in 1984. The country is divided into 26 administrative districts, each of which is headed by a people's council. The Albanian Labor Party, with a strongly communist ideology, is in full control. Under each people's council is a health section, which has immediate responsibility for the health program and services in the district.

In each district there is one major hospital, usually several smaller hospitals, and numerous polyclinics and health centers for ambulatory care. In the cities the hospitals and polyclinics are separate structures, but in rural areas they are often combined in one complex. One section of each polyclinic is usually open all hours of the day and night for emergency service, and an ambulance may be on hand for transportation of patients. Other health facilities in all districts include rural health centers with one physician and some other personnel, small maternity homes (for childbirths), maternal and child health examination clinics, units for health education, and in very small communities, village health posts staffed by a single nurse-midwife. As in the USSR model, there are many sanitary–epidemiological stations with staffs devoted to the promotion of hygiene and environmental sanitation. There are also dental clinics for children and adults.

Government is all-important in the Albanian health system; no voluntary health agencies are reported except the Red Cross, which is publicly subsidized. Likewise, no private market in health services is legally permitted in the country. Physicians, pharmacists, and other professionals are licensed only to work in the governmental framework. If any medical or dental service is sold privately, it must be done surreptitiously and this would doubtless be on a very small scale.

Health Resources

Most conspicuous among the achievements of the health system of Albania has been its great enlargement of the national supplies of every type of human and physical resource. Under a central plan, the Ministry of Health has systematically set out to train relatively large numbers of health personnel and to construct various types of hospital and facility for ambulatory care.

After national liberation in 1944, the first health personnel training school established was not in medicine, but in nursing. A school of nursing, with a 1-year curriculum, was founded in 1946, and then extended to a 3-year program in 1948. No school of medicine was started until 1952. The medical curriculum requires 5 years of study after secondary school, and in the 1980s there were about 150 graduates per year. Training for dentistry was added in 1959, and for pharmacy in 1970.

The growth of Albania's supply of physicians has been enormous. From 102 doctors in all Albania (trained abroad) in 1938, the supply increased to 3,840 in 1984. This meant an increase from 12 to 132 physicians per 100,000 population. With this expansion and the prohibition of private practice, it became possible to provide physician's services almost everywhere. (In 1980, some 1,400 doctors were reported to be stationed in small rural health centers.) Postgraduate medical education is mandatory in Albania. It is theoretically required of physicians for a few months every 5 years.

Virtually all other types of health personnel have also been greatly increased. Even by 1977, the World Health Organization reported 4,100 nurse-midwives, 2,860 professional nurses, 1,470 auxiliary nurses, and many hundreds of pharmacists, dentists, laboratory technicians, and others.

Hospitals and other health facilities in Albania have been expanded as much as health personnel. In 1950 there were 69 facilities with beds in the whole country, and these increased to 772 by 1982; various ambulatory care facilities were expanded from 362 in 1950 to 3,324 in 1982. Counting all types of structures—general hospitals, maternity homes, tuberculosis sanatoria, and so on—in 1982 there were 17,831 beds, or 6.4 per 1,000 population; such a ratio is usually found only in countries of much greater wealth. Moreover, health facilities were located in appropriate relationship to the distribution of populations; of the 4,096 units of all types in 1982, 85 percent were located in rural regions.

The relatively few large industrial enterprises in Albania have special polyclinics for the workers. The schools also have general clinics and dental clinics for children. The typical urban or rural polyclinic serves thousands of people; these are divided into geographic "sectors" of 3,000 to 4,000 people, linked to a team of general physician, pediatrician, and nurse-midwife.

After 1944, pharmaceutical production and distribution was gradually nationalized and expanded. By 1982 a central government pharmaceutical enterprise was producing 900 drugs and cosmetics, although antibiotics and several other essential drugs still had to be imported. A central Drug Control Laboratory was organized in 1965 to test all imported as well as domestically produced drugs. The Institute of Folk Medicine also does research on medicinal herbs. More than 4,000 pharmacies are located throughout the nation, and of these 2,000 are in rural areas. Pharmacies all come under the Ministry of Health, in addition to the pharmacy departments of hospitals and larger polyclinics.

Some Health Outcomes

Nearly all health services are available to the people of Albania free of charge. Relatively small charges are made only for drugs (outside of hospitals) and for dental replacements. Great emphasis is put on prevention. Screening for chronic disorders is widely promoted and general health education is regarded as a function of all health workers. In addition, each of the 26 districts has a "house of health

education," which distributes educational material on health problems.

Few data are available on the volume of health services provided in the Albanian health system, but the trend of childbirth attendance is probably significant. In 1938 fewer than 1.0 percent of all births were attended by a midwife or any other trained person. By 1960, childbirth attendances by qualified personnel were up to 38 percent. By 1970 this rate was 76 percent and by 1982 it was 99 percent. With its relatively small population, Albania has not encouraged contraception, but it is available. The birth rate has remained high—26 births per 1,000 population in 1986—although it had been 35 per 1,000 in 1965.

Malaria was rampant in Albania before 1944. It is now said to be absent or rare, as a result of the work of the sanitary–epidemiological programs. Tuberculosis has also been greatly reduced. In 1951 there were 296 newly reported cases, and in 1981 such cases numbered 35. Smallpox, syphilis, and cholera, common before liberation, have been wiped out. Safe water was reported to be available to 92 percent of the Albanian population in 1984.

The infant mortality rate in Albania declined from 112 per 1,000 live births in 1960 to 40 per 1,000 in 1987. By that year life expectancy at birth had reached 72 years. All of these achievements, of course, cannot be attributed solely to the health system, but considering the generally low level of living suggested by Albania's per capita GNP, the health services have surely had significant effects.

DEMOCRATIC PEOPLE'S REPUBLIC OF KOREA

The Korean peninsula in northeast Asia was dominated by Japan around 1907, and remained largely under Japanese control until the end of World War II. After the defeat of Japan, the northern half of the country became dominated by the Soviet Union, and the southern half (below the 38th parallel) by the United States. In 1950, war broke out between the northern and southern halves, ending in a truce in 1953. In that year national reconstruction started in the north, with a socialist 3-year plan (1954–1956) and then a 5-year plan

(1957–1961). North Korea became known as the Democratic People's Republic of Korea, which in most sectors including health, looked to the Soviet Union for both advice and assistance. Over the next two decades, the country was transformed from a predominantly agricultural economy in 1953 (66 percent agriculture and 34 percent industry) to an economy based only 26 percent on agriculture and 74 percent on industry in 1972.

A new Constitution in 1972 divided North Korea into nine provinces and four major cities with provincial status. Below these were several jurisdictions under provincial control: 152 counties, 17 cities, 152 towns, and 36 urban districts. At the most local level are 228 workers' districts and 4,151 villages or small urban areas. The health services are entirely governmental and their administration and organization correspond esseentially with these general political jurisdictions. The Constitution calls for free availability of health services, including pharmaceutical products, to every resident.

In 1985, North Korea had a population of 20,400,000. With considerable industrial development—supported by substantial investments from the Soviet Union, China, and other socialist countries—the culture became dynamic and urbanized. The GNP per capita was $1,134, much less than Cuba's but much more than in the People's Republic of China. The literacy level of adults had reached 96 percent by 1985.

Production of Health Resources

With the end of hostilities in 1953, great efforts were directed to the expansion of basic health resources. Between the defeat of Japan (in 1945) and 1950, three medical schools were established. Over the next 20 years, seven more medical schools were developed, so that by the 1984–85 academic year 2,200 young doctors were being graduated from 10 schools. The medical curriculum requires the customary 6 years of university study after completion of secondary school. All graduates must enter government service.

In 1979 there were 40,750 doctors (including a small percentage of stomatologists) in North Korea, or a ratio of 233 per 100,000 population. Their distribution throughout the country was determined largely by the location of health centers and hospitals, essentially proportional to the distribution of the population.

The capacity of hospitals also increased rapidly. In 1946 there had been 85 small hospitals in North Korea with about 2,100 beds. By 1979, there were reported to be 210,000 beds in hospitals and in larger health centers; this meant 12 beds per 1,000. Health facilities for both in-patient and ambulatory care had been developed in the main cities of all provinces and in virtually all 152 counties. At the 4,400 local rural or urban community areas, there are usually small health stations. Many of these local units are staffed by *associate doctors* who have been trained for only 2 years after secondary school. Finally there are more than 400 rest homes or "vacation homes" for workers, miners, and fishermen, whose working records are deemed to entitle them to a period (about 1 month) of rest and rehabilitation. Some 25,000 persons can be accommodated in these places at one time.

A modern pharmaceutical industry has been developed in North Korea, capable of producing most of the modern drugs needed; other drugs are imported. Traditional herbal medications also play a large part in the health services, and the herbs required are grown throughout the country. Ancient shamanistic medicine, involving magical procedures, has been repudiated as superstitious, but therapy with herbal preparations is widely advocated. It is reported that the majority of drugs used in North Korea are of herbal origin. There is an Institute of Oriental Medicine, devoted to careful study of these substances.

Delivery of Health Services

The North Korean health system stresses preventive medicine, health education, and continuing surveillance of all individuals and families. The basic structure was initiated in 1963, but it took some time to develop. The principles were spelled out in a Public Health Law of April 1980, as the *section doctor* program. Under this, small population groups of about 600 people are assigned to one physician at a local health station, health center, or even a small hospital. He or she is expected to travel around the section as frequently as once or twice a week. A "health card" is kept on every resident, and all health problems are recorded on it. Complex disorders that cannot be handled by the local unit are referred to a county or provincial hospital. Identification of a pregnant woman calls for notification of the nearest hospital-based obstetrician, who then visits the home. The section doctors visit workshops and farms, as well as homes. As a North Korean health leader expressed it: "patients do not look for doctors, but doctors look for patients." Medical and surgical specialists from the county hospitals (sometimes also from the larger provincial hospitals) make general rounds of households once or twice a year.

Since all these health services are available without any personal charges, they are financed by general government revenues. Salaries must be very low, or the data may not be reliable, but in 1983 total government health expenditures were reported as only $17 per capita per year, which amounts of only 1.5 percent of GNP. The health achievements, however, were remarkable. The infant mortality rate declined from 85 per 1,000 live births in 1960 to 26 in 1987. Life expectancy at birth in 1984 was reported to be 68 years and 70 years in 1987. The North Korean government reported in 1984 that 100 percent of the population had access to safe drinking water and that the average food intake was 134 percent of daily caloric requirements. It also reported that 99 percent of childbirths were attended by trained personnel. Immunizations, however, were less impressive; DPT vaccinations were stated to have reached 62 percent of children, polio 70 percent, and measles only 35 percent. These modest levels of immunizations reported (probably because of shortages of the vaccines) perhaps increase the credibility of the other more impressive statistics.

SUMMARY COMMENT

The similarities among the health systems of Cuba, Albania, and North Korea should not be surprising. As small socialist nations, taking shape in recent decades, all three modeled their health systems on that of the Soviet Union. Having much lower per capita GNPs and more frugal living conditions than the USSR, in fact, some of the rigidities of the Soviet model were perhaps less objectionable than they proved to be in the Soviet European homeland.

The overwhelmingly govermental character of the health system in each of these three countries has generated no significant reactions. The abundant availability of health services, compared both with earlier days in the countries and with conditions in other countries of similar income level today, has more than satisfied almost everyone. The remarkable national development of health resources, their efficiency of utilization, and the effectiveness of the health systems in advancing the well-being of the populations in all three countries have won the plaudits of the World Health Organization and other international groups.

REFERENCES

Cuba

Cuba Resource Center, "A Promise Kept: Health Care in Cuba." *Cuba Review,* 8(1):3–37, 1978.

Danielson, R. S., *Cuban Medicine.* New Brunswick, N. J.: Transaction Books, 1979.

Editorial de Ciencias Sociales, *Diez Anos de Revolucion en Salud Publica.* Habana: Instituto del Libro, 1969.

El Centro Nacional de Informacion de Ciencias Medicas, *Revista Cubana de Administraction de Salud,* 10(1), January–March 1984.

Gomez, Manuel R., "Occupational Health in Cuba." *American Journal of Public Health,* 71(5):520–524, May 1981.

Grundy, Paul H., and P. P. Budetti, "The Distribution and Supply of Cuban Medical Personnel in Third World Countries." *American Journal of Public Health,* 70(7):717–719, July 1980.

Guttmacher, Sally, "The Prevention of Health Risks in Cuba." *International Journal of Health Services,* 17(1):179–189, 1987.

Hamilton, Nora, "The Cuban Economy: Dilemmas of Socialist Construction," in W. A. Chaffee, Jr. and G. Prevost (Editors), *Cuba: A Different America.* Totowa, N.J.: Rowman & Littlefield, 1989, pp. 36–53.

Harrison, Paul, "Cuba's Health Care Revolution." *World Health,* pp. 2–7.

Huberman, Leo, "Cuba: A Revolution Revisited." *The Nation,* 2 August 1965, pp. 51–54.

Lockwood, Lee, *Castro's Cuba, Cuba's Fidel.* New York: Macmillan, 1967.

Long, William R., "Cuba Shifts Priority from Social

to Economic Issues." *Los Angeles Times,* 31 December 1984.

Ministerio de Salud Publica, *Revista Cubana de Administracion de Salud.* 10(1), January–March, 1984.

Ministerio de Salud Publica, *Salud Publica en Cifras 1970.* Habana, 1971.

Navarro, Vicente, "Health, Health Services, and Health Planning in Cuba." *International Journal of Health Services,* 2:397–432, 1972.

Navarro, Vicente, "Workers' and Community Participation and Democratic Control in Cuba." *International Journal of Health Services,* 10(2):197–215, 1980.

Nelson, Harry, "Huge Gains: Cuba's Health Care Reaches Its People." *Los Angeles Times,* 16 June 1980.

Oberg, L. R., *Human Services in Postrevolutinary Cuba.* Westport, Conn.: Greenwood Press, 1984.

Ordonnez Carceller, Cosme, and Pedro Pons Bravet, "Prevalencia de Factores de Riesgo Coronario en Area de Salud del Policlinico Communitario Docente 'Plaza de la Revolucion'." *Revista Cubana de Administracion de Salud,* 10(1):15–21, February–March 1984.

Republica de Cuba, Ministerio de Salud Publica, *Informe Anual 1982.* Habana, 1983.

Republica of Cuba, "Reorganisation of Social Security Scheme." *Bulletin of the International Social Security Association,* April–May 1961, pp. 258–259.

Roemer, Milton I., "Health Development and Political Policy: The Lesson of Cuba." *Journal of Health Politics, Policy and Law,* 4(4):570–580, Winter 1980.

Roemer, Milton I., *Cuban Health Services and Resources.* Washington, D.C.: Pan American Health Organization, 1976.

Rojas Ochoa, F., "El Policlinico y la Asistencia a Pacientes Ambulatorios en Cuba." *Revista Cubana de Medicina,* 10:207–255, March–April, 1971.

Rojas Ochoa, F., "La Red Hospitalaria del Ministerio de Salud Publica en el Periodo 1958–1969." *Revista Cubana de Medicina,* 10:3–42, January–February 1971.

Rosenberg, J. D., "Health Care and Medicine in Cuba," in W. A. Chaffee. Jr. and G. Prevost (Editors), *Cuba: A Different America.* Totowa, N. J.: Rowman & Littlefield, 1989, pp. 116–128.

Smith, H. M., "Castro's Medicine." *MD Magazine,* 27:144–163, 1983.

Stuhrenberg, Michael, "Pulling Cuban Soldiers Out of Angola." *World Press Review,* December 1988, pp. 30–33.

Ubell, Robert N., "High-Tech Medicine in the Caribbean: 25 Years of Cuban Health Care." *New England Journal of Medicine,* 309(23):1468–1472, 8 December 1983.

United Nations Fund for Population Activities, *Review of the Population Situation in Cuba and Suggestions for Assistance.* New York, Spring 1979.

World Health Organization, "Cuba," in *First Report of the World Health Situation 1954–1956,* Geneva, May 1959, pp. 177–178.

Albania

Anon., *40 Years of Socialist Albania.* Tirana: State Planning Commission, 1984.

Bland, William B., *A Short Guide to the People's Socialist Republic of Albania.* Bristol, England: The Albanian Society, 1981.

Cikuli, Zisa, *Health Services in the People's Socialist Republic of Albania.* Tirana: 8 Netori Publishing House, 1984.

Keefe, Eugene K., et al., *Area Handbook for Albania.* Washington, D.C.: American University, Foreign Areas Studies, 1971.

North Korea

Anon., "Socialized Medicine in the DPRK." *Korea Focus,* 2(4):24–25, April–May 1974.

Anon., "Universal Free Medical Service in Korea." *Reunification of Korea* (Bogota, Colombia), No. 4, pp. 12–13, 1983.

Brun, Ellen, *Socialist Korea: A Case Study in Economic Development.* New York: Monthly Review Press, 1976.

Bunge, Frederica M., *North Korea: A Country Study.* Washington, D.C.: American University, Foreign Area Studies Program, 1981, pp. 102–104.

Lee, Mun Woong, "Rural North Korea under Communism: A Study of Sociocultural Change." Houston, Tex.: *Rice University Studies,* Vol. 62, No. 1, pp. 1–176, Winter 1976.

Salisbury, Harrison, "Reporter's Notebook: Isolated North Korea Isolates Visitors Too." *New York Times,* 7 June 1972, p. 12.

World Health Organization, *World Directory of Medical Schools.* 6th edition. Geneva: WHO, 1988.

PART FOUR

VERY POOR COUNTRIES

CHAPTER FOURTEEN

Entrepreneurial Health Systems in Very Poor Countries

Many countries are less economically developed and have substantially lower GNPs per capita than those whose health systems have been reviewed in the last several chapters. They may be described as very poor countries, although the poverty of the vast majority of their populations is attributable to different causes. The GNPs per capita of these countries have been under $500 through most of the 1980s, although some have risen above this level in the later years of the decade. The greatest proportion of these very low income countries are in sub-Sahara Africa, but some are also located in southern Asia.

The health system characteristics of these very poor countries correspond in large part to the dominant political ideology. While the differences are less conspicuous than in countries of higher economic levels and, because of the sparsity of data, they cannot be as readily identified, many variations may still be observed. In this chapter, we analyze the health systems of several very poor countries, in which the health policies have markedly entrepreneurial characteristics. Systems with more socially oriented health policies are considered in the following chapters. Three of the entrepreneurial systems are in African countries and two in Asian. All five countries are former colonies of European powers, which achieved their independence only after World War II. As self-governing nations, therefore, all are relatively young and undergoing continuous political changes. The first health system, analyzed in some depth, is that of Kenya.

KENYA

Kenya is one of several former British colonies on the coast of East Africa that won its na-tional independence in 1963. This was 4 years after the violent Mau Mau uprising, led by Jomo Kenyatta, who became the new nation's first president. In 1984, Kenya had a population of 19,717,000 and had acquired a reputation of political stability, in contrast to most African countries. This reputation was shaken in 1982 by an attempted military coup, led by young officers in the air force, but soon subdued.

Basic Socioeconomic Features

The economy of Kenya is mainly agricultural (coffee, tea, cereals, cotton), although significant shares of its income are derived from light industry, tourism, and mining. Production and trade are dominated by an ideology of free private enterprise, and this is reflected clearly in Kenya's health system. The nation's gross national product per capita in 1984 was $322, putting it at a very low level among the world's national economies.

As in most African countries, Kenya's people are members of some 47 distinct tribes that no longer play an official role in governing the nation, but doubtless influence interpersonal relationships and loyalties. Most important among those are the Kikuyus, constituting about 20 percent of the population. Since the midnineteenth century, Christian missionaries (mainly from Europe) have had great influence; currently, some 60 percent of the population is Protestant or Catholic. In the conversion strategy, mission medical services have played a significant part. Since independence, the literacy of the population has improved markedly, although in 1984, it was estimated at only 59 percent of adults (much lower in women), with 62 percent of children enrolled in schools. More than 90 percent of the Kenyan population are of black African background, but the small balance, divided between Asians (mostly from India) and Europeans, earn a disproportionately high share of the national income.

Kenya is divided into seven provinces, plus the large capital city of Nairobi (nearly 1,000,000 population). The provinces are further divided into 41 districts, which play an important part in the organization of health services. Governance of the provinces and districts, as in the colonial period, is not entrusted to the local people, but is in the hands of commissioners appointed by the central government. At independence the major political party was the Kenya African National Union (KANU), and in 1981 the president declared this to be the only legal party. Some 84 percent of Kenya's total population live in rural areas.

Organizational Structure of the Health System

In the formal structure of the Kenyan health system a central Ministry of Health plays the major role. This authority is responsible not only for all preventive "public health" services, but also for establishing and operating public hospitals, registering health practitioners, training many types of personnel, and performing various forms of environmental and pharmaceutical regulation.

Ministry of Health. The top technical officer of the Ministry of Health is the director of medical services, under whom are deputy directors in charge of hospitals, rural service development, training, medical research, administrative matters (financing and personnel), and other functions. In each of the seven provinces, the minister appoints a provincial medical officer, who is assisted by administrative personnel, nurses, sanitary officers, and others. In Nairobi and three other cities, the medical officer is appointed by the Ministry of Local Government. Within each province the districts are headed by a district medical officer of health (DMOH), also appointed centrally. In 1982, all 41 of the DMOH posts were staffed with a physician (a few being expatriates), the-

oretically responsible for all health activities (public and private) in his district.

The DMOH may be assisted by a nursing officer, a hospital secretary (administrator), a sanitarian, a health educator, a nutritionist, and others. Most districts, however, do not have full complements of such personnel as yet; they remain to be trained. Only a small fraction of the DMOHs, furthermore, have had public health training, and it is not surprising that they spend most of their time giving clinical service in the district hospital or in various rural health centers.

Below the level of the district, the Kenya Ministry of Health since 1972 has been developing a network of rural health units (RHU), intended to provide general primary health care to the rural population. The plan calls for 254 RHUs, or about 6 per district, each serving about 75,000 people (varying from 10,000 to 100,000). The headquarters of the RHU would ordinarily be in a health center, around which there might be several small dispensaries or health posts. The unit is headed by a *clinical officer,* who is not a physician, but typically a young man with 12 years of basic schooling and 3 years of training in a hospital on elementary diagnosis and treatment. The RHU staff also includes *enrolled nurses,* sanitary technicians, family health educators, and others. To learn cooperative teamwork for primary health care, all these personnel receive a 3-month training course at one of the Rural Health Training Centers established around the country.

As of 1984, about 120 of the contemplated 254 rural health units were reported to be staffed and operating. A full staff included about 24 health workers. It was estimated that these units brought primary health care within reach (i.e., within 4 kilometers distance) of about 30 percent of the rural Kenyan population. The staffs in the health centers are reported to be well-motivated, but their performance has frequently been handicapped by shortages of drugs and other basic medical supplies. Peripheral to the health centers are many small dispensaries, mainly for maternal and child health services, and staffed by briefly trained community health workers.

Other Ministries with Health Functions.
Other ministries and nonministerial entities of
the government of Kenya make various contributions to the nation's health system. Pre-
eminent is the University of Nairobi, which is
financed almost wholly by the national government but has a semiautonomous status in the
Office of the President. In 1985, the national
President, Daniel Moi, served as chancellor of
the university—a position that, though hon-
orary rather than administrative, symbolized
the university's importance. Since 1967, the
university has had a Faculty of Medicine. In
1974, university programs were also established to train pharmacists and dentists, and in
1980 a graduate course for registered nurses,
leading to a university diploma, was established.

Major responsibilities in environmental sanitation are carried by a separate Ministry of
Water Development. Its work is largely in the
cities and small towns, where public water systems are feasible. (Small-scale rural water supply units and latrines are developed by the subdivisions of the Ministry of Health.) The
Ministry of Agriculture operates a modest extension education program, which includes education on family nutrition. The Ministry of
Education operates all public elementary
schools, in which health education is part of
the curriculum. (Personal health services for
school children have not, however, been generally developed as yet.) The Ministry of Social
Services operates a few custodial facilities for
the disabled and the aged.

Still other health-related functions in government come under the Ministry of Labor.
Factory inspectors attempt to visit plants with
five or more workers at least once a year, to
identify occupational hazards. Safety problems
get the greatest attention, but fumes, dusts, and
toxic substances are supposed to be monitored
by an industrial hygiene unit. Since in Nairobi
alone some 7,000 factories or workplaces are
registered with the Ministry of Labor, the degree of surveillance by that ministry's small
staff could hardly be adequate. Finally, there is
a worker's compensation program for industrial injuries, administered by the Ministry of
Labor. Financial compensation to the disabled

worker is paid by an insurance fund, but medical services are a responsibility of each enterprise; if a government facility is used, no payment is necessary, but if the employer wishes
to have the injured worker treated in a private
hospital, he must pay the costs.

It is the Ministry of Local Government that
bears the greatest official health responsibilities, outside the Ministry of Health. This ministry oversees and subsidizes Kenya's four
major cities, which maintain significant health
services. Under the Nairobi City Council, and
not included within the program or budget of
the Ministry of Health, health activities are
substantial. A 350-bed maternity hospital is
highly utilized. In addition, there are 11 sub-
sidiary maternity units with 24 beds each. The
city also operates 24 health centers for preventive and curative services, plus 22 dispensaries
for emergencies and other treatment services.
To staff this large establishment, there are
posts for 120 full-time doctors, although 40 of
these posts were not filled in 1982. In addition,
the city of Nairobi provides its own environmental sanitation surveillance services, communicable disease control, and health services
for school children. A staff of community
health nurses and sanitary inspectors do most
of this work under the direction of two medical
officers of health. Not surprisingly this health
program absorbed 60 percent of the Nairobi
City Council budget in 1982.

Kenya's three other major cities are also responsible for much of their health services.
They operate health centers and dispensaries,
mainly at municipal expense, with some subsidy from the Ministry of Local Government.
Technical standards in these units are theoretically supervised by the Ministry of Health.

Finally, within the governmental sector of
the Kenyan health system, two other health activities are loosely linked to the Ministry of
Health but for all practical purposes are autonomous. One is the Medical Research Institute,
established with foreign funding. It is physically housed in the major health facility of the
nation, the Kenyatta National Hospital, and is
devoted principally to research on tropical diseases in collaboration with the global program
of the World Health Organization.

The other autonomous but government health program is the National Hospital Insurance Fund, a form of social insurance for financing all or part of the costs of private hospital care. Though legally under the Ministry of Health, the fund is administered wholly independently and its financial operations (both revenue and expenditures) are entirely separate. All Kenyans, employed or self-employed, who in 1982 earned 1,000 Kenyan shillings (K.Sh. 1,000) or more a month, were required by law to pay K.Sh. 20 per month into the fund. In 1982, the fund had slightly more than 500,000 contributing members, amounting to some 2,000,000 covered people, with dependents (12 percent of the national population). Employers make no contribution on behalf of their employees, but they are obligated to see that qualified workers pay their premiums. A small proportion of the covered persons were individuals earning less than K.Sh. 1,000 per month who wished to enroll voluntarily.

The basic objective of the National Hospital Insurance Fund is different from that of the usual social insurance program. Its focus is on the more affluent, rather than the poorer, members of society. As stated in a lecture by the fund's director, "It is intended that the scheme should provide for the largest possible number of people in Kenya the opportunity of occupying the hospital beds available in Kenya, for which charges are made, by providing daily allowances to contributors towards meeting those charges." In other words, the Hospital Insurance Fund is oriented toward increasing the use of private hospitals, or private beds in public hospitals, for those whose earnings are high enough to qualify. The benefits payable by the fund are somewhat less than the usual charges for private hospital care; therefore the individual ordinarily pays extra (unless he or she has supplemental private hospital insurance, which is also marketed in Kenya). Moreover, coverage is limited to 180 days of hospitalization per family per year, although this can be extended by special request from the doctor.

In 1980–81, the National Hospital Insurance Fund collected K.Sh. 71,500,000 from its members, but paid out only K.Sh. 43,500,000 in benefits (including administrative expenses), leaving a surplus of K.Sh. 28,000,000. Since the fund is entirely separate from the Ministry of Health budget, these moneys were expected to be used for increasing future hospital benefits.

Organized Nongovernment or Voluntary Programs. Outside of government, there are several organized activities in the Kenyan health system, aside from the purely private sector of medical care. Some 15 parastatal enterprises are engaged in numerous activities related to transportation (railroads, port authority, airline) or agriculture—the Tea Development Authority, the Coffee Board, and others. The Ministry of Transport and Communication has certain responsibilities for the enterprises in its field, and the Ministry of Agriculture for the others. These semipublic enterprises provide relatively broad health services for their employees and their families. In the sugar industry, some estates and processing plants are parastatal, and others are purely private.

Private enterprises with 500 workers or more also generally have their own clinics, staffed by nurses and doctors, either full-time or part-time. About 10 enterprises were large enough in 1982 to have such health services. These in-plant health services treat acute illness, whether work-related or not, but if a chronic disorder develops, the case is referred elsewhere for care.

Voluntary nonprofit agencies are another significant part of the organizational structure of the Kenyan health system. Most important by far are the religious missions, Catholic and Protestant, which have operated hospitals and clinics in Kenya since about 1900. Christian missionaries from Europe and America learned early that their religious messages were more effective if they were accompanied by treatment for the physical ailments of people. Most highly developed are the Catholic missions, which in 1980 operated 27 hospitals (having resident doctors) with 3,565 beds, another 55 health centers with 1,293 beds, plus 135 dispensaries and special clinics. Coordinating all the Catholic missions is the Kenyan

Catholic Secretariat, which has a medical department.

Protestant missions in 1980 operated 14 general hospitals with resident doctors that had 1,731 beds, another 29 health centers with 366 beds, and 38 other ambulatory care clinics. These activities are coordinated by the Protestant Churches Medical Association. It is noteworthy that nearly one-fourth of the overall budgets of the mission medical facilities has been supported by subsidies from the Kenya Ministry of Health. The ministry obviously looks on the missions as providing services complementary to its own and attempts to coordinate the two types of resources geographically. In the 1980s, the Catholic mission leadership claimed that its emphasis was shifting from hospitalization to primary health care.

Other nonreligious voluntary health agencies in Kenya include the Red Cross, the Leprosy Society, the Child Welfare Society, and the Catholic Relief Fund for Malnutrition. These organizations also receive subsidies from the government. The Lion's Club has operated a health care program for children.

The Private Health Care Market. Finally, as elsewhere, there is a purely private market for medical care in Kenya, a substantial part of the total health system, especially ambulatory care. Oldest are the traditional healers, who are still major providers of health care in all of sub-Sahara Africa. These practitioners are of many types, classified by one observer as trance-healers, soothsayers, black magic doctors, herbalists, and bone setters. They may offer these healing services full-time or part-time, and they charge fees. They practice in both cities and rural areas, although in the latter, where other health services are less available, they play a relatively larger role.

The herbalists and sometimes the other healers dispense drugs, which may consist of a combination of traditional and modern remedies (such as penicillin). Drug peddlers, who have acquired stocks of contraceptive pills, vitamins, and sometimes antibiotics, sell them at busstops and street corners. In addition, many nonprescribed drugs are purchased at almost any general market. In the cities, private pharmacies sell modern drugs, both on medical prescription and over-the-counter.

Most visible in the private market of medical care in Kenya are the private physicians. Though estimates differ, it was agreed in 1982 that at least 70 percent of all doctors in Kenya were in full-time private practice, mainly as general practitioners. In addition, of the 30 percent of doctors working in government posts the great majority also engaged in private practice, when official hours were finished. There are relatively few dentists in Kenya, but the great majority of these are entirely in private practice.

Finally, there are growing numbers of private proprietary hospitals, over and above the mission hospitals, supported by insurance or patient fees. Government hospitals also have some private beds. Miscellaneous private vendors, such as opticians and sellers of prosthetic appliances and sickroom equipment, complete the private market for health care in Kenya.

Production of Health Resources

The organizational structure of the Kenyan health system, of course, depends on many types of resources, produced both inside and outside the country.

Health Manpower. In 1981 there were 2,057 physicians recorded on the official Medical Registry of Kenya (in the Ministry of Health), but not all of them were in the country and actively engaged in medical work. Adjusting for those away or retired, there were estimated to be 1,685 active physicians, or about 10.5 per 100,000 population. Geographic distribution of doctors is extremely uneven; about 53 percent in 1981 were located in Nairobi, where fewer than 6 percent of the national population lived. The great majority of the rural population do not have reasonable access to a modern physician.

Until independence all physicians working in Kenya had to be trained elsewhere. In 1967, the University of Nairobi established a Medical Faculty, which in 1984 turned out about

100 medical graduates a year. The course lasts 5 years, after which a 1-year internship is required, plus 2 years of mandatory work in a government hospital. These 3 latter years are spent in the relatively large provincial general hospitals, or the Kenyatta National Hospital, and are not used (as in some countries) to provide medical coverage for rural populations. Of the 1,685 doctors in the country in 1981, about 1,200 were Kenyans (trained at home or abroad) and 485 were expatriates.

Dentists in 1981 numbered 197, and trained pharmacists 84. Most drug dispensing is done by briefly trained pharmaceutical technologists, who numbered 326. The most numerous type of qualified health personnel were enrolled nurses, who are trained for 2 years after elementary school. There were 9,190 of these nurses in 1981. Fully trained registered nurses (with 3 years of training after secondary school) numbered 6,892, or 43 per 100,000 population.

An especially important manpower resource in Kenya is the *clinical officer,* who heads the staff of all of the rural health centers. Always male, he has received 3 years of training in elementary medical diagnosis and treatment after completing secondary school. These essential health workers, particularly for rural areas, are trained in large hospitals, with emphasis on out-patient work. There were 1,100 of these personnel in 1978.

The Ministry of Health's program for nationwide coverage with rural health units (RHUs) includes a major training component. Many of the enrolled nurses have been trained as "community health nurses" in 12 schools operated by the ministry; this training includes midwifery for home deliveries. The ministry also operates six Rural Health Training Centers (in six provinces) with several manpower objectives. They offer basic training for *public health technicians,* who receive a 3-year course in environmental sanitation (670 in 1978). They train *family welfare field educators,* who promote family planning and other preventive health practices. (These personnel, nearly all women, are also known simply as *community health workers.*) Most important, the training centers offer 13-week courses on managerial

concepts and practical problems, designed to help the basic teams of rural health personnel to work together harmoniously in rural health centers and posts.

Other health personnel in Kenya are engaged principally in urban posts, including 192 laboratory technologists, 196 rehabilitation technologists, 120 radiographers, and 230 nutrition field workers. Voluntary agencies, such as the Kenyan Catholic Secretariat, have also trained primary health care workers, known as *public health aides.* In 1981 there were 61 of these at 27 posts; they were trained for 5 months to provide mainly preventive services for mothers and children.

The number of traditional healers in Kenya, important as they are, is not known. Law does not call for their registration. Since they are very widely available in rural areas, a rough estimate might suggest one healer per 1,000 people, or about 19,000 in all (considering both full-time and part-time practitioners)—much more than the number of physicians. Knowledgeable observers report that the magical healers are gradually declining, but not the herbalists or drug-peddlers.

Health Facilities. Both government and nongovernment bodies sponsor hospitals in Kenya. In 1981 there were 221 hospitals in all, with 28,108 beds. This meant a ratio that year of 1.77 hospital beds (including infant bassinets) per 1,000 population.

The various sponsorships of these hospitals may be estimated through reports from different sources. In 1977, the Ministry of Health reported a total of 80 government hospitals (including those for the armed forces) with 11,941 general beds. Reports from the Catholic and Protestant missions for 1980 indicated a total of 6,955 beds (located mainly in hospitals, but 30 percent were in health centers). The remainder of hospital beds are in purely private facilities, although some of these are attached to industrial establishments. A report of the National Hospital Insurance Fund categorized 41 hospitals as "private" in 1982. Making adjustments for the different dates of these figures, and for some expansion of resources, one can estimate the 1981 distribution of hospital beds in Kenya by sponsorship approximately as follows:

Sponsorship	Hospital Beds	Percentage
Government	13,000	46.3
Religious missions	7,000	25.0
Private	8,100	28.8
Total	28,100	100.0

Thus, broadly speaking, about 46 percent of Kenyan hospital bed resources are public, and this includes beds for the military establishment. About 54 percent of the beds are in the private sector, somewhat more than half of which are proprietary.

Other health facilities in Kenya include health centers, subcenters, dispensaries, and health posts—essentially for ambulatory care. In 1981 a total of 262 health centers were reported to be in operation, of which 84 were sponsored by missions and an indeterminate number by enterprises or agricultural estates. The balance of 178 were undoubtedly governmental and were staffed by at least a clinical officer, who treated sickness and injuries. Health subcenters and dispensaries, also mainly but not exclusively government-sponsored, numbered more than 1,200 in 1986. These units are staffed only by auxiliary personnel who can offer preventive services (including family planning), first aid, and referral to other facilities when necessary.

Health Commodities. Virtually all medical equipment, supplies, appliances, and drugs used in Kenya are imported. For certain drugs, foreign firms have established plants in Nairobi, where tablets or other preparations are made and packaged from imported chemical products. As for traditional herbals, some are imported from Asian countries and some are prepared domestically. Since modern drugs are relatively expensive, requiring scarce foreign currency, there are frequent shortages, especially in government hospitals and health centers.

Some reflection of the importance of drugs in the entire Kenyan health system is shown by data from Ministry of Health expenditures in 1977–78. In that fiscal year the ministry had budgeted K.Sh. 72,587,860 for drugs in all its facilities. Actual expenditures, however, proved to be K.Sh. 111,557,120, or 54 percent higher. With total recurrent expenditures of the ministry that year of K.Sh. 518,000,000, drugs alone absorbed 21.5 percent of overall MOH operating expenditures. (In a developed country, the equivalent expenditure would probably be between 5 and 10 percent.)

Health Knowledge. The Medical Research Institute, based in the Kenyatta National Hospital, is doing research on certain tropical diseases. It is supported partly by the World Health Organization. Almost all health-related knowledge used in Kenya, however, is acquired from abroad through journals and books. The great bulk of medical literature comes from Great Britain or the United States. Each year, a number of Kenyan medical and public health personnel are sent to Europe and America for specialized studies, principally through funding from international health agencies or bilateral aid programs.

The overall picture of health resources in Kenya is one of a meager supply in all categories. Considering the great poverty of the people, one might logically expect most of the resources to be in the public sector. In fact, the great majority of physicians serve a small minority of the population as private patients, and a majority of the hospital beds are in facilities requiring private payments for care. The human and physical health care resources in the public sector for most of the Kenyan people reflect a lower standard of capabilities. The population is 84 percent rural, but the medical resources are heavily concentrated in Nairobi and three other urban centers.

Economic Support

The economic support for the Kenyan health system, as in all countries, comes from various sources. For several of these, only estimates can be made.

Ministry of Health. For the fiscal year 1980–81, the total budget of the Ministry of Health was K.Sh. 1,131,000,000, counting both recurrent (operating) and development (capital) expenditures. About 75 percent of this was for operating purposes and 25 percent for capital purposes, mainly to construct health facilities. The total amounted to 6.2 percent of the overall national government budget. Of the ministry's total budget, about 11 percent of the funds came from multilateral or bilateral foreign aid.

In 1980–81, the MOH budget went for various purposes in the following distribution:

Purpose	Percentage
Central and provincial hospitals	43.0
District hospitals	26.1
Subsidies to mission hospitals	3.8
Rural health centers, etc.	11.8
Preventive services	6.7
Supplies and equipment	1.9
Training	6.4
All purposes	100.0

The heavy expenditure on hospitals (almost 73 percent of the total budget) is quite evident, in spite of the official policy emphasis of the MOH on the importance of primary health care. It is obviously difficult to reduce the historically major role of hospitals and medical specialists in the policy making of a national health system.

Other Government Sources. The MOH budget does not include the expenditures of the National Hospital Insurance Fund, which in 1980–81 were K.Sh. 43,500,000. The Nairobi City Council had health expenditures of K.Sh. 75,000,000. Other municipal councils in 1980–81 spent about K.Sh. 12,000,000 for health services.

Health expenditures by other ministries and agencies are estimated at about K.Sh. 23,500,000, distributed as follows:

Agency	Percentage
Ministry of Water Development	42.6
University of Nairobi (health science schools)	21.3
Ministry of Education (health education)	8.5
Ministry of Agriculture (nutrition education)	6.4
Ministry of Labor (factory inspection)	12.8
Ministry of Social Services	4.3
Medical Research Institute	4.3
All agencies	100.0

Organized Nonpublic Sources. Most important among these sources are expenditures for the health activities of religious missions. Data from the Kenya Catholic Secretariat and from the Protestant Churches Medical Association permit estimates for 1980–81. The calculation is complicated by the fact that funds spent for operating these health facilities come from several sources, and one must avoid "double counting."

The Catholic Secretariat Medical Department spent K.Sh. 72,000,000 in 1980–81 (about 52,000,000 for hospitals and the balance for other units). Based on the approximate proportions of the two programs, the Protestant Church medical activities probably cost about K.Sh. 25,000,000, or a total for both of K.Sh. 97,000,000. Although the Catholic organization does not break down the sources of its funds, the Protestant organization publishes such data for each of its hospitals. Based on a sample of three of the major Protestant hospitals, the sources of financing were distributed as follows:

Source of Support	Percentage
Patient fees (in-patient and out-patient)	59.9
Training fees	0.6
Government (Ministry of Health) grants	23.5
Overseas income	2.5
Value of donated services	8.7
Other sources	4.8
All sources	100.0

It should be noted that patient and training fees are privately paid, and belong under "purely private spending," considered later. The government grants have already been included in the expenditures of the Ministry of

Health. These sources account for 84 percent of mission medical expenditures. The other charitable and miscellaneous sources account for only 16 percent. The latter amounted to K.Sh. 15,520,000 in 1980–81.

Regarding other organized nonpublic voluntary sources for health expenditures, crude estimates can be made as follows. For each of the 15 parastatal enterprises in 1980–81, one can estimate annual health expenditures to average K.Sh. 200,000, or a total of K.Sh. 3,000,000. For the 10 large firms with in-plant medical services, one can estimate annual expenditures of K.Sh. 120,000 each, or a total of K.Sh. 1,200,000. Similarly, other estimates, shown later, lead to the following tabulation:

Source for Voluntary Support	K.Sh. (millions)
Religious mission charity	15.52
Parastatal enterprises (15)	3.0
Large business enterprises (10)	1.2
Agricultural estates	2.0
Voluntary health agencies (Red Cross, etc.)	6.0
Total	27.72

One might expect the total for voluntary health agencies to be higher, but most of these agencies in Kenya receive government subsidies. Altogether then, organized voluntary sources contributed about K.Sh. 27,720,000 to support health services in 1980–81.

Purely Private Spending. Financial support of the health system from purely private sources in Kenya is the most difficult to estimate. On the basis of studies done in other developing countries, however, it is probably substantial. In Kenya, it is possible to make estimates using three methods.

One method is based on the findings in a household survey of family expenditures done in 1974. Adjustments must be made for inflation, population growth, and persons per household. Accordingly, a per capita health expenditure was derived that yielded an annual national estimate of private health expenditures in 1981 of K.Sh. 1,130,240,000.

A second method of estimating private health expenditures is based on the *percentage* of household spending devoted to purchasing medical care and drugs; in 1974 this was 1.5 percent. Several social trends in Kenya suggest a rise in this percentage to an estimated 1.8 percent in 1981. Applying this to the 1981 average per capita income yielded a national estimate of K.Sh. 1,152,000,000.

A third method of deriving private health expenditures is through a series of estimates of the gross earnings of all types of private health care providers in Kenya. Gross earnings of doctors from private medical practice, for example, came from the fees paid by private patients. From several sources, one may learn the approximate average gross income of Kenyan doctors in full-time private practice (K.Sh. 30,000 per month in 1981), and also the earnings of government doctors from part-time private practice. Equivalent estimates could be made for other health care providers. This process yielded the following tabulation for 1981:

Private Health Care Providers	Gross Earnings in K.Sh. Millions
Private medical practitioners (1,180)	424.8
Government physicians (505) at 25 percent of private	45.5
Private hospitals (15,000 beds) at 60 percent occupancy	330.0
Drugs purchased in pharmacies	118.0
Dentists (150) in private practice	45.0
Traditional healers (16,000) at K.Sh. 1000 per month	192.0
Traditional birth attendants at K.Sh 30 each for 640,000 deliveries	19.2
Other miscellaneous private health expenditures	20.0
All private health care providers	1,194.5

Table 14.1. Health Expenditures in Kenya, by Source, 1981

Source	Kenyan Shillings	Percentage
Ministry of Health	1,131,000,000	
Other governmental agencies	154,000,000	
Public sector	1,285,000,000	52.0
Organized nonpublic agencies	27,720,000	
Private households	1,158,913,000	
Private sector	1,186,633,000	48.0
All sources	2,471,633,000	100.0

Source: Field study by M. I. Roemer, 1982.

In the opinion of several knowledgeable health leaders in Kenya, the preceding estimates of private professional earnings in 1981 were deemed to be conservative. Nevertheless, the resulting estimate was higher than estimates from the other two methods. To be cautious, one can take the average of the three methods, as follows:

First method	K.Sh. 1,130,240,000
Second method	1,152,000,000
Third method	1,194,500,000
Average	1,158,913,300

One could then estimate that, in 1981, health expenditures from all sources were distributed as shown in Table 14.1. In summary, 52 percent came from public sources and 48 percent from private sources. Relating the sum of expenditures in Kenyan shillings to Kenya's overall gross national product showed health spending to absorb 4.8 percent of GNP.

In spite of the numerous rough estimates required to yield the data for 1981 in Table 14.1, the results were generally confirmed in a study made for the Kenyan Ministry of Health by a British research team in 1986. Additional data had become available from a household expenditure study made in 1982. Based on slightly different categories, and examining only recurrent expenditures (i.e., excluding capital spending, which is a relatively small share), the findings are shown in Table 14.2. Since most capital spending is done by government, its inclusion would probably increase the public sector and yield proportions of about 50 percent public and 50 percent private for total health expenditures in 1983–84. Also, the relatively much larger private expenditures for drugs, reported in the later British study, were important; if this proportion for drugs had been estimated in the 1982 study, the net public/private sector relationship would likewise have been about 50–50.

The 1986 British study also provides valuable information on the income levels of households responsible for private health ex-

Table 14.2. Recurrent Health Expenditures in Kenya, by Source or Type of Private Service, 1983–84

Source or Type of Service	Kenyan Shillings	Percentage
Ministry of Health	1,210,400,000	
Municipalities	160,600,000	
Other government agencies	33,800,000	
Public sector	1,404,800,000	49
Religious missions	168,900,000	
Other voluntary agencies	36,800,000	
Private enterprises	11,400,000	
Private households:		
Institutional care	264,800,000	
Medical practitioners	216,000,000	
Drugs	680,000,000	
Other	93,300,000	
Private sector	1,471,200,000	51
All sources	2,876,000,000	100

Source: Bloom, G., M. Segall, and C. Thube, *Expenditure and Financing of the Health Sector in Kenya.* Nairobi: Ministry of Health, 1986.

Table 14.3. Private Health Expenditures: Percentage Distributions by Place of Residence and Family Income Level in Kenya, 1981–1983

Family Income Level	Urban	Rural	Total
Upper	52	4	56
Middle	29	8	37
Lower	2	5	7
All income levels	83	17	100

Source: Bloom, G., M. Segall, and C. Thube, *Expenditure and Financing of the Health Sector in Kenya.* Nairobi: Ministry of Health, 1986.

penditures in a generally poor developing country. It found that in the period 1981–1983, of all private expenditures, 56 percent came from a small proportion (perhaps 5 percent) of families with high incomes. Moreover, 83 percent came from the residents of cities that had 15 percent of the national population at the time. The details are presented in Table 14.3.

Management of Health System

The overall management of the Kenyan health system reflects its colonial past; its pattern of controls is highly centralized.

Health Planning. The major planning for health services is done by a unit within the Ministry of Health; its chief concern has been to cover Kenya's rural areas with health centers and health posts. Although the rural coverage plans, put forward in 1972, were less than half implemented by 1982, efforts have continued along the lines of the original blueprint. The planning is done entirely at the central government level but is based partly on reports from the provinces and districts. The weakness of the general health information system would seem to be reflected by the fact that the ministry had not issued an annual report of its resources, activities, and so on between 1968 and the mid-1980s.

Kenya also has a Ministry of Economic Planning and Development (MEPD), which includes a subdivision concerned with health and social services. The scope of this concern, however, is limited essentially to the program of the Ministry of Health. It is noteworthy that

health planning in both the MEPD and the Ministry of Health is not concerned with the health services of Kenya's private sector, which absorbs some 50 percent of total national health expenditures.

Within the MEPD is the Central Bureau of Statistics, which has conducted the surveys of household expenditures, including spending for health purposes. This bureau also issues such valuable compendia as the *Economic Survey 1982,* which contains data on the Kenyan national supply of health facilities and hospital beds. As noted earlier, some 73 percent of the Ministry of Health budget is devoted to supporting hospital services (half goes to the Kenyata National Hospital in Nairobi), in spite of the espoused priority of primary health care for the rural population.

Another discrepancy exists between planning objectives and reality in the magnitude of the private market in medical care. Of the modest supply of physicians, 70 percent are in full-time private practice and most of the remainder are in private practice part-time. Less than half of the hospital beds are in governmental facilities. As stated in a MEPD document on "Development Prospects and Policies" (1982): "Since Independence it has been the policy of Government to promote the private sector as a major vehicle for development." It is difficult, however, to reconcile such a policy with the planning objective of achieving universal population coverage with primary health care, or with the promise of the Kenyan Constitution for universal medical service to all citizens at no cost. As stated in 1978 in an evaluative report of a project supported by USAID: "Uncontrolled growth of a private fee-for-service system of medical care in Kenya will have lasting and negative effects on the cost, quality and access to basic health services for most of the people most of the time."

Health Administration. From the preceding account of Ministry of Health programs, it is evident that authority is exercised mainly from the top. This has been particularly true since a change of government policies in 1970. Both provincial and district medical officers are appointed by the central health authorities, and it is their duty to carry out national policies. Since 1970, policy decisions even below the district level have been made essentially by the central MOH. Drugs and other supplies are distributed from the center to the seven provincial health offices, then to the 41 districts, and from there to the operating local health units. Under this pyramidal logistical system, shortages are common at the local level.

At the provincial and district levels, the administrative responsibility of medical officers theoretically includes both hospital and primary health care services. The district and provincial hospitals, however, come under the technical direction of the central ministry. The hospitals of religious missions are entirely independent, although the subsidies they receive from the Ministry of Health implies a certain degree of coordination with the public facilities. Poor roads and insufficient vehicles and fuel make general supervision weak throughout the whole pyramidal structure of MOH facilities. Appointments of supervisory personnel in the MOH program are theoretically governed by the rules of a civil service or public personnel system, but it is generally recognized that tribal affiliations play a large part in such selections.

Throughout Kenya's 120 operating rural health units in 1982, community participation of local residents was rare. In selected projects, supported by external funding, such participation was actively encouraged, as in the Kibwezi Rural Health Scheme of the African Medical and Research Foundation (AMREF), financed mainly by USAID. With the very low educational level of the rural population in Kenya, as in most African countries, the involvement of people in the management of local health or other social services usually requires strong encouragement from higher authorities. Some observers see one legacy of years of colonial domination as a sense of dependency on government in most of the people.

Evaluation has been used as a tool of health administration in Kenya on a very limited basis. The flow of information on vital health events and the utilization of services is too irregular to permit such evaluation on a regular basis. Occasionally outside agencies have made evaluative studies on selected health needs, such as malnutrition in children or the effectiveness of family planning programs.

Insofar as mortality data reflect the outcome of national health systems, in 1986 life expectancy at birth in Kenya was 57 years, compared with 61 years in other countries of comparably low income (GNPs of $400 per capita or less that year). On the other hand, progress has been shown in the decline of Kenyan infant mortality from 124 deaths per 1,000 live births in 1960 to 73 infant deaths per 1,000 in 1987.

Regulation. Aside from registration in the MOH of physicians, dentists, fully trained nurses, pharmacists, and certain other health personnel, the regulation of professional performance is negligible. Likewise, private hospitals are theoretically required to have ministerial permission for their construction, but their operation is not subject to surveillance; the same applies to mission hospitals. Legislation on the sale of drugs has existed in Kenya since colonial times, but resources for its enforcement are very weak. Except for narcotics, for all practical purposes almost any drug can be purchased from a pharmacy or an unlicensed drug-peddler, with or without a medical prescription. There is no regulation at all of traditional healers or of the remedies they sell.

Probably the most significant regulation in the Kenyan health system takes place within the hierarchical program of the Ministry of Health. Since official policy encourages the development of the private medical market, private providers of care are essentially unfettered. The weak enforcement of factory regulations on health and safety, because of insufficient inspectors, has been noted.

Legislation. The basic Public Health Act in Kenya was initially carried over from colonial times, but in 1972 it was extensively revised. The law of 1972 defined the broad authorities of the Ministry of Health, under which programs for both prevention and treatment of disease, including the reduction of environmental hazards, are carried out. Special legislation was enacted in the 1970s on pharmacies, dangerous drugs, and the scope of work of nurses, midwives, and health visitors.

Since Kenya has only one legal political party (the Kenya African National Union), debates in the national Parliament on health legislation concern only minor aspects of administrative procedure. The president's views are strongly dominant.

Delivery of Health Services

The reference earlier to access of only 30 percent of the rural population to MOH primary health care gives a general idea of the inadequacy of health service delivery in Kenya. The majority of people almost certainly depend on self-care or on traditional healers for most of their day-to-day health needs. For childbirths, at least 70 percent of the deliveries are done by traditional birth attendants. Pure and safe water is inaccessible to the majority of people, and outside the two main cities sanitary excreta disposal is rare.

The pattern of delivery of personal health service in Kenya varies with the source from which it is sought. A study in one rural district identified some 6,800 complaints of illness occurring in a 2-week period. For most of these, which were actually minor symptoms, no action was taken, and for the next largest fraction the response was self-medication. The overall percentage distribution of responses in this field survey (published in 1981) was as follows:

Response to Illness	Percentage
No action taken	37.5
Self-medication	35.2
Government health center or hospital	13.8
Church facility	3.5
Private physician	3.5
Traditional healer	4.1
Other or unknown	2.4
All responses	100.0

Because many rural people think that it is illegal to consult traditional healers, these responses are probably underreported. In fact,

out of the 35.2 percent of responses categorized as "self-medication," 5.3 percent involved use of traditional herb remedies; added to the percentage consulting traditional healers, this amounts to 9.4 percent of the total responses.

Of the various sources of health care, those from government and church facilities can be considered organized to some extent. The health teams in MOH health centers have been described, and in the church mission units there are also usually nurses, working with or backed up by physicians. The use of mission facilities requires payment of fees. The principal provider of care in the government health centers, it should be recalled, is not a doctor but a clinical officer.

Regarding the types of illness that lead individuals to seek ambulatory services at government health facilities in Kenya, as one would expect, they are principally infectious and parasitic diseases. The Ministry of Health tabulates major diagnoses (relatively crudely) for patient-visits to district hospital out-patient clinics, health centers, and dispensaries. In 1978, there were about 19,000,000 such visits (slightly above 1 per person per year), predominantly for the care of young children. Their diagnostic distribution was as follows:

Diagnostic Category	Percentage
Acute respiratory infections	31.2
Malaria	23.4
Diseases of the skin	17.3
Diarrheal diseases	8.8
Intestinal worms	6.0
Accidental injuries	5.9
Gonorrhea	2.7
Measles	1.5
Pneumonia	1.5
Other	1.7
All diagnoses	100.0

Individual and nonorganized care is the normal mode of service delivery by a traditional healer, typically rendered in the patient's home. The private physician, on the other hand, typically sees patients in his office (which is often attached to his home). This may be the same physician who, during official hours, works in a district hospital. In rural areas, medical fees are very low, to be affordable by rural patients. The rural or small-town physician typically maintains his own supply of drugs, which he dispenses directly to patients. In Nairobi, on the other hand, where a middle-class population has been developing, the fees charged by private specialists may be very high, as is suggested by the high percentage of private health expenditures by urban families, shown in Table 14.3.

The delivery of medical services in both government and mission hospitals is by organized staffs of salaried physicians. Only the purely private hospitals have open staffs, in which private physicians are paid by fees. The general staffing of public hospitals, however, is very frugal, particularly nurses and ancillary services personnel. To discourage excessive length-of-stay in public facilities, nevertheless, the patient is required to pay a moderate personal fee for each day of care. Mission hospitals tend to be better staffed and equipped, but their charges for in-patient care are much higher. Purely private hospitals are luxurious, compared with the other types. It was to make the private and some mission facilities financially accessible to middle-class families that the National Hospital Insurance Fund was established in 1966.

Before national independence, bed facilities in both public and private hospitals were generally separate, and of higher standards, for the small population of Europeans and Asians. Special private hospitals were built for Asians in the main cities. At the large mental hospital in Nairobi, the public expenditure per patient-day for care in the European/Asian wards was five times that in the African wards. Conditions of the latter wards were described in a 1946 colonial government report as resembling a "totally unsuitable prison environment." Such segregation is no longer tolerated on racial or ethnic grounds, but a nearly equivalent separation now occurs based on wealth and social class.

Tertiary-level medical care is provided mainly at the large Kenyatta National Hospital in Nairobi, and at some of the eight provincial general hospitals. Many of the physicians and surgeons on the medical staffs have had specialty training in Europe and America and carry on very lucrative practices in their own private clinics after official hours. Even during official hospital hours, 10 percent of their time may be spent seeing private patients; in-patient care for private patients, however, is usually given at a private hospital.

Finally, note should be taken of the organized general health services available to employees (and sometimes their families) in the parastatal enterprises. In large private factories, some health care is also provided, though only for the worker and for work-connected conditions. The Kenyan military services, of course, are also served by an organized program of comprehensive health care.

All in all, health care and development in Kenya reflect the social policies of a low-income African country, recently liberated from colonial rule but committed largely (though not entirely) to a free-market economy. Sustaining the private sector are policies that encourage investments by foreign corporations, provide government subsidies to the health facilities of private religious missions, authorize (even encourage) private medical practice by government doctors, mandate insurance to support private health facilities, and so on. The private health sector is inevitably enhanced by the growing demands of a slowly expanding middle class, the meager salaries paid to public medical officers, and the obvious inadequacies of the government health services.

On the other hand, public sector health services—preventive and therapeutic—are sustained by a program of national health planning that aims to make primary health care increasingly accessible to the population, by the hard work and dedication of many public health leaders and the concern of government for human welfare, if only in the interests of maintaining social stability. With Kenya's one-party political system, free expression is obviously inhibited and discontent among younger military officers and university students can be explosive, as it was in July 1982. Events of this sort may, in the long run, lead to a stronger public sector, which could ultimately promote greater health care equity for the Kenyan population.

GHANA

Ghana won independence from British colonial status as the Gold Coast in 1957. This was earlier than the liberation of most African colonies, and Kwame Nkrumah, the first national prime minister and president, soon became a symbol of African nationalism for the entire continent. In 1966, Nkrumah was overthrown by a coup of the military forces, which remained in power (except for short periods) throughout the 1970s and 1980s.

Ghana is on the coast of West Africa, with a population of 12,609,000 in 1984. Almost 70 percent of these people lived in rural areas. The country's GNP per capita in 1986 was $390, slightly higher than Kenya's, and its national health system has been dominated by an ideology of free private enterprise. In the 1970s, overall health expenditures, according to the World Bank, absorbed about 4 percent of the gross domestic product, of which 72.5 percent came from private spending. Throughout the years of military dictatorship, the nation's economic development has been extremely erratic, with difficulties caused for the health system along with all other social sectors. The adult literacy rate in 1984 was only 53 percent.

Health Resources

As in most developing countries of this very low economic level, the supply of health personnel in Ghana is extremely inadequate. Under British colonial rule, nearly all physicians had come from Great Britain or other Commonwealth countries. A small number of Ghanaians were sent to study medicine abroad, especially in England. After independence, in 1964 Ghana established a medical school at the University of Ghana. By 1970, out of 667 doctors in the country—about 8 per 100,000 population—51 percent were still expatriates. In 1976 a second medical school was established. In 1984 the supply of physicians was up to 15 per 100,000, but their distribution was all too typically characterized by great concentration in the national capital, Accra. More than 50 percent of all physicians were located in the capital city, where 8.3 percent of the population live.

Physicians serving in the government services—about half of the total—worked predominantly in hospitals. Health centers, health posts, and other public facilities for ambulatory care were staffed principally by nurses and various types of auxiliary health personnel. In 1981 there were 9,383 registered nurses, or 78 per 100,000. In addition, there were assistant nurses numbering 69 per 100,000, working mainly in rural areas. Male *medical assistants,* trained somewhat more thoroughly than professional nurses, were expected to provide stronger leadership in rural health centers, but only 209 of them had been trained by 1981. Other allied health personnel were available for work in hospitals, but in small numbers. In 1981 there were 257 laboratory technicians, 142 radiological technicians, 214 medical record technicians, and 71 physical or occupational therapists.

Pharmacists numbered 611 in 1981, or 5.1 per 100,000, and they worked predominantly in private pharmacies. The pharmaceutical services in health centers and hospitals were staffed mainly by 474 pharmacy assistants. There were only 95 dentists in Ghana in 1981, and chairside dental assistants numbered only 48. Trained midwives, who worked in both hospitals and health centers were more numerous, numbering 56 per 100,000 in 1981.

The major capital investments in Ghana's health system, during the colonial period, were devoted to hospital construction, and this continued after independence. By 1979 there were 329 hospitals of all types, with 17,026 beds. (This included the 1,276 beds in 180 small health facilities, with an average of 7 beds each.) This amounted to 1.5 beds per 1,000 population. Most of these beds were in eight large regional hospitals, a major central university teaching hospital in Accra, and in 35 district or other public hospitals. The principal military hospital, located in Accra, was especially well staffed and equipped. There were 36 hospitals of religious missions, all of which were subsidized by government. In 1979, the overall distribution of hospital beds in Ghana, by sponsorship, was as follows:

Sponsorship	Percentage
Government	76.1
Voluntary nonprofit	22.3
Proprietary	1.6
All sponsorships	100.0

With very bad economic conditions in the 1980s, and meager government revenues, public policy called for collection of fees, on a sliding scale, for services in all governmental hospitals, for both in-patient and out-patient service. Larger fees were payable in the 36 mission hospitals and in other voluntary nonprofit hospitals (numbering 16). In the proprietary hospitals (17 in 1978 but increasing since then), the patient must pay full costs; thus, only the most affluent families are served.

The investments in both construction and operation of health centers for primary health care in Ghana have been relatively small. Counting both health centers and small health posts, 118 units were reported by the Ministry of Health in 1978. These units were staffed entirely by auxiliary personnel. Small fees were payable by patients visiting the health centers, and their rate of utilization by the rural population has been low. A former director-general of health of Ghana suggested that the extensive use of traditional healers is attributable in part to the fees charged for government health unit services, which are perceived by many people as being no more effective than care by a traditional healer.

Traditional practitioners in Ghana, widely available in rural areas, are registered by the Ministry of Health. They are clearly a major resource for the large rural population. There has been a national Psychic and Healer's Association, since 1969, and the government's Center for Scientific Research on Medicinal Plants is well established. In many countries, the government provides hygienic training for traditional birth attendants, but in Ghana such training is also given to traditional healers.

They are taught not only about sanitary practices, but also about modern scientific measures, such as oral rehydration for diarrhea and basic methods of contraception for family planning. The course lasts 14 weeks. A study of local health practices in 1979 found that traditional practitioners, although widespread, served "as an adjunct to modern health care, not as an exclusive alternative."

Organizational Features

The Ministry of Health is clearly the major organized entity in Ghana's health system. Its authorities are highly concentrated at headquarters in the national capital. MOH administrative branches are established in the country's 10 political regions, and each region has two or three health districts, with a total of 24. One or more district hospitals are in each district, and the District Health Office is located in one of them.

At the national level, the MOH is subdivided into six directorates, the largest of which is for hospital, medical, and dental care, essentially for treatment services. At the regional level are four subdivisions, but all of them are notably for supportive activities, such as public relations, evaluation, training, and medical supplies; hospitals and major health centers are supervised from the top. At the district level, the major responsibilities relate to hospital out-patient departments and small health stations. Both regional and district levels have general health councils, but these are purely advisory.

Ghana's crude birth rate has long been very high—44 per 1,000 population in 1987. Much emphasis, therefore, has been put on family planning, to control population growth. To mobilize education and public information programs from several ministries (for Youth and Rural Development, Agriculture, Labor and Social Welfare, etc.), a Secretariat for National Family Planning was established, not in the Ministry of Health, but in the quite powerful Ministry of Finance and Economic Planning. Contraceptive practices are promoted in the various MOH maternal and child health clinics, but also through the various educational programs of the other ministries.

The 36 mission hospitals (1978) in Ghana are coordinated by national Christian agencies. Largest is the Catholic organization, which supervises 25 of the hospitals, while the others belong to several different Protestant sects. Some of the drugs and medical supplies imported for the mission hospitals come to the central body, from which they are distributed.

Ghana does not have a social security system, financing medical care, but a national Provident Fund was established by law in 1963. Under this, all employees in private firms with five or more workers, as well as government employees, must contribute to the national fund. The employee contributes 5 percent of earnings, the private employer contributes another 10.5 percent, but nothing comes from government. The benefits are linked to each person's individual contributions, however, and are not pooled, as under social insurance. All benefits involve wage replacement during sickness or disability, but not medical care. The entire program is administered by a Social Security and National Insurance Trust (really a misnomer), supervised by the Ministry of Finance.

Large industries and mining companies, employing more than 500 employees (of which there are only a few), are required to provide limited medical services for their workers. At mines in isolated locations, there are usually small hospitals that serve the workers' families as well.

The private market of health care in Ghana includes the services of private physicians, traditional healers and birth attendants, private pharmacies, and the private proprietary hospitals. Judging by the 72.5 percent of health expenditures coming from private sources, the general role played by the private market must be substantial. Except for the traditional practitioners, however, these providers of private care are located almost entirely in Accra and a few other large cities. Here, about one-third of Ghana's 1,900 physicians (in 1984) provide services in private clinics or offices, catering to a small middle-class of merchants and civil servants. (Other nongovernment physicians, of course, work in the religious missions or in large enterprises.) With a reduction in the percentage of the national government budget al-located to health, the proportion of doctors engaged in purely private practice has undoubtedly been rising. About the only private modern medical service available in villages and rural areas, however, is from the occasional government medical officer who practices privately in his off-hours. Private pharmacies or drugstores are a major source of self-prescribed (or pharmacist-prescribed) medication for low-income city-dwellers.

Management, Finance, and Delivery of Service

In 1975 a National Health Planning Unit was set up in the Ministry of Health, although a general Planning Commission for overall economic development had been established earlier. Regarding this commission, a high Ghanaian medical official wrote in 1973:

> In 1963 a Planning Commission including two doctors was set up, and a comprehensive national development plan was written. This plan, which was not implemented, was very ambitious. It aimed to provide for very rapid development of hospital services and at the same time for expansion of promotive, protective, and preventive services—an almost impossible task. . . . After the coup of 1966 this plan was shelved. . . . [A new Committee], reporting two years later, stated that the emphasis should be on the promotive and the protective services . . . and training of health personnel. Nothing was done to implement this committee's report. In 1971 another committee was set up [for] devising a health-sector plan. . . . This committee reported towards the end of 1971 . . . when the Government which ordered it was overthrown by another military coup. . . . Thus the latest attempt to produce a health plan can be regarded as stillborn.

Whether or not the newer MOH Health Planning Unit was more effective is not clear. Its intention was to shift the priorities in Ghana's health system from hospital construction and specialty services to primary health care, especially in its preventive aspects. Examining Ghana's central government expenditures for health, between 1975 and 1982 they declined from 8.3 to 5.8 percent of the total budget. Adjusting for inflation, a World Bank analysis shows the decline to be substantially greater. Within these government expenditures, much the greatest proportion has continued to be spent on hospitals. A World Health Organization report, published in 1983, states that 88 percent of the central health budget was used for "curative services."

With respect to general administration of the MOH program, the high degree of centralized authority has been noted. Studies at the local community level in Ghana have found very weak supervision of health center or health post personnel from the district and regional levels. Most primary health care workers have been trained to perform very specific tasks, and show little initiative to help in functions outside their narrow spheres. Drugs and other supplies are frequently lacking at the local unit, although they may be lying in storage in a district hospital; transportation logistics are deficient.

As a result, the ultimate impact of the MOH services on rural populations has been weak. A careful evaluation of primary health care in two typical districts of Ghana, carried out in 1976, found only 14 to 20 percent of children under 5 years to be receiving child care. Immunizations were extremely inadequate. DPT vaccine (at least two doses) reached hardly 10 percent of children, and measles vaccine was given to 4 to 17 percent. Of all childbirths in the two study districts, only 21 percent were attended by trained personnel. At government health units, "the quality of care was considered poor." The reasons for these difficulties are summarized as being due largely to poor training programs in 1979. In these programs, "problems included methods of selection of trainees, inadequate preparation of teachers, lack of supervision of field training, shortages of all types of resources at training schools, including transport and teaching materials, and lastly irrelevance of much of the curriculum to priority tasks and functions."

Considering Ghana as a whole, the percentage of children fully immunized with DPT vaccine actually declined from 22 percent in 1981 to 14 percent in 1985–86. Safe water was accessible in 1984 to only 49 percent of the national population, and doubtless to a lesser proportion of the rural population. In the period 1980 to 1986, according to UNICEF, only 45 percent of rural people were estimated to be within an hour's travel of any type of modern health service.

In 1985, the Ghanaian MOH decided to adjust to its budgetary constraints by substantially increasing charges for curative services at the rural health centers. Allowances were supposed to be made for very indigent persons. Part of the funds collected could be retained locally and part had to be sent to the national headquarters. A field study made in 1988 showed the utilization of services in rural health centers to have declined markedly.

Here and there in the impoverished developing countries of Africa, there are "demonstrations" of model health programs, usually with foreign financial and technical assistance. Such a program was conducted in Ghana from 1970 to 1979, at the Danfa District, not far from the national capital. The University of Ghana Medical Faculty was deeply involved, and the input of foreign funds, personnel, and equipment was very high. An experimental design was applied, so that various types of health care interventions in several districts could be evaluated.

After several years of work, it was possible to demonstrate substantial improvements in the population coverage of child care and prenatal health services. Rates of morbidity in children or mothers could not be shown to have declined, but child mortality declined significantly. Family planning services, measured by the percentage of families adopting contraceptive practices, were quite effective, and the birth rate declined. Maternal mortality, however (very high in Ghana—1,074 maternal deaths per 100,000 live births in 1980–1984), was not demonstrably improved. More important, the entire Danfa health service model, though educational to the Ghanaian health authorities, could not be replicated elsewhere in the country; it was much too expensive.

Reflecting the outcome of deficient health services in Ghana, the infant mortality rate in 1987 was 91 per 1,000 live births, even though this constitutes a great improvement over the rate of 132 infant deaths per 1,000 in 1960. Average life expectancy at birth in 1984 was 53 years. The handful of upper-class merchants, landowners, high public officials, and military personnel in Accra can doubtless obtain an adequate amount and good quality of medical care, but most of the population in the rural areas and periurban slums accept either very deficient health service or none at all.

ZAIRE

Zaire is another very low income country, with a largely entrepreneurial national health system. Located in south central Africa, with a population in 1985 of about 30,000,000, of whom 39 percent were urban, Zaire occupies a very large territory (905,000 square miles). The country won independence from Belgium in 1960. As a colony, it was known as the Belgian Congo, and the language of the government was French. Through missionary influence, the population has become 70 percent Christian. Ethnically the people are predominantly Bantus, divided among more than 200 tribes.

The first decade after independence saw great internal strife among political and ethnic groups. General stability was not attained until about 1970, and in 1971 the country's initial name (Republic of the Congo) was changed to Zaire, as part of a general policy of Africanization of the society and culture. Since 1971, although it is ostensibly a republic, government power has been essentially in the hands of the military forces, led by President Mobutu Sese Seko. The adult literacy rate in Zaire was 61 percent in 1984.

Health Resources

Perhaps the most conspicuous aspect of Zaire's health system has been its very deficient stock of human and physical resources, especially personnel. Before independence, there were hardly 200 physicians in the country, all of them European. Since then, the Zairian government has greatly expanded both health personnel and facilities, but in relation to the needs of the rapidly growing population, the resources are still extremely inadequate.

Health Manpower. One medical school was established by the Belgians in 1954 at Leopold-

ville (now Kinshasa, the capital). It included faculties of medicine, dentistry, and pharmacy, and the curricula were based on typical European models. After independence, the courses were modified to fit somewhat more closely the requirements of Africa. Two more medical schools were established in 1983, away from the capital. Qualified teachers, however, have been in short supply for the relatively large numbers of students accepted each year. The costs of higher education are met principally by the government, and most students receive fellowship support for their living expenses. After graduation, 7 years of public service is required of every new doctor.

A health manpower survey was conducted in 1973, when a total of 818 physicians were identified. Of these, 61 percent were still foreign, but 39 percent were Zairian. Of the total, 71 percent were employed by government and 29 percent by the private sector. The latter were working mainly in religious missions and in private mining or industrial enterprises. Only a handful were entirely in private practice, although most government physicians spent part of their time as private practitioners to supplement their meager official salaries.

Since 1973, health manpower has increased in virtually all categories. In 1984 there were more than 2,000 physicians, or 7.4 per 100,000 (one doctor to 13,510 people). They were still predominantly appointed in government posts, although they also engage in private practice. The largest category of health personnel in Zaire, by a wide margin, is nurses. Counting both graduate and auxiliary nurses, in 1981 there were 57.5 per 100,000; more than three-quarters of these were auxiliary nurses.

The auxiliary nurse has theoretically completed primary school (8 years), and had a 2-year course of nurse's training. Both the Protestant and Catholic missions operate training schools, which attempt to meet standards of the Ministry of Education. A greater number of schools for auxiliary nurses, however, have sprung up throughout Zaire as purely commercial enterprises. Their training programs are deficient both in scientific education and in clinical practice. They are not accredited by the government, and yet they are allowed to operate, simply because the demand for these personnel is so great.

Auxiliary nurses are the mainstay of the health services in rural areas throughout Zaire. In the 1973 survey, 88 percent of auxiliary nurses were working outside Kinshasa but only 59 percent of physicians, most of the latter being with the medical missions. Often a young auxiliary nurse is the only health worker available in a rural dispensary. Auxiliary midwives also serve mainly in rural areas.

Traditional healers are abundant throughout Zaire, and some observers claim that the great majority of the population depend on them for the treatment of some or all of their ailments. There are two types of *guérisseurs,* or healers, in the villages; most are herbalists, who use local plants as remedies, along with some simple incantations. Others are *witch doctors,* who tend to be older men; they apply elaborate magical techniques to withdraw the "curse" or evil spirit believed to be responsible for the patient's disorder. Herbalists are usually consulted for simple or acute complaints, and witch doctors are sought more often for chronic conditions. Both types of healer charge fees. The Ministry of Health has a Department of Traditional Medicine, which works with the Zaire Healers Association to attempt to mobilize healers for limited medical training. Some research on traditional remedies is being done by the national Institute for Scientific Research.

Health Facilities. In 1979, Zaire had 79,244 beds in all types of health facility; of these, 75 percent were in 351 general hospitals, and the balance were in maternity homes and small health centers (591 facilities). The ratio of 2.8 beds per 1,000 population is probably misleadingly high; beds in general hospitals alone amounted to 2.1 per 1,000, and the equipment and general conditions in these facilities under government auspices were extremely rudimentary. The distribution of total beds by sponsorship in 1979 was as follows:

Sponsorship	Percentage
Government	48.8
Voluntary nonprofit	33.3
Proprietary	17.9
All sponsorships	100.0

This relatively large hospital bed supply in a low-income developing country reflects the past priorities of the health system. Patients would come to medical attention only when their disorders were highly advanced, requiring care in a hospital bed. In 1979 there were 330 small maternity hospitals, with an average of 35 beds each. Three-quarters of these units were private, operated mainly by religious missions.

Health facilities for ambulatory care in Zaire consist mostly of small dispensaries, staffed principally by auxiliary nurses. There were 2,930 of these units in 1981, meaning that each served about 10,000 people. Nearly all of these units belonged to the Ministry of Health, and they come under the limited supervision of the Regional Health Offices. Some were satellites to mission hospitals, from which somewhat greater medical supervision was provided.

Zaire must import about 90 percent of pharmaceutical products. For the whole country, one-fourth of the drugs are stored and distributed to government health facilities through a central depot; three-fourths are handled by commercial pharmaceutical companies, about 45 of which come from Europe and the United States. These companies supply the private pharmacies, the medical missions, and private physicians. In the government units a drug shortage is the usual situation.

Patients are expected to pay small fees for each visit to a health facility, whether governmental, religious, or private. (The charges made in private and mission facilities are much higher than those in government units.) The same applies for each day of hospital care. For childbirth in a hospital, unless payment is made, the mother is not given the baby's birth certificate (required for various official purposes). The prevailing viewpoint in Zaire is that health services are not properly valued by individuals unless they pay something for them.

Organizational Features

The health system of Zaire is structurally an outcome of many years of European colonial rule, along with the influence of religion and an ideology of free private enterprise.

Public Sector. In the government, health authority is highly centralized. The national Ministry or Department of Health in Kinshasa has five principal directorates for (1) general services and studies (including planning, coordination, and legislation), (2) general administration (including laboratory services, pharmaceuticals, blood transfusions), (3) epidemiological and environmental sanitation services (including epidemic diseases, tuberculosis, malaria, urban sanitation), (4) medical and health services (including maternal and child health, development of health centers, occupational medicine), and (5) central medicine (with unclear functions). The organization chart of the ministry is difficult to understand; there seems to be little scientific or managerial rationale to the arrangment of various subdivisions.

Below headquarters are eight regional health offices, each headed by a regional medical inspector, plus the capital city of Kinshasa. Each of these offices also has five subdivisions, which seem somewhat more reasonable than those at headquarters; they are concerned with (1) general administration, (2) medical facilities, (3) pharmaceutical and laboratory services, (4) epidemiology and sanitation, and (5) medical–social services. Below the level of the region there is no further echelon of health administration; each regional authority is responsible for MOH activities affecting about 3,000,000 people.

Quite independent of the MOH is the *Fonds Medical de Coordination* (FOMECO), in the Office of the President. This agency is responsible for essentially all government health services in Kinshasa, including the operation of the enormous Mama Yemo Hospital. This hospital has 1,800 beds and handles about 150 obstetrical deliveries per day, possibly the largest number for any single facility in the world. In addition, FOMECO operates three maternal and child health centers, another hospital, a school of nursing, a tropical medicine laboratory, and an elaborately equipped hospital ship. FOMECO's annual budget, supported by the government, has been about equal to that of the entire MOH; with this generous funding, it has been able to attract many competent physicians, largely foreign.

Another somewhat health-related government agency is the National Social Security Institute (INSS). Workers employed in private industry are entitled to partial compensation for wage-loss due to sickness, but no provision is made for medical care. The INSS is controlled by the Ministry of Labor, which is also supposed to inspect mines and factories for occupational safety and health.

There are several large parastatal organizations in Zaire for scientific research (including food chemistry and medical microbiology), general rural development, health surveys, and other purposes. These bodies may be attached to the Office of the President, the Ministry of Health, or other public agencies. They usually provide health services of above-average quality to their workers and families.

Finally in the public sector is a National Council of Health and Welfare, established in 1974 to coordinate all government health activities and to undertake national health planning. A major objective of the council initially was to involve local leaders in determining and implementing health policy in their communities.

Private Sector. Nongovernment religious missions providing health services in Zaire have already been noted. These services are especially important in rural areas, where they have been estimated to provide 75 percent of the modern medical care. There are three types of medical missions. Largest are the 18 Protestant missions that, as of 1975, operated more than 400 health facilities and 14 health personnel training schools. Second are the Catholic missions that function in numerous towns and cities, through 46 dioceses. Third is an unusual sect named Kimbanguist after its founder, which attempts to apply certain magical or miraculous cures; in 1975 it operated 28 dispensaries in rural areas.

A typical Christian mission in Zaire has a hospital at its center, with several outreach clinics for maternal and child health services and general primary medical care. In a rural region not far from Kinshasa is the Vanga Mission, operated by North American Baptists, which serves as a sort of model for the whole country. Based in a 200-bed general hospital, there are several outlying clinics, mobile health teams, a tuberculosis-control program, and even a network of *animateurs,* or health promoters doing educational work in the villages. The missions generally advocate involving local people in making decisions on their programs, in contrast to the highly centralized policies of the government of Zaire.

The major industrial and mining companies of Zaire, largely under foreign management, operate hospitals and clinics to provide workers and their families with health care. This is required under the National Labor Code, but it is doubtless also motivated by commercial interest in having a healthy work force, especially under poor environmental conditions.

Purely private medical service is provided in the main cities of Zaire by a handful of private physicians, but mainly by government doctors in their off-duty hours. Since few people, except high civil servants and other elite, can afford private fees, the extent of private practice is probably not great. For hospitalization, a small well-equipped public hospital is maintained on a hill near the presidential palace for top officials and friends of the president. In rural areas, of course, the many traditional practitioners are part of the private sector. Drugstores in the cities are also an important part of the private health care market.

Trends and Health Outcomes

Zaire is one of the few countries in the world in which the GNP per capita has been declining. The World Bank reported it to be $260 in 1979, $190 in 1982, and $160 in 1986. Whatever the cause of this decline is, its impact on the national health system must obviously be great. It has naturally affected the ability to maintain a sound physical and social environment for the population, educate and provide housing for people, train health personnel, construct health facilities, purchase pharmaceuticals and vaccines, and provide all needed health services.

It is not surprising that national government expenditures for health also declined from 2.3 percent of the central budget in 1972 to 1.8 percent in 1985. Overall public and private health expenditures in Zaire are not known, but judging by some of the health outcomes,

they are probably a very low percentage of GNP.

Although international agencies have promoted family planning in Zaire, it has been extremely ineffective, and the population has grown rapidly. The crude birth rate in 1960 was 47 per 1,000 population, and in 1986 it was 46 per 1,000. The number of women (or men) of child-bearing age using contraception in the mid-1980s was estimated at 1 percent. The caloric value of food consumed by Zairians in 1984 was estimated to be 97 percent of average daily requirements. For the period 1986 to 1987, the coverage of children with DPT immunizations was only 36 percent. In 1984 safe water was considered accessible to only 19 percent of the population. General personal health service was considered accessible to 26 percent of the people.

Under such circumstances, measurements of health status of the population are understandably poor. In spite of improvements since colonial days, the infant mortality in 1987 was reported to be 99 per 1,000 live births (from 148 per 1,000 in 1960). Maternal mortality in the early 1980s was 800 per 100,000 live births. Life expectancy at birth improved greatly from 1960, when it was 42 years, but in 1987 it had reached only 53 years.

PAKISTAN

In the southern part of Asia, just west of India, is a very poor country of 111,000,000 people (in 1987) with an entrepreneurial type of national health system. Pakistan took shape as a nation in 1947, after liberation from British colonial status along with India. While under British rule, this territory, with a majority Moslem population, was part of India, but with independence the land was partitioned between predominantly Hindu India and predominantly Moslem Pakistan, separated into a West and an East part. (In 1971 East Pakistan broke away as the sovereign nation, Bangladesh.) For some years after 1947 there was much violence, and millions of Moslems fled from India to Pakistan, while millions of Hindus fled from Pakistan to India.

Pakistan is overwhelmingly agricultural,

with 69 percent of its population being rural in 1987. The GNP per capita in 1986 was $350. The literacy level has been very low—40 percent for adult males and 19 percent for adult females in 1985. Of all primary school-age children, only 44 percent were enrolled in school (in 1985). In 1977 national government authority was seized by a military coup, replacing a duly elected president. Throughout the 1980s, government was under military control, and progress was slow. In 1984 public expenditures for military purposes were approximately 12 times those made for health purposes. The mass of the people have survived at a bare subsistence level.

Health System Organization

Several government agencies function in the Pakistani health system, although the private sector is especially strong. Within government, the major public authority for health is the Ministry of Health and Social Welfare (MOHSW).

Ministry of Health and Social Welfare. Overall health policy formulation is shared by this ministry and two other powerful general agencies—the Ministry of Planning and Development and the Ministry of Finance. The federal MOHSW is, in a sense, supported by equivalent authorities at lower administrative levels (provinces and districts), although at these levels the agencies have considerable autonomy.

At the federal level, the MOHSW functions include control of communicable diseases, provision of health services for government employees, maintenance of standards in education of health personnel, regulation of drugs, external relationships in health matters, services for mental illness, and general coordination of government health activities. Supervision and provision of general health services by hospitals and other health facilities, however, are responsibilities of the semiautonomous governments of the four large provinces, into which most of Pakistan is divided. (There are also three territories, in which the central government has greater responsibility.)

The Provincial Health Departments have a wide scope of responsibilities. They are directly in charge of teaching hospitals and other facilities and indirectly of local health services, through district health offices. Programs for controlling the principal communicable diseases, malaria and tuberculosis, are conducted vertically from the national level, but much responsibility is also delegated to the provincial level. With only four provinces for some 100 million people, the population of each is quite large, and vertical programs are directed from the provincial level for immunizations, health education, and drug distribution.

Within the districts, the District Health Office is responsible for all day-to-day government medical care below the level of the district hospital; the medical superintendent of that hospital reports directly to the provincial health officer. There are about 75 districts in Pakistan, each of which is divided into subdistricts or *tehsils.* The tehsil hospitals come under the District Health Office, as do the rural health centers (serving about 100,000 people) and the smaller basic health units. Each rural health center was designed to back up 4 to 10 basic health units, which are expected to provide general primary health care.

The basic health unit (BHU) is intended to be staffed by one physician and several health auxiliaries. In the villages of a BHU area there are additional health personnel—community health workers (CHWs), trained for 3 to 6 months. As of 1983 about 50,000 of these CHWs were needed to cover Pakistan's villages, but only 10,000 had been trained. Health personnel at the rural health centers, the basic health units, and in the villages serve as local agents for the various vertical disease control programs, as well as for the direct provision of primary health care.

Other Public Agencies. Significant health functions are performed by divisions of other national ministries. These include the Population Planning Division, formerly in the Ministry of Health and Social Welfare, but transferred in 1979 to the Ministry of Planning and Development. Family planning services are still provided through MOHSW resources at the local level, but in the capital and at the provincial and district levels there are separate Population Welfare Offices.

Another agency (within the Federal Ministry of Housing and Works) is the Environmental and Urban Affairs Division, which oversees water supplies and sanitation in the municipalities. Cities large enough to be designated as municipalities are responsible for all their own public health services. Overall environmental sanitation work is carried out in different ways in each province through variously designated departments. At the federal level, the states and frontier regions and the Kashmir Affairs Division has health responsibilities in these territories of the far northern part of Pakistan. The Labor Division is responsible for a limited health program of factory inspection for the health and safety of workers.

Other health functions relevant to medical research are performed in the Science and Technology Division. Several semipublic organizations provide relatively broad health services to their employees. Also some cities have municipal corporations that provide health care for their workers.

For certain employees of private industry in three provinces, a social security program provides a broad scope of health services. Dependents are also covered, except that their hospital services are limited to obstetrical care (maternity), surgery, and treatment of cancer. In 1982, this program covered 2,724,000 persons, or about 3.1 percent of the national population at the time. To be eligible, the worker must earn less than a certain wage (1,500 rupees a month in 1987). Services are provided either in health facilities of the social security body itself or in other existing public or private facilities under contract. The program is administered separately in each province by a Provincial Employees Social Security Institution, under supervision of the Provincial Labor Department.

Finally, there are separate but relatively limited health care insurance programs for employees of government agencies, especially the railroads. The military establishment, of course, has its own organized health service.

Private Health Care Market. The private health care market throughout Pakistan has a greater impact than all the government programs combined. This market has three principal components: modern or allopathic medical practice, traditional healing, and modern pharmaceuticals. In addition, there are a small number of nongovernment but nonprofit health activities performed by religious missions and voluntary agencies.

Modern medical service was provided privately on a full-time basis by about half the scientifically trained physicians of Pakistan in 1984. Most of the other half, who worked in government health programs, also engaged in private practice after official hours to supplement their low salaries. Although the Ministry of Health offers its doctors a small "nonpracticing allowance," this does not compare with the private income they can earn. As expressed in one international document on Pakistan:

> There is considerable promotion of private practice by government doctors—for example through persuading patients attending government facilities to go to a private clinic after regular official hours. Patients are thus made to pay for a private consultation on the understanding that they will then receive better and faster treatment [especially if they require admittance as an in-patient in a government hospital]. . . . There are three other constraints in the private health sector in Pakistan. First, because of . . . financing on a fee-for-service basis, doctors have no incentive to provide comprehensive (especially preventive) health care, nor minimize the number of attendances/procedures per patient. Second, there is a serious lack of quality control over the curative care provided. And third, there is little control over the fees charged.

As we will see in more detail later, the money spent on private doctors and private hospitals in 1982 was much more than the health expenditures by government at federal, provincial, and local levels.

Traditional healing in Pakistan takes many forms. There are descendants of two derivatives of the ancient Unani cult, and there are the relatively modern homeopaths; altogether, these were estimated in 1982 to exceed 55,000 practitioners. This was more than the total number of physicians, although not all traditional healers practice full-time. About 65 percent of the population were estimated to consult healers at some time, especially because modern doctors are so rare in rural areas. Pakistani government has given official recognition to the *tibb* form of Unani medicine, approving eight tibb training schools in 1977. Government research is also done on the medicinal plants of Unani and homeopathic practice.

Aside from the commercial private medical market, there is a small voluntary nonprofit sector in Pakistan's health system. The principal component consists of religious missions, which operate some hospitals and clinics, even though most patients must also pay for services. There is a Red Crescent society and also associations for the health protection of children and for people with tuberculosis and certain other diseases.

Health Resources

Since the country's origin in 1947, human and physical resources in the health system have greatly expanded, but by the 1980s the supplies were still much smaller than needed.

Manpower. In 1984, Pakistan had 38,300 physicians on its Registry, which was a ratio of 40 per 100,000 population; not all of these, however, were in the country. About 17,000 doctors were employed in government or in nongovernment but organized settings. The rest were entirely in private practice. At the time of independence, Pakistan had two medical schools, and by 1984 it had developed 17, all but one of which were public. In the 1980s these schools altogether were graduating about 4,000 doctors a year, approximately half of whom became employed in the government health service. There was, however, no legal obligation for a period of public service.

Pakistan's supply of nurses (all grades) increased from 10.1 per 100,000 in 1965 to 17.0 in 1981. That year pharmacists numbered 1,770, or only 2.1 per 100,000, and dentists just 1.2 per 100,000. The government was appropriately emphasizing the preparation of auxiliary level personnel, with the operation of 50 schools for drug dispensers (instead of uni-

versity-trained pharmacists), 46 schools for midwives, and 26 schools for *medical technicians.* The latter are not laboratory workers, but rather general health service personnel who provide primary health care in rural health centers. By 1983 some 2,000 had been trained, but much greater numbers were planned.

Pakistan is one of several developing countries that have described their medical manpower as constituting a "surplus." This has been based on the fact that many of the graduates of their medical schools are not employed in government or any other organized program, and yet cannot succeed in private practice; the people are too poor to provide a market. One interpretation of this problem of "unemployed doctors" has been that the output of physicians by medical schools has been excessive. Another judgment is that government priorities for health are much too low, since the population is seriously in need of more health service.

Facilities. The number of hospitals, and especially ambulatory care facilities, in Pakistan has also greatly increased since independence, but the supplies are still much less than the needs. In 1983 there were approximately 800 hospitals with some 51,000 beds; this meant a ratio of only 0.47 beds per 1,000 population. These beds were controlled mainly by units of government—81 percent of them. Only 3 percent of the beds were under voluntary nonprofit sponsorship, and 16 percent were proprietary.

The facilities for ambulatory health service are designated in different ways. Small units, usually in the cities, for treatment of certain disorders are called dispensaries; these numbered 3,275 in 1983. More comprehensive curative and preventive services are provided by networks of rural health centers (RHCs) and basic health units (BHUs). In 1983 there were 1,715 BHUs, each staffed with one doctor and 4 to 6 health auxiliaries; each unit was intended to serve about 10,000 people. For every 4 to 10 BHUs there was expected to be one RHC with 3 doctors, 8 auxiliaries, and 10 to 20 short-stay patient beds. There were 374 RHCs in 1983, plus 632 subcenters (presumably facilities below RHC standards). Counting all three types of ambulatory care center, there were 2,721 structures in 1983. For a population of 90 million that year, if each structure served 10,000 people, some 9,000 should have been required.

Other ambulatory health care facilities in Pakistan included 867 maternal and child health clinics and 679 immunization clinics in 1983. The staffing of all these facilities, however, is far from accomplished. By 1983 some 363 integrated complexes of RHCs, BHUs, and community health worker stations in villages were to have been established, but only 12 were completed. The majority of facilities were open only in the mornings, and their use was generally light.

Pharmaceuticals. The consumption of drugs in Pakistan is high, accounting for about 28 percent of total expenditures in the health system. Approximately 6,500 drug preparations were registered for domestic sale in 1983, and each year another 25 percent are added. Some 225 enterprises are licensed to produce pharmaceuticals in the country, and 10 of these, belonging to multinational corporations, control about 65 percent of the market.

This domestic production accounts for 75 percent of Pakistan's drug consumption, and 25 percent is imported. Out of this total output, more than 90 percent is consumed in the private market and only 8 percent by govern-

ment. Each of the provincial health agencies and the federal government make their purchases independently. Distribution of the drugs to local health facilities seems to be inefficient, and at the local level shortages are frequent. For the private purchase of drugs, pharmacies abound in the cities and towns, and most preparations can be bought with or without a doctor's prescription.

Economic Support

Data available on expenditures in Pakistan's health system for the 1981–82 fiscal year show vividly the overall character of the system. In that year the total health system absorbed the equivalent of $13.30 per capita, which was 3.2 percent of the GNP. Of this amount 19 percent was spent for capital construction purposes, supported mainly by some level of government or foreign aid (76 percent of capital costs).

Day-to-day operating expenditures of the health system accounted for 81 percent of the total, and this money came predominantly from private sources. Of these expenditures, government at all levels (including semipublic organizations and social security) accounted for 27.8 percent and the private sector accounted for 72.2 percent. More details are shown in Table 14.4. The very large proportion of total health expenditures derived from private individuals and going to private doctors (including private hospitalization) and pri-

Table 14.4. Operating Health Expenditures in Pakistan: Percentage of the Total, by Source of Finance and Provider of Service, 1981–1982

	Source of Finance						
Provider of Service	Federal Government	Prov. Governments	Local Governments	Employers	Donations	Private Persons	All Sources
MOHSW	1.8						1.8
Other ministries	0.4						0.4
Provinces		8.6					8.6
Local governments			6.8				6.8
Employers				8.8			8.8
Social security	0.8			0.6			1.4
All public							(27.8)
Voluntary bodies					1.1		1.1
Private doctors						46.0	46.0
Private pharmacies						25.1	25.1
All private							(72.2)
Total	3.0	8.6	6.8	9.4	1.1	71.1	100.0

Source: World Bank, *Pakistan Health Sector Report.* Washington Report No. 4736-PAK, 30 September 1983.

vate pharmacies can only mean that the health services organized by government are not satisfying the population. Of course, only those persons who can afford to pay for private service can obtain it, and this adds to inequities by concentrating scarce health resources on service to the more affluent sections of the population.

The difficulties of Pakistan's health system are reflected in various measurements of mortality. The infant mortality rate was a very high 163 per 1,000 live births in 1960, and it has been reduced substantially. In 1987, however, it was still high at 110 infant deaths per 1,000 live births. Between 1983 and 1987 only 24 percent of births were attended by a trained health person, and the maternal mortality rate in 1985 was 600 per 100,000 live births.

The birth rate in Pakistan has long been high and it remains high. In 1960 there were 49 births per 1,000 population and in 1987 the birth rate was 47 per 1,000. Only 11 percent of women of child-bearing age were known to be using contraception in 1985. Life expectancy at birth in 1986 was 52 years.

INDONESIA

Another very poor country, yet with an entrepreneurial health system, is Indonesia. Its vast population of 166,400,000 people (as of 1986) is spread out over 10 major islands (the largest being Java) and more than 13,500 smaller islands south of Southeast Asia. The economy is predominantly agricultural, and in 1985 the country was 75 percent rural. Some 90 percent of the people are Moslem.

Indonesia's GNP per capita in 1986 was $490. The income distribution was extremely uneven. A household survey in 1976 showed the wealthiest 20 percent of family units to have 49.4 percent of the total national income, while the poorest 20 percent had 6.6 percent. The literacy level, nevertheless, has greatly improved over recent decades and in 1984 reached 74 percent among adults.

The Dutch East Indies, as the thousands of islands were previously called, were under the control of the Netherlands from the seventeenth century until the end of World War II.

In 1949, most of the islands attained independence, but relationships with the former colonial power were not stabilized until about 1960. In the early years of the newly liberated Indonesia, great turbulence and bloodshed occurred among domestic political and ethnic groups, perhaps linked to various foreign powers. In 1965, some 300,000 people were slaughtered in a systematic massacre carried out in the name of "anticommunism." In 1968 a conservative military group acquired power, and proceeded to shape national economic policies along lines strongly favorable to private enterprise.

A free-market ideology became dominant in the health system, as in other aspects of Indonesian society. The major exception in health matters was the program of organized services necessary to support the military forces and certain other population groups linked to the national power structure. Analysis of the Indonesian national health system, therefore, departs from our usual paradigm; first we consider its private market aspects and then its other features.

Private Health Care Market

Although the size and character of the private health care market in Indonesia must, in large part, be analyzed indirectly, there is much evidence that it is the predominant sector. This is in spite of the fact that the great majority of people are very poor and government also sponsors a wide range of health programs.

Most conspicuous among Indonesia's general health resources are its physicians in public or private medical practice. In 1981 these numbered about 12,200, or 8.1 physicians per 100,000 population. Even though this was a great improvement over the colonial period (when the ratio was less than 1 doctor per 100,000), the supply was still very meager. Medical care maldistribution was extreme, with 25 percent of the doctors being located in Jakarta, the national capital, where 3.6 percent of the population lived. Sixty percent of the doctors were in cities with 25 percent of the people, and another 10 percent of doctors served the armed forces. The 75 percent of Indonesians in rural areas had to depend on the remaining 30 percent of the doctors, plus various auxiliaries and drugstores. New medical graduates are theoretically obligated (as the Dutch colonial government had required) to spend 3 to 5 years in government service, but this has evidently done little to correct the maldistribution.

Almost all Indonesian doctors are appointed to a government position of the Ministry of Health or another agency, but virtually all of these engage in private practice some hours of every day. In Jakarta and other main cities, experienced doctors with good reputations engage entirely in private practice. Purely private group practice medical clinics also developed in the 1980s to serve upper-class families.

Although not sanctioned legally, many nurses and other non-medical health workers engage in private practice. While they do not presume to make specific diagnoses, they dispense drugs and give injections. In 1981, Indonesia had 43.5 nurses (of all grades) per 100,000 population.

Traditional practitioners practice legally throughout Indonesia, making use principally of treatment with medicinal herbs. Their fees are typically low, and in 1985 they were found to absorb an average of only 6 percent of private household expenditures for health services. Some 25 private pharmaceutical companies are registered with the Ministry of Health to manufacture traditional drugs in Indonesia.

Even the education of physicians in Indonesia is, to a significant degree, in private commercial hands. In 1979 the country had 28 medical schools, of which 13 were in public universities, supported by government, and 15 were private. Because tuition charges were relatively high at the private schools, their enrollments were small, and they graduated only about 50 doctors a year, compared to 400 to 500 coming from the public schools. The quality of private medical education was generally regarded as poor, although it was subject to surveillance by the Ministry of Health. (Government medical schools are supervised by the Ministry of Education and Culture, as part of that ministry's oversight of the universities.)

Even in the licensure of physicians, private interests play a significant part. While medical licenses are granted formally by the Ministry of Health, they depend on recommendation by the private Indonesian Medical Association. One can appreciate the pressure on a young physician to conform strictly with professional orthodoxy if he or she expects to be recommended for licensure.

In dentistry, there were seven dental schools in 1979, of which two were also private. Such private schools functioned in other health fields as well. Out of 290 schools for training nurses, about 30 percent were privately operated, as were 25 percent of the 36 schools for pharmacy assistants. Altogether in 1985–86, out of all health-related expenditures in Indonesia, 2.8 percent went for the education of health personnel. Most of these expenditures were, of course, public, but 36 percent were private, an increase from 21 percent in 1982–83.

In hospital facilities of Indonesia, the private sector is also substantial. As of 1985 there were 1,600 hospitals, with 110,000 beds, or a ratio of 0.67 beds per 1,000 population. Of the hospital structures, 55 percent were private, either nonprofit or proprietary. With the exception of one type of hospital, however, public hospitals were larger and had more beds. In 1985 government controlled 65 percent of the beds, although the trend was toward expansion of the privately owned beds. Maternity hospital beds, even in 1979, were 96 percent in private hands. In the late 1980s, furthermore, MOH policy called for privatization of public hospitals through conversion of 10 percent of beds or more to use by private patients.

In private hospitals, patients are attended by private physicians, who are paid on a fee basis; the fee is divided between the doctor and the hospital. Since the medical staff pattern is "open," professional discipline is limited. In Jakarta (1988) there were 66 hospitals, of which 45 were private and keenly competitive with each other.

Although most hospital beds are in public facilities, expenditures for hospital care are quite the reverse. In 1985–86, hospital care accounted for 30.4 percent of total health expenditures in Indonesia. Of this amount 63.4 percent came from private families and individuals—an increase from 49.2 percent in 1982–83. A small fraction of private expenditures are for personal charges made in public facilities, but more than nine-tenths of this spending went to finance the private hospitals. Their amenities, as well as most of their technical services, are much better developed than those in the public hospitals, which most people must use.

Drugs and medical supplies are a major component of the total health system of Indonesia, and especially of the private sector. In 1985–86, more than 40 percent of overall national health expenditures went for drugs and supplies. Of this large amount, 73.2 percent came from private sources for the purchase of items in Indonesia's thousands of private pharmacies. In addition, a good proportion of the fees paid to private physicians or traditional healers is really for drugs that they dispense directly.

There are a number of quasi-governmental companies in Indonesia that manufacture drugs; these companies furnish 57 percent of the pharmaceuticals used in government health programs and 16 percent of privately purchased drugs. The balance of private sector drugs (84 percent) come from purely private domestic companies or are imported. As of 1979, Indonesia had only 1,800 fully qualified pharmacists but more than 20,400 pharmacy assistants, many of whom worked in private drugstores.

Aside from traditional healers, traditional birth attendants (TBAs) are part of the private health sector in Indonesia, and are registered with the Ministry of Health. In 1979 54,400 TBAs were registered—far more than the 22,100 trained midwives at the time. Some TBAs may have received a little hygienic orientation from the MOH, but they can hardly be considered trained. In the period 1983 to 1987, only 43 percent of all Indonesian childbirths were attended by a trained midwife or a doctor; the remainder were unattended or were served by privately paid TBAs.

The implications of the private sector for the total health system of Indonesia were summarized by an international expert in 1982:

> According to the World Bank, since the mid-1970s the private market for medical care in Indonesia has been growing more rapidly than the public sector. This shift is attributed to the dissatisfaction of patients with public sector services, leading them to seek care privately. . . . The strength of the private health market in Indonesia obviously creates difficulties for the public sector. The limited supplies of health manpower, drugs, and other resources are significantly drained away from the program of the Ministry of Health, which is oriented to serving all the people—particularly those large numbers who cannot afford private health care.

Nongovernment but Organized Sector

A relatively small sector in the Indonesian health system provides organized services that are still outside the sphere of government. These can be described in only very general terms.

A number of religious missions operate small hospitals and dispensaries in rural areas of Java or on some smaller islands. They come principally from churches in the Netherlands. Since their external support is small, they must charge patients for their services, and they also receive subsidies from the Ministry of Health.

Most quasi-governmental and private economic enterprises in Indonesia usually take responsibility for health services for their employees and families. Illustrative of a highly favored population of this type is the manpower of the quasi-public National Oil Company (Pertamina), established under law but largely owned and managed privately. In 1988 there were 250,000 employees in this enterprise, plus 20,000 retirees and all of their dependents. To provide these people with complete health services, there was a staff of 3,000 health personnel, working at 18 hospitals and other facilities with 800 beds. The rate of health care utilization was reported as 7 doctor contacts per person per year—far higher than that in the general population of Indonesia.

Other industrial firms provide their work forces similar, if not as highly developed and organized, health services. These industrial programs are usually considered health insurance, although employees theoretically make no contributions and the programs are not mandatory. Each firm decides voluntarily if it wishes to enroll its workers. The health services are sometimes provided, especially in smaller firms, by private physicians paid by fees, but usually by doctors on salary. The Ministry of Manpower provides very general supervision over these health insurance schemes.

Compulsory health insurance is an entitlement of active or retired civil servants. Each government agency is responsible for its own employees and their dependents, and all the public schemes are coordinated by the Ministry of Health. Services must initially be sought at MOH facilities (for which each public agency pays the MOH), but they may be obtained on referral from private providers, whom the MOH pays fees. Altogether, about 4.5 percent of the Indonesian population have health insurance protection, public or private.

Voluntary health agencies provide certain charitable services in Jakarta and other main cities. The Red Cross is well developed and there are several agencies in the field of family planning. Help for patients with crippling conditions, tuberculosis, blindness, and other disorders is supported through private donations, with some government subsidies.

Government Health Sector

In 1986–87, government at all levels in Indonesia contributed 30.7 percent of the total costs of the nation's health system; this was exactly the same as the government share in 1982–83. Government health officials show the strong dedication to duty found in most other low income developing countries, but they express frustration for lack of the funds needed to reach health objectives.

Ministry of Health. The administrative framework of the Indonesian Ministry of Health parallels the political structure of the country. The seat of central government is in Jakarta, a city of more than 6,000,000 on the major island of Java. The 13,500 islands were divided among 27 provinces, each of which has a provincial health office, whose head is appointed by the provincial governor but is responsible to the national minister of health. Health policy decisions, in general, are made by the central

government. The provinces are divided into districts, numbering 233 in all; each district has a small hospital, the director of which is regarded as head of MOH activities in the district.

The most peripheral jurisdiction is the subdistrict, of which there are 3,177 (12 to 15 per district). Each subdistrict is served by at least one health center to provide primary health care. In 1979, half of these units had a full-time or part-time physician, and the total staff usually consisted of about 10 health workers, including a nurse, a midwife, a sanitary inspector, communicable disease workers, clerks, and others. Altogether there were about 5,000 health centers in 1986, and each was expected to serve 30,000 to 40,000 people. These would have reached no more than 14 percent of the national population at the time. In the villages of a subdistrict there may be small health posts, staffed only by two or three auxiliary health personnel, and devoted largely to maternal and child health (MCH) service. These posts are also called subcenters, of which some 15,000 were operating in 1985.

It has been widely reported that most Indonesian health centers are seriously underutilized. One United Nations agency report of 1979 states that "It is not uncommon for there to be fewer than 10 visits per day to some centers. In some rural areas, fewer than 10 percent of the people surveyed have ever been examined by a doctor, less than 40 percent have ever been to the health center, and only 20 percent of mothers have ever attended an MCH center. Most people in these areas seek care from more readily accessible and supporting traditional practitioners, or from the local equivalent of a drugstore." In 1985, the use of health centers was reported to be somewhat greater, but still relatively low.

General hospitals of the Ministry of Health are of four classes. At the district level are usually Class D hospitals with 50 to 100 beds, staffed by general practitioners. Larger districts may have a Class C hospital of 100 to 200 beds, with specialists in surgery, medicine, pediatrics, and obstetrics. In provincial capitals there are usually Class B hospitals with around 500 beds and specialists in cardiology, orthopedics, and other subspecialties. Class A hospitals are still larger and more sophisticated in medical staffing and equipment; there were only two such hospitals, both located in Jakarta, in 1985.

Based on 1985 data, all types of government hospital beds in Indonesia numbered about 72,000, or 0.44 beds per 1,000. It is these relatively few beds on which the great majority of people, who are very poor, must depend for hospital care. Since this ratio of government beds includes some outside the MOH—for example, in quasi-governmental enterprise facilities, limited to certain employees—the bed supply for the general population is even smaller.

Other Government Agencies. Aside from the MOH, several government agencies play roles in the Indonesian health system. The Ministry of Education has ultimate responsibility, through a Consortium of Medical Sciences, for the planning and development of medical schools in the universities. Theoretically this ministry works jointly with the MOH to coordinate the training of physicians with national needs for medical services.

The Ministry of Manpower, as noted, supervises various nongovernment health insurance schemes in a general way. This ministry also provides general supervision over compensation and medical care for industrial injuries, which are a direct financial responsibility of each employer of 25 workers or more.

The military establishment in Indonesia is served by an especially well-developed program of its own organized health care resources. Though no data on military health facilities are available, one can note that overall Indonesian military expenditures in 1984 were $23 per capita, compared with government expenditures for health of $4 per capita. This meant a ratio of 5.8:1, which can be compared with equivalent ratios of 1.8:1 in Mexico, 1.0:1 in Great Britain, or 0.5:1 in the Netherlands.

In 1983, a new government agency was set up—the Ministry of Population and Environment. Within this is the National Family Planning Coordinating Board, which had formerly been chaired by the minister of health. Indonesia's family planning efforts have, in fact, been quite successful, with reduction of the na-

tional birth rate from 43 per 1,000 population in 1965 to 28 per 1,000 in 1986. In 1985 an estimated 40 percent of women of child-bearing age were using some type of contraception. Family planning education in the late 1980s was extended beyond MOH facilities into almost every village; mobile teams, based at sub-district offices, were widely used. Unlike most medical treatment services in Indonesia, family planning services are provided free.

Other ministries have indirect relevance to the Indonesian health system. There is a Ministry on the Role of Women, which naturally supports family planning in the interest of women's welfare. A Ministry of Home Affairs encourages community participation at the local level, which is relevant to health service programs. In 1983, out of 64,000 villages, 26 percent were considered "modern" with regard to population participation.

The Overall Health System

In summary, the health system of Indonesia is heavily oriented toward the private sector. Even though a Ministry of Health supervises a large pyramidal framework of services, both preventive and curative, in the provinces, districts, and subdistricts, their use by the people is relatively small. Despite widespread poverty, the greatest proportion of health services involve self-medication (with personally purchased drugs), traditional healers, and private physicians.

A field study made throughout Indonesia in 1978 showed dramatically the distribution of health services, by income groups. In Table 14.5, one can see the percentage distribution of various sources of treatment for any illness occurring in the week before a household interview. (It does not indicate the general rates of health services received by different income groups, which are undoubtedly lower for the poor.) The greater dependence of lower-income families on self-care, usually meaning self-medication, is clear. Higher-income families obviously made the greatest use of physicians, who were almost certainly in private practice. Of the four types of health care source inquired about in this survey, only the "auxiliary" was manifestly part of the government

Table 14.5. Illness Treatment by Source and Household Income Level: Percentage Distribution in Indonesia, 1978

Source of Care	Household Incomes		
	Lowest 40%	Middle 40%	Highest 20%
Urban Java			
Self-care	58	20	12
Healer	10	7	1
Auxiliary	19	23	14
Physician	13	50	72
Rural Java			
Self-care	45	35	32
Healer	6	10	7
Auxiliary	34	34	20
Physician	16	21	41
Outer Islands—Urban			
Self-care	28	40	18
Healer	15	9	0
Auxiliary	39	20	17
Physician	18	31	64
Outer Islands—Rural			
Self-care	29	25	21
Healer	27	15	15
Auxiliary	32	42	25
Physician	11	18	39

Source: Chernichovsky, Dov, and Oey Astra Meesook, *Poverty in Indonesia: A Profile.* Washington, D.C.: World Bank (Staff Working Papers No. 671), 1984.

health sector; out of the 12 population groupings analyzed, only rural residents of the outer islands used such auxiliaries for more than 40 percent of their illness episodes.

The distribution of health expenditures in Indonesia may reflect even more clearly the characteristics of the overall system. In 1986–87, the principal sources of these funds were distributed as follows:

Source	*Percentage*
Government	30.7
Quasi-government enterprises	5.7
Private sector	63.7
All sources	100.0

Within government, seven-tenths of expenditures came from the central level (a small fraction of this came from foreign aid) and three-tenths were divided between provincial and district levels. Within the private sector, 95.2 percent of spending was by personal households and the balance by private companies.

Total Indonesian health system expenditures in 1986–87 amounted to 2.2 percent of GNP. Data on the distribution of services received and the sources of funds indicate that health expenditures go mainly to support care for families with the money to spend. If they are higher-income families, the money is likely to be used for the services of private physicians; in lower-income families, it is likely to be used to purchase drugs in a private pharmacy. Some low- and middle-income families, of course, use services of MOH health centers, hospitals, and other facilities.

Aside from family income, other circumstances favor certain groups in Indonesia. Health services for military personnel and dependents, especially in officer ranks, are very well developed. Services are also abundant for the employees (and families) of quasi-governmental enterprises. Central government civil servants and their families are another favored population, sometimes through public reimbursement of private health care providers.

These favored population groups, however, are a small minority of the national population. More generally prevalent health conditions are reflected by an infant mortality rate in 1987 of 85 per 1,000 live births, although this was a substantial decline from 139 per 1,000 live births in 1960. Maternal mortality between 1980 and 1987 was 800 per 100,000 births—an exceptionally high rate. In the same time period, only 36 percent of the population had access to safe water. The life expectancy of an average Indonesian at birth in 1986 was 57 years, compared with 70 years in Malaysia, a nearby country with an ethnically similar population.

SUMMARY COMMENT

The health systems of all five countries reviewed in this chapter reflect strong entrepreneurial policies, in spite of the general level of poverty. In all five systems, the ministries of health have developed nationwide frameworks of preventive and curative health services, but their support with personnel and supplies is very weak, and the programs have relatively little impact on the people. Ambitious plans have been made repeatedly, but for various reasons they are not carried out. As a percentage of national government budgets, the ministry of health share has been generally declining.

In Kenya, a large majority of the modern physicians are entirely in private practice, and in Pakistan about half are. In the other three countries most physicians have government appointments, but the majority of these also spend substantial time in private practice. Private pharmacies dispense large quantities of drugs, without prescription, directly to the people. Of all health expenditures in all five countries, therefore, the greatest proportion is derived from private sources—72 percent of the national total in both Ghana and Pakistan.

The people in these countries tend to make relatively little use of government health centers, preferring to seek care instead at the outpatient department of a hospital or to consult a private resource. Payments must usually be made for using public as well as private resources. Purely private health facilities are so actively promoted in Kenya that health insurance is mandated only for *higher* paid employees, to encourage their use of proprietary hospitals. In Indonesia, 55 percent of hospital structures are private, as well as more than half of the 28 medical schools.

Religious missions, which make significant personal charges for their services, play a strong role in all these countries, and they are subsidized by the government. The ministries of health themselves report that only a minority of the national population—30 percent in Kenya, 26 percent in Zaire—has access to modern health services. As a reflection of the poor health care in these systems, not to mention the general living conditions, life expectancies at birth vary from 58 years in Kenya down to 52 years in Zaire.

REFERENCES

Kenya

African Medical and Research Foundations, *AMREF in Action,* Nairobi, 1981.

Bloom, G., M. Segall, and C. Thube, *Expenditure and Financing of the Health Sector in Kenya.* Nairobi: Kenya Ministry of Health, 1986.

Family Health Institute, "A Working Paper on Health Services Development in Kenya: Issues, Analyses, and Recommendations," Washington, D.C.: USAID, 1978, processed.

Kenya Catholic Secretariat, Medical Department, Summary, "Catholic Health Care, Facilities and Services January–December 1980." Nairobi, 1981, processed.

Mburu, F. M., "Socio-political Imperatives in the History of Health Development in Kenya," *Social Science and Medicine,* 15A:521–527, 1981.

Mburu, F. M., "Rhetoric—Implementation Gap in Health Policy and Health Services Delivery for a Rural Population in a Developing Country," *Social Science and Medicine,* 13A:577–583, 1979.

Ministry of Economic Planning and Development, *Economic Survey 1982,* Nairobi, June 1982, pp. 213–217.

Ministry of Economic Planning and Development, *Kenya Development Plan 1979–83.* Nairobi, 1979, pp. 33–34.

Ministry of Finance, Central Bureau of Statistics, *Consumer Price Indices, Nairobi.* Nairobi, March 1977.

Ministry of Health, Kenya, *Outpatient Services for Rural Health.* Nairobi, 1979.

Ministry of Health, Kenya, *Rural Health Services.* Nairobi, 1978.

Ministry of Health, Kenya, *Health Information Bulletin.* Vol. 3, Nairobi, November 1979.

Nordberg, Erik, *On the True Disease Pattern in Kibwezi Division.* Nairobi: African Medical and Research Foundation, November 1981.

Republic of Kenya, Ministry of Health, *Proposal for the Improvement of Rural Health Services and the Development of Rural Health Training Centres in Kenya.* Nairobi, 1972.

Were, Miriam H., *Organization and Management of Community-Based Health Care: National Pilot Project of Kenya Ministry of Health.* Nairobi: UNICEF, 1978.

World Health Organization, "Kenya," in *Sixth Report of the World Health Institution 1973–1977.* Geneva, 1980, Part II, pp. 20–22.

Ghana

Anon., "Primary Health Care Is Not Curing Africa's Ills." *The Economist* (London), 31 May 1986, pp. 91–94.

Cole-King, Susan, G. Gordon, and H. Lovel, "Evaluation of Primary Health Care—A Case Study of Ghana's Rural Health Care System." *Journal of Tropical Medicine and Hygiene,* November/December 1979, pp. 214–228.

Faruqee, Rashid, *Analyzing the Impact of Health Services: Project Experience from India, Ghana, and Thailand.* Washington, D.C.: World Bank (Staff Working Paper No. 546), 1982.

Kaplan, Irving, et al., *Area Handbook for Ghana.* Washington, D.C.: American University, 1971.

Republic of Ghana, *Report of the Committee Ap-*

pointed to Investigate the Health Needs of Ghana. Accra: Ghana Publishing Corporation, 1968.

Sai, F. T., "Ghana," in I. Douglas-Wilson and Gordon McLachlan (Editors), *Health Service Prospects: An International Study.* London: The Lancet and Nuffield Provincial Hospitals Trust, 1973, pp. 125–155.

U.N. Fund for Population Activities, *Ghana: Report of Mission on Needs Assessment for Population Assistance.* New York, July 1984.

U.S. Office of International Health, *Syncrisis-Dynamics of Health: Ghana.* Washington, D.C.: June 1974.

Warren, D. M., "Ghanaian National Policy Toward Indigenous Healers." *Social Science & Medicine,* 16:1873–1881, 1982.

World Health Organization, "User Charges and Utilization in Ghana," in *The Challenge of Implementation: District Health Systems for Primary Health Care.* Geneva (WHO/SHS/DH/88.1), 1988, processed.

Zaire

Bureau du President de la Republique du Zaire, *Profils du Zaire.* Kinshasa, 1971, pp. 390–398.

Hiltzik, Michael A., "Zaire's Veneer of Affluence Undermined by Reality of Poverty." *Los Angeles Times,* 2 January 1989.

Lashman, Karen E., *Syncrisis: The Dynamics of Health—Zaire.* Washington, D.C.: U.S. Office of International Health, 1975.

Nelson, Harry, "Cuts, Inflation Sap Zaire Health Care." *Los Angeles Times,* 20 December 1980.

Republique du Zaire, *Synthese Economique 1981—Deuxième Partie: Etudes Sectorielles.* Kinshasa, October 1982.

Pakistan

Furnia, Arthur H., *Syncrisis: The Dynamics of Health—Islamic Republic of Pakistan.* Washington, D.C.: U.S. Public Health Service, June 1976.

Roemer, Milton I., "Judging Doctor Supply—Market or Health Criteria," *World Health Forum* 9:547–554, 1988.

Siraj-ul-Haq, M., *Primary Health Care in Pakistan.* Islamabad: Government of Pakistan Planning Commission, 1978.

Siraj ul Haq, Mahmud, *Health Manpower Management System in Pakistan.* Geneva: World Health Organization (working paper for Expert Committee on Health Manpower Management Systems), 1987.

United Nations Fund for Population Activities, *Pakistan: Report of Second Mission on Needs Assessment for Population Assistance.* New York: Report No. 71, August 1985.

World Bank, *Pakistan Health Sector Report.* Washington, D.C.: Report No. 4736-PAK, 30 September 1983.

Indonesia

Brotowasisto et al., "Health Care Financing in Indonesia." *Health Policy and Planning,* 3(2):131–140, 1988.

Bunge, Frederica M. (Editor), *Indonesia: A Country Study.* Washington, D.C.: American University, 1983, pp. 113–115.

Chernichovsky, D., and O. A. Meesook, *Poverty in Indonesia: A Profile.* Washington, D.C.: World Bank (Staff Working Papers No. 671), 1984.

Fulop, T., and U Mya Tu, "Cooperation Between the Republic of Indonesia and WHO." New Delhi: World Health Organization, South-East Asia Regional Office (mission report), August 1982.

Malik, A. Ridwan, *Health Expenditure and Financing in Indonesia.* Jakarta: Ministry of Health, Bureau of Planning, 1987, processed document.

Ministry of Health, Bureau of Planning, *Health Sector Profile.* Jakarta, 1986, processed document.

Ministry of Health, Republic of Indonesia, *National Health System.* Jakarta, March 1982.

United Nations Fund for Population Activities, *Indonesia: Report of Mission on Needs Assessment for Population Assistance.* New York: Report No. 20, August 1979.

United Nations Fund for Population Activities, *Indonesia: Report of Second Mission on Needs Assessment for Population Assistance.* New York, Report No. 74, June 1985.

World Health Organization, Regional Office of South-East Asia, *Experimental Country Profile: Indonesia.* New Delhi, India, 30 December 1976, processed document.

CHAPTER FIFTEEN

Welfare-Oriented Health Systems in Very Poor Countries

Several countries with a general economic level as low as that of countries reviewed in Chapter 14 have developed health systems oriented to greater promotion of social welfare. For various reasons, primarily political, their governments have assigned higher priority to providing health services to the general population, composed overwhelmingly of very poor families. Four such national health systems, two in Asia and two in Africa, are considered here.

BURMA

In the 1980s this ancient land in Asia was known as the Socialist Republic of the Union of Burma. By 1987 its population had grown to 39,100,000 people. For centuries the country just east of India was dominated by competing monarchies. Around 1600 Portugal took colonial control, and in 1886 Burma was brought into the British Empire.

Social Background

With the onset of World War II, the Japanese army occupied Burma from 1941 to 1945. During those years a nationalist and anticolonial movement arose, and after the war national elections led to the independent Union of Burma in 1948. The first years of independence were marked by many internal ethnic and political conflicts, until in 1962 a military group seized power. It set up a Revolutionary Council that in April 1962 declared that people would not "be set free from social evils as long as pernicious economic systems exist in which man exploits man and lives on the fat of such appropriation. The Council believes it to be possible only when exploitation of man by man is brought to an end and a socialist economy based on justice is established. . . ."

Under this manifesto of the Burmese Way to Socialism, the Revolutionary Council ruled the country for 12 years. Foreign businesses were nationalized, and almost all major enterprises were taken over by the government. A new Constitution was adopted in 1974, following a nationwide referendum. In March 1974, the Revolutionary Council was disbanded, and the Socialist Republic of the Union of Burma was born. National leadership became firmly vested in the single Burma Socialist Programme Party, which had a network of branches down to the smallest villages. Except for a violent period of student-led rebellion in 1988, one-party military rule has persisted in Burma.

In light of its troubled past—colonialism followed by military domination—it is not surprising that the people of Burma suffer from great poverty. In 1986 the annual GNP was $200 per capita, significantly lower than that of India or Tanzania. The principal base of the economy is agriculture, mainly rice and teakwood, with limited manufacture of textiles and furniture. The population settlement is 76 percent rural and 24 percent urban, with three principal cities. In 1985, the people of Burma, however, consumed food with a caloric value averaging 117 percent of normal daily requirements.

Burma's political jurisdictions were developed under the Constitution of 1974. Beyond the national capital in Rangoon, the first echelon contains 14 regions, known as divisions for those populated mainly by ethnic Burmese, and as states for those with mostly other ethnic minorities; there are seven of each. The divisions/states are subdivided into an average of 22 townships each, for a total of 314. Township government plays an especially important role in providing and managing health services.

Each township is further composed of small villages, which are clustered into *village tracts.* The average township contains abut 240 villages, and five or six villages make up a village tract. (Large cities have the equivalent units, known as urban wards.) Altogether, Burma has 13,751 village tracts and 75,327 villages.

At every jurisdictional level, formulation of general social policy and its enforcement are delegated to People's Councils, whose membership is dominated by the Burma Socialist Programme Party. Within each council there is normally a health committee, involved in establishing health facilities and similar matters.

In spite of the name of the ruling party, business enterprises in Burma have become predominantly private. Out of some 42,000 establishments (mostly small shops) in 1985–86, 94 percent were private, 2 percent were cooperatives, and only 4 percent were governmental. (Of the relatively few large enterprises with more than 50 workers, however, one-third were governmental.) The distribution of household incomes also does little to suggest a socialist ideology. In one typical township, a 1984 survey found families with low income to constitute 59 percent, marginal income 30 percent, and adequate income 11 percent of all families.

Literacy has greatly improved in Burma since independence; by 1984 the rate was 70 percent among adults. Education is complicated by the existence of 67 ethnic groups speaking an estimated 242 distinct languages. Some of the ethnic minorities have given rise to insurgent movements. Buddhism, however, is the dominant religion or (for many) philosophy of 85 percent of the people; sacred pagodas and temples are everywhere.

In 1989, the military government decided to change the country's name from the Socialist Republic of the Union of Burma to the Union of Myanmar. This was designed to reduce the antagonism of the nation's many ethnic groups (e.g., the Kachin, Karen, Mon, Chin, or Shan minorities) that do not consider themselves to be Burmese. "Burma" had been the designation of the British colonial rulers. The change of name was also designed to abandon the country's pretense at being socialist. In the account that follows, however, the country's familiar name, Burma, is still used.

Health System Organization

The central pillar of government organization for health in Burma is the Ministry of Health, with its branches throughout the country. The Constitution of 1974 declared a "right to medical treatment," and the Burmese Socialist Programme Party soon formulated six major policies for health advancement: (1) to raise the health standards of the working people and provide efficient treatment for all diseases within the country; (2) to give priority to preventive measures; (3) to narrow the gap between rural and urban areas in the availability of health services; (4) to achieve progressive improvement in health facilities with more cooperation from the public; (5) to extend and improve social welfare services, including those of health, which are commensurate with the economic progress of the country; and (6) to establish more hospitals, dispensaries, and rural health centres, extend curative, preventive, and disease eradication programs, improve water supply, and sink more tube wells.

In the late 1970s, the central government formulated a sequence of 4-year People's Health Plans. In summary, these included (1) community health care, (2) hospital care, (3) disease control, (4) environmental health, and (5) support services (laboratories, health education, health manpower development, etc.).

Ministry of Health. At the ministry headquarters in Rangoon, the national capital, four major departments operate under the minister, each headed by a director-general. These are the Departments of Health, of Medical Education, of Medical Research, and of Sports and Physical Education. The first of these, the Department of Health, employs 93 percent of the 45,000 personnel in the ministry and accounts for 75 percent of all MOH expenditures. This department is responsible for virtually all of the MOH's personal health services, preventive and therapeutic. Its scope includes supervision of all the division/state and township health offices throughout the nation.

Traditionally activities for the control of malaria, tuberculosis, and other communicable diseases were directed from the MOH headquarters and managed vertically throughout the nation. Since the first People's Health Plan in 1978, these programs have been decentralized and integrated horizontally into work at the township level. Specialists may be available for advice at the divisional level. Large hospitals in the principal towns of the divisions/states still come under the direct control of MOH headquarters. Small hospitals with fewer than 100 beds are supervised by township medical officers.

The health director of each division or state is appointed by the minister of health and has the rank of a deputy-minister. He is technically responsible to the minister (and his staff), but administratively responsible to the People's Council of the division or state. Assisting the health director are specialists in diverse fields, such as tuberculosis and maternal and child health, as well as midwives, nurses, and environmental inspectors. There may also be an officer for personnel training. This state/divisional office is responsible for the work of all Township Health Offices.

Each of the 314 townships in Burma has an average population of about 115,000 people. The average village in 1986 had 84 households, with about 420 people. Heading the township Health Office is a township medical officer, who is always supposed to be a physician. None of these posts was reported to be vacant in 1986, except in some of the 50 townships with local insurgency movements. In most, but not all jurisdictions, the township medical officer (TMO) is assisted by a township health officer (THO). The adminstrative office is typically located in a small township hospital, in which both the TMO and the THO are the clinically responsible physicians.

The township health officer is principally responsible for preventive health activities, when he is not assisting the TMO. In the Township Health Office, there may also be a *lady health visitor* (senior midwife), a senior sanitary inspector, a dentist, and occasionally a senior nurse. Each township has some four or five rural health centers, which are the major MOH facilities for providing primary health care (PHC). Each health center is expected to serve about 27,000 people.

Rural health centers are staffed entirely by nonmedical personnel. In charge is a male *health assistant,* who has been trained for 27 months at a special school. He is aided by midwives, sanitarians, and other auxiliary-level personnel. Urban health centers in the main cities sometimes have a physician on staff. Beyond the rural health centers in the villages, the MOH program has volunteer PHC personnel—community health workers, and auxiliary midwives—who work under the supervision of the health center staff.

All these PHC services come under the direction of the Township Health Office. Some health centers with a small number of beds are considered to be *station hospitals.* About 80 of the 314 townships in 1986 had school health teams of a doctor and a nurse. Some urban townships have dispensaries for traditional medicine, sponsored by the MOH. All these special services also come under TMO or THO supervision, although very few of these physicians have had formal public health training. Their usual preparation has been a 4 to 6-week orientation course at MOH headquarters before they start work. Township and divisional health offices have no responsibility for health activities outside MOH jurisdiction.

Other Government Agencies. Several government agencies in Burma, besides the MOH, perform health-related functions. While these may be secondary to the main objective of each agency, they still contribute to the national health system.

The Ministry of Labour supervises Burma's Social Security Law, enacted in 1954. Under this ministry, a Social Security Board manages a program of medical care for industrial and certain other types of manual worker in private or public enterprises with five or more employees; dependents are not covered. In 1986, some 343,000 workers were covered, constituting less than 1 percent of the national population. Of those covered, 52 percent worked in one of Burma's three main cities. Small as the coverage is, it has been slowly expanding.

The major social security benefits are medical care and cash compensation during sickness. Funding comes 75 percent from employers and government, and 25 percent from the workers. Medical services are provided by salaried physicians and other personnel employed by the Social Security Board. Care is given in two relatively well-developed hospitals (in Rangoon and Mandalay) and a network of 85 social security clinics throughout the country. Unlike the MOH, the Social Security Board does not use health assistants or other auxiliary types of personnel. Initially social security health personnel received premium salaries (to attract the best qualified manpower), but since 1970 all salaries in government health services have been equalized. The overall resources and quality of service provided for social security beneficiaries, nevertheless, are clearly superior to those available to the general population.

The Ministry of Cooperatives is another public agency with important health functions. This ministry monitors the activities of local cooperative societies, many of which operate general medical clinics. Cooperative societies, have operated in Burma since colonial times, but the Ministry of Cooperatives has been promoting an expansion of their functions to include social services, such as medical clinics. (The societies are nongovernmental, and their clinics are discussed later.)

The Ministry of Transportation and Communications supervises several quasi-public corporations that provide general health services to employees and their families. These include the Burma Railways Corporation, Burma Airways, and several others. The railways, for example, employ 28,000 workers who, with their families, amount to 115,000 people. These people are served by a salaried staff of physicians and others, working in a network of 30 special clinics and two small hospitals.

Still other public agencies operating special health facilities are the Ministry of Mines, the Ministry of Heavy Industry, and the Ministry of Light Industry. The Ministry of Planning and Finance has a special hospital for its own employees. The Ministry of Social Welfare operates numerous institutions for children, the disabled, and delinquent youth and provides health services for these groups.

Important aspects of environmental sanitation are responsibilities of several ministries other than the MOH. Public water supplies in rural communities (mainly through drilled wells) are developed by the Ministry of Agriculture and Forests. In large towns and cities, public water and waste disposal programs are often developed by the Minstry of Home and Religious Affairs. In some towns the Ministry of Construction establishes these programs.

Regarding pharmaceutical products in Burma, other ministries play a part. After the Revolutionary Council was formed in 1962, numerous foreign-owned drug companies were expelled, and the government set up a single large drug-producing organization, called the Burma Pharmaceutical Industry (BPI), put under the jurisdiction of the Ministry of Light Industry. The BPI has had difficulty in manufacturing needed drugs, largely because of inability to purchase pharmaceutical equipment and basic chemicals (due to lack of foreign currency). The available foreign currency has been used mainly to import finished drugs, through the Ministry of Trade. That agency has a Medicine and Medical Stores Trade Corporation for distribution of drugs throughout Burma, largely to private pharmacies, while the Ministry of Health has its Central Medical Stores for drug distribution to its own facilities. Drug shortages are common, however, giving rise to a large black market in drugs, which are smuggled across national borders.

Nongovernment Agencies. Nongovernment cooperative societies play a large role in Burmese community life, especially in the marketing of rationed food and other supplies. There are 21,000 local societies, of which 589 operated medical clinics in 1986. These clinics were started in 1972 in the main cities, and they have now been extended to about 100 townships. The clinics are open to anyone who can pay the small registration fee; they are not limited to cooperative society members, nor are they financed on a cooperative or group pre-payment basis. Patients pay for each service through fees, calculated to cover the cost of drugs and the doctor's time. Clinics are usually staffed by doctors on part-time salary and are open 3 to 6 hours per day. Nurses, drug dispensers, and other personnel may also be employed.

The Burma Red Cross is another voluntary society, with the usual functions of maintaining ambulances and providing disaster relief. There are branches in every township, but ambulances are located only in Rangoon. Most of the funding comes from personal donations and foreign aid, and a little from government subsidy.

Virtually every township of Burma also has a voluntary Maternal and Child Welfare Society, typically led by the wife of a local political leader. Though nongovernmental, these societies ordinarily accept the guidance of the Ministry of Health. Most MCW societies have two major functions: the operation of small nutrition centers for malnourished children and the establishment and operation of maternity shelters for childbirth deliveries by trained midwives.

Finally, there are health promotion activities of the general mass organizations of Burma, devoted to broad socioeconomic objectives. The Workers' Asiyone (Association) is important in the cities, the Peasants' Asiyone (Association) is important in the rural areas, and the Lanzin Youth Organization is important in all places. The latter groups of young people often give volunteer help in road construction and in building latrines at public places such as schools. They also help in general village clean-up campaigns. Medical student branches of the Lanzin Youth Organization may provide voluntary help in hospitals, in household data collection for surveys, and in treatment campaigns, such as those for trachoma or malaria.

Private Market. In spite of the constitutional guarantee of a "right to medical treatment," no attempt has been made to prohibit or diminish private medical service in Burma. The private health care market has four major components. Oldest, of course, is traditional medicine.

Traditional healing in Burma has been much influenced by Ayurvedic concepts from India and by Buddhist doctrine. For centuries before the entry into Burma of European powers, the entire population depended only on indigenous healers. Then, in the nineteenth century, the British introduced Western medicine in some of the main cities. Traditional medicine, however, remained the only source of help for sick people in the rural areas. Today, traditional practitioners are still very active throughout the country, but they are most significant in rural communities where modern scientific medicine is weak.

Because of the great dependence of people on traditional practitioners, actions to give them official recognition date back to 1928, when a British Committee of Enquiry studied the matter; it recommended formal classes in traditional medicine and the establishment of indigenous hospitals. No action was taken, however, until after national independence was won in 1948. In 1953, the Burmese Indigenous Medicine Act was passed by Parliament, and government-supported indigenous dispensaries were opened in Rangoon and Mandalay. Government registration of traditional practitioners was also established. This was later discontinued, but then reinstated by the Revolutionary Council in 1963, with a requirement that formal examinations be passed.

The number of traditional practitioners in Burma is explored later, but here it should be noted that the great majority are in private practice. Some accept only gifts for their services, but small fees, mainly for traditional drugs, are the general rule. Western drugs are also sometimes dispensed.

Still, the great anthropological interest in traditional medicine should not lead to exaggeration of its importance in the health care market. A nationwide study of 12,000 households in a random sample of 12 townships throughout Burma in 1982 found that, for all illness episodes during the previous 2 weeks, some type of help was sought in 77 percent of the cases. Of the patients who sought help, just 23 percent consulted a traditional practitioner. The population surveyed, furthermore, was predominantly rural.

Another whole category of traditional healing in Burma is the service of traditional birth attendants (TBAs). These typically older women handle a large share of the childbirths throughout the nation, and most of this work is part of the private market. The payment is often in goods (food or other commodities) rather than money, but it is still a private economic transaction. TBAs are gradually being trained, however, and integrated into the official MOH program.

The private market for modern professional medical care is of greater importance in Burma. The offices of private practitioners of medicine and dentistry are found in the main cities and most small towns everywhere. The principal form of work of Burmese physicians in 1982 was in government employment (52.1 percent), but 10.9 percent worked mainly in cooperative clinics, and 37.0 percent were exclusively in private practice. The vast majority of government and also cooperative clinic physicians, moreover, engaged in private practice part of the time every day. There is no regulatory or legal objection to this; it is generally recognized as a reasonable way to compensate for low public salaries. Assuming part-time private practice to be done by 80 percent of employed doctors for approximately 20 hours per week, the private market absorbs about 62 percent of physician time in the Burma health system.

About 90 percent of privately practicing physicians are general practitioners, with very modest offices. There are rarely nurses or other auxiliary personnel, and medical equipment is very limited. The fees charged are low, mainly for drugs dispensed or injected, and all but the very poorest people can afford them. In contrast to MOH facilities, which serve mainly pregnant women and small children, private medical clinics serve a full range of patients—male and female, adults and children. Private clinics are also more widely dispersed than MOH and other organized clinics, so that they are accessible to larger numbers of patients.

Private clinics come under little, if any, surveillance from public authorities or the Burmese Medical Council. They must register annually with the Health Office of the division/ state, and sometimes (if there is a complaint) they are inspected for sanitary conditions.

Private dental practice is very similar in character to private medical practice, except on a smaller scale. In 1986, of the 630 dentists in Burma, 229 were in purely private practice or working in cooperatives. Also a good share of the time of the 401 dentists in government service is spent in private practice. More than physicians, dentists are concentrated in the large cities, and their services are limited largely to extractions and fillings.

The private market for pharmaceutical products is particularly large in Burma. It arises fundamentally from the inability of the government health programs, despite their great efforts, to respond sufficiently to the needs of patients. The pharmaceutical market includes the direct dispensing of drugs by physicians and the sale of drugs by private drugstores for the use of private buyers or of patients in a public facility (in which the drug supply is often inadequate).

The doctor who dispenses drugs purchases them (at wholesale rates) either from a township drug shop, supplied by the Ministry of Trade, or from a private drugstore. Most of these drugstores are simply small commercial shops, staffed only by a clerk without any pharmaceutical training. Only a few of the buyers come with medical prescriptions. Most of the drugs sold have been obtained in the black market (smuggled from neighboring countries), and their prices are extremely high.

Finally, it is widely recognized in Burma that certain types of misconduct occur in official health programs and contribute to the private health care market. Although it is officially forbidden, paramedical and ancillary personnel in many villages, make private charges for "medical" services to patients after their official working hours.

Health Resources

Though greatly improved from the situation in colonial times, Burma's supply of resources is still much below the needs.

Health Manpower. Under British rule and even up to 1960, most physicians in Burma came from other countries, principally India. Medical education in Burma started in 1923, when the Rangoon Medical College was launched as a branch of the University of Calcutta in India. Only after independence did this become a medical faculty of the University of Rangoon, with the first graduates coming out in 1953. Then in 1954 and 1962 additional medical schools were founded. Soon the three schools were removed from the universities and made separate medical institutes, coming under the control of the Ministry of Health in 1973.

Medical institute enrollment gradually increased, with about 550 graduates per year in 1986. Except for specialty training, graduates rarely leave Burma; if they do, they must pay the government back for the costs of their medical education. Medical training requires 7 years after secondary school, plus a mandatory 1-year internship. After this, specialty training at a teaching hospital (23 in the state or divisional capitals) may be undertaken in numerous fields. MOH policy in the 1980s, however, was to emphasize studies in primary health care, rather than the usual medical and surgical specialties. Accordingly, the Department of Preventive and Social Medicine has a major role in each of the medical institutes; the training includes field visits to rural health programs. Faculty salaries are quite low, however, so that most professors are part-time and also engage in private practice.

In 1986 there were just over 10,000 physicians in Burma, or about 26.5 per 100,000 population. In 1965 the ratio was 8.4 doctors per 100,000. If physicians in cooperative clinics are considered private, roughly half are mainly in private practice and half are mainly in government service. Since most government doctors also engage in private practice, as noted, more than 60 percent of the medical time available is spent in the private sector. Despite the customary urban concentration, medical fees are quite low, and private practitioners are widely distributed in the small towns.

In Burma, distinctions are made among paramedical, basic, and primary health care personnel. Paramedical personnel are those who work under the orders of a physician, assisting him or her in the diagnosis or treatment of patients. These personnel have not been extensively trained in Burma; in 1984 they included, for example, only 83 radiographers and 95 physiotherapists. They are trained in one Paramedical Training Institute at the Rangoon General Hospital.

Professional nurses, also counted as paramedical personnel, numbered 5,560 in 1985, or 15.0 per 100,000. They are trained at one of seven hospital-based nursing schools, and they work almost entirely in hospitals. There are also relatively large numbers of midwives and auxiliary midwives in Burma, but there are no formally trained assistant nurses. (In hospitals, untrained young women may serve as nurse aides.)

So-called dental nurses are paradental workers, trained for 2 years after tenth grade, for the dental care of children. Only about 100 of these personnel were trained from 1975 to 1980; training was then discontinued (due to lack of dental equipment) but resumed on a small scale in 1986.

Basic health personnel are those who render "basic health services" at health centers in rural areas and cities. The leader among these personnel is the health assistant, who is always a man trained at the relatively well-developed Health Assistant Training School (HATS) near Rangoon. HATS was founded in 1953 and has a full-time faculty of 17 teachers. The curriculum lasts for 27 months, and includes not only health sciences, but also instruction in the structure of government, planning, and management. In 1986 there were 1,350 health assistants in Burma—barely enough to staff the nation's health centers.

Other basic health personnel include midwives and sanitary officers. The 8,200 midwives, as of 1986, had been trained in 16 midwifery schools, located in teaching hospitals. The course lasts 18 months after 10 years of schooling. The Burmese midwife is trained to provide preventive services for small children, as well as midwifery. After several years of experience, the midwife may undertake an additional year of study to become a *lady health visitor* (LHV). In the structure of health centers, the LHV is considered deputy to the health assistant, and she takes charge if the health assistant is away. There were 1,570 LHVs in 1986.

Personnel for environmental sanitation in Burma are known as *public health supervisors.*

These are typically young men who had worked previously in single-purpose health campaigns, such as immunizations or malaria control. They have had only 6 to 8 years of elementary school, and about 3 months of special training. They perform miscellaneous tasks at the health centers, in addition to environmental surveillance. After several years of experience, a public health supervisor can take 9 months of additional training to acquire greater responsibilities and a higher salary. In 1986 Burma had 675 of the elementary supervisors and 485 of those at a higher level.

Primary health care workers, in Burma's terminology, are volunteer personnel who serve in the villages. As volunteers, these personnel are not employed by the MOH or any government agency, but are appointed by the Village People's Council. Since 1978 auxiliary midwives have been prepared, and since 1982 community health workers for somewhat broader functions. Their training, at the nearest township hospital or health center, lasts only a few weeks, and their duties are mainly to educate villagers about available MOH services. While theoretically volunteer, most of these PHC workers receive gifts or small salaries from the villages or may earn a small profit from the sale of drugs (furnished by the township Health Office).

A third type of volunteer has been the *ten household health worker* (THHW), who has no special training, but simply encourages prenatal care for any pregnant woman in 10 surrounding households, and promotes latrine construction. Altogether in 1985, there were 10,200 THHWs, 10,150 auxiliary midwives, and 36,000 community health workers. As volunteers, they were all expected to work for only about 2 hours per day. The performance of volunteers is supposed to be supervised by the basic health personnel at the closest health center.

Traditional practitioners in Burma have been estimated to exceed 30,000, although only about 5,000 were registered with the MOH in 1986. The MOH employed 369 healers that year in public hospitals and dispensaries (numbering 89) of traditional medicine. Since 1976, the MOH has operated an Institute of Traditional Medicine, with a formal

training program of 3 years, after 10 years of schooling. While supported by the ministry, traditional healers are not brought into the general MOH program. Traditional birth attendants, however, are given some training and integrated with other MOH activities; by 1986 this applied to 17,320 TBAs.

Health Facilities. Before independence, there were many small hospitals in Burma, usually operated by religious missions in rural communities. In 1965, after the Revolutionary Council was in power, these were nationalized, except for a leprosarium and three small Buddhist and Moslem hospitals. The vast majority of hospitals are now controlled by the Ministry of Health under the Directorate of Medical Care; a few, founded since the 1960s, are under other public auspices. No purely private hospitals exist in Burma.

In 1984–85, there were 635 hospitals in the country with 25,960 beds, of which 98 percent were controlled by the MOH. The distribution of these facilities and beds was as follows:

Sponsorship	Hospitals	Beds
Ministry of Health	620	25,379
Cooperative Societies	3	30
Social security	1	150
Public corporations	11	400
Total	635	25,959

For the 36,392,000 people of Burma, reported for 1984–85, this meant about 0.71 bed per 1,000 population.

With such a relatively small supply of hospital beds, it is no surprise that many facilities, especially the larger ones, are seriously overcrowded. These data apply to "sanctioned" or officially approved hospital beds, but the number of beds actually set up (by increasing the beds in a ward, using lobbies and corridors for beds, etc.) and available is much larger. The Rangoon General Hospital, with 1,500 sanctioned beds, for example, has had to make 1,700 beds available for patients. The Mandalay General Hospital with 800 sanctioned beds has had to accommodate 1,400 patients. A study in 1981 found that nationally the number of beds actually in use was 23 percent greater than what was officially sanctioned, meaning a ratio of 0.87 bed per 1,000 population in use.

This overcrowding is less noticeable in the smaller hospitals, where the medical staffing is solely by general practitioners. Larger hospitals are usually staffed by better qualified medical and surgical specialists. With the heavily rural character of the population, however, the great majority of Burma's hospitals are small. In 1984–85, out of 620 MOH hospitals, 548 or 88 percent had under 50 beds each and only 12 percent had 100 or more beds. Of the 548 small hospitals, 295 were known as *station health units,* having been upgraded from former rural health centers. The gravitation of patients to larger hospitals certainly suggests a strong preference for the treatment of significant illness by specialists.

Hospitals are ordinarily constructed by the Ministry of Construction, according to specifications of the Ministry of Health or the few other bodies responsible for funding. Financial support for construction of small rural hospitals (usually 16-bedded), however, is usually given jointly by the Ministry of Health and the Ministry of Home and Religious Affairs, along with voluntary donations from the local community.

More recently established facilities in Burma are rural and urban health centers, which provide organized ambulatory care. They are the key resources for implementing Burma's devotion to the WHO-promoted principle of primary health care (PHC). Most health centers are located in rural areas, but a number of similar units are in the cities. The rural centers are staffed entirely by ancillary personnel. The urban facilities, some of which are called *dispensaries* and, unlike the rural units, are usually staffed by at least one physician plus other health personnel. Considering both rural and urban facilities, their types and numbers in 1985–86 were as follows:

Rural health centers	1,337
Cooperative clinics	589
Maternal and child health centers	348
Indigenous medicine dispensaries	89
Social security clinics	85
Urban health centers	64

Special dispensaries	47
Railway dispensaries	29
Other corporation clinics	15
Total	2,603

Among these nine types of ambulatory care unit, the MOH has put greatest emphasis on the rural health centers, each of which has been expected to serve about 20,000 people—although this is more than the number of people usually accessible to each one. As with hospitals, construction costs are usually shared between a government ministry and the local community.

Commodities. The different sources of pharmaceutical products used in Burma have been noted. For the period 1984 through 1986, these sources can be estimated approximately as follows (measured by expenditures):

Source	Percentage of Expenditures
Burma Pharmaceutical Industry (BPI)	24
Imports by Ministry of Trade	18
UNICEF and other foreign aid	5
Open market	53
All sources	100

Thus, the BPI has produced a much smaller share of total drugs than was intended. These several sources provide drugs for MOH facilities, cooperative clinics, the military establishment, the social security program, private medical practitioners, and drug sellers or drugstores dispensing items to the general population. The open market, of course, which accounts for more than half the total drug expenditures, is largely a black market of drugs smuggled into Burma illegally. Medical equipment and supplies is almost entirely imported, mostly from Japan.

Knowledge. Most of the scientific knowledge relevant to health and medicine has been acquired from abroad, but medical research is important enough in Burma to warrant a major department in the Ministry of Health. The Department of Medical Research has divisions doing studies in 16 fields, including immunology, nutrition, and indigenous drugs. A substantial share of this research is supported by foreign aid, mostly bilateral.

Some research has even been done on the operations of the health system. Modest medical and public health libraries are located in the two main cities, but such facilities are very weak elsewhere. The Burma Medical Association publishes a journal, in which clinical experiences are reported.

Economic Support of the Health System

The major sources of economic support for Burma's health system are government and private households. Buddhism encourages many charitable donations, both in money and in labor, although the measurable extent of these in the health system seems to be relatively modest. The currency of Burma is the kyat (K), which in 1986 had a value in international exchange of approximately K7 = US $1.

Government Health Expenditures. The principal government expenditures are by the Ministry of Health. For the 1985–86 fiscal year, these came to K621,000,000, or about $89,000,000. Of this amount, 36 percent was for capital purposes and 64 percent for program operations. Moreover, 23 percent of the overall budget came to the MOH from foreign aid.

As a share of total government expenditures, those by the MOH have fluctuated. They were 7.7 percent of the total in 1974–75, falling to 6.8 percent in 1979–80, and rising to 8.7 percent in 1983–84. Adjusting for both inflation and population increase, the World Bank estimated that real MOH expenditures between 1970 and 1985 were virtually constant.

MOH expenditures have been dominated by the costs, both capital and operating, of hospitals. In 1984–85, hospital spending accounted for 62 percent of the total. Of the balance, 22.4 percent went for primary health care, 7.3 percent for disease control campaigns, and 8.3 percent for support and administrative functions.

Foreign Aid. The share of MOH expenditures coming from foreign aid has been noted. Such aid was not accepted by Burma from 1962 to 1978, but since 1979 it has been welcomed. The United Nations Development Program (UNDP) has tabulated the amount of foreign aid from both multilateral and bilateral sources, but assistance from Japan was not reported—at least not for 1985. In that year, adjusting for substantial aid from Japan, health-related foreign aid amounted to $20.4 million, of which 56 percent came from multilateral agencies and 44 percent from individual countries. The largest multilateral donor was UNICEF and the largest bilateral donor was Japan.

Other Public Agencies. The medical care aspects of the social security program entailed expenditure of about $3 million in 1985–86. For rural water supply schemes, the Ministry of Agriculture and Forestry spent about $1.26 million in 1985–86. For the health-related expenditures of other ministries very crude estimates can be made. Considering the quasi-public corporations, the military forces, the Ministry of Cooperatives (not the local cooperative clinics), and foreign aid to agencies other than the MOH, about $6 million was spent in 1985.

Charitable Donations. Under Buddhist philosophy "merits" are earned for a peaceful future life through charitable donations. Furthermore, peasants in Burma are not subject to direct taxation. For both these reasons, when community leaders call on people to make donations for health purposes, virtually everyone responds, in rough proportion to family wealth.

Studies made by Burmese social scientists suggest that in the 1980s the average charitable donation in Burma amounted to between K0.5 and K1.0 per person per year. (Even this small average is heavily influenced by a handful of very large donations from rich families.) Donations are given mainly for the construction of health centers and sanitation equipment. Reports by government agencies on various construction projects indicated that almost exactly one-third of these capital costs were contributed by local community people. Donations to voluntary health agencies (Red Cross and the Maternal and Child Welfare Society) have been relatively small. Altogether in the 1980s, charitable donations in Burma amounted to about $4.4 million per year. In addition, some nongovernment and charitable donations are received from abroad, amounting in 1985 to a value of about $2.9 million.

Private Households. Expenditures for health purposes by families and individuals in Burma may be estimated from both the demand side (household surveys) and the supply side (provider incomes from private service). On the demand side, several urban and rural household surveys showed average health expenditures of K24 per person per year in 1985; of this amount 46 percent was for drugs. Nationally this came to private health expenditures of K871.2 million, or $124.5 in 1985.

Calculating private health expenditures from the supply side requires estimating the gross incomes from private practice of physicians, traditional practitioners, drugstores, and other providers. With various adjustments for part-time work, physicians were estimated to have average gross incomes from private service of about K50,000 each per year in 1985. Somewhat similar estimates can be made for other principal providers of private health care in Burma, resulting in an estimated national expenditure in 1985 of K839,440,000, or about $127.8 million. This gross income was distributed approximately as follows:

Health Care Provider	Percentage
Physicians and dentists	38
Drugstores and drug sellers	35
Traditional practitioners	11
Cooperative clinics	9
Village health workers	7
All providers	100

It should be noted that the supply side estimate of K839.44 million in health expenditures for 1985 is remarkably close to the demand side estimate of K871.2 million—providing some

confirmation of these two different analytical approaches. The somewhat higher figure for the demand side estimate (based on household surveys) might be a result of payments made to illegal practitioners, such as health assistants or lady health visitors, reported by families.

Summary of Economic Support. Based on the several figures for health expenditures, reported or estimated earlier, the overall economic support for Burma's national health system in 1985 amounted to about $231,975,000. The sources of these funds were distributed approximately as follows:

Source	Percentage
Ministry of Health	29.3
Foreign aid to MOH	8.9
Other government agencies	4.4
Foreign aid to other agencies	1.5
Charitable donations	1.9
Foreign charity	1.2
Private households	52.7
All sources	100.0

The total expenditures in the Burma health system may be related to the gross national product. For 1985, this came to 3.43 percent. If domestic charitable donations are combined with expenditures by private households, then 54.6 percent of health expenditures in 1985 came from the private sector. Moreover, because a significant portion of government health activities have been supported by foreign aid, the relative burden carried by the private sector in Burma would actually be somewhat heavier. The share of total health system costs borne by all parts of government in Burma in 1985 was 33.7 percent.

Health System Management

The management of Burma's national health system reflects a somewhat unusual combination of certain concepts of conventional socialism with the authoritarian principles of a military government.

Planning. The Burma Socialist Programme Party has theoretically been dedicated to a policy of planning in all social sectors, including health. Overall national social and economic planning is the responsibility of the Ministry of Planning and Finance, probably the strongest ministry in the government. The first general 4-year plan started in 1970, and 1987 marked the beginning of the fifth such plan.

For health, there is a responsible subdivision in the Ministry of Planning and Finance, but the initial work starts in the Ministry of Health. Here the Directorate of Planning, Administration, Budget, and Training (PABT) has the main responsibilities. In earlier years, health planning was devoted principally to the expansion of health manpower and to mounting campaigns against malaria and other endemic diseases. In the 1980s, plans were more explicitly focused on extending population coverage with primary health care. It was this planning that called for the training of volunteer health care workers in the villages, described previously.

Regarding all health planning in Burma, the role of the general population, as distinguished from the health professionals, is important. Little can be accomplished in any aspect of planning without the concurrence and support of both the numerous People's Councils and the several levels of the Burma Socialist Programme Party. The BSPP is especially important because it holds the decisive political power at all levels, from the national capital outward to the smallest village.

Administration. Health policy determination is highly centralized in Burma, consistent with a long tradition, going back even before the dominance of the BSPP. The hierarchy of authority in the BSPP usually ensures that any decision made at the top will be acted on throughout the nation.

Nevertheless, the initial preparation of budgets begins at the local level. Each township medical officer submits an annual budget, reflecting his perception of the needs, to the State/Divisional Health Office. Here it is reviewed, and usually adjusted, before it is submitted to Rangoon. The semifinal decisions are then made by the Minister of Health, and the final decisions by the full Council of State,

on advice from the Ministry of Planning and Finance. This entire process also applies to the Ministries of Labour, Cooperatives, Agriculture, and other public authorities with health-related programs.

Supervision is, of course, an important aspect of health system administration. The township medical officer and township health officer have the main responsibilities for primary health care in the villages, but so much of their time is absorbed by clinical work in the township hospital and perhaps in an urban health center, that little time is left for supervisory or consultative work.

Evaluation is an aspect of administration that has been relatively well developed in Burma. Numerous studies have been made by university social scientists, in cooperation with the Ministry of Health. The coverage of populations with MOH personnel and the rates of utilization of various services have candidly revealed strengths and weaknesses. Mortality and morbidity rates have been used as simple indicators of the results of health services, although changes may be due as much or more to overall standards of living.

Legislation. In a single-party political system like Burma's, most policy decisions are made directly by the government and its ministers, rather than through parliamentary legislation. Certain actions, however, which have major impacts on the behavior of people (that is, the regulation of society) have been the subject of legislation. Many of these regulatory laws in Burma have simply been carried over from British colonial times, and a few were enacted since independence.

Some of the major laws affecting health policies in Burma, in spite of their early origins, are listed here:

1897	The Epidemic Diseases Act
1898	The Leprosy Act
1908	The Vaccination Act
1912	The Lunacy Act
1915	Burma Medical Act
1917	The Ghee Adulteration Act
1930	The Food and Drug Act
1931	The Dangerous Drugs Act

1953 Indigenous Burmese Medical Practitioners Board Act
1972 Public Health Act
1974 Narcotic Act

The postindependence Public Health Act of 1972 has probably had the most sweeping affect of all these laws. It gives wide authority to the Ministry of Health and its subdivisions, and it authorizes the enforcement of various procedures (e.g., the notification of infectious diseases) by local People's Councils.

The regulation of medical practice under the Burma Medical Act of 1915 establishes basic requirements for the registration or licensure of physicians. It requires all medical practitioners (public or private) to affiliate with the Burma Medical Council (modeled after the similar British Council), whose members are chosen half by the profession and half by the government, for the purpose of ethical surveillance; unethical behavior of a doctor may lead to his loss of registration. Official registration with the state/divisional health office is also required of all private medical clinics, as well as public physicians. Maintenance of this registration requires annual renewal, permitting clinic inspection regarding minimum standards, and payment of a fee. Similar state/divisional registration is required of dental surgeons, graduate nurses, and midwives. Medical specialization is also certified by the Burma Medical Council.

A general Conscript Law of the early 1960s has relevance to medical practice. Under this law, in 1964 new medical graduates were required to serve for a time in rural areas. Then in 1969, this requirement was ended, since its objectives were theoretically achieved through the public employment of doctors.

The 1953 legislation on indigenous medical practitioners requires the registration of these persons with the Ministry of Health. This has not been strongly enforced, however; the great majority of these practitioners have not been registered, for which there is evidently no penalty. Since traditional practitioners have been engaged by the Ministry of Health to work in official dispensaries, they are required to pass an examination in three fields: (a) Buddhist concepts of body structure, (b) Ayurvedic medicine, and (c) astrology. Only those who pass this examination with high scores are engaged by the MOH.

An especially important type of legal regulation is that concerning pure food and proper drugs. Several of the laws listed earlier concern this, but their implementation has been seriously deficient. Authority in this field is now vested in the MOH Laboratory Directorate, where work has been done on designing an extensive new regulatory program. The widespread sale of illegally "imported" drugs in Burma, discussed earlier, adds special urgency to this problem.

Delivery of Health Services

Emphasis by the World Health Organization on the importance of primary health care has had a significant influence on policies of the Ministry of Health in Burma.

Primary Health Care. MOH responsibilities for supervising primary health care (PHC) in communities are carried by the township health offices. A nationwide field study in the early 1980s examined exactly how the TMOs and THOs spent their working days. It was learned that they spent only 4.4 and 4.3 hours per day, on the average, in official activities. (Most of the remainder of the working day was presumably spent in private medical practice.) Analysis of these activities in a random week showed the following distribution of official time:

	Percentage of Working Time	
Activities	Medical *Officer*	Health *Officer*
Hospital service	85.3	27.2
Field work	0.0	4.5
Travel	12.4	24.4
Office work	1.9	43.8
Other	0.4	0.1
All activities	100.0	100.0

Noteworthy is the very high proportion of time spent by the TMO in clinical service to hospital patients, although this official is supposed to be in charge of all health activities in the township. Even the THO, supposedly devoted to preventive services, spends substantial time in the hospital and only 4.5 percent of his time in field work.

The principal channels through which the MOH provides ambulatory basic health services (BHS) are urban and rural health centers. Both types of health center serve an average of about 20,000 people, but services are naturally more accessible in the cities. A major distinction is that the urban units are nearly always staffed with one or more doctors, while the RHCs are headed by health assistants and staffed by BHS personnel. The medically staffed urban centers are limited mainly to Burma's three largest cities: Rangoon, Mandalay, and Moulmein.

The greatest proportion of patients attending MOH health centers, both urban and rural, are small children and pregnant women. The most numerous personnel are midwives, including lady health visitors (essentially, senior midwives). At rural health centers, the dominant staff member is clearly the supervising male health assistant. When health records are good, weight charts are kept on infants, to alert mothers to the child's development.

Field surveys of a number of RHCs in several divisions offer more precise data on the performance of key personnel. In the early 1980s, it was found that health assistants spent 6.4 hours per day on their jobs, and lady health visitors spent 6.2 hours per day. This time was distributed as follows:

	Time Spent (percent)	
Activity	Health assistant	Lady health visitor
Work in the health center	30.5	11.8
Field activities	42.7	47.1
School health service	6.7	0.0
Travel	20.1	41.1
All activities	100.0	100.0

Another form of analysis was made in 1985 on RHC staff in two centers of one township.

From direct observation, the time spent by personnel during several days was classified as "productive" or "nonproductive." The findings were as follows:

Type of Personnel	Time (percent)	
	Productive	Nonproductive
Health assistant	38.9	61.1
Lady health visitor	37.7	62.3
Midwife	48.3	51.7
Sanitation supervisor	25.3	74.7

These disappointing findings can perhaps be explained by the relatively low rate of attendance of patients at the RHCs.

According to statistical data reported to the national People's Assembly for 1983–84, there were 19,900,000 attendances at all RHCs, urban health centers, MCH centers, and related general clinics. For the 260 days these units were open during the year, 76,538 patients were attended per day. The total number of health care units in 1983–84 was 1,712, with an average attendance at each of 44.7 per day. On the other hand, a report of the MOH on the People's Health Plan for 1983–84 indicates a total of 15,019,981 overall attendances. The same calculation suggests an attendance rate of 33.7 patients per day. With these diverse figures, it is probably safest to estimate a daily attendance at RHCs and UHCs of 30 to 40 patients. Considering the population theoretically served and the staff available, this is not a very high rate of use.

An opinion often heard in Burma is that the urban and rural health centers are not heavily used by patients because they often lack the necessary drugs. For this reason, most patients with disturbing symptoms prefer to go to a private physician, a cooperative society or other special clinic, or an open-market drug seller. As a result, the persons attending the UHCs and RHCs are largely pregnant women and small children, who get routine preventively oriented MCH care, seldom requiring medication. A study of RHC use, reported by UNICEF in 1986, found that patients coming to RHCs were demographically distributed as follows:

Type of Patient	Attendance (percent)
Women	61.2
Children under 5 years	17.9
Children 6–14 years	13.1
Adult men	7.8
All patients	100.0

In spite of this strong emphasis on MCH work, family planning service is not an official part of the program. (One can understand that, being surrounded by several large and powerful nations, the government of Burma wishes its population to increase.) Contraception and sterilization are not illegal, but they are not actively promoted. Contraceptive advice and materials are available from private physicians, and contraceptive pills are readily purchased (by those who can afford them) at open-market drug shops. Sterilization procedures are performed in hospitals, if a special hospital committee finds them to be medically justified. If a woman has had an excessive number of children, and wishes greater spacing between pregnancies, the midwife may refer her to the TMO; he may give contraceptive advice, which could include insertion of an intrauterine device (IUD). Contraceptive pills, however, are available only in open-market shops.

Abortion, on the other hand, is illegal in Burma, unless a hospital committee of physicians decides that it is necessary to save the life or preserve the health of the woman. In fact, therapeutic abortions are rarely performed in hospitals, although incomplete abortions or miscarriages are a very frequent cause of hospital admission. (In many hospitals there is one complicated abortion case for every two childbirths.) The evidence suggests that, as in many other countries, illegal abortions are frequently performed or attempted on women with unwanted pregnancies, perhaps done by a TBA, the woman herself, or someone else. Only those cases that are poorly handled, causing serious hemorrhage, end up in a hospital.

In one township of central Burma, Ayadaw, a special model primary health care program was developed in the 1980s. The township, with a 1986 population of about 150,000, was made up of a central town of 8,000 and 158 villages. Having earlier been a scene of insurgent action, Ayadaw was one of 30 townships chosen by the central government for priority development. Strong local organizations of peasants, workers, youth, and veterans were promoted, an ample township hospital and five rural health centers were established, and special efforts were made to provide all facilities with full complements of trained personnel. Numerous community health workers and auxiliary midwives were trained and posted in the villages, receiving modest local salaries (despite their "volunteer" status). No less than five Cooperative Society medical clinics were organized, and three physicians operated private clinics. The local Maternal and Child Welfare Society built a nutrition center and the local Burma Red Cross Society was particularly active. Exceptional energies, supported with foreign aid, went into the drilling of tubewells, so that by 1985, 141 were in operation, providing safe water to nearly every village.

The health accomplishments of the model PHC program in Ayadaw township were demonstrable in vastly improved environmental sanitation, the reduction of endemic diseases (such as trachoma and leprosy), vastly safer childbirths, better nutritional status of small children, dramatic reductions in diarrheal morbidity and infant and maternal mortality rates, a high rate of day-to-day medical care for adults in the cooperative clinics (whose doctors were well paid and pledged to refrain from private practice), and many other health and social conditions. In a word, the Ayadaw PHC model demonstrated what Burma's health system could achieve with the deliberate application of technical guidance, community leadership, economic support, and political will. In recognition of these achievements, carefully documented by a young MOH official, the township was awarded the International Sasakawa Prize on Primary Health Care of the World Health Organization for 1986.

Special Ambulatory Care Patterns. Aside from the MOH network of health centers, several other programs in Burma provide ambulatory health service.

Cooperative society clinics are open at least 6 days a week and sometimes 7. Based on the report of 8,090,000 attendances at 589 cooperative clinics in 1985, this would mean an average of 44 patients per day—higher than the number of patients coming to MOH health centers. These clinics are always staffed with at least one physician and usually with a nurse and certain other personnel, even in rural locations. They are open not only on Saturdays and often Sundays, when MOH facilities are closed, but often in the evenings for the special convenience of working people.

Many people prefer cooperative clinics over private physicians because they are less expensive. The drug costs are especially reasonable, since the cooperative societies are entitled to a specified share of each township's quota from the Trade Corporation, while most of the private doctor's drugs must be purchased from open-market shops. Cooperative clinic doctors are also reported to take an adequate amount of time with each patient, unlike busy doctors in the free but typically overcrowded hospital out-patient departments and urban health centers. The cooperative clinic doctor's time is preserved by the assistance of a nurse, who gives all injections and assists in other ways. In the larger cities, cooperative clinics are sometimes staffed by specialists. Almost all these physicians also maintain private practices after clinic hours.

The Social Security clinics are exceptionally well staffed with doctors, nurses, and other personnel. In the large cities, they are called Type A and are staffed with two or three doctors, and in the smaller towns the Types B and C clinics are also staffed with at least one physician. The 85 Social Security clinics are obviously busy places; there are 200 to 300 attendances a day in the Type A clinics, 100 to 150 in the Type B clinics, and fewer attendances only in the Type C clinics. In contrast to MOH facilities, the patients are principally adult men, indicating that these individuals do indeed seek health service when they feel confident that they can get it. Specimens for laboratory tests are sent to the Worker's Hospital in Rangoon.

Small wonder that the workers covered by Social Security use their health services at the high rate of 9 attendances per person per year. Social Security physicians, who are paid the same modest salaries as MOH medical personnel, are also free to engage in private practice after hours, and nearly all do so. Regulations require, however, that no socially insured workers may be seen in their private clinics.

The special clinics maintained by quasi-public corporations are also staffed with physicians. Unlike Social Security, they serve families as well as workers. In 1985, the Burma Railways Corporation clinics had 3.04 attendances per eligible person per year.

With its official recognition of indigenous medicine, the MOH operates 89 clinics of this sort, in both cities and rural areas. Based on data reported for 1985, and assuming that they are open 6 days a week, these clinics serve about 80 patients per day. The clinics are open for long hours, and three practitioners serve every day. A major feature of each of these dispensaries is the supply of traditional drugs. Under MOH influence, each clinic keeps a standardized inventory of 57 drugs. A few of these are provided by the Trade Corporation, but the great majority must be purchased in the open market, usually by the practitioner but sometimes by the patient. In addition to dispensing drugs, the traditional healer advises on diet, exercise, bathing, and so on. In cases regarded as mental in origin, he offers personal counseling. MOH policy recognizes that many people have faith in traditional healers, and the government must offer "free choice of doctor."

Finally, throughout Burma there are the thousands of private clinics, where general practitioners provide ambulatory medical care. Although they do little in the way of prevention, private GPs are probably the largest source for day-to-day curative service in the country. The large number of private practitioners was discussed earlier. Assuming that private clinics serve an average of 20 patients per day (a conservative estimate) or about 6,000 patients per year, the 6,240 FTE private practices provide 37,440,000 attendances annually—much more than the attendances at all MOH health centers and dispensaries.

Very much like private shops selling food or merchandise, the typical private clinic is very small, modestly furnished, and not particularly sanitary. It is rather conspicuous, however, on the main streets of almost every Burmese town and city, because of a distinctive sign with a large red cross symbol. The doctor's room is usually small, with space for an examining table and a little desk. The waiting room may be so small that patients must await their turn by standing outside. A small cabinet holds some drugs, purchased mainly in the open market, and dispensed directly to patients. Most of the charge to patients is for drugs, while the consultation costs less. It is estimated that private general practitioners, seeing some 20 patients a day, spend around 15 minutes with each. Services are available 6 or 7 days a week.

Village Volunteer Health Services. The training and posting of part-time volunteer health workers in the villages have been discussed. These included community health workers (CHWs) and auxiliary midwives (AMWs). According to several studies, however, the volume of services provided by these village health workers has been quite low. One study in 1983–84 reported that CHWs had an average of 286 personal health contacts per year, or about 0.8 contact per day. In 1984–85, the average contacts were even fewer, or about 0.4 contact per day. Environmental sanitation contacts of CHWs, reported only for 1983–84, were 14.7 per year or 1.2 such contacts per month. The decline in personal health contacts was associated with a shortage of drugs.

The performance of AMWs has been expressed in terms of the number of home deliveries that they supervised per year. These were reported as only 16.6 in 1983–84 (1.4 per month) and 18.0 in 1984–85 (1.5 per month). On the brighter side, it has been reported that in certain villages studied, the work of the AMW influenced the beliefs of mothers. Before the AMW was assigned, the majority of mothers (62 percent) expressed preference for the use of TBAs; after the AMW was at work, only 13 percent of the mothers expressed preference for the TBA, and the rest stated they would use trained personnel for deliveries.

Overall Ambulatory Care Utilization. In 1986, when rural health centers in Burma were estimated to serve some 20,000 people each, MOH officials regarded these units as covering about 30 percent of the rural population. This assumed a 1-hour walk for accessibility; if a 2-hour walk were acceptable, the rural population coverage would have been 60 percent. It

was this deficiency in coverage that led to the training of community health workers for the villages.

A major household survey was made in 1982 on all sources of ambulatory health care in Burma. Persons were interviewed in some 12,000 households of 12 randomly selected townships, located in the four main geographic regions of the country (delta, dry, coastal, and hilly). Respondents were asked about their illness experience in the previous 2 weeks, when memory is bound to be reliable. It was found that one-quarter (24.8 percent) of the people had some illness. Of these, 23 percent did nothing or acted on their own judgment with self-care. Of the 77 percent who sought attention for their illness, the distribution of health care providers consulted was as follows:

Provider Consulted	Percentage
Physician	38.4
Basic health service worker	35.2
Traditional practitioner	23.0
Volunteer health worker	3.2
All providers	100.0

We do not know where the "physicians" were located, whether in some organized program or in private practice. It is noteworthy, nevertheless, that the largest share of people sought help from physicians (and the sample studied represented the rural population in its proper nationwide proportion).

The same household survey inquired about deaths occurring during the last full year. Families were asked about any health care received by the decedent in the 7 days before death, with the following findings:

Health Attendant Before Death	Percentage
None	12.8
CHW or AMW	1.5
Basic health service worker	23.6
Traditional practitioner	29.8
Physician	32.3

Although almost one-third of dying patients were seen by a modern physician, two-thirds were not.

Hospital Services. The overcrowding of larger MOH hospitals, noted earlier, places a heavy burden on the personnel, whose numbers are based on the "sanctioned" beds, not the beds actually in use. The beds on a ward or in some other room (intended perhaps as a lobby) may be so close together that a nurse can barely walk between them. With such overloaded staffs, relative to the number of patients, it should not be surprising that hospitals, both large and small, do not give the bright and hygienic impression people everywhere have come to expect in these facilities. The shortages of strong cleansing agents and of paint in Burma doubtless contribute to the problem.

Hospitals in Burma, as in many low-income countries, provide meals for only a fraction (about 35 percent) of the patients—those who come from far away or who have no family nearby. The majority of patients must get meals from families or friends, who bring in the food once or twice a day. The toilet facilities for each ward are quite rudimentary. With such crowded conditions, patients are discharged as soon as possible; the average length-of-stay in large hospitals is only about 5 days, and slightly longer for surgical cases. Overall staffing, even in large and more technically developed MOH hospitals, is less than 1 health personnel per occupied bed.

Drug shortages were a common problem in the smaller hospitals throughout Burma in the 1980s. The only solution was for the patient's family to purchase needed drugs in the open market, at very high prices, of course. Laboratory and x-ray equipment is found in the larger state/division hospitals, but is usually lacking or in disrepair in the small township hospitals. Many small hospitals have no mattresses for the beds, and patients lie on wooden boards.

MOH hospitals are furnished drugs periodically by the Ministry's Central Medical Stores (CMS), but in 1986 only 60 to 70 percent of the needs could be satisfied. Normally the hospitals submit their requests to CMS three times a year, but the responses are seldom adequate. About 60 percent of CMS supplies come from the Burma Pharmaceutical Industry and 40 percent from overseas purchases by the Ministry of Trade.

One 25-bed Indigenous Medicine Hospital in Mandalay is exceptionally well maintained. It has no provision for laboratory or x-ray services or for surgery, but extensive supplies of traditional herbal medications are on hand. The clean and attractive atmosphere seems to serve political purposes.

Another unusual public hospital in Burma is the 150-bed Social Security facility in Rangoon. The Worker's Hospital was opened in 1964, and soon became overcrowded with insured workers. Its occupancy in 1986 was more than 100 percent, and there were 1.4 hospital personnel per patient—much higher than the ratio in MOH hospitals of similar size. There were 18 medical and surgical specialists. Also in contrast to MOH facilities, the wards were clean and orderly, with mattresses and linens on each bed. The x-ray department and laboratory were well staffed, with new equipment from Japan. All patients had charts and were served three meals a day. It should not be surprising that the cost per patient-day in the Social Security hospital has been approximately double that of costs in an equivalent 150-bed hospital of the MOH.

Personnel in the Worker's Hospital are officially on the same salary scale as staff throughout the Ministry of Health. (There may be some subtle form of supplementation.) As elsewhere, all the specialized physicians engage in private practice, after their hospital hours, although they are not allowed to accept any insured patients. The superior conditions of this hospital, compared to others of the same or larger size, seem to be attributable to (a) much greater funding from Social Security for capital purposes (equipment, beds, furniture, etc.), (b) more funds available for the purchase of food, supplies, paint, and drugs, and (c) a much higher personnel-to-patient ratio than that of other comparable hospitals. All of these factors doubtless contribute to high morale among the hospital personnel, medical and other. They also show the capabilities of Burma's health personnel, given more nearly adequate economic support.

Other exceptionally attractive amenities are provided in military hospitals for the care of high-ranking officers. In the Rangoon General Hospital, the nation's largest facility, about 50 special beds are reserved for persons of social importance. To some degree, of course, such policies are found in almost all countries.

Other Special Services. Burma's accomplishments in the immunization of children have been somewhat uneven, but they have improved with progress in maintenance of the "cold chain." By 1984, 79 percent of children had been vaccinated with BCG against tuberculosis by 6 years of age. For DPT (diphtheria, pertussis, and tetanus), however, only 23 percent of infants had received a full course of injections by 1986–87. For oral poliomyelitis vaccine, only urban infants have been targeted, and 35 percent of these were reached by 1984. The MOH policy has been to expand coverage of immunizations in about 18 additional townships per year.

Attendance at childbirths in Burma was studied, by place of delivery, in 1980. A survey in 146 towns found this distribution:

Place of Childbirth Delivery	Percentage
At home	57.7
Government hospital	39.5
Private clinic	2.8
All places	100.0

The same childbirths, analyzed by type of attendant, showed the following distribution:

Childbirth Attendant	Percentage
Trained midwife or nurse	46.3
Physician	39.3
Traditional birth attendant (TBA)	4.1
Other	10.3
All types	100.0

Thus, in 1980 trained personnel handled 85.6 percent of childbirths in Burmese towns. A later report by UNICEF (for 1980 through 1987) claims that 97 percent of total childbirths in Burma were attended by trained personnel.

The coverage of Burma's population with safe drinking water is difficult to quantify. A report of the World Health Organization esti-mated in 1979 that 75 percent of people in the capital city, Rangoon, had use of a public water supply. Among the other 296 towns, only 20 percent had public water networks, and population coverage was considered to be about 12 percent. Safe water was even less available to the rural population. Deep tube-wells were extensively drilled in the 1980s, although a 1985 survey found that, even when they were accessible, only 43 percent of households used the tube-well as their main source of water.

Regarding excreta disposal, the MOH strategy since 1982 has been to promote latrine construction in 12 additional townships each year. By 1986 about 375,000 sanitary latrines had been built in 50 townships. Plastic molds were provided to the villages, where local masons prepared the squatting slabs that households could purchase. About 80 percent of the latrines constructed were reported to be regularly in use. The MOH calls on every rural health worker to promote the construction of 10 new latrines per year.

Some Health Status Outcomes

While recognizing the countless influences on health outside the health system, one should still note certain health status data for the population of Burma. In 1974 the life expectancy at birth had been reported as 58.5 years, and by 1987 it was 61 years.

The infant mortality rate has been a subject of special controversy in Burma. Official government registration records indicated 130 infant deaths per 1,000 live births in 1961. During the years 1981 to 1985 various methods of calculation yielded four different rates, ranging from 45.1 to 60.1 infant deaths per 1,000 live births per year. For 1987, however, UNICEF reported an infant mortality rate of 71 per 1,000 live births. (Since infant births warrant a ration card and deaths cancel it, some under-reporting of infant deaths may be expected.) In any case, a substantial decline in the infant death rate has been clear.

The maternal mortality rate has also declined in Burma. In 1961, it was officially reported as 3.8 maternal deaths per 1,000 live births. For 1986–87 UNICEF reported a rate of 1.4 such maternal deaths per 1,000 births per year. The crude birth rate has also declined, in spite of the government's passive policy on contraception; it went from 42 per 1,000 population in 1960 to 31 per 1,000 in 1987.

Regarding morbidity trends in Burma, only a few comments can be offered. Malaria has been reduced but not eliminated; because of mosquito resistance to pesticides it remains, but has been stabilized at a lower level in the rural areas. Venereal disease has been reduced, but remains a problem in large cities. Trachoma has been greatly reduced in endemic areas, thanks to the treatment of cases. Judging by the record of cases seen at hospital out-patient departments, among the five leading causes of morbidity in 1981, three conditions were prominent throughout the country: fever of unknown origin, intestinal infections, and anemia. One can only speculate on the diagnoses behind these conditions.

The severe economic and political difficulties of Burma in the 1980s had obvious effects on the structure and operations of the national health system. With the inadequacies of support for the public sector, a substantial private sector of doctor's care and particularly drugs inevitably flourished. In spite of the resultant inequities, the health services provided have evidently had some effect in counteracting the countless diseases of poverty. Further progress in Burma will obviously depend mainly on socioeconomic and political developments.

INDIA

Very different from Burma is its previous neighbor to the west, India, the huge country of 802,100,000 people (1987) that won its independence from British rule in 1947. With relatively slow urbanization, by 1987 some 73 percent of the Indian people still lived in thousands of small rural villages. Although the country's principal economic foundation has long been agriculture, a slowly increasing share of productivity has come from the manufacture of textiles, steel, and chemicals, and other industries. The GNP of India in 1986 was $290 per capita.

Socioeconomic Background

Because of its great geographic size and the vast numbers and diversity of its population, the Union or Republic of India is frequently described as a "subcontinent." Civilizations of many types have occupied this large territory for at least 5,000 years. After a period of religious/philosophical domination by Buddhism several centuries before Christ, the religion and culture of Hinduism became dominant a few centuries A.D. Much later, in the period A.D. 700 to 1200, Arab and Turkish invasions brought the influence of the Moslem faith, which eventually led to division of the people into two conflicting populations—Hindu and Moslem.

Colonization of India by European powers started with the Portuguese around 1500, followed by the Dutch, and then the British in 1609. The British government assumed full political control in 1830, curbing the authority of local kings or rajahs. After World War I, a movement for national independence arose, culminating in British authorization of locally elected provincial parliaments, and also of a federal legislature in 1937. The power of these bodies, however, was limited in many ways, and the nonviolent resistance campaign led by Mohandas K. Gandhi, mounted. Finally in 1947, under the British Labour Party, foreign rule was ended, but only with the creation of two separate nations: predominantly Hindu India and predominantly Moslem Pakistan.

The previous structure of princely domains was inevitably carried over into the delineation of India's provinces or states. Today the large population is divided among 22 states and 9 "union territories" (the latter coming under principal control of the central government). The Indian Constitution of 1949 establishes a federated republic, in which many responsibilities, including those for health service and health protection, are vested in the states. The central government, nevertheless, establishes general policies throughout the nation, provides a substantial share of the financing of public services, and coordinates activities among the states. The compliance of states with national policies in various fields is ensured through the appointment of state governors by the national president. Unlike in various other federated republics, the governors responsible for administration of local affairs are not elected by the populations they serve.

As reflected in the very low GNP per capita ($290 per year in 1986) life in India, both urban and rural, is marked by extreme poverty. For centuries, Indian society has been dominated by the concept of *caste,* which combines considerations of occupation, biological race (color), and social position. There have been four main groupings—priests, warriors, merchants, and cultivators—but Indian culture has defined as many as 3,000 castes, into which all individuals are born. The lowest castes, or *untouchables,* have constituted a majority of the population, destined to do all sorts of menial and "unclean" work and to serve the higher castes. Religion reinforced all of these forms of segregation and inequality, which were deemed to be a requirement for the very survival of society and the universe.

After independence, through the influence of Gandhi and his followers, in 1949 the concept of untouchables was officially outlawed in functions of government or general social relations. Observation of everyday affairs in India, however, suggests some survival of the concept, if not the explicit labels, of the ancient castes. While there are now many exceptions, leadership is still largely in the hands of *brahmans,* and this word has become a symbol for the elite almost everywhere. Ancient Hindu religious practices, incorporated in various dietary rules and in the extravagant protection of cows ("sacred cows") are still almost universally observed.

The extreme inequalities of Indian society are indicated in data from national household surveys in 1975–76. Of all households in India at that time, the poorest 20 percent accounted for only 7 percent of the total income. Meanwhile, the upper 10 percent of households had 33.6 percent of the total income. Expressed another way, the upper tenth of households, with 33.6 percent of the national income, earned more than the bottom 60 percent (that got 30.1 percent of the total income). This massive poverty is evident in miserable housing conditions for the great majority of people, extensive homelessness in the cities (with thousands of families living and sleeping on the streets), and widespread illiteracy. While schooling has improved since colonial times, in 1985 literacy in any language could be claimed for only 57 percent of adult men and 29 percent of adult women.

The Congress Party, founded in the 1930s, has been in control of the government of India (except for the years 1977 through 1980) since independence. Its principal leaders are from the merchant and professional classes, which are dedicated to the preservation of private enterprise. At the same time, leaders naturally want to heighten the world position of India, increase production, and enhance the welfare of the people. In agriculture, for example, cooperatives among small farmers have been encouraged, with limited success, but there are no large "collective farms" such as exist in socialist countries. Charitable religious missions are encouraged to promote education and village industries, as well as health services.

With its huge population, India's structure of government is subdivided into several levels below that of the 31 states and territories. Each of the states is divided into districts—about 10 or 15 each and 408 in all. Each district is further divided into *development blocks,* numbering 5,011. Within the development blocks are 3,301 towns and nearly 576,000 villages. The health services of government, of course, are based on this hierarchical structure.

Perhaps from observation of the experience of the Soviet Union, in 1951 India started a sequence of 5-year plans to develop the entire socioeconomic order, including the health system. The USSR emerged from World War II as the friend of former colonial countries, and its general emphasis on planning was adopted by India (and many other countries) in spite of the nation's overall attachment to a free-market economy. Central planning became a prominent feature of the health system of India.

Health Planning

Very broadly oriented planning of health services in India was actually started in 1943, while the British were still in control. In that year the Health Survey and Development Committee was appointed, and it issued its report in 1946; this soon attracted worldwide attention. The Bhore Report, named after the

Committee's chairman, presented a vast and comprehensive analysis of health conditions and the existent organized health services in British India. It called for radical reorganization of the entire health system, with government taking responsibility for complete health services for the entire population. The recommendations were immediately supported by the Congress Party, and after independence they were formally adopted by the new government of India.

More specifically, the Bhore Committee recommendations advocated (1) development of a nationwide network of primary health center complexes, (2) provision of integrated preventive and curative health services for everyone, (3) extensive health education, with full participation of the people, (4) provision of all needed medical care, regardless of the individual's ability to pay, (5) training of all necessary health manpower and construction of all necessary facilities, and (6) implementation of all proposals to be entrusted to the ministers of health of each state.

The First Five-Year Plan for overall socioeconomic development of India (1951–1955) incorporated the Bhore recommendations within it. Each *primary health center* was intended to serve 100,000 people, with a staff of one physician, one nurse, and various other personnel. In addition the first plan called for health programs to control malaria, extend preventive services for mothers and children, promote health education, increase the output of drugs and equipment, disseminate family planning advice, and improve water supplies and sanitation. The goals were obviously very ambitious, and both human and physical resources were extremely limited. By 1956 some 725 primary health centers, not all of them fully staffed, had been built. Assuming that each center covered 100,000 people (which was most unlikely), these units were reaching 18 percent of India's 400,000,000 population at the time.

The Second Five-Year Plan (1956–1960) understandably put greater emphasis on the construction and staffing of health facilities. By 1961 the number of primary health centers increased to 2,800, theoretically meaning coverage of 63 percent of India's 440,000,000 people

at the time. Everyone realized, however, that with extremely meager transportation, only a fraction of 100,000 people could be expected to reach a primary health center for services; the real population coverage was much less.

The disappointing performance of government during the first two 5-year plans led to appointment of another major Health Survey and Development Committee, this one chaired by Dr. A. L. Mudaliar. The Mudaliar Report, submitted in 1961, referred not only to the inadequate coverage of primary health centers but also to the poor services provided even to those patients who came to a center. It recognized realities by regarding each primary center as serving only 40,000 people. Furthermore, the report recommended that no further primary centers be constructed, but that those in operation should be substantially upgraded in their staffing. Health center medical officers, it said, "should not be allowed private practice but should be given non-practicing plus public health allowances, together with residential accommodation."

To extend health service coverage, the Mudaliar Report recommended that mobile clinic units be organized at district hospitals, more physicians should be trained to staff these, and rural service should be required of all new medical graduates. These latter recommendations, however, were not implemented by the government. Instead, many small *subcenters* were established to serve 15,000 to 20,000 people within the larger areas served by primary centers. Then in the late 1960s, largely in response to external pressures for control of India's great population explosion, the major attention of health authorities was shifted toward large-scale birth control or family planning.

The relationships of family planning to general health services, specific maternal and child health (MCH) programs, hospital care, medical education, and so on occupied the attention of additional national health planning committees. Reports on various forms of integration of this work were issued in 1963, 1968, and 1970. In 1973, a Committee on Multipurpose Health Workers (chaired by Kartar Singh) recommended restructuring all specialized vertical health programs into locally integrated horizontal programs at the district level. Of course, this required extensive training of new types of auxiliary but broad-scope health workers.

In 1978, still another health planning group was formed as a joint committee of the Indian Council of Social Science Research and the Indian Council of Medical Research (ICSSR/ICMR). This committee's report, issued in 1980, emphasized the importance to health of overall economic development, gainful employment for women, universal education of children, improvement of housing, extension of democratic participation of people in all policy matters, and other factors. Regarding personal health service, the report urged departure from an urban-centered hospital-focused health care framework to a community-based one strongly oriented toward health promotion and disease prevention. *Community health volunteers* and middle-level personnel would be more numerous than physicians and nurses.

To implement these sweeping ICSSR/ICMR recommendations, greater authority would have to be delegated by the central and state governments to the 408 district authorities. Voluntary agencies would be encouraged, but only within the overall health policies of government. Financial support for the health system would have to increase from a level of about 3 percent of GNP in the mid-1980s to some 6 percent by the year 2000. These ambitious recommendations of the ICSSR/ICMR joint committee were incorporated in the Sixth Five-Year Plan of the government of India, for 1980 through 1985.

Like public health leaders in many other countries, the well-educated professionals in India have, over the years, prepared sophisticated analyses of health problems and made various proposals for solving them. These proposals have contributed substantially to overall official 5-year plans, and to some extent have been implemented through large programs for training personnel, constructing health facilities, and organizing health services in various ways. For many reasons—the loftiness of the goals, the poverty of resources, the weakness of political will, or all of these—the achievements of each 5-year plan have fallen very short of expectations. Yet since independence was won in 1947, India's health system has shown vast improvement.

Health System Organization

With all the changes and complexities of its past development, the structure of India's health system in the 1980s incorporates inputs from many sources and periods. Carried over from colonial times is the framework of 31 states and union territories that bear the main responsibilities in the operation of almost all government health programs. The major public authority, known formerly as the Ministry of Health, changed its name in the early 1970s to Ministry of Health and Family Welfare, reflecting the great importance attached to population control.

Ministry of Health and Family Welfare. At the national capital, in New Delhi, the MOHFW is a relatively small organization, since its principal functions are the formulation of national health policy, the publication of reports, and the coordination of state health ministries. The central ministry also operates certain national research and training institutes, regulates the health professions and pharmaceutical products, and oversees certain direct health services only regarding family planning. Almost all other personal and environmental health services of government are carried out by the 31 state and union-territory ministries of health and family welfare (MOHFW). About two-thirds of the financing of MOHFW health activities also comes from the states and one-third from allocations of the central government. On the other hand, almost all of the large budget for family planning is supported by the central MOHFW.

Within the states and territories, the 408 districts are the principal units for MOHFW administration. Districts vary greatly in geographic size and population, although the statistical average unit includes nearly 2,000,000 people. Each district is headed by a medical health officer, appointed by the state minister of health; he is responsible for all local MOHFW activities, including a district hospital. The ministry's most important mechanisms for providing general ambulatory health service are the primary health centers, numbering around 8,000 in 1988, each then regarded as serving about 30,000 people. Primary centers are supposed to be staffed by one or two physicians and several other personnel (including a pharmacist and a laboratory technician). Much more numerous are small subcenters, staffed only by auxiliary health workers, and expected (in 1987) to serve only 5,000 to 10,000 people. Finally, in the villages are *community health volunteers* or *health guides,* trained for a few weeks mainly to encourage sound health practices. All of these MOHFW activities below the district level were in process of development in the late 1980s, and not yet available everywhere.

The overall structure of the MOHFW in each state of India has been designed to have the customary pyramidal hierarchy of health administration. In the villages are volunteer health guides, theoretically supervised by health auxiliaries in subcenters (serving 5 to 10 villages). Several subcenters come under a primary health center, with one or two doctors and others (serving 30,000 to 40,000 people). Numerous primary centers are under the direction of a district health officer, with technical backup from the specialized medical staff of a district hospital. All district health officers report to the state health officer at the state headquarters of the MOHFW. The State Health Office comes under the general direction of the governor but is required to carry out health policies of the central MOHFW in New Delhi. The realities of health administration in India, however, seldom correspond tidily to the ideal model.

Social Security. Two major social insurance programs provide medical care for selected persons in India. The Employees State Insurance Corporation (ESIC) has operated for employees of private industry and their dependents since 1948. ESIC's population coverage has gradually increased, and in 1987 it provided or financed relatively complete medical and hospital care for about 28,000,000 people (workers and families). Coverage applies only to low-paid employees of firms with 20 or more workers, using electrical power. Although these workers and dependents consti-

tute only 3.5 percent of India's huge population, the pattern of organization of services may have larger implications.

Medical care under ESIC is given through a national network of the agency's own hospitals and dispensaries, with salaried doctors and others, as well as through regular MOHFW facilities of the state governments with which ESIC contracts. At sites with substantial local industry, ESIC constructs facilities, and elsewhere it makes contracts, for example, to reserve a certain number of hospital beds. General practitioner medical services are also arranged in large cities by contracts with private doctors, paid by capitation.

The second social security program providing medical care in India is for employees of the central government and their families. The Central Government Health Insurance Scheme (CGHIS) covered about 3,300,000 persons in 1987, providing services in its own facilities or through both private and public resources under contract. About half of these government employees were in New Delhi, the national capital, and the other half were located throughout India. Of the 293 dispensaries that CGHIS operated, it is noteworthy that 28 percent were based on Ayurvedic, homeopathic, or other healing concepts, differing from conventional modern scientific medicine (see later).

Other Government Agencies. Health-related functions are carried out by several ministries at both national and state levels in India, aside from the MOHFW. The social security programs come under the general supervision of the central and state ministries of labor; these agencies also supervise medical benefits for work-connected injuries in certain industrial centers. The ministries of labor have long conducted factory inspections, in the effort to ensure safe and proper working conditions, but the inspectors are few and the power to enforce is weak.

Ministries of education are responsible for all universities in India, but since independence their constituent colleges for training physicians, dentists, and pharmacists have come under the Directorate of Medical Education and Research of the MOHFW. This directorate maintains liaison with the ministry of education of each state. Of the 125 modern medical schools in 1987, all but a few were linked to universities, even though many of them functioned somewhat independently. Although much finanical support for some medical schools may come from nongovernment sources, their performance is subject to MOHFW approval. On the other hand, a few schools, supported entirely by private money, operate without official recognition.

The Ministry of Defense in the central government of India operates a well-developed health service for military personnel. Many features of this service were carried over from the period of British rule. The central and state ministries of social welfare promote rehabilitation of the disabled, through both public and private activities. The development of improved water supplies in rural villages is a responsibility shared by two major public authorities: the Ministry of Works and Housing and the Department of Rural Development in the Ministry of Agriculture.

The Ministry of Cooperatives has sponsored the organization of thousands of small cooperatives in the rural areas. Their function is principally to provide credit to small farmers (for seeds, fertilizer, etc.), and a few operate small dispensaries with salaried doctors.

Voluntary Health Agencies. Hundreds of diverse voluntary agencies provide health services to small population groups in India. Most numerous are religious missions from Europe and North America, missions that spread the Christian gospel, while operating small hospitals and clinics. Although most of the cost of mission health services must be supported by fees from patients using them, the foreign missionaries bring human and physical resources to India that supplement those available domestically.

Scores of special "experimental projects" have also been launched in India, to test certain health service ideas in selected areas. These have been supported by foreign governments, philanthropic foundations, universities (both from India and elsewhere), affluent corporations, and even rich individuals. The objective of population control has, since the 1960s, spawned a large variety of local health projects, providing family planning service, along with combinations of other types of health intervention. Such projects usually operate for 5 to 10 years, and typically cover populations between 10,000 and 100,000 (sometimes more).

Some voluntary health agencies in India have nationwide scope, with scores or hundreds of local branches. Among these is the Indian Red Cross Society, organized in 1920 to help soldiers and veterans from World War I, and gradually broadening its functions since then. The Indian Council of Child Welfare and the Tuberculosis Association of India are also nationwide agencies, deriving their chief support from donations by relatively wealthy families. The Family Planning Association of India works closely with the government family welfare programs, and gets support from various international sources; in 1985 it had more than 1,200 local volunteer groups providing family planning service and education. The United Nations Fund for Population Activities has listed 16 international nongovernment organizations that significantly assist India in the family planning field alone.

Private Health Care Market. The residual private market for health care in India, through which people purchase many types of curative medical and related services, is substantial. Its vast proportions are best reflected in the economic data offered later, but here we can consider simply its main characteristics.

The principal components of the private health care market in India are the services of traditional practitioners, of modern physicians and dentists, and of private drugstores. Exact data on the amounts of each of these are not available, but we can infer their general proportions from statistical information on health resources.

Practitioners of traditional medicine in India are principally followers of Ayurvedic doctrine (discussed later), and smaller numbers are devoted to the doctrines of Unani and Siddha. Altogether, in 1975, these practitioners were reported to number about 400,000— more than the supply of modern physicians. Nearly all Ayurvedic and related practitioners are in private practice. They are widely distributed in the cities and rural villages, and their fees are low; generally they charge the patient for the Ayurvedic drugs dispensed, while the consultation is regarded as free. They are respected and trusted by millions of people.

Scientifically trained physicians, registered with state medical councils in India, totaled 331,000 in 1987. The proporation of these in full-time private practice can be estimated from reports made by 7 of the 31 states and territories. In these states, the share of doctors employed by government agencies amounted to 41 percent. Another 12 percent worked principally in nongovernment organizations (NGOs). Private medical practice occupied the full time of 47 percent. We know, however, that government and some NGO physicians, especially in rural areas, see private patients when their official duties are ended. This may not be officially permitted but the practice is widely recognized. Doctors engaged exclusively in private practice are concentrated in the large cities, but in India as a whole it is commonly estimated that 60 percent of all available physician time is devoted to private patients paying fees for their care.

In 1981, India had 156,000 licensed pharmacists, working in both public facilities and private drugstores in the cities. Most drugstores, however, are operated by Ayurvedic practitioners and by persons without any training in pharmacy. For the low-income patient, purchasing self-prescribed medication in a drugstore is less expensive than consulting a physician or even a traditional healer.

Production of Health Resources

Since independence, both the human and physical resources for health services have been enormously expanded in India. Although the rate of population growth has been high, the rate of production of health manpower and facilities has been even greater.

Health Manpower. At the time of independence (1947), there were 26 medical colleges in India, turning out fewer than 2,000 graduates per year. By 1987 there were 125 medical schools, 85 percent sponsored by state governments, and graduating about 10,000 young doctors annually; one-third of these were women. "Lady doctors" have special importance in India, since many Hindu women object to being examined by a male doctor. A large proportion of new medical graduates settle in the large cities as private practitioners; there is no legal obligation in India to devote a period of time to government service or to work in a rural area. The great majority of Indian physicians are in general practice, although an increasing fraction undertake specialty training. During the years 1947 to 1979, when other affluent countries (like Great Britain and the United States) welcomed foreign medical graduates, some 13 percent of doctors educated in India emigrated. After 1980, to avoid this "brain drain," the output of Indian medical schools was actually reduced.

Nationally, India's stock of physicians in 1987 was about 41 per 100,000 population. Variations are great not only between the cities and rural areas but also among the different states and territories. To distinguish modern or Western-type physicians from the greater numbers of traditional doctors in India, the former are often called *allopathic*. This separates them also from *homeopathic* doctors, who numbered 151,000 in 1978. Homeopathy is a medical cult, originating in nineteenth-century Germany, which in other countries has greatly declined or entirely disappeared.

The Ayurvedic and other traditional practitioners in India are numerous and important in the health system. Although not integrated in the framework of government health centers and hospitals, they are officially recognized and supported by government as a separate and parallel program. In 1975 there were 102 indigenous medical colleges (91 Ayurvedic and 11 others), admitting 7,000 students per year. The duration of training varies, and may be as long as 5 years after secondary school. Most of these training programs teach elements of modern medicine, as well as the ancient, somewhat metaphysical doctrines originating 3,000 years ago.

It has been estimated that in the mid-1970s about 200,000 traditional practitioners were officially registered with state governments. Of these, 50,000 were graduates of a government-approved training school, and therefore knew a little about modern as well as ancient therapy. Another 200,000 practitioners were estimated to be selling their services mostly in rural areas, without being registered or formally trained; they learned their skills simply by working with older practitioners. Only the institutionally trained practitioners are appointed to government-supported hospitals and dispensaries.

Professional dentists in India are trained in 40 dental colleges that had about 650 graduates in 1987. That year there were 9,800 professionally qualified dentists in the entire country. With so few trained dentists, most of the people go completely without dental care. A larger number of meagerly qualified "denturists" extract inadequate teeth in older patients, replacing them with full artificial dentures. Only small numbers of dental auxiliaries, who do restorative work for school children, have been trained.

Professional nurses are less numerous in India than physicians. In 1986 there were 207,000, or 26 per 100,000 population; 85 percent of these were "senior grade," having had more training than the "junior grade" nurses. All these nurses completed secondary school before they were trained, typically in a hospital-based school. Almost all nurses work in hospitals, while in health centers less thoroughly trained auxiliaries render equivalent types of services.

Professionally trained midwives are important in India; they perform most of the deliveries in hospitals. In 1986 there were 185,000—nearly as many as professional nurses. In addition, there were 108,000 auxiliary nurse-midwives, prepared by the MOHFW to work in health centers or subcenters. The medical supervision of hospital midwives is quite limited.

The Sixth Five-Year Plan for 1980–1985, as noted, called for a major shift of health manpower emphasis from doctors and nurses to very briefly trained community health workers (CHW). In India these CHWs (male or female), who staff thousands of subcenters, are also known as *multipurpose health workers;* their 3-month training is done in a primary

health center. By 1987 about 88,000 male and 85,000 female workers had been trained.

Even less training is provided for *health guides,* who do educational work in the villages. By 1987 some 387,000 guides, three-quarters men, had been trained. The task of handling childbirths in the villages of India is so enormous that the government has made no attempt to furnish professional or even auxiliary midwives. Instead, the MOHFW has a large program to briefly orient traditional birth attendants or *dais* in hygienic procedures. Between 1974 and 1987, nearly 560,000 dais were given such short courses.

The education of personnel for public health work and for efficient management of India's large and complex national health system has long been a difficult challenge. In 1921, under the British a small School of Tropical Medicine for highly technical work was established in Calcutta. In 1932, a more comprehensive All-India Institute of Hygiene and Public Health was organized, also in Calcutta, with foreign assistance. Physicians were provided postgraduate training here for various aspects of public health work. In addition, some 30 of the regular medical colleges have come to offer postgraduate training in public health (mainly for physicians), through their departments of preventive and social medicine.

In the 1960s and later educational and research institutions, focusing on health service administration or management, were set up in India. One was the National Institute of Health Administration and Education in New Delhi; another was the Indian Institute of Health Management Research in Jaipur. These were linked to the MOHFW, and provided training for many types of university graduates, in addition to physicians.

Health Facilities. The British established hospitals in all the main cities of India, and these have been greatly expanded since independence. In 1987, there were nearly 7,800 hospital structures with 550,300 beds. This amounted to 0.71 beds per 1,000 people, including hospitals of all types.

The great majority of hospital beds are in governmental facilities; nearly 70 percent of the beds in 1987 were in hospitals of the central and state governments and another 4.6 percent in hospitals built by local authorities. Voluntary nonprofit (mostly religious) bodies and purely private individuals or groups controlled 26 percent of the beds. The central and state government hospitals tend to be larger, with an average capacity of 102 beds, and local authority units average 61 beds. The voluntary and private hospitals have about 40 beds on the average. Under all types of sponsorship, some hospitals give entirely Ayurvedic care— 195 of them in 1978 with 9,000 beds.

Often associated indirectly with hospitals, as small outlying units for ambulatory medical care, are quite rudimentary *dispensaries.* In 1988, India had 27,500 such dispensaries. About 50 percent of these were sponsored by central, state, or local governments and 50 percent by voluntary or purely private bodies. Most people using dispensaries are expected to pay small fees, although the very poor may be treated without charge. After 1980, some dispensaries were upgraded to subcenters in the MOHFW program for primary health care.

For implementation of India's several Five-Year Plans, the most important facilities are the primary health centers, first launched following release of the Bhore Report in 1946. After a slow beginning, by 1988 some 8,000 primary centers had been built, nearly all staffed with one physician and sometimes two (a woman and a man). In 1981, nearly 9,200 physicians were working in the network of primary health centers, along with much larger numbers of general health assistants, auxiliary nurse-midwives, health visitors (equivalent to public health nurses), sanitary inspectors, health educators, clerks, and others. Although originally expected to reach 100,000 people, each primary center has eventually come to be recognized as serving about 30,000 people; this means approximately 240,000,000, or 30 percent of India's huge population.

To extend primary care coverage more effectively, in the 1960s after the Mudaliar Report was published, India began to establish subcenters. Each of these was intended to reach 5,000 people without access to a primary center. Subcenters would be staffed entirely by auxiliary health personnel, principally the male and female multipurpose health workers and sometimes the more thoroughly trained health assistants and drug dispensers. By 1967, the end of the Third Five-Year Plan, about 5,000 subcenters had been established throughout India, and this was increased to 103,000 by 1988. If each of these units served 5,000 people, this meant coverage of 64 percent of India's population.

Furthermore, to provide stronger technical backup to the subcenters, certain primary health centers have been upgraded to *community health centers*—facilities with a few medical specialists on staff and up to 30 hospital beds with diagnostic equipment. In 1987, there were 1,250 of these upgraded centers, each of which was regarded as serving a population block of 200,000. Unlike the hospitals, community health centers were regarded as part of the framework of MOHFW preventive and therapeutic primary health care.

These data on health resources in India have all been presented as national totals, but, in fact, major differences exist among the states and union territories. Since so much manpower training and facility construction must be financed principally by the states, the extent to which national policy can be implemented depends very much on state wealth. One of the higher-income states, for example, is Maharashtra (including Bombay), with 63,000,000 people in 1987. That year, this state had a ratio of 58.2 modern physicians per 100,000 people. Of much lower income level was the mountainous state of Uttar Pradesh (including Lucknow), with a 1987 population of 111,000,000 people. Its supply of modern doctors was just 6.0 per 100,000. Other health resources show essentially the same relative disparities between states.

Drugs. With respect to one resource, pharmaceutical products, India has achieved a remarkable degree of self-sufficiency compared with other very low income developing countries. After independence, the central government set out to develop a domestic pharmaceutical industry to meet the needs of its people, without dependence on foreign imports. Government production of drugs, along with domestic private enterprise, both play a part. Technology in drug manufacture would, of course, be brought in from abroad, and even foreign investment would be sought to help firms under private Indian ownership.

By 1972, domestic drug production had increased enormously, and it was largely but not entirely under the control of Indians. In terms of the value of finished drug products, 39 percent was produced by 50 firms owned entirely or principally by private Indian businesses. Two large government enterprises produced 34 percent of the drugs (in terms of their value). Twenty-seven firms, dominated by foreign ownership but located in India, accounted for 27 percent of the value of all drug products. Raw chemicals had to be imported for a great deal of this drug production, but it is noteworthy that imports of finished formulations (tablets, solutions, etc.) were virtually eliminated.

Several branches of the central government of India are involved in carrying out this drug production program. The State Trading Corporation (STC) is responsible for importing raw materials and distributing them to domestic manufacturers, both private and public. Other raw materials are produced inside India by a government enterprise (known as Indian Drugs and Pharmaceuticals, Ltd.) under the Ministry of Industry. This ministry is also responsible for drug pricing in both private and public sectors. Finally, the Ministry of Health and Family Welfare is responsible for registering all new drugs and for quality controls.

In spite of the successes in Indian drug production policy, the output of vast numbers of nonessential and even harmful drugs has become a problem (as in many industrialized countries). Some 20,000 drug combinations (e.g., antibiotics plus vitamins) have been put on the market at high prices, despite the lack of therapeutic value. Between 1952 and 1983, bulk drug production in India increased 18-fold, but in 1980 only 28 percent of the drugs produced were "essential," by the World Health Organization definition. Also, in spite of the great drug output, WHO estimated that in 1984 only 6 percent of the Indian population could afford to purchase modern drugs that they needed, and another 25 percent had only limited access to essential drugs. The remainder of the people—in rural areas and urban slums—had to depend on traditional compounds of unproven value or do without any medication.

Knowledge. As a basic resource for its health system, most health-related scientific knowledge in India has been acquired by transmission from Europe and North America over the centuries. Ancient Ayurvedic medicine, however, has contributed certain therapies, which objective investigation has shown to be effective; the best known is the plant *Rauwolfia serpentina,* used originally for the treatment of "insanity," but found in 1952 to yield an alkaloid effective in reducing hypertension.

Several specialized research centers have been developed in India for generating new scientific knowledge. In New Delhi is the National Institute of Communicable Diseases and in Kasauli is the Central Research Institute for rabies surveillance and studies of salmonella infections. Various types of focused microbiological research are done by the Haffkine Institute in Bombay, the Pasteur Institute in Coonoor, and the National Institute of Virology in Pune. The latter institutes also produce large quantities of vaccine for national use. At most medical colleges, some limited clinical research is undertaken.

Economic Support

Total expenditures for the health system of India in the early 1980s were approximately 3 percent of the GNP. The proportion of this derived from private sources is undoubtedly high, although the most recent available figure applies to 1970. A World Bank publication in 1984 indicates that in 1970, of all health expenditures in India, 84 percent came from the private sector. Government health activities at all levels, in other words, accounted for only 16 percent of total health expenditures. The further development of public programs since 1970 suggests that the public share may have increased, but one must realize that the private health care market in India has also continued to be robust. In neighboring Pakistan, data for 1982 show the private side of the health system to account for 71 percent of total expenditures.

Examining government expenditures, the share of total public spending that is allocated for health has declined somewhat over the years 1950 to 1980. In the Sixth Five-Year Plan (1980–1985) the Ministry of Health and Family Welfare received 2.9 percent of the total funds. Improvement of water supplies and sanitation received even more—4 percent of the total—a greater share than the 1.2 percent spent 20 years earlier. (The strong emphasis on environmental improvement in the 1980s may constitute adjustment for previous neglect.)

Within the public sector, spending by the MOHFW has been about two-thirds by the states and territories and one-third by the central government. Central expenditures have been largely for the family planning programs. The latter has shown the most dramatic increase over the years. Expenditures rose from Rupees 700,000 nationally in the First Five-Year Plan (1951–1956) to Rupees 516,000,000 in the fifth plan (1975–1980). A major portion of these funds for population control came through foreign aid, especially from the United States.

A breakdown of the government portion of health system expenditures has been reported for the years 1975 through 1980. In that period public spending for health was distributed as follows:

Purpose	Percentage
Water supply and sanitation	44.3
Family planning	22.4
Personal health services in hospitals, dispensaries, and health centers	19.4
Communicable disease control	7.3
Education and training	4.9
Traditional medicine (government)	1.2
Other services	0.4
All purposes	100.0

This distribution includes expenditures by both the central government and the states. The relatively modest proportion of public spending going for *personal health services* suggests the likelihood of very large expenditures for medical care and drugs in the private sector.

Delivery of Health Services

The patterns of delivery of health services to the people of India vary enormously according to their social class. There are also great variations between cities and rural areas, among the different states, and between higher- and lower-income districts within any state. Any generalization, therefore, must be qualified by these socioeconomic circumstances.

Personal Health Service. The great majority of Indian people, who are very poor, must depend for ambulatory medical care on the services of Ayurvedic and related traditional practitioners. These healers, located everywhere, are consulted in their small shops, where they dispense various herbal medications and sometimes give advice on diet, rest, and exercise. If a patient is very sick and disabled, practitioners sometimes visit the home. Proponents of Ayurveda, who are critical of modern medicine, like to say that "allopathic medicine treats the disease while Ayurvedic healing treats the patient." A desperately ill poor person who has not been helped by a traditional practitioner may consult a higher-priced private physician, if one is accessible; this is more likely to be done in a city. Alternatively, the frustrated low-income patient may go to a modern drugstore for self-medication.

If a government health facility is accessible, and if its staff has acquired a reputation for being kind and considerate to impoverished patients, the poor person may go there for primary care. The most likely such facility to be visited is a subcenter, staffed entirely by auxiliary health personnel. These very briefly trained health workers, of course, have limited knowledge and respond to various disorders with symptomatic treatment. Sometimes this is adequate (since much disease is self-limited) and sometimes not.

If a primary health center or a hospital outpatient department (or dispensary) is accessible, the poor person may be able to consult an MOHFW doctor. Sociological studies have revealed, however, that the patients who see physicians in public facilities are concentrated in the higher castes; even though they are poor, they are seldom among the untouchables. Even so, studies at primary health centers have shown that 60 percent of doctors estimate that the time spent with each patient averages less than 2 minutes, and 90 percent estimate that it averages less than 5 minutes.

Just above the level of extreme poverty, families with slightly more education and somewhat higher standards of living are likely to consult a private doctor as their initial response to sickness. This would be most likely in a large city, where such physicians—allopathic or homeopathic—are relatively numerous. The doctor's private clinic is small and very modestly equipped, and he dispenses medications from his own supplies. This less impoverished social class in India also includes many families covered by the social insurance programs for private employees and central government civil servants. It is noteworthy that the insurance-financed clinics serving these people are staffed essentially by physicians and allied professional personnel; auxiliaries are not used, except for minor delegated tasks.

The small percentage of Indian people with high incomes are provided health service entirely in the private sector, and particularly in a special portion of it. The large cities of India, as in most countries, have upper-class neighborhoods, where the homes of the rich are clustered. In or near those sections, there are usually small structures accommodating the private clinics of well-trained medical and surgical specialists. The quarters are not only attractive and well-equipped, but also staffed with professional nurses and other personnel. Affluent families in these private settings can even obtain the preventive services for small children—periodic checkups and immunizations—provided free at public facilities.

The patterns for delivery of hospital care correspond roughly to those for ambulatory service. Fortunately, nearly three-quarters of India's hospital beds are in government facilities, mostly at the state level, but some under central or local governments. These beds are accessible to everyone, regardless of income level, and naturally they serve the great majority of people. Except for a few rooms for isolating patients with communicable disease, public hospital beds are typically in large, rather dismal wards, with few amenities for patient comfort. Sanitary facilities are usually rudimentary.

The one-fourth of hospital beds in facilities under voluntary agency or religious sponsorship are typically of higher standards, both technically and in terms of patient care. They are less crowded with patients, and the nurses and other personnel available are more plentiful. Basically, they are better financed, because of endowments and donations and also because the majority of patients must pay for the service. These nongovernment hospitals can afford to engage larger staffs, offer higher salaries, and acquire more modern medical equipment and supplies. The patients, of course, belong predominantly to higher socioeconomic groups, even though some beds may be reserved for "charitable service" to the very poor.

The medical staffs of both public and private hospitals in India are predominantly qualified in some specialty, and employed by the institution on salary. For younger physicians, the salaries are expected to be full-time, but senior specialists or consultants may be free to spend some time each week or even each day in outside private practice. Service to out-patients is given by the same doctors who serve the in-patients. In the relatively few small hospitals that are purely proprietary (operated for profit), the specialists may see private patients in the outpatient department.

Special Health Programs. A great deal of the organized health service in India is oriented toward attacks on special disease problems. Before about 1970, many categorical disease-control programs were administered vertically by each state government, but even since the integrated approach of the 1970s and 1980s, certain specialized strategies continue.

The reduction of diarrheal diseases, for example, has led to programs for greatly extending the use of oral rehydration therapy (ORT).

This has required pharmaceutical production of ORT salts, their wide distribution, the training of health personnel in ORT methods, and the widespread education of mothers of small children. Both public and private firms were entrusted with the production of millions of packets of ORT salts annually in the 1980s. Of course, the more rapid development of safe water supplies is recognized as basic. To cope with the diarrheal diseases occurring, nevertheless, some 400 *sentinel centers* for promoting this work were established throughout India, mainly at the district health offices.

Malaria control has long been another special program in India. Between 1953 and 1965, the incidence of malaria was greatly reduced by clearing swamps, which bred mosquitoes, spraying houses with pesticides (mainly residual DDT solution), and treating patients carrying the malaria parasite with drugs. The anopheles mosquito then developed resistance to the chemical pesticide, and by 1970 the rate of malaria cases rose steeply again. In 1977 a new antimalarial strategy was developed, essentially with the use of different insecticides in different ways. This has required field and laboratory research by special teams that work with the personnel at primary health centers. Laboratories at the district level examine patient blood specimens. Antimalarial drugs are distributed to "fever cases" by volunteer health guides in more than 325,000 villages. Even when the services are integrated, the need for specialized efforts is apparent.

Leprosy control is another focused program. In 1983, there were 390 leprosy control units in the health districts and 243 temporary hospitalization wards. Leprosy training centers that teach the use of special drug combinations, as well as reconstructive surgery, were established at 42 facilities.

The expanded program of immunization (EPI), promoted by the World Health Organization, is part of India's maternal and child health (MCH) efforts. The central MOHFW supplies the states with vaccines and equipment for maintaining the cold chain. The immunizations are conducted through the regular network of hospitals, dispensaries, and MCH clinics in the cities and through primary health centers and subcenters in rural areas.

Special EPI program leaders have been trained for work in the state and district offices, to coordinate local efforts.

Tuberculosis control has been spearheaded by specially trained personnel in 350 district health offices. These personnel do TB casefinding, ambulatory treatment, and distribution of BCG vaccine, produced in India at one government laboratory. There are 44,000 beds for tuberculosis, reserved in hospitals throughout the country.

Family planning (contraception) and measures for improving the nutrition of children and women in the child-bearing years are other special activities incorporated generally in the MCH programs. The high priority assigned to population control in India was dramatized in the 1970s by the change of name of the health authorities at both central and state levels to Ministry of Health and Family Welfare. Major family planning (FP) financial support went to the states through grants from the center. In every state and district, there are physicians, specializing in FP procedures, who carry out training programs for personnel in the primary health centers and the subcenters. Training is also provided for health guides and traditional birth attendants in the villages. Great educational efforts are also conducted through the mass media.

The most extensively used method of birth control in India in 1981 was female or male sterilization, requiring a relatively simple surgical procedure by a physician. This applied to 63.5 percent of FP users; much less frequently used were condoms (11.8 percent of families), contraceptive pills (2.7 percent), intrauterine devices (1.3 percent), other modern methods (0.3 percent), and traditional or "natural" methods (20.4 percent). However, only 35 percent of eligible couples in India were using any FP procedure in 1981.

Some Health Status Indicators

In spite of the enormous health and social problems of India, and the apparent slowness of advances against them, the available data suggest that some improvements have occurred.

Average life expectancy at birth in India was

44 years in 1960, and in 1987 it was 59 years. The infant mortality rate in 1960 was 165 infant deaths per 1,000 live births, and this declined to 100 infant deaths per 1,000 live births in 1987. The crude birth rate, contributing to India's huge population, was 42 per 1,000 people in 1960, and it went down to 32 per 1,000 in 1987. None of these more recent rates, of course, can be considered satisfactory, but all of them signify improvements in standards of living, in the health system, or both.

Data for the 1980s show that only 33 percent of childbirths in India were attended by a trained health person, and even fewer occurred in a hospital; the great majority of births took place at home, managed by a traditional birth attendant who usually had no training. The maternal mortality rate in the 1980s was still as high as 500 deaths per 100,000 births. In the early 1980s about 30 percent of newborn infants were reported to have low birth weights.

In 1985, of all boys of primary school age in India, 100 percent were reported to be attending school, but this applied to only 76 percent of the girls. Also only 29 percent of adult women were literate in 1985, compared with 57 percent of the adult men.

Access to clean water was claimed for 54 percent of India's population in 1984, and for fewer in rural areas. In 1988, the central government regarded the water supplies of 231,000 of the country's 574,000 villages to be unsatisfactory—either not accessible or definitely unsafe.

One state in the south of India, Kerala, with a 1981 population of 25,500,000 and a per capita wealth lower than the national average ($160 per person in 1980, compared to the national figure of $190) has a remarkably superior health record. The state of Kerala had an infant mortality rate in 1980 of 41 per 1,000 live births in rural areas, when India's rural rate was 124 per 1,000. Kerala's urban infant mortality rate was 34 per 1,000 live births in 1980, when India's urban rate was 65 per 1,000. For each age group, furthermore, from 0 to 4 years to 70 years and over, the Kerala general death rate has been much lower than the national average. For males of all ages in 1975, the death rate was 8.2 per 1,000 population in Kerala, compared to 15.5 per 1,000

in India as a whole; for females, the comparison was 8.8 per 1,000 in Kerala and 16.3 per 1,000 in India. Life expectancy for females at birth in Kerala was 64.4 years in 1979, when it was 51 years in all of India.

The reasons for Kerala's remarkable health record, in spite of its poverty level being even lower than the Indian average, have long been debated. Certain historical facts seem relevant. As far back as 1865, the Maharajah controlling the region was renowned for his charitable policies. In 1900, the state of Travancore (part of current Kerala) already had 22 hospitals and 20 dispensaries, when these were uncommon in the rest of India. By 1935, government medical facilities had increased to 85. By 1958, when the state of Kerala was established, modern (allopathic) medical facilities had increased to 318, and to 557 by 1976. In 1981, there were 144 hospitals, 563 dispensaries, and 163 primary health centers; there were 30,200 hospital beds, which meant 1.19 beds per 1,000 people, when the national ratio was about 0.6 per 1,000. Personal preventive services, such as immunizations and infant examinations, were also developed early in the Kerala region, although village water supplies have been poor—even worse than the national average.

Modern physicians were settled in Kerala in 1987 at a ratio of 54 per 100,000 people, compared with 41 per 100,000 for all of India. In addition, there are a roughly equal number of Ayurvedic practitioners, but Kerala residents are reported to consult both types of doctor regularly, rather than using traditional doctors exclusively.

A pervasive social influence on the people's health in Kerala has been an exceptionally high level of education. Since earlier centuries and under British rule, partly through Christian missionary influence, government in the region has put a high priority on the education of children, especially girls, who were grossly neglected elsewhere in India. In 1978, of all Kerala girls 6 to 10 years of age, 86 percent were enrolled in school, compared to 55 percent in all India; for girls 11 to 13 years, the enrollment was still 74 percent compared to 32 percent nationally. In 1971, adult literacy of men in India as a whole was 40 percent and 67 percent in Kerala; for women it was 19 percent in India and 54 percent in Kerala. Educational expenditure data from 1961 showed the government of Kerala to be spending 35 percent of its total revenue on education, compared to 19 percent in India as a whole. The emphasis in Kerala was greatest at the elementary school level, and this has persisted through the 1970s and 1980s.

Educational attainments in Kerala have been linked (perhaps as both cause and effect) with socialistically oriented government policies. In the first general elections after the state of Kerala was formed in 1956, the Communist Party of India (CPI) was elected to power. The first legislative act of the new government was to protect agricultural tenants from eviction. Although the CPI was removed from authority by a national presidential decree in 1959, subsequent state governments in Kerala have included various left-wing parties in coalitions, and land reform strategies have been continued. Land redistribution has been only partially implemented, but it has achieved some more effective equalization of family incomes than is found in other states of India. Overall per capita income, nevertheless, has remained lower in Kerala than in India as a whole.

The greater relative equality and higher educational level of people in Kerala evidently contribute to high rates of utilization of the health facilities that exist. Government expenditures for health (both prevention and medical care) in 1975–76 were Rupees 14.1 per capita in Kerala, compared to 10.6 in India nationally. In 1977, there were 11 subcenters for each primary health center in Kerala, compared to 6.2 in the somewhat similar state of West Bengal (containing Calcutta). The catchment area of each subcenter in Kerala was 22 square kilometers in 1978, compared to 99 square kilometers for subcenters in West Bengal. Many observers stress the high consciousness of their "social rights" among rural people in Kerala, in contrast to a rather passive, fatalistic attitude in most of India. If a primary health center loses its physician, for example, there is a great popular clamor (with political overtones) until the post is filled. Childbirths in Kerala in 1980 were attended by trained personnel in 81 percent of the cases, compared with 33 percent in all of India. Furthermore,

nearly half of the deliveries in Kerala took place in hospitals.

Though the issue is debated, Kerala's remarkable health achievements can hardly be attributed to any single cause. Education seems to play a large part, but its effects are intertwined with those of political ideology and land reform legislation; these social forces, in turn, strongly influence the development of health resources, for both treatment and prevention, and their active use by the people. Since the great majority of Kerala's people remain very poor, one may well conclude that education and health service have enabled them to compensate for some of the worst consequences of their poverty.

ZIMBABWE

One of the youngest of the newly independent countries of Africa is Zimbabwe, a nation of 8,700,000 people (1986) in southern Africa, which achieved sovereignty in April 1980. Formerly a British colony, known as Southern Rhodesia, Zimbabwe demonstrates an outcome of racial conflict very different from that evident in South Africa. Complex and painstaking efforts to achieve a peaceful settlement had failed, and guerilla warfare arose in the 1970s, leading to many thousands of deaths. Then in April 1979 a general election was called, and independence was achieved a year later.

Unlike in South Africa, the black people of Zimbabwe (95 percent of the total population) have won clear control of the government. They live peacefully, however, with the small percentage of Europeans and others, who still own much of the land, mines, and other sources of wealth, and still carry much managerial responsibility in the society. With major mineral resources, productive agriculture, and light industry, Zimbabwe's GNP per capita in 1986 was $620—above that of India or Tanzania. The population was 24 percent urban and 76 percent rural, with adult literacy being exceptionally high—81 percent for men and 67 percent for women in 1985. Under a single political party, originally the United African National Council, the government has been stable, in spite of serious problems of inflation and debt developing in the mid-1980s. Personal wealth has still been concentrated in the families of the small minority of Europeans, and the standards of living of Africans are still extremely low by comparison.

For many years, the territory of Zimbabwe and its antecedent Southern Rhodesia has been divided into provinces—originally five and after independence eight. In independent Zimbabwe, each province was subdivided into districts, which have been important in the structure of the health system. More significant under British rule were the Tribal Trust Lands (TTLs), reserved for communal grazing and agriculture of the Africans, and also small Purchase Areas (PAs) for African farms. This poor-quality land was occupied by 68 percent of the Rhodesian Africans. Much better quality land was occupied by 17 percent of the Europeans on larger farms and plantations. However, 82 percent of the Europeans lived in the cities, and only 16 percent of the Africans. All this racial segregation of land and people was changed after independence, but not all of the many inequalities could be eliminated overnight.

Rhodesian Health System Background

Before national independence was won, the health system of Southern Rhodesia had many characteristics similar to those of other colonies of European powers. The health system was highly centralized and yet administratively fragmented, which can be described in five main parts.

The central pillar was a Ministry of Health in the colonial government (headquartered in Salisbury, later known as Harare), oriented principally to the operation of hospitals in the main cities. Separate facilities were reserved for each racial group, with the better ones for the whites. In 1978, there were four central MOH hospitals in the national capital, nine general hospitals in the other cities, and five special hospitals (for mental cases, tuberculosis, etc.). There were also 60 small rural health centers, which sometimes had beds.

After 1948, the British began developing certain preventive services that were managed as separate vertical programs directed from the top. A provincial medical officer of health (PMOH) followed central orders to implement preventive campaigns (against malaria, tuberculosis, etc.), and was granted direct responsibility only for well-baby clinics, health education, and local sanitation. He had no connection with hospitals, which absorbed 90 percent of the MOH budget, while prevention used under 10 percent.

The second component of Rhodesian health services consisted of numerous small clinics operated by local authorities; some were in the cities, but most were in rural areas, sponsored by rural councils. In 1977 some 363 static and mobile rural clinics had been established, although many were closed down in the period of rebellion before independence. Services at these clinics required payment of small fees.

Industrial medical services were a third type of services in Rhodesia, including 18 clinics in 1977 and 10 hospitals with 1,380 beds. These served the employees of mines and usually their families, and they were financed by the managements of mines and other enterprises.

A fourth health system component came under the control of religious missions. In 1978 there were 82 hospitals and clinics, predominantly rural, sponsored by foreign Catholic and Protestant missions. These provided some 32 percent of the country's total general hospital beds and 66 percent of the beds in rural areas. Most patients had to pay fees for the services received, as both in-patients and out-patients.

A fifth and very important part of Rhodesian health services was the private sector of modern medical care. In 1977, there were 771 physicians on the register of the Rhodesian Medical Council, of whom 36 percent were entirely in private practice. These 280 practitioners were settled in a few large cities, serving predominantly white patients; many of these were economically protected through small voluntary medical aid insurance schemes. The effective supply of physicians for the urban white population in colonial Rhodesia was estimated to be one doctor for 830 people. For the much larger rural black population, there was one doctor for 45,000. (By 1981 Zimbabwe had a larger stock of physicians but, as noted later, an even greater proportion of them were probably in private practice.)

The private market of Rhodesia also included large numbers of traditional healers, estimated to be about 11,000 at the time of independence. At one point the new government spoke of "incorporating" them in the official services, but such action has not been reported.

For decades these enormous inequities were accepted in Rhodesia until, after World War II they fueled a liberation movement that led to national independence in 1980. When the new Zimbabwe government took control in April 1980, many physicians and others had left the country, and many physical resources (hospitals and clinics) had been destroyed or damaged in the struggle for freedom. Still, Zimbabwe began its period of reconstruction with an infrastructure of resources somewhat greater than those of many newly liberated colonies of Africa.

Health System of Zimbabwe

The Ministry of Health of the new government of Zimbabwe declared that the injustices of the colonial era would be corrected and a policy of Equity in Health would be instituted. This would be based on application of the WHO concept of primary health care (PHC), emphasizing services in rural areas where the great majority of people lived.

To implement these policies, the operation and costs of all local health services (under both municipalities and rural councils), as well as the services of religious missions, would be integrated under a strengthened Ministry of Health. Furthermore, everyone earning less than 150 Zimbabwe dollars (about U.S. $100) per month, rural or urban, was entitled to complete health service without charge; this meant some 97 percent of the population. The remaining 3 percent would purchase health care privately. To administer this massive expansion, the MOH centrally developed a major Rural Health Care Division. Another large new central MOH unit was a Mental Health Care Division.

Of much greater importance than the restructuring of the central MOH headquarters was the action taken at provincial and district levels. The country's former five provinces were reorganized as eight provinces, each headed for health affairs by a provincial medical director (PMD). Since preventive and curative services were to be integrated, the PMD was responsible for all hospitals and clinics, as well as all preventive campaigns or other activities, within his jurisdiction. (No longer were hospitals and disease control campaigns directed entirely from the top.) To integrate further all health activities at the local level, each province was subdivided into 5 to 8 districts (55 in all) each of which was headed by a district health team (DHT). District populations varied from 20,000 to 300,000, averaging about 100,000. The DHT usually, but not always, included a physician, depending on the availability of one from the district hospital. Planning, however, theoretically called for a district medical officer, based in the district hospital, as the head of each DHT. If this hospital had only one doctor, he was usually too occupied with clinical duties to permit any administrative work.

Of greatest importance for PHC delivery in the districts was the rural health center, of which 274 had been established (about 3 to 5 per district) by 1987, and 50 more were being planned. The typical center was staffed by a professional nurse-midwife, a second registered nurse, an assistant nurse, an environmental health technician, and a general maintenance worker. Some rural health centers had male *health assistants,* trained in all aspects of preventive health service for 3 years (after 12 years of basic schooling). There might also be *medical assistants,* trained briefly for simple curative work.

At the village level, or a "ward" of several villages (3000 to 6000 people), there were village health workers (VHWs), chosen by local ward development committees. VHWs were nearly always young women, trained for 3 months to motivate families in sound living habits and use of the local health center. They also carried a simple health kit with medication for treating malaria, cleansing wounds, relieving aches (aspirin), and so on. VHWs got small salaries from district councils, and by 1986, some 7,000 had been trained.

With this pyramidal structure of MOH health services—from village to health center to district to province to capital—integration of the former vertically directed health programs would be the guiding policy in Zimbabwe. A mother and child visiting a rural health center would be provided a package of all needed services: examinations, immunizations, nutrition education, instruction on oral rehydration (in case of diarrhea), and treatment of any illness present. Environmental work for the control of malaria and schistosomiasis, previously managed from the national capital, has been decentralized to the health offices of the provinces and districts. Tuberculosis control (case-finding, treatment, contact-tracing, etc.) has also been decentralized to the district hospitals.

To cope with the technical problems of all these responsibilities at the district level, the office of the provincial medical director might include special consultants. Since Zimbabwe did not yet have an adequate number of such specialists, in most fields they were available only at the national level, but they helped the districts through the provincial offices. Of the 55 districts, all but two had a district hospital in 1988; of these 53, however, only 26 were considered satisfactory, and 27 required major improvements. The importance of district hospitals in Zimbabwe transcends their role as places for in-patient care; they are also a basis for attracting and holding doctors and other health personnel in rural areas.

After a few years, the initial reorganization of the central MOH of Zimbabwe was modified a second time. Around 1985, as provincial and district health organization were developed, the central establishment of a Rural Health Care Division was changed. The central ministry instead simply set up a Health Care Services Division, to promote local services in both urban and rural areas. Also the Mental Health Care Division was abolished, and its functions were absorbed by all health programs at provincial and district levels. The central MOH headquarters arranged its various consultant functions under two main divisions: (1) health care services for environmental health, maternal and child health, communicable disease control, and so on, and (2) health support services for health manpower, pharmaceuticals, laboratory services, management, and other factors. Both of these divisions are concerned with relevant aspects of the four large central referral hospitals.

Several other changes were made in the health system after Zimbabwean independence. Water supplies and sanitation in many African communal areas (the Tribal Trust Lands of Rhodesia) were much improved. The expanded program for immunization (EPI) was strengthened, as was the instruction of mothers on use of oral rehydration therapy (ORT) for infant diarrhea. Official MOH drug use was restricted to a WHO-recommended essential drugs list.

The education of physicians at the nation's single medical school of the University of Zimbabwe was recast from the British model to a more appropriate African curriculum. Enrollment was increased and a greater emphasis was put on primary health care. One month is devoted to field work in a rural community, each year from the very first of the 5-year sequence. On qualifying, every new medical graduate is required to enter the government health service (apparently until no longer needed). Equivalent adjustments have been made in the education of nurses, pharmacists, and others. Rehabilitation assistants have been newly trained, and the output of broad-gauged *health assistants* has been increased to improve the staffing of rural health centers.

Health Expenditures and Commentary

Overall expenditures (public and private) in the health system of Zimbabwe have been reported only for the very first year of independence, 1980–81; in this period they amounted to 156,000,000 Zimbabwean dollars, or 5.3 percent of the GNP. This was an exceptionally high share of national wealth for an African health system, but it may reflect a relatively strong welfare orientation, even in the colonial period. In the 1979–80 fiscal year, central government spending for health was 4.6 percent of the total central government budget. Significantly, by 1986–87 this share of central government expenditures had risen to 5.9 percent.

Over the first 6 years of independence, furthermore, the allocation of MOH funds for different health purposes changed. In 1980–81, only 7.6 percent of the MOH spending was earmarked for preventive services, with the balance going for curative services (88 percent), research (0.8 percent), and administration (3.5 percent). By 1985–86, preventive efforts received 14 percent of MOH funds, and the balance went to medical care, administration, and research.

The economic magnitude of the private sector in Zimbabwe can be reported only for 1980–81, but it reflects the proportions of various health system subdivisions, discussed earlier, so well that it should be noted. In Table 15.1, we see that, even before the Zimbabwe government could have implemented new policies, expenditures for health came substantially from organized sources rather than private individuals. Within "organized" sources, some were private but the lion's share (60.1 percent) was governmental.

The distributions shown in Table 15.1 include both recurrent and capital expenditures. Since the figures identify sources (rather than place of expenditure), the large share for the MOH includes its allotments to municipalities, district councils, missions, and other bodies; it does not include relatively small revenues collected from patients using MOH facilities. On the other hand, the small share derived from religious missions reflects the fact that most of the financing of their services comes from patient fees.

Regarding its total health resources, Zimbabwe was relatively well supplied at the time it won its independence. Some physicians emigrated after the end of British rule, but larger numbers were soon trained. On the medical register in 1981 there were nearly 1,300 physicians, which meant 17 per 100,000 population. Only 31 percent of these, however, were in government or other organized health service (including missions and industry); the bal-

Table 15.1. Health Expenditures in Zimbabwe by Source: Percentage Distribution, 1980–81

Source	Percentage
Ministry of Health	51.2
Other ministries	4.2
Parastatal enterprises	2.9
Municipalities	1.4
Foreign aid	0.4
Subtotal government	(60.1)
Religious missions	0.4
Industry and mines	2.8
Voluntary agencies	1.1
Nongovernment organizations	(4.3)
Private insurance schemes	18.6
Families and individuals	17.0
Private commercial sector	(35.6)

Source: World Bank, *Zimbabwe: Population, Health and Nutrition Sector Review,* Vol. II. Washington, D.C. (Report No. 4214-ZIM), June 1983, p. 46.

ance of 69 percent were either in private practice in the main cities or could not be accounted for. (One may recall that in 1977 the physicians in private practice were only 36 percent of the total.) Registered nurses in 1980 numbered 71 per 100,000, and only 40 percent of these were in public or other organized employment. Dentists and pharmacists were known to be mainly in the private sector.

Health facilities were also relatively well supplied at independence. In 1980, hospital beds numbered 18,200, which meant 2.4 per 1,000 population—an exceptionally high ratio. These were distributed under the following sponsorships:

Sponsorship	Percentage of Beds
Ministry of Health (all levels)	60.1
Religious missions	32.2
Industry and mines	7.7
All sponsorships	100.0

Of the MOH beds, one-fourth were in four large central facilities and three-fourths were at the provincial and district levels. Because public hospital beds are more heavily utilized than beds in other facilities, the average length of patient-stay is quite short—6.3 days per case in public facilities and 10.2 days in the others.

The absence of purely private proprietary

hospitals in Zimbabwe or even in colonial Rhodesia is noteworthy, except for the impact of segregated health policies that previously prevailed. Under these policies, all hospitals, whether operated by government, missions, or industry, were reserved for white patients or black patients. The hospitals for whites were of much higher quality and their bed–population ratios were much greater. After independence, such racial policies were ended, but essentially similar delineation resulted from the use of beds by patients financed through private versus public funds (see later).

The substantial changes in the health system of Zimbabwe, compared to that of Rhodesia, have been clear; the new policies emphasize a stronger orientation toward primary health care, prevention, services in rural areas, and nondiscrimination based on race. The attainment of health equity, however, requires even greater intervention into the free market of Zimbabwe's health system than had been undertaken by 1988.

In spite of the large share of total health expenditures coming from the public sector, and the high proportion of hospital beds in public facilities, great inequities persist in the health system of Zimbabwe. The basis for these is not biological race, but socioeconomic status. The private sector clearly favors the wealthy, but in the sovereign nation that succeeded Southern Rhodesia, inequalities were already deeply institutionalized in the public sector as well.

Thus, at the time of independence government hospitals had some 1,500 private beds. The care of patients in those beds is not only luxurious, compared to the care of others, but it is subsidized by government. This is because charges for the use of private beds are only about one-third of their operating costs; two-thirds of costs come from tax funds. Even the commercial insurance schemes financing much of the private medical care are indirectly subsidized by government, insofar as the insurance premiums are not subject to taxation; they constitute revenue lost to government and tax-exemption for the fortunate 3 percent of people who have such insurance.

Most regrettably, serious economic difficulties in the 1980s affected Zimbabwe, like most developing countries, with great inflation of both prices and wages. The original criterion for entitlement to free government health service (earnings under 150 Zimbabwe dollars per month) was no longer meaningful. Instead of raising this threshold, economic pressures forced the government to require payments by most people for the use of public treatment (but not for preventive) services.

The purely private sector of Zimbabwe's health services promotes greater inequities. We have noted in Table 15.1 that 18.6 percent of total health expenditures comes from private insurance, covering 3 percent of the population. This means that insured families receive six times their proper share of health care financing. The 17 percent of health expenditures spent by families and individuals gives affluent persons further access to private health care providers, with little if any relationship to the extent of their health needs. Some of this, however, doubtless pays for drugs and traditional healing purchased by the poor.

The government of Zimbabwe is not unaware of these problems but has chosen to accept a substantial private sector, perhaps as a price for political stability. In the early 1980s, however, the government understandably decided to disallow certain requests for construction of new private hospitals. Physicians earn much higher incomes from private practice than in government service, and government has found it difficult to bar MOH physicians from seeing patients privately.

The overall health record of Zimbabwe has, in spite of persistent inequalities, shown substantial progress. The crude birth rate has been reduced from 55 per 1,000 in 1965 to 45 per 1,000 in 1986. The infant mortality rate has declined from 110 per 1,000 live births in 1960 to 73 per 1,000 in 1987. Life expectancy at birth was 55 years in 1979 and 58 years in 1986. In 1984, it was estimated that 52 percent of the national population had access to safe water. These improvements, of course, must be attributed to changes in the total society of Zimbabwe, as well as to the provision of both preventive and curative services in the health system.

LIBERIA

Another low-income African country of a very different background from Zimbabwe and with a somewhat welfare-oriented health system is Liberia. Having great political instability, the country's health system has also been highly unstable, but its main contours around 1985 are described. In 1980 a military group seized power, and many features of the health system ceased to advance or even declined.

Located on the northwest coast of Africa, Liberia had a 1988 population of 2,500,000. The nation was founded in 1822 by freed slaves from the United States (through the American Colonization Society), and became independent and self-governing in 1847; it was the first autonomous republic in Africa. Although the economy is mainly agricultural, urbanization has been relatively rapid, increasing from 23 percent of the population in 1965 to 37 percent in 1985. The annual GNP per capita in 1986 was $460.

Liberia is divided into 11 counties (plus two other territories), which serve, among other things, as the framework for its health system. Before 1963, much of the interior was under the control of 28 tribal chiefs, who still have influence in the large land areas not on the coast. County officials are not elected, but appointed by the several ministries in the capital, Monrovia. Even before the military government in 1980, the staffing of various administrative offices was especially large. The families of the original freed slaves, coming from America, constitute an elite 5 percent of the population, in relation to the 95 percent who are indigenous African people. Overall adult literacy in 1984 was 35 percent.

Health System Structure

The dominant organization in Liberia's health system is the Ministry of Health and Social Welfare, but several other groups and programs play substantial parts. There has been little evidence of coordination among these essentially autonomous programs.

Ministry of Health and Social Welfare. The official activities of the MOHSW acquired ministerial status as recently as 1953, and since then the ministry has been gradually evolving. Its central administrative structure in 1985 included three main departments, for (a) health services, (b) administration, and (c) social welfare. Under the Department of Health Services were a Division of Preventive Services and a Division of Curative Services. The Division of Curative Services was responsible for the operation of the 14 principal hospitals of the ministry. This did not, however, include the nation's largest tertiary-level hospital (the J. F. Kennedy Memorial Medical Center), which came under a semiautonomous special board, appointed by the head of state.

The Division of Preventive Services was responsible for all other peripheral services of the ministry, both preventive and therapeutic. These services were provided in the country's 11 counties through a network of MOHSW health centers and health posts. More peripherally, in 1985 the villages of three counties had briefly trained (6 to 8 weeks) teams of a village health worker and one or two traditional birth attendants. At the head of each county's MOHSW program was a county medical officer, theoretically responsible for preventive public health services as well as the county hospital; in fact, only in three of the counties was the staff sufficient to perform both these functions. In seven counties, the county medical officer functioned essentially as the hospital's medical director. In addition, the Division of Preventive Services was responsible for three largely vertical programs: (a) an expanded program of immunization, (b) tuberculosis control, and (c) leprosy control.

Under the Division of Curative Services was a major training institution of the ministry: the Tubman National Institute for Medical Arts. This is physically located on the grounds of the J. F. K. Memorial Medical Center, though it is administratively separate. The medical center was closed down for an extended period in 1983 and 1984, for lack of funds, but was reopened in 1985. The occupancy levels of all the county hospitals under ministry control have been extremely low, estimated at between 25 and 50 percent. The overall rate of MOHSW hospital utilization actually declined in the 1980s. Likewise, the ministry reported that utilization of its out-patient services declined nationally from 1,520,000 visits in 1979 to 863,000 visits in 1983.

Although the large J. F. K. Memorial Medical Center (300 beds) is not strictly under the Ministry of Health and Social Welfare, the minister serves as chairman of its semiautonomous board of directors. Its budget is handled separately from that of the ministry. When fully operational, the center employs a staff of nurses, doctors, and allied health personnel of about 1,900 persons, so its impact on the overall health manpower resources of the country is obviously great.

Other Government Agencies with Health Functions. Although the Ministry of Health and Social Welfare has major responsibilities for environmental sanitation in rural areas, other ministries play significant roles in developing both rural and urban water supplies. The Ministry of Rural Development assists villages in establishing both water supplies and waste disposal facilities. The Ministry of Lands, Mines, and Energy constructs many village wells. Most important is the Liberian Water and Sewer Corporation, a parastatal enterprise that constructs and maintains public water and sewerage systems in Monrovia and other major cities. Other parastatal enterprises furnish electrical power, transportation, and so on, and these enterprises also maintain special clinics for their employees and families.

Since 1980, Liberia has operated a limited social security program, managed by the National Social Security and Welfare Corporation. The initial health-related benefit has been cash compensation and medical care for work-related injuries. In 1985 about 103,000 workers in both public and private employment were covered. The corporation negotiates agreements with selected doctors and hospitals to treat injured workers for specified fees. Most of these providers are private, and relatively high fees are ordinarily payable.

The plans of the National Social Security and Welfare Corporation included the extension of benefits to pensions for the aged, as well as welfare assistance for the aged and disabled. The development of an insurance program for financing general medical care for the eligible population was also considered.

Religious Mission Health Programs. Important sources of health care in Liberia are the religious missions, representing overseas churches; these include several Protestant sects and Roman Catholicism. Though they originally were concerned only with curative services in hospitals, mission programs in the 1980s stressed the provision of various aspects of primary health care.

In 1985 the missions operated six hospitals, one health center, and 31 small health posts. The hospitals all had out-patient departments, and these as well as the other units had a high rate of utilization; in 1983, for example, they provided 353,000 clinic visits. The in-patient beds were also heavily used, with occupancy rates around 80 percent—much higher than those of MOHSW hospitals. A reflection of the high utilization of mission hospitals is their very short average length of patient-stay—only 5.2 days.

Mission health facilities in 1985 employed 43 physicians (about one-third expatriates and two-thirds Liberians) and a total staff of 748 health personnel. Many of these—nurses, midwives, laboratory technicians—had been trained by the missions, but the majority were graduates of training programs of the MOHSW. This apparently causes no difficulties, since the government of Liberia looks on the mission health services as complementary to, not competitive with, its own. In one county, in fact, the mission hospital serves as the county government hospital.

The cordial relationship between government and the missions is reflected in substantial public subsidies each year; in 1983, these amounted to 38.5 percent of total mission health expenditures. Another 46.1 percent of mission costs came from fees paid by patients, and only 15 percent was derived from philanthropic donations. It is generally recognized that mission facilities are better staffed and supplied with drugs than their governmental counterparts. The county medical officer is theoretically supposed to supervise the local mission, as well as all government units, but in practice this has had little meaning.

Voluntary Nonsectarian Health Agencies. Liberia has few voluntary health agencies unrelated to religious goals, but two are significant. The Family Planning Association of Liberia promotes the extension of contraceptive practices, in the attempt to reduce the nation's high birth rate (46 per 1,000 population in 1986). The association offers general education, as well as direct services to women. Family planning workers (nurses and others) operate special clinics, and also offer their services in cooperation with the maternal and child health program of the MOHSW. Most of the funding of the Family Planning Association comes from international agencies and overseas donations.

The Liberian Red Cross is a small organization, subsidized by the government, to assist in emergencies. It also operates a small clinical laboratory, which charges fees for various tests.

Commercial Enterprises (Concessions). The first modern health facility in Liberia was a general hospital established by an American rubber company (Firestone) in 1928. The objective was to provide health care to company employees and their families. Since the government conceded land for use by foreign companies (in agriculture, timber, or mining), with public entitlement to a share of the profits, they are known as *concessions.* In 1985 concession health facilities included 10 hospitals, 2 health centers, and 14 health posts. With their relatively abundant source of corporate funding, these facilities were especially well staffed, equipped, and supplied with drugs and other materials.

Concession health resources are financed entirely by the company, as are the houses occupied by the workers' families and schooling for the children. (On the other hand, the wages are relatively low.) Nonemployees of the concession, living in the same general area, may also use the health facilities, but they must pay fees. These charges are no higher than those made by mission facilities, and the services are considered of good quality, so that concession health services have been well used by neighboring people over the years. Concessions have no difficulty in recruiting health personnel, trained largely by the government, since their salary scales are high.

The Private Market for Modern Health Care. In Liberia, as everywhere, much medical and related service is provided by purely private practitioners and institutions. It is used mainly by upper-income families in the cities, but occasionally patients of low-income who are desperate will pay for private medical care, and the private purchase of nonprescribed drugs is commonplace in all income groups.

The extent of the private health care market in Liberia is difficult to estimate. (A household survey of all family expenditures, made in 1977, might provide some relevant data, but the findings were never tabulated.) Of an estimated 300 physicians in Liberia in 1985, about 89 were entirely in private practice, almost all in the national capital. In addition, most of the 130 doctors employed in the MOHSW and the Kennedy Memorial Hospital see private patients part of the time each day. Two large *private medical clinics* in Monrovia, each with 20 to 30 hospital beds, are staffed by specialists on the salaried staff of the Kennedy Hospital.

In 1985 there were 161 *medicine stores* selling drugs among other products in Liberia, although the entire nation had only 50 trained pharmacists (of whom six were Liberians). Registered pharmacies, staffed by pharmacists, numbered 42. Five large wholesale distributors sold imported drugs to most of these outlets, and about 10 large pharmacies imported their own drugs directly. A substantial share of the drugs consumed in the country are simply purchased over-the-counter, without benefit of a prescription by any trained person. Furthermore, many drugs prescribed in a health center or hospital out-patient department must be purchased in the private market, since they are not available in the health facility.

Finally, the private modern health care market in Liberia includes a number of urban "clinics," which give the impression that they are staffed by physicians. Actually, they are operated by nurses or physician assistants, who have left organized employment and are able to acquire supplies of drugs. With limited knowledge, these health personnel treat almost any patient who comes along, for a fee, making liberal use of drugs given by injection. Certified midwives, trained in official programs, occasionally also leave their government posts and set themselves up as private practitioners.

Traditional Healing. It is generally agreed that traditional healing plays a large role in the Liberian health system, particularly in rural areas. Traditional birth attendants are ubiquitous, and government policy calls for their recognition and upgrading through special training. Private fees are nevertheless payable for their services. For general medical care, there are typically untrained male healers. The Ministry of Internal Affairs maintains a registry of those who choose to register—about 600 in 1985. For each healer who registers, there are estimated to be two others, for a total of 1,800. (This correspond closely to the number of villages in Liberia, and there is usually one healer per village.)

Most healers are farmers or other rural workers who practice traditional healing part-time. It is said that 60 percent of rural people with a health complaint consult a healer first, before seeking care at a health post or other modern facility. For certain disorders, considered mental in origin, traditional practices are often believed to be more effective than modern. Certain healers are regarded as especially skillful in setting broken bones or treating snake bites.

Most traditional healers charge low fees for their services or, more accurately, for the herbal drugs that they dispense. Some traditional healers, who have acquired a reputation for great competence, make high charges for treatment—essentially the same fees as the modern physician charges.

Health Resources and Expenditures

The health manpower resources for staffing various programs in Liberia's health system have been meager. In 1984 there were about 300 physicians in the country, and most of these came from other countries. This meant 13.9 modern doctors per 100,000 population. Although this was an improvement over the 8.1 doctors per 100,000 in 1965, the great majority were concentrated in the national capital, and very few served the population in the outlying counties. A medical school was established in Monrovia in 1968, under the MOHSW, but it has been graduating only about 10 to 20 doctors per year (not all being from Liberia). New graduates must spend a year in a rural post.

The distribution of principal activities by the 300 doctors in Liberia in 1984 was roughly as follows:

Principal Activity	Percentage
Ministry of Health and Social Welfare	27
Kennedy Memorial Hospital	17
Religious missions	14
Enterprise concessions	13
Medical school faculty (full-time)	2
Exclusive private practice	27
All activities	100

Nurses of various grades have been trained at four hospital-based nursing schools in Liberia. The high rate of attrition among graduates, however, has actually reduced the ratio of nurses (of all grades) to population, from 43.7 nursing personnel per 100,000 in 1965 to 34.2 per 100,000 in 1981. In part, the decline of nurses may have been due to the training of *physician assistants* in a 3-year course, starting around 1975. These mainly male health workers replaced physicians on rural health center and clinic staffs.

Hospital resources in Liberia have been somewhat greater than manpower; the hospitals have been constructed largely with funds from foreign sources—religious, entrepreneurial, and bilateral public foreign aid. In 1973, Liberia reported to the World Health Organization a total of 41 hospitals, with 2,530 beds, or a ratio of 1.55 beds per 1,000 population at the time. Of these beds, 56 percent were in government facilities. The sponsorship of 44 percent of beds in nongovernment structures was divided among religious missions, business concessions, and private physicians.

Facilities for ambulatory care in Liberia include health centers, health posts, and some clinics. In 1983 there were 30 health centers, of which 27 were under the MOHSW, two were operated by concessions, and one was run by a religious mission. These facilities are supposed to be staffed by a physician plus other personnel. The MOHSW operated 212 health posts staffed only by health auxiliaries; another 14 posts were maintained by concessions and 31 by missions. Private medical clinics numbered 37 in 1983.

Estimates of the sources of economic support for all aspects of the Liberian health system may give better perspective on its character. In 1985 a field study was made in Liberia, and it was found possible to assemble information, directly or indirectly, on all the principal sources of health expenditures; these data are presented in Table 15.2, along with the methods used in obtaining or estimating the figures. Insofar as no exact data were available, estimates were on the conservative side.

Liberia uses the U.S. dollar for its currency, and in 1983–84 about $65 million were spent in the health system. If this is related to the gross domestic product of $980 million in 1984, it comes to 6.6 percent. This seems quite high for a low-income developing country, but it may reflect the large parts played in the Liberian system by business enterprises, religious missions, foreign aid, and the domestic private sector. Of the total health expenditure in 1983–84, about 42 percent came from government and 58 percent from private sources— roughly half of the latter coming from organized programs and half from individuals and families.

The Ministry of Health and Social Welfare accounted for only 23.3 percent of the total expenditures. The low rate of utilization of MOHSW facilities has been noted, and this would contribute to the high private expenditures for drugs, as well as traditional healers. At the same time, the rates of utilization of religious missions and business concessions have been generally high.

Conducive to private health spending in Liberia has been the sale in the 1980s of com-

Table 15.2. Health Expenditures in Liberia by Source: Percentage Distribution, 1983–84

Health Activity	Expenditure	Percentage
Ministry of Health and Welfare[a]	$15,106,000	
J. F. K. Memorial Hospital[b]	8,500,000	
State enterprise health services[c]	984,000	
University medical school[d]	500,000	
Other governmental bodies[e]	2,000,000	
Government subtotal	(27,090,000)	41.73
Religious missions[f]	4,291,000	
Voluntary health agencies[g]	250,000	
Business enterprises (concessions)[h]	14,103,000	
Private organized subtotal	(18,644,000)	28.72
Private institutions[i]	457,000	
Private medical and dental "clinics"[j]	1,089,000	
Privately purchased drugs[k]	10,200,000	
Traditional birth attendants[l]	750,000	
Traditional healers[m]	6,480,000	
Private individual subtotal	(19,176,000)	29.54
Grand Total	$64,910,000	100.00

Source: Based on a field study by M. I. Roemer in February 1985. Information was obtained from sources indicated in footnotes.
[a]Ministry of Health and Social Welfare.
[b]MOHSW.
[c]Derived from "Study of Health Care Costs and Financing," furnished by Office of United Nations Development Program (UNDP), Monrovia, 1984.
[d]Based on World Health Organization cost esitmate of $35,000 per graduate, for 15 graduates in 1984.
[e]Estimate of expenditures by three public agencies concerned with water and sanitation, plus medical and administrative expenditures of Social Security Program for employment injury.
[f]Christian Health Association of Liberia.
[g]Estimate of expenditures by the Family Planning Association.
[h]UNDP Office, Monrovia.
[i]UNDP Office, Monrovia.
[j]Data provided by the Commissioner of Income Tax, Ministry of Finance, with assumption of 25 percent underreporting.
[k]Based on estimate of Liberian Pharmaceutical Association that drugs imported cost $6,800,000 in 1984, and retail pharmacies plus "medicine stores" markup sales price 50 percent.
[l]Birth rate of nearly 50 per 1,000 means that in Liberia's 2,000,000 population there were 100,000 births in 1984. Assuming that half of these were delivered by traditional attendants, at an average of $15 per case, yields $750,000.
[m]The estimated 1,800 traditional healers are believed to collect an average of $300 per month, or $3,600 per year, which comes to $6,480,000.

mercial insurance for medical care costs. This has enabled both public and private white-collar employees in Monrovia to pay for care by private physicians. Liberia also holds a national lottery, the proceeds of which help support medical missions.

The declining trend in use of government health facilities has been noted. Government health expenditures have also declined, both absolutely and as a percentage of the total government budget. Between 1981–82 and 1985–86, the health expenditures of government fell from 10.6 to 8 percent of the total. Of these public moneys, about 80 percent went for hospitals and 20 percent for all other health services.

In summary, one can conclude that most of Liberia's health system—70 percent as reflected in expenditures—involves organized activities. Organization under the government, however, has evidently been declining, while organized services under private auspices (business enterprises and church missions) have been increasing. Continuation of this trend might alter the consideration of Liberia's health system as being "welfare-oriented."

Some indication of trends in Liberian health services is given by biostatistical data. The infant mortality rate did show a great decline from 153 per 1,000 live births in 1960 to 88 per 1,000 in 1987; most of that decline, however, occurred before 1980, when a military coup took over. The crude birth rate, reflecting the outcome of family planning efforts, on the other hand, has been stationary for years; it was 46 births per 1,000 population in 1965 and the same in 1986. In 1984, of the total population only 37 percent had access to safe water. The life expectancy at birth in 1987 was 55 years. Immunizations against measles were reported to have covered 99 percent of babies in 1981, declining to 55 percent in 1986–87. Over the same period the percentage of children who received DPT (diphtheria, pertussis, and tetanus) immunizations fell from 39 percent to 28 percent.

SUMMARY COMMENT

In spite of the low per capita GNPs in these four countries, all of them have made notable efforts to improve their national health systems. All except Liberia were former British colonies in which, despite the severe deficiency in health resources, there was a certain administrative discipline. The ministries of health of these countries, since their independence, have planned and partially achieved nationwide networks of reasonably well staffed hospitals, health centers, and health posts.

The three liberated British colonies have all designed broad health plans that, though not entirely fulfilled, have served to guide social policy. All have espoused a socialist viewpoint in the health system, although such ideas have not characterized the general economy. In spite of this health policy rhetoric, only half the physicians or fewer are employed in the government, and public doctors engage freely in private practice as well. In India, Ayurvedic doctors are abundant and almost entirely in private practice. As a result, most health expenditures in India, Burma, and Liberia (though not in Zimbabwe) come from private sources.

Hospitals and hospital beds, as well as health centers, are predominantly governmental in all four of these countries. Their medical technology and amenities are quite weak and their staffing is modest, however, although all hospitals have some full-time physicians. Ambulatory care units typically have trained auxiliary personnel. Many resources in India and Liberia are operated by religious missions, usually with higher standards than government facilities, though the patients served must pay.

Health programs funded by social security operate in India and Burma, implementing high standards but covering only very small percentages of the population. In Liberia, foreign enterprises provide good quality medical care to employees and their families. In Burma, nongovernment cooperative medical clinics, charging private fees, are important.

All four of these welfare-oriented health systems espouse primary health care as their top priority, but the achievement of full nationwide coverage with such service has been a relatively slow process.

REFERENCES

Burma

Aung Tun Thet, *Health Care Delivery the Cooperative Way: A Comparative Analysis.* Rangoon: Institute of Economics, February, 1984.

Aung Tun Thet, *Records of the National Seminars*

for Preparing Plan of Action for Implementing Strategies for Health for All by the Year 2000 (20–27 June 1983). Rangoon: Ministry of Health, 1983.

Aung Tun Thet, *A Study of Cooperative Health Clinics in Burma.* Rangoon: Institute of Economics, March 1981.

Aung Tun Thet, *Voluntary Health Workers: Evaluation Study.* Rangoon: Institute of Economics, January 1983.

Aung Tun Thet and Aye Aye Thwin, *Comparative Profile Analysis of Urban and Rural Community Health Workers: Evaluation Study.* Rangoon: Institute of Economics, September 1984.

Central Statistical Organization, *Household Expenditures and Expenditure Survey: Ye Sa Gyo Township.* Rangoon, February 1985 (Original in Burmese).

D. Khin Hlaing, *Experiences Through Different Mechanisms for Community Financing—Burma.* Rangoon: Ministry of Health, May 1985.

Department of Medical Research, *Research Programmes and Facilities,* Rangoon, 1985.

Health Assistant Training School, *Task-Oriented Curriculum for Public Health Supervisor Grade 1.* Aungsanmyo, Burma, May 1983.

International Labour Organisation, *Social Security Planning, Legislation and Administration: Socialist Republic of the Union of Burma.* Geneva, 1979.

Joint Committee on Health Policy (WHO/UNICEF), *Health Systems Management (Burma).* Rangoon, May 1985.

Joint Committee on Health Policy (WHO/UNICEF), *Development and Mobilization of Health Resources—Burma.* Rangoon, May 1985.

Khin Maung Thwin, *Household Survey on Morbidity, Mortality, and Health Care.* (Joint SRUB-USAID Study), Rangoon: Ministry of Health, Health Information Service, July 1983.

Khin Maung Thwin, *A Study on the Reliability and Validity of Demographic Indicators in Burma.* Rangoon: Ministry of Health, Health Information Service, 1 July 1986.

Klein, Wilhelm, et al., *Burma (Insight Guides).* Hong Kong: APA Productions, 1984.

Liberi, Dawn, *A Study of the Health Sector of Burma.* Washington, D.C.: U.S. Department of Health and Human Services, Office of International Health, December 1979.

Ma Sann Shwe, and Thein Maung Myint, *Work Study of the Health Personnel of Selected Rural Health Centres in Bassein East Township.* Rangoon: Ministry of Health, Department of Medical Research, February 1986.

Ministry of Health, *Community Health Programme: Report of Central Evaluation Workshop* (16–19 September 1985). Rangoon, 1986.

Ministry of Health, Department of Medical Educa-

tion, *General Information Booklet.* Rangoon, 1985.

Ministry of Health, Department of Medical Research, *DMR Research Findings Applicable to Health Care.* Rangoon, 1984.

Ministry of Health, Health Information Service, *Annual Report on Peoples' Health Plan Service Programme Activities (1983–84).* Rangoon, September 1985.

Ministry of Health, Health Information Service, *General Health and Health-Related Information in Burma.* Rangoon, August 1984.

Ministry of Health, Health Information Service, *Health Information Booklet.* Rangoon, 1985.

Ministry of Health, Health Statistics Division, *Extracts from Country Profile: Burma.* Rangoon, August 1983.

Ministry of Health, Task Force for Mid-Term Evaluation of PHP II, *Mid-Term Evaluation Report on Disease Control Project (1982–1984).* Rangoon: Health Information Service, October 1984.

Ministry of Planning and Finance, *Report of the Pyithu Hluttaw (People's Assembly) on the Financial, Economic, and Social Conditions of the Socialist Republic of the Union of Burma for 1986/87.* Rangoon, 1986.

Myat Thein, *An Evaluation of Rural Water Supply Project in Ayadaw Township, Burma.* Rangoon: Ministry of Health, March 1984.

Oot, D., A. Fairbank, and T. Baker, *A Review of AID's Health Sector Strategy in Burma.* Rangoon: USAID, February, 1985.

Roemer, Milton I., *Primary Health Care in Burma's National Health System.* Rangoon: U.S. Agency for International Development and Western Consortium for the Health Professions, August 1986.

Social Security Board, *The Social Security System in Burma.* Rangoon, 1977.

SRUB-UNICEF, *A Situation Analysis of Children and Women in Burma.* Rangoon: United Nations Children's Fund (UNICEF), April 1986.

Than Sein, *Health and Development: A Case of Ayadaw Township, Burma.* Rangoon: Ministry of Health, April 1985.

Thein Maung Mint et al., *Evaluation of Voluntary Health Workers.* Rangoon: Ministry of Health, May 1982.

U Ba Tun, *Maternal and Child Health Care Delivery System, Burma.* Rangoon: WHO/SEARO Inter-Country Meeting of Principal Investigators of Risk Approach in MCH Care, 30 December 1985.

U Tin Oo, "Traditional Medicine of Burma," in *Regional Seminar on Traditional Medicine Programme.* New Delhi: World Health Organization, SEA/OMC/Trad. Med./Meet. 2/1, April 1977.

United Nations Development Programme, *Annual*

Report on Development Cooperation with the Socialist Republic of the Union of Burma 1985. Rangoon: UNDP, July 1986.

United Nations Fund for Population Activities, *Burma: Report of Mission on Needs Assessment for Population Assistance* (Report No. 70). New York: (UNFPA) March 1985.

World Bank, *Burma: Policies and Prospects for Economic Adjustments and Growth.* Washington, D.C., World Bank, November 1985.

India

Banerji, Debabar, *Poverty, Class and Health Culture in India.* New Delhi: Pracki Prakashan, 1982.

Banerji, D., *Health Behavior of Rural Populations: Impact of Rural Health Services.* New Delhi: Nehru University, Centre of Social Medicine and Community Health, June 1974.

Bhattacharji, Sara, et al., "Evaluating Community Health Worker Performance in India." *Health Policy and Planning,* 1(3):232–239, 1986.

Bose, Ashish, and P. B. Desai, *Studies in Social Dynamics of Primary Health Care.* Delhi, India: Hindustan Publishing Co., 1983.

Deodhar, N. S., "Primary Health Care in India." *Journal of Public Health Policy,* 3(1):76–99, March 1982.

Faruquee, Rashid, and Ethna Johnson, *Health, Nutrition, and Family Planning in India: A Survey of Experiments and Special Projects.* Washington, D.C.: World Bank (Staff Working Paper No. 507), February 1982.

Government of India, Health Survey and Planning Committee, *Report, Vol. 1.* New Delhi: Ministry of Health, 1961.

Government of India, Health Survey and Development Committee, *Report, Vol. 1–4.* New Delhi: Ministry of Health, 1946.

Indian Council of Social Science Research and Indian Council of Medical Research, *Health for All—An Alternative Strategy.* Pune: Indian Institute of Education, 1981.

Indian Council of Medical Research, *National Conference on Evaluation of Primary Health Care Programmes: Proceedings.* New Delhi, 1980.

Jeffery, Roger, "New Patterns in Health Sector Aid to India." *International Journal of Health Services,* 16(1):121–139, 1986.

Jeffery, Roger, "Health Planning in India, 1951–84: The Role of the Planning Commission." *Health Policy and Planning,* 1(2):127–137, 1986.

Krishnan, T. N., "Health Statistics in Kerala State, India," in Scott B. Halstead et al. (Editors), *Good Health at Low Cost.* New York: Rockefeller Foundation, 1985, pp. 39–45.

Ministry of Health and Family Welfare, *Primary Health Care in India.* New Delhi, 1980.

Ministry of Health and Family Welfare, Government of India, *Health Information of India.* New Delhi: Nirman Bhavan, 1987 and 1988.

Ministry of Health and Family Welfare, Rural Health Division, *Rural Health Statistics in India.* New Delhi, December 1988.

Nag, Moni, "The Impact of Social and Economic Development on Mortality: Comparative Study or Kerala and West Bengal." In Scott B. Halstead et al. (Editors), *Good Health at Low Cost,* New York: Rockefeller Foundation, 1985, pp. 57–77.

Nayar, P. K. B., *Impact of Welfare Measures on Mortality: A Study in Kerala, India.* Trivandrum: Centre for Gerontological Studies, 1983.

Nehru University and Indian Council of Scientific and Industrial Research, *The Pharmaceutical Industry in India* (Case Studies in the Transfer of Technology). Geneva: United Nations Conference on Trade and Development, October 1977.

Panikar, P. G. K., "Health Care System in Kerala and Its Impact on Infant Mortality," in Scott B. Halstead et al. (Editors), *Good Health at Low Cost.* New York: Rockefeller Foundation, 1985, pp. 47–55.

Panikar, P. G. K., and C. R. Soman, *Health Status of Kerala: The Paradox of Economic Backwardness and Health Development.* Trivandrum: Centre for Development Studies, 1984.

Rajan, V. N., *Monograph on the Organisation of Medical Care within the Framework of Social Security: India.* Geneva: International Labour Office, 1968.

Ramasubban, R., "The Development of Health Policy in India," in T. Dyson and N. Crook (Editors), *India's Demography.* London: Asia, 1984.

Rao, M. N., and K. K. Radhalaxmi, *History of Public Health in India.* Calcutta, 1960.

Ratcliffe, John, "Social Justice and the Demographic Transition: Lessons from India's Kerala State." *International Journal of Health Services, 8(1):123–144, 1978.*

Seal, S. C., *Health Administration in India.* Calcutta: Dawn Books, 1975.

Takulia, Harbaus S., et al., *The Health Center Doctor in India.* Baltimore, Md.: Johns Hopkins Press, 1967.

Udupa, K. N., "The Ayurvedic System of Medicine," in K. W. Newell (Editor), *Health by the People.* Geneva: World Health Organization, 1975, pp. 53–69.

United Nations Conference on Trade and Development, *Case Studies in the Transfer of Technology: The Pharmaceutical Industry in India.* Geneva (TD/B/C.6/20), October 1977.

United Nations Fund for Population Activities, *Report of Second Mission on Needs Assessment for Population Assistance: India.* New York, May 1985.

World Health Organization, "India," in *Health Care in South-East Asia.* New Delhi: Regional Office for South-East Asia, 1985, pp. 91–110.

World Bank, *Determinants of Fertility Decline in*

India. Washington, D.C. (PHN Technical Notes RES 11), 1984.

World Bank, *Health, Nutrition, and Family Planning in India: A Survey of Experiments and Special Projects.* Washington, D.C. (Staff Working Paper No. 507), February 1982.

Zimbabwe

Anenden, H., "Zimbabwe: From Supermarket to Cafeteria." *World Health,* June 1987, pp. 21–23.

Faruquee, Rashid, *Social Infrastructure and Services in Zimbabwe.* Washington, D.C.: World Bank (Staff Working Paper No. 495), 1981.

Gilmurray, John, R. Riddell, and D. Sanders, *From Rhodesia to Zimbabwe: The Struggle for Health.* London: Catholic Institute for International Relations, 1979.

Government of the Republic of Zimbabwe, *Growth with Equity: An Economic Policy Statement.* Harare, February 1981.

Lamb, David, *The Africans.* New York: Vintage Books, 1984.

Sanders, David, "Reorganization of the Health Sector: The Way Forward in Light of Zimbabwe's Experience." Harare: University of Zimbabwe (unpublished report), March 1987.

Segall, Malcolm, "Planning and Politics of Resource Allocation: Promotion of Meaningful National Policy." *Social Science and Medicine,* 17(24):1947–1960, 1983.

United Nations Fund for Population Activities, *Zimbabwe: Report of Mission on Needs Assessment for Population Assistance.* New York (Report No. 50), October 1982.

World Bank, *Zimbabwe: Population, Health and Nutrition Sector Review, Volumes I and II.* Washington, D.C. (Report No. 4214-ZIM), June 1983.

Liberia

Development Consultants, *Republic of Liberia: A Study of Health Care Costs and Financing.* Monrovia, 1984.

Republic of Liberia, *Ten Year National Health Plan 1967–1976.* Monrovia, 1967.

United Nations Fund for Population Activities, *Liberia: Report of Mission on Needs Assessment for Population Assistance.* New York, August 1978.

U.S. Office of International Health, *Syncrisis: The Dynamics of Health—VII Liberia.* Washington, D.C.: U.S. Department of Health, Education, and Welfare, November 1973.

CHAPTER SIXTEEN

Comprehensive Health Systems in Very Poor Countries

Of the very poor countries in the world, two stand out for the exceptionally high priority they have put on the development of their health systems. Both are former British colonies—one in Asia and the other in Africa—in which postindependence events led to periods of dominance by semisocialist political groups. The Asian country is Sri Lanka, known under British rule as Ceylon. The African country is Tanzania, which combined the former British colonies: Tanganyika and Zanzibar.

SRI LANKA

The tropical island south of the southern tip of India was occupied by indigenous people and settlers from India until the sixteenth and seventeenth centuries, when colonists from Portugal and the Netherlands invaded. The British seized control in 1796, developing tea and rubber plantations along with a transportation network and an unusually strong program of education. An independence movement arose during World War I, leading to the Constitution of 1931, which granted universal adult suffrage. In 1931, government responsibility for health was also strengthened by integrating local government and health affairs under one new ministry. Demands for full independence, however, continued until it was declared after World War II in 1948.

Social Background

The first leadership of the free nation was oriented toward government's playing a major role in the economy and also toward strong social welfare programs for the entire popula-

tion. In 1951 the Sri Lankan Freedom Party was founded and, with a coalition of left-wing parties, it gained political power in 1956. When the elected prime minister, S.W.R.D. Bandaranaike, was assassinated in 1959, he was succeeded by his widow; under her, foreign corporations were nationalized. A more moderate socialist group won control from 1965 to 1970, but a three-party anticapitalist coalition regained power from 1970 to 1977. The country's name was changed from Ceylon to Sri Lanka in 1972.

In the final years of British rule, various welfare programs had already been introduced in Ceylon. Universal free public education was provided in 1945 up to university level. Subsidized food rations had been started during World War II, and the general health services for both treatment and prevention had been expanded. The number of small health stations serving expectant mothers and preschool children, for example, increased from 86 in 1935 to 503 in 1945.

After independence was won in 1948, the pace of all these social developments accelerated. Schools were built everywhere and the food distribution program was improved. Physicians in the government health services increased from 673 in 1950 to nearly 1,500 in 1965. Hospital beds were expanded from 15,000 in 1950 to more than 35,000 in 1965—a rise of 167 percent, while the population grew by 68 percent. The number of government nurses increased over this period from 1,300 to 3,600. Between 1950 and 1965, overall government expenditures for food subsidies, education, housing, and health rose from 5 percent to 12 percent of the nation's GDP. In this 15-year period, great reductions were achieved in smallpox and cholera (virtually eliminated), in hookworm disease, schistosomiasis, tuberculosis, and leprosy.

In 1977 a more conservative market-oriented government was voted into power in Sri Lanka. Foreign investments were encouraged, various government subsidies of consumer goods were ended, and the currency was devalued. Food rations were provided free only to the poorest families, but the "core of the welfare package" (as stated by one leading Sri Lankan social scientist) "was maintained intact." The free midday meal for school children was continued. Government health expenditures, which were 6.4 percent of the national budget in 1972, however, had declined to 4 percent in 1986.

Sri Lanka had a national population of 16,100,000 in 1986. The GNP per capita was $400. In spite of the health and education services, not conventionally counted as "household income," the distribution of income among families has still been extremely uneven; a household survey in 1980–81 showed that the wealthiest 20 percent of households earned 49.8 percent of the total income, while the poorest 20 percent earned only 5.8. Social programs obviously compensate, to some extent, for these great disparities. In 1987 the population was 21 percent urban and 79 percent rural. The level of adult literacy in 1985 was very high, 91 percent among men and 83 percent among women.

For purposes of governance, Sri Lanka is divided into 25 districts, each of which has several hundred thousand people. In 1971, district political authorities, headed by elected members of parliament, were set up, but in 1978 these were replaced by district ministers appointed by the central government. Members of district development councils, however, were locally elected. Within each district there are many municipalities and villages, although larger territorial jurisdictions are established for various administrative purposes, including health services.

Health System Organization and Resources

Government policy in Sri Lanka calls for the provision of complete health services, for treatment and prevention, which are free of charge to everyone. These services are provided by the Ministry of Health through its network of health facilities and personnel.

Ministry of Health. At the capital, Colombo, the MOH headquarters has major directorates for medical services (including hospitals), public health services, laboratory services, and planning, and a special department for Ayurvedic medicine. Each of the 25 districts is headed by a centrally appointed health official, known as a *superintendent of health services,* or SHS (a term carried over from an earlier period). The SHS is responsible for all health activities in the district, including hospitals, dispensaries, maternity homes, and certain vertical disease control programs (such as tuberculosis and leprosy control) other than malaria control, which remains a central responsibility. Certain Ayurvedic services also fall within the general MOH orbit, centrally and locally.

Public preventive services for mothers and children were developed in colonial Ceylon at a relatively early stage. In 1926, the Rockefeller Foundation, based in New York, developed at the town of Kalutara an exceptionally well-staffed health center for monitoring pregnant women and protecting the health of young children. Other smaller units for MCH service were soon developed throughout the country, usually as rural satellites to the numerous central dispensaries that the combined Ministry of Health and Local Government had set up for general medical care; by 1945 there were 250 such central dispensaries. Health education was also emphasized by the peripheral units. Small maternity homes were established in many rural towns, where expectant mothers could be treated for anemia and childbirths were safer. The original Kalutara Health Center was later developed into a general public health training facility.

The contemporary physical infrastructure of the MOH program has inevitably been influenced by the array of hospitals and dispensaries constructed over previous years. In 1981 there were 488 hospitals at several levels of complexity—large ones serving as nine provincial or "base" facilities, smaller district hospitals, and still smaller rural or peripheral hospitals. Altogether there were 44,000 beds, for a ratio of 2.9 beds per 1,000 population. The vast majority of these beds (around 90 percent) were in government facilities. Religious missions operated very few hospitals or clinics.

Hospitals generally have out-patient departments and, in addition, there were about 340 *central dispensaries* in 1981, staffed by assistant medical practitioners. Another 600 *branch dispensaries* and *visiting stations* were staffed by even more briefly trained auxiliary health workers, especially assistant midwives.

To arrange primary health care in a more orderly and efficient manner, the MOH took steps in 1982 to reorganize ambulatory services throughout the country. Each district was to be organized into divisions—about 10 per district, averaging a population of 60,000. In the division would be a divisional health center, staffed by a physician and numerous allied personnel. The division was to be further divided into three areas of about 20,000 people, served by a subdivisional health center; this facility would be staffed entirely by assistant medical practitioners (trained for 2 years) and other auxiliaries. Finally in the villages would be community or *gramodaya* health stations, staffed by volunteer family health workers, who were trained for only 2 weeks. As of 1983, it appeared from the MOH Annual Report that only a few district hospitals had been converted into the planned type of divisional health center and only a small proportion of the established dispensaries had been converted into small health centers at the subdivisional level. The facilities existed, but not with the newly planned relationships.

Other Government Agencies. Several parts of government in Sri Lanka, outside the MOH, are concerned with water supply and sanitation. The Ministry of Local Government, Housing, and Construction has a National Water Supply and Drainage Board. This ministry also has a Division of Public Health Engineering. The Division of Occupational Hygiene in the Ministry of Labor is responsible for inspection of factories for health and safety conditions.

In 1980, the government of Sri Lanka established a National Health Council, to promote interministerial cooperation for the advancement of health. The minister of health was responsible for convening meetings and providing staff support, but the chairman of the council was the prime minister. Other members were the ministers of education, agriculture, labor, and home affairs. The National Health Council plays a key role in the implementation of the entire decentralized program for primary health care described earlier.

Nongovernment Agencies. Among the older voluntary health organizations in Sri Lanka are the Red Cross Society, the Cancer Society, and the Family Planning Association. In the 1980s, greater emphasis was put on education for healthful living and self-help by broad organizations of women, youth, and local clubs known as *Saukyadana*. The latter emphasize certain types of nutrition.

For some years after independence, the Ceylon Planters' Association Estates' Health Scheme engaged doctors and nurses to provide medical care to workers on rubber and tea estates. By 1971 only about 50 percent of these workers and their families—about 1,200,000 people—were served by this nongovernment but organized program. By the 1980s, estates or plantation workers simply used the public medical services.

Professional associations play an especially big role in Sri Lanka, because of the coexistence of large numbers of doctors of Ayurvedic medicine and of Western-trained scientific physicians. There are also associations of nurses and of pharmacists.

Ayurvedic Medicine. The private market of Ayurvedic medical service is very large in Sri Lanka. In 1982 there were 10,700 Ayurvedic practitioners—far more than the modern physicians. About 62 percent of these were general practitioners and 38 percent regarded themselves as specialists. Only about 10 percent of these healers were graduates of one of the three Ayurvedic colleges in the country; these usually practice full-time, while the great majority practice only part of the time, working principally as teachers, priests, or in other ways.

Fewer than 300 Ayurvedic doctors are employed in official dispensaries, operated mainly by local municipalities. In 1980 about 120 were employed by the MOH in government hospitals. These hospitals had about 1,400 beds, out of the 44,000 in the country.

Private Modern Medicine. A count of the total number of modern physicians in Sri Lanka has been reported only for 1972. At that time there were 3,251 physicians, or a ratio of 25.7 per 100,000 population. Of these, 32 percent were entirely in private practice, but the great majority of government doctors also engaged in part-time private practice. In 1986 private practice by government doctors was reported to be so extensive it compromised the integrity of the official MOH program.

In 1981, the government health service employed 1,964 physicians; if the proportion of doctors in private practice was the same as in 1972, the country had a total of 2,890 physicians—an overall reduction. Several factors account for a net decline of Sri Lanka's stock of modern physicians in this period. Government employment of health personnel was reduced after the political change in 1977. Competition from traditional practitioners was great. A disproportionately large share of Sri Lankan physicians are ethnically Tamils, who suffer from various forms of discrimination. As a result many graduates of Sri Lanka's five medical schools left the country, mainly for Great Britain or America. The national stock of modern physicians, reported to be 17.2 per 100,000 in 1965, declined to 13.4 per 100,000 in 1981.

Expenditures and Health Outcomes

Overall health expenditures, excluding capital investments, have been reported by the Central Bank of Sri Lanka. Counting both public and private spending, in 1975 they amounted to 6.6 percent of total national expenditures. In 1982, 5 years after the change to a more market-oriented government, health expenditures rose in absolute amount but, as a share of the total, declined to 5.3 percent.

The proportion of the total Sri Lankan health expenditures that came from government was reported to be 60 percent in 1970, with 40 percent coming from private sources. (This was when the equivalent economic rela-

tionships in India were 16 percent from government and 84 percent from private sources.) In 1982, in spite of the change in government social policy, the proportion of health expenditures in Sri Lanka was still 60 percent public and 40 percent private. Expressed in rupees per capita, the health expenditures by government have been substantial, rising from Rs. 5.4 per capita in 1947 to Rs. 82.8 per capita in 1983.

Even though the reorganized and decentralized model for primary health care in Sri Lanka was hardly in place in the early 1980s, the country's health achievements have attracted worldwide attention. Closeness to India has naturally invited comparison, and Sri Lanka's infant mortality rate of 36 per 1,000 live births in 1985 is contrasted with India's rate that year of 105 per 1,000 live births. The Sri Lankan infant mortality rate had been 70 per 1,000 live births in 1960 and was down to 34 per 1,000 in 1987. Life expectancy at birth in Sri Lanka was 71 years in 1987, compared with 59 years in India.

The previously high birth rate in Sri Lanka has been brought down substantially. In 1965 it had been 33 births per 1,000 population, and by 1986 this was reduced to 24 per 1,000. In the period 1983 to 1987, about 87 percent of Sri Lankan births were estimated to be attended by trained personnel. The maternal mortality rate was still as high as 90 per 100,000 births in the 1980–1987 years, but far lower than India's 500 per 100,000 in that period.

The stock of physicians in Sri Lanka, as we have noted, declined between 1965 and 1981, but in this period the supply of nursing personnel (as well as community health workers) increased considerably. All grades of trained nursing personnel grew from 31.2 per 100,000 population in 1965 to 79.4 per 100,000 in 1981. Sanitarians, however, were relatively few—only 6.1 per 100,000 in 1981. It is not surprising that in the early 1980s only 36 percent of the population had access to safe drinking water.

What, then, explains the remarkably good health record of Sri Lanka, as reflected at least by customary mortality rate indices, since independence and even for several decades earlier? Three or four influences seem to be important. The policy on food distribution has undoubtedly been basic. Every family received a minimal ration of rice for many years. Even when this was ended in the 1970s, free food was assured for the very poor, subsidies were provided for marginal families through food stamps, and all school children got free lunches.

Education has had a high priority even during the period of British rule. Nearly all girls have gone to primary school, as well as boys. Some 67 percent of teenage children were enrolled in secondary school in 1985. Even university education became government-financed, and 39 percent of university students are women.

The free and almost wholly accessible health service, for both prevention and treatment, must be considered a third determinant of Sri Lanka's health achievements. In the mid-1980s the MOH reported that 93 percent of the population had ready access to health services, and this was probably a modest claim compared with that of other countries. The very extensive availability of health facilities for both ambulatory and in-patient care, without any user charges, suggests that by the end of the 1980s care may well have been accessible to virtually all the people. Not everyone, of course, takes advantage of free health service, if one judges from the DPT immunization coverage of only 61 percent in 1987.

Another possible health factor in the Sri Lankan story is the nature of the services given by Ayurvedic practitioners. Insofar as the Ayurvedic medical schools influence practices, these schools include a little Western medicine in their training; thus, among the thousands of these traditional healers, some use penicillin and other scientific drugs in their work. Private Ayurvedic services tend to be inexpensive and would, therefore, be used by low-income people not satisfied with or not using the public program.

The major attribution of Sri Lanka's health record to food and education is emphasized by the country's own public health leaders. *Intersectoral coordination* for health—that is, action by other sectors outside the health sector—has become a key slogan in the health field. This was shown concretely in the organization of the interministerial National Health Council set up in 1980 and chaired by the prime minister. Research and training in support of the council have been done by several standing committees, defined as a National Health Development Network (NHDN). Based on Sri Lankan experience, the World Health Organization has tried to promote NHDNs in other developing countries, as vehicles for achieving intersectoral coordination.

TANZANIA

The East African country that is now the United Republic of Tanzania was colonized by Germany in 1885. After Germany's defeat in World War I, it became a mandate of the League of Nations (1920) entrusted to British management; in 1946 after World War II, it became a United Nations trust territory, also under British control. In 1954, the Tanganyika African National Union (TANU) became a politically active force for independence, which was achieved in 1961. Then, after a revolution in the British colony Zanzibar, that island state combined with Tanganyika in 1964 to become the United Republic of Tanzania.

Under the unchallenged leadership of the country's first president, Julius Nyerere, the *Arusha Declaration* was issued in 1967. This major policy statement called for egalitarianism and self-reliance. Government was to be decentralized, banks and large industries were to be nationalized, and rural development was to be emphasized, with establishment of *ujamaa,* or cooperative villages and farms. (By 1973 about 2,000,000 rural people had been regrouped into 8,000 cooperative villages.) The economic productivity of these cooperative agricultural enterprises did not prove very satisfactory, but in the fields of education and health there were many benefits.

In 1986, Tanzania had a population of 23,000,000, with a GNP per capita of $250. The population was 14 percent urbanized (1985), an increase from 6 percent in 1965. Literacy was especially high—93 percent among adult men and 88 percent among adult women in 1985; this was an advance from 48 and 18 percent, respectively, in 1970. Primary school enrollment applied to 32 percent of children in 1965, rising to 72 percent in 1985. Ethnically the population is about 35 percent Moslem, 30 percent Christian, and 35 percent with various traditional tribal beliefs. The economic base is still mainly agricultural—sisal, cotton, coffee, tea, and tobacco. The TANU political party was still in control in the late 1980s, although less dedicated to its original socialist aspirations.

Health System Organization

When independence was won in 1961, a certain stock of physical resources for health care was available to the new government. The inequalities typical of colonial rule were obvious, but a number of health facilities for both hospital and ambulatory care had been established under the British authorities and even the Germans, to some extent.

Historical Background. In the last decade of the nineteenth century, the German military forces had set up small hospitals in the towns; these were intended to serve families of the military and the civilian administrative personnel, but not the African natives. After British control was established in 1920, the small government hospitals were expanded—from 30 in 1920 to 55 in 1930—and some of them provided separate wards for the Africans. Religious missionaries from Europe also developed hospitals, especially in the rural sections. By 1944, hospitals in Tanganyika had 6,600 beds, amounting to 1.2 beds per 1,000 population. Of these beds, 64.3 percent were government-sponsored, 31.3 percent were in mission facilities, and 4.4 percent were under industrial or private sponsorship. Classified by race, however, these beds were available to Africans at a ratio of about 1 per 1,000 and to Europeans at a ratio of 50 per 1,000.

In 1926, under the British colonial government, certain responsibilities were decentralized to tribal chiefs, designated as Native Authorities. Among other things, these authorities set up small dispensaries in rural

areas for first-aid and simple treatment. They increased from 35 dispensaries in 1926 to 314 in 1941. Small schools were also organized for training dispensary personnel. Financial support for the dispensaries, however, had to come from local Native Authorities—much weaker than the support for urban hospitals by the central government. The African personnel trained for hospital work were *hospital assistants,* who were much more thoroughly trained than the *rural medical aids* who staffed the dispensaries. Thus, although rural populations got some attention for health care under the colonial government, it was distinctly lower in quantity and quality than that provided in the cities.

After World War II, under the British Labour Party greater colonial support was extended to health services in Tanganyika, but the priorities remained heavily urban. Recognition of rural health needs was expressed mainly in advocacy of greater supervision over the rural dispensaries, not in enlargement of their resources. Hospitals continued to receive the major emphasis. Finally in 1956, the conversion of some dispensaries into rural health centers, offering both preventive and treatment services, was planned; by 1961 some 22 such health centers had been established. At the same time, 715 small and meagerly staffed and equipped dispensaries were being operated by local authorities.

With independence in 1961, both the rural health centers and dispensaries expanded rapidly. Over the next decade, by 1971, health centers were increased to 90 and dispensaries to 1,160. The training of medical assistants was upgraded, and in 1962 a medical school was organized in Dar es Salaam, the national capital. In 1964, a boost was given to the expansion of rural health centers; in the First Five-Year Plan (1964–1968), all dispensaries were regarded as satellites to a rural health center. With the Arusha Declaration in 1967, further health center development was embodied in the Second Five-Year Plan of 1969–1974. In the 1972–73 fiscal year, the health development budget was nearly tripled and, for the first time, rural health centers and dispensaries got greater support (38 percent of the total) than hospitals (29 percent). In the health system of Tanzania, the Arusha Declaration was clearly being implemented.

Ministry of Health. Major responsibilities in Tanzania for health, both prevention and treatment, are firmly vested in the Ministry of Health and its branches throughout the country. In 1985, the central headquarters included major directorates for preventive services, hospitals, and health manpower development. Regarding manpower, the MOH was training 30 categories of health personnel, in addition to its indirect control over the university training of physicians, pharmacists, and others.

Throughout the country the hierarchical framework of the MOH corresponds to the general political jurisdictions. There are 20 regions in Tanzania, each of which is headed by a regional medical officer. In addition to his responsibility for all disease control in the region, the RMO serves as director of the regional hospital and as supervisor of all district health programs. A World Health Organization review in 1984, however, reported that in practice many of the control programs for immunizations, tuberculosis control, and maternal and child health were still operating under central management. The RMO is technically responsible to the central MOH but administratively to the regional development director.

Each region has five or six districts, headed by district medical officers. The DMOs in the 104 districts are responsible for all health programs in their areas, as well as for directing the district hospital. They are technically under the RMO and administratively under the district development officer. A major responsibility is the DMO's supervision of the health centers in the district.

For administrative purposes, the districts are subdivided into divisions with populations of about 50,000 people each. In 1984 there were 360 such divisions, of which 239 were served by health centers. These facilities were staffed by medical assistants, who have completed secondary school and had 3 or 4 years of practical training in diagnosis and treatment of common ailments, assisted by several other health auxiliaries. The latter include rural medical

aids, trained for 3 years after elementary school, and assistant nurse-midwives, MCH aids, and others trained more briefly. The several specialized health programs are most well-integrated at the level of the divisional health center.

Each health center has 10 or 20 dispensaries, as satellites numbering 2,600 in 1984. These were staffed mainly by rural medical aids, and many of the physical structures were legacies of the colonial period; the majority, however, were newly built. A dispensary is expected to serve around 5,000 to 10,000 people in several villages, of which there are altogether about 8,500 in Tanzania. A few hundred of these villages have very briefly trained (a few weeks of lecture-discussions) *village health workers,* who are supposed to give health education on family planning, sanitation, and use of the local dispensary.

The posts of RMO and DMO had many vacancies in 1985; the single medical school in the country (University of Dar es Salaam) had only 67 graduates in 1984. In the MOH positions that were occupied, moreover, the young physicians were providing very little health leadership to the staffs of the health centers and dispensaries. At both the regional and the district levels, they were spending most of their time in clinical work in the hospitals; this work, of course, was demanding and it appealed to them professionally. Very few of these medical officers had training in public health or community health work. Tanzania's achievements (as well as its shortcomings) in health care must be attributed largely to the services of auxiliary personnel.

Voluntary Health Agencies. The health activities of religious missions were noted in the colonial period. In 1983 Tanzania had 61 such nongovernment hospitals, almost all located in rural areas. They were fully integrated with the MOH facilities, and 17 served as district hospitals. Because they receive special subsidies, they cannot charge for their services; the others levy small charges. The strength of the voluntary agencies in Tanzania is reflected by their large contribution to professional health manpower; in 1984 they accounted for 38 percent of the physicians and 54 percent of the graduate nurses in the country. Most of the schools that train grade B or assistant nurses are located in mission hospitals.

In 1979, out of 34,235 hospital beds in Tanzania, 11,600 or 34 percent were in voluntary agency mission hospitals. Missions also operated 390 dispensaries, 95 percent of which were rural.

A few enterprises are described as *parastatal,* since they carry out publicly essential functions but are managed by autonomous bodies. These provide health services to their employees through institutions with 655 beds, or 2 percent of the total.

Private Medical Market. Modern private medical practice has not been prominent in Tanzania. In 1980, as part of the government policy to provide free health care for everyone, private practice was legally prohibited. Perhaps the law is occasionally broken, but it is not a significant issue.

Traditional healing is also not prominent in Tanzania, although it has been used by some families. A survey of households found that in 1970–71, only 25 percent of families in the towns made any use of traditional healers, and those that did averaged just one visit per year; in rural areas the use was somewhat higher— 40 percent of households, averaging 1.8 visits each per year. A British law of 1928 outlawing witchcraft for healing or any other purpose may have had a suppressive effect. Nevertheless, a Traditional Medicine Research Unit is maintained in the MOH, to analyze plant, animal, and mineral substances used by healers.

Before 1980 some 400 hospital beds (1.2 percent of the total) were under private control, but these have presumably been converted to public or nonprofit sponsorship.

Health Expenditures and Outcomes

In 1977, it was reported that Tanzania spent a total of 3 percent of its GNP, from both public and private sources, on the health system. Of this amount, about 77 percent came from government and 23 percent from private sources.

(This can be compared with the approximate 50 percent of health system financing derived from private sources in Kenya in the early 1980s.) Within the central government budget, health expenditures rose from 5.2 percent in 1970–71 to 8.9 percent in 1973–74, but then declined to 5.5 percent in 1980–81.

In spite of its basic poverty, Tanzania has made clear progress in preparing health personnel of midlevel capabilities. The supply of physicians has barely kept up with the growth of population; in 1967 there were 4.2 doctors per 100,000 people and in 1984 the ratio was only 5 per 100,000. The numbers of other health personnel, however, expanded appreciably. Trained nurses and nurse-midwives increased from 1,372 in 1961 to 8,752 in 1982. Rural medical aids, the principal staff for dispensaries, grew in number from 380 in 1961 to 3,210 in 1982. Medical assistants, who provide day-to-day medical care in health centers, numbered 200 in 1961 and 1,950 in 1982.

Assistant medical officers are a somewhat uniquely Tanzanian category of health professional. After some 15 years of experience as medical assistants, they receive 2 years of further training in a special "medical college." If they then pass an examination they are registered as AMOs, with qualifications to serve in posts ordinarily reserved for physicians. These AMOs numbered 32 in 1961 and increased to 293 in 1982. Other quite briefly trained personnel in 1982 included 1,081 health assistants and 3,180 MCH assistants.

It is these allied health personnel who have been mainly responsible for the gains accomplished in Tanzania's health system. Largely because of the network of district hospitals, health centers, and dispensaries, the MOH could claim that 72 percent of the population in 1982 were within 5 kilometers of a resource for personal health care; if access were defined as being within 10 kilometers of a resource, the coverage would have been 93 percent of the population. An estimated 50 percent of the population had access to clean water in the early 1980s. Immunization with DPT vaccine increased from 58 percent of the children in 1981 to 81 percent in 1986.

Population control has not been a high priority in Tanzania, although family planning advice is available at health centers. The crude birth rate in 1960 was 51 per 1,000 population, and in 1987 it was the same. In the early 1980s it was estimated that 74 percent of childbirths were attended by trained health personnel. The maternal mortality rate, however, was still relatively high—370 maternal deaths per 100,000 live births.

The infant mortality rate in Tanzania in 1960, just before national independence, was 146 per 1,000 live births. By 1987 the rate was lowered to 107 per 1,000 live births—a level that doubtless reflects the persistently low general standards of living. The life expectancy at birth was 41 years in 1960, and was extended to 54 years by 1987.

These relatively modest improvements in Tanzania's health status probably demonstrate, above all, the inadequacy of health services alone—in the absence of equivalent advances in food consumption, environmental sanitation, housing, employment, and overall living standards—in reducing mortality rates. The expansion of health care resources, the continued provision of services to everyone without charge, and the banning of private medical practice have all doubtless meant an increasing volume of personal health service for people. But these factors alone seem to have had only a limited impact on infant and maternal mortality rates.

Under the leadership of Tanzania's first president, Julius Nyerere, a strong cadre of technical personnel were assembled in the central government. This has been conspicuous in the Ministry of Health and in the medical faculty of the University of Dar es Salaam. The medical faculty has even been relatively strong in the field of community medicine and public health, although not many medical graduates undertake specialized studies in this field.

Below the top, however, the organization of the TANU party has been reported to be weak. The inspiring goals of the Arusha Declaration were evidently not translated into disciplined and enduring programs of economic development in the regions and districts. During the period 1965 through 1980, agricultural production grew at the rate of only 1.6 percent per year, and from 1980 to 1986 it was virtually static (growing only 0.8 percent per year). Tanzania's efforts to develop industry showed a growth rate of 4.2 percent per year during 1965 to 1980, but actually declined by 4.5 percent per year in the 1980 to 1986 period.

In the late 1980s, reports from Tanzania suggested a new surge of economic development. With the relatively strong foundations of its health system, stressing primary health care in rural areas and principles of social equity, there may be grounds for greater optimism about future health status.

SUMMARY COMMENT

Both Sri Lanka and Tanzania are considered to be very poor countries with comprehensive health systems, but Sri Lanka's longer period of independence and somewhat higher GNP per capita have given it advantages over Tanzania. Soon after liberation, both of these former British colonies announced socialistic objectives, which shaped the structures of their health systems.

In both countries, extensive networks of health centers and dispensaries (health posts) have been established, so that primary health care is quite accessible to more than 90 percent of their populations. Sir Lanka has lost many physicians by out-migration, and Tanzania has never had many, but both systems depend heavily on medical auxiliaries trained for several years. Government health spending accounts for 60 percent of the total in Sri Lanka, where much of the private spending is for Ayurvedic practitioners. In Tanzania, public expenditures constitute 77 percent of the health total, and private medical practice has even been banned. All government health services in both countries are free of charge.

The exceptionally good health record achieved by Sri Lanka, especially in comparison with that of nearby India, has been attributed generally to very egalitarian policies on food and basic education, as well as to health service. Tanzania's overall economic development has not been very successful—an experience shared with many other African countries—but recent reports were more promising.

REFERENCES

Sri Lanka

American Public Health Association, *A Health and Population Brief: Republic of Sri Lanka.* Washington, D.C., May 1979.

De Silva, U. H. Susantha, *A Review of the National Health Development Network of Sri Lanka.* Colombo: Ministry of Health, 1986, processed document.

Gunatilleke, Godrey, "Health and Development in Sri Lanka—An Overview," in Scott B. Halstead et al. (Editors), *Good Health at Low Cost.* New York: Rockefeller Foundation, 1985, pp. 111–124.

Marga Institute, *Intersectoral Action for Health: Sri Lanka Study.* Colombo, 1984.

Namboodiri, N. Krishnan, et al., *Determinants of Recent Fertility Decline in Sri Lanka.* Washington, D.C.: World Bank, July 1983.

Perera, P. D. A., "Health Care Systems of Sri Lanka," inScott B. Halstead et al. (Editors), *Good Health at Low Cost.* New York: Rockefeller Foundation, 1985, pp. 93–110.

Roemer, Milton I., *A Health Demonstration Area in Ceylon.* New Delhi: World Health Organization Regional Office for South-East Asia, 1951, processed document.

Simeonov, L. A., *Better Health for Sri Lanka.* New Delhi: World Health Organization Regional Office for South-East Asia, 1975.

Tanzania

Hamel, J., *Health Care Delivery in Tanzania.* The Hague: Ministry of Foreign Affairs, August 1983.

Power, Jonathan, "Nyerere Leaves Flawed Legacy in Tanzania." *International Herald Tribune,* 24–25 August 1985.

Tarimo, E., "Another Development in Health: Ideas Based on the Tanzanian Experience." Uppsala: Dag Hammarskjold Foundation, June 1977 (unpublished report).

United Nations Fund for Population Activities, *Report of Mission on Needs Assessment for Population Assistance: Tanzania.* New York, May 1979.

United Republic of Tanzania, Ministry of Health, *Guide Lines for the Implementation of the Primary Health Care Programme in Tanzania.* Dar es Salaam, October 1983.

United Republic of Tanzania, Ministry of Health, *Evaluation of the Health Sector 1979.* Dar es Salaam, October 1980.

van Etten, G. M., *Rural Health Development in Tanzania.* Assen: Van Gorcum & Comp., 1976.

World Health Organization and Tanzanian Ministry of Health, "Joint PHC Review: Tanzania 1984." Geneva 1984, unpublished document.

CHAPTER SEVENTEEN

Socialist Health Systems in Very Poor Countries

In several countries of a very poor economic level revolutions occurred after World War II, resulting in the establishment of socialist governments. In every instance, the revolutions were directed against ruling elite classes who were directly or indirectly supported by foreign powers, European or American. The conflicts were long and complex, and inevitably had enormous influence on the national health systems—shaping them along socialist lines.

The most far-reaching revolution occurred in China, the world's largest country, in which the Chinese Communist Party won national power in 1949. Health system developments in the People's Republic of China have been especially complex, as different ideologies have gained ascendancy in the new society. Somewhat simpler expressions of socialist principles in health system development are seen in another Asian country, Vietnam, and an African country, Mozambique, both of which attained national independence in 1975. The systems of these two very poor countries are examined first.

VIETNAM

In the great Asiatic peninsula south of China—known formerly as Indochina—is the long narrow country known since 1975 as the Socialist Republic of Vietnam. This land was settled by people from central China a century before Christ. It was invaded by European (Portuguese, Dutch, English, and French) traders from the sixteenth century onward, and in 1858 the French gained control. Vietnam, as well as neighboring Cambodia and Laos, re-

mained firmly under French rule until occupation by Japan in 1940. At the end of World War II, in 1945 the League for Independence of Vietnam (the Viet Minh) won control in the northern half of the country, but bitter opposition of the French continued until 1954, when the French were defeated (at the battle of Dien Bien Phu) and the Democratic Republic of Vietnam was established in the 22 northern provinces.

A "temporary demarcation line" was established, separating north and south Vietnam at the 17th parallel, to be eliminated after a general election in 1956. This election, however, was never held; instead, a staunchly anticommunist government was installed in the south (the Republic of Vietnam) in 1955. South Vietnam had 39 provinces and the highly developed French capital city, Saigon. Hostilities soon developed between the two Vietnams, with U.S. aid going to the South and Soviet and Chinese aid going to the North. In 1964, the United States intervened directly on the side of the South, launching high-powered military action by land, sea, and air. Hundreds of thousands of people, mostly Vietnamese, were killed before the United States and South Vietnamese forces were defeated, and a Provisional Revolutionary Government assumed control in 1975. In 1976, an officially unified Socialist Republic of Vietnam was established.

Social Background

With this extremely violent background of colonial repression, war, revolution, and renewed war, Vietnam in the late 1980s is naturally a land of extreme poverty and austerity. Attempting to rebuild a society along socialist lines, with only very limited international assistance (mostly from the Soviet Union) and virtually complete economic isolation by the great Western powers, has been enormously difficult. Only great fortitude and discipline, coming from 30 years of war and suffering, have enabled these people to cope with their countless tasks.

In 1987, the population of the Socialist Republic of Vietnam was estimated to be 63,000,000. As of 1984, about 81 percent of the people were rural. National wealth in 1980 was reported to be $161 in GNP per capita. The estimate for 1987 set this figure at $180 per capita. The economy is based mainly on agriculture (rice, corn, sugar cane), but there is some manufacturing of textiles, fertilizer, and cement, and some mining of coal, iron, and other minerals. The traditionally dominant religion was Buddhism, which is no longer encouraged but is by no means repressed.

Political unification of the formerly socialist North Vietnam (1945–1975) and the colonial and capitalist South Vietnam (before 1975) has naturally been difficult. Between the two regions there were 61 of the formerly French-defined provinces, but after 1976 the unified country was divided into 40 new provinces. These vary in population from about 1,000,000 to 3,000,000. Each province is subdivided into some 10 to 15 districts, totaling 466 in all. Within each district there are further levels of organization. First is the commune, sometimes called a village. There are about 8,600 communes, with an average of 7,000 people each. Finally, each commune has some 5 to 10 production brigades, sometimes called hamlets.

The government of Vietnam has put a very high priority on education. In 1981 some 89 percent of children of primary school age (6 to 11 years) were enrolled in school (in the south 80 percent and in the north 99 percent). Literacy in adults has made tremendous gains. Before 1945, under the French, hardly 5 percent of Vietnamese people could read and write. By 1984, adult literacy was 84 percent. In 1978 a study of people between 12 and 50 years of age found 94 percent to be literate.

Health System Organization

As in other socialist countries, almost all major functions in Vietnam's national health system are lodged in the Ministry of Health.

Ministry of Health. The headquarters of the MOH in the national capital, Hanoi, contains some 15 principal departments. These include departments for epidemiology, medical care (therapy), traditional medicine, manpower training, and pharmacies, as well as political education, the health protection of government employees, and international relations. Separate from but linked to the ministry is a Union of Pharmaco-Chemical Enterprises, concerned with the production of modern and traditional drugs. Also centrally associated with the MOH are some 20 research institutes on epidemiology, nutrition, occupational disorders, maternal and newborn health, and other fields.

Parallel with the nationwide political structure, the Ministry of Health is represented in each of the nations's 40 provinces by a centrally appointed provincial health director, who is typically a physician, oriented with 3 or 4 months of special training in health care management. He is supported by a staff of other physicians, a pharmacist, assistant nurses, technicians, a training officer, and assistant doctors. The latter are important auxiliary health workers, carried over from the French period and playing key roles throughout the national health system (see later).

Each of the 466 district health services is headed by a district health director, appointed by the provincial health director. Most of these posts are held by physicians, who must usually divide their time between clinical work in the district hospital and administrative duties. In some small rural districts, the health directorship may be held by an assistant doctor with several years of experience. On the district health service staff are generally assistant doctors, assistant nurses, one or more technicians, a pharmacist, and perhaps additional physicians in selected fields, such as hygiene and epidemiology, maternal and child health, or infectious diseases. A traditional practitioner is also usually on the staff.

Within the districts, each of the 8,600 communes is expected to have an organized health service; this is headed by an assistant doctor, supported by a few other personnel. This staff is the responsibility of a Commune People's Health Committee, selected by the local Commune People's Council, which is popularly elected. At the production brigade level, there are usually local part-time health workers. The Commune People's Health Committee is responsible for reporting births and deaths, statistics that are important for rationing rice.

Other Organizations. Besides the MOH, in the communes there are Red Cross societies, started in the war years to help the wounded, and now mobilizing young people for general health promotion. These youth assist in immunization campaigns, encourage family planning, help in environmental cleanups, and so on. They are unpaid volunteers, and are estimated to number 100,000 nationally. (These activities are not tied to the national Red Cross societies, concerned with emergencies and blood donation.) Red Cross volunteers receive a few weeks of orientation at the commune level. In addition, certain peasants are trained briefly as *hygiene activists* for simple elements of primary health care; they receive "work points" from the production brigade for this part-time health service.

The military establishment of Vietnam is still substantial, and it has its own relatively well-developed medical services. Vietnam regards strong military protection against China and other possible invaders of continuing importance. In the mid-1980s an estimated 40 to 50 percent of the national government budget was devoted to military functions, counting military health services. A designated percentage of each medical school graduating class is assigned to military duties.

Private Health Care Market. Finally, in the structure of the Vietnam health system must be included the private market for medical care. The largest portion of this market is for traditional medicine. As noted, traditional practitioners are included within the official MOH health services, but the vast majority of these persons are in private practice, especially in the rural areas. In 1983, the MOH estimated 3,780 traditional healers to be active, part-time or full-time, in the country. Compared with other developing countries, this was a relatively small number—fewer than 0.5 practitioner per commune or village. Traditional drugs, however, are sold in MOH pharmacies, as well as by the healers. In fact, the patient seeing a healer is ordinarily expected to pay only for the drug, not for the consultation.

Growing in its proportion of the Vietnam health system, although it is still not great, is private medica' practice by modern physicians. Since the national economy suffered severe difficulties in 1986, MOH physicians were authorized by the minister to engage in private practice, when their official work was completed. The extent of private practice by government physicians cannot be very great, since few people have the money to pay private fees. Physicians are permitted to use public facilities for seeing private patients, since quarters for private clinics are not available. Retired physicians are free to spend all their time in private practice, usually conducted in their small homes. (Men retire at age 60, women at 55.)

Groups of MOH physicians may also form a *private group clinic,* which serves paying patients when their official work is done. This is most likely at a hospital in the larger cities. The fees are regulated; a share of the earnings is used for auxiliary personnel and "rent," with the balance going to the doctors. Private medical and dental practice is most prevalent in Ho Chi Minh City (formerly Saigon).

Resource Production

Soon after victory, Vietnam put great energy into the development of its health resources, both human and physical. Almost the entire physical infrastructure for health services and for health personnel training had been destroyed by the decades of war, and reconstruction was needed everywhere.

Health Manpower. In 1975 there were two medical faculties at Hanoi and Ho Chi Minh City, and six more were soon established in the center of the country. All of these were under the MOH, except the two smallest schools, which functioned as parts of universities under the Ministry of Higher Education. As in Europe, medical education in Vietnam requires 6 years of study and practical work following secondary school (12 grades). With serious shortages of teachers, equipment, books, and even paper, medical school conditions are naturally quite rudimentary. About half the medical students are women; there are many (up to 20) applicants of both sexes for each medical school opening. Higher education is entirely government-supported. Enrollment in each medical school averages about 200 students per class.

At a higher educational level, there are two faculties of pharmacy and one of dentistry, each requiring 5 years after secondary school. Formal training in traditional medicine is given by two faculties, requiring 3 years after secondary school. (Some principles of scientific medicine are included in the traditional medicine program, and a limited amount of traditional medicine is taught in the regular medical curriculum.) Noteworthy are two schools of public health, which offer both year-long and short courses in health service management and related fields.

Most widespread of health training institutions in Vietnam are the *secondary medical schools,* as they are called, in each of the 40 provinces. In addition, six such secondary schools are operated directly by the MOH, making 46 in all. Enrollment is about 1,000 students per school. These schools provide 3 years of training for assistant doctors and, in separate classes, for graduate nurses and graduate midwives. The professional nurses and midwives work almost entirely in hospitals, while the assistant doctors work both in hospitals and in health stations, providing ambulatory care at provincial, district, and commune levels. Two- or 3-year courses also prepare medical technicians (secondary level) and pharmaceutical technicians.

The secondary medical schools (or provincial health training schools) also train large numbers of auxiliary health personnel in 1-year programs following elementary school. These include elementary-level nurses, elementary-level midwives, assistant pharmacists,

and laboratorians. It should be noted that Vietnam, following policies established under the French, does not prepare any health workers specialized in environmental sanitation, although this subject is included in the education of assistant doctors and auxiliary nurses. About 30 percent of auxiliary personnel graduates of the secondary medical schools fail to work in their fields of training.

In 1984, there were reported to be nearly 18,000 physicians in Vietnam, or about 30 per 100,000 people. This was an enormous increase over the supply of doctors available under the French; aside from alien colonial physicians, in 1945 there were fewer than 100 Vietnamese doctors for 20,000,000 people in the country. Much more numerous are the assistant doctors, numbering 33,600 in 1983 or 61 per 100,000 population. Pharmacists, trained in universities, numbered 5,200 in 1983, or 9.4 per 100,000.

Nurses have also been trained in relatively large numbers. In 1983 there were 14,000 secondary-level or graduate nurses (25.6 per 100,000) and 65,500 elementary-level or assistant nurses (119 per 100,000). Midwives of secondary and elementary level were also available at ratios of 6.3 and 19.3 per 100,000, respectively.

The majority of Vietnamese physicians are general practitioners, nearly all working in the government service. Specialty status may be earned at two levels—"first degree" after 5 years of postgraduate work and "second degree" after two additional years at a medical facility.

Health Facilities. Hospitals in Vietnam were badly damaged by the war (especially from aerial bombing), but in 1980 there were 676 general and specialized facilities, with 128,000 beds. This meant 2.46 hospital beds per 1,000 population. In the commune health stations there are also small complements of five or six beds for maternity cases or urgent care, pending transfer to a hospital, amounting to another 1.32 beds per 1,000, or 3.78 beds per 1,000 in all. (The rate of occupancy of the commune beds, however, has been very low.) The use of straw mats, rather than mattresses, on hospital beds simply replicates normal conditions in homes. The national hospital network includes a provincial general hospital of about 500 beds in each province, and a district general hospital (sometimes two) with 150 to 250 beds in each district.

Every hospital has a relatively large out-patient department, at which the patient demand rate is relatively high. (As in other developing countries, many rural patients bypass the commune health station to seek care from a physician at the district hospital.) In some of the larger districts, where the district hospital may be distant from many people, a special polyclinic (staffed by internists and obstetrician-gynecologists) can be set up.

Other physical facilities are also part of the Vietnamese health system. In 1980 there were 103 *sanatoria* that offered rest periods for certain workers. Local MOH pharmacies numberd 472. Pharmaceutical factories, for packaging and sometimes fabricating drugs (modern and traditional), amounted to 55. Special clinical laboratories, linked to the National Institute of Hygiene and Epidemiology and serving general public health purposes, are located in all 40 of the provincial hospitals and in some larger district hospitals.

Government facilities for ambulatory health care are relatively abundant in Vietnam, and well distributed. Very simple and modestly equipped commune health stations have been set up in almost every commune—8,445 such facilities in 1980. Somewhat larger are 113 health centers for hygiene and epidemiological work, for maternal and infant care, and for antimalaria work. In addition there were some 101 dispensaries in 1980 for care of tuberculosis, venereal diseases, and eye conditions.

Regarding drugs and other commodities, the network of provincial factories has been noted. Except for very simple products, like aspirin, and traditional herbal medicines, however, domestic capabilities in Vietnam are very limited. Most antibiotics, antimalarial drugs, cardiac therapeutic agents, and the like must be imported—principally from European socialist countries—or acquired through donations. The shortage of essential drugs, even in hospitals, is a serious handicap of the entire health system. Medical equipment of all sorts is also in very short supply, and much is in disrepair for lack of spare parts. Cars are also scarce, so that the major form of transport, even for sick patients, is by crowded buses, bicycles, or pedicabs.

Finally, among resources must be counted the institutions producing and disseminating knowledge in Vietnam. There are 20 specialized research institutes, coordinated by the MOH National Medical Research Council. One of the largest is the National Institute of Hygiene and Epidemiology (formerly one of the French Pasteur Institutes), which conducts a diversified program of research in various bacterial and virus diseases and also prepares vaccines. Other institutes focus on nutrition, occupational disorders, malaria, maternal and newborn health, and other areas. Some medical research is also done in the larger provincial hospitals.

To help disseminate new medical knowledge throughout Vietnam, there is an Institute of Medical Information. It publishes monthly journals in medicine and in pharmacy, reporting Vietnamese research, and also issues bibliographic reports on relevant international medical literature. The institute maintains a library, built largely from donations of foreign medical books and journals, and it is helping in the development of small branch libraries in each province.

Economic Support

The major source of support for Vietnam's health system is the general revenue of the national government, but this is not the sole source. The Ministry of Health absorbs 3.2 percent of the government budget, which is unfortunately a decline from previous years because of economic difficulties and continuing high military expenditures. No breakdown of the national MOH budget is available, but a report on Ho Chi Minh City for 1983 shows 86 percent of those urban expenditures to be devoted to hospital maintenance.

Social security for medical care, in the usual sense, is not found in Vietnam, but two population groups have medical benefits in a comparable sense. Government employees are provided drugs and food in hospitals without charge (others are asked to pay small fees); these costs are paid by the employee's agency. Employees of state enterprises are entitled to similar benefits, at the expense of the enterprise; large enterprises can also operate special clinics for their workers. Dependents are not medically covered in either of these programs.

Another major source of health care financing is the commune. Virtually all of Vietnam's 8,600 communes maintain a cooperative fund, to which almost all households contribute. This fund, along with some contribution from the earnings controlled by the Commune People's Health Committee, is used for the financial support of health stations and for some of the drug costs of hospitalized commune members. The money finances the construction and maintenance of the health stations, while the salaries of local personnel are paid through "work points." District and provincial health workers are paid by MOH funds allotted to the provinces. Local sources of health financing contribute substantially to health system support.

Finally, the economic support of health services in Vietnam depends on private individuals and families of two types. Since the economic difficulties of 1985–86, charges for drugs and food have been imposed on most patients served in public hospitals, and commune cooperatives pay only part of these costs. Even before this policy change, it was customary for food to be brought to hospital patients by their families. In ambulatory care of illness, consultations are without charge, but drugs must also usually be paid for.

The second type of private payment is for care by a private doctor—either one who is retired or one in government service after official hours. Although this type of practice has been growing in the north, it is still not common, and in the south it is extensive only in Ho Chi Minh City. Private payments to traditional practitioners are doubtless most common in all parts of the country.

Eyeglasses are rarely seen in Vietnam, but when needed they must be purchased in a private shop. They are fabricated in two government workshops. The corrective lenses are prescribed, without charge, by ophthalmologists in a hospital out-patient clinic.

Health System Management

With little more than a decade since the revolutionary birth of the Socialist Republic of Vietnam, general management of the health system in 1987 was still quite centralized. At provincial and district levels, policies are clearly formulated at the top. Below the level of the district, policies are made by People's Health Committees in the communes, but even these are still expected to follow the general directives of the Ministry of Health.

Health system planning is the responsibility of a key department in the central MOH. Plans call for greater use of fully trained physicians at all levels and less dependence on assistant doctors. There seems to be no equivalent emphasis on graduate nurses, who work predominantly in hospitals. Major efforts are being made to enhance Vietnam's capabilities in the domestic manufacture of modern drugs.

Many developing countries require new medical graduates to serve in a rural post for 1 to 3 years, but in Vietnam the policy is different. On entry to medical school, each student simply agrees to serve on graduation wherever the MOH sends him or her. The most outstanding graduates have broad freedom in choosing a place, but the majority are usually sent to the area from which they originated. Applicants from rural areas, in fact, have priority for medical school admission. There are no formalities for medical licensure, beyond qualification assured by the medical faculty.

Health legislation is not yet well developed in Vietnam, although a Code for the Protection of Public Health has been drafted by the MOH and reviewed by the Ministry of Justice. Regarding drugs, the MOH issues regulations that govern the activities of drug-producing units in each of the provinces. The MOH also approves the quality of drugs that are imported. Abuse of narcotics has not been a serious problem, but a law, enacted shortly after the revolution of 1945 in the north, imposes criminal penalties for the smoking of opium.

Regarding human reproduction, the goal of Vietnam is a maximum of two children per family, with a 5-year interval between them. Some provinces imposed penalties on families who have a third child, but this practice has been discontinued. Family planning is widely encouraged, with IUD insertion by midwives being the most common method (about 30 percent of women of child-brearing age). Abortion has been declared legal during the first 3 months of pregnancy, and it is done free in almost all district and provincial hospitals.

Provision of Services

With the severe shortages of equipment and supplies and the general poverty of Vietnamese society, the overall setting of health care delivery is inevitably very humble. The quarters of health centers and hospitals are well maintained, but they lack the sparkle that depends on generous supplies of soap and water.

The MOH is committed to the World Health Organization concept of primary health care. With some modification to fit local conditions, a commune health station is reported to carry out 10 functions: (1) health education, (2) environmental hygiene, (3) improvement of water supply, (4) treatment of common diseases, (5) immunization against six infectious diseases, (6) combatting epidemics, (7) family planning, (8) growing medicinal herbs, (9) sports promotion, and (10) training of people in massage and self-care. Among these functions, notably weak are activities in environmental hygiene and water supply improvement; it will be recalled that Vietnam lacks personnel specializing in these areas. Also absent is reference to maternal and infant hygiene; the MOH does not encourage routine examinations of all newborns, but only attention to infants considered ill by the mother. Prenatal visits by expectant mothers, however, are encouraged.

The pattern of work at commune health stations appears to be divided about half for the treatment of ailments in patients and half for health promotion and prevention. In the mornings, most of the time is spent in serving patients, while community health visits are made in the afternoons. In the production brigades, hygiene activists and the Red Cross workers assist in reaching families.

At most commune health stations, ambulatory care is provided by traditional healers as well as modern personnel; the choice of practitioner is up to the patient. Traditional remedies are believed to be especially effective for minor respiratory infections, headache, weakness, and functional disorders. Treatment by traditional practitioners, however, is most often sought outside the MOH framework.

The district health officer is expected to supervise the commune health stations. This is more feasible when there is a deputy in charge of the district hospital, but most often hospital work requires about half of the district director's time. With only the remaining time available for field supervision and with difficulties in transportation, commune health stations are seldom visited more often than once a year. At these visits, moreover, the district physician may be called on to examine difficult clinical cases, rather than to oversee the commune health program. District health directors in larger towns and cities are also expected to make at least annual visits to the clinics of private medical practitioners, to determine whether they meet minimal sanitary standards.

Most commune health stations and district health centers have a few beds for maternity cases and emergencies. After a maximum of 5 days in such a bed, the patient must be transferred to a district hospital. These beds, however, are obviously little used. Evidently people use health stations and health centers for ambulatory care, but for bed treatment they usually prefer to travel the greater distance required to reach a district hospital. Pregnant women coming for prenatal checkups to some commune health stations are provided supplementary foods (rice, dried milk, cooking oil, fish powder, and sugar), if they are malnourished—weighing less than 45 kilograms.

Conditions in the district hospitals, and especially in the provincial general hospitals, are usually quite crowded. Since 1980, almost all childbirths in Vietnam have taken place in a hospital or other health facility. The same applies to abortions during the first trimester of pregnancy. As a result, there are often two postpartum mothers to a bed in a maternity ward of a provincial hospital.

Provincial and district hospitals maintain clinical laboratories and small x-ray departments. The laboratories appear orderly and well managed, but meagerly equipped.

A final aspect of health care delivery in Vietnam must be recognized. Almost all countries, of any ideology, maintain one or more special medical facilities for care of the national elite. Vietnam is no exception. In Hanoi, there is a facility with about 150 beds that has priority in obtaining the services of the best-qualified physicians and the most sophisticated equipment. This is the institution that serves the health needs of government leaders and the leading cadres of the Communist Party of Vietnam.

Some Health Outcomes

In spite of the extremely spartan conditions in Vietnamese life after 30 years of war from 1945 to 1975, the country's health achievements are notable. The broad egalitarianism, the rationing of food, the great extension of basic education, and the enormous self-reliance engendered by massive suffering are all responsible, as well as the health system.

The MOH estimated in the mid-1980s that 80 percent of the population had access to health services. Immunization with DPT vaccine was reported by UNICEF to cover 51 percent of the children in 1986. Provision for safe childbirth was especially good, with 99 percent of deliveries being handled by trained attendants, usually in hospitals, in 1986. Access to safe water was not as good, applying to about 41 percent of the population in the mid-1980s.

The crude birth rate in Vietnam was reduced from 41 per 1,000 population in 1960 to 32 per 1,000 in 1987. The maternal mortality rate in the mid-1980s was 110 per 100,000 births. The life expectancy at birth in 1984 was 63 years. The infant mortality rate was reported to be 156 per 1,000 live births in 1960,

and it was brought down to 65 per 1,000 in 1987.

MOZAMBIQUE

The land in southeast Africa that is now Mozambique was first settled by Portuguese traders in 1505. Over the centuries, Portuguese rule was violently contested by Africans and in the nineteenth century by other Europeans, but after World War II it continued until the 1960s. In 1962 several African nationalist groups united to form the Mozambique Liberation Front (FRELIMO), which started guerrilla warfare in 1964. After 11 years of struggle, FRELIMO prevailed and an independent nation was established in June 1975.

The People's Republic of Mozambique was explicitly dedicated to a gradual transition to socialism. Private schools were closed, businesses nationalized, and collective farms organized. (About 1,000 communal villages were established in 1977, and 1,300 by 1982.) Most of the country's white Europeans left, and soon internal armed insurgency arose with support of weapons and manpower from neighboring and hostile South Africa. This turmoil was compounded by severe drought and massive foreign debt. A meaningful analysis of Mozambique's health system, demonstrating socialist concepts in a low-income African country, must apply principally to conditions in the early 1980s, before the period of counterrevolutionary insurrection and chaos.

In 1986, Mozambique had a population of 14,200,00, of which 87 percent were rural people. The GNP per capita in 1986 was estimated to be $210. School attendance by children in 1984 was reported as 74 percent, and adult literacy had achieved a level of 72 percent. The entire national infrastructure of utilites, power, and transportation, however, was disrupted by the hostilities stemming from South Africa.

Health System Organization

The main principles of the health system in free Mozambique were drawn from the experience of FRELIMO during its 11 years of struggle for national independence. In the northern regions that it occupied, FRELIMO made health care a public service, entirely free and noncommercial, provided mainly by African equivalents of China's "barefoot doctors." The handful of trained professionals available supervised the primary care workers.

Nationalization of several social sectors was undertaken as soon as the new government was stabilized. Agriculture, housing, banking, education, and health were the main sectors. Eventually government control of agriculture and housing was reduced, but maintenance of health care as a public benefit, with legal prohibition of private medical practice, was continued. (Traditional healing was exempted from this rule.) Authority for virtually all aspects of the health system was vested in the Ministry of Health.

Ministry of Health. Many of the leaders of the FRELIMO cause were health workers, and the movement's first president, Samora Machel, had originally been a male nurse. The Ministry of Health, unlike those in most countries, occupied a strong position in the central government. Central direction of all government health services comes within the MOH under a national Directorate of Health, which combines three former departments for medical care, preventive medicine, and community health. In addition there are directorates for social welfare, for human resource development, for supplies, for planning, and for personnel discipline and control. The Maputo General Hospital in the national capital and the national pharmaceutical enterprise are semiautonomous bodies also attached to the MOH. Foreign health assistance is especially important to Mozambique, and this is coordinated by a Department of International Cooperation. Hundreds of personnel and much equipment and supplies come from international agencies and many countries of Europe, Asia, and Africa.

The work of the MOH is carried out through very modest staffs in the 10 provinces. Trained personnel are too few to permit any formal provincial health offices, but seven of the provinces have provincial hospitals with about 200 beds each. Provinces are divided into dis-

tricts—109 in all—but these also have no formal administrative authorities. The districts have rural hospitals, health centers, and health posts, discussed later.

No other agency of government has significant health functions. The medical school, attached to Eduardo Mandlane University in the national capital, Maputo, is controlled by the MOH. Only the armed forces have a separate medical establishment.

Voluntary Agencies. The Mozambican Red Cross functions as a channel for conveying foreign assistance to the country. As in other socialist countries, several mass organizations function outside of government but in support of official objectives. Women are grouped in the Organization of Mozambican Women, workers in the National Trade Union Confederation, youth in the Organization of Mozambican Youth, and there are other local communal groups, all participating in various environmental and other health campaigns.

Religious medical missions had played a significant role in colonial Mozambique, especially in establishing and operating rural hospitals and some health posts. When the entire sector was nationalized, within a month of independence, the mission facilities were taken over by the MOH, and virtually all the missionary personnel left the country. Some 17 percent of the population had been converted to Christianity (mainly to the Catholic faith), and many health personnel had been trained, but voluntary missions did not continue to operate.

Private Market. With FRELIMO nationalization of the health sector in 1975, virtually all private medical practice was ended. Out of 550 physicians in Mozambique, almost all European, 85 percent departed, leaving only a skeleton medical staff working in a few large hospitals.

Regarding traditional healers, or *curandeiros,* FRELIMO had a mixed attitude. Unlike many other African countries, it opposed any form of witchcraft or magical therapy as unscientific obscurantism, which misled and swindled the people. Yet empirical therapy with herbal drugs was accepted as possibly beneficial, and permitted even as a commercial transaction.

The major private sector activity in Mozambique, however, is that of the private pharmacy. The larger pharmacies were nationalized, but many small ones—about 60 percent of the total—have continued as small businesses. They obtain their drugs from the MOH pharmaceutical enterprise.

Certain joint public–private enterprises in Mozambique operate health facilities for their employees, in cooperation with the MOH. A sugar cane refinery and a large dam have such programs. Medical supplies and part of personnel costs are provided by the MOH.

Health Resources

Perhaps the most devastating effect of the FRELIMO revolution on the Mozambican health system was the massive departure of trained health personnel. As noted, the vast majority of European doctors left soon after independence, reducing the supply from 550 to 80, but fortunately other foreign physicians, sympathetic to the principles of the new government, came to help. By 1977, the supply was increased to 285 physicians, and by 1982 to 385. This meant about 3 doctors per 100,000 population in 1982. The single small local medical school in Maputo had been turning out only 5 to 10 graduates a year, and that output was greatly increased. In 1982 there were 35 Mozambican physicians, and this number increased to 135 in 1986. On graduation, 2 years of mandatory rural service is required of all young doctors.

Nurses are trained to a higher (grade A) and a lower (grade B) level, and there is also one grade of midwife. Training is done in two large hospitals. By 1982 there were 2,181 nurses, most of whom were male and of the grade-A level; there were 507 female midwives. This meant altogether 21.5 nurses and midwives per 100,000.

The *medical technicians* and *medical agents* are very important types of health personnel in Mozambique. These multipurpose personnel are the mainstay of health services in the rural areas. The medical technician is trained for 3 years, after 9 years of basic schooling, and is taught essentials of diagnosis and treatment as well as prevention. The medical agent has a more superficial training of similar scope, requiring 2 years after 6 years of elementary school. In 1984 there were reported to be 234 medical agents in the country and a somewhat smaller number of medical technicians. Almost all of these were working in health centers or health posts in the rural districts.

The most modestly prepared health worker in Mozambique is the *agente polivalente elementare* (APE), trained for a few months to work closely with the people. By 1982 some 1,200 APEs had been prepared, but their supervision was inadequate and many quit. By 1984 their training was discontinued.

Health facilities have been greatly expanded in Mozambique since independence. There are 3 major tertiary-level hospitals, with 500 to 1,400 beds each, 7 provincial hospitals of about 200 beds each, and 27 rural hospitals of 50 to 100 beds in the districts. All hospitals had been staffed with full-time physicians until the extremely disruptive effect of the counterrevolutionary insurrection in the 1980s. In 1982 there was a ratio of slightly more than 1 hospital bed per 1,000 people in the country.

Ambulatory care for both treatment and prevention is provided at health centers and health posts. Health centers are staffed by medical technicians, as well as nurses and midwives; they also usually have 10 to 20 beds. Health posts are staffed by the more briefly trained medical agents. At the time of independence, these units numbered 426 altogether. By 1986, this increased to 1,326 units, of which 213 were health centers. The total number of units established had been 1,921, but 595 were destroyed by insurgent action or looted and forced to close.

Virtually all drugs must be imported into Mozambique and purchased with hard currency. This is done by the MOH pharmaceutical enterprise, with assistance from UNICEF and other international groups. Transportation of drugs from Maputo to the provincial and district facilities has been seriously impeded by the insurgent hostilities. Great economies and improved quality were achieved in pharmaceutical use, however, by the reduction of the registered list from 26,000 brand-name products in the colonial period to a national formulary of 343 essential substances in 1980. (Counting different dosages and strengths, there were 500 drug preparations.)

The destructiveness of the insurrection has not been limited to physical facilities and transportation. Many health personnel have been killed and kidnapped. An estimated 430 health workers have been robbed of their belongings and terrorized. In 1982 there were 82 physicians working in rural district hospitals, but by 1986 the number was down to 31, and most rural hospitals lacked a single physician.

Delivery of Services

With the expansion of human and physical health resources in Mozambique, the services provided to people increased. Services were more readily available, of course, in the capital city and the main provincial towns, but even including the total rural population, ambulatory contacts reached 0.62 consultation per person per year in 1982. Then with the insurrection, the rate declined to 0.4 consultation per person in 1986. The MOH estimated that in 1983 about 30 percent of the national population had access to modern health services.

From the outset the FRELIMO government put high priority on preventive services. In 1979 the MOH started to prepare briefly trained *preventive medicine agents* for work on immunizations, latrine construction, and general health education. After a few years the ministry found that this preventive work was done better by the medical technicians and medical agents, with the cooperation of women and youth from the mass organizations. In 1986, DPT immunization had reached 51 percent of the children. Around 1985, childbirths were attended by a trained health worker in 28 percent of the cases. Mass screening tests are done, whenever possible, for tuberculosis, malaria, and schistosomiasis.

The network of primary care posts and health centers, district (rural) hospitals, provincial hospitals, and central hospitals is intended to be regionalized. Patients were to enter the network at the most peripheral point and then be referred to more technically developed facilities as necessary. In practice, the supply of

drugs and the staffing is often inadequate at the peripheral units and even in the district hospitals, especially with the difficulties caused by the war. As a result patients often bypass the nearest places and go directly to provincial and even central hospitals, which then become very congested.

The drilling of wells and laying of pipes for clean water have been greatly handicapped by lack of equipment and supplies. Safe water in 1984 was accessible to only 13 percent of the people.

With all of these difficulties, Mozambique has been able to make very limited progress in its health status record. The infant mortality rate was 190 per 1,000 live births in 1960 and was still as high as 170 per 1,000 in 1987. The life expectancy at birth was a scant 47 years. No special effort has been put into family planning, and for many years the crude birth rate has remained 45 per 1,000 population.

Economic Support

Considering its severe economic problems, Mozambique's expenditures on the health system have been relatively high. Government expenditures for health rose (in U.S. dollars) from $1.50 per capita in 1974 before independence to $4.70 per capita in 1982; this meant an increase from 3.3 percent of the national budget to 11.2 percent. Public expenditures for health declined in 1986, however, to $3.80, or 7.8 percent of the budget, though they were still much higher than in 1974.

Because of Mozambique's desperate need for external assistance, in 1987 the government decided to comply reluctantly with demands of the World Bank and International Monetary Fund; these called for reduction of government spending for health and greater shifting of costs to the private sector. Enterprises were required to pay the full cost of health services for workers and their dependents, and at all health units fees had to be charged well beyond the nominal amounts previously expected. Government held fast, however, on the prohibition of private medical practice. Even though some collectivized land had been sold to private farmers, the "reintroduction of private medicine in Mozambique [was] something quite unacceptable" to the FRELIMO movement.

In 1986, a beginning was made in restoring the war-ravaged health infrastructure. Some 27 peripheral health posts and health centers were reopened and 54 new health posts were built. By the end of 1986, a total of 186 closed health posts had been reopened. The vaccination program was accelerated. Training courses for health workers were held by the provinces and the MOH. Plans were developed in 1987 to equip 200 health posts, 4 health centers, and 5 rural hospitals. Even though certain private financial constraints were introduced in the health system, as a price for international economic aid, the FRELIMO government was making every effort to sustain and advance its health system along socialist lines.

PEOPLE'S REPUBLIC OF CHINA

In the late 1980s China, with a population of well over 1,000,000,000 people, was by far the largest country in the world. The social revolution that triumphed in 1949, to establish the People's Republic of China, marked a monumental change in all aspects of that society, among the most dramatic of which was the development of a modern national health system. In the centuries before this watershed event, China's history had been extremely rich and complicated, and virtually every chapter of it has left some imprint on the health services observable today.

Historical Background

Evidence of human civilization in the northern regions of what is now China has been dated to some 20,000 years ago. For centuries, since the second millennium B.C., a characteristic Chinese culture had spread over almost all of this vast territory. The linguistic and ethnological attributes of this culture were subject to influence by various conquering "barbarians" from outside, with a succession of ruling dynasties. The first such dynasty lasted for 500 years, from 1523 to 1027 B.C. (Shang). The

great philosopher Confucius lived in the subsequent Chou dynasty, from 1027 to 256 B.C. The years A.D. 220 to 265 began a period of warfare among petty states, lasting for four centuries. This era, however, saw the entry of Buddhism, Confucianism, and developments in medicine (transmitted from India). Feudalism began to govern land holdings. The centuries after A.D. 618 brought some unification of government civil service policies, and the invention of printing.

European infiltration into China began with Portuguese settlement on the southern coast at Macao in 1557, and this provoked a strong antiforeign policy. Meanwhile Manchu peoples from the northern region advanced south in the sixteenth and seventeenth centuries, ending with their complete conquest of China by 1644. Under this dynasty, China achieved its greatest territorial sovereignty, with a succession of emperors. The last of these was Emperor Puyi (of the Ch'ing Dynasty), whose power was ended by the triumph of the first Chinese Revolution in 1911, led by Sun Yat-sen, an intellectual who was trained as a physician.

The enormous complexities of events in the political and cultural history of China, after it became a republic in 1912, are beyond the scope of this book. We simply note that, following centuries of monarchy and the semifeudal control of most agriculture, the persistence of several major influences, from both inside China and the outside world, thwarted the peaceful development of a modern democratic society. Within the country, many large districts were dominated by owners of vast resources of land and local industry; these "warlords" commanded their own armies, and they resisted any control by a central public power. Also, inspired by the success of the Russian Revolution of 1917, a Chinese Communist Party was organized by Marxist intellectuals in Shanghai in 1921, and it gained supporters rapidly.

To implement the reforms called for by the 1911 revolution, a parliamentary party was organized. Known as the Kuomintang, its leaders were largely merchants, professionals, and intellectuals, dedicated to Chinese nationalism and opposed to foreign intervention. Claims by European countries to favorable conditions for trade with China—an "open door" policy—had been made since the early nineteenth century. Great Britain had provoked the Opium War in 1939 through 1942, resulting in freedom for British merchants to import opium into China, the ceding of Hong Kong to British control, and eventually similar permission for the "extraterritorial" sovereignty of foreign powers in Shanghai and other coastal cities. China's military weakness forced it to make all sorts of concessions to European commercial interests.

Japan had invaded China with military forces in 1894–95, and early in World War I it seized German holdings in one Chinese province. Then in 1931 after the birth of the Republic, Japan invaded northern China, setting up the puppet state of Manchukuo. The Kuomintang government, initially joining with the expanding Chinese Communist Party, fought to oust the Japanese invaders. General Chiang Kai-shek, leader of the Kuomintang Armies, then turned against the Communists, concentrating hostilities on them rather than the Japanese. In the mid-1930s the Communist forces (People's Liberation Army) undertook their famous "Long March" from their southeast base to the northwest province of Shensi, setting up permanent military headquarters at Yenan. There were further periods of alternating unity and hostility between the Kuomintang and the Communists, until Japan brought the United States into World War II with its attack on Pearl Harbor (Hawaii) in December 1941.

During and after World War II, power and territory fluctuated between the Communists, in the northern, more industrialized parts of China, and the Kuomintang in the south, in spite of American military support for the Chiang Kai-shek Nationalists. Finally in October 1949, the Communist Red Armies under Mao Tse-tung prevailed, declaring a new central government of the People's Republic of China, with headquarters at Peking (later Beijing). The new government was immediately recognized by Great Britain, the USSR, India, and other countries, but not by the United States. General Chiang Kai-shek and the Kuomintang leadership fled to the island of Taiwan, to establish a Chinese government-in-exile.

This is only the sketchiest summary of the complex events leading to the consolidation of power by the Communist Party of China. Our focus on the national health system of this large country can consider only the broad political background, in which health-related activites played a relatively small part. After 1949, orderly steps could finally be taken to design and implement a network of health resources and services for extension of needed health care throughout this vast country. The four decades from 1949 to 1989, however, were far from smooth sailing in the development of the health system and the general social order.

In the first postrevolutionary decade, the Communist government brought the soaring inflation under control and introduced massive land reforms. An initial 5-year plan was launched for 1953 to 1957, during which most agriculture was collectivized and industry was nationalized. Great assistance was received from the Soviet Union, and long railroads were built. Some severe setbacks were encountered, when the Great Leap Forward (started in 1958) failed to develop small village industries on a cooperative basis, as intended. For a combination of political reasons, Soviet economic aid ended rather abruptly in 1960, and the People's Republic was left on her own. But Soviet health system advice and standards from 1949 to 1960 had made their mark.

Internal power struggles in the Communist Party of China came to a climax in 1965, with the outbreak of the nationwide Cultural Revolution. Initiated by rebellious students at Peking University, the GPCR (great proletarian cultural revolution) called for an end to central political domination and an emphasis on local self-reliance in all matters. This meant construction of small factories in the countryside and energetic development of agricultural communes. The intense spirit of populism led to bitter opposition to "elitism" and intellectualism. Every intellectual had to spend some time working with his hands. Universities, factories, and government agencies were closed. This was the period that gave rise to the "barefoot doctor" and other health system features discussed later.

In 1971 the United States, for its own geopolitical reasons, withdrew its oppostion to recognizing mainland China, after 22 years of recognizing only the government-in-exile on the island of Taiwan. Soon after this, the United Nations and its specialized agencies, including the World Health Organization, welcomed back the government in Beijing to occupy the seat of China in these international bodies. After more than two decades of isolation from most of the world's powerful nations, the People's Republic of China returned to the world community. The island of Taiwan became regarded as one province of China that had not yet been "liberated."

In 1976, the great leader of the Chinese Revolution, Mao Zedong (formerly spelled Tsetung) died. In his declining years, Mao had supported, and even encouraged, the Cultural Revolution and its young Red Guards; the excesses of this movement, however, had led not only to the closure of most universities, but also to retarded development in both industry and agriculture. The Communist Party group that gained power after 1977, therefore, condemned the Party leaders, one of whom was the widow of Mao Zedong, who were deemed largely responsible for these difficulties. They were branded as the "Gang of Four."

The national leadership of China from 1977 to the end of the 1980s was oriented to technical and pragmatic change, rather than Marxist ideology. The new slogan became achieving progress through "four modernizations"; this meant techincal advances in industry, agriculture, science and technology, and military affairs. Scores of elderly men—veterans of the revolutionary movement of the 1930s and 1940s—retained the leading positions in the Communist Party of China, and the most important of these was Deng Xiaoping. The views of Deng and his associates were oriented toward greater free-market dynamics in economic affairs and greater pluralism in culture and daily life. The dominance of Communist Party controls, however, continued, as shown tragically in the reaction to mass student dem-

onstrations in Beijing's great Tienanmen Square in June 1989.

With this relatively brief historical background of modern China, we can examine its national health system in terms of the major contributions that can be traced to various historical periods. Current characteristics have inevitably been influenced most intensively by recent events, but the overall development is considered under five major periods: (1) Imperial China, before 1911; (2) the Kuomintang years, 1912 to 1949; (3) the period of Soviet influence, from 1949 to 1960; (4) autonomous China and the Cultural Revolution, 1961 to 1975; and (5) post-Mao modernizations, from 1976 to 1989. Then, with the most recent period, we examine the major components of the health system in greater depth.

Imperial China (before 1911)

The most prominent contribution of ancient imperial China to the national health system of modern China is the large domain of traditional Chinese medicine, which still plays a substantial role. With Western influence on medical services in China traceable to the seventeenth century, however, this must also be regarded as an aspect of Imperial China.

Traditional Chinese Medicine. A vast literature has been produced on the development of concepts about disease and its treatment in ancient China. Only some highlights need be noted here.

The major doctrines of ancient Chinese medicine are usually traced to the Chou Dynasty (1121–255 B.C.) and the Han Dynasty (206 B.C.–A.D. 221). These were philosophical ideas attributing disease to imbalances in various basic forces of nature, expressed within the human body. Best known is the doctrine of *yang* (meaning male or sunny principle) and *yin* (meaning female or shadowy principle). Another philosophical doctrine related disease to changed relationships among "five elements"—wood, fire, earth, metal, and water. The greatest written classic expounding these theories is known in English as *The Yellow Emperor's Classic of Internal Medicine.* It has been dated to about 200 B.C., but various modified editions appeared over subsequent centuries. This work contains references to physical therapy interventions, such as acupuncture and massage, but makes little reference to drugs. It is likely that these philosophical doctrines about disease were applied mainly to treatment of persons in the royalty and upper social classes.

Quite separate from this philosophical type of medical concept were the principles of popular healing used by the masses of common people of ancient China. These were based mainly on magical and religious doctrines, associated largely with Taoism (sixth century B.C.) and in some degree with Buddhism. The plebeian healers, who applied magicoreligious concepts, also sometimes gave their patients drugs made from local herbs; such empirical therapies, however, were rejected by the elite philosophical doctors. There were also empirical specialists in disorders of the eyes, ears, and teeth, as well as barber-masseurs.

Over the centuries, these two schools of traditional healing—each associated with different social classes—became intermingled. The importance of acupuncture declined and herbal therapy grew stronger. A "Great Pharmacopoeia," compiling all traditional herbal drugs was issued in the year 1596. On the other hand, acupuncture and moxibustion were virtually banned by the Great Imperial Medical Board in 1822.

Thus, the whole field of traditional Chinese medicine that plays so great a part in the health system of contemporary China is by no means a clear and unified discipline. It is built from diverse theoretical foundations, and its practitioners may have been trained according to varying educational regimes. As reflected in numbers, until the time of the Communist Revolution (1949), traditional Chinese doctors were vastly more important than Western-trained physicians. The former were estimated to number about 400,000, compared to 12,000 of the latter. Educational programs for traditional medicine in the People's Republic eventually became much more standardized.

Early Western Influence. The earliest impact on China of Western medical ideas was made by Jesuit priests, who had been trained in medicine, and came to spread the Christian gospel in the seventeenth century. At about the same time, physicians employed by the British East India Company extended some of their services to Chinese patients. Somewhat later, the American Board of Commissioners for Foreign Missions from the United States took organized steps to offer Western medical care as an aid to the spreading of Christianity. Western medical ideas became strongly influential in China, however, only after the great European scientific breakthroughs of bacteriology and pathology in the late nineteenth century.

Medical missionaries had come to China from Great Britain or the United States, as individuals, as early as 1820, when one of them (John Livingstone, a surgeon) established a dispensary for the poor in Macao, the early Portuguese settlement. In 1835, Dr. Peter Parker, a medical graduate of Yale University in Connecticut, opened the Canton Ophthalmic Hospital, where many operations for cataracts were performed. Parker also trained Chinese young men as dispensers and dressers. In 1838 the Canton Medical Missionary Society was organized with the explicit objective of extending Western medicine to China through basic education of the Chinese. Not until 1863, however, was a 3-year program for training medical apprentices organized in Canton. In 1881, a formal program of medical education was started by a Scottish missionary group in Tientsin, and soon missions set up other small medical schools elsewhere, giving lectures in Mandarin to small classes of fewer than 10 students. A survey in 1897 reported 39 such mission medical schools, with a total of 462 students and graduates.

In 1897 a Charitable Medical Society was organized along Western lines by a Chinese upper-class medical reformer. The first action for public health objectives had been taken in Shanghai in 1873, and then in other coastal cities, to establish quarantine against cholera that had broken out in Thailand and Malaya. A national public medical organization, however, was not set up until 1905 in the Ch'ing dynasty, and its work was devoted to some sanitary measures in the areas of the coastal cities occupied by foreign concessions.

An early, relatively extensive program for

public health purposes in Imperial China was the Manchurian Plague Prevention Service, organized in 1910 to combat a large plague epidemic. This body was unable to control the epidemic, but it prevented its spread to other areas. A public health action had been forced on the weak imperial government by Japan, Czarist Russia, and the United States, which wanted to seize Manchuria. Once established, however, the service extended beyond epidemic control to provision of some general hospitals for the poor (in the European manner) and limited preventive maternal and child health work. The same Ch'ing government set up a small Peking Special Health Station and a National Epidemic Prevention Bureau.

In the last years of the nineteenth century and the first decade of the twentieth, medical education was the major vehicle for Western influence in the health field of China. Much leadership was taken by foreign universities, as well as religious missions. In 1887, the Hong Kong College of Medicine was opened for Chinese in that great coastal city, after it had become a British colony. In 1906, several missionary societies of different Christian denominations combined to found the first "union" medical college in Peking, and soon additional union schools were started in eight other cities. Around 1908, three American universities established still other small medical schools. Later, as national pride developed in China, with hostility to foreigners, several of these schools died out.

The Kuomintang Years— 1912–1949

When Imperial China came to an end in 1911 and the first Republic of China was born in 1912, the first serious attempts were made to extend modern health services beyond the large coastal cities, to the vast inland provinces where most people lived. In spite of the generally pervasive anti-Western feelings, the value of Western medical science was recognized by Chinese leadership, and numerous actions were taken to apply these foreign concepts in medical education, public health work, and the provision of general medical care.

Nationalist Government Health Developments. In 1914, the Rockefeller Foundation of the United States put major support into strengthening the union medical college that had been started by groups of missionaries in Peking. This Peking Union Medical College (PUMC) soon became the most highly developed center for education on modern medical science in China, in a sense serving as a model for the organization of other schools throughout the country. (The image of PUMC as a center for training doctors to serve the urban elite, rather than the masses of Chinese people, arose much later.) Then in 1920 PUMC added a school for educating female nurses, in place of poorly trained male apprentices, who had previously given most nursing service. In 1921, an academic Department of Public Health (headed by John Grant) was added to the PUMC, with a small health center in the city—the Peking Special Health Station—for demonstration and teaching purposes. Tied to the Special Health Station, a North China School of Midwives was opened in 1929, the first such training program to prepare successors to the 200,000 untrained birth attendants then functioning in China.

On a broader scale, the Nationalist government of China established a Public Health Department in the Ministry of Interior in 1927. A year later, this function was separated as an independent Ministry of Public Health, with five major departments: (1) general affairs, (2) medical administration, (3) health service, (4) epidemic prevention, and (5) statistics. In addition, for policy determination there was a Central Public Health Committee. Personnel to staff these programs were drawn largely from PUMC graduates—about one-fourth of whom had focused their studies on public health. A few years later, however, in 1931 public health functions in government were deprived of ministerial status and returned to an office in the Ministry of Interior. This arrangement continued until the end of the war with Japan in 1945; during those chaotic years, the adminstrative headquarters for public health work were moved several times. Only in 1945, was a Ministry of Public Health reestablished at Nanjing, the capital city of the Nationalist government.

In its various administrative forms, the national authority for public health extended modern medical services well beyond their level in Imperial China (before 1912). In relation to the enormous health needs of this vast impoverished population, the accomplishments may have been small, but they still constituted progress. Services were largely developed in major cities (in the interior as well as on the coast), but they contributed to the beginnings of an infrastructure for modern medical care (mainly in hospitals) and medical education, on which the later revolutionary government could build. In addition to the health services intended for the general population, the Nationalist government organized military medical services, a Factory Inspection Office (for workplace hazards) in the Ministry of Industry, a Health Office in the Ministry of Railways, and a Medical Education Commission in the Ministry of Education.

The first well-developed local health authority was the Office of Public Health Affairs, established within the Police Department of Beijing in 1925. It was modeled largely on a typical local public health agency of the United States, but it also offered some curative service to the poor. After 1928, similar public health offices, stressing prevention, were set up in several of the larger provinces (under provincial supervision) and in major municipalities. By 1937 there were 52 health offices—for communicable disease control, maternal and child hygiene, health education, environmental inspection, and so on—under provincial control, and 82 under municipal control. By 1945, some 70 health organizations were operating in 16 provinces of China. During the war with Japan, most of the major coastal cities were occupied, and municipal health offices actually declined. After the war ended in 1945, Kuomintang services improved, and in 1947 a survey reported 105 health offices under provincial supervision and an equal number under municipal governments.

In 1932, the Kuomintang government set out to establish hospitals at the county level, to serve the rural population. Previously such a rural orientation had been shown only by certain missionary groups. A survey in 1934 had found only 17 *rural health organizations* in the whole country. By 1947, the new hospital initiative had resulted in establishment of 40 public hospitals at the county level in 11 provinces.

Over the same years, from 1932 to 1947, the Nationalist government encouraged the construction of other types of health facility in most of China's 2,046 counties (then delineated), which by definition were predominantly rural. (Cities or municipalities are jurisdictionally separate from counties.) Difficulties in translation from Chinese to English must be appreciated, but a report of China's Ministry of Public Health, published in English in 1986, reported that in 1949 the country had 2,600 "hospitals" with 59,614 beds. It is very likely that the great majority of these structures were actually health centers mainly for ambulatory care, with small complements of perhaps 10 to 20 beds, for maternity cases or acutely ill patients awaiting transportation to a proper hospital. They might have served the population of a county or municipality. Another report from the Chinese Medical Association, published in 1944, stated that the country had about 500 "hospitals."

Still another official report, published in 1960, stated specifically that 1,775 county health centers had been built between the mid-1930s and 1945. In addition, 125 provincial hospitals had been constructed, plus 26 "provincial medical centers." Outside of government, by 1945 there were 307 missionary and other private hospitals.

For training personnel, by 1945 there were 30 medical colleges, of which 15 were national, 5 were provincial, and 10 were private. Modern pharmacists were being trained in 5 schools, dentists in 3 schools, midwives in 22 schools, and nurses in 317 schools, attached to hospitals under both government and religious missions. Much of the leadership for these Chinese developments in health care and education came from foreign professionals, and the outputs barely scratched the surface of the vast rural needs, but these efforts under the Kuomintang had two significant results for the national health system: (1) they helped China's leaders and many people to accept many Western ideas as scientific and beneficial, and not merely foreign and negative; (2) they launched the beginnings of a national infrastructure for medical care, preventive health service, and health manpower education, to serve the extremely backward population of Imperial China.

As a result of all this activity under the Nationalist government, health manpower with some scientific training were greatly expanded in China. A report from 1930, 19 years after the first revolution of 1911, stated that only 705 modern physicians existed in all of China, and of these 304 were foreigners (mostly missionaries). By 1945, modern doctors had been increased to 12,946, of whom the great majority were Chinese. In addition, there were 353 modern dentists, 918 drug dispensers, 5,189 trained midwives, and 5,972 trained nurses. In relation to China's many hundred million people, of course, these personnel stocks were still woefully inadequate.

Because of its policy to Westernize the entire health system, Kuomintang attitudes toward traditional Chinese medicine were negative and hostile. In 1919, attempts were made to virtually wipe it out, but nationwide opposition compelled the government to compromise. Efforts were made to regulate traditional medicine practices—banning, for example, the use of syringes. A special committee for traditional Chinese medicine was finally set up in the Ministry of Education in 1936. Stores dispensing herbal drugs were widespread in the cities; in 1941 there were 250 such traditional pharmacies in Beijing alone.

Health Services in Communist Territory. During this entire period of general Kuomintang domination, the Communist Party of China and the Workers' and Peasants' Red Army were mobilizing as a separate movement. The Second National Party Congress in 1922 formulated policies on health protection. In 1927 the first Red Army Hospital was established in an abandoned school. As large areas of northwest China came under the control of Communist Party forces, after about 1931, a formal program of health services was organized in the Communist-held territory. Unlike policies of the Kuomintang government, those of the

Communist authorities, headquartered in Yenan and led by Mao Zedong, called for combining Chinese traditional medicine with Western medicine in combatting all diseases. Health committees were set up at provincial, county, and municipal levels in the occupied territories; their major task was to prevent disease by improving environmental sanitation and general hygienic education.

The Red Army tried to help local people dig wells and generally clean up their villages, wherever soldiers were stationed. In 1934 a Central Antiepidemic Committee was established to formulate and promote policies on disease-reporting, isolation of cases, and environmental sterilization. A central Health Bureau organized public clinics to treat the sick and also to form some cooperatives for dispensing herbal drugs.

Hospitals were established principally to treat the wounded soldiers of the Red Army. After 1931, a general hospital was organized in each major military command. By 1934 there were 10 such hospitals, each of which was surrounded by five or six small clinics; in addition there were three hospitals for the seriously disabled or convalescent. Altogether about 20,000 wounded men could be accommodated. Even a military medical school was founded at Yenan in 1931, preparing "Red doctors who are sound politically and competent technically." The course of study was for 1 year. Up to 1934, this school trained 181 "doctors," 125 health care officers, 300 nurses, and 75 drug dispensers.

The policy of "combining traditional and Western medicine" was implemented by assigning principal responsibility for general disorders (internal medicine in the West) to traditional doctors, and principal responsibility for surgical conditions to Western doctors. These lines, however, were not too sharply drawn. It must be recalled that in the 1930s, the sulfa drugs and powerful antibiotics were not yet generally known even in Europe and America. Furthermore, traditional Chinese medicine, as noted earlier, was a polyglot mixture of practices. After 1937, with the mounting of serious military resistance to the Japanese invaders, the Communist Party Central

Committee called for elimination from traditional medicine of "witchcraft and other superstitious practices." In other words, herbal drugs and other empirical measures were to be encouraged, but not magic.

In 1944, the Communist leadership called for organization of a general clinic in each of the 1,000 townships of the northwest border region. The several military hospitals organized in the early 1930s broadened their role, as hostilities mounted in the period 1937 to 1945. At this time, the Communists were battling against the Japanese, as well as against the armies of the Kuomintang. The out-patient departments of Red Army hospitals began to treat local people, and often to admit them to beds. In 1941, at a military hospital of 150 beds in the northwest border region, 25 percent of all the patients treated were civilians.

In 1941 the Border Region Government Council had formulated a 3-year program for health service development, including general inspection of hygienic conditions, research on traditional Chinese medicine, and mass health propaganda (education). Great progress was also made in the education of professional health workers. The Red Army Medical School, founded at Yenan in 1931, was greatly strengthened in 1938, and in 1946 was converted into the China Medical University. Its training curriculum for doctors was lengthened from 1 to 4 years, and it eventually was moved to the city of Shenyang in 1948. Courses were also offered for nurses and pharmacists. During these years of the war with Japan, moreover, as many as nine other small medical schools were organized in eastern and central China. More than 3,000 medical and health personnel were trained by these rapidly assembled schools.

The 10 military hospitals developed for the Red Army up to 1934 gradually evolved into hospitals for the general population, as the war against Japan continued. By 1939 an additional military hospital had been established, plus six regular civilian general hospitals. In the last months of the war against Japan, health services for the Red Army were extremely difficult to organize; incredible hardships were endured, as wounded soldiers were hidden in mountain caves, secret tunnels, and the simple homes of peasants.

Following the atomic bombing of Japan, the war against the invaders from that country was soon ended, but intense hostilities broke out between the Communist forces and the armies of the Kuomintang. This period, from 1945 to 1949, brought other developments to the health system of China. In 1945, a General Health Department was set up by the Communists, to oversee all military as well as civilian health activities. If only to protect the strength of the fighting forces, epidemic prevention in each locality had high priority. Civilians were also mobilized to provide first-aid and transport for the wounded. The schools for training doctors, nurses, and others, described earlier, continued to function during the civil war between the Communists and the Kuomintang; by the time of national liberation in 1949, some 6,000 doctors and dispensers had been trained, as well as thousands of nurses.

Early Postliberation China—1949–1965

The victory of the Chinese Communist movement, and the establishment in October 1949 of the People's Republic of China is described by most Chinese people as the time of liberation. In the first decade of the new China, this great war-torn nation was almost wholly isolated in the world—except for the strong friendship and technical advice of the Soviet Union. The first postliberation developments in the national health system, therefore, were naturally substantially influenced by the Soviet model.

In the early 1950s, Soviet consultants came to China in great numbers. As in the first years after the Russian Revolution of 1917, the initial strategy was to expand rapidly the number of educated health personnel—not only physicians (trained along Western scientific lines), but also *middle medical personnel,* as the Soviet consultants called them. The latter included nurses, midwives, and drug dispensers and, most important, assistant doctors, who were essentially like the Russian *feldsher.*

By 1957 the supply of Western-trained doctors had been increased from about 13,000 claimed under the Kuomintang in 1945 to an estimated 70,000. In 1966, the total stock of Western-trained physicians was estimated to be about 150,000. These were trained in medical faculties, organized along Soviet lines into "specialties," of adult medicine, pediatrics, hygiene, and stomatology. Soviet-type incentives were also provided through much higher salaries for professors and hospital department chiefs, but rather modest salaries for others. Also, as in the USSR, the medical schools were independent of general universities and, in fact, were often termed *medical universities* (insofar as they prepared various types of personnel beyond physicians). In 1957 there were about 35 medical schools, and the rapidly expanding output of doctors was achieved mainly by greatly enlarging the enrollment of each of them.

The development of middle or secondary medical schools in the postliberation years was even more impressive. By 1957 there were estimated to be 170 such schools, and 230 by 1965. Their output, along with the equivalent personnel surviving from the Kuomintang period, yielded an overall supply of 170,000 assistant doctors, 185,000 nurses, 40,000 trained midwives, and 100,000 drug dispensers. The latter are not to be confused with higher-level professional pharmacists, who numbered about 20,000 in 1966.

This strong Soviet influence in health manpower policy should not imply any lack of creativity by Chinese health leadership. Soon after liberation in the early 1950s, a National Health Congress in Peking formulated four basic principles to guide policy developments for many years: (1) medicine must serve the people—the workers, peasants, and soldiers; (2) prevention must have priority over curative medicine; (3) Chinese traditional medicine must be united with Western medicine; and (4) all health work must be integrated with mass movements. If these principles are broadly interpreted, it may be said that they have continued to apply in China up to the present time.

In 1966 there were estimated to be 500,000

practitioners of traditional Chinese medicine, and the directive on combining their work with that of Western-trained doctors was implemented in many ways. There were 21 colleges training traditional doctors, but many of the latter were also prepared simply by apprenticeship to a seasoned practitioner. These healers, in whom millions of people had great confidence, were posted in virtually all health facilities, for both in-patient and ambulatory care, throughout China. In general, the patient was free to consult whichever type of doctor he or she preferred, and also to change from one type to the other. In government health facilities, however, the great majority of health personnel were usually of the Western type, and the great majority of traditional doctors were entirely in private practice.

Health facilities were expanded after liberation almost as rapidly as health manpower. Between 1949 and 1957 some 860 hospitals, with an average capacity of 350 beds each, were constructed—a total increase of more than 300,000 beds. Thousands of additional hospital beds were built after 1957, so that by 1965 a Ministry of Health official could report in the *Chinese Medical Journal* that every county in China had at least one modern hospital. The hospital doctors, like all other hospital personnel, were on full-time salaries.

Perhaps the main impact of Soviet advice on China's health system in the first postliberation decade was the development of the pyramidal administrative framework for health care delivery. The main towns of rural sections or in municipal districts had health centers, which are principally for ambulatory care (although usually with a few beds); many of these were staffed, like Soviet polyclinics, with adult generalists, pediatricians, and gynecologists. At a second level in each county were one or more county hospitals for patients requiring surgery or other relatively simple specialized treatment. At the third level, in the provincial capital or in large municipalities, were larger highly specialized medical centers for complex cases, as well as for teaching and research.

In parallel with these facilities for personal health service, at the county level a public health authority or bureau was established, which was responsible for the local health centers as well as county facilities. Also at the county or large municipal levels, were separate antiepidemic stations, obviously modeled after the Soviet sanitary–epidemiological stations. Some 1,400 of these were reported to be operating in 1961. At the provincial level there were Provincial Public Health Bureaus, which came under the direction of the Ministry of Public Health in Peking.

In northern China, where the Communist forces had controlled affairs for many years, health care organization at the most local level, below the sphere of county government, was more highly developed. As early as 1960, local production units here in agriculture and even in village industry, were organized into *people's communes*. These groupings of families had not only economic functions, but also provided education and health services for their members. The commune, in turn, was divided into *production brigades* for specific tasks.

It is not clear how extensively this commune pattern of production, along with health service, was implemented within the nearly 2,300 counties of China in 1960. A report published in *Public Health* in 1960, however, describes one such health service near Honan Medical College in detail. There were 40,121 people in the commune, divided into 17 production brigades. A central commune health center had 16 doctors (9 modern and 7 traditional), 10 nurses, 11 technicians, and others; there were also 25 patient beds. Each of the 17 production brigades had a small health station, staffed by three or four doctors (modern or traditional) plus one nurse for maternal and child preventive health work. The article reporting these arrangements comments that the health services of many other people's communes, even in the northern China regions, were usually not as good as in this one, because of staff shortages.

Another important strategy developed in the postliberation decade was a clear reflection of Soviet influence, and even to some extent concepts from Japan. This was the initiation in 1951 of health insurance for central government employees and for workers in government enterprises. As in the USSR, the insurance contributions came entirely from the government and the enterprise management; there were no deductions from the wages of

workers. Also, as in the USSR, services could be obtained at special facilities attached to the workplace or, if the worker preferred, elsewhere in the community. As in Japan, however, benefits for dependents were much less than those for the primary worker, and none at all for the dependents of government employees. All this insurance facilitated medical care essentially for city-dwellers, and similar programs for rural people were not developed until much later. These economic support mechanisms are discussed more fully later.

In one important respect, health services in China differed markedly from the Soviet model. Although the resources, both personnel and facilities, were public rather than private, the care was not provided free; most patients had to pay small fees for all services. It is likely that these fees paid for only a portion of the true costs of service, and they did not go to the doctor or anyone else personally, but rather to the support of the service; the economics of China's whole health system are explored later. As a very poor country, China's leaders hasten to explain, the government has not yet been able to provide free health service for everyone. Certain sections of the population, as just noted, are protected by social insurance for medical costs, but each health facility is supposed to be largely self-supporting.

Accomplishments in the reduction of infectious disease in China, made during the first postliberation decade, were very impressive. Before liberation, it was estimated that schistosomiasis afflicted 10 million people. Through a combination of strategies that involved mobilizing millions of peasants to kill snails, early detection and chemotherapy of cases, more sanitary handling of human excreta, and other measures, the prevalence of this crippling disease was greatly reduced. Concerted actions to fight this endemic disease started about 1955, with national government leadership and local direction at the county level. By 1960, 4,000,000 fewer cases of schistosomiasis were reported.

Similar strategies, involving the mobilization of people in massive campaigns against vectors of disease, were applied to malaria, filariasis, and even enteric disease spread by flies. In the early 1950s, health workers called on peasants to help eliminate the "four pests"—mosquitoes, flies, rats, and sparrows; children were paid small rewards for jars filled with killed flies. (Sparrows were to be killed because they consumed a great deal of grain, needed by the people.) Later the movement called for destroying flies, cockroaches, fleas, and snails. In back of these specific targets was the encouragement of a general attitude toward promoting a more sanitary physical environment. Foreign missionaries, who knew the old Imperial China and returned for visits in the late 1950s, reported astonishing improvements in the general appearance of cities and towns everywhere. "Countless old refuse dumps and stagnant pools," it was said, "have been transformed into parks and recreational areas throughout the country."

In spite of all this progress in China's health system—resulting from a harmonious interaction of the vast energies mobilized by the Communist Party of China and the organizational advice of consultants from the Soviet Union—ir. the late 1950s political tensions developed between the top leadership of China and the Soviet Union. (Josef Stalin tended to regard China as a satellite, while China felt large and strong enough to develop socialism in its own way.) In 1960, therefore, thousands of Soviet consultants departed from China.

The next few years were a period of intense discussion and debate within the Chinese Communist Party. The ultimate causes of this turbulence are still not certain, but the climax in the Great Proletarian Cultural Revolution, starting in 1965, was broadcast around the world. In the health system, quite aside from the larger social scene, the Cultural Revolution had many consequences.

The Cultural Revolution— 1965–1975

Started by rebellious students at Peking University, the Cultural Revolution was openly supported by Communist Party Chairman Mao, and soon spread throughout the country. It became a sweeping attack by young Red Guards against the established leadership of almost all enterprises in industry and agriculture, in the universities and theaters, in com-

merce and transportation, in the entire organizational framework of the Communist Party itself, and in all health and health-related institutions. Millions of executives, professionals, and intellectuals were removed from their posts, denigrated, and humiliated. An estimate in late 1980 suggested that 400,000 people had been killed.

In a famous statement of 26 June 1965, Chairman Mao singled out the health authorities for criticism with the following statement:

> Tell the Ministry of Public Health that it only works for fifteen percent of the country and that this fifteen percent is mainly composed of gentlemen, while the broad masses of the peasants do not get any medical treatment. First they don't have any doctors; second they don't have any medicine. The Ministry of Public Health is not a Ministry of Public Health for the people, so why not change its name to the Ministry of Urban Health, the Ministry of Gentlemen's Health, or even the Ministry of Urban Gentlemen's Health?

This bitter criticism of the Ministry of Public Health was clearly an extreme exaggeration, and yet the validity of its basic objective, to demand much greater concern for health services to China's large rural population, could not be denied. As Victor and Ruth Sidel have commented, despite the great rural improvements by 1965, the cities still received disproportionate funding. Despite the accomplishments of prevention, curative medicine still got most attention. Despite efforts to integrate Western and traditional medicine, the latter was still of low status. Too many organized health patterns were slavishly copied from the Soviet Union. Despite education of the people, top management was still unresponsive to popular demands. There was allegedly more concern with "raising quality standards" than with extending minimal service to everyone. Intellectuals were still honored more than manual workers.

To act on his criticisms, Chairman Mao called for reduction of all medical education to 3 years after basic primary school; the balance of education should come from practice. Medical research should focus on the prevention and treatment of the common diseases, and not on the rare complex disorders. As for health service, all doctors should go to work in the rural villages, except for the incompetent ones, who could remain in the cities. Coming from the nation's top political and philosophical leader, these formulations had a profound impact in the entire health system.

During the Cultural Revolution, the medical schools admitted no new classes, and students already enrolled were accelerated. Faculty members, researchers, and others left their urban posts to do manual work and give some medical service in the countryside. As many as one-third of the staff of an average city hospital were away at any one time. By 1971, the administrative leadership of virtually all hospitals and health organizations had been changed, to put authority in "revolutionary committees"; these were tripartite, with one representative of the government (a "cadre" member), one from the People's Liberation Army, and one of the local health workers (who might be a doctor or nurse or other such person).

The most enduring contribution of the Cultural Revolution, however, was not in these policies, most of which were modified as the political passions of the period came to an end (see later), but in the nationwide development of auxiliary health workers, who came to be known as *barefoot doctors.* The concept had actually been developed in some peripheral rural sections of Shanghai municipality in the late 1950s, but it did not spread and, in fact, was virtually terminated by 1965. With the new emphasis of the Cultural Revolution, the idea of preparing elementary health workers from the village people, with very brief periods of formal training, spread like wildfire. No national schedule of education was promoted. Every county and every commune, of which there were about 27,000 in China around 1970, was free to prepare barefoot doctors in its own way. As a result, relatively young men and women, who were usually but not always graduates of middle school (seven grades), were selected by their villages for training. The instruction was given at a health center or hospital. The duration of training was usually 2 to 6 months, but varied between 1 month and 2 years.

The content of barefoot doctor training was a blend of elementary modern medicine and traditional herbalist medicine. Political concepts of Mao and Marx were incorporated throughout. Prevention was supposed to be emphasized, along with medical care. This included immunizations, how to educate people about sanitation, and the dispensing of contraceptive pills. Periodically the barefoot doctor was supposed to return to the health facility for a day or two of continuing education. Most important, the barefoot doctor in most communes was regarded as part-time; he or she still did other work as a peasant or worker and spent only the time necessary for medical activities.

Although small fees were charged for the services of the barefoot doctor, they were passed along to the leaders of the commune or the local production brigade within it. This money was used mainly to purchase both modern and traditional drugs. Remuneration for the medical service was by "work points," the value of which depended on each commune's overall productivity each year. Payment for health work was essentially the same as for agricultural or other work, to avoid undue attraction away from production labor. It must be emphasized that during the Cultural Revolution, there was no program for accreditation or licensure of barefoot doctors. Such credentialing was regarded as breeding elitism and to be avoided. Naturally, there was some turnover among these health workers, often because of changes in their family situation.

The total number of functioning barefoot doctors, according to an estimate in 1972, was about 1,200,000—far more than any type of "professional" health personnel. Some estimates of barefoot doctors went as high as nearly 3 million by the end of 1973. In addition, many barefoot doctors at busy health stations had *health aides,* trained on the spot for about 2 weeks, who were estimated to number some 3,000,000 in 1978.

In the cities, the equivalent of barefoot doctors were prepared to serve the people in an urban "lane," usually by training housewives. They were called *red medical workers* and, because modern health facilities were usually nearby, their scope of work was not as broad as in the communes. Some of these personnel were simply factory workers. Their training was usually even shorter than 3 months. Family planning education was an especially important function of the red medical workers in cities, as well as the rural barefoot doctors. Since the 1970s, a policy of favoring one-child families has been promoted in China, and community health workers regard the dissemination of contraceptive education and materials as their political responsibility.

With political changes, the political and geographical jurisdictions in China have changed from time to time, especially in the terminology applied. At the end of the Cultural Revolution in 1975, the national structure, with which the health system was largely parallel, was as follows: there were 22 provinces, of which one (Taiwan) was regarded as not yet liberated; the average provincial population was about 40 million. In addition there were five autonomous regions and three centrally administered cities (Beijing, Shanghai, and Tientsin). Provinces were divided into counties—about 100 each with populations of about 300,000 to 400,000—amounting to nearly 2,300 counties in all.

Within counties, during the 1965–1975 decade some 27,000 communes were organized—about 8 to 14 per county with populations of 20,000 to 60,000. Being so large, communes were further divided into *production brigades* of approximately 3,000 to 5,000 people each. Sometimes, varying with the local terrain and type of production, these brigades were further subdivided into small production teams with 50 to 500 adults.

Urban municipalities are organized differently, and somewhat less uniformly than the rural counties. Municipalities may vary from perhaps 50,000 people to more than 10,000,000 in Shanghai. (The central city of Shanghai and other large municipalities can be surrounded by rural counties within the jurisdiction of the municipality.) If the municipality is large, it is divided into districts, and these are further divided into neighborhoods or urban communes of around 40,000 population. The most local unit for various social purposes, including health, is the "lane" with 1,000 to 5,000 people. As we will see, many

changes in these jurisdictions were made after the Cultural Revolution.

Soon after the People's Republic of China was accepted as the proper occupant of China's seat in the United Nations, worldwide attention was drawn to the great advances in health it had achieved since preliberation days. The date of this major change was 1971, when the Cultural Revolution and its vast output of barefoot doctors were still in process. With world attention on the barefoot doctors, many other developing countries set out to replicate this Chinese health manpower model. The U.S. government published an English translation of *A Barefoot Doctor's Manual,* prepared originally by the Institute of Traditional Chinese Medicine of Hunan Province.

The major contents of this nearly 1,000-page manual are worth noting: (1) understanding the human body, (2) hygiene, (3) introduction to diagnostic techniques, (4) therapeutic techniques, (5) birth control planning, (6) diagnosis and treatment of common diseases, and (7) Chinese medicinal plants. The long chapter on "Diagnosis and Treatment of Common Diseases" contains the following 10 sections: first-aid, other medical emergencies, common symptoms, common infectious diseases, parasites, medical illnesses, surgical conditions, gynecological and obstetrical diseases, common pediatric ailments, and diseases of the sense organs. Within each of these sections, treatment is outlined both by Chinese traditional methods (usually herbs) and by Western methods. The longest chapter (more than 400 pages) in the manual is the final one on "Chinese Medicinal Plants."

The heightened recognition of traditional Chinese medicine was, indeed, probably the second major impact of the Cultural Revolution on China's health system. There had long been a handful of higher colleges of traditional medicine, but around 1970 they were increased to 24, and their enrollments were enlarged. The course of study was eventually standardized at 5 years after middle school (the same length as most Western medical schools). Meanwhile the Western medical schools were reduced generally in length from the conventional 6 years (after secondary school) to 4 years or even 3, and a certain amount of traditional medicine was incorporated in their curricula. (The traditional medicine schools also taught various principles of Western medicine.) The departments of traditional medicine in virtually all hospitals and health centers were strengthened and, of course, all barefoot doctors were encouraged to use medicinal herbs as much as possible, growing their own plants whenever feasible. Research institutes on methods of diagnosis (for example, study of the tongue, the pulse) and methods of treatment (acupuncture, herbs, etc.) were also strengthened.

All in all, the Cultural Revolution clearly led to extension of health services in the vast rural areas of China. With some 27,000 people's communes organized, subdivided into 500,000 or more production brigades, the latter groupings of around 3,000 to 5,000 people each were virtually all served by a small health station. The barefoot doctor or doctors and their health aides at these stations had extremely modest equipment, and only a small supply of traditional and Western drugs, but they were typically well-liked and respected by the villagers. Their educational efforts on environmental sanitation and personal hygiene, their encouragement of private plots to grow nutritious food, their dissemination of family planning information, their giving immunizations to children, and their winning the people's confidence through treatment of their common ailments had measurable impacts on the health of the rural population. Permeating rural health service during the Cultural Revolution was a political spirit, affirming that cleanliness and cooperation in various health programs (such as destroying vectors of disease), signified "patriotic" behavior and personal virtue.

Post-Mao Modernizations— 1976–1989

With the death of Mao Zedong in 1976, and the tapering off of the Cultural Revolution, there were bound to be further changes in China's health system. The four "modernizations" did not refer specifically to health service, but this was clearly one aspect of science and technology. "Modern" strategy called for

returning medical education to the conventional Western schedule of 6 years after secondary school (10 grades). It also called for the upgrading of barefoot doctors through additional education, with credentialing based on examinations. Attempts would be made to acquire better medical equipment and larger supplies of Western pharmaceuticals for health centers and hospitals.

The step-by-step changes in the health system after 1976 mirrored political debate, but one overriding trend was a movement to encourage private initiative and competition in all social affairs. A free market for producing goods and services, formerly condemned as the wrong "capitalist path," was not only accepted but actively promoted. In agriculture, this meant the gradual termination of the people's communes, with collective ownership of almost all land, and their conversion to townships, as simple local units of government within counties. The production brigades became simply villages or village clusters. If there were production teams, the new term might be translated as "hamlet." Cooperation in agricultural production might, in fact, continue among the farmers in a township, but each farmer was ultimately independent.

In the cities, many retail shops or restaurants were opened and operated by individuals or partnerships. Small factories for manufacturing garments, furniture, tools, cosmetics, and so on were organized privately or, if moderate numbers of working people and others were involved, were considered as "collectively owned" enterprises. Large enterprises, such as coal mines, steel mines, railroads, or electrical utilities usually remained governmental. In both urban and rural schools, education about Marxism–Leninism and the Thoughts of Chairman Mao was gradually reduced. Political posters and billboards were taken down, and sometimes replaced with commercial advertisements. Communist party cells, which had previously held meetings every week or more often, still existed but they met infrequently. The *People's Daily,* organ of the Communist Party of China, continued to be published, but its stories emphasized individual successes rather than major social achievements.

In light of the many decades of development of China's health system we have reviewed, the situation in the current period obviously embodies the impacts of several distinct periods. Keeping these periods in mind, the characteristics of the system in the late 1980s may be summarized according to our customary health system components. But first a few basic statistics are in order.

In 1986, China's population was reported to be 1,054,173,000—by far the largest of any nation on earth. Occupying the great land mass of southeastern Asia, it has a very long coastline, along which large cities developed and became the bases for trade and exploitation by foreign powers in previous centuries. Its territory is slightly larger than that of the United States, but two-thirds of this is mountainous or desert, and only one-third is cultivated. Urbanization has been gradually increasing, but in 1985 it had reached only 22 percent (which was 232 million people), while 78 percent remained in rural locations.

In spite of its rapid industrial development, extraction of natural resources, and improvements in agricultural productivity since liberation in 1949, the nation's GNP per capita was still low in 1988, reported by the World Bank as $300 that year. Gross domestic production was growing at the high annual rate of 10.5 percent between 1980 and 1986. The population engaged in industry and services (rather than agriculture) rose from 19 percent in 1965 to 26 percent in 1980.

Ethnically, the population of China is quite homogeneous—94 percent of Han ethnic background and the other 6 percent (still, 60 million people) distributed among 54 minorities, located largely in the five autonomous regions. Religion has not been a strong force in China, even before the Revolution in 1949. Although the several versions of the Constitution guarantee "freedom to believe in religion and freedom not to believe in religion," after 1949 the government ceased to subsidize any religious activities. Relatively small populations of Buddhists, Taoists, and Moslems still practice their faith, with monks and temples. The foreign missionaries spreading Christianity, however, were asked to leave, and by 1953 almost all had departed. Their church buildings, as well as schools and hospitals, were converted to general community use. The doctrines of Confucius (who lived about 500 B.C.) are not regarded as a religion, but rather as a set of ethical and behavioral concepts that emphasize personal self-effacement and obedience to authority. These doctrines were strongly condemned after liberation.

A special accomplishment of the People's Republic has been the extension of adult literacy. While female handicaps are still prominent, in 1985 literacy was reported to be 85 percent for men and 56 percent for women—enormous advances over preliberation days.

Health Resources in China

Resulting from the first (1911) but especially the second Chinese Revolution (1949), the availability of human and physical resources for health purposes in modern China has been enormously expanded and its quality has improved.

Health Manpower. The largest group of health personnel in China before both twentieth-century revolutions was the traditional Chinese medical practitioner. With changes in policy over the years since 1911, the number of these doctors has fluctuated, but in 1986 it was still substantial. The Ministry of Public Health (MOPH) stated their number to be 336,224 in 1986, which amounted to 31.9 per 100,000 population. Thousands of these were in salaried posts of governmental health facilities, but the majority were probably mainly in private practice, in both cities and rural villages. Over and above these practitioners in 1986, there were some 151,000 dispensers of traditional herbal drugs, trained in secondary medical schools (discussed later).

There were 24 colleges of traditional Chinese medicine in 1986, usually offering a 5-year training program. Students usually entered this training after middle school (seven grades), but this prerequisite has not been rigid, and some colleges enroll applicants after primary school (four grades). These colleges are usually linked to hospitals of traditional medicine, described later. They may be sponsored by the national MOPH, the provincial health authorities, or sometimes the counties. The curriculum content recommended by the Division of Traditional Medicine of the MOPH devotes about 70 percent of the teaching to traditional concepts and about 30 percent to principles of Western medicine. Thus, a traditional practitioner may be free to use penicillin, digitalis, and other "modern" pharmaceuticals if his herbal preparations do not seem to be working. If a case is believed to require surgical intervention, it is supposed to be referred to a Western doctor, since the traditional field does not include surgical techniques. An uncertain number of traditional doctors, however, have learned their calling only by apprenticeship to an older practitioner, and have not been exposed to such broadly designed education.

Expansion of the output of Western-type physicians in China has been phenomenal. As previously noted, under the Kuomintang government the stock of Western physicians had been increased to reach nearly 13,000 by 1945, and the MOPH reports that by the time of liberation in 1949 the number had reached 38,000. By increasing the medical colleges and enlarging the enrollments of most of them, the national census of medical students in 1985 exceeded 157,000 in 86 colleges or medical universities. These centers of higher education were founded and operated predominantly by provincial governments, associated with large provincial hospitals, but some came directly under the national MOPH, and some belonged to municipalities, county governments, or even enterprises (such as the railroads).

The duration and content of medical education have fluctuated in the various changing political periods since 1949, and general uniformity had not been achieved even by 1988. The most common schedule became a 5-year program of higher medical education, usually after completion of secondary school (about 10 grades altogether). Several medical colleges, however, provided training for 6 years, and one—the rehabilitated Peking Union Medical College—still aimed to train an elite medical leadership with a curriculum of 8 years. All modern medical schools give some instruction in the basic principles of traditional Chinese medicine. Medical education is essentially free to all students admitted, although about $12 a month must be paid for food and for some books (charges waived for very poor students.) All medical students are required to live in dormitories provided by the school.

By 1986 China had a total of 602,200 Western-type physicians, or 57.1 per 100,000 population. Because of the country's huge size and population, these doctors were located mainly in hospitals and large health centers in towns or cities, but not only in the few coastal cities to which modern medicine was confined in preliberation days. In 1977, China had 53 cities, located throughout all the provinces, with populations of 100,000 or more, and 48 of these had more than 300,000 people. As elsewhere, the urban population continues to grow, although China's policy of decentralized industrialization may slow down urbanization below the rate occurring in other large countries.

Although it is not frequently discussed, China's health system depends substantially on a large supply of assistant doctors, first developed in the postliberation decade under the influence of the Soviet Union. These are not to be confused with the very briefly trained barefoot doctors or with nurses; they are modeled essentially after the Soviet feldsher. They are trained in *secondary medical schools,* organized mainly by the county governments and numbering 550 in 1985. Entry usually requires middle school qualification (about seven grades), but this varies. The training typically takes 3 and sometimes 4 years, and includes instruction in diagnosis and treatment of common ailments as well as all forms of prevention; even minor surgery is taught. In spite of the ending of Soviet collaboration after 1960, these personnel have still been trained and numbered 473,000 (45 per 100,000) by 1986. Assistant doctors are the mainstay in staffing township health centers, rural hospitals, and various types of clinics throughout China.

Of special interest is the multiplicity of functions of the 550 secondary medical schools just noted. In addition to training Western-oriented assistant doctors, 79 of these schools in 1985 were also training assistant doctors of traditional medicine. Technicians for laboratory work were trained in 83 of these schools, and many schools trained pharmaceutical assistants or drug dispensers. The secondary medical schools also train nurses, who have an important role in China. The nurse is trained for 3 years after middle school, and her functions are especially well-developed for services to children and on the reproductive problems of women, aside from the usual bedside care of patients in hospitals. In 1986 China had 637,000 nurses and an additional 75,500 trained midwives, with a total of 67.6 per 100,000. Also, the stock of trained health manpower includes pharmacists, prepared in higher medical institutions, and pharmacy assistants or dispensers, trained at the secondary medical schools; there were 33,000 pharmacists and nearly 90,000 dispensers in 1986.

Finally, China's health personnel in 1986 included the post-Mao successors to the barefoot doctors, so abundant during the Cultural Revolution. After 1976, government policy called not for elimination but for upgrading the quality of work of these briefly trained peasants. Their training was increased by a few months and strengthened with more intensive continuing education, sometimes for a whole year. Supervision from the township (formerly the commune) level was increased. Examinations were given, and those who passed (perhaps 60 to 80 percent) were designated *village doctors* or *rural doctors* (varying with the translation from Chinese to English). Examinations could be repeated once, but those who continued to fail would be considered rural health aides or orderlies, authorized to do preventive work but not treatments. The total number of village personnel declined from a peak of 1,800,000 barefoot doctors in 1975 to 1,247,000 village doctors in 1989 (according to the estimate of one MOPH official). In the village, at the former level of *production brigades,* these personnel are still clearly important.

Health Facilities. All types of health facilities in China continued to expand and improve in the Period of Four Modernizations. Although translation of *hospital,* in contrast to *health center,* presents problems, if we recognize hospitals as facilities at the level of a county or municipality and above, by 1985 these had been increased to 11,500 structures, with 1,487,000 beds. In addition, there were patient beds in almost every health center for ambulatory care, bringing the total bed supply in 1985 to 2,229,000. This meant an overall ratio of about 2.1 beds per 1,000 population—an enormous increase over preliberation days.

Almost all hospitals in China have been controlled, since 1949, by some unit of government, mainly the counties and provinces. Missionary hospitals were taken over after the revolution. Since about 1980, the government has encouraged groups of doctors and other health personnel to take full responsibility for running hospitals as private enterprises, but the extent of such management is not clear. In addition to general hospitals, which are most common in the larger cities, there are special hospitals for infectious diseases, cancer, mental illness, maternity, children, and so on. Of the total, 1,414 hospitals (12 percent) are oriented mainly to traditional medicine.

Quite separate from hospitals are convalescent sanataria, operated mainly by labor unions and industrial enterprises, developed in the period of Soviet influence. During the Cultural Revolution, most of these "rest homes" for workers were closed down, but in the 1980s they were reopened and by 1985 numbered 640, with places for 106,000 occupants. As in the USSR, physical therapy is emphasized in these facilities. On the other hand, China is just beginning to study institutional needs of the elderly and chronically ill, for whom very few special facilities exist.

Also stemming from the period of Soviet influence, throughout the counties and municipalities of China there are special small units for sanitation and antiepidemic work. These have been gradually increased to 3,410 such units in 1985. At the county level, there were also 2,724 special facilities for maternal and child care in 1985. These structures handle childbirths and offer simple primary care, preventive and therapeutic, to expectant women and small children. They numbered 4,600 in 1957, but as their work was absorbed into the programs of general hospitals and health centers, they declined to 2,000 units in 1975; since then they have increased to 2,724 specialized maternal and child health facilities.

Below the county level, for each of the former 27,000 communes (now townships) and the municipal districts, there is nearly always at least one (sometimes two or three) health center for general primary health care, preventive and curative. These structures usually have a few short-stay beds, but their principal service is to the ambulatory patient. In 1986 there were about 48,100 such facilities, averaging one per 22,000 people. Those in larger cities were usually staffed with both Western and traditional doctors, as well as assistant doctors, nurses, and others, averaging 18.6 personnel in each. In the small towns that serve as trade centers for rural townships, they might be staffed only by assistant doctors, both Western and traditional, plus other personnel.

Another health facility, reflecting the period of Soviet influence, is the emergency or first-aid station attached to hospitals in large cities. Because of China's lack of motor vehicles, they are not equipped with ambulances, but 75 such specialized stations are prepared to handle disaster problems in the main municipalities. In addition, one or two hospitals in each city, without a fully developed first-aid station, have out-patient departments capable of helping in major disasters.

Finally, in China's thousands of villages or the village-clusters, formerly called *production brigades,* there are small extremely simple health stations or clinics. In 1985 these amounted to 126,600 structures. Sometimes they are newly built places with two or three rooms, but more often the units are simply developed from converted houses, stores, or former schools. Here the village doctor and his or her aide see local patients, give treatment for minor ailments, and offer immunizations, family planning advice, and other preventive service. A crucial role of these units is to serve as the point of entry to the entire health system, from which the patient may be referred to a health center or hospital.

Commodities and Knowledge. Regarding various pharmaceutical products, the situation with China's pattern of combined Western and traditional medicine is very complex. Since 1949, the country has developed 800 pharmaceutical plants with 360,000 employees, producing virtually all types of modern drugs (antibiotics, oral contraceptives, anticarcinogens, etc.) amounting to some 3,000 compounds. Not only has China managed to meet its own modern drug needs, but more than 300 types of drugs are exported to other countries. Relatively few modern pharmaceuticals have to be imported.

In addition, more than 480 factories have been developed in China to manufacture some 3,800 kinds of traditional herbal drugs. These are distributed throughout the country and sold to more than 80 foreign nations. These medicinal herbs are grown not only in small plots everywhere, but also on large mechanized farms.

For distribution, the central Ministry of Commerce maintains six national drug and chemical reagent depots. The provinces, autonomous regions, and major municipalities maintain pharmaceutical warehouses, which numbered 360 in 1985. In the counties there are also some 3,000 pharmaceutical companies for the wholesale handling of drugs. Finally, at the point of contact with patients are pharmacies or drugstores, which function either as independent units (about 20,000) or as part of hospitals or health centers (about 50,000).

The exact ownership of these drug production and distribution resources in the current post-Mao years is not clear. After liberation, in the period of Soviet influence, drug production was largely under the central Ministry of Petroleum and Chemicals, even though in the provinces the provincial government also participated in the management process. The central Ministry of Commerce was responsible for general drug distribution, but retail outlets, where patients purchased drugs, were operated or supervised by the Ministry of Public Health. Since 1976, with the emphasis on private or cooperative ownership and free-market processes, the management of pharmaceutical affairs has been turned over in large part to the private sector.

A final resource in China's health system is the production and dissemination of medical and related knowledge. In the first postliberation decade a central Academy of Medical Sciences was established, with ties to the MOPH, under which several research institutes investigated major disease problems. Gradually, the Ministry of Public Health found it helpful to organize a separate Academy of Traditional Chinese Medicine and also an Academy of Preventive Medicine. In 1985, therefore, there were three central academies, with 16 research institutes attached to the first, and 8 to each of the other two. In addition, separate research institutes on selected health problems are associated with medical schools and major hospitals throughout China, 307 discrete medical research institutes in the country altogether, with nearly 23,000 research personnel, in 1985. The content of Chinese medical research need not be explored, except to note the remarkable development of general anesthesia by acupuncture, in which worldwide interest has been aroused.

Since 1977, China has shown exceptional interest in "learning from the West." Thousands of the brightest young men and women have been sent abroad to study in all aspects of basic sciences, medicine, and public health. Foreign journals and books are imported copiously, and almost all medical students study a foreign language, especially English. Professors from America and Europe are invited to Chinese universities to teach entire courses, and countless foreign publications in the health sciences are translated into Chinese. National conferences on health subjects, addressed by foreign experts, typically invite representatives of all provinces and major municipalities to attend. In contrast to its earlier nationalistic pride, in matters of science and technology China has clearly adopted an open door policy.

Organizational Structure

From the previous account, it is evident that the major organization for all aspects of China's health system has been and remains the Ministry of Public Health (MOPH). The headquarters in Beijing, however, by no means functions as a monolithic central authority, but rather as a center of policy leadership to the provinces and autonomous regions, which have considerable autonomy, especially since the changes in 1977. Beside the MOPH, cer-

tain other government bodies are also concerned with health, as well as various health activities outside of government, including a purely private sector.

Ministry of Public Health. The structure of government agencies inevitably changes with evolving problems, but in 1984 the principal divisions of MOPH headquarters included (1) health and epidemic prevention, (2) medical administration, (3) science and education, (4) maternal and child health, (5) pharmaceutical administration, (6) traditional medicine, (7) planning and finance, and several other divisions concerned with supportive administrative and personnel matters. In addition, there were a high-level General Office for Patriotic Health Campaigns, several especially important medical colleges, the three research academies, one large hospital in Beijing, and offices for several health publications.

In each of the 21 mainland provinces (leaving Taiwan aside), 5 autonomous regions, and 3 centrally administered municipalities there is a Department or Bureau of Public Health, responsible for almost all health activities within its jurisdiction. General policies of the central MOPH are supposed to be followed, but the very wide leeway in their implementation is underscored by the fact that some 90 percent of government financing of health services must come from within each province, and hardly 10 percent from the national level (see later). The organized subdivisions for health work in the provinces are not uniform but vary with the nature of local problems and the interests of provincial political and health leaders.

Each of the counties within the provinces also has a Bureau of Public Health, responsible for the county-level hospitals, antiepidemic work, patriotic health campaigns, distribution of pharmaceuticals, operation of secondary medical schools, supervision of township health services, and so on. Most of the 2,300 counties of China have populations of more than 200,000 people, so their health administrative responsibilities are substantial. The health director is nearly always a Western-type physician, but he tends to be one who commands general respect among doctors and is politically acceptable, rather than one who has had formal training in public health or health care management.

Below the county level, in the townships, usually served by health centers with a small number of beds, there is ordinarily no public health administrative office. If the county public health authority requires cooperation on a problem at this level, help is sought from the staff of the health center. At the next most local level in the villages, equivalent help is sought from the staffs of village health stations.

In cities, and especially in the 53 municipalities with more than 100,000 population, there are also typically Bureaus of Public Health. The largest cities—of which at least 20 have populations of over 1 million people—have districts, some of which have their own health administrative organizations. Municipal public health authorities have special responsibilities for maintaining safe water and sanitary waste disposal.

Other Government Agencies. For certain aspects of the health system, other government agencies play a part. As noted, the production of pharamaceutical products concerns the Ministry of Petroleum and Chemicals, and the distribution of drugs concerns the Ministry of Commerce. Medical equipment is produced under the supervision of the Ministry of Light Industry. Standards for safe conditions in the workplace are issued by the Ministry of Labor, in cooperation with the MOPH.

In the elementary instruction of students in public schools, education about personal hygiene plays a significant part in China; standards for such instruction are established by the Ministry of Education nationally and its counterparts in the provinces and lower local units. The school authorities also work jointly with the public health personnel to ensure hygienic school environments and perform physical examinations of school children. Although China has made enormous progress in the education of its children, deficiencies in rural areas are still serious. As of 1986, of all school-age children in the nation only about 55 percent were reported to be enrolled in school.

Most of the medical colleges, for training both Western-type and Chinese traditional doctors, are financed by provincial bureaus of higher education, although they are all expected to abide by MOPH standards.

The military forces of the Ministry of National Defense are substantial in China, and they maintain their own medical resources and services. In 1986, the People's Liberation Army (PLA) and associated groups in the air force and navy were reported to have nearly 3,000,000 troops; the medical facilities for this large a number of men must be substantial. Chinese leaders emphasize that PLA personnel are not restricted to military functions, but participate in general construction projects, popular education, and other aspects of national development.

Another important government function concerns insurance for medical care costs—known generally as *health insurance*—which involves responsibility by the Ministry of Finance, the Ministry of Labor, and numerous government enterprises. The economic aspects are discussed later, but here we note that, unlike most of China's population, certain sections are collectively protected for the costs of various types of medical care. Four such insurances exist, each managed by a separate agency or type of agency: (1) insurance for central government employees (but not dependents), handled by the Ministry of Finance; (2) insurance for the workers in national or provincial government enterprises and their dependents, handled by each enterprise and supervised generally by the Ministry of Labor (MOL); (3) insurance for workers in enterprises run by the counties, municipalities, townships, or other local levels of government, with some protection for dependents, supervised by the MOL; and (4) health cooperatives for farm families working in the former communes and current townships. Each of these medical care insurance programs has numerous limitations in benefits, which are considered later. The fiscal aspects of their operation are quite outside the jurisdiction of the MOPH.

Nongovernment Organizations. Outside of government at some level, there are relatively few organized programs in China. Those relevant to health are of two principal types: associations of professional health personnel and agencies devoted to tackling specific disease problems.

The Chinese Medical Association was founded in 1915, soon after the first revolution ending the empire. Its activities have been largely related to the continuing education of physicians on advances in medical science, international relations with the profession in other countries, and recommendation of certain health policies to government. In 1986, the association had 42 special societies and 360 local branches with 110,000 members.

Equivalent professional associations exist in traditional Chinese medicine (21,000 members), pharmacy (21,330 members), nursing (about 170,000 subscribers to its journal), and the Combination of Traditional Chinese Medicine and Western Schools of Medicine. The latter society had 9,200 members in 1985, but it published a journal that went to 60,000 subscribers at home and abroad. The major professional associations have branches in every province.

Among voluntary agencies oriented to disease problems in China, the Anti-Tuberculosis Association, founded in 1933, is important. Its function is mainly to educate both the people and health personnel. In 1985 it had some 10,000 members, with branches in all provinces. A Mental Health Association, started in 1936, was quiescent until its recent growth to 4,000 members. In the 1980s, an Anti-Cancer Association and an Anti-Leprosy Association were started. Relatively new also are an Anti-Smoking Association and a Family Planning Association. The two latter groups, which promote educational objectives of the MOPH, receive small financial subsidies from the central government. Similarly an old Chinese Red Cross Society has been reactivated, to help in emergencies and collect human blood for banking, and branches exist in most provinces.

The Chinese Communist Party. Theoretically outside of government, the Chinese Communist Party (CCP) is obviously crucial to determination and implementation of official pol-

icy in all aspects of Chinese society, including the national health system. The background and mode of operation of this organized movement have been explored extensively elsewhere, and here we simply note that since 1949 China has been essentially ruled by this single major political party, although its dominant ideology has fluctuated over the several historic periods reviewed in this chapter. In 1977, after the death of Mao Zedong, the predominant viewpoint, shaped largely by Deng Xiaoping, favored substantial enlargement of private management and market principles in all aspects of economic and social life. This had an obvious influence on the health system.

The CCP organization is roughly parallel with the structure of government, with a National Party Congress, a Central Committee, committees at provincial, municipal, and county levels, and in townships, urban districts, and villages. In addition, at virtually all large and medium-sized places of work, including health establishments, small CCP branches may exist. Since 1945 the CCP has had five constitutions to guide policy, the most recent one being adopted in 1977 after the death of Mao. The latter document stresses the importance of full and free discussion of all issues before decisions are reached, while still prescribing review of decisions of lower-level bodies by higher echelons and emphasizing general discipline. Membership in the CCP is by election of the local branch or committee, and has generally included no more than 4 percent of the population. It has doubtless been the pervasive influence of the CCP organization throughout the entire society that has been responsible for the relatively rapid implementation of China's health policies, such as the patriotic campaigns on pests, the extensive establishment of health centers, the training of barefoot doctors, or the combining of Western and traditional medicine.

The Private Market. In the post-Mao "modernization" years, a private market for health service has not been considered a residual part of the system structure, as in so many other countries. Rather, it has been deliberately encouraged. In China, both before and after liberation, personal payments were required for public services, as well as for the private services of traditional practitioners. The new emphasis since about 1980 has been to expect private payment for services of Western or modern character—services given by personnel engaged entirely in private practice or by government professionals (even assistant doctors or village doctors) who do this after their official duties are completed. The extent of the latter is not known, but an MOPH report for 1989 states that there were 138,000 private practitioners, presumably meaning exclusively private. Since the same MOPH publication refers to a total of 1,482,000 "medical doctors . . . of both Western and traditional Chinese medicine" in China, this suggests that about 9.3 percent of the total are exclusively private. This figure probably also includes private stomatalogists or dentists.

Another form of private provision of health service in China is the sale of drugs by pharmacies, owned by private individuals or perhaps partners or cooperatives. Since this sort of small business does not require a major investment to start, it is probably extensive in China's cities, especially for the sale of herbal medications, but statistics are not available.

As of 1989, purely privately owned or even cooperatively owned hospitals were not known to exist in China. Hospitals may be operated by "collectively owned" productive enterprises, which operate at a county, municipal, or even more local echelon. Such entities may earn a profit (or suffer a loss) for their members, but they are not private in the usual sense. Likewise, health centers at the township level have sometimes come predominantly under collective or local control, although they cannot be considered private.

The most important aspect of private exchange in China's health system is not in the delivery or provision of services, but in the payment for services rendered by public resources. Except for persons protected by the medical care insurance programs noted earlier, almost everyone must pay for health services—with certain exceptions, such as contraceptive materials. The nature and extent of these payments and expenditures are discussed below.

Economic Support

From the onset of the People's Republic of China, this socialist country differed from other such countries in regarding health services like food or other commodities, customarily requiring payment. Government at the national, provincial, and lower levels took extensive action to develop health resources, to mount campaigns for preventing disease, to educate the population on personal hygiene, and so on, but the delivery of services was not made a government obligation and it had to be paid for. Through extensive social and economic planning, the prices were carefully regulated and kept relatively low, but individuals and families were still charged fees.

A remarkably comprehensive study of the health sector in China was issued by the World Bank (for official use) in 1984. This study estimated that total health expenditures in 1981 constituted 3.3 percent of GDP, of which 95.3 percent was for recurrent purposes and 4.7 percent for capital construction. The costs of construction of hospitals, health centers, and other health facilities are derived entirely from funds of the central, provincial, or lower levels of government. The various sources of the 95.3 percent of health expenditures, devoted to recurrent costs, which are calculated to include health personnel education as well as health services, are worth analyzing.

Overall Recurrent Expenditures. In spite of the policy that health services must be paid for, soon after liberation actions were taken to support those costs for selected groups in the population. In 1951, the central government decided to cover the costs of general health service for government employees at the national and provincial levels (but not their dependents). University teachers and students were also covered by this scheme. In the same year, government enterprises at national or provincial levels also took action to support "labor insurance" for their workers and partially for their dependents. Somewhat later, enterprises at lower echelons (counties and townships, municipalities and districts) began to institute similar medical care insurance schemes voluntarily. Still later, during the Cultural Revolution, production brigades often organized *health care cooperatives* to help finance certain medical expenses.

In the meantime, the national government continued its partial support of personnel salaries in urban and rural health facilities, most preventive service, health manpower education, certain pharmaceuticals, and medical research. Provincial governments covered most of these costs. A substantial balance remained to be paid by the individual patient or family.

For 1981, the World Bank estimated the percentage distribution of these sources of China's recurrent health expenditures to be approximately as follows:

Source	Percentage
Government: national or provincial	30
Enterprise labor insurance	31
Commune or village cooperatives	7
Private individuals	32
All sources	100

Estimates could also be made on the health purposes for which these recurrent expenditures were made in 1981. Their percent distribution was as follows:

Purpose	Percentage
Western pharmaceuticals	48.7
Traditional herbal medication	9.2
Salaried health personnel	20.3
Hospitalization (except salaries)	13.0
Medical equipment	4.9
Barefoot doctors, aides, and birth attendants	3.9
All purposes	100.0

Especially conspicuous, of course, is the high proportion of expenditures devoted to Western pharmaceuticals, even though practically all of these are manufactured in China rather than imported.

Health Insurance. The several types of insurance or equivalent financial protection noted earlier differ in their operational features. The protection for government employees at national or provincial levels, often called *Government Insurance,* is nearly comprehensive in scope of services financed, although it omits dependents. In spite of the term *insurance,* entitlement to cost protection is not linked to any employee or even payroll contribution. The funds simply come to each government agency from the general revenues of the Ministry of Finance, and are considered a line item in the budget of the Ministry of Public Health at central or provincial levels. No copayments are required from government employees, except for the cost of meals in hospitals, which in China are customarily regarded as the responsibility of the patient or his or her family.

Medical care is delivered for persons with government insurance at facilities maintained by the agency, equivalent to those in a military unit. Otherwise the patient can seek care at any convenient health facility, where he or she must pay the charge and then seek reimbursement from the official department.

Labor Insurance in national or provincial-level enterprises is essentially the same for the primary worker. Large plants, with more than 100 workers, may have a clinic at the workplace, but the employee is free to seek care outside, for which he or she must pay and then be reimbursed. In large cities, the enterprise often has contracts with certain hospitals, to which the cost of the worker's care is paid directly by the enterprise. Dependents are covered, but reimbursement is received at only 50 percent of the official rate. To discourage overutilization, as well as to collect additional funds, under labor insurance the patient, both primary worker and dependent, is required to pay a small *registration fee* for access to any ambulatory service. At lower levels of enterprise, such as employment by a county or a township, the benefits available to dependents are sometimes less than 50 percent of charges.

The health insurance schemes at the level of smaller townships or villages, usually known as *rural health cooperatives,* have been the least stable and provide the most uncertain benefits. In 1981, when the comprehensive Health Sector study of the World Bank was applicable, there were 714,700 *production brigades,* of which 58 percent still had rural health cooperatives (after a peak of 85 percent in 1975). Although it was theoretically voluntary for families, when the leadership of a commune decided to have such a cooperative, with annual membership premiums from each family, virtually every family joined. The financial benefits, however, varied with the general income level of the commune. For the services of village doctors at the local health station, the cost protection was usually complete, but for the use of a township health center, a county hospital or higher-level facility, the reimbursement was seldom complete and might be as low as 40 percent for everyone (primary worker and dependents).

After the responsibility policy in the early 1980s led to the termination of communes and their conversion to townships, these rural health cooperatives gradually declined, to probably under 10 percent of townships by 1988. In the late 1980s, many other changes occurred in the spectrum of economic support for health services in China.

Commentary and Economic Trends. As a reflection of the overall priorities for health in China, the trend of expenditures reflects strikingly the changing policies. Resource inputs in 1957 suggest that at this time, in the first post-liberation decade, all health spending amounted to 2.3 percent of GDP. We have noted that by 1981, this had increased to 3.3 percent. Studies in the late 1980s showed that health spending was rising more rapdily than the growth of GDP, so that by 1987 total spending for the Chinese health system had reached about 4.0 percent of GDP.

In spite of the greater attention to health care in the rural areas, analysis of data reported in 1983 showed that government expenditures (central and provincial levels) for health per capita were still much higher for city residents than for country-dwellers. In cities, government subsidies supported more than three-quarters of health expenditures, but less than one-third in rural areas. The total amount of money spent for health purposes, furthermore, was much higher per capita among city resi-

dents than among rural. Of course, comparisons are complicated by the fact that many rural people seek medical care in city hospitals. Even so, the rural peasant must use more of his modest personal income for health care, which in urban families is much more generously financed by government subsidy or social insurance.

Considering the economic support for China's health system as a whole, the strong emphasis after 1980 on personal responsibility, rather than collective action, was bound to modify the proportions of health funds derived from various sources, as well as the purposes for which these funds were spent. Data that have not been published suggest that, as of about 1987, the proportion of health expenditures coming from both government insurance and labor insurance at large enterprises rose both absolutely and in relation to the total. Funding from rural health cooperatives declined sharply, as these communal projects came to an end. Large numbers of uninsured rural people, as a result, were required to pay greater amounts out-of-pocket for medical care.

Regarding China's policy toward health insurance, the practice of maintaining separate funds for different socioeconomic groups seems to be accepted without question. Yet, as many other countries have found, social insurance can give equitable protection only by pooling contributions from all types of people—the old and the young, the rural and the urban, the sick and the well, the worker and the professional, and so on. Commercial insurance, concerned with profits, divides its subscribers into risk groups, but social insurance or social security is based on maximum pooling of risks. It is by such principles of social solidarity that health care benefits in countries have been adjusted to diverse personal health needs.

Governmental support (central and provincial levels) of health services has continued to rise absolutely, but not as a proportion of the total. Between 1981 and 1987, greater attention was given to the modernization of medical technology in hospitals, especially the largest ones, at the expense of the basic preventive programs (sanitation, immunizations, health education), from which modern China had made such impressive health gains. Very rough data comparing the source of China's health system expenditures (both recurrent and capital) between 1980 and 1987 helps clarify these post-Mao trends:

	Percentage	
Source of Health Funds	1980	1987
Insurance (all forms)	48	50
Government revenues	35	19
Individuals (patient fees)	17	32
All sources	100	100

A glimpse at these changed proportions inevitably raises questions about the equity of health service distribution in China during the late 1980s, compared with earlier periods.

Health System Management

With all the changes in policies of China's national health system from liberation in October 1949 to the Tiananmen Square "crackdown" on demonstrators in June 1989 (some 40 years) it is not easy to describe and analyze the patterns of health system management. One feature, however, has been clear in all periods—the dominant role played by the Chinese Communist Party (CCP). As noted earlier, from the headquarters of the Central Committee in Beijing to Party cells in the smallest villages, this organization serves to guide and promote policies in the health system, as in all other aspects of society.

But how are those policies formulated in the first place? In contrast with the world pioneer of socialism, the USSR, the political ideology of the CCP is said to emphasize decentralized authority or "local self-reliance." This distinction may be valid with respect to the exact manner in which a policy is implemented. But the general contours and objectives of the policy still appear to be centrally determined. This seems to apply to planning as well as to the administration of programs.

Planning policies for the development of general hospitals in every county, the establishment of health centers for both curative and preventive service in every commune (later township), the training of barefoot doctors to staff small health stations in production brigades (later clusters of villages), the mounting of campaigns against disease vectors such as snails, and so on, these planning decisions were made by the national health leadership. Plans and strategies to carry them out, as we have seen, have allowed wide variations among provinces and, within provinces, between counties. As noted, economic support from the central government has been small; more than 90 percent of funding depends on the economic strength of each province and county. As a result, there are substantial differences in the health resources developed and services rendered in different parts of China. To cope with natural or environmental handicaps, the dominant political slogan is that "hard work can overcome difficulties."

In the Ministry of Public Health, as noted, there is at the central headquarters a Division of Planning and Finance, within which there are sections for statistics, planning, capital construction, and materials. This office must give technical guidance to the provinces, which in turn help the counties. The population of each province of China is so large that for most resources in the health system—building materials for facilities, trained health personnel, or pharmaceutical products—the planning required can be done within the boundaries of the province. Special equipment, of course, such as x-ray machines (produced at only a few places), would require planning on a nationwide scale.

The health system consequences of the Cultural Revolution gave a striking indication of the impact of national leadership on administrative methods. In the drive against elitism and the previously customary forms of authority, the direction of every hospital, health center, and epidemic control station was quite abruptly changed from its former pattern of a single director to control by a revolutionary committee. The composition of this committee, as noted earlier, was quite explicitly prescribed—even though the actual members were locally elected. Previous directors were almost routinely humiliated or punished in some way.

Virtually every component of the health system of China varies in its detailed manner of local implementation. The variations in training personnel from barefoot doctors up to specialists in, say, Western surgery are countless. The methods of operating health insurance schemes in industrial enterprises or in rural communes may vary widely. The rigor with which occupational hygiene standards are enforced differs greatly among different Chinese cities.

Yet the MOPH became aware in the late 1980s of the need for more orderly and effective management of hospitals. It formulated Principles for the Organizational Set-up of General Hospitals, and specified duties of the director, the head nurse, the department heads, and so on. A Hospital Management Society was organized to promote education in modern management methods. Large hospitals are expected to help smaller ones in both clinical and administrative activities.

Regarding *regulation* in the health system, general policies on the control of personnel have been conspicuously different from those in most other countries. China's health leaders stress that they are concerned about a person's capabilities, not his or her formal credentials. Hence, very little is required in the way of licensing or registration. The term *doctor* is applied to personnel educated for various lengths of time and with quite different content of instruction. The same applies to *nurse* and other types of health professional or health workers. Mobility between provinces and even counties is not as great in China as in other large countries, but there has been no need for "reciprocity" in credentials, as long as the person can explain what tasks he has been performing and is capable of doing.

Only as recently as 1986 were provisional regulations issued by a "Central Leading Group on the Medical and Health Professions" in the National People's Congress. (This was not the vote of a parliamentary body.) To put some slight order into a confusing situation, this regulation stated that "Medical and health personnel must cherish a love for the motherland, support the leadership of the Chinese Communist Party, carry out the Party's policies governing medical and health work, observe professional ethics, serve the people

whole-heartedly, and endeavor to contribute to socialist construction and modernization of the country." For specific posts in a health facility, this 1986 regulation called for graduation from a certain sort of school (duration of training not specified) and a defined number of years of practical experience. The latter was especially emphasized, with such formulations for Associate Chief Physicians as "They should make outstanding achievements in work and have fairly rich clinical and technical experience and be capable of solving complicated and difficult problems. . . ."

Regarding standards for food hygiene and the regulation of drugs, there seems to be special concern at the national level in China, with several actions being taken by a Standing Committee of the National People's Congress. A 1982 Provisional Law of this committee stated, for example, that "Undertakings involved in food production and handling must have buildings or premises that are suitable for treating raw materials and for processing, packing, and storage of foods in accordance with the quality of products concerned." The enforcement of such broad national regulations must obviously depend on performance by the bureaus of public health of the provinces, counties, and municipalities.

Regarding drug control, a national law, adopted by the Standing Committee (on health) of the National People's Congress in 1984, specified that "A new drug will be approved for clinical use and a license issued by the Ministry of Public Health, if the clinical trial or clinical verification has been completed and an appraisal of its efficacy has been made."

Below the top, at provincial, county, and municipal levels, people's congresses are also elected. These bodies, or their standing committees, have two functions: (1) to enact any local legislation necessary to implement the directives of the national government, and (2) to adopt any other legislation or regulation consistent with national policy that could be helpful in tackling a uniquely local problem. The latter might be illustrated by the need to control an insect vector of disease, concentrated in certain provinces because of their climate or terrain.

The dominant role of the CCP in determining policy throughout the health system has been emphasized, and an unusual study published in 1988 shows this dramatically. The decline in rural health cooperatives has been noted, and the conventional wisdom in China attributed this to changes in the economic structure of the communes, popular demand for more sophisticated health services, and financial deficits. A field study was made in three randomly selected counties, however, from 1978 to 1986. Using measurements of both process and outcome, it was found that over this 8-year period, the personal health expenditures of families increased, while health consultations and childhood immunizations decreased. With a general elevation of living standards, nutritional status improved and the rate of infectious disease declined. The infant mortality rate, however, in two of the three counties (the two poorest) increased. The researcher concluded that the decline in the rural health cooperatives was not due to any of the three alleged causes listed previously; the county residents were actually favorable to the health cooperatives. Their termination was due, instead, to political directives passed down from above.

Delivery of Health Services

The diverse ways that health services are provided in China, by various types of personnel and in various places, are evident. Here we consider some general features of the delivery of primary health care, hospitalization, and certain other types of service.

Primary Health Care. To most of the world, the prominent achievement of China's health system has been its provision of primary health care (PHC) to almost all of its huge population. Much of this achievement has been equated with the innovative training and development of barefoot doctors, and subsequently the somewhat better trained village doctors and their aides. Effective PHC must also be attributed to the services of more thoroughly educated assistant doctors in thousands of rural health centers and to the work of fully prepared physicians, both Western and traditional, in municipally located health centers

and in the out-patient departments of county hospitals and maternal and child health units.

Below the level of the province, China's health care delivery is often described as a three-tier network—the county hospital, the commune or township health center, and the brigade or village health station. At each of these levels PHC is provided by the appropriately trained type of health workers, with referrals made for cases beyond the local person's ability. At the county hospital, of course, treatment may call for a specialized medical or surgical skill, constituting secondary care. Some observers have noted relatively low rates of use of health stations and even township health centers, when people bypass these facilities to see better-trained personnel at county hospitals—that is, if they can afford the higher charges.

Much of the primary care at the village and township levels, however, is preventive. Family planning guidance, immunizations, education about personal and environmental hygiene, all figure prominently. Family planning is more than a matter of contraceptive devices, however, as we will discuss later. Campaigns against pests or vectors of disease are also important.

Considering expenditures as a rough proxy for services, we have noted that pharmaceuticals, mostly Western but partly traditional, accounted in 1981 for 58 percent of recurrent national health system activities. Some of these drugs were, of course, used in in-patient hospital care, but the great majority were probably consumed by ambulatory patients. Contributing to the huge consumption of drugs in China is a very widespread use of "tonics" by millions of adults, especially in their later years; these may be compounded from traditional herbal materials, from modern synthetic drugs (such as vitamins), or both. On the whole, pharmaceutical expenditures are made largely in support of primary health care.

The traditional practitioner, in both health centers and private practice, is of course a major source of primary health care. Psychosocial symptoms in China, as in many other cultures, tend to be defined as physical ailments. For these, the traditional practitioner and his herbal drugs are often more effective than the remedies of Western medicine. Traditional treatments are also much less expensive—a major consideration, in light of the high expenditures for drugs.

The local and convenient availability of a village health station, according to many observers, creates a sense of well-being in the local population, in spite of the modest technical resources. People know that some type of help is nearby, if needed, and that appropriate referrals can be made to a better-staffed health center or hospital, if necessary. In the late 1980s, the local village doctor was often paid a small salary, and could earn some money from the sale of drugs, in place of the former pattern of remuneration by "work points."

Hospitalization. The relatively low percentage of health expenditures for hospitalization reported earlier (13 percent) may be misleading, since it covers only overhead costs exclusive of salaries and drugs. If one were to make some crude estimates to take account of the latter elements (counting also the 4.9 percent spent for medical equipment), perhaps the overall national expenditure for hospital services would come to 35 to 40 percent of the total. Even this proportion is relatively low, compared with those of many developing countries that were analyzed along these lines. Yet the Four Modernizations, which characterized policy after 1977, have clearly led to an increasing emphasis on hospitals and probably less attention to primary health care.

The delivery of services in the hospitals of China varies, of course, with the size and hierarchical level of the facility. Large urban tertiary hospitals, affiliated with medical schools, are naturally more fully staffed and equipped than small county hospitals in the town serving as trade center for a rural population. The MOPH has reported the professional health personnel for all hospitals in urban districts as of 1985. That year there were 174 such personnel per 100 hospital beds; in rural hospitals the comparable ratio was 137 professional health personnel per 100 beds. Of these personnel, 41 percent were full-time salaried doctors (counting both Western and traditional), 19 percent were nurses, and the remaining 40 percent were technicians and others. Compared with other countries, even of similar low-income level, this staffing seems quite frugal. Such modest staffing may help explain the long average patient-stays, which in urban hospitals of China have typically been more than 20 days.

A tertiary Chinese hospital, studied by American observers in 1980, was found to have a remarkably egalitarian spirit among all the members of its staff. Even 5 years after the end of the Cultural Revolution, it was difficult to distinguish between top-level physicians (who might be men or women), nurses, custodial attendants, and others; they all wore similar white garments and caps. In decision-making on patient care, the views of even the most junior doctor or nurse were solicited at informal sessions. Patients were also invited to express any complaints they might have. Apropos of the medical malpractice issue in other countries, one patient admitted to the tertiary hospital had a strange abdominal tumor; on surgery, her abdomen was found to contain a sponge overlooked after a previous operation at a county hospital. When informed of his negligence, the county surgeon apologized, but no legal action was taken because he had not "intended" to make this mistake.

In light of the low earnings of most Chinese people, especially in rural areas, the cost of hospitalization is very high. The charges for a hospital case are typically equivalent to several times a person's monthly earnings, even up to the annual income of some peasants. As a result, uninsured people, mainly rural, are seldom hospitalized, unless they have an infectious disease (such as malaria or schistosomiasis), for which no charge is made. In one tertiary hospital, intended to serve a large territory, 72 percent of the patients were from the adjacent urban sections and only 28 percent from the large surrounding rural areas where most of the people lived. Distance, of course, is an obstacle, but the impediment of costs is clear. Since the demise of rural health cooperatives, few rural people have insurance coverage.

Health Insurance Coverage. Since insurance protection is so important for providing access to health care in China, as elsewhere, what is the degree of population coverage? Only rough estimates are possible.

As of 1987, the Government Insurance covered about 22,000,000 employees. The benefits were quite comprehensive, without any copayments required. The Labor Insurance scheme for government enterprise workers, at both national and provincial levels, provided services or cost protection to about 71,000,000 workers, plus 50 percent reimbursement to their dependents. A household survey in 1981 found only 0.77 dependent per primary worker (since most spouses are also workers), thus, these dependents, with partial protection, would add another 55,000,000 people.

"Collectively owned" enterprises, essentially at the county level, have been estimated to provide insurance coverage for 36,000,000 workers. Enterprises (nonagricultural) at township or even village levels may provide health care coverage for another 90,000,000. Adding dependents, even though their benefits are typically much weaker, brings this unevenly insured population to about 223,000,000.

Remnants of the old rural health cooperatives are found in the Shanghai region and some other parts of China. As a percentage of the peasant population, one might guess no more than 5 percent, or perhaps 30,000,000 people.

Altogether, insurance for medical care costs—ranging from complete to very partial—around 1987 was approximately as follows:

Type of Health Insurance	Estimated Number (millions)
Government employees	22
Government enterprises	71
Dependents of enterprise workers	55
County enterprises	36
Township and village enterprises	90
Dependents of local workers	97
Rural agricultural cooperatives	30
All types of insurance	401

In relation to China's 1987 population, this amounts to about 40 percent of the total with some degree of health insurance protection.

We know, however, that the benefits for dependents are very limited, and even the insurance coverage of primary workers at the level of townships and below is seldom complete and dependable. In light of these factors, it is probably safest to estimate that in 1987, for China's huge population exceeding 1 billion people, insurance protection for medical care costs was approximately as follows: (1) comprehensive benefits—20 percent; (2) limited benefits—20 percent; and (3) no significant insurance benefits—60 percent. These are, of course, not only crude estimates, but they change from year to year. As in other countries, however, it seems highly likely that access to treatment services in China is directly proportional to health insurance protection. The uninsured people, mainly rural, are forced to spend greater shares of their meager personal incomes on health care costs, but they still receive less care than the insured.

Regarding preventive health services, even these must be paid for since the economic "reforms" of the 1980s. If a person has insurance, fees must be paid for immunizations and prenatal examinations. (For persons without any insurance the requirement is not clear.) Studies of health expenditure trends between 1981 and 1987 show that the greatest increases have occurred in spending by insurance funds and in personal payments, and the least change in spending by general government revenues. Government support for the antiepidemic stations seems to have declined relatively. All of these trends, though they show increased health expenditures in China both absolutely and as a share of GDP, also point to a less egalitarian distribution of services in relation to needs, an erosion of principles of health equity.

These economic trends, linked to the enrollment in health insurance and to modified spending from the general government budget, point to changing priorities in health care delivery. Most dramatic has been an increasing share of support for larger higher-level hospitals, and a decreasing share of support for township health centers and antiepidemic stations. The demands made on higher-level hospitals by well-insured urban people only add to the pressures for them to acquire more sophisticated technology.

Family Planning. Efforts to slow the rate of population growth in China have undergone various swings in policy since liberation in 1949. The first 4 years, Chinese leadership rejected any idea of a population problem, and actually encouraged fertility. From 1954 to 1962, the policy changed for and against birth control several times. Then in 1968, national policy crystallized in a strong position to limit further population growth. Once this position was firmly reached, China pursued a policy of family planning vigorously throughout the nation, a policy unequalled in its effectiveness by that of any other large developing country in the world. From the national government headquarters, through the provinces and counties down to the villages, there are official Birth Planning Committees to supervise this entire program.

Notable in China's family planning (FP) program is its very broad social approach. The details have changed from year to year, but the strategy includes much more than promoting contraceptive techniques. It includes such policies as (1) encouraging relatively late marriages: 23 years for men and 20 years for women; these and older ages were made legal requirements for marriage; (2) incentives for a maximum of two children (later one child) per family: priorities in access to housing, for example, went to the smaller family; (3) extensive dissemination of knowledge and devices or pills for contraception (see later); (4) legalization of abortion, essentially on request; and (5) the general emancipation of women, so that they see their role as broader than that of raising children.

The implementation of FP strategies on contraception has involved far-flung activities in national planning. Intrauterine devices are widely used, and these had to be properly manufactured. Many women prefer the contraceptive pill, and the Chinese pharmaceutical industry produced billions of these, in a dosage calculated to minimize complications. In contrast to other pharmaceutical products, these pills are distributed free of charge. To simplify recourse to abortion, if necessary, the woman is entitled to time off from work with pay. Distribution of contraceptive pills and education are functions of every barefoot doctor or his or her successor. Insertion of intrauterine devices is done at any health center. Health education to dramatize the advantages of a one-child family is widespread throughout China.

Other Services. A few other features of health care delivery in China are worth noting. With the emphasis on small families, every effort is made to ensure complete safety in childbirth. In 1986 it was reported that 97 percent of childbirths were attended by some type of trained personnel, and most of these occurred in MOPH health facilities. Inability to pay the official charge is never an impediment to an inpatient delivery. Breast-feeding was declining in the cities, but it is being widely encouraged. As noted, hundreds of facilities specialize in maternal and child care, including childbirths.

Occupational health work has been attracting greater attention in China, as the country has become increasingly industrialized. In the first two decades after liberation, the haste to develop factories often resulted in neglect of precautions for worker safety. After the onset of the Four Modernizations, large government industrial projects under construction were reduced from around 1700 in 1978 to 600 in 1981, while smaller enterprises, owned collectively at the county or township levels, were greatly expanded. The latter are lighter industry, producing furniture, clothing, appliances, and other goods, and quasi-private in ownership, although often helped by government loans. Strictly speaking, they are outside the sphere of government, and less likely to observe standards of industrial hygiene. Accordingly, the need for surveillance of working conditions to protect the worker has become more conspicuous, and efforts are underway to reduce the major hazards: occupational lung disease, chemical intoxication, physical hazards, and occupational cancer. On many problems, progress has not been clear, but for silicosis there is strong evidence of its substantial reduction in mines and industrial plants since 1960.

The great ingenuity of China's health workers is well illustrated by the response of barefoot doctors to infantile diarrhea. Apparently before the well-packaged salt–suger mixtures, distributed by UNICEF for oral rehydration therapy (ORT), were available, mothers were being advised to prepare simple salt and sugar solutions for their sick infants at home. Measurements of the ingredients were not accurate, but the treatment was evidently effective. County hospitals, on the other hand, were using intravenous infusions, since these were considered to be more "scientific." This was reported in 1984, and indicates the continuing need for education in China, to distinguish science from pseudoscience.

Some Health Status Outcomes

As an outcome of all these developments of the health system of China and, more important, the general socioeconomic development of China after its emergence from the semifeudal society existing before 1911, the health status of the Chinese people has shown amazing improvements. The gains have clearly been greatest since the socialist liberation of 1949, and they have continued to show further advances through all the periods of political change since then.

The rampant infectious disease, malnutrition, opium addiction, and general human misery in preliberation China have been reported by countless observers. Even without exact numbers on malaria, plague, tuberculosis, schistosomiasis, syphilis, leprosy, cholera, typhoid fever, smallpox, trachoma, and more, the incidence and prevalence of these pestilential diseases earned Old China the epithet of being "the sick man of Asia."

Health status changes, for which statistical data are available, apply to more recent decades. Even so, the infant mortality rate declined from 150 infant deaths per 1,000 live births in 1960 to 33 per 1,000 in 1987. The mortality rate under 5 years of age declined from 202 per 1,000 in 1960 to 45 in 1987. The life expectancy at birth in China before 1949 is not known, but it is usually estimated at under 40 years. By 1960 it was 47 years. In 1979, it had been extended to 64 years, and life expectancy at birth in 1987 was 70 years.

The crude birth rate in China in 1960 had been 37 per 1,000 population. By 1987 it was reduced to 20 births per 1,000. The use of contraception was reported in the period 1981 to

1985 to be 74 percent of women in the childbearing years—a rate higher than that in the United States. The maternal mortality rate in China in the late 1980s was 44 per 100,000 (when in India, with approximately the same GNP per capita, it was 500 per 100,000).

Leading causes of death in any country reflect a good deal about the accomplishments of its health system and its general social order. Such data are available for a sample of 36 cities and 72 counties throughout China, on which the MOPH has collected vital statistics. In 1985, the major causes of death were as follows:

		Deaths per 100,000	
Rank	Cause of Death	Cities	Counties
1.	Heart diseases	131.0	165.8
2.	Cerebrovascular diseases	117.5	101.3
3.	Malignant tumors	113.9	98.8
4.	Respiratory diseases	50.9	79.7
5.	Digestive diseases	23.3	35.5

Noteworthy is the absence of any communicable diseases among the five major causes of death, in both cities and counties (which are substantially rural). The five leading causes of death in cities accounted for 78 percent of the total of such deaths, and in counties the five leading causes accounted for 74 percent of the total. The basic mortality profile is like that of an affluent developed country.

With the more recent emphasis on modern technology in China and the policy that each local health facility must be largely self-supporting, the priorities for primary health care and prevention may eventually change. It remains to be seen whether such changes will alter the remarkable health indices in China's population achieved up to now.

TAIWAN—A NOTE

The island of Taiwan, east of People's China and south of Japan, to which the Nationalist government of Kuomintang China fled in

1949, has developed a prosperous society. Known formerly as Formosa (a Portuguese term), the island was ruled by Japan from 1895 to 1945, when the World War II settlement returned it to China. The People's Republic regards Taiwan as its last "unliberated" province, but efforts at reunification have not yet been successful.

Taiwan's population in 1988 was about 20,000,000, of whom some 72 percent were urban. The GNP per capita was $3,000, as of 1984 (at least 10 times that of the People's Republic), and was growing rapidly. The Taiwanese economy has been vigorously industrializing, especially with the benefit of massive investments from the United States and other Western powers during the 22 years from 1949 to 1971, when mainland China was essentially "quarantined" by the capitalist world. As a favored little land, with less than 2 percent of the population of mainland China, Taiwanese society strikingly demonstrates the possibilities of great economic development of a former Asian colony under conditions of generous external economic support, internal peace, abundant free trade of commodities and ideas, and a very hard-working population. Only 15 percent of these people, it should be noted, are ethnically of Chinese background and 85 percent are native Taiwanese. While strongly anticommunist, Taiwan is like the PRC in being ruled by a single political party. The dynamic overall development of the society is also reflected in its strong health system.

Health System Structure and Resources

As in the People's Republic of China (PRC), the principal government authority is headquartered in the capital of Taiwan Province, known as Taipei. The agency, called the Department of Health (although before 1971, it was a unit in the Ministry of Interior), has some 15 major operating divisions or offices and several standing committees. The island is divided into 21 counties and two centrally administered cities, each of which has a health bureau that carries out central DOH policies. Within every county are about 10 to 15 townships, 363 in all, each of which has a small health station staffed by one or two nurses.

Nurses are the most numerous type of personnel in Taiwan, numbering 26,270 in 1986; they are trained either to the full professional nurse level in 10 paramedical junior colleges or to the vocational nurse level in 14 paramedical vocational schools. This amounts to 131 nurses of all types per 100,000 people. There are 15,910 Western physicians, or 80 per 100,000, and another 2,000 traditional Chinese doctors. There are eight medical colleges training Western physicians, half of which are governmental and half private (with substantial tuitions payable for enrollment). Of the junior colleges and vocational schools training other personnel, the great majority are privately owned.

This strongly private management of educational institutions is also found in the ownership and mangement of health facilities in Taiwan. Both hospitals and clinics are abundant (clinics being mainly for ambulatory care, but usually containing some beds as well). In 1986, there were 835 hospitals, with 71,173 beds. Of these, 90 percent of the hospitals with 58 percent of the beds were privately owned. In addition, there were 11,202 clinics, of which almost 96 percent were private physician premises and only 4.3 percent public; the latter (487 structures) are, indeed, known as *public clinics,* rather than *health centers.* Clinics also have many patient beds, bringing the total to 81,500 or 4.1 beds per 1,000 population.

National health policy in Taiwan is manifestly oriented toward a private health care market, and yet one can observe certain trends in the other direction. In 1963, some 83 percent of all physicians had been in private practice, but by 1985 this figure had declined to 45 percent. This trend has evidently been due mainly to the engagement of an increasing number of physicians on full-time salaries in public hospitals. While such hospitals are only 10 percent of the total, their average size is large (350 beds), and they have 42 percent of the total beds. Since hospital physicians are typically specialists, their earnings are usually higher than those of community doctors, who are mainly general practitioners, but not as high as earnings of specialists in private practice.

Likewise, the public clinics, though only a small share of the total, tend to be expanding their medical staffs, in response to popular demands. Another strategy for improving access to medical care in rural areas of Taiwan has been a DOH requirement that teaching hospitals establish *group practice centers,* staffed by resident physicians-in-training, in small towns serving rural populations. There were 60 such group practice centers in 1987, and they came under the supervision of the Department of Health.

With its high per capita income and an obvious political will to exceed the performance of the communist mainland in every possible way, Taiwan has attached top priority to its health system. This has been expressed in many ways. It has emphasized the most modern quality of health service, with acquisition of high-technology equipment at every health facility, public and private. Health promotion is stressed, with energetic campaigns against smoking and excessive use of alcohol and for sound dietary habits and early case-detection. The DOH has doubled its efforts to promote immunizations, tuberculosis control, food sanitation, nutrition education, and so on. Pharmaceutical production and distribution have been closely regulated.

Economic Support, Health Services, and Trends

Not surprisingly, Taiwan has been devoting an increasing proportion of its total wealth to the health system, since its establishment as an independent province in 1949. Expressed in Taiwan dollars, the Taiwan population was spending $41 per capita for health in 1952, and this rose steadily to $2,948 in 1983. Much of this increase was due to general inflation, but as a percentage of total national expenditures for all purposes, this represented an increase from 2.6 to 5.5 percent for health purposes between 1951 and 1986. Considering health expenditures solely within the government budget of Taiwan, they rose from 1.34 percent in 1951 to 3.60 percent in 1986.

Much of the economic support for personal health services in Taiwan is buffered by health insurance schemes. As in the PRC, the principal schemes are for government employees and employees of large firms. Both schemes

are operated by government, through the Labor Insurance Bureau and the Ministry of Interior, but the entitlements of dependents are different. In Taiwan, dependents of government employees have full benefits, but not those of labor dependents—essentially the opposite of policies in the PRC. There are also small government health insurance schemes in Taiwan for university students, teachers and other staff of private schools, and some farmers. There is a strong military department, with its own medical resources. No private health insurance is available.

The pattern for delivering care to eligible persons under the health insurance programs in Taiwan differs strikingly from that in the PRC. Regarding contributions, government employees put in 35 percent of the premiums, and workers pay 20 percent. The government insurance program operates three of its own polyclinics but most services are purchased, through contracts, with public and private hospitals, and contracts with public and private clinics. Payments are made by negotiated fees, sent from the insurance agency to the provider. (There are no copayments.)

Labor insurance was initially only for hospital cases (from 1956 to 1970), but since 1970 has provided comprehensive benefits. These services are also provided in both public and private hospitals and clinics, under contract. Fees are paid by the agency according to negotiated schedules. To attract these insurance contracts, both hospitals and clinics tend to maximize their technological resources, but this naturally escalates costs to both the insurance programs and other patients.

Altogether about 25 percent of the Taiwan population have insurance protection, and household studies have shown that insured persons make much higher use of physician services than the uninsured, with a rate of 9 contacts per person per year among the insured and 5 such contacts among the uninsured. Moreover, judging by their lower net income level, it is likely that the uninsured have a higher prevalence of illness.

Taiwanese health leaders have been aware of these inequities and have been exploring the possibilities of developing a government health insurance program that would protect the entire population. The planners are encountering difficulties, however, in resolving ideological differences between the wishes of private sector doctors and hospitals for maximum free market competition and the concern of the DOH for achieving the broadest coverage at a politically acceptable cost.

In spite of its problems, the Taiwan health system has achieved many gains for its population. With the unusual economic prosperity, the standard of living of the people is relatively good, there is a high level of employment and adequate housing for nearly everyone. Adult literacy rose from 63 percent in 1956 to 92 percent in 1986. The nutritional status is reflected by an average food consumption of 2,890 calories per person per day in 1986, compared to 2,260 calories in 1956.

By customary indices of health improvement, Taiwan's gains have been remarkable. The overall infant mortality rate was brought down from 44.7 per 1,000 live births in 1951 to 6.3 per 1,000 (close to a world record) in 1986. Life expectancy at birth rose from 57 years in 1951 to 76 years in 1986. The Taiwan health story is a dramatic demonstration of the capabilities of a society that, while accepting many inequities of the private market, has (with vast foreign and domestic investment) developed a strong basic economy, and has devoted an increasing share of it to its health system.

SUMMARY COMMENT

The socialist health systems in these three countries of very low GNP per capita have certain features in common, but many more features that are different. They have all trained relatively large numbers of health personnel, especially at auxiliary, or middle-medical, levels. They have blanketed their territories with public facilities for primary health care and, except in Mozambique, for hospital care also. Within their limited economic capacities, all have put a high and increasing priority on the health system.

All three countries began their socialist regimes only after lengthy revolutionary struggles, so that major initial periods of reconstruc-

tion were necessary. The orderly health system developed in Vietnam, with provinces, districts, and communes, was very similar to that of China at the beginning, and this model was retained after it was changed in China. Also as in China, an official place was made for traditional medicine in Vietnam. Both countries accorded favored treatment to central government employees and to workers in state enterprises.

The great poverty of Mozambique, the flight of its European physicians, and the continuing hostilities from foreign enemies have compelled this country's health system to rely almost wholly on medical assistants trained for 2 or 3 years. To acquire international loans, the government has been forced to impose charges on patients, to reduce public spending. A policy of charging patients for health services in public facilities has prevailed in People's China from the very outset, on the grounds that government could not bear the full burden of the health services.

The major strategy of China, to facilitate the economic access of people to medical care, has been to develop insurance for special population groups. Altogether about 40 percent of the people have good or partial health insurance protection, but these are concentrated in the cities, so that the large rural population is very weakly insured and receives much less modern health service. Insurance is also promoted for certain groups in Taiwan. Purely private family health expenditures account for about one-third of the total in People's China, but probably a lesser share in the other two socialist systems.

REFERENCES

Vietnam

Glazunov, Y. (Editor), *Vietnam.* Hanoi: Van Hoa Publishers, 1986.

Ladinsky, Judith L., and Ruth E. Levine, "The Organization of Health Services in Viet Nam." *Journal of Public Health Policy,* June 1985, pp. 255–268.

Lee Hung Lam, "Leadership in Primary Health Care, Role and Training" (a case-study prepared for the World Health Organization). Hanoi, 1983, unpublished document.

McMichael, Joan (Editor), *Health Care for the Peo-*

ple: Studies from Vietnam. Boston: Alyson Publications, 1980.

Ministére de la Santé, *Le Service de Santé dans la République Socialiste du Vietnam.* Hanoi: Editions Médicales, 1981.

Ministry of Health, "Health Service in the Socialist Republic of Viet Nam." Hanoi, 1981, unpublished document.

Quinn-Judge, Sophie, "Shortages Confront Vietnam's Health Care." *Indochina Issues.* Center for International Policy, Washington, D.C., Vol. 65, April 1986.

United Nations Fund for Population Activities, *Viet Nam: Report of Second Mission on Needs Assessment for Population Assistance.* New York: UNFPA Report No. 53, March 1983.

"Viet Nam Facts and Figures." Hanoi, March 1985, unpublished document.

World Health Organization, *Country Health Information Profile: Socialist Republic of Viet Nam.* Manila: WHO Western Pacific Regional Office, August 1982.

World Health Organization, "Health Manpower Development (HMD) Review of Viet Nam." Geneva, August 1983, unpublished document.

Mozambique

Hanlon, John, *Mozambique: The Revolution under Fire.* London: Zed Books, 1984.

Jelley, Diana, A. Epstein, and Paul Epstein, "Mozambique," in R. B. Saltman (Editor), *International Handbook of Health-Care Systems.* New York: Greenwood Press, 1988, pp. 197–214.

Lowther, Kevin, "Mozambique: The Struggle for Development." *Progress: Reports on Health and Development in Southern Africa,* Fall/Winter 1988, pp. 22–23.

Marzagao, Carlos, and Malcolm Segall, "Drug Selection: Mozambique." *World Development,* 11(3):205–216, 1983.

Mozambique Business Council, *Notes from Report of the Minister of Health* (Mocumbi Report). Washington, D.C., June 1986.

People's Republic of Mozambique, Ministry of Health, *The Impact on Health in Mozambique of South African Destabilization,* 2nd Edition. Maputo, December 1987.

Sheppard, Samona, "Mozambique: Progress Toward Health Care for Everyone." *Journal of Health Politics, Policy and Law,* 6(3):520–527, Fall 1981.

Walt, Gill, and Julie Cliff, "The Dynamics of Health Policies in Mozambique 1975–85." *Health Policy and Planning,* 1(2):148–157, 1986.

Weir, Andrew, "Only 135 Mozambican Doctors." *Africa Now,* July 1987, pp. 28–29.

WHO/UNICEF Joint Committee on Health Policy, *Country Decision-Making for the Achievement of the Objective of Primary Health Care: Report from the People's Republic of Mozambique.* Maputo, June 1980.

People's Republic of China

Agren, Hans, "Patterns of Tradition and Modernization in Contemporary Chinese Medicine," in Arthur Kleinman et al. (Editors), *Medicine in Chinese Cultures: Comparative Studies of Health Care in Chinese and Other Societies.* Washington, D.C.: Fogarty International Center for Advanced Study in the Health Sciences, 1975, pp. 37–60.

Blendon, Robert J., "Can China's Health Care Be Transplanted Without China's Economic Policies?" *New England Journal of Medicine,* 300:1453–1458, 28 June 1979.

Bowers, John Z., "The History of Public Health in China to 1937," in M. E. Wegman et al. (Editors), *Public Health in the People's Republic of China.* New York: Macy Foundation, 1973, pp. 26–45.

Chen Haifeng, "Brief History of Public Health in China," in Chen Haifeng (Editor), *Chinese Health Care: A Comprehensive Review of the Health Services of the People's Republic of China,* Vol. 3. Beijing: People's Medical Publishing House, 1984, pp. 13–50.

Chen, William Y., "Medicine and Public Health in China Today." *Public Health Reports,* 76(8):699–711, August 1961.

Christiani, David C., "Occupational Health in the People's Republic of China." *American Journal of Public Health,* 74(1):58–64, January 1984.

Committee on Scholarly Communications with the People's Republic of China, *Report of the Medical Delegation to the People's Republic of China.* Washington, D.C.: National Academy of Sciences, 1973.

Cooper, John A. D., and Lin Yin-gang, "Medical Education in People's Republic of China." *Journal of Medical Education,* 62:287–304, April 1987.

Cui Yueli (Chief Editor), *Public Health in the People's Republic of China (1986).* Beijing: People's Medical Publishing House (Ministry of Public Health), 1986.

Dimond, E. Grey, "Peking Union Medical College: Born-again Elitism." *The Pharos,* Spring 1988, pp. 19–22.

Dobson, Allen, "Health Care in China After Mao." *Health Care Financing Review,* Winter 1981, pp. 41–53.

Faundes, A., and T. Luukkainen, "Health and Family Planning Services in the Chinese People's Republic." *Studies in Family Planning,* 3(7):165–176 (supplement), July 1972.

Fogarty International Center, *Topics of Study Interest in Medicine and Public Health in the People's Republic of China.* Washington, D.C.: U.S. Public Health Service (DHEW Pub. No. NIH 74-395), 1973.

Fogarty International Center for Advanced Study in the Health Sciences, *A Barefoot Doctor's Manual* (Translation of a Chinese Instruction to

Certain Chinese Health Personnel). Washington, D.C.: U.S. Public Health Service (DHEW Pub. No. NIH 75-695), 1974.

Fox, T. F., "The New China: Some Medical Impressions." *The Lancet,* 9, 16, and 23 November 1957, pp. 935–939, 995–999, 1053–1057.

Fu, Xingzhi, *A Brief Introduction to the Policy and Development of Health Service in China.* Beijing: Ministry of Public Health, 1989, processed document.

Henderson, Gail E., and Myron S. Cohen, "Health Care in the People's Republic of China: A View from Inside the System." *American Journal of Public Health,* 72(11):1238–1245, November 1982.

Henderson, Gail E., and Myron S. Cohen, *The Chinese Hospital: A Socialist Work Unit.* New Haven, Conn.: Yale University Press, 1984.

Hinman, A. R., R. Parker, et al. (Editors), "Health Services in Shanghai County." *American Journal of Public Health,* 72(9)(Suppl), September 1982.

Honan Medical College (Department of Public Health), "A Survey of the Basic Organization of Medical Care in the People's Commune System—Mee Hsien, Honan." *People's Health,* 2:219–222, April 1960.

Horn, Joshua S., *Away with All Pests: An English Surgeon in People's China 1954–1969.* New York: Monthly Review Press, 1969.

Hu, Teh-wei, "The Financing and the Economic Efficiency of Rural Health Services in the People's Republic of China." *International Journal of Health Services,* 6:239–249, 1976.

Kaplan, Fredric, et al. *Encyclopedia of China Today: An Updated Edition.* New York: Harper & Row, 1979.

Kleinman, Arthur, "The Background and Development of Public Health in China: An Exploratory Essay," in Myron E. Wegman et al. (Editors), *Public Health in the People's Republic of China.* New York: Josiah Macy, Jr. Foundation, 1973, pp. 5–25.

Li Wang, Virginia, "Motivating the Masses for Family Planning in the People's Republic of China." *Bulletin of the Pan American Health Organization,* 9(2):95–111, 1975.

Li Wang, Virginia, "Training of the Barefoot Doctor in the People's Republic of China: From Prevention to Curative Service." *International Journal of Health Services,* 5(3):475–488, 1975.

Liang, Matthew, et al., "Chinese Health Care: Determinants of the System." *American Journal of Public Health,* 63(2):102–110, February 1973.

Lou, Jie-zhu, and Chen Zhou, "The Prevention of Silicosis and Its Future Prevalence in China." *American Journal of Public Health,* 79(12):1613–1616, December 1989.

Mechanic, David, and Arthur Kleinman, "Ambulatory Medical Care in the People's Republic of China: An Exploratory Study." *American Journal of Public Health,* 70(1)62–66, January 1980.

National Academy of Sciences, Institute of Medicine, *Report of the Medical Delegation to the People's Republic of China.* Washington, D.C.: National Academy of Science, 1973.

Orleans, Leo A., "China's Science and Technology: Continuity and Innovation," in Joint Economic Committee of the U.S. Congress, *People's Republic of China: An Economic Assessment.* Washington, D.C., 1972, pp. 185–219.

People's Republic of China, Ministry of Public Health, *A Brief Introduction on China's Medical and Health Services.* Beijing, 1979.

Pickering, Errol, and Stephen Duckett, "The Organization of Hospitals in the People's Republic of China." *World Hospitals,* 16(3):31–33, August 1980.

Prescott, Nicholas, and Dean T. Jamison, "Health Sector Finance in China." *World Health Statistics Quarterly,* 37(4):387–402, 1984.

Quinn, Joseph R. (Editor), *Medicine and Public Health in the People's Republic of China.* Washington, D.C.: Fogarty International Center for Advanced Study in the Health Sciences, 1972.

Sidel, Ruth, and Victor W. Sidel, *The Health of China.* Boston: Beacon Press, 1982.

Sidel, Victor W., and Ruth Sidel, *Serve the People: Observations on Medicine in the People's Republic of China.* New York: Josiah Macy, Jr. Foundation, 1973.

Sidel, Victor W., and Ruth Sidel, "Shoes for the Barefoot Doctor." *U.S.–China Review,* 6(2):11–13, March–April 1982.

Snow, Edgar, *The Other Side of the River: Red China Today.* New York: Random House, 1961.

Taylor, Carl E., "Oral Rehydration in China." *American Journal of Public Health,* 76(2):187–189, February 1986.

U.S. Senate, Subcommittee on Health of the Committee on Labor and Public Welfare, *Health Policies and Services in China, 1974.* Washington, D.C.: U.S. Government Printing Office, 1974.

United Nations Fund for Population Activities, *China: Report of Mission on Needs Assessment for Population Assistance.* New York (Report No. 67), May 1984.

Veith, Ilza, *Huang Ti Nei Ching Su Wen: The Yellow Emperor's Classic of International Medicine.* Baltimore: Williams & Wilkins, 1949.

Wen, Chi-pang, and Charles W. Hays, "Health Care Financing in China." *Medical Care,* 14(3):241–254, March 1976.

World Bank, *The Health Sector in China.* Washington, D.C. (Report No. 4664-CHA), 13 April 1984.

World Health Organization, *Organization and*

Functioning of Health Services in China. Geneva (CPD/78.1), 1978.

World Health Organization, *Primary Health Care: The Chinese Experience.* Geneva: WHO, 1983.

Zhu, Naisu, Zhihua Ling, Jie Shen, J. M. Lane, and Shanlian Hu, "Factors Associated with the Decline of the Cooperative Medical System and Barefoot Doctors in Rural China." *Bulletin of the World Health Organization,* 67(4):431–441, 1989.

Taiwan

Chiang, Tung-liang, "Health Care Delivery in Taiwan: Progress and Problems," in *Conference on Economic Development and Social Welfare in Taiwan,* Taipei: Institute of Economics, January 1987.

Department of Health, Republic of China, *Health and Medicine in Taiwan Area: Republic of China.* Taipei, 1987.

Hsu, Shih-chu, "Observations on the Government Free Medical Care Program for Workers and Public Employees and the Hospitals Operating under the Program." Taipei: Joint Commission on Rural Reconstruction, unpublished document, March 1971.

Lan, C. F., "Development of Health Insurance and Its Coordination with Health Care System and Health Resources: The Case in the Republic of China," in *Proceedings of the North-Eastern Asia Symposium on Health Insurance.* Taipei, September 1982.

PART FIVE

COMMENTARY

CHAPTER EIGHTEEN

Health Systems of Oil-Rich Developing Countries

Several countries in which economic and technical development was weak acquired sudden wealth in the mid-twentieth century from the discovery of oil. In a relatively few years, their per capita wealth shot upward from levels typical of most countries of Asia and Africa to levels found in the highly industrialized European nations or even higher. This rapidly acquired economic bounty, which elsewhere required centuries to accumulate, gave rise to health systems with unique characteristics.

These oil-rich countries are located predominantly in the Middle East, but not entirely so. To illustrate their health systems, we examine conditions in four of them: Gabon in sub-Sahara Africa, Libya in North Africa, and Saudi Arabia and Kuwait in the Arabic Middle East region. The governments in all four countries have made substantial use of their earnings to extend and improve health services for the general population. None of the health systems, therefore, can be considered entrepreneurial, in the sense that this term has been applied to other countries. Also none of the systems is socialist. The health systems of Gabon and Libya may be classified as welfare-oriented. These countries have developed various schemes of social insurance to extend the coverage and quality of health services to large sections of their people. The systems of Saudi Arabia and Kuwait may be classified as universal and comprehensive; they use general government revenues to provide complete health services to everyone.

GABON

Gabon is a small country on the west coast of central Africa, occupying territory colonized and controlled by France around 1840. Independence was achieved in 1960, with establishment of a republic headed by an elected president. The Gabon Democratic Party soon came to power, repressing all opposition.

Mineral and timber resources had long been exploited, and in the early 1970s oil was discovered. This brought rapid prosperity and transformed national life. Foreign investment was encouraged, and major energy and transportation projects were developed. New schools and hospitals were built and old ones renovated. A limited social security scheme for industrial workers, in operation since 1963, was greatly expanded in its coverage and benefits for both monetary and medical services.

Gabon is divided into nine provinces, each headed by a governor who is appointed by the central government. The provinces are divided into 50 districts, or *départements,* for various administrative purposes. The national capital is Libreville, and nearly 50 percent of the population are located in three principal cities.

The population of Gabon was 1,700,000 in 1988. The GNP per capita was $3,773 in 1984—somewhat lower than a few years earlier (when world petroleum prices were more inflated), but much higher than that of any other sub-Sahara African country. School was attended in the mid-1980s by 72 percent of the children, and the adult literacy rate was 62 percent. With its relatively small population and limited geographic size, combined with very high earnings, Gabon has been able to develop relatively abundant resources for its health system.

Hospital resources are especially great. In 1983 there were facilities with more than 5,000 beds, not counting institutions for tuberculosis and leprosy. Some 80 percent of these beds were in government hospitals, about 10 percent were in three special social security facilities, and the balance were under private auspices (nonprofit religious or proprietary). One of the religious mission hospitals, expanded to 375 beds, is the rural unit founded by the legendary Belgian medical missionary, Dr. Albert Schweitzer. The overall hospital bed supply was 7.1 per 1,000—extremely high.

Organized units for ambulatory care are also well developed, although their numbers have been reported only for 1974. At that time 123 general dispensaries were under the Ministry of Health, nine units for specific diseases and 15 for social security beneficiaries.

Physicians numbered about 300 in 1982, or about 38 per 100,000 population. A medical school was founded in 1973 at the University Center for the Health Sciences, but the great majority of doctors in the 1980s had to be drawn from other countries. In 1978 about 35 percent of the doctors were mainly in private practice, but virtually all physicians spent some time each day in private activities. All Gabonese medical graduates (about 25 percent are foreign) are obligated to serve 10 years in the government health service. Nurses and midwives are trained in several large hospitals in numbers adequate to provide a trained birth attendant for 92 percent of the childbirths in 1985. The maternal mortality rate at that time was 120 per 100,000 live births.

A notable feature of the Gabon health system is the social security program (CNSS), operating since 1963 and with greatly extended health services after oil was found and exported in the 1970s. The number of persons covered, as employees and their dependents, has steadily increased. Then, a separate social insurance scheme was organized for government civil servants. In 1981, total beneficiaries of both schemes came to nearly 60 percent of the national population. In 1983, a third social security program was established for the self-employed (including farmers), nonestablishment government employees, and the indigent. It was put under a National Social Guarantee Fund (NSGF), which was within the government, although the CNSS was semiprivate.

Medical services under the social security schemes are provided in 15 special medicosocial centers (for ambulatory care) and 3 hospitals with 450 beds, sponsored by the CNSS, or under contract in the network of facilities operated by the MOH. If the latter resources are used, the social security program reimburses the ministry. For higher-income enrollees in the NSGF program, copayments of 15 to 25 percent of medical expenses are required.

In 1985 about 50 percent of the Gabonese population were estimated to have access to safe water. To heighten this proportion the central government installed pumps during the late 1980s in 355 villages with more than 200 inhabitants. Access to general health services in the mid-1980s was estimated to apply to 90 percent of the population. About 48 percent of children were immunized with DPT vaccine.

The birth rate in Gabon has been unusually low, apparently because of a great deal of infertility among women. In contrast to policy in many other African countries, MOH efforts have been directed to increasing the birth rate. This increase has occurred, from 31 births per 1,000 population in 1960 to 38 per 1,000 in 1987. The infant mortality rate was reduced from 171 per 1,000 live births in 1960 to 104 per 1,000 in 1987. Life expectancy at birth in 1987 was 52 years.

LIBYA

Libya, bordered by the Mediterranean Sea in North Africa, was occupied by European powers for centuries. In 1912, Italy got control and after World War II authority was assumed by France and Great Britain. A few years later, in 1951, an independent monarchy was proclaimed—the United Kingdom of Libya. Then in 1969, Colonel Muammar al Quaddafi led a bloodless military coup, and the Libyan Arab Republic was established.

Under the control of Col. Quaddafi, the Arab Socialist Union became the only recognized political party in 1971. Oil had been discovered in 1958 and became increasingly important in the Libyan economy. Under Quaddafi, much of the oil industry, the banks, and almost all other business enterprise were nationalized; only agriculture remained largely in private hands. Internationally, Libya became vehemently opposed to Israel and was linked to terrorist activities, but domestically its new wealth was used for developing an infrastructure of social services in education, housing, and health.

In 1988, the population of Libya was estimated to be 4,200,000, of which 76 percent were concentrated in a few metropolitan centers and 24 percent were rural. The GNP per capita in 1984 was $7,892. Of all school-age children, 80 percent were attending school in the mid-1980s; adult literacy was 67 percent.

After 1971 the Arab Socialist Union party pledged to provide free health services for every citizen of Libya. The core of the health infrastructure was two large hospitals in the coastal cities, Benghazi and Tripoli, the national capital; these were operated by the central Ministry of Health, through its Department of Curative Medicine. Other departments of the central MOH were for preventive medicine, endemic disease, medical equipment and supplies, planning, and administration and finance.

Libya is jurisdictionally divided into 10 governorates, which contain 46 municipalities altogether. For health administration purposes, there are 29 *health control districts,* each headed by a health controller. Seven governorates are close to the Mediterranean in the north and contain the great majority of the population; three are large desert areas, very thinly settled (with many nomadic people) in the south. Each governorate has one relatively large MOH hospital, and usually a few small local or rural hospitals. The more densely populated northern governorates have health centers for preventive and therapeutic services, and many small health posts.

Libyan health leaders put great emphasis on hospitals. In 1976, the Ministry of Health operated 47 general and specialized hospitals, with many more being planned. The social security program (see later) operated two large facilities, and two very large teaching hospitals were under construction for the two medical schools. Three small hospitals were under private sponsorship and a fourth small one was owned by an oil company. Altogether in 1977 the MOH controlled 85 percent of the beds, so-

cial security controlled 13 percent, and the private sector 2 percent. This meant a ratio of 4.4 beds per 1,000 population.

By 1982, hospital beds had been expanded under all three sponsorships. There were altogether more than 16,000 beds, amounting to 5 per 1,000 population, and planning called for increasing the ratio to 7 beds per 1,000.

Ambulatory care facilities in Libya are also numerous. In 1976 the MOH operated 16 polyclinics, 78 health centers, and 678 health posts. The social security program had 4 polyclinics, 27 health centers, and 83 health posts. In addition, there were 14 private medical clinics under contract with the social security program.

Much emphasis has also been put on health manpower development. In 1965, Libya had only 26 physicians per 100,000, mostly expatriates under contract, mainly from Egypt, Pakistan, and India. In 1970 a medical school was established in Benghazi and in 1974 a second medical school in Tripoli. With relatively large enrollments, the number of physicians was rapidly increased, and by 1982 there were 163 per 100,000 people. Every medical graduate must spend 3 years in government health service. The faculty at Tripoli prepared dentists and pharmacists, as well as physicians. The supply of nurses was also greatly increased, from 118 per 100,000 in 1965 to 278 per 100,000 in 1981.

Outside the MOH, since 1957 Libya has had a social insurance program, including medical care, for industrial employees and their families. Since 1973 the self-employed and government civil servants have also been covered. The program is operated by the Ministry of Social Security, which has great autonomy in raising and spending funds. With the gradual extension of coverage, by 1975, 52 percent of the national population were covered, and by the 1980s it was likely that the social security program for medical care protected a substantial majority of the total population. Health services were provided by salaried personnel in the special hospitals and ambulatory care units of the Ministry of Social Security or in the regular facilities of the Ministry of Health, under contract.

In periurban slums around the large cities

and in the thinly settled rural areas of Libya are many very poor people who make little use of government health services, despite their legal entitlement. They consult religious or magical healers, even though payment of small fees is required.

For the general population the Libyan health system has accomplished a great deal. In the mid-1980s, of all childbirths 76 percent were attended by trained personnel. The maternal mortality rate was down to 80 per 100,000 live births. DPT immunizations were given to 62 percent of the children. The MOH estimated that 90 percent of the population had access to safe water.

The birth rate in Libya in 1987 was 44 per 1,000 population, down from 49 per 1,000 in 1960. Infant mortality had occurred at a rate of 160 per 1,000 live births in 1960, and was reduced to 84 per 1,000 in 1987. Life expectancy at birth in 1987 was 62 years. Much of the wealth acquired from Libya's oil resources, it would seem, has been applied effectively to advance the health of its people.

SAUDI ARABIA

The great Arabian peninsula came under the control of Arabian monarchs in the 1920s, after centuries of domination by Turkey. The Kingdom of Saudi Arabia was established in 1926, with the king advised by a Council of Ministers. In 1936, oil was discovered, bringing sudden wealth to this barren desert land. The explorations for oil were undertaken by foreign corporations, mostly American and British, but majority control of these enterprises was taken over by the monarchy in the 1970s.

In 1988 Saudi Arabia had a national population of about 12,400,000, of which 72 percent lived in cities and only 28 percent in thinly settled and nomadic groups. The GNP per capita in 1986 was $6,950, lower than its previous level because of the decline in world petroleum prices. Of school-age children, in the mid-1980s, 46 percent attended school, and adult literacy was only 34 percent. The Moslem faith is followed by 99 percent of the population, and strictly enforced by government in everyday life.

Although there is no parliament or any legal constitution, the Saudi Arabian monarchy has regarded health service as an obligation of government and an entitlement of every resident. The criterion is residency, rather than citizenship, since the majority of people are not citizens but "guest workers" (and their families) from other countries who have gladly come for good wages. Their entitlement to health care is the same as that of citizens.

The Ministry of Health has been made responsible for developing a national framework of physical and human resources for health care, and is generously funded to do so. General hospitals with modern equipment have been constructed in 11 health directorates, designed to cover the country's 14 provinces. Hospital beds, numbering about 9,000 in 1970 were expanded to 31,000 in 1985—an increase from 1.4 to 3 beds per 1,000 population. Since money was virtually no constraint, high technology was emphasized everywhere. For example, the MOH constructed the world's largest hospital for eye diseases (a major problem in Saudi Arabia) in Riyadh, the national capital; it is staffed by 30 specialists in ophthalmology and has 12 surgical operating rooms. Almost all the country's hospitals are equipped with the most advanced medical technology.

Aside from the MOH, the Ministry of Education is responsible for large teaching hospitals attached to each of the four medical schools. The Ministry of Interior has its own health service for the police, as does the Ministry of Defense and Aviation for all military personnel, and their dependents. The major nongovernment health agency is the Red Crescent, which has 60 branches, providing ambulance transport and emergency services. Also, private enterprises with more than 50 employees (such as Aramco) are legally obligated to provide health services for their employees; this may be done through agreements with the MOH or directly through the company's own health facilities.

In spite of the abundant free government health services in Saudi Arabia, there is a private medical care market for the significant number of people who can afford private attention. The proportions of the private market are shown in the following tabulation for public and private sector affiliation of health personnel in 1985:

| Health Personnel | Total Number | Percent with | |
		Government	Private Sector
Physicians	16,969	79	21
Nurses	35,590	85	15
Technical assistants	17,527	87	13

Regarding the 176 hospitals with 31,000 beds in 1985, nearly 13 percent of the beds were in facilities outside of any government program and under purely private sponsorship.

To develop its generous health resources, Saudi Arabia has drawn on capabilities throughout the world; this has applied to both the construction and equipping of facilities and the provision of health manpower. Close to 90 percent of physicians and 80 percent of other health personnel have been brought in from abroad. With the development of four medical schools between 1969 and 1983, this will surely change, as Saudi physicians are trained; no period of government service, however, is required of new medical graduates. The ratio of physicians was increased from 10.6 per 100,000 population in 1965 to 140 per 100,000 in 1985.

For ambulatory service, more than 2,000 health centers and clinics were developed throughout the country by 1984. About 63 percent of these were under the MOH, and the balance under other public agencies or industrial enterprises. In contrast to conditions in low-income developing countries, virtually all of these units were staffed by physicians along with auxiliary personnel.

In the rural desert regions of Saudi Arabia, there are still nomadic Bedouin people, who do not make use of the public facilities for health care available to them. Many of these people are deeply fatalistic about health and disease. Home is considered the appropriate place for childbirth; if the mother encounters difficulties, they say "God will save her or she dies." Abortion is illegal in Saudi Arabia, and even contraceptive practices are prohibited.

The crude birth rate in Saudi Arabia in 1987 was 42 per 1,000 population—somewhat lower than the rate of 49 per 1,000 in 1960. In the mid-1980s, of all childbirths 78 percent were attended by trained personnel. The MOH estimated that 97 percent of the national population had access to modern health services. Some 93 percent had access to safe water. Of all children, 89 percent were immunized with DPT vaccine in 1986–87. Life expectancy at birth in 1987 was 64 years. The great progress in Saudi Arabia's health system is perhaps shown most dramatically by the decline in its infant mortality rate from 170 per 1,000 live births in 1960 to 72 per 1,000 in 1987.

KUWAIT

In the northeast corner of the Arabian peninsula is the small independent state of Kuwait, also distinguished by great wealth acquired from oil. Kuwait is a constitutional monarchy, with an elected National Assembly. Although the monarchial dynasty goes back to 1759, Great Britain controlled foreign relations and defense from 1899 until 1961, when full independence was achieved.

Oil was discovered in the 1930s and exported in 1946. From the outset a percentage of the profits of foreign oil companies came to Kuwait, and in the 1970s the kingdom gradually acquired complete financial control. The enormous earnings, especially high per capita because of the small population, were used to build up the social infrastructure for education, housing, public utilities, and health services rapidly.

Kuwait's population in 1988 was 1,900,000, the majority of whom were guest workers and dependents from other countries. All but 7 percent of these people lived in urban circumstances, essentially in a small modern city-state. The GNP per capita in 1986 was $13,890, almost all of which was derived from oil. In the mid-1980s some 65 percent of the school-age children attended school, and adult literacy was 70 percent.

As in Saudi Arabia, health services in Kuwait have been made an entitlement for everyone, free of charge. The financial support comes simply from government oil revenues, without resort to social insurance or any other special form of fundraising. To implement its health policy, the government has constructed an impressive network of hospitals and clinics, and has developed an ample stock of health manpower, by both training and recruitment of personnel from abroad.

In 1983, Kuwait had 2,835 physicians, more than 80 percent of whom came from other countries, principally Egypt. This was a ratio of about 177 doctors per 100,000 population. Of these, 92.5 percent worked in the government health services (including some attached to the oil extraction enterprises), and only 8.5 percent were in private practice. Since government salaries were quite high, there was very little tendency of public physicians to engage in private practice part-time. A medical school was established in Kuwait University in 1976, to increase the number of Kuwaiti physicians in the 1980s. Other professionally qualified health personnel were also numerous—6,700 graduate-level nurses in 1983 and 900 laboratory technicians. The most privately oriented profession was pharmacy, with 614 pharmacists in 1984 and 57 percent of these doing private work.

Kuwait had 23 hospitals in 1984 with about 6,200 beds; of these, 15 large facilities with 90 percent of the beds were public and 8 small facilities with 10 percent of the beds were private. This meant an overall ratio of 4 hospital beds per 1,000 population. Since government was committed to provide comprehensive health services for everyone, it also operated a network of general and special clinics for ambulatory care. In 1983 there were 56 polyclinics, making general primary care and some specialty care conveniently accessible to everyone. In addition, there were 137 dental clinics, 49 maternal and child health care centers, 23 preventive health centers, and 517 school clinics.

Since Kuwait occupies such a small geographic area, it has no territorial subdivisions for health system management. The country has four governorates for certain administrative purposes, but the Ministry of Public Health directs health affairs simply from a central headquarters. There are major departments of curative medicine and of preventive medicine, under each of which are numerous special divisions. Other ministries with health

responsibilities include those for education (schools for the handicapped), social welfare (care of the elderly), and planning. The major nongovernment organization in the health field is the Kuwait Society for the Handicapped.

Because of the enormous public revenues, the very generous health service program of government can be financed with only a small fraction of the national budget. In 1983, it was 6.9 percent. As a share of GNP, public expenditures for the health system amounted to 2.8 percent in 1983. The private sector in Kuwait's health services is known to be rather small, because of the highly developed public services available. If private spending accounts for one-fourth of the total, overall health expenditures in Kuwait would constitute 3.7 percent of its large GNP.

With all this development of a health system for less than 2 million people in a small city-state, it is not surprising that the health record is remarkably good. In 1983, a Joint Committee of the Government of Kuwait and the World Health Organization concluded that 100 percent of the population had access to safe drinking water, as well as hygienic waste disposal. The entire population also had access to primary health care and to health services generally. Immunization with DPT vaccine was accomplished on 94 percent of the children. For 99 percent of childbirths, there was a trained attendant.

The crude birth rate in Kuwait was 33 per 1,000 population in 1987, down from 44 per 1,000 in 1960. The infant mortality rate was reduced from 89 per 1,000 live births in 1960 to 19 per 1,000 in 1987. Life expectancy at birth in 1987 was 73 years. In spite of the lavish life-style of some families in Kuwait, the enormous earnings of this oil-rich kingdom have developed and sustained a health system bringing great benefits to its people.

SUMMARY COMMENT

These four countries all have relatively small populations and high per capita incomes because of their great oil resources, in spite of other characteristics of developing countries.

Each has developed health system policies designed to provide substantial services to their populations, even without distinction between citizens and aliens.

Gabon and Libya have developed schemes of social insurance, protecting the majority of their population for medical care. The service is provided through salaried medical and allied personnel, working in public polyclinics and hospitals. These health systems are essentially welfare-oriented.

Saudi Arabia and Kuwait have used their vast earnings from exporting oil to establish fully staffed government health facilities, where all services are free to the total population. Doctors, nurses, and other skilled personnel are brought in from abroad and, in addition, large numbers of local young men and women are being trained in the health professions. Since in the recent past, money has seemed to be no constraint, highly sophisticated equipment and supplies are imported, for use in the newly constructed health facilities. These two national health systems are comprehensive.

Private medical and dental practice is allowed in all four of these countries, and the very wealthy upper-class families use these practitioners for most of their own personal care.

REFERENCES

Gabon

Blanc, L., and M. Blanc, "The Role of Utilization Studies in Planning of Primary Health Care." *World Health Forum*, 2(3):347–349, 1981.

Fulop, Tamas, and Milton I. Roemer, *International Development of Health Manpower Policy.* Geneva: World Health Organization, 1982, pp. 127–129.

"Gabon," in *The Europa Yearbook 1987: A World Survey, Vol. I.* London: Europa Publications, 1987, pp. 1119–1131.

Gruat, J. V., "The Social Guarantee in the Gabonese Republic: A New Kind of Social Protection in Africa." *International Social Security Review*, 2:157–171, 1985.

Gruat, J. V., "The Extension of Social Protection in the Gabonese Republic: Consolidating the Development Process." *International Labour Review*, 123(4):457–471, July–August 1984.

Vasquez, Videla, *La Situation Hospitalière au Gabon.* Brazzaville: World Health Organization, African Regional Office (AFR/OMC/5), 30 June 1973, processed document.

Libya

Annabal, Ahmed Bascir, *Proposal for a National Health System in Libya and Design of a Primary Health Care Center.* Los Angeles: University of California, School of Architecture and Urban Planning (Master's Thesis), 1979.

El-Farrah, Abdul Razzak Ali, *Health Care Facilities Planning and Design in Libya.* Los Angeles: University of California, School of Architecture and Urban Planning (Master's Thesis), 1980.

"Libya," in *The Europa Yearbook 1987: A World Survey, Vol. I,* London: Europa Publications, 1987, pp. 1747–1760.

Schulz, Rockwell, *Preliminary Report on Study of and Recommendation for Libyan Arab Republic Public Social Security Institution.* Madison: University of Wisconsin, March 1977.

Saudi Arabia

Kingdon of Saudi Arabia, *Achievements of the Development Plan: Facts and Figures 1970–1984.* Riyadh: Ministry of Planning, 1987.

Kingdom of Saudi Arabia, Ministry of Health, *Annual Report.* Riyadh, 1985.

McHan, Eva Jane, "Saudi Arabia," in Richard B. Saltman (Editor), *The International Handbook of Health-Care Systems.* New York: Greenwood Press, 1988, pp. 255–266.

Nyrop, Richard F. (Editor), *Saudi Arabia: A Country Study.* Washington, D.C.: American University, March 1984, pp. 126–130.

Royal Embassy of Saudi Arabia, *Saudi Arabia: Health and Social Services.* Washington, D.C., 1988.

Sebai, Zohair A., "Health Services in Saudi Arabia, Part I: An Overview." *Saudi Medical Journal,* 8(6):541–548, 1987.

Sebai, Zohair A., *Health in Saudi Arabia, Vol. I.* Riyadh: Tihama Publications, 1985.

Kuwait

Kurtz, Richard A., "Changing Characteristics among Medical Doctors in Kuwait." *Journal of Kuwait Medical Association,* 18:5–21, 1984.

State of Kuwait, Ministry of Planning, "Health Services," in *Annual Statistical Abstract,* 1984, pp. 319–333.

State of Kuwait, Ministry of Public Health, *Health Services in Kuwait.* November 1981.

World Health Organization, *Report of Joint Government of Kuwait/WHO Programme Review of Technical Cooperation,* Geneva, 1983, processed document.

CHAPTER NINETEEN

Health Systems in Society

We have examined national health systems in 68 countries—some in depth, others only their significant highlights. Among the approximately 165 countries in the world, those selected for review are believed to illustrate all major types of health system.

OVERVIEW

Along an economic dimension, the health systems are in countries of four levels: (1) affluent (24 countries); (2) transitional (26); (3) very poor (14); and (4) oil-rich (4). According to their health policies, scaled by the degree of market intervention, the national systems are distributed as follows: (1) entrepreneurial (11 systems); (2) welfare-oriented (27); (3) comprehensive (16); and (4) socialist (14).

The matrix combining these two conceptual dimensions, as shown in Chapter 4, has 16 cells within it, but as of the 1980s, only 14 cells had any countries and national health systems in them. If one were to insert every country on earth in the appropriate cells, rather than selected examples, some cells would be very crowded and others occupied by only a few countries. The dispersal of health systems selected, in any case, may be great enough to stimulate some useful questions about strategies employed in diverse countries to provide their populations with health services.

In this closing chapter, we examine certain general questions on which insights may be derived from study of diverse national health systems.

First, are there any generalizations on the performance and tendencies in national health systems, as observed and analyzed in the 1980s, that we may safely draw? Do certain broad social influences affect health systems everywhere? A scientific generalization must be sufficiently broad to apply to all or virtually all the specific cases, and it can enable one to predict the future, with some caution. Thus, planning resources and services in the health system, at least in the short term, can be undertaken with some degree of confidence.

Second, the political dimension in our entire analysis of health systems—the ideology of health policies as reflected in the degree of market intervention—is inevitably dynamic. The relative position of a health system on this scale is changing all the time. What can be said about the balance of forces, driving the system toward the private end of the policy spectrum or the public?

Third, does a study of national health systems lead to any general theory about (a) their future development or (b) a major underlying force determining their character? Under what assumptions about world affairs should one set out to classify the health systems of countries into different types?

Fourth, returning to a crucial issue posed first in Chapter 2, what do we know about the impact of health systems on human health or on the health status of populations? More than other questions, the answer to this one depends on exactly when and where it is asked. The answer must surely differ for the 1980s and for the 1930s or the year 2030. The answer, furthermore, must depend on the general social setting in which it is asked—in a country with high basic standards of living or in one with very poor general standards defining the physical and social environment of the people.

A fifth general question to be addressed is the relevance of national health systems to the entire issue of human rights. Are there any relationships between widespread discussion, in many countries, of a "health care crisis" and the concept of access to health care as a basic human right?

The thrust and various ramifications of these five questions are addressed in this closing chapter of Volume One.

SOCIAL TRENDS AND THEIR IMPACTS

Several broad social trends that have substantial affects on national health systems are observed almost everywhere in the world. They differ in degree, of course, but the directions are clear. Six such major social influences are conspicuous.

Urbanization

Countries at all stages of economic development have become increasingly urbanized. Between 1965 and 1985, affluent industrialized and capitalist countries increased from 70 to 75 percent urban, socialist countries from 52 to 65 percent, middle-income developing countries from 37 to 48 percent, and low-income (or very poor) countries from 17 to 22 percent urban. The squalor and misery of large city slums are all too well known—the central-city slums in the megacities of affluent countries and the periurban slums around the metropolitan clusters in developing countries. Yet, urban life in the long run yields many advantages over miserable rural villages for employment, education, transport, energy, health care, and other social services.

Industrialization

Parallel with urbanization, almost every country has, to some degree, increased the proportion of its labor force working in industry and services in contrast to agriculture. Between 1965 and 1980, this was obvious in all the industrialized countries—under both free market and centrally planned economies. Even in the developing countries this was the trend. In the middle-income countries, the percentages of nonagricultural workers rose from 44 to 57 percent between 1965 and 1980. In the lowest-income developing countries, this percentage rose from 23 to 28 percent.

These trends doubtless reflected the decolonization occurring after World War II in Asia, Africa, and elsewhere. They imply much more than a change in type of work. They mean that many countries are playing smaller roles as sources of raw material for industrial powers and greater roles as producers of their own goods and services. They have contributed to a spirit of pride in national independence. They have led to trade unionism, to social class consciousness, and to all sorts of democratic demands for self-determination and social advancement.

Education

The effects of strengthened educational systems almost everywhere in the world have been enormous. The advances have been greatest in the primary school years, but even in the secondary school years and at university level, progress has been measurable. The achievements of certain countries, with strong political commitment to popular education, have been spectacular, but the levels of adult literacy have risen almost everywhere. The literacy level of women is still generally lower than that of men in all but the most highly developed countries, but even in the developing world advances have been great. In 1986 average female literacy levels in Latin America were 81 percent, in the Middle East they were 38 percent, in the Far East they were 65 percent, and in Africa they were 37 percent. Poor as some of these rates still are, they are a vast improvement over the past. Male literacy rates, for many cultural reasons, are invariably higher. Education, of course, maximizes all sorts of democratic participation in social and political affairs.

Government Structure

Since decolonization and the extension of self-government, the infrastructure of public authority has been strengthened. Even though many of the developing country governments fell under military dictatorships, this did not always obstruct (sometimes it even facilitated) the development of a framework of governance. Out of 113 major developing countries in 1987, 59 (or 52 percent) were essentially under military control. This usually meant forceful repression of human rights, the elimination of democratic voting procedures, and various sorts of corruption. At the same time, in these countries and in the other 48 percent of developing nations, some framework of central as well as regional and local government was usually established. Whatever the principles of authority may have been in the health system—highly centralized, decentralized, or some combination of these—a viable government infrastructure can usually be helpful.

International Trade

When countries engage in international trade, it can generally benefit their social and economic development, although judgment on the exact consequences is always complex. World Bank reports indicate that developing countries, on the whole, have engaged in foreign trade that seems to have contributed to their development. Thus, between 1965 and 1986, all middle-income developing countries reduced their imports of food from 15 to 10 percent of their total imports; meanwhile they increased their imports of machinery and transport equipment from 30 to 33 percent of the total. Data for China and India are unfortunately lacking, but in the other low-income developing countries, food imports also declined from 19 to 14 percent of the total between 1965 and 1986, while machinery imports rose from 29 to 32 percent of the total. (Over these years, we know that China and India increased their food production immensely, and also imported machinery on a vast scale.) In the industrialized countries, the same differentials favoring the import of machinery were even more striking.

This sort of international trade has many implications for health systems. Machinery includes equipment for drilling wells and making pipes for environmental sanitation. Agricultural equipment contributes to better nutrition and construction equipment multiplies human dwelling units. Machinery also includes equipment for manufacturing and packaging pharmaceutical products. All sorts of basic diagnostic and therapeutic instruments in hospitals and health centers can be fabricated, if the proper equipment is available. This should not imply excessive technology, but even the simplest primary health care requires certain basic instruments for clinics and laboratories.

Most international trade also spreads ideas. Many of these ideas have special relevance to the health system, and are discussed later.

Demographic Changes

The worldwide reduction in infant mortality, and in most places a concomitant reduction in the crude birth rate, have resulted in an important change in the proportion of elderly people in the population of countries. Described often as the *demographic transition,* increasing shares of the babies born live on to the later years of life. Prevention and treatment are, of course, also effective in keeping many people alive after they have reached adult life. Even at age 65 years, for example, the average American born in 1986 could expect to live to about 82 years of age, whereas someone of age 65, born in 1950, could have expected to live only to 79 years.

This "graying" of the population is most extreme for the highly industrialized countries, and for certain regions it is not true at all, except for the absolute numbers of elderly found in all very large populations. Calculating the percentage of persons 65 years and over, in relation to those in the "working years," 15 to 64 years of age, we find the following rates:

	Old-age Dependency Percent	
Region	*1950*	*1980*
Northern America	12.5	16.7
Europe	13.2	20.1
USSR	9.5	15.3
East Asia	5.9	8.5
Oceania	11.9	12.7
Latin America	6.0	7.6
South Asia	9.2	5.9
Africa	6.7	5.9

Thus in six of these eight large global regions, the nature of society, and especially the types of disorders to be faced by the national health systems, are quite different for the population in 1980, than for that of 1950. The same trend to an aging population can be expected, even at an accelerated rate, in the coming decades. The health systems of the 1980s and onward must be prepared to deal with health problems of the elderly, therefore, to a much greater degree than was true in 1950.

All six of these basic social trends, quite prominent in the modern world, have significant implications for health systems, although some are indirect. In addition, several other major developments may be identified within the conventional boundaries of national health systems. The precise form and extent of these trends vary tremendously, of course, across systems. Yet, if we conceive of them very broadly, one finds numerous developments or tendencies that have shaped the characteristics of virtually all national health systems over the course of recent decades.

HEALTH SYSTEM DEVELOPMENTS

Applying a perspective of roughly half a century, from 1940 to 1990, all national health systems have been changing significantly, some, of course, more rapidly than others. The forces responsible for these changes have been discussed throughout this book, and here we summarize the general nature of these principal health system developments.

General System Organization

Perhaps the most overriding attribute describing the development of health systems over the last half-century has been their mounting organization. Viewed from almost any vantage point—the resources, the financing, the management, the provision of services—health activities are being increasingly arranged in various sorts of programs or organizations. Even if the policy objective is to reduce centralized authority and enhance local participation in health system operations, organization is required. The inherent complexities of human society make organized actions inescapable.

Probably the oldest form of enduring organization for health purposes was the founding and management of hospitals, which mobilized funds and brought together various types of personnel to care for the seriously sick. Internal hospital organization in all types of national health system has become increasingly complex. Teams of personnel have also come to be organized for the care of ambulatory patients in dispensaries, health centers, or polyclinics. In large geographic areas, the array of hospitals and facilities for ambulatory care have often become interconnected through publicly supervised schemes of regionalization. Regionalized networks of health facilities often correspond to general jurisdictions of government.

Resource Expansion

The vast topic of health system resources throughout the world is explored in Volume Two, but here we note that virtually every type of health resource in almost all national health systems is being increased. The priority assigned to health systems within larger political settings, of course, varies greatly and determines the extent and kinds of health resource expansion (types of personnel, facilities, equipment, etc.), but some enlargement of health resources at rates exceeding the population growth has characterized virtually every health system. This has been true in countries at all economic levels and in systems of every ideological type over the last half-century. In lower-income countries, briefly trained health workers and facilities for ambulatory care have multiplied the most. Many countries have taken deliberate actions to attain more balanced distribution of physicians and hospitals between cities and rural areas.

Increased Utilization of Health Services

For reasons associated with the six basic social trends reviewed earlier, as well as other movements within the health systems themselves, the demands for and use of health services by populations have been rising steadily. The increases vary greatly, of course, with social classes, age groups, urban or rural settings, and other factors, but in almost all subsets of people utilization of health care has been rising. The elevations may partially reflect perceived need and demand induced by providers (mainly doctors or their equivalent) as well, but the result is the same. Greater pressures are put on the health system to produce various services for people in greater quantities.

The precise mix of rates of utilization for hospital services, primary health care, pharmaceuticals, preventive modalities, and other services varies with health system policies. Pressures for certain types of service, however, are inexorable in certain social environments. Deliberate attempts to modify the technical mix of diverse types of service are always difficult to carry out.

Rising Expenditures

Because of the mounting utilization rates of health services, whatever their roots, expenditures are rising almost everywhere. Different national health systems have responded to cost escalation in different ways, with varying results. To one degree of another, however, health-related expenditures are climbing at rates greater than the growth (if any) of the nation's overall wealth. This is also aside from general inflation, insofar as prices for health service rise at the same or usually a higher rate than the rise in overall prices. As a result, health expenditures in virtually all systems absorb increasing percentages of the GNP. Thus, in purely economic terms they become more important.

The percentage of GNP devoted to the health system is typically greater in the more affluent than in the lower-income countries. Cross-national comparisons are explored in Volume Two. In both high-income and low-income countries, nevertheless, the magnitude of this percentage has been rising over the last several decades, since such economic measurements were made. The sources of these in-

creased expenditures, as between public and private sectors, reflect complex dynamics in national health system policy.

Collectivized Financing

Because the costs of health service tend to become so high, are regarded as important for the preservation of life and well-being, and are still almost unpredictable in the individual, virtually all national health systems have devised methods of spreading the risk of incurring health expenditures over groups of people and periods of time. The various mechanisms by which this may be done are numerous and in many ways reflect the political ideology dominating the health system. That some type of action is taken to buffer the impact of health costs on individuals, however, may be regarded as a general rule. The relationship to utilization rates, moreover, seems to be circular; higher use generates collective financing, and collectivized financing facilitates higher utilization of health services.

Cost-Control Strategies

The higher expenditures for health care, generated by both higher utilization of services and collectivized financing, have induced governments and other organized bodies to develop strategies for controlling health care costs, often euphemistically termed *cost-containment.* Spending more money in a national health system usually means that less can be spent on some other goods or services, which may or may not coincide with the preferences of many people.

Therefore, countless strategies have been developed to reduce or limit medical expenditures, at least from collectivized sources. Health planning has tackled the problem from the "supply side" by restricting the quantity of physicians or hospital beds. Probably the most common approach has been to reverse the allowance of collective responsibility for certain charges, through various forms of personal cost-sharing (copayments, user fees, deductibles, etc.) and indirectly through other strategies to improve health system efficiency.

Improving System Efficiency

The variety of strategies applied to improve the efficiency (that is, the output for a given input) of health systems are too numerous to catalog fully here. One should take note of only the most frequently used approaches, namely (1) the substitution of low-cost auxiliary health personnel to perform tasks previously done by high-cost professional personnel, but not requiring professional skills; (2) the maximum use of ambulatory care of low cost, to replace hospital care of high cost when the latter is not medically necessary; and (3) the dispensing of low-cost generic pharmaceuticals, on which patent rights have expired, in place of high-cost pharmaceuticals whose prices are protected by patents. Many other strategies to reduce or contain health care cost escalation have been employed in national health systems, and are reviewed in Volume Two.

Higher Technology

Advances in the health sciences and collectivized financing to pay for their use have heightened demands for higher technology in the diagnosis and treatment of disease. This has been most prominent, of course, in the health systems of the more affluent countries, but even in low-income countries high technology apparatus and materials are widely acquired. All too often, weakly financed and inequitable health systems invest scarce funds in elaborate medical machines (such as computerized tomographic scanners) that serve only a few patients—usually of high family income—while large sections of the population go without elementary low-cost services, such as immunizations. This type of problem has led the World Health Organization to call for appropriate technology in all countries.

It should not be assumed that all advanced technology is more costly than older methods of coping with disease. X-ray images that rapidly yield an exact diagnosis may, in the long run, reduce expenditures for medical care. Pharmaceutical products are a form of technology, and the discovery and use of antibiotic drugs have undoubtedly reduced the costs of treating pneumonia, syphilis, osteomyelitis, and many other bacterial diseases. The same applies to drugs for treating diabetes, heart disease, certain psychoses, thyroid problems, and many other disorders. In any case, the application of new technologies adds to the complexity of any national health system.

Prevention and Primary Health Care

Partially in reaction to undue emphasis on advanced technology, much of which is linked to hospitals, and partially in recognition of the vast potentialities of prevention, since about 1970 most health systems have given renewed attention to preventive services and elementary forms of medical care. The 25 years from the end of World War II (1945) to 1970 saw enormous extension of collectivized financing, in support of increasingly complex medical services, throughout the world. As we noted earlier, the proportions of GNP devoted to the health system in virtually all countries climbed steadily. People's natural psychological and political reactions were to extend greater efforts to preventing disease and promoting health through deliberate actions.

The evidence that prevention saved money was, in fact, based largely on short-term considerations for certain infectious diseases. The cost of immunizations against diphtheria in 1,000 children, for example, was demonstrably less than the cost of hospital treatment of even a few cases occurring in unimmunized children. But extension of this economic reasoning to the prevention of heart disease or cancer or other disorders of later life is not so clear. Prevention of the early onset of these diseases—or, indeed, of almost any disease—means that people will live longer. In those additional years, individuals may incur numerous disorders, the treatment of which is costly. In the long term, therefore, disease prevention and health promotion may entail greater expenditures in a health system. Prevention, in other words, can save lives and save years of life, which have enormous value, but it does not necessarily save money in the long run. This seems to be the case, and the gradually increasing expenditures of most health systems are probably due, in part, to the successes of prevention in the early years of life and even of effective medical care in the middle years.

This reasoning, of course, is not intended to denigrate strategies for prevention and primary health care. It is intended only to stress recognition of the benefits of prevention in human terms, not as fiscal economies. This should be realized in spite of the rhetoric about "prevention being cheaper than cure" that is so frequently articulated.

Quality Assurance

Another response of health systems to the increasing expenditures for medical care in recent decades has been heightened concern that the money, especially when raised collectively from the whole population, be spent wisely. Professional licensure laws have long been in effect in nearly all countries, but in recent years they have been made more rigorous through regulatory measures. Increasing malpractice suits against physicians and others in some countries have reflected greater sophistication of patients (and their advocates) about proper standards of medical performance. Quality standards are also being set increasingly for hospitals, laboratories, and other facilities. The regulation of pharmaceuticals is being extended almost everywhere under law, if not always in practice.

If an individual wastes his or her own money on some worthless medical procedure, that is unfortunate; if similar waste applies to a whole population, the problem is more serious. Therefore national health systems, providing extensive medical care to people at social security or general revenue expense, have taken steps to be assured that the service is of good quality. This has involved supervisory discipline in hospitals and clinics, schemes for systematic review of medical claims under health insurance programs, arranging for "medical audits" of patient charts, establishing norms for various interventions to identify extreme deviations, and so on. Such procedures are more likely to be applied in sophisticated health care programs of the more affluent

countries, but even in the less elaborate systems, quality assurance strategies have been designed.

Scope of Public Responsibilities

All of these trends, the actions and reactions in national health systems, have had the effect of widening the scope of public responsibilities for diverse aspects of those systems. Many, though not all, responsibilities come to ministries of health, widening their role at different administrative levels. Even when other ministries or agencies are involved—for education, labor, the environment, agriculture, commerce—the reach of government is extended in health affairs. In time, many such public functions are transferred to ministries of health or linked with those bodies in some way.

A broadened scope of public responsibility for health system operations tends to draw increasing political attention to the overall efficiency of the system. It tends to demonstrate that formerly conventional concepts about the role of government in health affairs, often restricted to certain preventive activities for the reduction of environmental hazards and control of communicable diseases, are rapidly being extended to include issues concerning health manpower, the construction and regionalization of hospitals, the regulation of pharmaceuticals, rehabilitation of the physically and mentally ill, the assurance of health services in rural areas, and virtually every other aspect of a national health system. The planning of total health systems and the regulation of their component parts are increasingly evident in countries at all points on the political spectrum.

The extent to which any of these functions is performed directly by government, or by private sector entities under public contract or surveillance, is discussed later. The basic fact remains that throughout nearly all national health systems, the component parts are becoming increasingly organized and subject to some sort of social influence, usually through government. The scope of social, as against purely personal, responsibility for health services, and all the necessary antecedent activities that make those services possible, is steadily broadening in virtually every country.

Popular Participation in Policy Determination

People outside the medical and health professions have long participated in health system organization. Hospitals were founded by church leaders, sickness insurance schemes by industrial workers, visiting nurse services by private philanthropists, public health agencies by nonmedical social reformers. All of these innovations were launched before the twentieth century, however, when the capabilities of medical science were limited and not widely accepted.

Since about 1900 the capacity of the health sciences has increased enormously, and the voice of the medical profession, in particular, has become much stronger. As a result, in almost all countries great authority has been entrusted to physicians, as both individuals and members of the profession. High officials in most national health systems are usually expected to be physicians, whatever other attributes may be demanded. In a substantial share, probably most, of the cases, these physicians in various positions of administrative authority have had no special training or even orientation in the theory or skills required for health system management.

In response to this "medical dominance," many health systems have developed strategies of "community participation," "consumer input," or "popular involvement" in health policy decision making. Early health programs under voluntary auspices in Europe, as noted, were started by ordinary citizen groups, rather than by health professionals. But the movements of the period from 1940 to 1990 applied to the management of government health programs. Health planning bodies were required to include representatives of farmers, workers, women, and others along with the technical experts. The same applies to various municipal or district councils of citizens, to whom public health or hospital administrators must report. Such a voice for the average citizen, of course,

is more likely to be specified in countries dominated by democratic, rather than highly authoritarian, ideologies.

All 12 of these features of national health systems developing in recent decades add up to a central attribute—namely, their *growing importance* in the social and political affairs of nations. Compared with the place of health services, and all the factors leading to their establishment, in the world of a hundred years ago (say, around the midnineteenth century), they were significant social movements by the decades from 1940 to 1990. Their development, of course, has been stronger in nation-states stressing broad human values than in those bent on military conquest or glory for the benefit of a small social class.

PUBLIC/PRIVATE DYNAMICS IN HEALTH SYSTEMS

The enhanced social importance of national health systems in recent decades has obviously been manifested in different ways among the world's 165 countries. A major factor in the variation has been the relative strengths of activities in the private sector and the public sector.

Historical Background

The contours of national health systems from 1940 to 1990 were shaped by developments in knowledge and in society going back several centuries. Discoveries in the basic sciences not only affected the modes of treatment and prevention of disease but equally influenced the organization of hospitals, the design of medical schools, the scope of health insurance programs, and the role of ministries of health. The evolution of economic orders and the methods of exchange of money for goods and services have likewise had enormous impacts on the nature of health systems.

With the decline of feudalism, and the rise of free trade, medical care became one of many commodities and services sold in the market. This process of exchange initially had distinct benefits for health systems everywhere. By providing physicians, apothecaries, and various healers with a source of income, it attracted many gifted persons to these callings, and gave them incentives to work diligently. It also yielded health services for many people in the emerging cities—people who lacked the protection of a feudal estate. The growth of science and the universities, of course, led to great expansion of knowledge and skills in the practice of the healing arts.

As industry grew, and as democratic and parliamentary forms of government took shape in various regions of the world, the concept of health service as a social or public responsibility also developed. However, this conception often led to consequences at variance with the normal objectives of free trade. Examples of some of these consequences were noted in Chapter 4 and also in numerous accounts of the evolutionary background of national health systems. A commercial transaction to purchase treatment for sickness or injury confronted individuals with many problems not associated with purchases of other kinds. The health need was usually unpredictable and might have no relationship to the ability of an individual to pay for the service at the time.

As a result, social mechanisms were developed to provide health service to people on the basis of their personal needs and outside the exchanges of a marketplace. These mechanisms included the founding and operation of general hospitals for the poor (later for everyone), the organization of insurance programs to pay for the costs of sickness (both the medical expenses and compensation for lost earnings), and development of long water pipes and sewers that were beyond the capability of most individual families. Such altruistic social actions were undertaken above and beyond various measures for community protection against common hazards, such as the construction of "pest-houses" to isolate persons with contagious disease or the organization of public health agencies to combat or prevent epidemics. Both types of social action constituted fundamental departures from market dynamics.

Since the early nineteenth century, these two concepts of health services—that is, as market commodities and as social undertakings—have developed side by side. In many national settings, the two ideas have come in conflict, representing a clash in ethical values. Increasingly the concept of health service as something for market transaction has led to results widely perceived as problems, such as a severe shortage of physicians in rural areas, the performance of unwarranted surgery for the surgeon's profit, the sale of worthless drugs at high prices, the death of a child whose family could not afford necessary care, and countless other such events.

To avoid such consequences of regarding health service as a market commodity, all countries have intervened in this market and taken certain actions to organize, finance, regulate, and provide health service as a social good. The extent of this market intervention obviously varies greatly among national health systems and at different times within any one system. Various forms of intervention can be observed within each of the five main components of all health systems, outlined in Chapter 3. In a very general way, the extent of market intervention has become greater in most health systems over time, but for special reasons there are certain exceptions and the trend line is by no means straight, or "linear." The proportionate strengths of market and social concepts or, as more often expressed, of the private and public sectors, are subject to continual change in the cauldron of social affairs.

Private/Public Sector Expenditures

So many aspects of health systems have, over the decades, been removed from marketplace dynamics, that one may take the situation for granted, not realizing the long evolutionary process that led to various health policies. Most social initiatives of government or other group entities intervening in the private market of health care have been confronted with opposition of various types. Innovations have been attacked politically, by rumor or innuendo, and even by violence. Regulations to protect people against harm have been assailed as bureaucratic interference with personal freedom. Social insurance has been condemned as encouraging indolence. Public programs have been widely stigmatized as inherently deficient in quality.

An examination of private and public sectors in national health systems, however, reveals defects as well as assets in both domains. If public sector health programs are meagerly financed, in spite of large populations to be served, they can hardly be expected to provide the high-quality care feasible in well-funded private sector programs that serve small affluent groups. Meager compensation to government health personnel leads to bribery and corruption, not very different ethically from the various inequities, deceptive marketing practices, and superfluous "therapies" bred by free trade and competition in a medical marketplace.

Whatever may be the political and social causes, when the public sector in any national health system is weak, relative to the population's perceived needs, the private sector grows stronger; if the public sector is strong, the private sector is likely to be small. The exact proportions of this equilibrium tend to vary with the overall wealth of a country and the general equality among its social classes. The basic impetus, however, is clear; at any given level of wealth, if government programs do not respond adequately to health needs, people will spend their own money to get help. Severe illness drives even poor families to pay for private medical care, if at all possible. When government programs seem to respond properly to health needs, the demand for private services tends to be slight.

Such dynamics are evident in countries at various economic levels, as illustrated in Table 19.1. At each of the three economic levels, the first country listed derived well under half of its health system expenditures from public sector sources; most of its health funding, therefore, came from private sector sources. The second country listed at each economic level, on the other hand, derived most of its health system expenditures from public sector sources, so that less than half came from private sources.

In the lowest-income-level countries, where the vast majority of people are extremely poor,

Table 19.1. Total Health System Expenditures by Public/Private Origin for Selected Countries, 1976–1983

Country	Percentage	
	Public	Private
Affluent level		
United States (1983)	42	58
Canada (1983)	73	27
Transitional level		
Philippines (1980)	26	74
Mexico (1976)	69	31
Very poor level		
Indonesia (1982)	38	62
Sri Lanka (1982)	55	45

Sources: Organization for Economic Cooperation and Development, *Measuring Health Care 1960–1983.* Paris: OECD, 1985; deFerranti, David, "Strategies for Paying for Health Services in Developing Countries." *World Health Statistics,* 37(4):428–450, 1984.

the health effects of a weak public sector are especially distressing. Up-to-date data on this question are not easily available, but one should note for several other very low income countries the following distribution of health expenditures:

Country	Percentage	
	Public	Private
Bangladesh (1976)	13	87
Ghana (1970)	27	73
Pakistan (1982)	29	71
Uganda (1982)	20	80

One of the few studies examining the various purposes of private health expenditures among different families within a very poor country, was made in Indonesia in the early 1980s. Judging by the findings of this survey, private health expenditures for physician's services come mainly from a relatively small number of upper-income families; private expenditures for drugs are derived from the relatively large number of impoverished families. There is some crossover of these spending patterns, of course, in both directions.

The balance or interaction between public and private sectors in national health systems is manifested in other ways, besides overall systems expenditures. Some of these relationships can be quantified.

Private/Public Mixes of Resources

Relatively large proportions of medical schools to train physicians are privately owned and operated in the entrepreneurial health systems of countries at different income levels. This type of health system in the affluent United States had 127 medical schools in 1985, of which nearly 50 percent were under private control. Of the 23 medical schools in the entrepreneurial health system of the Philippines (at a transitional economic level), 87 percent were under private auspices in 1984. Even in Indonesia, a very poor country, the entrepreneurial ideology of the health system is reflected in the mix of medical schools; in 1979, of 28 medical schools in the nation, 54 percent were under private auspices. The capacities of the private schools were, indeed, small—not surprising for such a low-income country—but the government actually encourages the establishment of medical schools as private enterprises.

Within welfare-oriented health systems, medical education is predominantly under government control in countries at all economic levels. Of the 16 medical schools in Canada, 87 percent belong to provincial governments. In Malaysia at a transitional economic level, there are three medical schools, all government-sponsored. Likewise in Peru, at the same economic level, of the seven medical schools, 86 percent were governmental in 1985. In the welfare-oriented health system of Burma, a very poor country, there are three medical schools, all of which are public.

On the other hand, the irregularities of health system dynamics are illustrated by Brazil, a transitional-level country with a welfare-oriented health system. In 1960 there were 31 medical schools, which were almost entirely under public auspices. Then in a period of military control, private enterprise was strongly encouraged in all fields. Medical schools multiplied, mainly under private management. By 1985 Brazil had 76 medical schools, of which only 43 percent came under government auspices.

In the comprehensive-type health systems of countries at all economic levels, medical education is almost entirely government-sponsored. This applies to the four medical schools

of affluent Norway, the four schools of transitional-level Israel, and the single school of low-income Tanzania. An exception occurred in low-income Sri Lanka when, in 1981 under a national government strongly oriented to free enterprise, one private medical college was established; four of this country's five medical schools, however, are government-sponsored.

In the socialist health systems of countries at all economic levels, medical education is exclusively in government institutions. As a general rule, moreover, medical schools are governed by ministries of health or their subdivisions, rather than by authorities responsible for other aspects of education.

Comparable public/private proportions are generally identifiable in the distribution of the control of hospitals or hospital beds. Approaching the issue differently from that of medical education, one can observe that among industrialized countries, with different types of national health system, the proportions of hospital beds under the control of some level of government in the late 1980s were as follows:

Type of Health System	Hospital Beds, Percent Governmental
Entrepreneurial (United States)	38.3
Welfare-oriented (West Germany)	52.3
Comprehensive (Sweden)	94.5
Socialist (Soviet Union)	100.0

In the different types of health system of countries at the transitional economic level, also for the late 1980s, the following proportions of hospital beds under public control are reported:

Type of Health System	Hospital Beds, Percent Governmental
Entrepreneurial (Philippines)	45.4
Welfare-oriented (Argentina)	68.6
Comprehensive (Costa Rica)	98.1
Socialist (Cuba)	100.0

Among very poor countries in the same decade, the supplies of hospital beds in different types of health system were government-controlled in the following percentages:

Type of Health System	Hospital Beds, Percent Governmental
Entrepreneurial (Kenya)	46.3
Welfare-oriented (India)	69.8
Comprehensive (Tanzania)	66.0
Socialist (Vietnam)	100.0

The deviation of Tanzania from the expected ranking is more apparent than real; most of the 34 percent of nongovernment hospital beds were in facilities run by religious missions. These were government-subsidized and functioned very much like public hospitals.

Patterns of Health Service Delivery

It is not as easy to quantify public/private sector proportions in the patterns of delivery of health care under different types of health system. Some general observations, however, can be made for services rendered by physicians.

In the entrepreneurial system of the United States, the most common pattern of physician's care is through private practitioners—in solo or group medical practice—working in private quarters and paid by fees for units of service. This pattern is customary, whether the source of payment is the individual patient, a voluntary insurance program, or a government agency. Other patterns exist, but private fee-for-service practice is the most common.

In affluent countries with welfare-oriented health systems, such as in West Germany or France, the U.S.-like pattern is also predominant for ambulatory medical care. Because payments come predominantly through government-supervised insurance programs, however, medical practice is subject to somewhat greater regulation. More important, payment of the physician for service in a hospital is mainly (though not entirely) by salary; the physician is employed by the hospital administration.

In affluent countries with comprehensive health systems, such as Sweden, the great majority of physicians providing both ambulatory and hospital service are engaged by public

agencies on salary. (There are variations among systems of this type, but the trend is clearly in this direction.) In socialist health systems of affluent countries, almost all physicians are government employees for all types of service. Some may also engage in private practice, but this has usually been regarded as a supplemental activity, subject to regulation.

In entrepreneurial health systems of transitional-level countries, such as the Philippines, of all physicians in 1981 some 59 percent were entirely in private practice, and nearly all of the 41 percent in public employment practiced privately part of the time. In a welfare-oriented system like that in Guatemala, in the early 1980s full-time private practice occupied about 38 percent of the physicians and public employment about 62 percent, although most of the latter also did some private work part-time. In comprehensive systems of this economic level, such as Nicaragua, about 91 percent of physicians in 1986 worked in the government service and only 9 percent worked exclusively in private practice; many government doctors, however, spent a little time seeing private patients. In socialist health systems, such as that of Cuba, virtually 100 percent of physicians work for government full-time until retirement; after retirement, some private practice is possible.

Among very poor countries, the health system of Indonesia would probably typify the entrepreneurial ideology. Here in 1982 about 70 percent of physicians were estimated to be entirely in private practice; of the 30 percent working in government, the majority also practiced privately on the side. In the welfare-oriented system of India, reports of 1987 indicated that 47 percent of physicians were entirely in private practice, 12 percent worked for nongovernment entities, and 41 percent were in full-time public service. (This did not count the large number of Ayurvedic practitioners, who were mainly in private practice.) The comprehensive-type health system of Tanzania is almost unique in its 1980 legislation, which officially prohibited any private medical practice; all physicians must serve in a public program. (How fully this law has been implemented is not clear.) The socialist health system of Vietnam does not prohibit private practice, and in the metropolitan center of the southern region (Ho Chi Minh City) it is relatively common; in the northern region, virtually all physicians work in the government, but some engage in private practice after official hours.

In all the types of health system discussed here, at all economic levels, private medical practice refers to the pattern of care provision, not to the source of funding. Payment for private services may come from either private or public sources. On the other hand, government-provided services may be financed by government or sometimes wholly or partly by the payment of private fees (frequently so, for example, in China). Whether or not personal payments are required, medical services in government programs are typically rendered by teams of health personnel, working in some type of organized framework. Private services to the ambulatory patient are most often provided by individual practitioners, perhaps with the assistance of a nurse or another type of health worker. Medical services in hospitals are intrinsically furnished in organized settings, under any type of health system. In all types of health system, furthermore, a trend toward greater organization of the settings for providing more ambulatory care is evident.

There are many more policy implications in the mix of public and private sector responsibility within national health systems that cannot be explored here. Much of Volume Two of this book explores this issue, as it relates to the numerous components of health systems. As noted earlier, the conventional wisdom in some countries considers private management of any enterprise, including health service provision, as inherently more effective and efficient than public. Yet, when scientifically objective studies are made, examining truly comparable situations, this assumption is often not confirmed.

In the United States, general hospitals operated for profit have been carefully compared with others of nonprofit sponsorship; performance has been found to be essentially similar, except for higher prices charged by the for-profit institutions. Extensive study of immunization programs in Canada has found those under public sponsorship, compared with pri-

vate services, to "offer theoretical advantages . . . with respect to accountability, standardization of procedures, vaccine handling practices, manpower utilization, records management, cost, ease of program evaluation, and levels of coverage." In Cuba, the abrupt transformation of the health system from a predominantly private character to an almost wholly public character, after the revolution of 1959, was associated with vastly increased rates of health services and spectacular improvements in the population's health status. The great health achievements of Sri Lanka, compared with India, are well known, though both countries have about the same GNP per capita. In Sri Lanka public expenditures for health in 1982 accounted for 55 percent of the total, while in India this share was only 16 percent (though reported only for 1970), and the private share was 84 percent. Even in 1982, the public share of national health expenditures in neighboring Pakistan, with somewhat poorer health status indices than India, was only 29 percent.

An ingenious comparison of private with public management of general hospitals was made in California in the late 1970s. Seven county governments had turned over the management of their general hospitals to private firms, in the hope of achieving greater efficiency and saving public funds. After several years of trial, and careful study of the hospital services and expenditures, no evidence of reduced unit operating costs or improved efficiency could be found. Indeed, after a few years five of the seven "private management" contracts were terminated by the counties.

The many subtleties, implicit in the equilibrium between public and private sectors of most national health systems, warrant further discussion in Volume Two. In any case, we should try to avoid oversimplification and stereotyped images of the character of one sector or the other in a national health system.

A Privatization Movement

After the many decades of a swing toward public sector dominance in the health systems of most countries, it is not surprising that in the 1980s reactions set in. In Europe, North America, and even some developing regions, political voices were raised against the "welfare state," especially in its health service aspects. Market-oriented governments in several countries actively encouraged the "privatization" of various health programs, that had long evolved under public auspices. Where hospital structures were firmly under government control, private insurance was promoted to permit their use by private patients. This has been especially prominent in Great Britain, where private beds are available in public hospitals. To a lesser degree, it has been happening in West Germany, Switzerland, Australia, and elsewhere. Multinational corporations, based principally in the United States, have constructed relatively luxurious private hospitals in these countries to serve well-to-do private patients. Even in developing countries, such as Brazil, Ecuador, and Malaysia, private hospitals have been set up by these corporations to cater to the small minority of wealthy families.

Controversy has been vigorous on the consequences of the privatization movement for equity in health systems. Individual private medical practitioners have long functioned with profit motives, even under social insurance legislation, but the involvement of distant corporations controlled by stockholders concerned *only* with profits raises ethical issues of a different order. The operation in many countries of at least two subsystems of health care—one for the vast majority of people dependent on the government and the other for an affluent minority who can pay their own way—raises serious ethical questions in modern nations. The rationing of medical services, whether by age, physiological condition, or by social criteria, may ultimately be necessary in any public system (since resources are never infinite), but a second subsystem, in which money can buy service cuts through all principles of equity.

In some countries, such as Canada, reactions occurred to the privatization movement in the 1980s; as a result, the regulatory powers of government have been extended to minimize the scope of private financial transactions within the national health insurance program. In Chile, economic trends have been instructive, with the acquisition of power by a military and strongly market-oriented government

in 1973. Health system expenditures derived from public sources promptly declined from 51 percent in 1970 to 34 percent in 1980. Yet limited public services remained available to the very poor, who could not afford private care; as a result, life expectancy at birth continued to increase in Chile, from 64 years in 1973 to 70 years in 1985. A long-delayed popular election in 1989 led to the rejection of military rule and reinstatement of parliamentary government. Health system developments remain to be seen.

A pendulum swing in health policy between a social-welfare approach with market intervention, on the one hand, and rugged individualism with maximum free trade, on the other, may be expected in national health systems for some years. The trends of the last century have clearly been toward social solidarity and greater market intervention in most countries. In 1989 a general review was published on health service privatization throughout the world. Its editor, Joseph L. Scarpaci, points out that privatization has been defended as widening the individual's choices. He concludes that "The luxury of truly having free choice in the health care field remains confined to a small group of privileged consumers in industrial societies. The historical record to date suggests that the pendulum will gradually shift to more state control, as the conceptual and methodological lessons of health services privatization are learned." The timing of such a policy shift will obviously depend on larger political forces in a turbulent world.

A GENERAL THEORY OF HEALTH SYSTEM DEVELOPMENT?

Does our study of national health systems in 68 countries permit the formulation of any general theory on the development of such systems? As we explained in Chapter 4, the analysis and classification of health systems have been based on a conceptual matrix of two dimensions: the economic level of the country, as measured by its GNP per capita, and the estimated degree of societal (usually government) intervention in the traditionally private market of health services. The exact scaling along both dimensions has been somewhat arbitrary, but four steps marked along each axis result in 16 theoretical cells, into 14 of which national health systems fall. The two dimensions in this matrix are regarded as important (not necessarily exclusive) determinants of the nature of the health system in each country.

Previous Approaches

Other investigations have sometimes sought more sharply defined determinants of the nature of national health systems. With a special influence identified, a classification of system types follows. The proximate causative influence in virtually every classification has been political, but in back of this a deeper underlying cause is deemed to be responsible.

In the early 1950s my own work for the World Health Organization required preparation of a monograph on "Medical Care in Relation to Public Health: A Study of Relationships Between Preventive and Curative Health Services Throughout the World." The major objective of this study was to clarify the extent and manner of involvement of public health authorities (typically ministries of health) with responsibilities for any aspect of medical care. In attempting to address this objective, it seemed helpful to categorize countries into four types, described as follows:

> One pattern is that in which the predominant form of procurement of medical services is a direct relationship between private professional personnel and individual patients. . . . A second pattern is that in which medical service has become predominantly, though not entirely, a responsibility of the government, with the mass of the needy population theoretically entitled to it without personal cost. Private practice nevertheless persists for a small upper-income segment of the population. . . . A third pattern is that in which action has been taken to make the financial support for medical service a collective responsibility. . . . Insurance for medical care is associated with this pattern, but the health professions remain es-

sentially independent. . . . A fourth pattern is that in which all medical service has been completely organized by government as a public service, financed from general revenues and available free to all persons.

In 1960, I categorized these "health service programs of different countries" in a slightly modified way as (1) free enterprise, (2) social insurance, (3) public assistance, and (4) universal service. Every country's health system was believed to fall within one of these four types; almost all the developing countries belonged within the "public assistance" pattern. Aside from the relative crudeness of these categories, the basis for their classification was essentially their method of financing medical care for the population. In 1980, this classification was simplified still further by Milton Terris into three "basic systems of medical care: public assistance, health insurance, and national health service." These were regarded as corresponding with three basic economic systems in the world: precapitalist, capitalist, and socialist.

Another early classification of the main types of systems for health services was offered by the great Norwegian health leader, Karl Evang, in 1960. He wrote of (1) the Western European type, (2) the American type, (3) the Soviet Russian type, and (4) "the type gradually taking form in the so-called technically underdeveloped countries."

In the 1970s, Vicente Navarro wrote that social class and the class struggle, as formulated by Marx, were "the main determinants of social and medical legislation." He did not propose any scheme for classifying national health systems on this basis, but argued that within any country the relations between working class and bourgeoisie, with some influence from the upper and lower sections of the middle class, determined the type of national health system that would develop. National insurance for medical care, protecting the entire population, he argued, could be expected only where there was a strong and effective political party representing the working class. In developing countries, health system difficulties were attributed mainly to the international effects of imperialist exploitation.

The role of organized labor in the development of social insurance for health care is widely recognized, but this has not been the only influence. In Japan, for example, there are labor unions, but they have played no special part in the enactment of that country's several health insurance laws. The same applies in Canada, where prairie farmers, with a tradition of agricultural cooperatives, were the motor force leading to nationwide health insurance. Marxian concepts can also be mechanistically distorted, as has been done when organized health services are defined pejoratively as leading to "the proletarianization of physicians." Malcolm Segall has tried to discourage sectarian stereotypes of health systems, by observing that a socialist country system may exhibit "a doctor-dominated model of health, popular passivity, lack of democracy, corruption, and privileged access" while in a capitalist system there may be "a national health service with universal access, distributive resource allocation, strict health sector legislation, and elements of democracy and popular participation."

A broader application of Marxian concepts to the classification of health systems in the world has been attempted by Ray H. Elling. He has categorized nation-states and their health systems under five types, ranked largely (but not entirely) according to the strength of their workers' movements:

1. Core capitalist—illustrated by the United States, Switzerland, and West Germany.
2. Core capitalist, social welfare—illustrated by Canada, Great Britain, Sweden, other Scandinavian countries, and perhaps Japan.
3. Industrialized socialist-oriented—illustrated by the USSR, East Germany, and other East European countries.
4. Capitalist dependencies in periphery and semiperiphery—illustrated by Brazil, India, Indonesia, Guatemala, Haiti, Philippines.
5. Socialist-oriented, quasi-independent of world system—illustrated by People's Republic of China, Cuba, Nicaragua, Tanzania.

Elling emphasizes that these five categories of national health systems are meant to be "working" or transitional and subject to change. He regards them as helpful, nevertheless, in suggesting "countries that have undergone significant transformation toward socialist forms of production, giving priority to the development of all human beings, rather than profits for the few."

Another less global approach to analysis and classification of national health systems has been put forward by Mark G. Field, on the basis of study of several industrialized countries. He emphasizes the convergence of all such systems to a common pattern because of the basic social forces of industrialization, urbanization, and technology. Yet he also recognizes the influence of particular cultural factors, unique to each country, which combine with the universal social influences. Within this theoretical framework, he classifies industrialized country health systems into five types as follows:

1. Emergent—no illustrative countries.
2. Pluralistic—illustrated by Switzerland and the United States.
3. Insurance/Social Security—illustrated by Canada, France, Japan, New Zealand, Spain, and Yugoslavia.
4. National Health Service—illustrated by Scotland and Great Britain.
5. Socialized—illustrated by the USSR.

The book in which this typology appears examines health systems from four of these five types, showing that in the 1980s each had serious problems of costs, bureaucracy, access of the population to care, or other difficulties.

Still another theoretical approach to conceptualizing national health systems has been based on a "typology of state intervention" along two dimensions: (a) the form of government control over medical services, and (b) the basis for eligibility of the population for health care. This approach by J. Frenk and A. Donabedian results in a matrix of 12 system types.

Perhaps it would be more accurate to describe the types as programs, since various health schemes within the United States appear in four separate cells, some cells refer to "many countries" or to "several Western European countries," and two of the 12 cells are blank. This contribution, nevertheless, clarifies two significant dimensions along which organized health programs may be analyzed.

Finally, Paul Basch writes of different kinds of medical care systems that may exist and co-exist in various countries. Without linking them to any *national* system, he distinguishes seven types, according to their source of funding, as follows: (1) general revenue or taxation, (2) specifically earmarked contributions, (3) various employer and employee payments, (4) employer and employee contributions, (5) donations and some fees, (6) various contracts, fees, and personal payment, and (7) fees, donations, and payment in kind.

Sociopolitical Functionalism?

In the light of our analysis of the national health systems, or major aspects of them, in numerous countries, is there anything more to be said about the general determinants of the character of those systems? The typology of 12 major system types (and two special types for the exceptional oil-rich countries) followed in this book and explained in Chapter 4 may appear simple and even superficial. Can anything more be inferred about the determinants of or the reasons why a health system falls into one cell or another at a particular time in world history?

A comprehensive answer to such a question must be extremely complex. Determinants of the economic development of countries constitute a mixture of political, geographic, historical, cultural, and social factors that have challenged social scientists and philosophers for centuries. Determinants of political ideologies, which play a large part in setting the degree of market intervention in a health system, are even more complex. The Marxian contributions on social class and class struggle are doubtless enlightening to some extent, but the endless ramifications in health system structure and operation can hardly be explained by

any such unitary force. To meet the objective of improving health systems to meet the needs of all people, with optimal equity, efficiency, and effectiveness, given the physical and social realities of any time and place, one must know much more about the internal dynamics and the external environments of these systems.

As discussed earlier in this chapter, numerous social developments have compelled all component parts of national health systems to become increasingly organized. We have identified six basic social trends, observable in virtually all countries (to differing degrees, of course) that drive health systems to be more complex and organized. There is no mystique about these influences; they are readily observable and quantifiable. We have identified 12 attributes, observable within virtually every health system to one degree or another, that have characterized system dynamics over the half-century 1940 to 1990; all of these have also contributed to heightened health system organization. Directly or indirectly this organization usually constitutes intervention in health care as a market process.

The ultimate character of a national health system depends largely on the material resources of the country and how these are shaped and developed by the prevailing political will. No health system is "pure" and homogeneous. It always embodies the impacts of various social and political forces of different origins and periods. But we can still try to characterize the system by its *predominant* effects in the national population at a certain time. Because of the complexities, almost any generalization about a health system is bound to be oversimplified.

Despite the focus of this book, and many others, on national health systems, one must avoid a health care–centered view of any country. In the larger society, the entire health system is typically a relatively minor issue. Much as it is shaped by political forces, it is usually a marginal topic in political debate. It seldom attracts the attention of issues such as inflation, unemployment, agricultural output, industrial production, crime, social unrest, foreign policy, or war and peace. Therefore, the ideology reflected in a health system, or in the degree of market intervention in that system, may not always correspond exactly with the larger political ideology of the nation. Several other social and historical forces influence the consistency of this relationship.

Thus, a very capitalistic nation, like Great Britain, can have the highly "socialized" British National Health Service. The People's Republic of China, ruled by a Communist Party, can have a health system with extensive obligations for personal payments by patients, even under Chairman Mao Zedong. An extremely elitist monarchy, like Kuwait, can offer free health care to all its people, domestic and alien. And socialist-oriented Zimbabwe can allow 3 percent of its people with private insurance to have access to 18 percent of the nation's health resources. These ideological inconsistencies (and many others could be cited) can all be explained by special circumstances, but they may serve to dictate caution before one attributes the character of all health systems to any single cause.

A health system feature, growing out of one political setting, can become established and endure, even when political configurations change. This has been evident in Costa Rica, which abolished its army and organized strong health and education services in 1948; these services were then continued even after the government changed. The same has applied in Sri Lanka, where high priority for the health system, established after independence in 1948, was retained when a very different type of government acquired power. Of course, every government makes system changes to embody its own ideas, but usually not so extensively as to threaten its popularity. Furthermore, health care demands may change as a result of technology or demographic developments, while the old health system is resistant to adaptation.

Being a marginal social issue, the contours and capabilities of the national health system may be manipulated by the main centers of power for various purposes. We have seen how the very birth of social security in Germany during the 1880s was motivated, not by socialist, but by antisocialist objectives. The rural health service developments in Malaysia were instrumental to the campaign against left-wing guerilla groups. The establishment of manda-

tory health insurance in the Philippines in 1969 was designed to strengthen private medical practice, as the hospital insurance law in Kenya was intended to support private hospitals. Socialist health systems, in spite of their vast accomplishments, have been found by their official leaders to be rife with mediocrity and corruption.

Within the boundaries of health systems—in the annals of medicine, the nursing profession, hospitals, the public health movement, and so on—there is no lack of ideals and worthy social objectives. Much health service is motivated solely by altruism. Yet a goal of money and power can be the driving incentive for some individuals in all health systems. One system may constrain personal gain more effectively than another, but the realities of any health system are seldom as glowing as the rhetoric of its defenders or as bad as the slander of its opponents.

Whatever the declared objectives of a health system, as articulated by its leadership, they can seldom be achieved without adequate economic support, especially from social sources. Spokespersons in many developing countries may declare health care to be a human right for all people, but such words are hollow if the funds to develop the needed resources and to provide the needed services are not forthcoming. The several successive health plans of India have been classics of literature much more than of social implementation. The same has been true in some industrialized countries, even those with welfare-oriented health systems, when economic support has been seriously deficient. Inadequacies in the public sector may be compensated by purchases or even bribes in the private sector, but seldom with satisfactory results. On the other hand, a health system may be extravagant in the use of funds, as seen in the United States, with serious gaps in the protection of its population.

All in all, it seems wisest to regard health systems as a *partial,* but certainly not a completely accurate reflection of the social settings in which they are observed at any particular time. That setting combines an economic level, a political ideology influencing market intervention in the system, a past history, and a complex array of cultural influences. To define this formulation, we may say that national health systems tend to be *sociopolitically functional* at every time and place. No health system is static; it is always being modified by pressures from the larger society, as well as from within the dynamics of the system itself. Ultimately these pressures may be considered materialistic, but this does not deprive them of conceptual or ideological meaning. National health systems in every country are intended, with greatly varying degrees of political will, to advance the health of the population.

HEALTH SYSTEMS AND HUMAN HEALTH

Health systems may be marginal issues in the larger social scene of countries, but most people would say that they play a substantial role in determining human health. In Chapter 2, we discussed the enormous influences on health status of physical and social conditions, quite aside from the health services. The great impact on health of all the concomitants of poverty have long been recognized—poor housing, malnutrition, unemployment, limited education, accident hazards, excessive childbirths, deficient sanitation, and all the physical/mental stress that comes from these miseries. Compounding these external influences are the attributes of any individual—his or her personal life-style (habits regarding tobacco, alcohol, sex, diet, etc.), genetic endowment, demographic position, and so on. An attempt to summarize these dynamics was made in Figure 2.1.

In this section we explore what can be learned from relatively simple statistical relationships between measurements of the health of a country's population and data on its general physical/social environment, as well as its national health system. Both of these types of relationship are relatively crude, but they may shed some light on a central issue of health policy throughout the world.

Life Expectancy in Countries

The best overall measure of a population's health status, available currently for nearly all countries in the world, is the life expectancy at birth. This figure, expressed in years, gives some reflection (not exact) of the mortality rates of persons in all age groups, not solely of infants, as the commonly used infant mortality rate does. Thus, the life expectancy at birth is defined as "The number of years a newborn infant would live, if patterns of mortality prevailing for all people at the time of its birth, were to stay the same throughout its life." These data are assembled from virtually all countries by the United Nations Population Division, sometimes supplemented by the World Health Organization or the World Bank.

The global life expectancy at birth in 1986, used as a general indicator of the health status of populations, was 64 years. In all developed (or mainly industrialized) countries, the figure was 73 years and in all developing (or mainly agricultural) countries it was 61 years—a contrast that immediately implies a great deal about the dependence of health on many influences. Which of these influences seem to be most important?

As a first approach to answering this question, data were assembled on 142 countries, with life expectancies reported (countries with less than 1 million people were excluded), with respect to six well-recognized variables. Three of these variables reflect important aspects of the national society (S), and three reflect significant aspects of the national health system (H). None of the six variables may be the most ideal indicator of these influences, but these variables are features of the country on which generally accepted international data are available.

The three S variables were (a) the country's GNP per capita, (b) the percentage of adult women (usually 15 years of age and over) who are literate, and (c) the percentage of the national population with access to safe drinking water. (The last variable might well be considered as part of the health system, but it is so strongly affected by urbanization, industrial development, and geography that it belongs more with "society," as defined here.) The three H variables were (a) the government's (all levels) expenditure for health purposes as a percentage of GNP, (b) the number of active physicians per 100,000 population, and (c) the number of hospital beds per 100,000 population. All data apply to 1986 (or sometimes another year close to this), and have been gathered from official international agencies.

Simple correlations were first calculated between each of these six variables and the life expectancies in all 142 countries (or a slightly smaller number, when values were missing for certain countries). In rank order of the resulting coefficients of correlation, the findings were as follows:

Society (S) or Health System (H) Variable	Coefficient of Correlation with Life Expectancy
Female literacy (S)	0.877
Access to water (S)	0.862
Doctor supply (H)	0.754
GNP per capita (S)	0.658
Government health expenditure (H)	0.635
Hospital bed supply (H)	0.582

Thus, as reflected in simple correlations, the strongest relationships to life expectancy, in almost all countries in 1986, were found to be two variables reflecting social conditions—the literacy of women and access to safe water. Nevertheless, all six of the variables, considered independently, are rather strongly related to life expectancy, and all six relationships were found to be statistically highly significant ($P = <.001$).

The same six variables were then examined together against the life expectancies of countries by stepwise regression. (This calculation determines which among a group of independent variables has the strongest correlation with the dependent variable; it then adds other independent variables in rank order of their further "explanatory" impact.) With this statistical procedure, the explanatory power of female literacy and access to safe water remain very strong. The coefficient of determination (R^2) of female literacy was 0.780 and the second influence, safe water, elevated the R^2 to 0.883. All four other S and H variables raised the R^2 only to 0.893.

There are, of course, statistical problems of multicollinearity among variables in any multiple regression of this type. These statistical artifacts must lead us to recognize that all six variables examined here are, to some degree, interrelated. Each of them, nevertheless, is independently associated with life expectancy, but the two strongest relationships involve aspects of society as a whole, more than specific features of the health system.

One may speculate about the social, political, geographic, cultural, and economic factors that lie behind the level of literacy of adult women and also the people's access to safe drinking water in any country. Statistical correlations and regressions, of course, indicate only an association and not a direct causation. Yet these relationships cannot be dismissed as merely numerical accidents. They suggest features of the physical and social environment of countries that have been found in countless observations to be associated with people's health.

Some Contrasting Health Systems

In the type of relationships explored previously, health system attributes may be hidden or obscured by the overwhelming "influence" of societal factors, such as female literacy and access to safe water. Identification of the special impact of national health systems can be attempted by examining selected pairs of countries, in which many (though not all) features of the society are similar, but where the health systems are demonstrably different. Insofar as the general social orders within the pairs of countries also differ, a reasonable reflection of the differences would be the GNP per capita. Then, making some allowance for differences in GNP per capita, if necessary, one can compare the life expectancies in the two otherwise largely comparable countries.

Data of this sort for five pairs of roughly comparable industrialized countries are given in Table 19.2. The several dichotomies of health systems are designated simply as "more weakly" or "more strongly" organized, since the situations are too complex to warrant more specific designations. Corresponding pairs of developing countries are presented in Table 19.3.

Table 19.2. Life Expectancies at Birth in Weakly and Strongly Organized Health Systems: Selected Industrialized Countries with GNPs per Capita, 1986

Weakly Organized Systems		Strongly Organized Systems	
Country (GNP)	Life Expectancy (years)	Country (GNP)	Life Expectancy (years)
United States ($17,478)	75	Canada ($14,124)	77
Switzerland ($17,808)	77	Sweden ($13,734)	77
Australia ($12,454)	76	New Zealand ($7,115)	74
Belgium ($9,298)	74	Netherlands ($9,861)	76
West Germany ($12,049)	74	East Germany ($8,808)	73

Source: Sivard, R. L., *World Military and Social Expenditures,* 13th Edition. Washington, D.C.: World Priorities, 1989.

Comprehensive interpretations of the various life expectancies (at birth) in each of the pairs of countries, in relation to their health systems and their general social settings, would require lengthy analyses. Statistical comparisons of the sort made here are bound to be oversimplifications. Yet a few comments may be offered on the possible meaning of the data in these tables.

The United States and Canada have many social, economic, and political similarities, although the United States is somewhat more affluent. One would expect the greater U.S. average GNP per capita (24 percent higher than Canada's) to be associated with a longer average life expectancy at birth. Yet, the Canadian life expectancy is 77 years, compared with 75 years in the United States. One cannot ascribe this, as some have done, to the racially mixed population of the United States. The GNP figures include all races in both countries, and Canada also has ethnic and racial minorities in its population. The Gini coefficients, reflecting household income distribution (as explained in Chapter 2) for 1980–1981, were virtually identical in the two countries. There is no inherent reason, furthermore, why a heterogeneous population should suffer health disadvantages, except for inequities in social policy. It seems plausible, therefore, that this difference in the two life expectancies is attributable largely, if not entirely, to their different types of national health system.

Regarding Switzerland and Sweden, both European countries have been prosperous, both were neutral in World War II, both are rather restrictive of immigration, but Sweden had a GNP per capita 30 percent lower than Switzerland's in 1986. The household income distribution in Sweden for 1978 through 1981, in fact, showed slightly greater inequality than that in Switzerland. One can therefore probably attribute the similarity in life expectancies largely to the highly organized Swedish health system, in which everyone has access to virtually comprehensive health services.

Australia and New Zealand are both former British colonies in the South Pacific Ocean, with many cultural and social similarities; they are both 84 or 85 percent urbanized, and they both have small populations of aboriginal people. Their household income distributions for 1976 through 1981 were virtually identical (although Australia had a slightly larger share of

Table 19.3. Life Expectancies at Birth in Weakly and Strongly Organized Health Systems: Selected Developing Countries with GNPs per Capita, 1986

Weakly Organized Systems		Strongly Organized Systems	
Country (GNP)	Life Expectancy (years)	Country (GNP)	Life Expectancy (years)
South Korea ($2,418)	69	North Korea ($1,231)	69
Venezuela ($2,922)	70	Cuba ($1,999)	73
Uruguay ($1,900)	71	Costa Rica ($1,458)	74
Arab Yemen ($707)	50	Democratic Yemen ($414)	50
India ($272)	57	Sri Lanka ($400)	70
Ghana ($496)	54	Tanzania ($284)	53

Source: Sivard, R. L., *World Military and Social Expenditures,* 13th Edition. Washington, D.C.: World Priorities, 1989.

wealthy families). The life expectancy in Australia is greater than that in New Zealand by 2 years—76 years to 74 years. The relative GNP per capita of New Zealand, however, is 75 percent lower than that of Australia. One may speculate that New Zealand's highly organized comprehensive health system compensates for its considerably lower average living standards reflected in the GNP per capita.

The comparison between life expectancies in Belgium and the Netherlands involves many subtleties. In 1986 Belgium's GNP per capita was slightly (6.1 percent) lower than that of the Netherlands, although in previous years the opposite was true. (In 1980, Belgium had a GNP per capita 5.5 percent higher than that of the Netherlands.) In effect, the standards of living in these two adjacent countries, insofar as they are reflected by the GNP per capita, have been virtually the same. The household income distributions for 1979 through 1981 were also almost identical. The greater life expectancy in the Netherlands, by 2 years, therefore may well be attributable largely to differences in the two health systems. Although both countries have extensive social insurance protection for medical care, the Belgian system has much more entrepreneurial, even commercialized, characteristics. Belgian physicians are paid on a fee-for-service basis for both ambulatory and in-hospital care; significant copayments are also required, which may be burdensome for the poor. The health care benefits in the Netherlands insurance program are more comprehensive. Primary care physicians are paid by capitation, and almost all specialists work in hospitals on salary. Preventive services have exceptionally high priority in the Netherlands. Altogether in 1983 the Netherlands spent 8.8 percent of GDP on the health system, compared with 6.5 percent in Belgium.

Finally, among the industrialized countries, the comparison of West Germany and East Germany in 1986 has special interest. Although the GNP per capita in West Germany was appreciably higher than that in East Germany, by 36.8 percent, the life expectancy was just 1 year longer. Despite the frugality of living standards in East Germany, it seems that the highly organized, indeed, fully socialized, health system yielded noteworthy benefits for the health of the general population.

The comparisons of life expectancies in six pairs of developing countries shown in Table 19.3, are in some ways more striking. Differences between the national health systems, designated as "weakly organized" or "strongly organized" in 1986, were certainly sharper.

The highly entrepreneurial health system of South Korea was in a country with nearly double the GNP per capita of North Korea's, with its socialist health system. Nevertheless their life expectancies of 69 years were identical. We have no data for the household income distribution in North Korea, but in South Korea this was reported for 1976. At that time the highest 20 percent of South Korean households earned 45.3 percent of the total income, while the lowest 20 percent earned only 5.7 percent; it is probable that household incomes in North Korea were more evenly distributed. Aside from this, the relatively long life expectancy of North Korea seems to be related to its health system.

The comparison between Venezuela and Cuba is especially significant. In spite of Venezuela's GNP per capita being 46.2 percent higher than Cuba's its life expectancy was 70 years in 1986, compared with 73 years in socialist Cuba. A quite similar contrast is evident in the comparison between Costa Rica and Uruguay. Despite a GNP per capita 30.3 percent lower in Costa Rica, the life expectancy was 74 years in 1986, compared with 71 years at that time in Uruguay. The unusually comprehensive health system in Costa Rica surely seems to be relevant.

The two Yemens present a contrast similar to that of the two Koreas, although at a much poorer socioeconomic level. Although Democratic Yemen (in the south) had a GNP per capita 70.8 percent below that of Arab Yemen (in the north), the life expectancies of both were the same in 1986. An expectancy of 50 years of life at birth, of course, is especially low, but one might expect the inferior economic status of democratic Yemen to make it even lower than that of its northern neighbor.

The contrast between the health records of

India and Sri Lanka was discussed earlier in this book. Both countries were former British colonies, winning independence about the same time after World War II. Their economic levels were previously almost identical, although in 1986 Sri Lanka's GNP per capita was 47.1 percent higher than India's. It is also relevant that adult female literacy in Sri Lanka was 83 percent, compared to 29 percent in India. The difference in life expectancies of the two countries is greater than that for any of the other pairs of countries analyzed in this chapter—a gap of 13 years in 1986. We know that the population's access to health services in Sri Lanka is especially high, much higher than in India, so this small country's health system doubtless has a substantial influence on its life expectancy.

Both Ghana and Tanzania were former British colonies in Africa that gained their independence in 1960 to 1961. Since about 1970 Ghana has been politically oriented toward free private enterprise, while Tanzania has leaned toward a socialist ideology. The GNP per capita of Ghana in 1986 was nearly 75 percent higher than that of Tanzania, but Ghana's adult female literacy rate was 43 percent compared with 70 percent in Tanzania. One can only speculate on the relative impacts of these several factors to explain the nearly similar life expectancies—54 years in Ghana and 53 years in Tanzania.

These 11 sets of life expectancies in roughly comparable countries with contrasting types of national health system are at best, only suggestive. Taken together with the statistical analyses of both societal and health system variables in some 140 countries, however, they may warrant some cautious conclusions.

Influences on Life Expectancy

The preceding analyses have attempted to distinguish between different types of influence on a population's health status, especially between aspects of the national health system and various features of the general society. As a quantitative indicator of health status, we have used the average life expectancy at birth (in years) in 1986.

The inherent difficulty of making this distinction between influences must be appreciated. The percentage of literacy (ability to read and write at an elementary level) among adult women was, for example, found to be highly correlated with the average life expectancy of national populations. This is regarded as a societal influence, since it obviously reflects the educational system, the position of women, urbanization, political will, and other factors. At the same time female literacy surely influences the use of health services, especially for infants; the literate mother is better able to care for her children, if only to read instructions about hygiene, food, or medication. Access to safe drinking water is another societal factor highly correlated with life expectancy and this, too, may simultaneously reflect access to various elements of primary health care.

Viewing the issue from the health system side, overlapping influences are equally great. The two-country comparisons attempt to select contrasting health systems, and other features in the country differ besides the per capita GNP. Cuba differs from Venezuela in countless ways beside the health systems, in ways not necessarily reflected by the GNP per capita, and the same applies in some degree to all the comparisons. Other investigators have compared "quality of life" indicators in countries of a given economic level, according to their "capitalist" or "socialist" characters, perhaps even less rigorous traits.

The relative crudeness of life expectancy at birth, as a measure of health status, need hardly be explained. Everyone realizes that healthful life—the ability of people to function effectively and happily in society—involves far more than being alive or dead. One can pose theoretical measures of human well-being that are much more refined—for example, days of illness or disability per person per year, as discussed in Chapter 2. Such measurements are available, however, for only a few countries, and even these entail disparities in the definition of *disability days*. Measurements of positive health are even more elusive. At this stage of international health studies, we must be satisfied with life expectancy as an approximate indicator of health status.

One may conclude, therefore, that observation of countries throughout the world in the 1980s suggests that the health status of populations is determined by the country's total socioeconomic and political character in general, as well as its national health system in particular. The relative impacts of these two sets of influences cannot be generalized for all countries or all types of health system, but must vary with circumstances at each time and place. If improvement of a population's health is the main objective, social policy calls for strategies to strengthen *both* the operation of national health systems and people's overall standards of living.

HEALTH CARE AND HUMAN RIGHTS

Whatever the precise influence on human health of modern health service, compared with general social conditions there is no doubt that it is valued by people in all countries. Health resources vary greatly, and political wills to mobilize them for health goals may vary even more, but virtually every country on earth has accepted the principle that health services *should* be available to everyone. Availability may command a price, but inability to pay that price is not a socially acceptable obstacle to obtaining the service. Whether or not disease may be cured—or better, prevented—the actions to eliminate it, or at least to reduce the distress it may cause, are regarded as a proper obligation of society.

In public policy terms, this has meant the affirmation of health service for everyone as a human right. Insofar as this principle is in conflict with the earlier notion of health care as a market commodity, by the twentieth century the conception of health care availability as a basic human right had gained ascendancy throughout the world, at least in theory.

After World War I, the Versailles Treaty gave birth in 1919 to the International Labour Organisation (ILO), based on the principle of "peace through social justice." The ILO became the major world body to promote social security for the protection of people against various hazards, including sickness and injury. After World War II, the United Nations went further. A principal purpose of the UN, defined in its charter, is to "promote and encourage respect for human rights and for fundamental freedoms for all, without discrimination as to race, sex, language, or religion."

To elaborate on this broad purpose, in 1948 the UN adopted its Universal Declaration of Human Rights, which provides that "Everyone has the right to a standard of living for the health and well-being of himself and of his family, including food, clothing, housing and medical care and necessary services, and the right to security in the event of unemployment, sickness, disability, widowhood, old age or other lack of livelihood in circumstances beyond his control."

Many other international statements have reaffirmed the right to health protection. The Constitution of the World Health Organization, adopted by its First World Health Assembly in 1948, established as its objective the attainment by all peoples of the highest possible level of health. It also stated that "Governments have a responsibility for the health of their people which can be fulfilled only by the provision of adequate health and social measures."

In 1968, the Proclamation of Teheran provided for the protection of the family and children. In 1974, the Universal Declaration on the Eradication of Hunger called for the elimination everywhere of hunger and malnutrition. In 1975, the Declaration of the Rights of Disabled Persons affirmed the right of such persons to full rehabilitation.

In 1978, 30 years after the founding of the World Health Organization, in Alma-Ata, a city in the south-central region of the USSR, WHO, UNICEF, and WHO member states reaffirmed that "health ... is a fundamental human right" and that "a main social target of governments, international organizations, and the whole world community in the coming decades should be the attainment by all peoples of the world by the year 2000 of a level of health that will permit them to lead a socially and economically productive life." And still other international statements have elaborated on the concept of health as a human right and on strategies for implementing this.

One may question, of course, the practical value of all these international legal instruments. Are they just words that do not reflect reality? They are statements, however, that record social values and policy goals, not of poets and intellectuals, but of the established leaders of virtually all countries. They affirm principles for social action, shape political strategies, and influence the features of national health systems in many subtle ways.

At various times in the 1970s and 1980s, the health systems of many countries—both industrialized and developing, and at various points in the political spectrum—were regarded as being "in crisis." They have been faced with serious problems of costs, access to care, waste, inefficiency, and so on. But these problems are identified only because society has expectations of much better performance of systems. If people did not expect health services to be provided to the entire population effectively and efficiently, they would not be so aroused, personally or through politicians, by the failure of the health system to perform its role.

Even if the declared health principles of the United Nations and the World Health Organization are far from being implemented, they remain as inspirational goals. "Health for all by the year 2000" is less important as an explicit objective than as an affirmation of the crucial principle of equity in the development of health systems and the myriad other conditions contributing to health. No country's health system has yet achieved the social justice advocated by world health leaders. But the very formulation of this concept is significant. It is a further step in the long evolution of health service from a market commodity to a human right.

REFERENCES

Abel-Smith, Brian, *An International Study of Health Expenditure.* Geneva: World Health Organization (Public Health Papers 32), 1967.

Ashworth, W., *Short History of the International Economy Since 1850.* London, 1975.

Bankowski, Z., and J. H. Bryant (Editors), *Health Policy, Ethics and Human Values: An International Dialogue.* Geneva: CIOMS, 1985.

Banta, H. D., "Medical Technology and Developing Countries: The Case of Brazil." *International Journal of Health Services,* 16:363–373, 1986.

Basch, Paul F., *Textbook of International Health.* New York: Oxford University Press, 1990, pp. 39, 294.

Becker, Carl, *Modern History: The Rise of a Democratic, Scientific, and Industrialized Civilization.* New York: Silver, Burdett & Co., 1935.

Berliner, H. S., and C. Regan, "Multinational Corporations of U.S. For-Profit Health Chains: Trends and Implications." *American Journal of Public Health,* 77:1280–1284, 1987.

Bryant, John H., "WHO's Program of Health for All by the Year 2000: A Macrosystem for Health Policy Making—A Challenge to Social Science Research." *Social Science and Medicine,* 14A:381–386, 1980.

Callahan, Daniel, *Setting Limits: Medical Goals in an Aging Society.* New York: Simon & Schuster, 1987.

Centre for Human Rights, *Human Rights, A Compilation of International Instruments.* New York: United Nations, 1988.

Ceresto, Shirley, and Howard Waitzkin, "Economic Development, Political-Economic System, and the Physical Quality of Life." *Journal of Public Health Policy,* 9:104–120, Spring 1988.

Chen, L. C., "Primary Health Care in Developing Countries: Overcoming Operational, Technical, and Social Barriers." *The Lancet,* 2:1260–1265, 1986.

Chernichovsky, Dov, and Oey Astra Meesook, *Poverty in Indonesia: A Profile.* Washington, D.C.: World Bank (Staff Working Papers No. 671), 1984.

deFerranti, David, "Strategies for Paying for Health Services in Developing Countries." *World Health Statistics,* 37(4):428–450, 1984.

Elling, Ray H., "The Comparison of Health Systems in World-System Perspective," in *Research in the Sociology of Health Care,* Vol. 8, Part IV, JAI Press, 1989, pp. 207–226.

Elling, Ray H., "The Capitalist World System and International Health." *International Journal of Health Services,* 11(1):21–51, 1981.

Elling, Ray H., *Cross-National Study of Health Systems.* New Brunswick, N.J.: Transaction, Inc., 1980.

Evang, Karl, *Health Service, Society and Medicine.* London: Oxford University Press, 1960.

Field, Mark G., "Introduction," in Mark G. Field (Editor), *Success and Crisis in National Health Systems: A Comparative Approach.* New York: Routledge, 1989, pp. 1–22.

Foege, William H., "Public Health: Moving from Debt to Legacy." *American Journal of Public Health,* 77(10):1276–1278, October 1987.

Frenk, Julio, and A. Donabedian, "State Intervention in Medical Care: Types, Trends, and Variables." *Health Policy and Planning,* 2(1):17–31, 1987.

Fried, Bruce J., R. B. Deber, and P. Leatt, "Corporatization and Deprivatization of Health Services in Canada." *International Journal of Health Services,* 17(4):567–584, 1987.

Goodrich, L. M., et al., *Charter of the United Nations: Commentary and Documents,* 3rd Edition. New York, 1969.

Greenberg, W. (Editor), *Competition in the Health Care Sector: Past, Present, and Future.* Washington, D.C.: U.S. Federal Trade Commission, 1978.

Gunatilleke, Godfrey, "Health and Development in Sri Lanka—An Overview," in Scott B. Halstead et al. (Editors), *Good Health at Low Costs.* New York: Rockefeller Foundation, 1985, pp. 111–124.

Kleczkowski, B. M., M. I. Roemer, and A. Van Der Werff, *National Health Systems and Their Reorientation Towards Health for All.* Geneva: World Health Organization (Public Health Papers No. 77), 1984.

Light, D. W., "Corporate Medicine for Profit." *Scientific American,* 255(6):38–45, December 1986.

March, J. G., and H. A. Simon, *Organizations.* New York: John Wiley & Sons, 1958.

McIntyre, Lynn, and Franklin White, "Canadian Immunization: Public Programs or Private Enterprise?" *PAHO Bulletin,* 22(4):355–363, 1988.

McKeown, Thomas, *The Role of Medicine: Dream, Mirage or Nemesis.* Oxford: Blackwell, 1979.

McLachlen, Gordon, and Alan Maynard (Editors), *The Public/Private Mix for Health: The Relevance and Effects of Change.* London: Nuffield Provincial Hospitals Trust, 1982.

Mountin, Joseph W., "Medical Care: A Private Enterprise or a Social Service?" *Public Health Reports,* 59(43):1405–1411, 27 October 1944.

Navarro, Vicente, *Class Struggle, the State, and Medicine: An Historical and Contemporary Analysis of the Medical Sector in Great Britain.* New York: Prodist, 1978.

Navarro, Vicente (Editor), *Imperialism, Health and Medicine.* Farmingdale, N.Y.: Baywood Pub. Co., 1981.

Palen, J.J., *The Urban World.* New York: McGraw-Hill, 1981.

Pattison, R., and H. Katz, "Investor-Owned and Not-for-Profit Hospitals." *New England Journal of Medicine,* 309:347–353, 1983.

Perlman, M. (Editor), *The Economics of Health and Medical Care.* London, 1974.

Raynor, G., B. Griffith, and J. Mohan, *Commercial Medicine in London.* London: Greater London County Council, 1985.

Roemer, Milton I., "Health Developments and Medical Care—A World Scanning." *American Journal of Public Health,* 50(2):154–160, February 1960.

Roemer, Milton I., *Medical Care in Relation to Public Health: A Study of Relationships Between Preventive and Curative Services Throughout the World.* Geneva: World Health Organization (WHO/OMA/25 Rev. 1), 7 December 1956.

Roemer, Milton I., "Political Ideology and Health Care: Hospital Patterns in the Philippines and Cuba." *International Journal of Health Services,* 3(3):487–492, 1973.

Roemer, Milton I., "Priority for Primary Health Care: Its Development and Problems." *Health Policy and Planning,* 1(1):58–66, 1986.

Roemer, Milton I., "Proletarianization of Physicians or Organization of Health Services?" *International Journal of Health Services,* 16(3):469–471, 1986.

Roemer, Milton I., "The Public/Private Mix of Health Sector Financing: International Implications." *Public Health Review* (Israel), 12:119–130, 1984.

Roemer, Milton I., "Resistance to Innovation: The Case of the Community Health Center." *American Journal of Public Health,* 78(9):1234–1239, September 1988.

Roemer, M. I., and C. Montoya-Aguilar, *Quality Assessment and Assurance in Primary Health Care.* Geneva: World Health Organization (Offset Pub. No. 105), 1988.

Roemer, Milton I., and John E. Roemer, "The Social Consequences of Free Trade in Health Care: A Public Health Response to Orthodox Economics." *International Journal of Health Services,* 12(1):111–129, 1982.

Scarpaci, Joseph L. (Editor), *Health Services Privatization in Industrial Societies.* New Brunswick, N.J.: Rutgers University Press, 1989.

Segall, Malcolm, "On the Concept of a Socialist Health System: A Question of Marxist Epistemology." *International Journal of Health Services,* 12(2):221–225, 1983.

Shonick, William, and Ruth Roemer, *Public Hospitals under Private Management: The California Experience.* Berkeley: University of California, 1983.

Tabibzadeh, I., A. Rossi-Espagnet, and R. Maxwell, *Spotlight on the Cities: Improving Urban Health in Developing Countries.* Geneva: World Health Organization, 1989.

Terris, Milton, "The Three World Systems of Medical Care: Trends and Prospects." *World Health Forum,* 1(1&2):78–86, 1980.

U.S. Public Health Service, *Healthy People: The Surgeon General's Report on Health Promotion and Disease Prevention.* Washington, D.C.: DHEW-PHS-Pub. No. 79-55071, 1979.

Weller, Geoffrey R., and Pranlal Manga, "The Push for Reprivatization of Health Care Service in Canada, Britain, and the United States." *Journal of Health Politics, Policy & Law,* 8(3):495–518, Fall 1983.

Wilensky, H. L., and C. N. Lebeaux, *Industrial So-*

ciety and Social Welfare. New York: Russell Sage Foundation, 1958.

World Health Organization and United Nations Children's Fund, *Primary Health Care* (Report of the International Conference on Primary Health Care). Geneva, 1978.

World Health Organization, *The First Ten Years of WHO.* Geneva: WHO, 1958.

World Health Organization, *From Alma Ata to the Year 2000: Reflections at the Midpoint.* Geneva: WHO, 1988.

World Health Organization, *Financing of Health Services.* Geneva: WHO Study Group (Technical Report Series No. 625), 1978.

Epilogue

National health systems throughout the world have obviously been changing constantly. Each system component responds in some way to the dynamic political, economic, and social circumstances around it.

In early 1990, when this text was completed, many national governments were in especially great political and economic turmoil. The cold war, which had shaped both international and domestic policies in countries for decades, was tapering off. Relationships between countries and priorities within countries were transformed, as military budgets were adjusted to the new situation.

Most dramatic were the changes in Eastern Europe, where one country after another brought to an end the dominance of the Communist Party. As free expression was increased, the economic frameworks, modeled after that of the Soviet Union, were transformed. In countless ways, market dynamics gradually replaced central planning for the allocation of resources.

Privatization, competition, and other market features have been found in socialist health systems to varying extents for many years. Their influence has been marginal, however, and one may only speculate on the effects of their development as central tenets in the economies of Eastern European countries.

Both in private and public sectors of health systems the trend everywhere has been toward increasing organization. Even in a health system as entrepreneurial as that of the United States, highly organized innovations have arisen in the private sector. Health maintenance organizations (HMOs) and preferred provider organizations (PPOs) were developed in such a setting. Payment to hospitals according to the patient's "diagnosis-related group" (DRG) arose in response to the perverse incentives of a profit motive.

Thus, whatever may be the proportions of public and private sectors, the complexities of technology and of society generate regulatory responses. It is very likely, therefore, that health system changes in Poland or Hungary, for example, will involve replacing socialist patterns with highly regulated markets. Individual freedom may be subject to no fewer constraints than before.

The extent of organization in a national health system depends on the political will mounted to achieve objectives, on which consensus is wide. The bureaucratic requirements of the Soviet Union's health system are no greater than those of the United States health system. In many ways the extensive use of private fee-for-service remuneration in a free market setting generates greater bureaucracy than does simple salaried employment in a socialist setting.

The advocacy, since the 1970s, of a lifestyle conducive to health, illustrates the dynamics. In the democratic societies, where this emphasis is strongest, all sorts of social organization have developed to promote it. There are national associations, conferences, academic courses, campaigns in mass media—all intended to spread the message of healthy personal lifestyle. Laws are passed on advertising of cigarettes, on labeling the ingredients in packaged food, on the use of seat belts in vehicles—all designed to influence individual behavior. Greater pressures are mounted to ensure minimum standards of work and living, and to prevent environmental pollution.

Changes also mark health system development outside of Europe. In China, more vigorous political education is launched to counteract the "democratic" rebellion of students in June 1989. The Sandinista government of Nicaragua is replaced, after an election, by a conservative coalition of antisocialist political parties. The two Yemens, capitalist and socialist, become united. Several military dictatorships in Latin America are replaced by newly elected governments.

The massive political convolutions going on in socialist countries are still in process, as this book goes to press. We are still much too close to these changes to identify their impacts on health systems. If regimented social orders are indeed replaced by democratic societies, we may expect that "health for all" will remain a global objective. The structure and functioning of national health systems of all types will become increasingly organized to attain both efficiency and equity.

Scholars and politicians have debated the accuracy of obituaries on socialism. Some have said that the essence of socialism lies in public rather than private ownership of the means of production. With this there could be political democracy rather than thought control, and distribution through a market rather than through centralized planning. Events of the 1990s would determine the subsequent direction of the world's diverse national health systems.

Index

This index should be used along with the contents *section. Under the countries and other headings shown in the contents, several major subjects are usually listed, and these are not repeated in the index. The index is oriented mainly toward subjects or topics within national health systems. Under each heading are listed, in alphabetical order, the countries on which the subject or topic is discussed.*

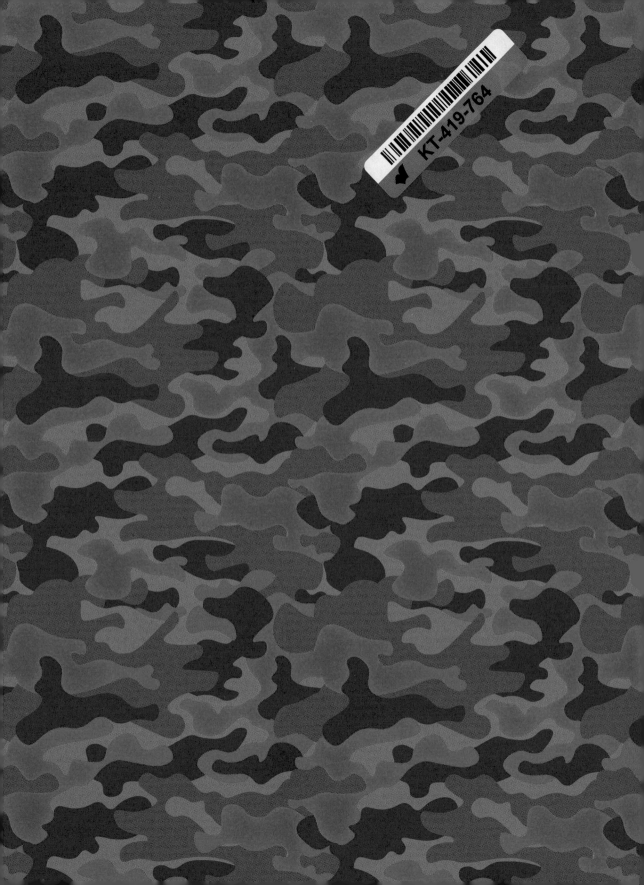

skin
care

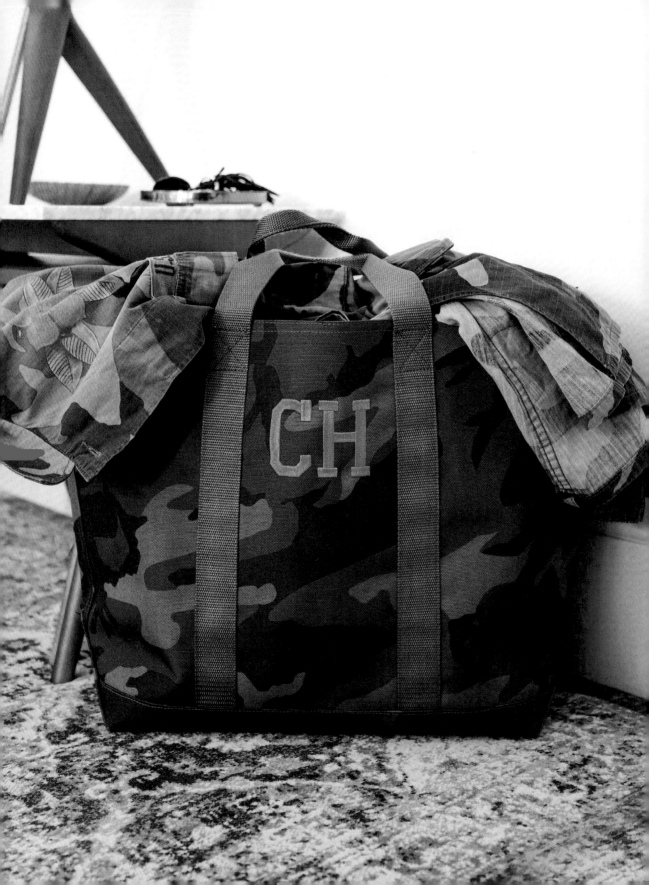

CAROLINE HIRONS.

skin care

THE ULTIMATE NO-NONSENSE GUIDE

Photography by Christopher Oakman

HQ

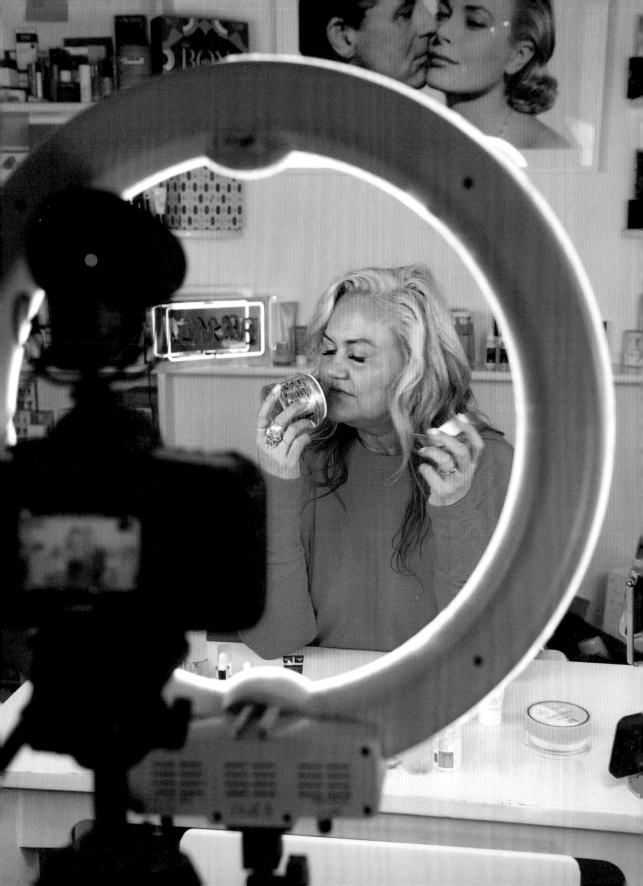

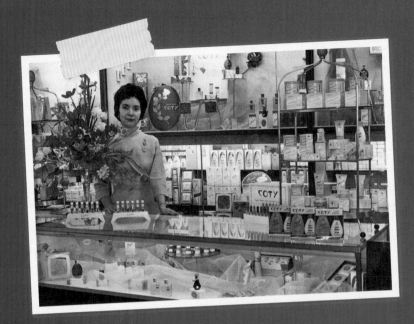

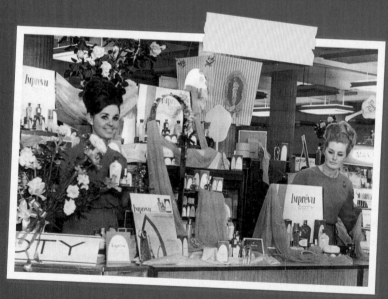

This book is dedicated to my
mum and nana.

INTRODUCTION

> I feel like I grew up in the industry.
> It's literally in my blood.

Some of my earliest memories are of my grandmother religiously removing her makeup before bed. It was as hypnotising as it was methodical. Eyes first, in her bedroom mirror, then a full facial cleanse at the bathroom sink. The message was always the same: take care of your skin. It was non-negotiable. That message was passed down to my mum, who in turn made sure I heard it loud and clear. The first time I asked if I could buy some makeup, Mum said, 'Yes, once you've shown me you can take care of your skin.' That seemed a fair deal to get my hands on my first pot of Bourjois blush.

My nana started working on beauty counters in Liverpool in the 1960s, for Coty, then for Guerlain. We would go and meet her for lunch and the counter girls always looked immaculate, with their crisp uniforms, perfect makeup and styled hair. And they smelled amazing. My mum Cathy followed in her mother's footsteps, working for Coty as a teenager and going on to work for Helena Rubinstein in the 80s. As a teenager, I tried everything from white lipstick to blue eyeshadow, and Mum never batted an eyelid (though the black crimped hair and pale lipstick did make her look twice) – all she said was, 'Make sure you wash that off properly.'

It hadn't occurred to me to work in beauty until I'd had my first two children. I needed a part-time job and called my friend Lorraine, who at the time was working on the Aveda counter in Harvey Nichols. She'd always been the mate that I'd follow around London to buy my Clarins (I used Clarins pretty much throughout my late teens and early 20s). As it turned out, Aveda had a vacancy for a Saturday/Sunday salesperson. I went for the interview, got the job and never looked back. I realised on day two that not only was I good at the job, but that I loved it: I loved the interaction with customers, the banter on the shop floor, and the general retail environment. On reflection, I think I felt like I was also keeping up the family tradition. I discovered that I had a particular affinity with the skincare section. It made sense to me.

One of my first staff training sessions sealed the deal: some of the tips and techniques that the trainer mentioned I still use to this day.

As much as I loved the shop floor, I knew I wanted to take my passion for skincare further. The Aveda counter had a beauty room attached to it and we were all trained in mini-treatments. I found I was trying to spend all of my time in the treatment rooms; it added another dimension to skincare that I found more interesting, to see it in action on someone's skin. I knew I wanted to qualify as a beauty therapist and that I had to go to the best training school available, with the highest qualification. I've always been annoyingly Type A.

> I started working for Space NK in London and knew 100 per cent that skincare was my thing.

And thanks to sitting through brand training sessions that would be either brilliantly informative or 'kill me now' dull, I learned how to talk to people if you want them to listen.

After doing my research and finding out what courses were available, I signed up to the prestigious Steiner Beauty School in Central London. They offered the best courses for me at the time, as they ran night classes, which meant I could keep working in the job I loved (and needed). I went to work as normal, then on Monday and Tuesday evenings I would go straight to class at Steiner, knocking up regular 50+-hour weeks while still being a wife and mother.

Steiner was brilliant. It had floral divider curtains, pink waffle blankets, a hideous uniform, and a picture of the Queen in the main training room, which was the first thing you saw when you walked in – it always cracked me up.

It was so old-fashioned, but the training – intense and in-depth – was excellent. They did not play: they were really strict and no-nonsense, and I loved it. I knew I had made the right choice. It took me longer to graduate than planned, as I had another two children while I was training. I would train as long as I could to clock up the required hours, go off and have a kid, then return to work full-time and head back to Steiner in the evenings, until I got the certificate that, without a doubt, sealed the direction that my career would eventually go in. It was hard, but when you're obsessed with what you're doing, and have an end goal, and support, it's fun. It also helps if your parents instilled a borderline-psychotic work ethic in you, which mine did. Thankfully.

I left Space NK and went on to work for Chantecaille and Liz Earle (among others), and at one point even did a stint at my beloved Clarins. The training was great – the uniform, not so much.

Eventually realising that I was a square peg in a round corporate hole, I started my own consultation business in 2009. My (at the time undiagnosed) ADHD would frequently land me in hot water as an employee, but as an independent consultant I was paid to tell brands what they needed to hear, not what they wanted to hear. As my husband once said, 'Who would have thought that being gobby and opinionated would become a career?'

When I started my blog in 2010, no one was really talking about skincare, and if they did, it was only to mention a new product release. The focus was on makeup and nails. My blog stood out. I could never have planned how successful it would become – you can't 'make' something go viral.

I quickly gained a trusted audience by saying things like: 'Actually, I wouldn't advise that. Don't do that. Do this.' 'Don't put that on your face.' 'Wipes are horrible.' And so on. My followers are incredible, and insane about skincare. I couldn't do this without them.

The blog has now had over 120 million page views and has opened up a whole new world for me.

Through my Skincare Freaks Facebook group, I've seen every fad, heard every myth, and witnessed with my own eyes what works and what doesn't.

I've handled thousands of faces and tested so many products, and I'm lucky enough to count leading cosmetic scientists, the best dermatologists, expert doctors and especially my fellow aestheticians, as friends.

Skincare covers all issues for all ages, ethnicities, budgets, skin tones and skin types, from your daily routine to spots to dryness, and how to care for your skin when you're ill. You'll find tips to help you deal with pigmentation, dehydration, and lines and wrinkles, too.

I've taken everything I've learned from my years in the industry and my time on the blog to help you navigate the world of skincare simply and succinctly, tell you what you need and what you don't, and where not to waste your time and energy.

If I rave about a product or an ingredient, it's because I know it genuinely works.

Equally, if I tell something to get in the sea and get lost, it's because I know it's a waste of your hard-earned cash. If you already follow me, you'll be aware that I never kiss or blow smoke up anyone's arse — I haven't done it before and I'm not about to start now. And if you're new, come and join us.

Thank you so much for reading. Skin Rocks™ 🤘.

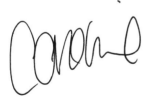

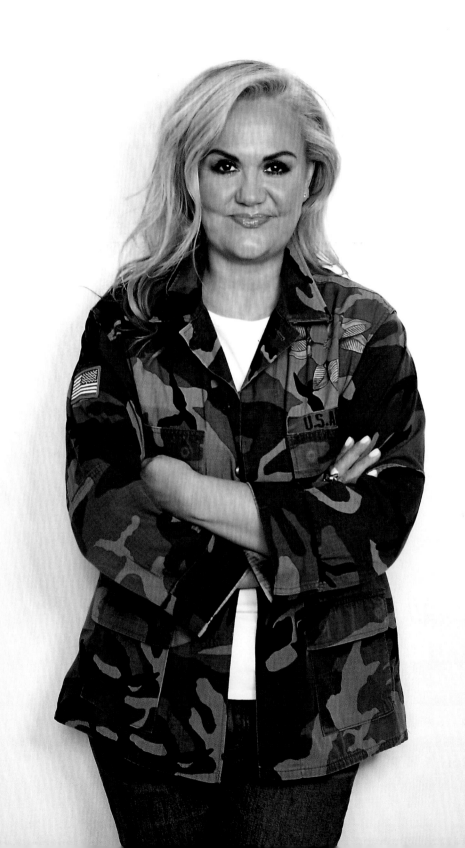

HOW SKIN WORKS

Your skin is incredible. Whether you're a bright young thing without a wrinkle in sight, someone who's struggled with acne their entire lives, or an older person in the first flushes of menopause wondering what the hell's going on with your complexion, your skin is still a miracle of nature. It's hard at work every day underneath all the grease, sweat, dirt, pollution, makeup and gunk.

In fact, **your skin is the biggest organ in your body.** It's a living, breathing mechanism and it's working overtime for you. These are just a few of the jobs it's doing, 24 hours a day:

- Acting as a waterproof shield so that vital nutrients don't leak out of your body (gross).

- Regulating your temperature, by opening and closing blood vessels, and perspiring to allow sweat to evaporate and cool us down.

- Acting as a barrier between your insides and the many harmful toxins and microorganisms in the environment.

- Sweating out waste products including salt and ammonia.

- Helping protect you from sun damage by producing melanin.

- Synthesising vitamin D for strong bones and healthy organs.

- Patching itself up against the various cuts, bruises, grazes and burns that we get day to day.

- Giving us that little thing known as the sense of touch, which we'd be pretty screwed without.

It's complex, and it deserves respect. To understand how your skincare products work, it can help to have a basic understanding of what goes on beneath your skin.

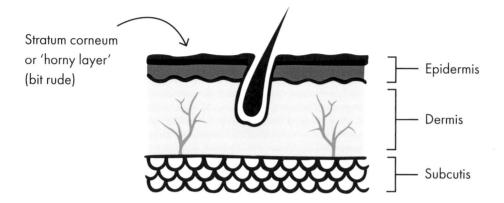

Stratum corneum
or 'horny layer'
(bit rude)

Epidermis

Dermis

Subcutis

EPIDERMIS

This is the outermost part of the skin, and the bit that you see. It's made up of keratinocytes (our skin cells), and is the part of you that keeps bacteria at bay. It's your first line of defence.

Your epidermis is constantly renewing and regenerating, with new cells made in the lowest layer, the basal cells, and travelling, over the course of about a month, to the top. The 'living' layers of cells are known as the 'squamous cells', which eventually become a layer of dead keratinocytes that are constantly shedding in the stratum corneum. This process slows down as you get older. So, making sure you're keeping your skin clean and exfoliated is important if you don't want your complexion to look dull and lifeless.

The bottom layer of the epidermis also produces melanin, which helps protect you from UV rays and gives your skin its colour. When you tan, your skin is actually producing more melanin in an attempt to shield you from the sun.

Over-the-counter skincare will only ever treat the epidermis. If you want to go deeper, you'll need a prescription or a needle.

THE DERMIS

This thicker layer of your skin contains the blood vessels and nerves that give you your sense of touch. The connective tissues are made up of two proteins: collagen, which gives skin its fullness and shape; and elastin, which gives skin its resilience and its ability to 'snap' back into shape. The cells that make these proteins are bathed in hyaluronic acid, a cellular lipid that holds water and gives your skin its bounce and texture.

When you are young, the dermis is so full of collagen and elastin that it can bounce back into shape, but as we age, they break down faster than our cells can replace them, and this leads to wrinkles and dry skin.

The dermis also contains your hair follicles and oil glands, as well as the beginning of your pores, which push hair, sweat and oil to the surface.

SUBCUTANEOUS TISSUE

This is a layer of fat and tissue lying between your skin and muscles. It protects your muscles from the beating your skin gets every day, and insulates and regulates your body's temperature too.

The subcutaneous tissue layer tends to thin as we age, and when this happens our skin looks less smooth, and the underlying veins show through. It also results in cellulite in other areas of the body.

Nobody's asking you to go back to biology class, but if you understand the basics of how your skin works, you can start to understand the claims that the skincare industry is making, what works, and what's totally impossible, what it does for you, and what you can do for it.

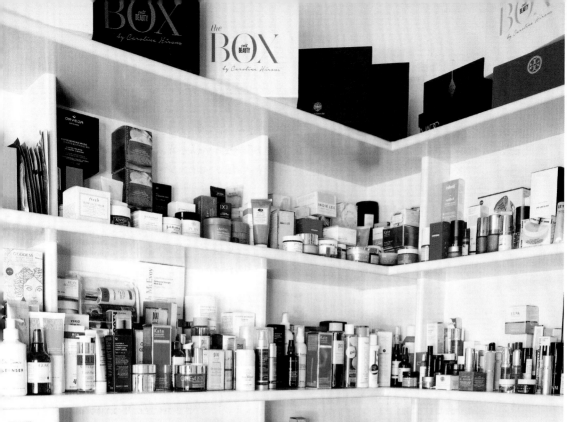
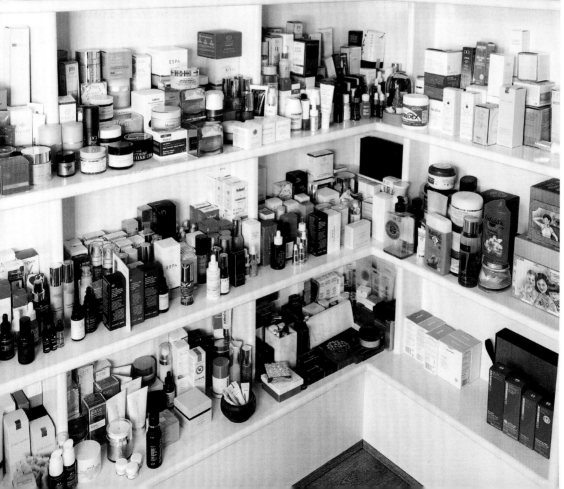

SKINCARE FOR ALL SKIN TONES

The skincare world is still way behind where it should be when it comes to showing darker skins. Ads, packaging and magazines still don't feature as many non-white faces as they should. And don't get me started on the white-washing of the 'wellness' brigade. The advice in this book is mostly for all skin tones, however there are a few, but significant, differences across skin tones when it comes to taking care of your skin day-to-day.

THE DIFFERENCES BETWEEN DARKER AND LIGHTER SKIN TONES:

- The obvious difference is the dispersion of melanin in darker skin tones. Darker skin has more melanocytes producing melanin, which, as we've seen, is what gives your skin its colour.

- The skin barrier of darker skin can be more prone to disruption through a process of trans-epidermal water loss (TEWL), because of lower levels of ceramides in the stratum corneum. This means skin can feel rough and dry. When choosing moisturisers, those with darker skin may find it helpful to use products that contain natural moisturising factors (NMF), or are labelled as 'barrier repair' or 'ceramide' cream.

- As melanin offers protection from UV rays, darker skins have a natural SPF of around 13.3 compared to white skin's 3.4 SPF. This does not mean that if you have darker skin you do not need to use SPF. You do.

- Studies show that the stratum corneum is not thicker on darker skins, but it is more compact. This is good news for the elasticity and tone of darker skin.

- A darker skin tone is more prone to hypertrophic or keloid scarring (see Glossary), where excess collagen creates a raised scar.

The skin barrier function (see Glossary) is mentioned frequently in this book. A soft, smooth-to-the-touch, plump skin is a sign of good barrier function. A compromised barrier function will present as a dull skin that feels rough and/or dry.

- Post-inflammatory hyperpigmentation (PIH) can also be an issue in darker skins. The discolouration (caused by an increase in melanin) can occur during the wound-healing process and remain after the skin has healed. When checking ingredient lists on products, look for the following to help combat this pigmentation:

  – vitamin C
  – kojic acid
  – arbutin
  – licorice extracts
  – mequinol
  – niacinamide
  – azelaic acid
  – N-acetyl glucosamine
  – hydroquinone
  – cysteamine cream
  – tretinoin

  And I can't say it enough – GET YOUR SPF ON.

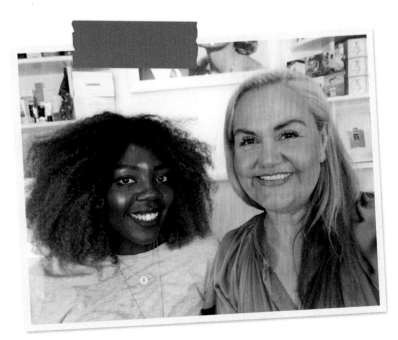

Dija Ayodele, founder of the Black Skin Directory and an incredible facialist.

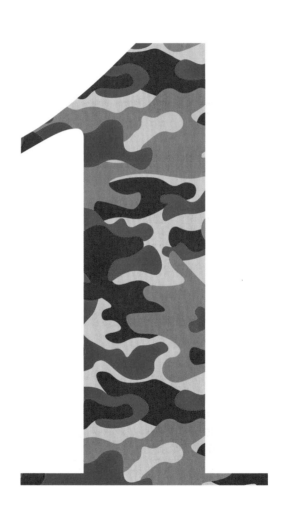

A GOOD SKINCARE ROUTINE !?#

"

SKIN IS THE FOUNDATION

"

WHERE TO START

Our skin is the biggest organ in your body, and it deserves a bit of attention. But that doesn't mean we all need to be scientists. Get into a few good habits with a daily routine and you'll soon see the benefits. A routine is the foundation of everything. And if you get it right, you can set your skin up for life. Make it a habit. Morning and evening, for 2–3 minutes, or longer if you want to take the time to enjoy it. Make sure you take the time.

It's easy to see how your skincare routine can be a little overwhelming. We are sold so many products these days – there is something for everyone – but if you have more than two serums, which do you use first? And what about eye cream? And double cleansing and, and... stop. Chill. These pages explain exactly what needs to happen at each stage of your routine.

SOME BASICS:

- You're going to need to buy some flannels or washcloths (see page 27).
- There is no mineral oil anywhere in my routine. I don't like it on my skin. Companies use it for two reasons: 1) it's not likely to cause an allergic reaction, and 2) it's cheap.
- There's nothing foaming.
- There's nothing 'mattifying' (see page 32).
- I don't recommend using wipes unless you have no access to water (hospitals, fannies, flights, festivals – emergencies only, you get the idea).
- All stages are suitable for all skin types, unless otherwise stated.
- When I talk about 'bookends' in this chapter (and in skincare in general), I mean cleansing and moisturising. Start with a good cleanse to prep your skin, and finish with an appropriate moisturiser to seal it all in and protect your skin.

BEFORE WE BEGIN:

If it ain't broke, don't fix it. If you have a product that you've known and loved for a long time, and it works for you, I'm not telling you to change it. You know your skin best.

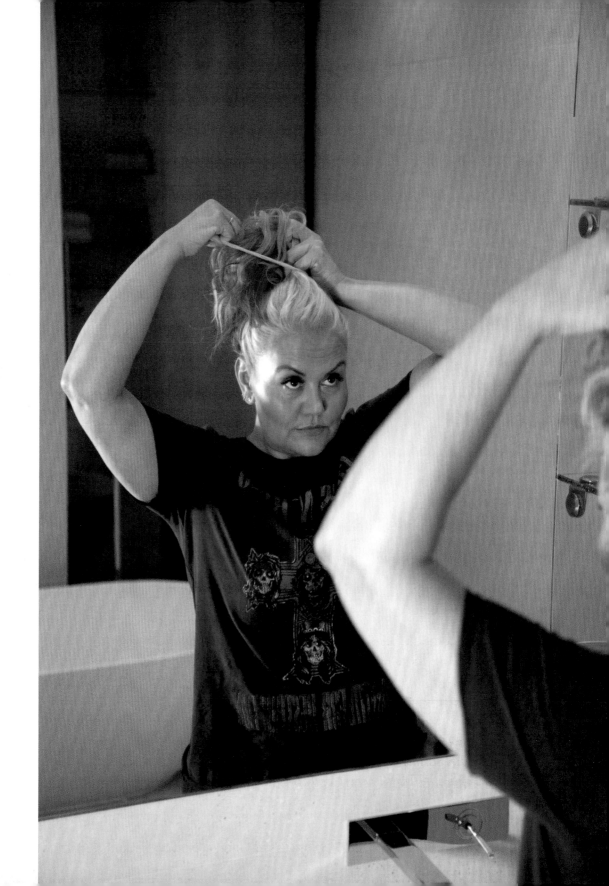

TOP TIPS FOR GREAT SKIN

Obviously everyone is different, but, *in general*, these are your basics if you're wondering where to start.

- **Cleanse your skin every night without fail** – cleanliness is next to Godliness. Double cleanse if you are wearing makeup or sunscreen, or both (which applies to most of us).

  A **little tip** for those of you that say you have no time: either take your makeup off **as soon as you get home** OR **take your makeup off before you take your bra off** (if you sleep in your bra or don't wear one, then follow the first tip!).

- **Cleanse your skin every morning.** It obviously doesn't have to be as intense as the night-time cleanse, but a quick warm flannel and milk/balm/gel wouldn't go amiss to get rid of the overnight shedding. I know some brands say you don't need to cleanse your skin in the morning. That's okay. They're wrong.

- **Wash your face properly.** A clean canvas makes everything better. There is no point in spending your hard-earned cash on expensive serums if you are using wipes or winging it when it comes to cleansing. See page 41 for more on cleansing.

- **Do not smoke.** That's really the beginning and end of it.

- **Get some sunshine.** The term 'everything in moderation' really applies here. I work indoors all day and live in the northern hemisphere. I don't get a lot of sun so I supplement with vitamin D (under doctor's advice). I don't use skincare with SPF: I apply it separately **in between** moisturiser and foundation or primer. SPF is too active an ingredient and can interfere with other anti-ageing ingredients, making all of your expensive moisturisers potentially redundant.

  Yes, obviously too much sun *is* damaging to the skin, but so is too much chlorine. And too much pollution. Get out there and get *some* sunshine. Some brands would have us believe the sun is the ultimate enemy. That's only true if you don't respect it. Get *some* sun. Not a lot, some. *Just don't be stupid about it.*

"

IF YOU WOULD SPEND MORE ON A BAG THAN YOUR FACE, YOU'RE READING THE WRONG BOOK

"

- **Use a high SPF** (30+) and encourage your kids to use it. You will save them a lot of time trying to repair sun damage in later years.

- **Use good-quality skincare.** I'm not talking about creams that cost more than your monthly food budget; I'm just suggesting you step away from the cheap packet of wipes and moisturisers in the chemist or supermarket and step it up a gear.

- **Equate your skincare spending to what you would spend on a handbag or shoes.** I'm not saying you *should* – I'm saying you *should be willing to*. (See the Your Kit section on pages 172–237.)

- **Get enough sleep.** When you are not getting sufficient rest, it shows on your face.

- **TITTT: take it to the tits.** Your neck and décolleté, which is a fancy French term for your upper chest and shoulder area, are part of your facial skincare, too.

- **Try to eat well.** I'm not being a killjoy – a little of what you fancy definitely does you good – just don't go overboard. Gut health is linked to healthy skin function: for example, taking probiotics is thought to support a healthy skin.

- **Drink enough water.** This is important not only for the normal functionality of your skin, but for your general good health, too. If your urine is dark and you suffer from a lot of headaches, you would do well to up your H_2O levels.

- **Try to avoid stress.** I know it's much harder than it sounds, but do whatever you need to do to keep your stress levels low.

MORNING ROUTINE

The main point of the morning routine is to prep your skin for the day.

Taking care of your skin in the morning is no different to having a shower before you put clean knickers on.

You may think this is obvious, but I am contacted regularly by people who say, 'Do I really need to cleanse in the mornings?' Yes.

I don't know about you, but I wake up with a lovely glow in the mornings – maybe you do too?

It's called sweat. Please wash your face.

SHOWER FIRST

I have never put my face under the shower. The water is too hot for your face (well, my choice of water temperature certainly is). You also have the surfactants from your shampoo running all over your face. Stand with your back to the shower and your chin raised – like the shower has greatly offended you.

Cleanse when you get out of the shower, not before.

FLANNELS

Flannels get your skin CLEAN. Think of your parents: how did they wash you when you were a kid? They used a flannel.

They are more substantial than wipes or muslin, are far more effective at removing dirt, and help exfoliate the skin, too.

Buy eight flannels minimum and use one a day (you'll need the eighth flannel as a spare on wash day): start with a fresh, clean flannel for your morning cleanse and use the same flannel for your evening cleanse, chucking it in the washing basket when you're done.

You don't have to spend a fortune on the plushest, fluffiest flannels. Any will do. But go for white so you get the satisfaction of seeing the muck come off.

Machine-wash your flannels so they get properly clean, but avoid using fabric softener, as traces can end up on your skin.

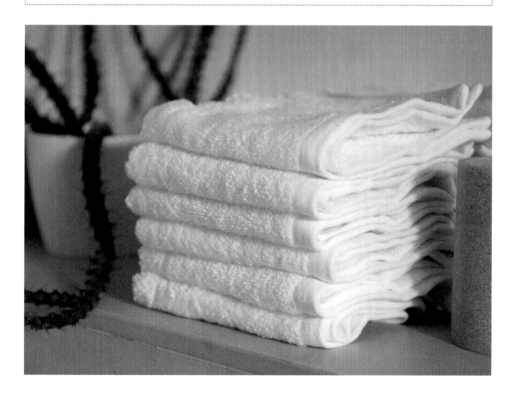

#CLEANSE

Any non-foaming cleanser is fine – milk, balm (a little), gel – as long as it doesn't turn your face into a foam bath, carry on. Yes, you can absolutely use the same product in the morning that you use in the evening if you want to, but you're only cleansing once.

Use a clean flannel.

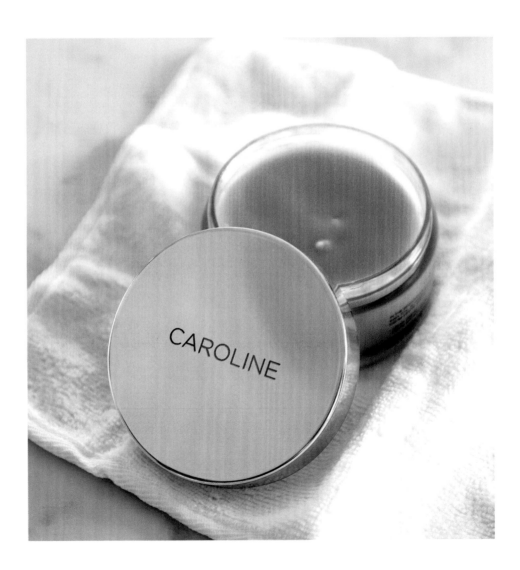

#EXFOLIATE

Rather than harsh scrubs (which are thankfully going out of fashion), acids are about taking off the layer of dead skin cells and, depending on the type of acid, stimulating the skin. **Your skin's surface is naturally acidic, and acid toners lower your skin's pH.** They have the effect of blowing a trumpet in your ear. Your skin is forced into action.

Most brands make exfoliating/acid products that you use at the traditional 'toner' stage. To call them a 'toner' is to do them a great injustice – these are the 'toners' of the 21st century.

Try to have a couple of exfoliating/acid products if you can: a milder version and a more 'active' one. There's no point in having two of one type. Alternate them daily. There are lots of different types of acid (see pages 189–193) but the main ones are glycolic, lactic and salicylic. If you can only afford one, either buy a mild one and use it twice a day, or a stronger one and use it in the evenings only. If you have sensitive skin, or you are just concerned about using acids, start by using them twice a week and see how your skin reacts.

All packaging for *anything* with *any* acid in it will legally have to say 'avoid eye area'. Unless you are using a prescription strength, dermatologist-prescribed hardcore acid, it's fine. Apply the acidic toners on cotton pad or gauze then take it around the eyes – full circle – upper brow to corner brow and under eye to inner eye – and reverse.

Caveat: using acids twice a day or even daily may be too much or unnecessary for some skins, especially if you are also using active ingredients in other products, such as strong retinoids in the evenings. If you're new to acids, start slowly and follow your skin's response.

> Go easy and listen to your skin. If you have overdone it or your skin feels like you've gone too far, acid is the first thing you should drop. Actives are the second.

#SPRAY HYDRATE

I love this step. It's the start of the hydrating process and it wakes me up. Use whatever hydrating flower mist or water you like. Any spray should have glycerin or hyaluronic acid in there somewhere, but something like a good-quality rosewater is fine. I mean *good* quality – i.e. the INCI (International Nomenclature of Cosmetic Ingredients – see Glossary) list is proper rosewater, not fragrance (parfum) and colouring. Check your ingredient labels.

You can also use your traditional 'toner' at this stage, as long as its main function is to hydrate. Some traditional toners are designed to 'mattify' or strip back sebum (see Glossary) and this is not what we want. If you are using toner in this way, decant it into a spray bottle and keep it as a spray, too. Try to avoid alcohol at this stage.

#APPLY EYE PRODUCT

Do not apply your eye product last. No matter how carefully you apply your serums and moisturisers you will always get some in the eye area, and then your eye product won't be absorbed where you want it to be. Pointless.

Apply eye products to the orbital area (the area covered by your sunglasses) before serum, moisturiser and SPF (you can put these on top of the eye product if you fancy it and it's not a contraindication).

APPLYING YOUR EYE PRODUCT LAST IS LIKE WEARING YOUR KNICKERS OVER YOUR TROUSERS

#APPLY SERUM/OILS

This step is what I am asked about the most. I use a mixture of oils and serums, and application goes by texture.

Serums – especially water-based ones – go on first. Next, a couple of drops of facial oil (if you are using one), topped off with your moisturiser. In the case of a heavily siliconed serum, I would probably skip the oil and go straight to moisturiser. Spending 20 seconds 'warming' your serum in your hands by rubbing them together is a complete waste of time, money and product, unless your intention is to have fabulously soft palms (see pages 62–63 for my 'therapist hands' technique for dispersing product in the palms and onto the fingers).

There will *always* be exceptions, so if what you are doing works for you, don't change it on my account.

#MOISTURISE

Choose your moisturiser according to your skin *type*, not skin *condition*. Your moisturiser is your coat/protection. People tend to spend far too long choosing their moisturiser and far too little time taking care of what goes on beforehand: for example, using a quick swipe of a wipe, slapping on an expensive face cream and then wondering why their skin isn't great.

Remember to avoid anything 'mattifying' – a promise that's often made on products for oily skin. Skin is not designed to be 'matte'.

> Your skin has plenty of time to be matte when you're dead.

If your skin is excessively oily, just go for light hyaluronic acid serums, which help lock in moisture, and oil-free moisturisers. No need to force the issue. Leave that to your makeup.

Whatever moisturiser you are using that is right for your skin, whack it on now.

YOUR SKIN 'SLEEPS' DURING THE DAY

No. Your skin does not, will not, and has never 'slept' during the day.

The other argument for using different products in the evening is that your skin 'may' relax a little while it's not busy fighting off free radicals (see Glossary). Funnily enough, free radicals are not particularly conscious of time and are, in fact, around us 24/7, but that's apparently by-the-by for some marketing people. If you wanted to really annoy someone you could argue that as soon as you breathe out carbon dioxide, your face is surrounded by a cloud of free radicals.

You use different products at night because you don't need SPF (or thicker 'protecting' moisturisers), which means you can use lighter, more effective formulations – serums/oils/retinoids etc. – to target and treat skin issues.

AM: Protect
PM: Treat and repair

'Your skin is your biggest organ.' Replace the word 'skin' in this sentence with 'heart', 'brain', 'lungs', 'kidney' or 'liver' and see how long you would be alive for.

'Your skin sleeps during the day'?
Right, well, that's me dead then.

#APPLY SPF

I always recommend using a walnut-sized dollop of a separate SPF. A moisturiser with added SPF will not benefit the skin as much as two separate products will. I mean, it's better than nothing, but wouldn't you rather be safe than sorry?

> Do not use an SPF instead of a moisturiser.
>
> That's like going out all day with a raincoat on and only bra and knickers underneath.

Unless that is your everyday outfit of choice, I suggest you wear actual clothes (moisturiser) underneath your raincoat (SPF). You should always use a broad-spectrum sunscreen (see page 217) that protects against UVA rays, which damage your skin's elasticity, and UVB rays, which can cause skin damage and alter the structure of cells, potentially leading to skin cancer. I would always recommend an SPF30 or higher.

Make sure you apply it everywhere, including the back of your neck and the top of your ears. Women typically apply their SPF before they hit the beach and put their hair in a ponytail the minute they hit the sand. EARS! Even if you aren't on holiday.

To achieve the SPF on the label, you need 2 milligrams of sunscreen per square centimetre of the area (see pages 61 and 86 for advice on product quantities). The official recommendations change regularly, but current thinking is that for the face, it's a good amount more than you are used to applying as a moisturiser. Double it.

IF YOU HAVE OILY SKIN YOU DO NOT NEED TO MOISTURISE

The biggest mistake people with oily/combination skin make is to try to 'strip' the skin during the cleansing stage – to the point where it squeaks *faints* – and then not apply anything else on top and just go.

Your face is not a shampoo advert. You cannot just 'wash'n'go'.

For the more lubricated among us:

#1 Cleanse your face with a good non-foaming cleanser (oil, cream, milk or gel – no mineral oil and no bubbles).

#2 Exfoliate with an acidic toner.

#3 Spray hydrate.

#4 Apply a light serum to target specific skin conditions (ageing, pigmentation, scarring/dehydration etc.) if that is a concern.

#5 Apply either a hyaluronic serum, a moisturiser, or even a facial oil designed for your skin type.

Use serums to treat your skin **condition**. Use moisturisers or facial oils to treat your skin **type**.

Washing your face and going out with nothing on it is akin to leaving the house butt naked.

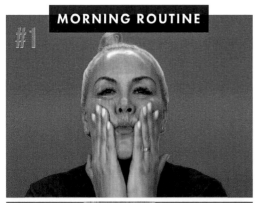

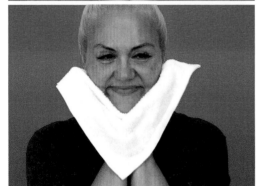

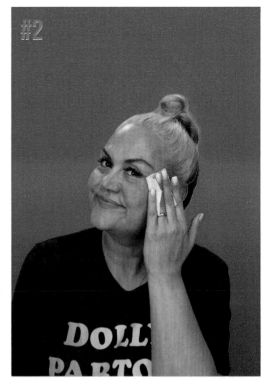

#1

#2

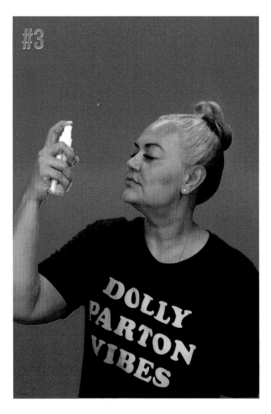

#3

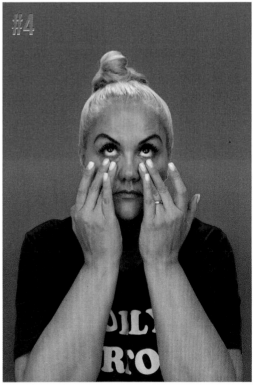

#4

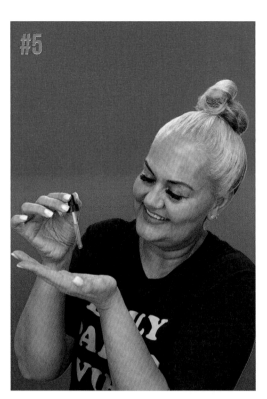

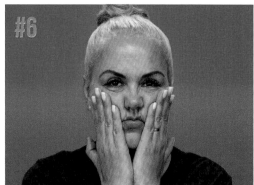

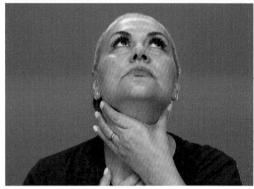

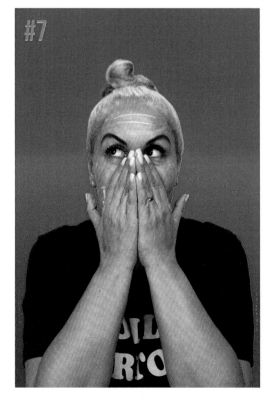

STEP-BY-STEP

1 Use your hands to apply a non-foaming cleanser. Wipe off the cleanser with a clean, warm, damp flannel.

2 Exfoliate your skin with an acid toner or wipe.

3 Spray your skin with a hydrating spray.

4 Put a little cream on the edge of your ring finger, blend it with the other ring finger, then apply to the eyes. You need enough to cover the entire orbital area, over and below your eye.

5 Put a couple of drops of serum or facial oil on your palm, then use the fingertips of the other hand to apply immediately.

6 Apply moisturiser all over your face, neck and décolletage: take it to the tits. Your skin should feel comfortable, not 'wet'.

7 Apply SPF after your moisturiser, and make sure you use enough.

SPF: MY MOST-ASKED QUESTIONS FROM READERS

- **Do 'once-a-day' sunscreens work?**
Personally, I would not dream of using a 'once-a-day' sunscreen on holiday, *especially* on my children. It gives a false sense of security. According to some once-a-day SPF websites, if I use their SPF50 with my skin type, I can 'safely' stay in the sun for ten hours. TEN. HOURS? No. Where once-a-day formulas *might* come in handy are...

Young children going to school. If, as mine do, your young children attend a school where the teachers are not allowed to touch the children, even with your permission, a once-a-day formula may be a good option. Your children may sweat a little, but they aren't in the sea so should still be protected until the end of the day. In *theory*. It makes me uneasy nonetheless, but it's better than applying a typical 'kids' SPF15 first thing and that's it for the day... It's your judgement call as a parent or carer. Remember the backs of their necks and the tops of their ears.

If you are wearing SPF under your makeup and going to work.
You will probably not be covered by lunchtime so you either need to reapply (not likely, I know), use a once-a-day product – these are far better suited to city living than beach in my opinion – or buy yourself a big hat and be done with it.

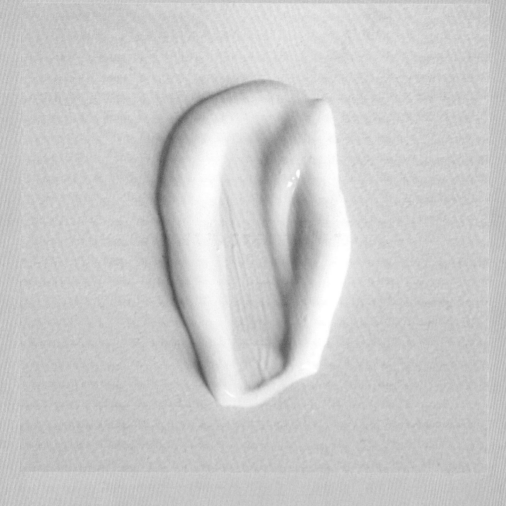

- **Do you recommend sunscreen sprays?** Here's the thing with sprays: you have to make sure you have covered the entire area thoroughly and that is unlikely unless you are applying it to your child, in which case most of us show more due diligence than when we are applying to our own bodies. Use a spray over your makeup if you know you have applied it evenly and feel protected, otherwise, go down the once-a-day route or make like Jackie O and enjoy a hat and sunglasses. There is also cause for concern when inhaling sprays – something you will invariably do if the point is to apply it over your makeup. Your judgement call.

- **Is it safe to use acids and vitamin A products in the summer?** Yes – just make sure you are also using your SPF.

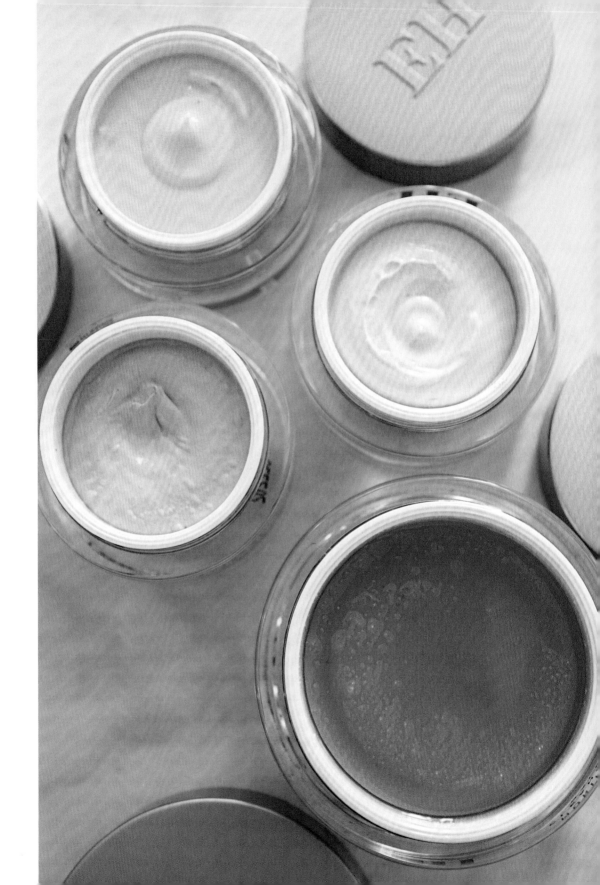

CLEANSING LOWDOWN

Cleansing is **by far** the most important step of your routine.

If you are consistently 'cleansing' with wipes (aka moving the dirt around your face) and then applying a really expensive serum or moisturiser on top, you are wasting your money. And your time.

'Double cleansing' may be something that you are doing already in the evenings, this is just what I call it.

Essentially, if you are using more than one product to remove your makeup in the evenings, you are double cleansing.

For example, if you remove your eye makeup with a micellar water or eye-makeup remover before you cleanse, that is your first cleanse. You follow with a proper cleanser to remove everything else. That was your second cleanse.

NOTE: a micellar water is not your second cleanse. Stop that nonsense.

Let's be clear on something — there is no double cleansing in the mornings. Wake up, cleanse once, you're good to go. You have no makeup or SPF to remove. Crack on.

There is a trend for 60-second cleansing, meaning you apply all your cleanser, massage it around for 60 seconds, and remove. And you only do this once. That's fine if you want to do it in the mornings, but for the evening? I'm not a fan. If you are wearing makeup and SPF it is far less irritating to the skin to do two quicker cleanses than one long one. Loosen and remove the topical makeup/SPF with your first cleanse and clean your skin with the second one.

MORNING CLEANSE

Use any of the following:

- Non-foaming gels
- Milks
- Lotions
- Balm cleansers
- Oils
- Clay-based cleansers

Basically, *anything* except:

- Wipes
- Micellar water

The morning cleanse routine is dependent on how your skin feels when you wake up and what you are doing with the rest of your day. For example, if I have a long day ahead of wearing makeup, I will probably use an oil to cleanse. My skin feels soft and holds moisture for longer afterwards, which has a knock-on effect on the rest of my routine and stops my makeup going patchy by the afternoon.

If I'm based at home for the day I'll use something slightly more 'active', follow with a strong acid toner and apply some treatment serums and heavier moisturisers.

If you know you are going to be based at home for the day and not wearing makeup, treat your skin as if it's a spa day: **cleanse**, **exfoliate**, **treat**, **repeat** (repeat the treat, not the entire routine!).

This is why my skin looks great if I've had a few consecutive days working from home, and looks merely 'okay' if I've had appointments in town every day of the week. And do not get me started on travelling… that's a whole other subject (see pages 80–81).

Wipes and micellar water are not suitable for mornings because you use them in an emergency or when removing makeup, and you won't be wearing makeup to bed, will you?

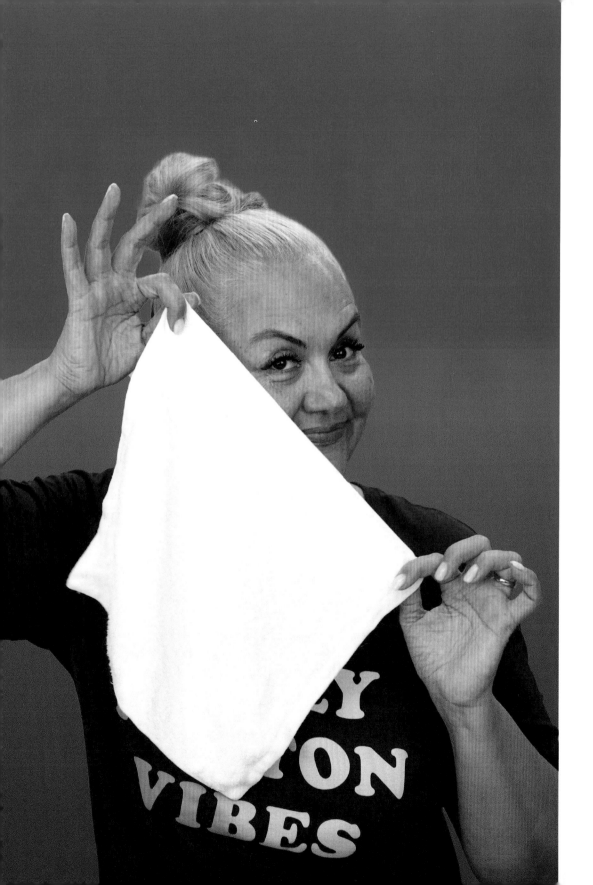

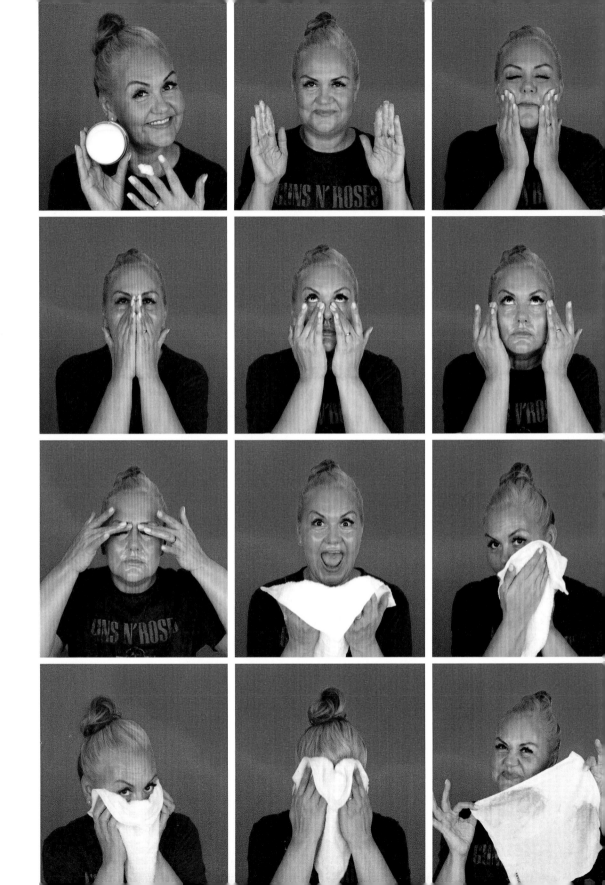

EVENING (DOUBLE) CLEANSE

Do what *you* need to do to remove what you've put on your face. You know your face/routine better than anyone on a beauty counter. Or me.

Wearing a ton of eye makeup? Remove it first.

Slathered in SPF? Take care of that first.

Both? Go in with grease. **When in doubt, go in with grease.** Think of all the old Hollywood movie stars and the footage of them removing their face with grease. It works. Just look at the last picture on the grid opposite – you know you're going to need to go in again with more cleanser and a rinsed-out cloth.

FIRST CLEANSE:

- Eye-makeup removers
- Micellar waters
- Greasy balms – not necessarily expensive ones, just ones that do a great job of removing makeup
- Cleansing creams – preferably thicker ones with a good oil content
- Oils – oils are great for removing makeup, but you don't have to pick a really expensive one for the first cleanse

SECOND CLEANSE:

This is where you use your most expensive cleansing product. This one is your skin cleanser more than your makeup remover. Its job is to make sure your skin is clean, balanced and comfortable and ready for everything else that you are applying afterwards. It's time to use your good stuff.

Some people are saying that double cleansing means using oil followed by foam. No.

You can obviously use one cleanser for both cleanses if you have budget concerns. We've all been there. Well, I certainly have. Just buy the best that you can afford, when you can afford it.

If you are using one product, apply a small amount for the first cleanse mainly to loosen eye makeup and product on cheek areas (where we tend to apply the most SPF). Remove with a flannel and go in again with another round.

The second cleanse is the massage stage, not the first. Don't spend a lot of time on your first cleanse. It's loosening the dirt, not vacuuming it all up.

The best products for second cleanse are:
- Cleansing balms: good ones. Gorgeous, plant-based, greasy ones. Greasy in the best way.
- Cleansing milks
- Cleansing gels: non-foaming (i.e. without sodium lauryl sulphate)
- Cleansing creams
- Cleansing clays
- Cleansing oils: oils and balms are easily my favourite choice for skin cleansing. They are brilliant for ensuring that everything is off and don't disturb the acid mantle (see Glossary) in an aggressive manner.

See page 181 for my recommendations of brands and products.

That is really all there is to it.

The important part is to remember to cleanse properly every single day without fail.

'PAT DRY'

This may seem like a strange one, so the context is important. I am always asked about routines and what order products should be used in.

There are some things that make it onto packaging purely because NPD (new product development) and marketing departments regurgitate the same advice time and time again, just because it's what they've done before.

One of the main culprits is on cleanser packaging, or in cleansing routines when it says that after cleansing, you should 'rinse off, then pat dry'.

If you're soaking wet after a shower, you may want to lightly dry your face, mainly so you can see, but here's the thing: in an ideal world, you want a damp face.

If you use your flannels and follow my routines, your skin will be damp once you've cleansed. You need to go from there right to the next stage. Whether that's acids or spritzes. There's no need to pat dry first. Go straight in – a damp skin is a great skin to work on. Seal in the moisture with your following products.

▌ There is one big exception: vitamin A.

Retinoids, especially prescription-strength ones, should be applied to dry skin after cleansing. I cleanse, use a flannel, then leave my skin to air-dry for a few minutes (usually just the time it takes to make tea; not hours) before I apply the retinoid, then I put other products on top (see pages 52–53).

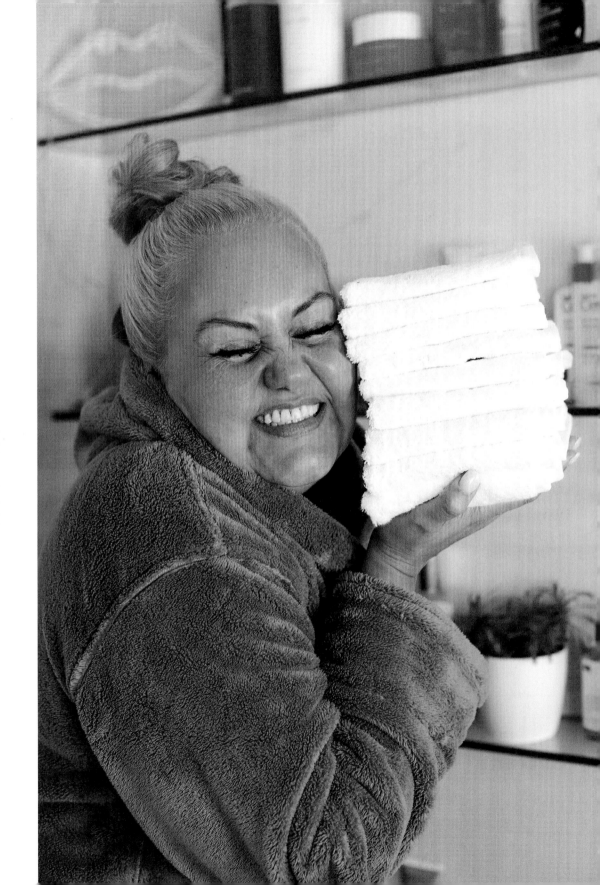

EVENING ROUTINE

| At home? Bra off. Hair up.
| Clean your face.

The main point of your evening routine is to help your skin help itself.

Repair and correct.

Your face is not being bombarded with sunlight, dirt, aggressors etc. at night, so you can get the treatments in while they actually have a better chance of being effective.

'Your skin repairs itself at night' is the biggest old wives' tale out there in skincare. It's nonsense. And please don't get me started on **'your skin sleeps at night'**. No. YOU sleep at night. Your skin does not have an on/off switch like your heating. **Your skin is repairing itself 24 hours a day** – the reason you use treatments while you sleep is *because you have the full attention of your skin.*

#CLEANSE

'Do I need to double cleanse?' is my most frequently asked question about the evening routine. The only time I don't double cleanse is if I have been indoors all day and have applied neither SPF nor makeup. Otherwise, I go straight in with an oil-based product to hit the grease, dirt, makeup and general gunk on my face after a day in Central London.

If you wear SPF you need to double cleanse. A lot of people who think they are allergic to SPF because it breaks them out are simply not taking the time to wash it off properly. (Please don't take it personally if you genuinely are allergic to SPF – I'm clearly not talking to you.)

SPF is designed to stay on your face.
Take the time to remove it.
Makeup is designed to stay on your face.
Take the time to remove it.

Using the flannel from the morning is fine. I usually use two out of the three products below.

- Pre-cleanse oil or eye-makeup remover
- Oil/balm cleanser
- Milk/gel cleanser

NOTE TO MICELLAR WATER USERS: if you prefer to take your makeup off with a micellar water before you cleanse, that is your first cleanse. But if you are wearing an SPF or heavy makeup you still need to go a couple of rounds with a flannel. Don't be lazy. Your skin will thank you.

#APPLY VITAMIN A

If you are using vitamin A (see pages 52–53), apply it onto dry skin after cleansing. Leave it for about 20 minutes, then follow it with your eye product. If you need it, apply your moisturiser afterwards. If you are new to vitamin A, or are using a strong vitamin A product, the effects can be quite extreme at first so you may need to buffer it by applying a moisturiser or mild facial oil around 20–30 minutes after applying it.

SKINCARE MYTH

IT'S OKAY TO SLEEP IN YOUR MAKEUP

Enough already.

STOP SAYING that it is okay to sleep in your makeup. It is not. The average woman wears a mix of the following:

SPF
primer
foundation
powder
concealer
blusher
bronzer
eyeshadow (multiple)
eyeliner
mascara
brow pencil
lip liner
lipstick
lip gloss

That is a LOT of product on your face. SPF, in particular, is designed to stick to your face; that's its job. Add to that all the dirt and pollution from being outside and you have the perfect storm brewing for spots, dehydration, dullness – a whole plethora of issues.

**Wash your face at night.
Do not sleep in your makeup.**

If your partner prefers you with makeup, get a new partner. 😉

HOW TO USE A VITAMIN A PRODUCT

Brands all provide instructions on the packaging. While there will always be exceptions, the key things to remember are:

- Vitamin A products, most commonly known as retinoids, go onto the skin **after cleansing**.

- **You can use other products**, but they go on after the vitamin A.

- **Don't apply a lot, thinking it will work faster.** It won't. Save your money, and your skin. Apply a small, pea-sized amount, or in the case of an oil, a few drops, not an entire pipette. The results can be very alarming (in a good way – you may notice the difference almost overnight). Do not be tempted to think more is more. It isn't. In the case of vitamin A, and especially if you have not used a vitamin A product before, less is more.

- **Use it every third night,** moving to more regular use when you know your skin is tolerating it (unless a brand specifically says differently). This analogy might be helpful: if you're in your 30s, try to use it 3 times a week; if you're in your 40s, go for 4 times a week; and in your 50s, aim for daily use.

I have been using vitamin A products for a long time. If I know I'm using an OTC (over-the-counter) vitamin A product in the evening, I cleanse, sometimes acid tone (although less so if I am using a high-percentage retinoid), spritz, leave a gap for my skin to be touch-dry, then apply my retinoid. If, however, I'm using a prescription-strength retinoid, I cleanse and then apply the cream. If in doubt, apply your retinoid after cleansing, leave it on for 20–30 minutes by itself, then follow with either a soothing moisturiser or facial oil.

I love retinoid products. They are easily the best products for fighting signs of ageing. Everyone should use one. They are worth the faff. Just use them correctly.

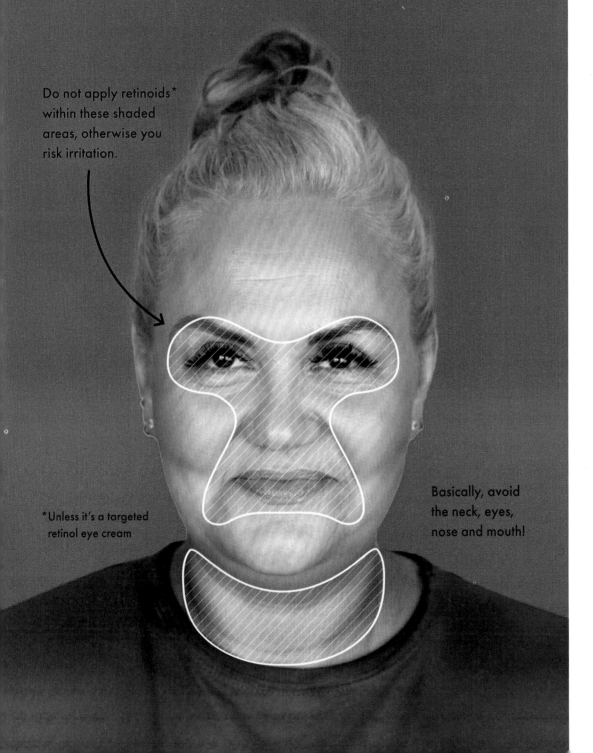

WHERE *NOT* TO PUT IT

Do not apply retinoids* within these shaded areas, otherwise you risk irritation.

*Unless it's a targeted retinol eye cream

Basically, avoid the neck, eyes, nose and mouth!

#APPLY EYE PRODUCT

As in the morning routine, if you typically wake up with puffy eyes, move to a lighter texture and use a serum or gel. Avoid rich creams.

#APPLY TREATMENT PRODUCTS (USUALLY SERUMS) OR FACIAL OILS

This is my favourite step. This is where you can really go to town. **Treatment products should be your main expense skincare-wise.** Try to have at least three products you can use, depending on your skin's needs. *At least.*

Use a good facial oil, a good serum or treatment – whatever you need for your skin. And before you ask me what you need, really think about it. You know your skin.

Whether or not you use a night-time moisturiser depends on what treatment you use. If your treatment is IN your moisturiser, you're done. If you are using a lovely night-time oil, you may not want/need anything else. Personally, I am a fan of the 'piling it on lightly' approach.

> All this 'cleanse and then just let your skin breathe' is daft. Your skin is always breathing. If it wasn't, you'd soon know about it. In the morgue.

Your skin will breathe regardless of whether you put product on it or not.

My PM routine is literally: pre-cleanse, cleanse, acid, spray hydrate, eye product, oil/treatment and night treatment/oil/cream (not all three!).

Sometimes less is really not more. Having one cleanser and one moisturiser is like having one pair of shoes or one bra. If you can afford more than one pair of shoes, you can afford more than one cleanser and more than one moisturiser.

'WARM PRODUCT IN HANDS BEFORE USE'

This is another thing that brands have got into the habit of putting on their packaging.

A good formulation will be ready to go as soon as it comes out of the bottle or tube, so warming a product in your hands will only put most of the product on your hands. Oil doesn't need to be warmed to be absorbed. If you want to rub it in your hands and inhale it before you apply it, that's your choice, but it won't change the way it works.

> I prefer to put it on my face and smell it while it gets to work on my face – not my hands.

If your product is such that it needs to be 'warmed', I probably wouldn't bother. As always, there are some exceptions: Weleda Dry Skin Food, for example, needs a little help.

My 'therapist hands' technique (see pages 62–63) shows you how to apply your product so you see the benefits on your face, rather than your hands.

EVENING ROUTINE

#1

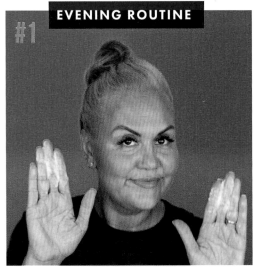

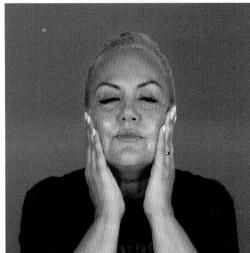

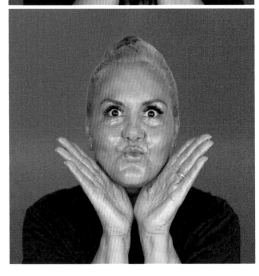

#2

#3

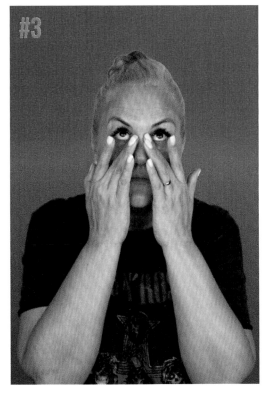

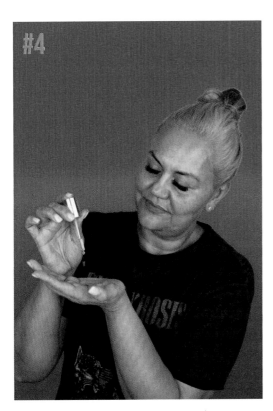

#4

Don't forget to
put your flannel
in the wash!

STEP-BY-STEP

1 If you have been wearing SPF and/or makeup, you need to double cleanse.

If you're wearing lots of eye makeup, swipe around the eyes with a cleansing oil, using your fingertips, or use a dedicated eye-makeup remover on cotton pads if you're wearing lash extensions or a lot of mascara.

Get your cleansing oil or balm straight on and around the eye area first, then spread it out across the rest of the face. To take it off, hold a flannel under a warm running tap, squeeze out excess water, then wipe away makeup. (Don't fill the sink bowl with water – this cleansing stage will not splash off.)

If you have only done one cleansing step at this stage, finish with a quick going over of a lighter milk or gel cleanser geared for your skin type. Get it straight onto the skin, then off with a warm, damp flannel.

2 Apply vitamin A (optional) onto dry skin after cleansing, leave it for about 20 minutes, then follow with eye product.

If you're not using a vitamin A product, proceed as in the morning routine (without SPF).

3 Apply eye product (and moisturiser, if using), as in the morning routine.

4 Apply your favourite treatments or facial oils.

HOW MUCH PRODUCT SHOULD I USE?

Take this as a rough guide, not hard-and-fast rules: everyone's face is different in size (mine is huge!). Remember the mantra: *grip, not slip.* Your face shouldn't feel greasy or slippery.

CLEANSER

Because we're not talking about foam, I would break it down by the formula and what are you using the cleanser for – either makeup removing or skin cleansing.

First cleanse/makeup removal – balm: either a big fat grape or two grapes if they're smallish [1].

First cleanse/makeup removal – milk: a heaped teaspoon or two pumps (if applicable) [2].

Second cleanse/AM cleanse – a level teaspoon (or one pump, if applicable).

ACID TONING

Dampen a flat cotton pad (not cotton-wool balls) until two thirds of the pad is wet. Use both sides. Always. For pre-soaked pads, use one pad on both sides.

EYE PRODUCT

I usually use about a 'pine nut' per eye. If your eyes are dry or showing signs of ageing, then you may want slightly more. But for younger skins, one pine nut on the edge of your ring finger, blended with the opposing finger then applied to the eyes, is sufficient. You need enough to cover the entire orbital area, over and below your eye.

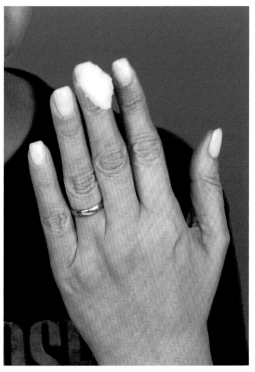

CLEANSER 1

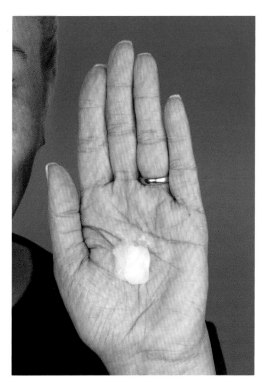

CLEANSER 2

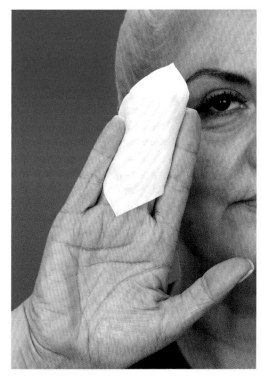

ACID TONING

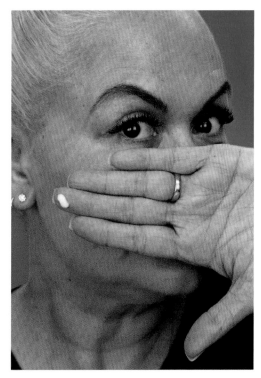

EYE PRODUCT

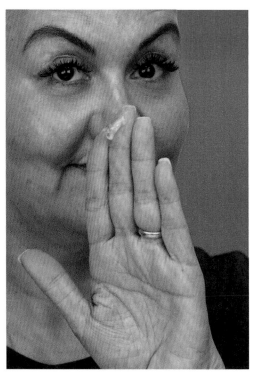

SERUMS

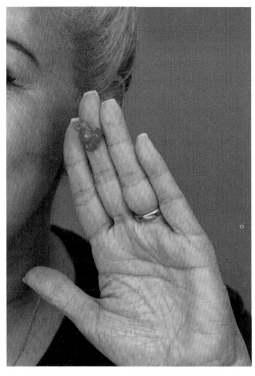

MOISTURISER / NIGHT CREAM

SPF

SERUMS

Serums are easy to gauge because the majority of them are in a bottle fitted with a dispensing pump and are designed to be dispensed at one pump per application. Ergo, if you have a large face, use two pumps, and for a smaller face, use one pump. For comparison purposes, about the size of an almond.

There has, however, been a huge increase in the use of pipettes for serums (I hate them – they are messy to use, you're more likely to drop them and waste product, and they allow air into the formula). If yours has a pipette, start with half a pipette maximum, adding a little more if you need it.

MOISTURISER AND NIGHT CREAM

Depending on your skin and face size, two blueberries, or three if you're a dry pumpkin head. Think almond-size again.

SPF

It is suggested that, on average, people apply one fifth of the amount of product required to actually reach the SPF level listed on the bottle.

At the time of writing, to achieve the SPF on the label, you are advised to use 2 milligrams of sunscreen per square centimetre of the area.

The official recommendations change regularly, but current thinking is, for the face, it's a good amount more than you are used to applying as a moisturiser. Double it. For your body, it's a teaspoon per limb. A *teaspoon*. One for each leg and arm, one for your trunk, one for your back, and if you're wearing skimpy swimwear or going nude, then good for you! You need to add one lotion allowance for your bottom, hips, thighs etc. See page 86 for more information.

APPLYING PRODUCT

One of the things I see time and again is people spending ages warming and rubbing skin products into their hands rather than putting them to work on their face! Why?! This technique makes sure the product gets onto your face. I call it 'therapist hands' because no professional would put expensive product on their hands and spend time rubbing it into their palms before applying it. You should not need to warm a product in your hands to make it work (see page 55).

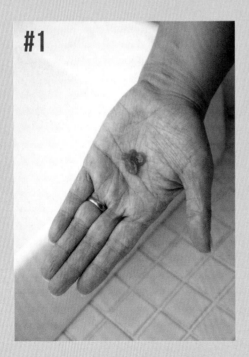

#1

Deposit product into the centre of your palm.

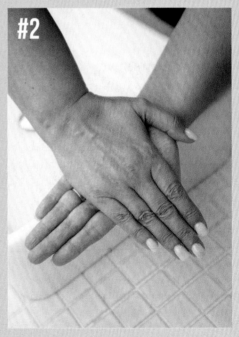

#2

Put your palms together in an 'X'.

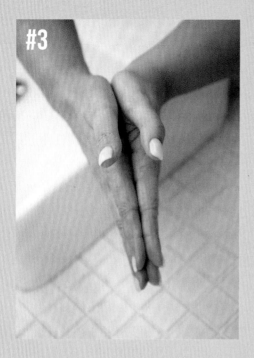

#3

Twist the hands 90 degrees so that your palms are facing.

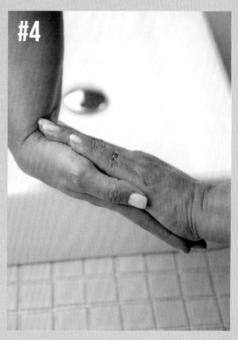

#4

Twist the hands a further 180 degrees so that your palms are opposing.

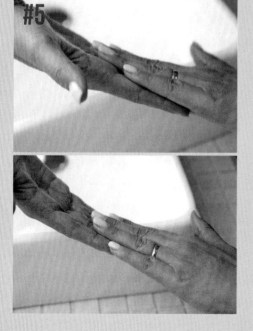

#5

Pull your hands apart smoothly.

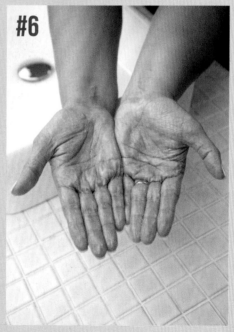

#6

The product should be evenly distributed across your fingers and palms ready for application.

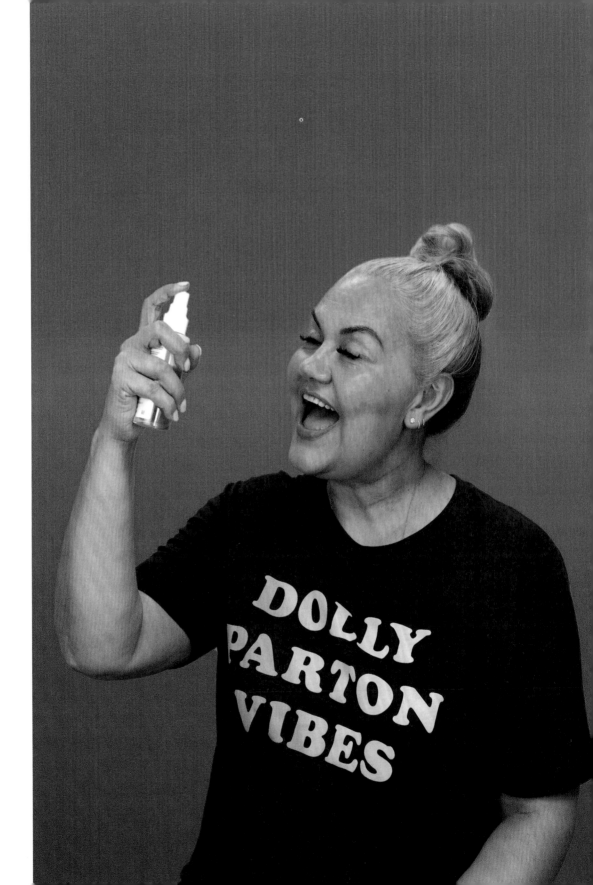

ROUTINE FOR DRY, DEHYDRATED OR PARCHED SKIN

Now you have the basics for a good routine sorted, here are some situations where things may need to be tweaked. Dehydrated skin can seem like it would need a whole new routine, but actually the foundations are exactly the same. These are the situations and products you'll want to focus on to help quench your skin's thirst.

#CLEANSER

Stay away from foaming cleansers. I know I say this all the time, but it's particularly important when your epidermis already resembles a prune. Stick to cleansing milks, oils or creams. They will help plump up your skin and enable it to retain moisture from your very first step. Using a foaming cleanser on a dry, parched, dehydrated skin is akin to skin torture and is a skincare crime of the highest order. Please bear that in mind whenever you see the term 'recommended by dermatologists' or 'approved by dermatologists'. Derms don't do that for free. Someone is getting paid.

#ACIDS

Keep using acids, but consider switching to lactic acid, which is good for surface exfoliation.

#MISTS OR SPRITZ

This is key and your best friend. You'll be using these liberally until your skin feels better. Layer moisture between every step in your skincare routine to give the feeling that your skin is hydrated. 'Mist' or 'spritz' always means using a spray that contains hyaluronic acid, which locks in moisture, not just plain water in a spray bottle or tin.

■ Fake it 'til you make it.

#SERUMS/OILS

Apply a hyaluronic-based serum to your skin, let it soak in, spritz, and spritz again if necessary. If this isn't enough, you can apply an oil on top. I tend to use oil-based serums or full facial oils when my skin feels really dry and dehydrated.

With this skin situation, silicone-based serums tend to 'roll' more and don't feel like they are doing their job. Wait a week or so before introducing them. The easiest way to tell if your product is silicone-based without the aid of the ingredient list is to apply half a pump to the back of your hand. If it is absorbed immediately, it's silicone; if there is residue on the skin and the product seems to spread all over your hand, it's probably oil-heavy.

#SPRITZ AGAIN

I cannot say this enough. YOU CAN NEVER SPRITZ TOO MUCH.

#MOISTURISER

This is not a time to go oil-free. You need oil in your moisturiser to help lock in the moisture.

Think of the top layers of the skin as a sponge that is emerging halfway out of a bowl of water. The top part of the skin is drying out and exposed. A common mistake when treating dry, dehydrated or parched skin is to apply a thick layer of moisturiser. This is akin to applying a thick layer of cold butter to cold toast. It won't penetrate – it will sit on the surface of the skin and/or roll off. Don't waste your product. Apply just enough moisturiser on top of your oil or serum to give comfort to your skin. Wait a little while, *spritz again*, then reapply a little moisturiser. In scientific terms you would normally apply oil last, as the molecules are bigger than those in moisturisers. However, for ease of wearing makeup and a non-sticky feeling on the face, I like to apply my moisturiser last. And in this case, it's nice to seal in the oil or serum. If you're not weaing makeup, you can repeat thin layers of moisturiser throughout the day. Cleanse as usual in the evening and do your normal routine. Repeat as before, until your skin feels more comfortable.

LIPS

Include your lips in your entire routine when they're dry. Just be gentle…

Cleanse them, use your acid pads over them, even if it's just around the edges – if they are split it will sting like hell, so go with your instinct (a word of warning; I have yet to taste a nice acid), use your oil on them, and use your moisturiser on them. Reapply a little oil as needed throughout the day. They will improve quickly with a little TLC.

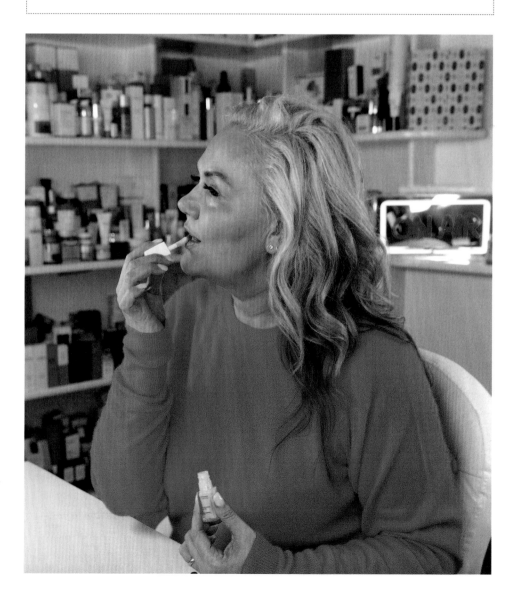

WHEN YOU'RE EXERCISING

I am frequently asked by people that exercise in all manner of ways about when they should schedule their skincare routines and what they should use. As there are SO many variations, I thought I'd try to cover all bases.

So, let's start with the 'skeleton' or bare bones.

JOGGING/RUNNING

Early-morning run:

COLD CLIMATE (ENGLISH WINTER FOR EXAMPLE)
Apply a little facial oil to protect your face before you pound the streets, go run, sweat, come home, do morning skincare routine.

HOT CLIMATE
Apply SPF before you hit the streets, go run, come home, do skincare routine.

After-work run:

Remove makeup, apply a thin layer of moisturiser (and/or SPF if outside and the sun is out), go run, sweat, shower, do your proper evening skincare routine.

GYM SESSIONS/WEIGHTS/CARDIO

Early-morning classes:

Get up, if you have dry skin apply a little moisturiser, go to the gym, sweat it out in your class/workout, shower, then do your proper morning skincare routine.

Lunchtime classes:

Go to the gym, remove your makeup, apply a minimal moisturiser (a thin layer), do your class/workout, sweat like a racehorse, shower, repeat your morning skincare routine.

After-work classes:

Go to the gym, remove makeup and apply a thin layer of light moisturiser, do your class/workout, sweat, shower, then do your full evening skincare routine – unless you're going out for dinner etc., in which case apply moisturiser, apply your makeup and remove it all before bed as usual.

SWIMMING

It's not great to swim in makeup, no matter how rushed you are. Equally, you don't want a ton of moisturiser (or other product) running into your eyes and blinding you while you do your laps.

Early-morning swim:

Get up, apply a thin layer of moisturiser (I avoid my forehead to prevent product dripping down into the eyes, but do what you feel your skin needs), swim, shower, do morning skincare routine.

After-work swim:

Remove makeup, put on a thin layer of something protective – I prefer a little facial oil, but light moisturiser works – swim, shower, do your full evening skincare routine, unless you're going out for dinner.

CYCLING

Whatever time of day you cycle, you want protection on a face that is being wind-bashed. Cycle with no makeup, make sure you have applied a protective moisturiser and/or SPF, and do your full skincare routine after your post-cycle shower. I would consider applying facial oil to the cheeks too, although you might end up covered in bug roadkill.

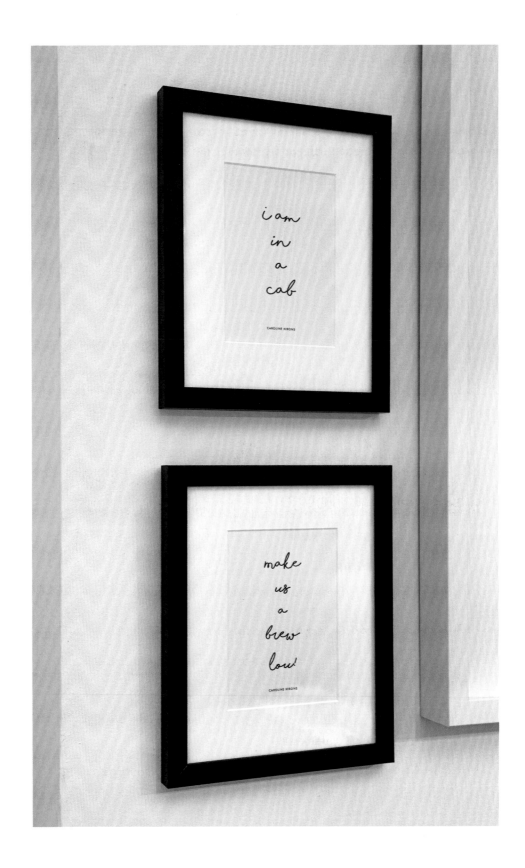
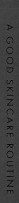

HOT YOGA

Being frank, hot yoga is not good for your face. The entire purpose of it is to make you sweat, however, unlike in other sports, you can't cool down because you're in a room where the temperature is maintained at 'scorching'. That healthy 'glow' will eventually lead to broken capillaries. Having said that, I know some of you are completely addicted to it, so your main concern is to keep the nose/cheek area under control.

Firstly, it should go without saying that you should not be wearing a full face of makeup for exercise, ever.

After the class, spritz as soon as you can with a floral water – not normal water – shower, then apply a hydrating serum AND moisturiser. You will be dehydrated afterwards, so if you regularly attend hot yoga classes I would keep spritzing bottles handy, and keep an eye on your face for signs of dehydration like fine lines and cakey makeup.

EXERCISE + SKINCARE TIPS

- Remove your makeup before you exercise. Yes, you can use micellar water if you have to, but you would be much better off using a good oil cleanser: it's more gentle and nourishing and kinder all round, especially if you exercise every day, or 4 or 5 times a week.

- Try to exercise with a light moisturiser on your face.

- If you are going to use saunas and steam rooms, have some facial oils on your face – heat and oils are lovely. Don't use a mineral oil-based product on this occasion – go for plant oils instead. (A paraffin wax mask done by a professional is great, but that's because it is done by a pro with a good plant oil underneath.)

- Protect the cheeks: those are the areas most prone to visible signs of damage from sport. Use oils, moisturisers and SPF where appropriate.

WHAT TO USE DAILY AND WHAT TO DIP IN AND OUT OF

Now that you have established the foundations of a good routine, you should have a better idea of which products you need to use when. And, of course, what to look out for if you have particular needs. Whether you're tweaking a routine you already had, or finally throwing out the face wipes and giving your skin the TLC it deserves, you may have identified some gaps in your routine and be looking for some new products.

The volume of products out there is huge, and when there's always something new and exciting on the market, sometimes you want to give it a try. But some products are designed to be used continually until you reach the end of the bottle, and won't benefit from being put back on the shelf too soon. So, what should you 'use up' quickly and when is it okay to mix and match?

In general, use up your middle (serums, oils) and dabble with your bookends (cleanser, moisturiser).

- **Cleansers.** You can mix up cleansers. Go by what you're wearing on your skin – makeup or SPF, whether it's a morning or evening cleanse, and your skin type or current skin condition (see Skin Types and Conditions chapter). Equally, it's totally and completely fine to own and use just one.

- **Eye products.** Choose one and use it up before buying another. Having said that, eyes are usually the first place to tell you if they aren't happy with a product. Eye products are not something you 'persevere' with. If it doesn't suit your skin, pass it on.

- **Acids** generally keep for a healthy period of time due to their preservative qualities, so using a couple of different ones a week shouldn't do any harm, although try to remember to use different types of acid as opposed to just different types of the same acid: most people, when asked, turn out to have 2 or 3 glycolic acids, but no lactic or salicylic. Lactic acid is a safe starting point for most people if you haven't used an acid before (see page 191).

- **Serums.** These should absolutely be used until finished up, especially vitamin Cs, retinoids etc. When they're empty, you can work out if your skin liked the product/you saw a noticeable improvement and if you need to step it up or move back a gear.

- **Moisturiser.** While it's nice to have lots of moisturisers, they're unnecessary. These days I tend to finish the moisturiser I'm using before moving on to a new one. I do have ones for dryer days, and ones for travelling, but generally I get through them in a pretty methodical fashion.

- **SPF.** The best SPF is one that you are going to use. Find one you like and use it daily. Don't 'keep' SPFs from one holiday to the next. They degrade.

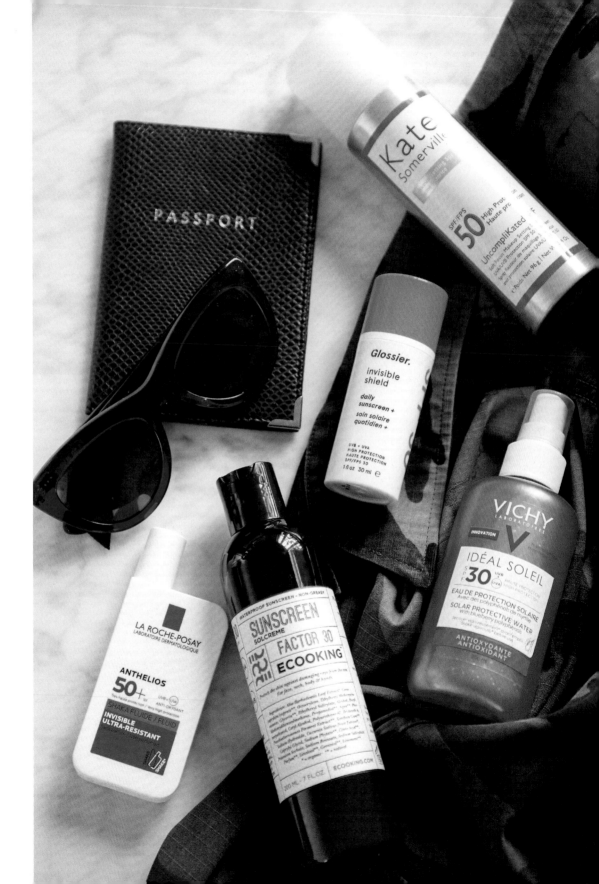

FESTIVAL SKINCARE

This was one of my most popular blog posts, so I'm bringing it out again for all those of you who *will* insist on sleeping in a tent in the pouring rain, drinking yourselves into oblivion and having, at best, questionable hygiene habits for the duration. This, we call 'entertainment'. Personally, I prefer a day ticket, VIP pass and a nice hotel with hot showers, but that's me. God knows what posesses you.

So, you're packed and ready for Glastonbury/Reading/Leeds/Download/ Coachella Festival etc. — what's in your skincare stash?

If you're the type of person that keeps their wits about them, you can do most of your normal routine. If, however, you know you're going to party non-stop for 3/4/5 days, I would just take wipes and SPF and deal with the carnage when you get home. At least you'll have a great time without adding sunburn into the mix.

WIPES

If you're going to use a wipe, now is the time. Bear in mind, like good tea and 80s rock bands, all wipes are not created equal (see 'Try These...' on page 78).

However: if you can, I'd go with a **micellar water/eye-makeup remover and cotton-wool pads**. They just do a better job.

I also love a good traditional milk cleanser in this situation, one that can either be washed off in the shower (literally going against my religion here, I know) or removed with cotton pads.

But still, if you're boozing, stick to wipes. And have the foresight to take two packets: one to keep in your bag (porta-cabin toilet horror) and one to leave in your tent/accommodation to remove your makeup.

ACID

Here's the thing. I would probably not bother with acid during the day at a festival. You're going to be outside all day, sitting in the sun (although if you're in the sun, you're probably not in the UK), you may be drunk/tipsy and forget to apply your SPF... is it worth it?

For the sake of three days, give it a miss. If, however, you're going for longer and want to use acids to 'back up' your wipes, use them in the evening and make sure you have your SPF for the next day. Ready-soaked acid pads are an obvious choice here.

Failing that, pre-soak your own cotton pads in your chosen acid toner and put them in a Ziplock lunch bag. It's what I used on flights before they made pre-soaked pads...

If you have time, can be bothered, and know you will use it, I would take some La Roche-Posay Serozinc with you. This face toner mist may help keep your skin hydrated, can be used to help remove wipe residue and is antibacterial. It also comes in a travel size. Well handy.

SERUM

There's really only one choice for festival serum and that's hyaluronic acid. You need it. Whether you're boozing or not, the weather (sun, wind or rain) will take its toll on your hydration levels, so the easiest way to keep it topped up is with a dose of hyaluronic acid. This is not the time for your expensive anti-ageing serums. Save your money.

My first choice would be a hyaluronic acid product in a plastic tube (avoid fiddly packaging or glass containers — not what you want in a tent or, God forbid, a shared cubicle shower monstrosity). You could also use a hydrating spray or hyaluronic acid mist.

66

WIPES ARE FOR FANNIES, FLIGHTS AND FESTIVALS ONLY

99

MOISTURISERS

For ease, if you have to, use one with SPF included. For safety, I'd personally use a good hydrating moisturiser and a high, broad-spectrum SPF on top. If you can take your normal moisturiser and it's not in any heavy/glass packaging, do. Tubes and pumps are obviously safer and more hygienic.

SPF

Take SPF50. Don't faff about with an SPF15 – it's pointless, especially in this scenario. Apply a cream to your face and body in the morning and carry a spray to top up throughout the day. For more on SPF, see pages 217–226.

WHERE TO DO IT ALL IN A ROUTINE

Assuming you're doing the festival in a fairly controlled manner and get up and go to the showers at a decent hour in the morning, cleanse with your micellar water or milk cleanser and flannel if you can (please). Make sure your skin is as clean as you can get it, apply your hyaluronic acid and your moisturiser, then your SPF. I know for a lot of you this will be your only cleanse of the day that goes anywhere near water.

If, in the evenings, you get back to your tent a little worse for wear and manage to wipe your face down a few times and apply a moisturiser on top, well done.

If you can, use your wipes or micellar water, then serum, then moisturiser. Just do your best. Let's face it, the point of a festival is not meticulous skincare.

TRY THESE...

- Clinique Take The Day Off Face and Eye Cleansing Towelettes
- Glossier Milky Jelly Cleanser
- La Roche-Posay Serozinc
- Indeed Labs Hydraluron
- The Ordinary Natural Moisturising Factors + HA
- La Roche-Posay Anthelios SPF50

!?#

CELEBS DON'T WASH
THEIR FACES

Here's the thing: if you don't want to use anything on your skin, don't. If you want to only use mānuka honey on your skin, do. If you don't want to wash your face ever, that's up to you.

The 'caveman' regimen trend has been aided and abetted by reports of certain celebrities who swear they 'only ever use soap and water' on their skin and are 'horrified' at the thought of washing their faces in the mornings.

Firstly, let's be clear. Celebrities telling us they don't wash their faces and saying they only use soap and water is not new. Some have always said that. It was utter bollocks then, and it is now.

The 'average' woman (you and me) feels enough pressure to be perfect without XYZ celeb saying they don't work out (lies), they eat 'everything in sight!' (lies) and now that they don't wash their face at all? Give me a motherflannel-loving break.

If it was just celebs being arses it wouldn't be that big of a deal, but there is a whole industry behind this caveman crapola. You can spend a lot of hard-earned cash to be shown how NOT to use any products on your skin.

pauses

Yes, of course you can use too much stuff on your face. I've always said do what you have to do for you – whatever that is. But please don't think that these people have perfect skin without skincare and/or without medical intervention. The jig is up, people. Enough.

Now, go wash your faces.

UP IN THE AIR: SKINCARE WHEN TRAVELLING

I travel a lot and take more than my fair share of long-haul flights. I always travel makeup free, covered in skincare products, and I have my in-air kit down to a fine art:

- **Tissues or wipes,** or both. I always need a small packet of tissues and I use face wipes on planes too, but mainly for my hands. I can't remember the last time I used a wipe on my face.

- **Hand sanitiser.** A no-brainer. If you're applying product to your face, your hands need to be clean, and when you're on a plane, there's not always a convenient time/place to wash them.

- **Hand cream or medicated/antibacterial cream.** Putting some hand cream just inside your nostrils when you're on the go – especially when flying – is a well-known travelling tip. The air on the plane is recirculated and really dehydrating to your skin, and the theory is that when your nasal hair is dried out it offers no protection against airborne germs. I used to always get sick after flying – usually getting a sore throat for a few days – but then I started doing the hand cream trick and it worked. Any hand cream will work.

- A small, refillable, plastic spray bottle from Muji filled with a **hyaluronic acid or glycerin-based mist.** I probably use this more than anything else.

- **Eye drops.** I haven't always travelled with eye drops and I don't know why. They're great for dry eyes, itchy eyes and again, help keep the warm, damp areas on the face from drying out. They are obviously totally optional, but I now take them on every flight.

- **Eye product.** Not vital, but I get dry eyes when I travel and I wear glasses. I am never more than 3 feet from my eye cream on a normal day, never mind in a dried-out, airless vacuum.

- **Facial oil.** I usually use a plain squalane oil, but you could use whatever your skin loves. My skin loves squalane. I can use it to calm it down, or to give it a layer of protection, applying it after or before other actives or serums (depending on the action of the other product), and it is hands-down one of my favourite facial oils ever. It works well under or over pretty much any product.

- **Moisturiser.** Which you use depends on your skin type (see pages 111 – 112). I like a hydrating emulsion as opposed to a thick occlusive cream.

- **Lip balm.** The lips are usually the first area of the face to dry out, especially on a flight. I love a hybrid between a lip balm and a gloss; this saves me carrying two separate items.

- I may travel without makeup as much as possible but there's no need to scare small children. I take a **concealer or a tinted moisturiser** to apply when they turn the seatbelt signs on – just enough to give a hint of some colour. And then I mist again. 😊

TRY THESE...

- Nivea Biodegradable Cleansing Wipes
- Ole Henriksen Truth On The Glow Cleansing Cloths
- O'Keeffe's Working Hands Hand Cream
- La Roche-Posay Toleriane Ultra 8

- Indeed Labs Squalane Facial Oil
- Lanolips Face Base – The Aussie Flyer
- Kopari Coconut Lip Glossy

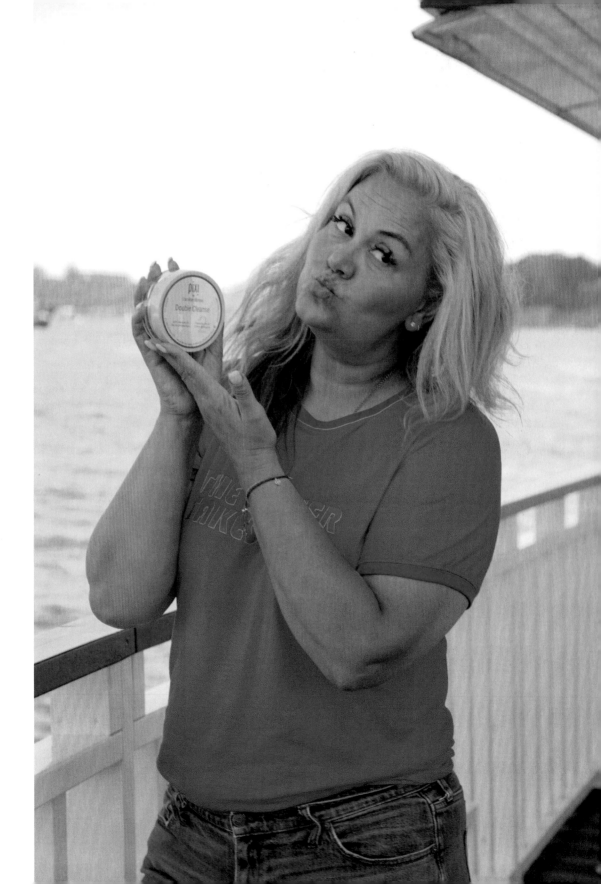

SUMMER SKIN

Sometimes the first warm day of spring or summer sneaks up on you and you find your makeup feels heavy, or your creams suddenly feel sticky.

The change from cold to warm, from using central heating to sitting in an air-conditioned office, means you need to make a few simple swap-outs to your routine. You will still be layering your skincare, but using less of your topical product and/or switching out a couple of key products for lighter options.

FIVE THINGS TO CHANGE FOR SUMMER

Here are five key things to consider changing in your skincare routine when you pack away your winter woollies.

#1 CLEANSING

Cleansing milks and gels are light and won't feel heavy in the heat. I use balms all year round, but I know a younger, more combination skin frequently finds them a tad heavy.

#2 SPF AND SUNBURN

As the days get longer, don't forget to up the ante on your SPF. If you enjoy sitting out in the summer evenings, and you last applied your SPF when you left for work, it's worth carrying a spray or mineral SPF so you can top-up throughout the day (neither are perfect for coverage, so just do your best). Don't go lower than an SPF30.

There is no such thing as a 'safe' tan. If you do get sunburned, strip back actives, take down the heat and keep the skin cool with regular cold showers and wet cloths. Take aspirin or ibuprofen and wear loose clothing that protects the burned areas.

#3 ACIDS AND SERUMS

Glycolic acid does make you more sensitive to the sun, however, it doesn't stop me recommending it or using it myself. Just make sure you are using your SPF.

In all its forms, hyaluronic acid (HA) is great for hot weather as long as you are using it alongside something else, whether it's a moisture-loaded mist or a light moisturiser. Some hyaluronic serums are actually hybrid moisturisers, if you are using a serum or a very light moisturiser that contains a good dose of HA, you may find it's enough.

#4 ANTIOXIDANTS

Vitamin C is a powerful antioxidant that helps protect against free radicals and encourages collagen production. It is of course recommended year-round, but it's worth another mention for the warmer months. You'll probably be outside more, in sunlight for longer, and who doesn't like the added glow?

#5 MOISTURISER

Oil-free moisturiser is obviously an option for oilier skins year-round, but it becomes a good option for the rest of us in higher temperatures. Your skin will be able to retain more of its own moisture in humidity, so if your products feel a little heavy, or greasy, switch to a lighter, and perhaps oil-free, moisturiser until the weather cools down.

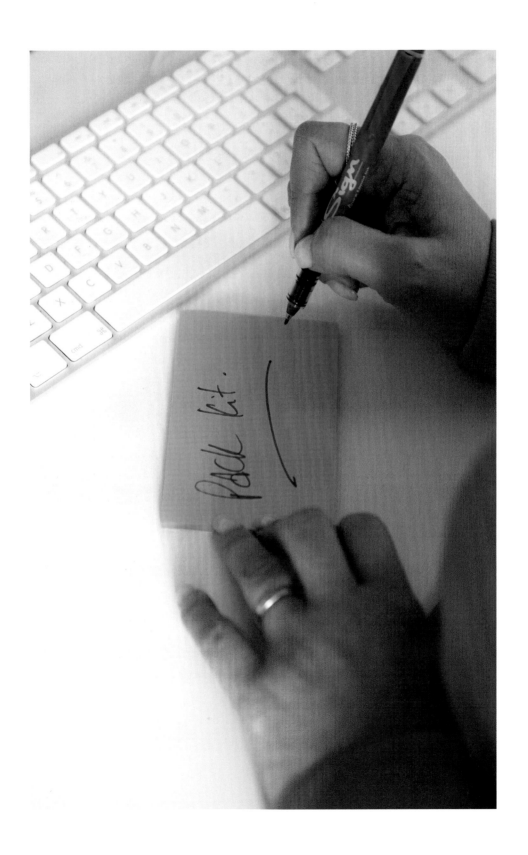

DON'T SCRIMP ON SPF

If you are sitting in the sun, you need to reapply sunscreen every 2 hours, no matter the factor.

Most people apply too little sunscreen. This results in sunscreen users achieving an SPF coverage of 50–80 per cent less than that specified on the product label.[1] You need at least a teaspoonful for each body part – arm, leg (tablespoon for me, thanks!), front, back and face – and don't forget your ears and neck.

- Apply SPF 15–20 minutes before you go in the sun.

- Apply 2 milligrams per square centimetre. This equates to approximately:

  FACE AND NECK: 1 teaspoon
  CHEST: 2 teaspoons
  BACK: 2 teaspoons
  ARMS: 2 teaspoons per arm
  LEGS: 2–3 teaspoons per leg, depending on your height, obviously

  If you are particularly tall, or have a large frame, obviously use more. I use a tablespoon altogether for face, neck and décolleté, but I've got a fat head – and I'm 5′11, so I use two tablespoons per body part. Don't be shy!

- Reapply SPF every 90 minutes to 2 hours, or more often if in water.

" SPF SHOULD ALWAYS BE THE LAST PRODUCT YOU APPLY TO YOUR SKIN "

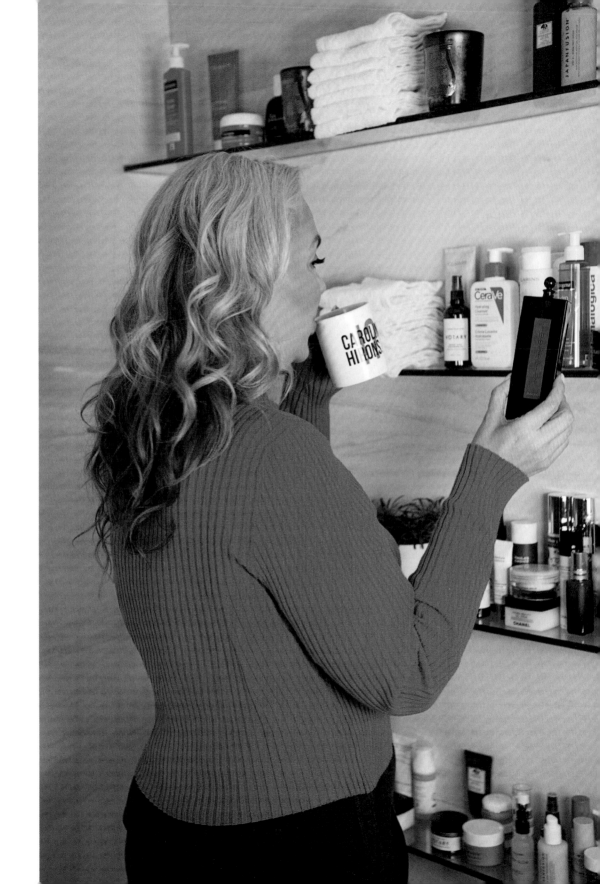

WINTER SKIN

The change from warm to cold, from central heating to cold, can really make your skin feel parched.

Here are a few tips that may help keep your skin feeling hydrated, plump and healthy.

- Treat the skin like you do your clothing. If you're layering clothing, **layer your skincare**. You need a skincare 'wardrobe' at this time of year more than any other. Cleanse, tone (acid/mist or both), serum, oil, cream, SPF and/or balm. How much and when you use all of these depends on your skin, but a general rule of thumb is to start with 'less is more' and if your skin is still absorbing the product, **keep going** (the only thing to be aware of is layering silicone products, as they don't always play well together and have the potential to 'peel' or 'roll', which feels grim).

- **Don't over-cleanse.** Your skin needs all the moisture it can get at this time of year. If your skin is dry/sensitive and you are using harsh cleansers suitable for the summer months, or even worse, overusing the electronic facial cleansing brushes (see pages 184–186), it may be very unforgiving.

- **Avoid alcohol-heavy products.** It's one thing to have a toner with *alcohol denat* at the very end of the INCI list (see Glossary), but it's another to have alcohol as the main ingredient. Acids can be an exception here, as alcohol is used to stabilise the formula.

- If you love a foaming face wash, try to **change to a cleansing milk** when the weather is cold. You can buy a milk for oily skin if you need it.

- **Oils and balms** can feel very comforting on the skin. Natural ones. If your skin is particularly dry, a heavy balm may actually be stripping it, so go easy. For oily skin, use an oil designed for its specific type.

- You should **NEVER** aim for 'squeaky clean' any part of your body, be it hair or skin. If you have this feeling after washing/cleansing, you really need to **stop and rethink** what you are using.

- **Exfoliate** your face and body regularly. Topical exfoliants in liquid form are far more effective than scrubs. Skin is acidic and it is receptive to acid products. Use toners or pads with AHA acids (see Glossary) twice a day and follow with a spray of a hydrating toner containing glycerin and/or hyaluronic acid before you apply your serum and you'll feel a difference after one day.

- Not everyone can use/wants to use liquid acids. For those of you that prefer a physical exfoliant, aim for gentle, naturally sourced granular scrubs that don't use beads. The ones that dissolve as you are rubbing them in are generally safest.

- Ensure you are taking **omega oils** to help your skin internally. Fish oils are the best – flax are a good second for vegetarians and vegans.

- Do continue to use face masks, but go for more **hydrating** ones as opposed to clay ones. If you have a combination skin, use your clay mask and go straight in afterwards with a hydrating one for a good boost.

- If you are a shower person, **do not** be tempted to stand under a hot shower to warm up. Your skin will not thank you for it. Keep it warm-hot, not boiling!

- If you suffer from psoriasis (see page 118) or eczema (see page 116) it is likely that you will experience a worsening of symptoms in the colder months. Make sure your shower/bath products are as irritant-free as possible, **avoid** tumble dryer sheets as they can also aggravate the skin, and remember to **moisturise.**

- And finally: **do not forget your vitamin D**. You can buy vitamin D supplements either as a spray or as tablets, though as with all supplements, always follow your doctor's advice.

"MOISTURISE, MOISTURISE, MOISTURISE!!!"

VITAMIN D

Vitamin D is crucial for your overall health. I tell anyone who will listen about all number of supplements, but vitamin D has been my obsession for a while.

Too much sun can be bad for you – *really* bad for you. So, too, can *too little* sun. Particularly in the northern hemisphere, where most people living modern life spend a larger proportion of their time indoors, and with most of their skin surface covered by clothing or sunscreen when outdoors, there is a growing deficiency in vitamin D. Vitamin D needs to be present in your system for the intestines to absorb dietary calcium.

Vitamin D is actually, in its truest form, a hormone, and it is essential for our wellbeing, yet the use of sunscreens prevents the development of vitamin D in the body. Vitamin D also degrades as quickly as it generates, creating another stumbling block to retaining it in our system.

- **Vitamin D can reduce your risk of the flu and health complications related to flu.** Vitamin D contributes to lowering the incidence of infections and inflammation during the autumn–winter flu season. The Canadian government has recommended increased vitamin D intake as part of their flu prevention strategy, including prevention of swine flu.[2]

- **Vitamin D can help reduce your risk of depression.**[3]

- **Vitamin D can reduce chronic muscle aches and pain.** Vitamin D helps to normalise blood calcium which is required in order for tight, shortened muscles to soften, lengthen and relax out of spasm.

- **Vitamin D can reduce your risk of cancer.** Low levels of vitamin D are associated with an increased incidence of many cancers.[4]

- **Vitamin D can reduce your risk of developing Type 1 diabetes.**[5]

According to NHS guidelines,[6] everyone (including pregnant and breastfeeding women) should consider taking a daily supplement containing 10 micrograms of vitamin D during the autumn and winter.

People with darker skin tones make less vitamin D than those with paler skin.

Ageing skin makes 75 per cent less vitamin D than young skin.

VITAMIN D AND DIET

Vitamin D-rich foods include cold-water fish such as wild salmon, wild cod and sardines and cod liver oil. However, you would need to eat mammoth amounts of these foods to build up your vitamin D stores. If you're shopping for supplements, look for vitamin D3 listed on the label.

FIVE THINGS TO CHANGE FOR WINTER

Here are a few key things to consider changing in your skincare routine when you swap your rain mac for something woolly!

#1 CLEANSING

If you worship at the altar of wipes and foaming cleansers, you might find your skin slightly more unforgiving in a colder climate. Switch to milks, creams and balms and you'll feel a difference in your skin immediately.

#2 TONERS

Keep up with the acids. Now is not the time to slow down. Acids are crucial for keeping your skin exfoliated and fresh, and ready to accept anything that follows them. Treat yourself to a new one and keep the skin challenged in a safe, non-aggressive way. If you can afford it, absolutely use more than one.

#3 FACIAL OILS

If you don't already use one, now is the time to consider investing. If you've already boarded the facial oil train, try two drops under your moisturiser in the mornings to keep your skin protected throughout the day. Skin shouldn't feel greasy when you do this; if it does, you're using too much product. Remember: **Grip, not slip.**

#4 CHANGE YOUR ROUTINE TIMES

Take advantage of the darker nights and perhaps getting home earlier and do your routine as soon as you get in from work/school run/college. Full cleanse, acid, serum/oil application. Go about your business, check your skin hourly until you go to bed, and reapply if you feel like your skin is still absorbing. The skin has done most of its repairing work by 11pm, so don't leave it until 10.30pm when you're going to bed – give it as much time as possible.

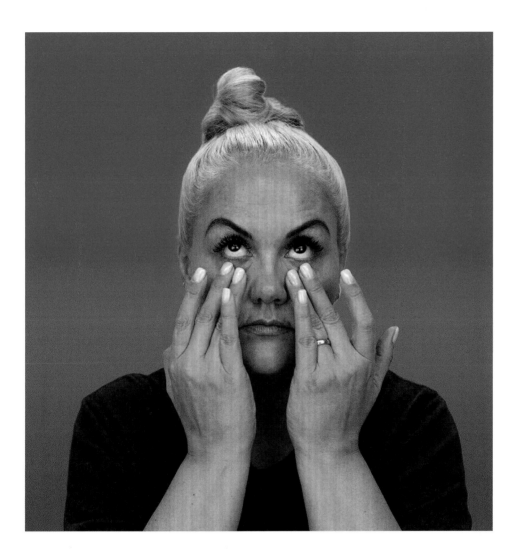

#5 UPGRADE YOUR SPRITZES OR ESSENCES AND USE THEM LIBERALLY

This is no time to be using spray water, like Evian in a can. You'll be dehydrated already and that will just make it worse. Use spritzes or essences that contain other ingredients, like minerals and oils. They work as an extra layer of hydration and hold everything that follows in place, including individual serums and oils.

FACE WIPE FIENDS: If all else fails, cleanse with a balm, remove with a flannel, then apply acid and oil. **That** is your bare minimum, not a wipe.

DIET AND THE SKIN

The following advice is exactly that, just a rough guide to what may potentially give you some hassle with your skin. You will never hear me utter the word 'clean' when it comes to food or skincare. The opposite of 'clean' is 'dirty', and eating food and taking care of your skin should be pleasurable, not guilt-ridden. That said, if you are having some skin concerns and you suspect that your dietary choices could be playing a part, the below advice might be a safe place to start.

> Inflammation is the root of all evil. Try to eat less sugar and take vitamin D supplements and probiotics.

SUGAR

The worst thing for the skin. And it's in *everything*. You need to think of sugar as the Devil. And fizzy drinks/soda as Liquid Satan. Avoid fizzy drinks, fruit juice, pastries, condiments such as ketchup, salad cream, brown sauce and steak sauce. Get into the habit of reading labels: fructose, sucrose, maltose, golden syrup, dextrose – these are all forms of sugar. Empty calories. Drink water. Sugar is the easiest addiction to stop – after a few days you won't even think about that mid-afternoon chocolate. Cutting out sugar from your diet is one of the best things you can do for your health and skin.

WHITE FOODS

If 'cooking' to you means piercing the film of a ready-meal packet, you are not cooking – you are reheating, and eating processed food, which has no benefit to your health or skin. Everyone laughs when I say it, but Mother Nature makes very little that's white. Avoid processed white foods. It's not rocket science. They have, for the most part, been completely bastardised by the food industry. Bread, pasta, cereals, sugar and cakes – if they are white they are not real food. Think how fast your car would break down if you used 'petrol substitute'.

DAIRY

Dairy is designed to take that cute calf and turn it into a 1,500 lb cow/bull in under a year. And it does a bloody good job of it. We are the only species that drinks the milk of another species. It's not natural and you don't need it. But again, it's in everything. Dairy contains hormones that can alter our endocrine system and can possibly in turn contribute to acne. That, sadly, yet obviously, includes cheese. If you eat or drink dairy, try to cut down your intake and go for organic, full-fat. Consider non-dairy alternatives.

FRIED FOODS/BAD FATS

Avoid all margarines, corn oil, sunflower oil, cottonseed oil, grapeseed oil, trans fats and hydrogenated oils. This obviously means by association that you should avoid crisps, chips (French fries) and deep-fried anything. Use olive, rapeseed or macadamia oil.

> If you're a parent and you won't let your toddler eat what you are eating, why are YOU eating it?

- Consider supplementing your diet. If you have problem skin and don't take fish oil, try it – in large doses.* If you are vegetarian or vegan, try the flax substitute (but in my experience it's not nearly as powerful).

- Watch your alcohol intake. It's extremely dehydrating and, again, is predominantly sugar. If you are disciplined and can have the odd glass of good red wine, fine. If not, you may want to reconsider altogether.

*as long as you are not contraindicated in any way. Always speak to your doctor before supplementing.

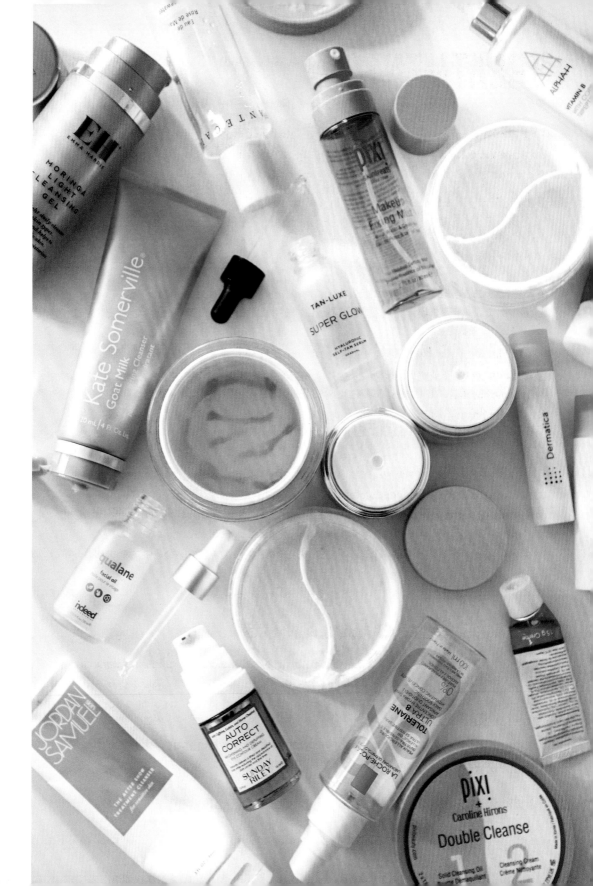

TREATMENTS

It is worth mentioning that although a good skincare routine will undoubtedly improve the quality of your skin, glowing, clear skin is different to facial structure. No amount of skincare will actually stop you ageing or change the *structure* of your skin. If you are more concerned about the signs of ageing such as a heavy brow, hollow cheeks, sagging jawline or hooded eyelids, you'll need either a needle or an operation. To be clear, I am not suggesting for one second that you actually *need* any interventions with your face; I am merely trying to manage expectations.

It would also be helpful to change the conversation around things like Botox and filler in the media. Saying things like 'of course they've got good skin, they've had Botox/filler' etc. is just not scientifically correct. Every time I speak to people in the media, they say 'what have you had done?', as if that negates years of a good skin routine. Yes, I've had filler twice (see overleaf), and will definitely have it again at some point, and I've had my eyelids done – they were so heavy that they were impairing my vision (I would highly recommend this if you are in a similar boat) – but I've also looked after my skin.

Botox and filler change the *structure* of your skin, not the *surface* of it. You may have plumper, higher cheeks, but you could still have acne, pigmentation, redness, dryness and the other conditions discussed in this book. That's where good skincare comes in. Having said that, sometimes you can have a good skincare routine and use the right products, but your skin either does not respond, it has a bigger issue that requires professional or medical intervention, or is simply showing natural signs of ageing.

COMMON COMPLAINTS

Outside of specific skin complaints, such as acne or dermatitis, the following signs of ageing are what often bring people to the clinic door, whether it be for treatments with a facialist, or more invasive options with a dermatologist or qualified doctor:

- More obvious lines on the face that do not improve when your usual products or topicals are applied.

- Skin is noticeably less firm as you move closer to, and through, menopause (see page 159).

- Pigmentation (see page 117): whether related to the condition known as melasma, post-inflammatory pigmentation or good old sun damage, this is an issue I am often asked about at my events and on my social media accounts.

- The fat pads in your cheek area shrink with age, giving you not so much a thinner face, more of a gaunt one.

- Sagging skin: this is caused by the ageing process and those fat pads in your cheeks diminishing.

- Dry, dull skin: this is a result of your inability to retain oil and water in the surface of the skin, and it can make your skin look 'flat' and lifeless. There is very little moisture in the skin to reflect the light.

- Alongside your cheek pads, bone recedes, most noticeably around the eye and brow area, causing the sunken appearance of older eyes.

- Broken capillaries or thread veins: general (and very common) signs of wear and tear on the skin.

'TWEAKMENTS'

In my 'Skincare Freaks' Facebook group, people post a lot of pictures pre- and post- treatment. They want to hear what others think, which is fine, but at the end of the day, the fact is that you should only do this for you. And if you see pictures of someone else after a treatment, don't just say they looked better before. Pay them a compliment or, as I love to tell them, get in the sea.

If you **do** feel like you want 'more', at what age should you delve into having treatments that go further than an over-the-counter serum or cream, and a standard 'facial'? This depends very much on your genes and lifestyle.

The goal is a healthy skin, not to make you look permanently surprised.

Ageing is a privilege not everyone gets.

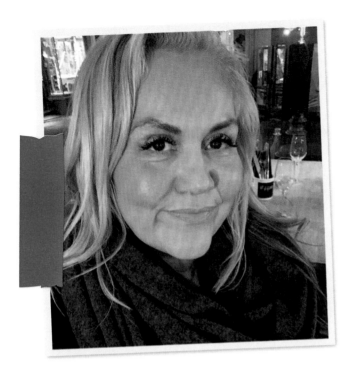

Me after my first round of a small amount of cheek filler.

If you are interested in having some slightly more invasive treatments, or are interested in what is possible with aesthetics, I highly recommend the book *The Tweakments Guide* by Alice Hart-Davis. Alice goes into the minutiae of what to expect, what to look out for, everything that is available on the market and how to find not only a treatment plan for you, but all-round best practice. As an aside, I think Alice's book is also an absolute must for any fellow beauty therapists out there. The book has an accompanying website with a 'tweakment finder tool'.

In the meantime, if you have good skin and are happy with it, excellent. If you are not happy with your skin, use the lists on the next two pages as a rough guide. They are not intended as a timetable or instructions, just a helping hand if you're finding the products you use in your daily routine aren't giving you the results you desire. I've arranged them by age, as 'tweakments' vary in strength and skin suitability.

Firstly, let us not discount the traditional machinery used in various types of facials that is still relevant and suitable for most ages and skins. Faradic and microcurrent (its newer version), galvanic, high-frequency, radio-frequency (see Glossary) — all of these treatments have led to more sophisticated options that are now available to all, such as laser, botox, fillers, PRP, ultherapy and thread lift.

20s:

- Prevention is always better than cure, so please don't stop using SPF. You won't see it now, but you'll be saving yourself a lot of time and effort when you're in your 40s and signs of sun damage start to show through.

- Facials can help with extractions, gentle resurfacing and longer-term issues such as light, fresh scarring and problem complexions.

- Light peels will help manage combination skins and are not contraindicated at any age. Salicylic or lactic acid are great at this age.

- If you have genetic lines on your skin that bother you at this stage, you might consider some superficial or 'baby' botox to help the lines from becoming static. Please only go to reputable derms/qualified practitioners for this – do not ever be tempted by botox 'parties', ever.

30s:

- Pigmentation caused by sun damage in your earlier years will start to come through at this age. Fractional laser and microneedling are all options at this point.

- You may appreciate slightly stronger peels in your 30s, and progressing into stronger acids is an option.

- Your forehead and eye area may be showing deeper lines and/or 'crow's feet'. This is the area I am most frequently asked about. Botox will nip this in the bud quickly and without pain (no, genuinely, a pin-prick on your finger is more painful).

40s:

- Your collagen and facial fat starts to deplete in your 40s, and that is impossible to replace without a needle, despite what some brands would have you believe. Well-placed filler will literally replace the structure lost in your face. It is worth remembering that filler merely aids the structure of the face; it does not affect the skin topically.

- Injectable moisture treatments are hugely beneficial at this age and beyond, and practically painless. Two treatments a year are recommended for very visible results.

- Stronger high-percentage peels are excellent for general skin tone, pigmentation issues and late-onset hormonal spots.

50s+:

- Loss of elastin and collagen are most noticeable now, especially during and after menopause. This age group will have the most visible and immediate results from the following treatments:

  Fillers, botox, laser, radio-frequency, PRP, ultherapy, thread lift... the options are endless and limited only to how much you want to tweak and, of course, how much you have to spend.

DERMATOLOGISTS

I am always asked for derm recommendations and when it's the right time to see a dermatologist. Dermatologists are the specialists you want to seek out if...

- You have severe acne (obviously try not to wait until it gets that bad, but if you have it on your face and back, please go down the medical route as a matter of priority).

- You have allergies or dermatitis. You will know if this has happened: your face will be hot, itchy, inflamed and potentially have small pustules. Go to your doctor in the first instance, then a derm if necessary.

- You have unexplained rashes. In the first instance go to your doctor, then depending on how happy you are with the treatment they prescribe, and the outcome, go to a dermatologist.

As with all roles in life, not all 'doctors' or their brands are created equal, or are as straightforward as they appear. Just because a product says 'Dr' on the label does not mean that the person who created it is qualified in dermatology. At the time of writing, basic medical training gives students very little training on the head and facial anatomy – I can't blame them, they have a lot to cover. In the UK, they get just half a day. *Half a day.*

As a potential patient, you need to do your research before visiting someone who may potentially be injecting you, lasering you, or operating on you.

Find out:
 – Are they specialists in their field?
 – Where did they train?
 – What level of training in dermatology do they actually have, if any?
 – Are they a consultant on the plastic surgeon register?

All this information should be included on their website. As with all things, if their training was good, they'll be shouting about it.

Outside of personal recommendations from someone whose opinion you trust, if you are ever unsure you can visit the General Medical Council's website, click on 'search the register', enter the doctor's name and gender and their registration will be there for you to check. Ideally, you're looking for 'this doctor is on the specialist register' and the 'specialist register entry date' will tell you what their speciality is. Similar registers are available in all countries, and by state in the USA. You may also see 'Registered as a GP with a special interest in dermatology'. There are *of course* extremely knowledgeable doctors that work in skin who, for whatever reason, did not take the full dermatology training route, but really know their stuff. This is where personal recommendation, reputation and trust comes into play. Do not be afraid to ask for credentials. (For some of my favourite dermatologists, see The Brands section on pages 282–292.)

DOCTORS AND SKIN

Do bear in mind that completing basic medical school means that someone can call themselves a 'doctor' (as can someone with a PhD in any topic). A board-certified dermatologist has been through a further 6–8 years of training, specifically in skin. There are over 3,000 diseases of the skin, and these are not covered in basic medical training. By all means go to qualified doctors and nurses for aesthetics, but I always go to a board-certified dermatologist for actual 'skin' issues.

There is one notable exception to the 'stick to derms' rule for aesthetics, and that is dentists that have moved into aesthetics. Outside of derms, specialised surgeons and ENTs, there are few medical people more well-trained in facial anatomy.

FACIALISTS AND AESTHETICIANS

Thankfully, not everything requires medical intervention, and this is where facialists and aestheticians come in.

As with the medical field, all facialists are not created equal. All qualifications in England are regulated by Ofqual (Office of Qualifications) on behalf of the Department for Education. The most basic level of training in the UK is considered an ITEC/CIBTAC Level 2 (even these vary slightly), which – at the time of writing – requires 390 hours training, 300 of which are under the guidance of a tutor. To become a fully qualified beauty therapist in the UK, the TQT (total qualification time) is 990 hours. After this, there's specialised training, where you will find lasers, IPL (intense pulse light), advanced radio-frequency, dermapen/needling and the like.

There is currently no central register for therapists in the UK, and the industry is still self-regulated. BABTAC (British Association of Beauty Therapy and Cosmetology) offers a directory and insurance to qualified and verified practitioners, but each borough requires individual registering before therapists can work.

Most reputable clinics/treatment rooms will have their licences and insurance certificates displayed prominently in reception.

The USA is different again, with the hours required for qualification varying dramatically across the individual states. Florida, for example, only requires 250 hours of training, whereas Washington requires 750 for your basic aesthetician licence, with a further 450 required for the Master Aesthetician qualification. Some states will allow you to inject under the guidance of a doctor's clinic, but others, like California, won't even let you break the skin with a lancet to remove milia or perform dermaplane on clients. It's a minefield.

You will need to check the qualifications in your home country, so always do your research. Seek recommendations and don't be afraid to ask questions. It's your face!

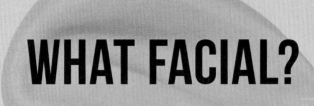

WHAT FACIAL?

Despite their popularity and the continued growth of spas and salons, the average woman in the UK has a facial as a 'treat' on only three occasions in their lifetime: a birthday, Christmastime/celebration, or their wedding.

There is nothing more frustrating than looking forward to something, paying out good money and coming away feeling dissatisfied. Here's a general guide of what's out there and when it might prove useful.

There are lots of different types of facials, yet most involve the following steps:

Cleanse
Exfoliation (sometimes with steam)
Extraction
Massage
Mask
Application of product

TYPES OF FACIAL

MAINTENANCE: Will include massage, extractions, steam and possibly machinery

PAMPERING: Lots of massage, possible steam and lots of masks or serums

CLEANSING: Massage, clay masks, steam, and usually extractions

ANTI-AGEING: Machinery such as FRAXEL, fractional laser (all lasers), light therapy, galvanic, Caci, microneedling and serums/massage

ACNE: Deep cleanse, exfoliation, extraction, masks, high-frequency treatment

GETTING MARRIED

You don't want to walk down the aisle on the biggest day of your life with a beetroot face or spots. If you want to gear up for your wedding and your skin needs a little help...

- Try to start around 4 months before – 6 if you can afford it.

- Have a couple of maintenance facials 6 weeks apart, then a pampering facial a couple of days before the big day itself.

- Avoid invasive machinery, extractions and anything you haven't had before on the last facial before the wedding. No 'last-minute' peels!

If the dress of your dreams is backless or low on the back and you're worried about spots on your back, speak to your facialist – they can treat it.

CELEBRATIONS

If you fancy a one-off treat for a special occasion, go for a pampering facial.

- You want something that includes plenty of massage, masks, serums and moisturisers to leave your skin plumped up and bouncy – something that will last for around 48 hours.

- Avoid extractions or *too much* steam, which can leave you red-faced and dehydrated.

- This is not the time to have a go at those spots.

MY FAVOURITE FACIALISTS

- Dija Ayodele (UK)
- Abigail James (UK)
- Andy Millward (UK)
- Pamela Marshall (UK)
- Jennifer Rock (Ireland)
- Olga Kochlewska (Ireland)
- Teresa Tarmey (US/UK)
- Nerida Joy (US)
- Candice Miele (US)
- Renée Rouleau (US)
- Jordan Samuel (US)
- Kate Somerville (US)
- Joanna Vargas (US)

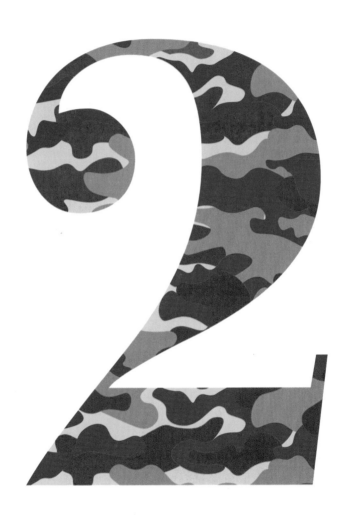

SKIN TYPES AND CONDITIONS

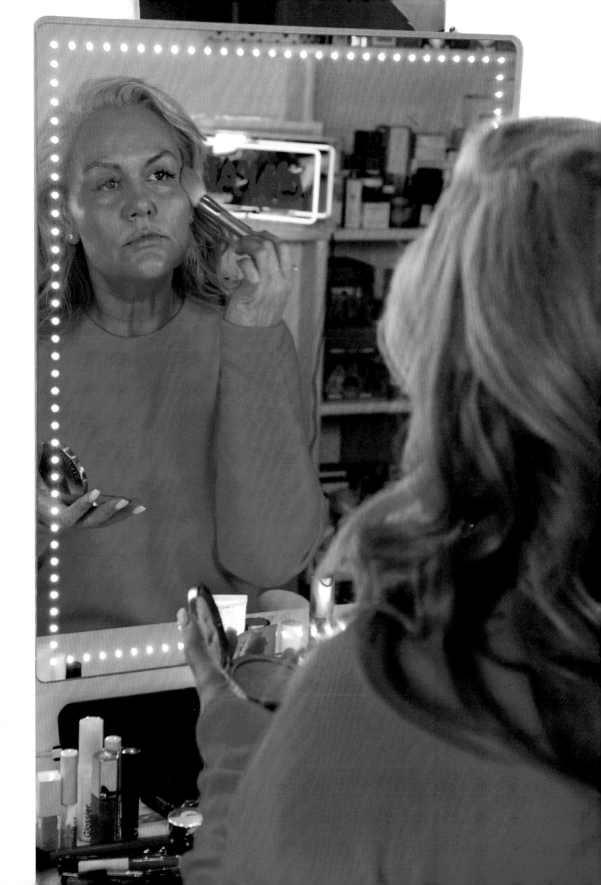

THE DIFFERENCE BETWEEN SKIN 'TYPE' AND 'CONDITION'

'Of the secrets of beauty there is but one,
and a simple one at that: make your skin work.'

— **HELENA RUBINSTEIN, 1930**

First of all, I want to clear up the difference between skin type and skin condition. The terms are often used interchangeably, but they are totally different things and you work with them in very different ways.

Your skin **type** is essentially the skin you were born with. It's what your parents gave you – it's your genes.

Most brands will try to sell you products based on your skin type when they should be targeting your skin condition. A skin **condition** generally occurs more as a result of your lifestyle or as a symptom of your skin type.

SKIN TYPE

Little did Helena Rubinstein know the effect that she would have on the skincare industry when she defined three skin types over 100 years ago. She classified skin as 'normal', 'over-moist (oily)' or 'dry', with each type determined by the level of secretions produced by the skin glands.

At its core, Rubinstein's classification is still very much relevant to today's skin 'types', which are down to your genes. However, the skincare industry now typically classifies skin into *four* types:

DRY SKIN

Usually has a lower-than-usual production of sebum, which is the oily substance your skin produces to help waterproof the skin. There may also be a lack of natural moisturising factors such as triglycerides, wax esters and squalane (see Glossary), and an impaired skin barrier. Skin will feel tight and can look dull.

OILY SKIN

Usually prone to excessive production of sebum, skin may appear shiny and thickened, and show larger pores. Blackheads and spots can be present.

NORMAL SKIN

Contains a good balance of sebum and moisturising factors. Pore size is not an issue and the skin texture is good.

COMBINATION SKIN

A mixture of skin types, and these days the most common skin type. Usually presents a slightly greasier T-zone (your forehead and nose) and dehydrated or dry cheeks.

> **NOTE:** It is entirely possible to have oily skin on the face and dry skin on the body. Your arms and legs lack sebaceous glands and therefore dry skin is far more prevalent in those areas.

It's important to identify your skin type before you invest in skincare so that the product is more likely to suit your skin. For example, a facial oil on a dry skin is lovely, but the same oil will feel heavier on an oily skin.

PORES

My followers and clients are obsessed with pores. They say they are HUGE, then send me a picture and I can SEE NOTHING. Nobody can see your pores. The only person who can see your pores close up is your opthalmologist or facialist (or your partner). Your opthalmologist is looking at your eyes. Not your pores. And if your partner is **thisclosetoyou** and notices your pores, it's time for a new partner.

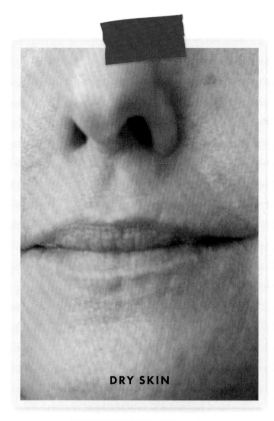

DRY SKIN

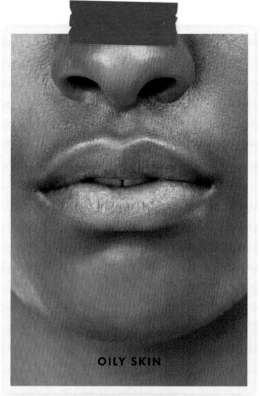

OILY SKIN

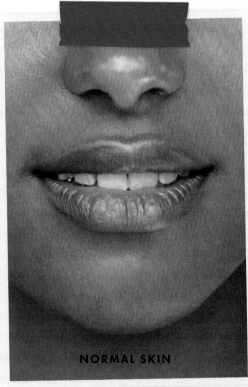

NORMAL SKIN

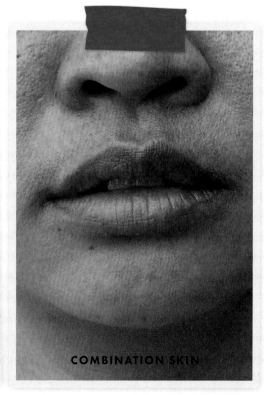

COMBINATION SKIN

SENSITIVITY

Sitting between skin 'type' and 'condition' is sensitivity. This can be genetic or lifestyle-led and it is important that you always have your skin's sensitivities at the forefront of your mind when choosing products.

SENSITIVE SKIN is increasingly common, and instances are shown to be more prevalent in women than men. Why? Men have a thicker epidermis, which seems to be a better barrier to allergens and irritants, but it is more likely that the increase is caused by the overuse of numerous products by women: as a rule, we tend to own and use more products than our male counterparts.

Dry skin will automatically be more prone to sensitivity because the barrier function (the skin's protective layer) is depleted. If your skin regularly reacts to products – for example, perhaps you've reacted to something, which has caused dermatitis (inflammation of the skin) – it will likely remain sensitised for some time afterwards, and your skin will need to be treated accordingly.

TRY THESE...

- Curel – entire range is for sensitivity
- Dermalogica UltraCalming Cleanser
- Jordan Samuel Skin The Aftershow Treatment Cleanser for Sensitive Skin
- Avène Skin Recovery Cream
- Sunday Riley Juno Face Oil
- DeliKate Recovery Cream
- Clarins Skin Beauty Repair Concentrate SOS Treatment
- REN Evercalm Overnight Recovery Balm
- Zelens Power D Treatment Drops
- Clinique Super City Block SPF40
- Pai Hello Sunshine Sensitive SPF30

SKIN CONDITION

> A skin 'condition' is something that can describe either a (hopefully) temporary situation that occurs as a result of lifestyle factors, or a more long-term problem that can occur for other reasons, such as illness or inherited diseases.

'SIGNS OF AGEING' is the all-encompassing term for the skin conditions most targeted by brands, for obvious reasons. This includes everything from wrinkles to uneven skin tone, 'smile lines' to lack of elasticity in the skin.

ACNE is characterised by pustules (spots that look ready to pop, filled with pus-like fluid), blackheads and whiteheads (comedones), nodules and cysts. They are painful to the touch, and are found on the face, back ('bacne') and chest. I have found acne to be the most mentally debilitating of skin conditions in clients. They used to be largely found in adolescents, though are now also extremely common in women over the age of 40. The cause is unknown and is being extensively researched by skincare brands and labs. See pages 128–134 on how to identify and treat acne.

DEHYDRATION, in my experience, is the most common skin condition and is a sign of water loss in the skin. Repair and support of the skin barrier function can aid the prevention of trans-epidermal water loss (TEWL). A healthy combination of fatty acids, cholesterol and ceramides, ideally in one formula (usually a serum or moisturiser), will help barrier recovery and thus prevent TEWL. Dehydrated skin absorbs moisturisers very quickly and may look dull in appearance. Products such as liquid foundations will always look uneven and patchy on a dehydrated skin.

If you suspect you have any of the conditions on the following pages, seek out a skin specialist or doctor to confirm diagnosis and suggest treatment. Where appropriate, I've suggested products that may help alleviate symptoms.

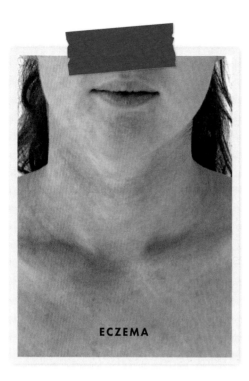

ECZEMA

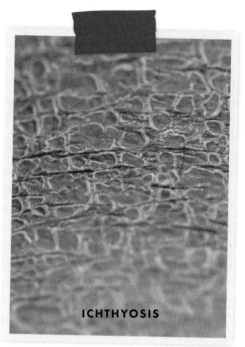

ICHTHYOSIS

ECZEMA, which can occur from birth, is itchy, inflamed and crusty skin that is sometimes sore to the touch, or swollen. Atopic eczema (atopic dermatitis) is part of a group of conditions that includes hay fever, asthma and food allergies. Sufferers generally have over-reactive inflammatory responses to environmental factors and products such as detergents, and it tends to run in families. If you suffer from eczema, you will gain some immediate relief from using rich moisturisers such as those listed below.

TRY THESE...

· Weleda Skin Food

· Eucerin

· Diprobase

· Avène

ICHTHYOSIS is the continual scaling of the skin (build-up of skin cells). It can occur on any area of the body and presents as extremely dry, cracked skin. There are many forms of ichthyosis, the most common being the inherited ichthyosis vulgaris. Sufferers of this type of ichthyosis are shown to have a gene defect in filaggrin, a protein in the skin that impairs the formation of a healthy skin barrier and the natural moisturising factors (NMF) that are key to keeping the skin hydrated. Seek out a skin specialist or doctor to confirm diagnosis and suggest treatment.

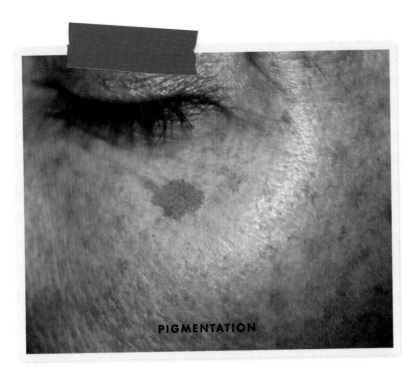

PIGMENTATION

PIGMENTATION issues arise either through age, sun exposure, hormonal changes or physical damage to the skin and are usually caused by a combination of factors. Pigmentation issues include melasma (see page 147) – also called chloasma and PIH (post-inflammatory hyperpigmentation) – or PIPA (post-inflammatory pigment alteration), which is extremely common in darker skin tones and usually happens after an injury to the skin. If you have pigmentation issues of any kind, you need to use a high SPF daily and invest in serums that target this condition.

TRY THESE...

- SkinCeuticals Advanced Pigment Corrector
- Zelens Z Luminous Brightening Serum
- The Ordinary Alpha Arbutin 2% + HA or Niacinamide 10% + Zinc 1%

KERATOSIS PILARIS (aka 'chicken skin') is thought to be associated with, or in the same family as, eczema and ichthyosis. It presents as bumps most commonly found at the top of your arms and thighs, giving the appearance of goose bumps. 'Pilaris' (from the Latin for 'hair'), and 'keratosis' (too much keratin), simply means that you have extra keratin accumulating in your hair follicles. It is harmless, and not contagious, but it can be annoying for the sufferer.

You can help remedy it by body brushing and using dedicated acid-based moisturisers on the area. My readers have found that taking their acid-soaked cotton pad over the areas of keratosis pilaris on a daily basis after using it on their face helped with the 'chicken skin' on their arms.

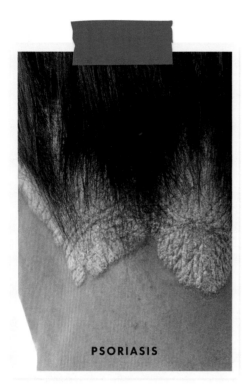

PSORIASIS

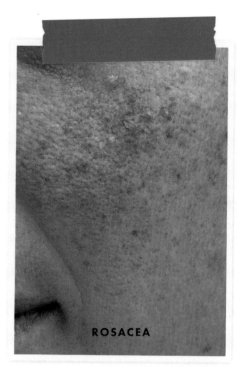

ROSACEA

PSORIASIS is an autoimmune inflammatory disease that presents with dry, red, itchy and scaly skin in patches, predominantly on the elbows, knees, lower back and scalp. Most skin cells take 3–4 weeks to move up through the layers of the skin. In psoriasis, that process takes 3–7 days, leading to the cells stacking on top of each other and giving a white, silverish effect to the skin's surface. You would be hard pushed to find an over-the-counter product that will fix psoriasis. Stick with the prescription goods.

ROSACEA is a much-recognised auto-inflammatory skin condition that has numerous symptoms and different levels of diagnosis. Symptoms can be as mild as flushing, and as intense as swelling, burning and stinging. It tends to be episodic, flaring up when aggravated, and will in all likelihood make you sun-sensitive. It can be triggered by alcohol consumption, extreme temperatures, stress, exercise and the consumption of spicy foods. Treatment for rosacea is unique to the individual, but using anti-inflammatories such as over-the-counter azelaic acid, along with SPF, is key. If you have rosacea you may prefer a mineral SPF, as they are usually tolerated better than chemical blockers. Early diagnosis is shown to help slow down progression. If you're a long-term rosacea sufferer, you should be under a clinician's care. OTC products may help relieve the symptoms of subtype 1. All the other types require the attention of a doctor, and prescriptions.

Rosacea is categorised medically by four subtypes (patients may suffer with more than one type):

Subtype 1: Erythemotelangiectatic rosacea. Sufferers may present with facial flushing, swelling and telangiectasis (broken capillaries/spider veins).

Subtype 2: Papulopustular rosacea. Sometimes misdiagnosed as acne, this is 'classic rosacea' and typically presents with persistent redness across the central panel of the face and occasional papules and pustules.

Subtype 3: Phymatour rosacea. Most commonly seen in older men, this affects the nasal area and can also present on the chin and cheeks. Skin will appear thickened and uneven, with a rough surface. It can be treated with lasers, isotretinoin and, in extreme cases, surgery.

Subtype 4: Ocular rosacea. Sometimes going undiagnosed for many years, this is literally rosacea around the eye area and can present as stinging, burning and watering of the eyes along with common occurrences of blepharitis and conjunctivitis.

Couperose sits in the rosacea family and is caused by small blood vessels on the cheeks, nose, forehead or chin expanding and losing their elasticity. It generally causes permanent redness and can be accompanied by a feeling of heat, burning or tingling. Bear in mind it's exacerbated by heat.

TRY THESE...

· Paula's Choice 10% Azelaic Acid Booster
· The Ordinary Azelaic Acid Suspension 10%

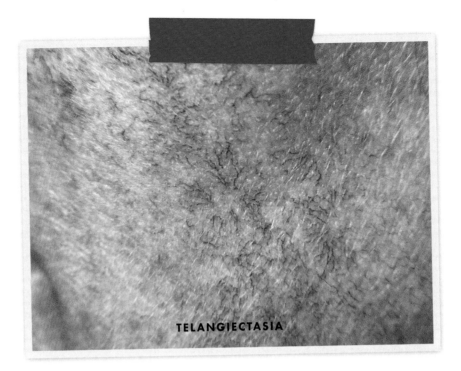

TELANGIECTASIA

TELANGIECTASIA is more commonly known as broken capillaries. You may be more prone to these if your parents have them. They are extremely common and appear more noticeable in paler skins. It is a common condition in skins with rosacea.

VITILIGO is a chronic condition that can start at birth and usually presents before adulthood. People with vitiligo have the same number of melanocytes (the cells that decide your skin tone) as a person without, but the melanocytes are inactive, leading to patches of paler/pinker skin. Vitiligo affects both men and women equally, but is more noticeable in people of colour. It is considered an autoimmune condition as the body's immune system appears to reject its own cells (in this case, melanocytes). Seek out a skin specialist or doctor to confirm diagnois and suggest treatment.

Darker skins are found to be more prone to the following two conditions:

PROBLEMATIC INGROWN HAIRS, known as *pseudofolliculitis* (and *pseudofolliculitis barbae* for the beard area), or more commonly as 'razor bumps' or 'shaving bumps'. This inflammation of the hair follicles and the surrounding area is due to hair being trapped in the follicle. It is caused when

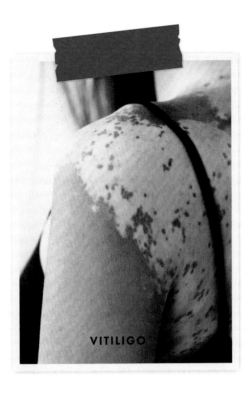

VITILIGO

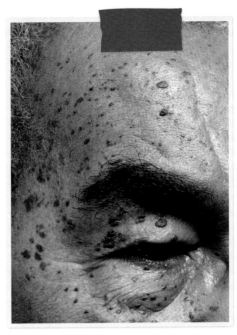

DERMATOSIS PAPULOSA NIGRA

fragile Afro hair is removed, most commonly by shaving, and retreats in on itself due to its helix-like shape.

DERMATOSIS PAPULOSA NIGRA (DPN). This affects black skins more than any other skin tone. It presents as small, benign skin lesions that can clump together on the skin, forming the appearance of bigger patches. They are thought to be genetic and are not harmful, although people with DPN may seek to get them removed. I would urge you to research all medical options and only consider treatment with doctors fully versed in the possible known side effects of treatment on darker skins, such as scarring, postoperative hyper/hypo skin pigmentation and the potential for keloid scarring. Surgical removal options include curettage (scraping), cryotherapy and laser therapy.

TRY THESE...

- CeraVe Hydrating Cleanser
- Elizabeth Arden Advanced Ceramide Capsules Daily Youth Restoring Serum
- Pixi Rose Ceramide Cream
- Paula's Choice Clinical Ceramide-Enriched Moisturiser
- Ecooking Sunscreen SPF30

IS YOUR SKIN DRY OR DEHYDRATED (OR BOTH)?

Dry skins and dehydrated skins can have very similar characteristics, but different underlying causes, and interestingly blur the line between skin type and skin condition.

DRY SKIN

Dry skin is normally a skin type *but* it *can* also be a temporary skin condition. It is caused by lack of oil in the skin. Characteristics of dry skin include:

- small pores
- skin feels 'tight'
- skin may be flaky
- milia, blackheads and spots may be present
- skin looks dull
- skin is not plump
- skin doesn't absorb products easily
- skin is easily irritated and more likely to suffer reactions to products
- skin is aggravated by poor skincare

DEHYDRATED SKIN

A skin condition such as dehydration can affect any skin type, including dry and oily skin. It is caused by lack of water in the skin (not lack of water taken orally!). Characteristics of dehydrated skin include:

- pores can be large or small
- skin feels 'tight' and dry, although confusingly, in the case of oily skin, it can still look shiny and have breakouts
- skin absorbs moisturisers really quickly
- blackheads and spots are still visible
- makeup disappears (and goes patchy) throughout the day as the skin is absorbing any water in your foundation
- skin looks 'ashen'
- a possibility of suffering from headaches

In normal circumstances, your hydrolipidic film (on the surface of the skin) acts as a regulator and barrier – retaining moisture and protecting your skin against germs. If, for whatever reason, that film's effectiveness is affected, the moisture in the epidermis evaporates too quickly and the normal, healthy state of the skin is compromised.

The reality is that most of us at one time or another have dehydrated skin. Any and all of the following can cause dehydration:

ENVIRONMENT: Wind, cold air, dry air, too much sun, air conditioning, central heating

DIET: Eating the wrong foods, consuming alcohol and caffeine, not eating enough water-heavy foods or not drinking enough water (see pages 96–97 for more on diet and the skin)

LIFESTYLE: Stress, poor skincare routine, using the wrong products, medication (including birth control) or smoking

GENETICS: Monthly cycle, pregnancy or hormones

A WORD ON SUPPLEMENTS

Omega oils found in either flax or fish oil supplements will help both dry and dehydrated skins, however you need to be using them for at least 3 months before you'll see the benefits on your skin.

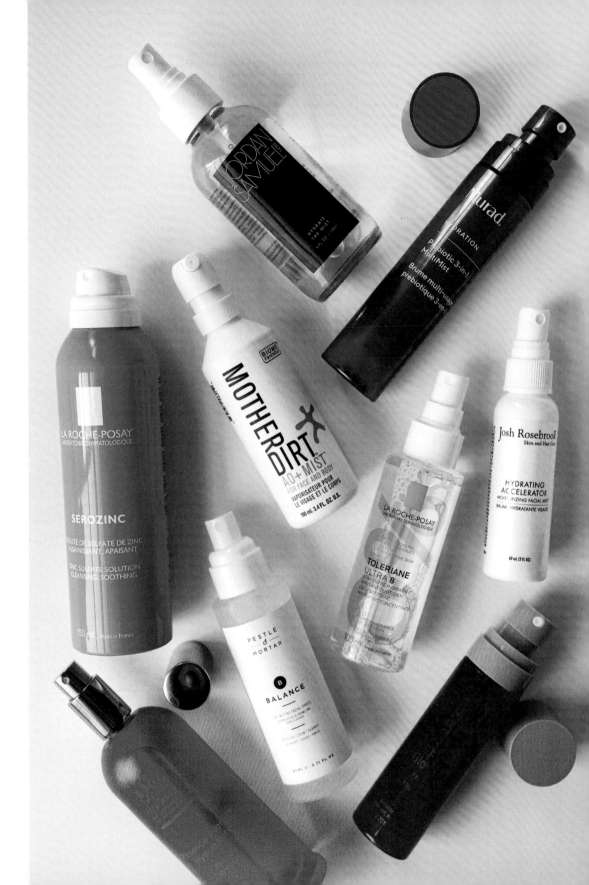

It is quite common to have skin that is both dry and dehydrated, but if the definitions above have helped you ascertain that your skin is either dry or dehydrated (or both), these dos and don'ts might help:

- **Do** upgrade your moisturiser to one suitable for dry skin if you recognise the signs – go for products using the words 'nourishing'.

- **Do** change your moisturiser to one labelled 'hydra' or 'hydrating' if you suspect you are dehydrated.

- **Do** use balms, oils and serums for dry skin.

- **Do** use milks, specified oils and treatments for dehydrated skin.

- **Do not** use products that are too harsh or too stripping.

- **Steer clear of foaming products** – keep the bubbles for your dishes.

- Whether your skin is dry or dehydrated, adding a little hyaluronic acid (see Glossary) to your routine won't hurt.

TRY THESE...

- Bioderma Hydrabio Cream
- Clarins Cleansing Milk with Alpine Herbs
- Darphin Rose Aromatic Care
- Weleda Skin Food
- Murad Hydro-Dynamic Quenching Essence

- Neutrogena Hydro Boost
- NIOD Multi-Molecular Hyaluronic Complex
- Hada Labo – range is made for dehydrated skins
- Zelens Daily Defence SPF30

HUNGOVER, PARCHED OR WEATHER-WORN SKIN

The three main culprits of dehydrated, parched and dry skin are over-indulgence in alcohol, salt and sugar.

The effects this has on the skin are similar to those experienced by many teachers, nurses and doctors who work in dry, warm, germ-festering classrooms and insanely hot hospitals. If you've overdosed on 'All I Want For Christmas Is You', you live somewhere with four seasons, or your professional environment is taking its toll, and you've noticed that your skin is not itself and/or that your lips are so dry that they feel like they may split, tackling these potential causes may help...

ALCOHOL

There are no two ways about it: booze is dreadful for your skin. It dehydrates you to the point of raisin-like status, and if you are slack in your skin-product usage because of the effects of alcohol, it will only get worse. If you are prone to reddening (see rosacea, pages 118–119), alcohol will give you a helping hand to the point where you could easily understudy for Rudolph.

SALT

Puffy/bloated and dehydrated? Those heavy dinners, gravy and salty snacks may have taken hold. And, if your indulgences are of the sweeter nature, blame...

SUGAR

This is the Devil for your skin and your internal organs. That's basically all. You may as well take a hammer and chisel to your collagen. Sugar causes glycation (see Glossary), which in turn makes it much harder for your skin to produce healthy collagen. It literally puts a spanner in the works.

Take all three of these culprits together and you may look in the mirror with some concern. Fear not. It's easily fixed: drink water like it's going out of fashion. First thing, on the hour every hour, and before bed (if you don't already). Rehydrate yourself.

WHAT IF YOUR WORKPLACE IS NOT HELPING YOUR SKIN?

I know this is particularly difficult for teachers. Do what you can, when you get a break. Nurses: keep a water bottle on your station and keep it filled.

Drinking water will give you clarity of mind and help prevent headaches, but how much water you drink sadly has little effect on the hydration levels of your skin. It won't hurt, but it's not the cure.

Follow my tips on a skincare routine for dry and/or dehydrated skin on pages 122–125.

ACNE

Acne is a skin condition that presents typically as a combination of blackheads, whiteheads and spots or cysts on the face and neck (and sometimes the back and chest). It can be severe and distressing, and the psychological effects it can have on sufferers should not be ignored.

We tend to associate acne with puberty and teens, but when I turned 40, **out of nowhere** I experienced adult-onset acne, along with food allergies. And it has become increasingly obvious to me that the same is happening to a lot of women. I had near-perfect skin for 40 years and then, suddenly, a face full of red, angry cysts. My doctor put me straight on antibiotics and I, in my desperation, took them unquestioningly.

Once I realised that the acne was more than likely hormonal, and that the antibiotics were doing me no favours, I decided to fix it myself: I stopped taking the antibiotics, adjusted my diet (I'm not going to tell you what I did and didn't eat, because I'm not a dietician) and changed my skincare. Where I'd previously used heavier moisturising products, I switched to more hyaluronic acid serums and oil-free moisturisers and this did the trick. The reason I am giving you so much background is because you need to give the same care to your skin.

There is **no magical 'cure'** for acne. There are different types, yes, but no one-dose-fits-all cure. Do read the below, but bear in mind that acne is different for everyone. You may have one type – or three types. You need to know your whole 'system' – skin, body and state of mind – to see results.

TYPES OF ACNE

HORMONAL ACNE: can occur if you're just starting periods, just finishing periods, experiencing perimenopause or menopause. Raging androgen in boys can also cause over-production of oil, slow shedding of dead skin cells, which all create the perfect breeding ground for acne.

SENSITIVITY-RELATED ACNE: can be related to allergies, an adverse reaction to a product, or reactions to foods (such as shellfish) or your environment.

"
YOU NEED TO KNOW YOUR SKIN, YOUR BODY AND YOUR STATE OF MIND INSIDE OUT TO TRULY SEE RESULTS

"

The two key cuplrits are **bacteria** and **inflammation**.

Propionibacterium acnes is the bacteria that gives our friend acne its name. All it needs is the perfect environment in order to spread.

Inflammation can be caused by illness, foods or stress – a system fighting illness is inflamed. Add medication and you are doubling your potential problems. Foods can cause inflammation (especially food allergies) and stress always causes inflammation – these are all breeding grounds for acne.

Looking at the above you may see where your skin fits in, and why antibiotics just will not work for some people (the exception is when they are prescribed as part of a full regimen from a dermatologist).

A WORD ON ANTIBIOTICS

Antibiotics can save your life. Literally. I'm not bashing the drugs. I'm bashing the over-prescribing of them by some doctors, specifically GPs (not dermatologists), who should know better. If you are taking antibiotics for a skin problem and they haven't 'done anything' – something I hear a lot – consider stopping taking them (in line with your practitioner's advice). They are bad for your digestive system and make you massively susceptible to severe sun damage. They wreak havoc on your tooth enamel, too, and can make you resistant to antibiotic usage for severe infections.

Instead of referring you to a specialist dermatologist, some GPs insist on giving out repeat prescriptions for skins that are not responding to them because they don't know any better. If your acne is really bad, ask for a referral to a hospital consultant or specialist unit. You may not get a referral unless it is visibly bad: a few hormonal spots once a month, requiring you to break out the heavy-duty concealer, is not on a par with the suffering of people with the severest cases. Ask for that referral if you need it, or pay to see a dermatologist. Invest in your skin.

MYTHS AND OLD WIVES' TALES

It seems that once something has been said in a glossy mag or seen on TV (or both) it becomes The Law. Sad but true. And this is not helpful to those of us with real problems that we want to fix. Here are a few untruths out there:

- **Acne is caused by dirty skin.** Not true. There is a massive difference between bacteria and dirt. Over-washing your face destroys the acid mantle that protects your skin (the very fine acidic film on the surface of the skin that is your first line of defence against bacteria and viruses), creates an alkaline environment, and makes your acne worse and your skin a dry, dull, sore breeding ground. Having said that, I highly recommend that you regularly change your pillowcases (at least once a week).

- **You can 'dry up' spots.** Not true. A spot is a mixture of oil, inflammation, bacteria and dead skin cells. There's no water in that list. All you are doing is drying the surrounding area in the hope that it will make the spot look smaller. What it actually does is put the spot on its own 'look at ME' platform.

- **You can use toothpaste or nappy/diaper cream to spot-treat acne.** A one-off spot may have its redness taken down — temporarily — by applying one of these, but they won't get rid of acne. If acne could be fixed by what you're using on your teeth or your baby's backside, all of our problems would be solved. Dude. **Stop putting toothpaste and bum cream on your face.**

THINGS THAT MAY HELP

Thanks to my friends, clients and readers of my blog, I've created a list of things that have helped some people with their acne over the years. It is not definitive, but rather a list of suggestions. They may not work for you or they may work brilliantly – unfortunately, there is no perfect solution.

- **Avoid too much alcohol in products.** A 'tingle' is okay, but 'burning' is not. Products where the main ingredient listed is alcohol will dry out the surface of your skin, destroy the acid mantle and make the perfect breeding ground for bacteria. However, alcohol in acids is the exception: alcohol is sometimes a necessary evil for suspending things like glycolic acid in a solution where they would normally not work as well.

- **Do not completely strip your skin of oil and moisture.** An acneic skin that sticks solely to foaming cleansers and oil-free products is nearly always – always – reddened with inflammation and sensitivity. Alkaline soaps and foaming washes that contain SLS will contribute to the breakdown of the acid mantle of your skin and take your skin to the wrong end of the acid/alkaline scale. It's called acid mantle for a reason. Remember litmus paper from science classes? Alkaline skin is the perfect breeding ground for bacteria.

- **Do not pick red cysts.** A whitehead can be popped in the correct manner (see pages 168–171).

> A cyst is going nowhere and will always, always prevail if you battle it. And then it will scar, just to teach you who is boss.

- **Avoid moisturisers made with good-quality, heavy shea butter.** Yes, it's natural, but it's harder than most oils for the skin to break down and thus tends to clogs pores and give you nice whiteheads. Buy moisturisers with water as the main ingredient for daytime use. You can use appropriate oils and balms at night.

- **Treat your skin gently and with respect.** You know what I mean. Abusing it with harsh products and getting angry with it as if it's a different person will make it worse.

> Your skin belongs to you. Do not try to disown it when it needs you.

- **Cleanse with good-quality oils and balm cleansers.** There is absolutely no reason to avoid oil when you have acne. Avoid mineral oil, yes, but good, light, plant-derived oils do not clog pores; they nourish the skin you are now pledging to take care of, and they do not cause breakouts.

- **Use topical exfoliants.** Using acids topically will help tackle blocked pores, remove dead skin cells, trapped hair follicles and reduce your acid mantle to the lower end of the scale – usually around a 3 or 4 – which is, in layman's terms, strengthening your first line of defence to the acne. Use glycolic, lactic or salicylic acid (see pages 189–194 for more information on acids).

- **You can use products containing benzoyl peroxide or sulphur,** found in spot treatments, to topically treat bad acne spots. It can penetrate the pore and kill off the bacteria specific to acne, but I prefer to use the acids I mention in the step above. A word of warning: both are extremely drying to the skin in high percentages. Go easy.

- **Hydrate your skin and consider that it might need facial oil in places.** You can have acne in some areas and be really dry or dehydrated in others.

- **Consider supplementation.** Probiotics are a must, especially if you are on antibiotics. Your skin is the first part of your body that will indicate if there's something going wrong in the gut. Keep your stomach and intestines as strong as possible. Go for the highest dosage of probiotics you can find and be aware that they have a short shelf life and may not be as effective as the label states. As always, speak to your consultant before supplementing.

Stress is the key to most flare-ups, whether they are acne, rosacea or eczema.

Practise relaxation. And not in some hippy-dippy way. Seriously. See the bigger picture.

Chill.

DIET AND ACNE

Unfortunately, there really is no definitive list of foods that cause acne, though some might like to claim they've nailed the 'no spots' diet. There *is*, however, awareness of foods that cause inflammation in the system (and therefore the skin) and are therefore best avoided. See pages 96–97 for more information on diet and the skin.

TRY THESE...

- Dermatica – online prescription service
- Sunday Riley Ceramic Slip Cleanser
- Skingredients Sally Cleanse
- Renée Rouleau Anti Bump Solution
- REN ClearCalm 3 Non-Drying Spot Treatment
- Paula's Choice Clear Regular Strength 2% BHA Exfoliant

- Kate Somerville Oil-Free Moisturiser
- La Roche-Posay Effaclar H Multi-Compensating Soothing Moisturiser
- May Lindstrom The Problem Solver
- Paula's Choice Skin Balancing Moisturiser SPF30
- Clarins UV Plus SPF50

SKIN PURGING

Your skin should not 'purge' (heavily break out) when using over-the-counter (OTC) acne products. Prescription-strength products given to you by a dermatologist for acne, for example, can cause purging, but these are drugs and the purging will happen under the care of a medical professional. For example, if you are put on a medical regimen to tackle acne, you may well purge for a good few weeks, even a couple of months (some patients find this the most trying part of a new routine, but eventually it is worth it).

However, if you start using a new OTC product and suddenly have a face full of spots, redness or swelling, it is likely that the product (or machine) is not for you. However, strong OTC retinoids (vitamin A treatments) can cause purging, and in that case, I would recommend down-scaling to a milder one until your skin adjusts. There may be a risk of slight exacerbation of spots if you are acneic and suddenly use a product high in salicylic acid, for example, but that should not last for weeks on end.

I often come across products that claim, 'this may make your skin purge for a while, but then it will be GREAT!'. The reality is probably closer to 'this may give you a face full of spots, either because the ingredients are comedogenic (block pores), or your skin does not like some of the ingredients'. The odd whitehead (i.e. a proper, traditional spot) appearing after using a new product is no big deal.

An angry red face with a mixture of swollen, won't-come-to-a-head spots, cysts, whiteheads and blackheads is not 'purging'. It's your skin begging you to stop whatever it is you are doing. Listen to it.

Personally, even if my skin was bubbling under the surface like a dormant volcano, I'd rather treat it gently. I do not want to use something that makes it erupt. Hey ho, that's just moi.

HAVING SPOTS MEANS YOU HAVE ACNE, OR OILY/COMBINATION SKIN

Most of the people I see have normal, dehydrated or sensitive skin with occasional spots. This is very different to acne. There are two vicious circles you can get into that can lead to occasional spots.

VICIOUS CIRCLE ONE

You had acne as a teenager and are now in your 20s, 30s or 40s+, and continue to treat your skin as if it is acneic. In fact, your skin moved on when you were 19 or 20. Underneath that redness and sensitivity is actually normal skin. The redness and sensitivity have been caused by years of using products for oily/combination skin that dry it out and 'mattify' it (*cries*), causing it to over-produce oil, give you angry red spots, burning cheeks and lead you to think that you are still an oily/combo skin and that your skin hates you. And usually this makes you hate your skin and despair.

VICIOUS CIRCLE TWO

You once had a few breakouts and you went to a beauty counter or had a facial where you were told you had oily/combination skin because your sales assistant or therapist's training led them to believe spots = acne = oily/combination = foaming = mattifying.

Your skin was actually pretty normal. Now it's oily because it's dried out and is desperately trying to replenish itself, so your skin is oily by midday or 3pm and you keep thinking that you have an 'oily' skin. You therefore think you are doing everything wrong and your skin hates you. And usually this vicious circle will also make you hate your skin and despair.

I'm not suggesting that occasional spots are not a serious condition and mentally taxing, I'm simply suggesting that we overuse the word 'acne' across the industry and do not train our people well enough to detect the difference between acne and hormonal breakouts, food intolerance spots, product reactions or other reactions. Most people I see with breakouts have a normal, slightly dehydrated or sensitised skin with spots. That is very different to acne. It can happen to anyone, at any time, for any reason.

So please, please, the next time you have breakouts – even if they are multiple or in different areas of the face, and at different times of the month – they are spots. Do not treat your entire face as if you have acne/combination skin. Think about what it could be. Have you done anything differently? Have you ever had intolerance tests for food groups? Is your period due? Have you been on a three-day bender? Are you using a sodium lauryl sulphate (SLS) shampoo in the shower and letting it run all over your face?

> Treat the spots by taking care of the skin. Your skin is not your enemy – do not treat it like it is. Spots and acne are two very different things.

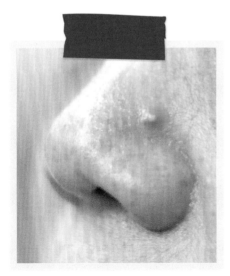

SPOTS

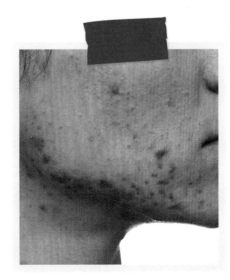

ACNE

PERIORAL DERMATITIS

(aka 'those red annoying spots that won't go away')

- You've had spots, redness, flakiness, or something that looks like (but isn't) eczema or acne, for ages, in one place around your mouth, nose or eyes. The spots are not particularly big, they don't seem to want to LEAVE and sometimes they appear to multiply.

- You have clusters of spots, redness or flaking around your nose or mouth that laugh at you and say, 'nice try!' when you apply spot treatment.

- Sometimes the spots sting or burn.

- Sometimes the spots flake over and literally peel off.

- Sometimes the spots disappear altogether and give you a sense of satisfaction, then POP BACK UP AS IF LIKE MAGIC.

- The thought of using something harsh such as an exfoliating acid on the area makes you feel a tad faint.

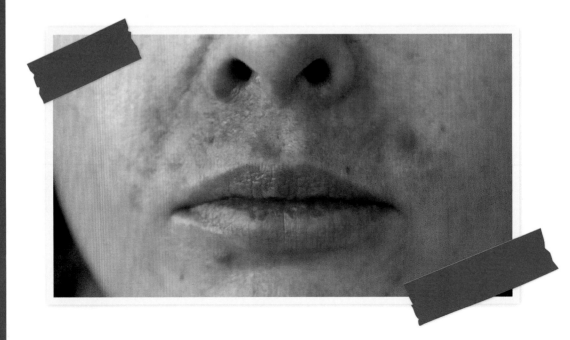

Does this sound familiar? You may have perioral dermatitis (or periorificial dermatitis if it's around your eyes). Do not panic or worry. It's very common and easily fixed. If you ignore it, however, it can spread.

While it occurs predominantly in women aged 20–45, giving it a possible hormonal factor, men and children can also be affected. The causes are multiple, and the triggers can be a combination of things:

- a reaction to some cosmetic products
- a reaction to steroid creams (often referred to as steroid rosacea)
- strong winds/UV light (think joggers and chapped skin)
- hormonal contraception
- dribbling in your sleep
- fluoride in toothpaste
- sodium lauryl sulphate (SLS) in toothpaste and cleansers

The parts of the face affected are near areas that are warm, dark and wet – the perfect combination for bacterial growth.

It's easy to treat. If it is a recurring problem, visit your doctor. You will be prescribed a topical cream, or oral antibiotics if it's really severe. Avoid applying active ingredients to the area until it subsides. Good, plain nourishing oils such as jojoba – or one that contains vitamin D – will help to stop the itchiness and remedy the dryness. **The biggest single difference for me personally was using toothpaste that did not contain any SLS. I avoid it completely now.**

MILIA

Stubborn, unsightly and annoyingly hard to get rid of, milia are found in people of all ages. Babies, kids and adults can all be affected. All races and genders. Milia do not discriminate. They generally affect the thin skin around the eyes and upper parts of the cheeks in adults, and are basically a mini cyst: a cyst full of keratin. We like keratin — we need it. It's what gives our skin, hair and nails structure. You just don't want it trapped under your skin and trying to get out.

The important things to remember are:
- they're NOT spots
- they have nothing to do with your pores — milia are under your epidermis
- they're not harmful
- they're not infectious
- they're not caused by germs or bacteria
- you can't get rid of them by taking an antibiotic or the contraceptive pill

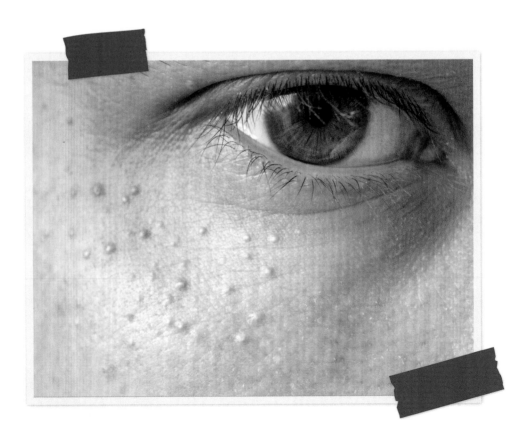

If you have a lot of them – and if your family also suffer with them – it's likely you're genetically predisposed to them. If you just get the odd one here and there you probably just need to up the ante on your skincare routine.

HOW TO GET RID OF LARGER MILIA

First of all, **don't bother trying to pick at milia**. You're setting yourself up for a whole heap of trouble. Essentially what this will do is pick a hole in your skin.

- **Get a professional to remove them.** Phone your nearest salon. Ask them specifically if they remove milia. Double check. Say, 'Do you *physically* remove milia?' We're talking manually – no microdermabrasion, no laser – just your therapist, her steady hand and a suitable needle. If they hesitate, don't go. You do not want someone who's not confident and well-trained poking around your eye area with a needle. Few salons offer the service – in some districts you're not allowed to 'pierce the skin' in a salon (this is down to old legislation relating to sex clubs in city centres, not facials).

- **Go see a dermatologist** – let them deal with them.

HOW TO HELP SHIFT SMALLER MILIA

Well, to start with, get into a routine every day that makes your skin work for itself.

- **Keep your skin well cleansed,** using flannels and warm water (see pages 41–46).

- **Exfoliate every day** (gently – don't go tearing at your skin or the area of milia) and do not – repeat after me – DO NOT use any of those apricot scrubs you can get in the chemist. EVER. END OF.

- **Alternate between a topical acid toner and a hydrating toner/ essence** (a really runny serum). Toners or toning lotions are essential for controlling milia. The acid toner – used on the area affected by the milia only – will help shift the surface layers of the skin quicker, the hydrating one will ensure you don't dry your face out at the same time. It takes 2 seconds. Use the acid toner first, the hydrating toner second.

- **Keep the milia moisturised.**

- You may like to **use a clay mask** occasionally, in the privacy of your own home. Just do your nightly cleanse, whack it on the area and have dinner/ watch telly/whatever – remove, tone, moisturise.

You should find that some of the smaller milia shift themselves doing this. Also, follow these general guidelines:

Do not pick at the milia with needles – if you don't know what you're doing you'll scar your face.

Do use a topical acid on the area, exfoliate regularly, moisturise normally, and use good-quality clay masks on the area regularly. If you wish, get the milia removed safely by a professional.

"

DO NOT COMPLAIN ABOUT TIME TAKEN TO TAKE CARE OF YOUR FACE.
IT'S YOUR *FACE*

"

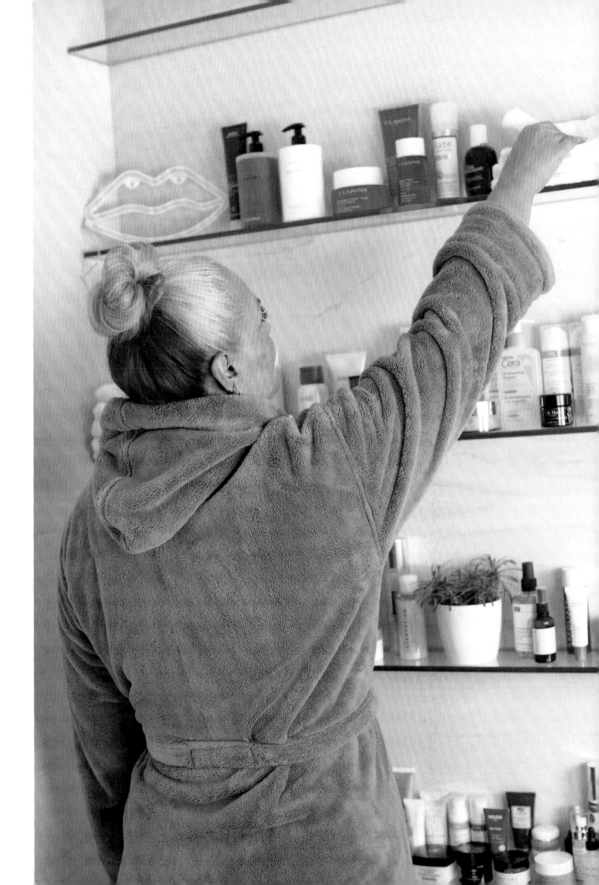

HOW TO TREAT YOUR SKIN

Now that you know a bit more about how your skin works, how do you treat it?

Very few of us have what could be termed 'normal skin', which is why I find it odd that there's a skin type called 'normal'.

For most of us, there are multiple issues to contend with: pigmentation, rosacea, dry skin, oily skin, combination skin, sensitive skin, dehydrated skin – you name it, you probably have at least one of them.

But, what if you have **more than one?** What if you have three skin issues? Or four?

'Normal skin' is far from the norm for most people. It's not uncommon, for example, to see a dehydrated, hyper-pigmented, sensitive, ageing skin with hormonal breakouts. Dr Leslie Baumann gave us her 16 skin types years ago, and she was spot on, although I think there are even more than that. Start by treating your skin according to the potential your issue has to cause pain and/or long-lasting damage, such as scarring or broken capillaries.

#1 First, take care of sensitivity or rosacea. Inflammation will exacerbate the other issues. For example, if you have rosacea and acne and use a traditional foaming acne 'wash', your cheeks will scream at you. That's not good. That's not what you need or want for your face.

Sensitivity is King. Best product choice: moisturiser or a fragrance-free facial oil designed for sensitive skin.

#2 Tackle dehydration. Dehydrated skin drinks anything you put on it, but you have to hydrate it repeatedly: your anti-ageing serums end up just filling a gap in your skin rather than actually doing their job.

If you are dehydrated, you can leave the house in the morning with perfectly hydrated, bouncy skin and it will be dehydrated to the point of it showing on facial machinery by mid-morning. No matter what you do, what you use, how old you are, or your lifestyle, you can be dehydrated just by waking up. You need to treat the dehydration.

Best product choice: those in the toning phase – use both acid and spritz, followed by serum. Use acid on cotton pads to gently strip back the skin and then spritz with a mist containing hyaluronic acid, glycerin (or both) and follow with hyaluronic acid serum. None of these products should irritate any of the other issues.

#3 **Now you can start to be more general.** As long as you are keeping your redness under control and your skin hydrated, you can tackle anything. Here are the best product choices for the following skin types or conditions:

DRY SKIN: use facial oils and oil in products including balm cleansers – no foam, ever. Dryness frequently overlaps with dehydration. If your skin is both dry and dehydrated, treat both issues simultaneously, and if you are unsure which you are, read pages 122–125.

AGEING SKIN: use targeted serums; think retinoids and peptides.

PIGMENTED SKIN: use dedicated serums for pigmentation, retinoids and SPF (I'm not suggesting you don't use SPF under normal circumstances; it's just the priority if you scar easily, get sun spots etc.)

OILY SKIN: use acid toners, and a suitable serum and moisturiser. Do not over-embrace oil-free and foaming products.

ACNE: the acid toning phase is key, as is your moisturiser. Please, please think carefully about how you will go about replenishing the oils in your skin if you use an oil-free moisturiser. If you want to try to keep your oil under control by mid-afternoon, use an oil-free moisturiser if you want to, but use a facial oil dedicated for acne/combination skin underneath it. I promise, a drop or two can make all the difference. We're ahead of the game now and the skincare market has plenty.

> The old 'foam wash, alcohol-laden strip-tone, oil-free moisturiser' routine is dead and buried. Or should be.

And, finally, a special mention to the sufferers of melasma – or chloasma, as it may be called by your midwife if you're pregnant.

Melasma and pigmentation are different things:

PIGMENTATION can be caused by sun damage, acne scarring, picking spots or inflammation, and can normally be treated with topical products – glycolic, kojic and azaleic acids, retinoids, and liquorice, for example – with some success.

Best product choices: peels, and targeted serums containing those ingredients and SPF.

MELASMA can be *triggered* by the same things that cause pigmentation but is also linked to hormones (hence the link to pregnancy, the contraceptive pill and perimenopausal women) and illnesses such as Addison's disease, lupus and celiac disease. Female sufferers outnumber male 9 to 1. It's basically your melanocytes throwing their toys out of the pram. In a skin with melasma the melanocytes are going off like fireworks.

Best product choice: time, a package of laser treatments, supportive products for pigmentation, and sun block. I had mild melasma with pregnancy: it eventually cleared up on its own, but some people aren't that lucky. Clinical peels can help, but if you want it gone, you need the laser. And the bad news is that even if you stay out of the sun and wear a complete sunblock, it will probably come back, because that's what it does. It is also heat-triggered, so stay away from saunas and steam rooms.

Make sure you know whether you have melasma or pigmentation before you part with your hard-earned cash.

TRY THESE...

- The Ordinary Alpha Arbutin 2% + HA
- Biologique Recherche P50 PIGM 400
- Zelens Z Luminous Brightening Serum
- Murad Rapid Age Spot Correcting Serum

- OSKIA Renaissance Brightlight Serum
- Renée Rouleau Advanced Resurfacing Serum

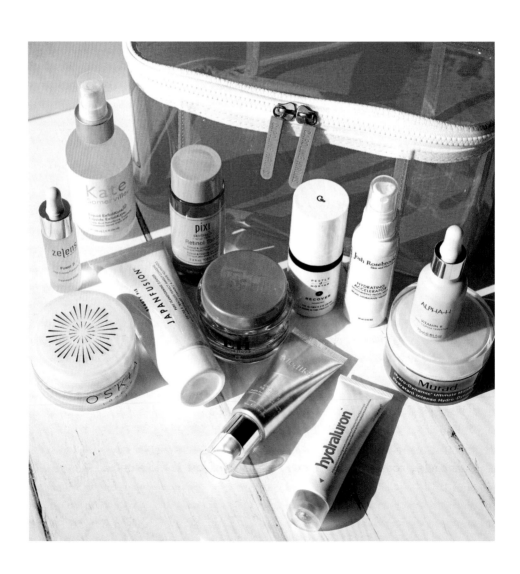

EYE PRODUCTS FIX GENETIC DARK CIRCLES

Are dark circles driving you mad? Have you tried everything under the sun to get rid of them?

> Your options are limited in terms of what you can do about them, and there are definitely things that can make them worse.

I'm talking specifically to my lovely Asian readers, darker-toned readers and even my lovely red-headed, extremely pale readers. If you can see dark circles under your eyes and, to your knowledge, there is no particular reason for them, look at your parents/immediate family. If they also have dark circles, they probably run in your genes, and there isn't a cream alive that will safely deal with that kind of dark circle.

Sure, there are excellent eye products that can take the edge off, and some brightening ones that will 'lift' the appearance of them, but anyone who looks you in the eye and says 'this cream will absolutely fix your dark circles' is either misinformed or not being completely straight with you. It's a little easier for those of us with occasional dark circles caused by things like illness, dehydration, or too much of a good (bad) thing, but genes are hard to mess with.

If you really hate the dark circles, you could talk to a dermatologist about trough filler: a non-surgical procedure, it involves injecting the area with hyaluronic acid filler, which sits just under the skin and essentially hides the dark circles. For most people, one treatment will last 12–18 months.

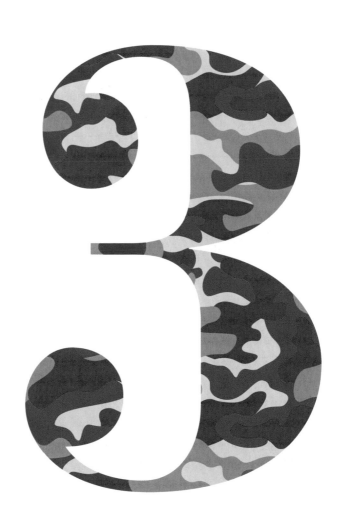

WHEN LIFE HAPPENS

!?#

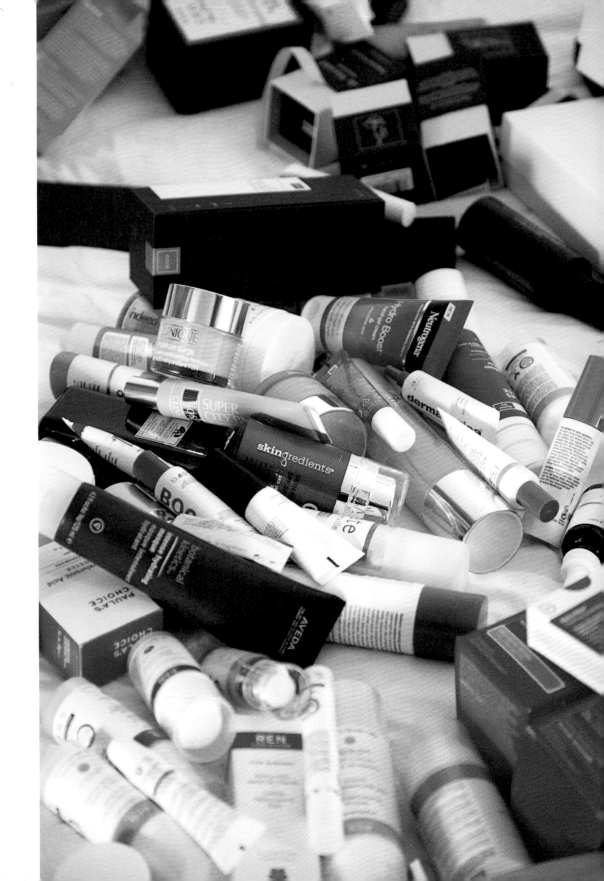

SKIN THROUGH YOUR LIFETIME

■ Work with your skin, not against it.

As you age, your skin changes, and your skincare routine and kit need to adapt with it.

The best thing you can do for your skin is get into good habits young (wear your SPF, people!), then tackle signs of ageing when you see them — skin starts to lose the ability to retain moisture in the face as you get older, your collagen is depleted and you need to step things up a notch.

Life throws many skin challenges our way, thanks to our hormones, habits, our environment etc. Don't let it blindside you: this section will make sure you're well prepped.

THE THREE WORST THINGS FOR YOUR SKIN

SUN: get a little, not a lot. Be sensible.

SUGAR: probably one of the best (and hardest) things you can do for yourself, your health and your skin is to cut out sugar. In a nutshell, sugar works to destroy your collagen — think of collagen as scaffolding for your face. Every time you eat/drink sugar it is like taking a piece of the scaffolding away — leading to saggy, baggy and drawn skin.

SMOKING: I was once able to tell a client how she blew her smoke out of her mouth (straight up her face from her bottom lip) because of the condition of her skin in the middle panel of her face. Smoking leaches the oxygen out of your face with every puff. Smokers have grey skin. If you smoke, try to get help and stop, as soon as you can.

THE AGEING TRIANGLE

Getting older should be seen as a privilege, not a problem. Some people don't get to see their 40th, 60th or 80th birthdays. Rather than whinging about ageing, let's be grateful that we're still here.

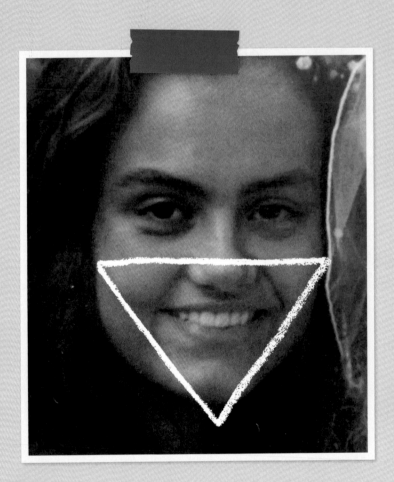

This photo was taken when I was in my early 20s, before my collagen decided to go on holiday. As you can see, all the definition is in the middle of my face. I have solid, high cheekbones, fat cheek pads and very few lines. My eyelids are not hooded and the area under the eye is full.

As you age, your face shape changes. The production of collagen in your skin decreases rapidly after 30. You can think about this like a triangle shape in the bottom half of your face. When you're younger, the base of the triangle is at the top, with the definition at the two corners of your cheekbones, moving to a point at your chin. As you age, the definition — the base of the triangle — moves towards your jawline with the point at your nose. So, the products you're applying need to go from protecting to repairing and supporting.

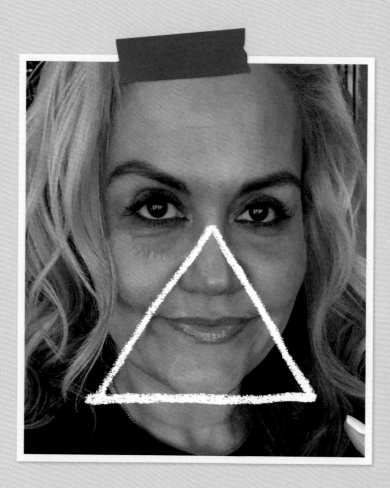

This photo is me in my 40s. The definition has all fallen towards my jawline. The collagen in my skin is massively depleted, therefore the structure of my skin has naturally altered. No amount of product will lift that cheek pad, no matter what the marketing on the packet says. The only thing that will lift this is a needle.

LIFE HAPPENS

Hormones are potentially the biggest skin disruptor of all.

Hormones, hormones, hormones. They have a lot to answer for, and at certain times of our lives they RAGE. When this happens, and when illness happens, there are things you can do to help tackle the effects they have on the skin. It just takes a few tweaks to your kit.

PUBERTY

Poor teenagers. Just as your hormones erupt, so do your moods and, in some cases, so does your skin. The best thing you can do when your skin is going through hormonal changes (whether you're a teenager, or an adult buying products for a teenager) is to take care of yourself, so:

- Buy gentle products and use them regularly. Getting into a routine is the hardest part.

- Change pillowcases regularly (at least once a week), as they harbour bacteria.

- Use light, oil-free moisturisers.

- Use spot treatments containing salicylic acid.

- Go for a professional treatment to encourage a good skincare routine and to pick the right products for your skin (not all teenage skins get spots!).

- LED light is great for acneic younger skins and non-invasive.

- Do not be afraid to seek medical advice (or seek it on a teenager's behalf). That is what doctors are for.

> **ADULTS:** Do not, under any circumstances, negate or dismiss their feelings if a teenager's skin is having a detrimental effect on their mental health. Take it, and them, seriously.

PREGNANCY

Hormones can wreak havoc with your skin, but there is no way of telling which way your skin will go, so:

- Invest in a hyaluronic facial mist to spray on your face when you are hot and flustered, or dry and dehydrated (or both). You'll love it when you're in labour.

- Buy a good-quality fragrance-free facial oil to apply if your skin is inflamed.

- Switch out your vitamin A for something like bakuchiol (see Glossary).

- Surges in hormones frequently result in breakouts, and despite old wives' tales, low levels of salicylic acid are completely safe for pregnant women. Doctors recommend using no higher than a 2 per cent product to tackle pregnancy breakouts, and most OTC products are sold at levels lower than 2 per cent.

All other acids are fine, although I wouldn't use anything that your skin is not accustomed to during this period.

157

PCOS OR ENDOMETRIOSIS

The effects of PCOS and endometriosis on the skin are best treated by causing no further harm. If you present with acne, follow the recommendations for that condition on pages 132–134.

In the meantime, try to avoid known skin irritants such as rough scrubs, fragrance (synthetic and natural), strong ingredients such as camphor, eucalyptus, mint and menthol, and stay away from high levels of alcohol in your skincare products.

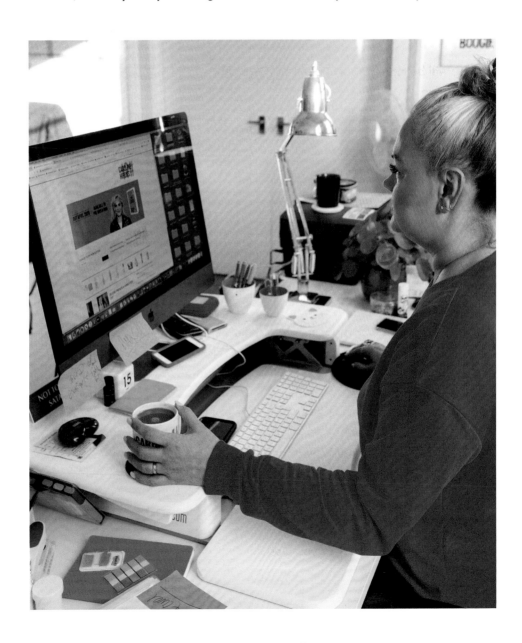

PERIMENOPAUSE AND MENOPAUSE

Perimenopause and menopause cause the biggest changes to the skin. The signs of ageing are accelerated, while the skin's ability to regenerate slows right down. Ceramides, collagen and hyaluronic acid levels are all depleted.

As well as treating your skin as a 'maturing' one (see page 179), be aware of the following:

- You must keep an eye on your moles, as pre-cancer and cancerous changes become more common. Check your skin (and your boobs) more regularly.

- You will be more prone to bruising due to falling levels of oestrogen. Your skin is now thinner.

- Your skin will be slower to heal. If you have an open wound that is not healing, and you suspect infection, seek medical help.

ILLNESS

If you have an auto-immune disease that causes skin inflammation and flare-ups such as multiple sclerosis or lupus or perhaps depression and/or ME:

- Go easy on stimulating ingredients such as acids and exfoliators.

- Use soothing cleansers, facial oils and moisturisers. You may be able to use slightly more active products if you are not in the middle of a flare-up/ episode, but you know your body and skin better than anyone else.

- Consider using fragrance-free products if you think fragrance is aggravating your skin. If you have broken skin as a result of your illness, fragrance may well irritate. Some people, however, find that the ritual of their self-care routine is vital to their wellbeing and is enhanced with fragranced products. If there is a scent you love, and it makes you feel better, don't deprive yourself. Do what feels good to you, both physically and mentally.

Treat your skin as delicately as you feel.

CHEMOTHERAPY

Chemo has a strong impact on your skin and will require changes to your usual routine. The job of chemotherapy is to kill your cancerous cells and prevent them from reproducing and growing. Unfortunately, it also has this effect on healthy cells, leading to very dry and fragile, and more sensitive, skin.

At a time when your immune system is already compromised, a damaged skin barrier can leave you even more prone to infection. Your skin barrier needs to be fortified and strengthened as much as possible in order to cope with chemotherapy's side effects.

Everything in your kit should be geared towards protecting your skin from the outside in. Think of it as fully closing a door that has been left slightly ajar.

Chemotherapy can leave the skin red, sore, irritated, itchy, blistered and extremely dry. This is a time for treating your skin delicately, and with the goal to nourish and protect, not stimulate.

- Cut out most of your active products, including anything like scrubs, acids and retinoids. Exfoliation is not required during this period.

- Avoid using alcohol, fragrance and essential oils directly on the skin. They can all be especially irritating on a disrupted skin barrier.

TRY THESE...

Some people going through chemotherapy have told me they've found the following helpful, but always check your product choices with your oncologist first.

- Zelens Power D Treatment Drops
- Indeed Labs Squalane Facial Oil
- Dermalogica Barrier Defense Booster
- Pai Rosehip BioRegenerate Oil
- Try the product recommendations for sensitive skins on page 114.

- Try to switch to a zinc oxide-based physical sunscreen and use SPF30+. Some chemotherapy drugs may also cause a sun allergy, so ensure that you are taking your doctor's advice and covering up well.

- Chemotherapy drugs can cause severe disruption to the nail bed. This can, again, leave you extremely susceptible to infection, so keep nails short and do not, however tempting it is, pick at your nails or cuticles.

- Avoid taking hot showers and baths. Ensure the water is warm, not hot.

- Try not to scratch or rub your skin. Wear loose clothing to prevent skin irritation and heat on the surface of your skin.

- Your skin will continue to be sensitised and vulnerable for a certain period after your last treatment finishes. Talk to your doctor before reintroducing your normal products to your routine. It is also common to be left extremely sun-sensitive for an extended period after treatment. Bear this in mind, go easy, and always listen to your doctor's advice.

CHILDREN AND SPF

If you have children, the best advice is to cover them up and keep them out of direct sunlight as much as possible.

- Reapply their SPF every 90 minutes, more frequently if they are getting wet.

- If you have children with short hair, remember the back of their necks and their ears. Every single person I have seen under a Wood's Lamp has significant sun damage at the tops of their ears and above the eyebrows – and it's always worse in my Australian clients.

THE BARE MINIMUM

The joy of doing in-person events is that I get to talk to a lot of you in a much more intimate fashion than via the internet. It's not unusual for up to five people each day to share that they would normally have struggled to attend something quite so loud/busy/frenetic due to various conditions such as ME, fibromyalgia, depression, anxiety or other serious illnesses such as MS.

> Honestly, the only reason I advocate attempting any kind of skin 'care' in all of these situations is purely for the self-care aspect.

On days where you think 'I can't face moving' – for whatever reason – do the absolute bare minimum and don't give yourself a hard time about it.

When you can't face much, but want to do 'something', keep these skincare routine tips to hand: they're affordable, easy and not too active.

CLEANSING

Wipes. Yes – there is the odd wipe that isn't atrocious (in this situation):

Water wipes are literally water, with a natural preservative to keep them fresh. If I still had small people these would be my wipe of choice. They're enough to freshen you up if you can't move. In 'all' areas.

RMS Beauty Ultimate Makeup Remover Wipes only contain coconut oil and shouldn't do any further harm if you need something to feel a little more substantial for your face than the water wipes. You need to hold the packet in your hand for a few minutes to heat up the coconut oil and ensure it's melted in the sachet before you open it.

Don't flush either of the wipes down the toilet.

MOISTURISING

Moisturiser-wise there are plenty of good, nourishing options for affordable, soothing, calming products that get to work on your skin without causing irritation: you can literally stick them on your face and forget about them.

> Just do what you can.
> When you can.

TRY THESE...

· **Squalane oil** is one of my first recommendations for anyone with a reactive, reddened, sensitised skin. It is a great light, moisturising facial oil for all skin types, and it's fragrance-free so won't irritate you if you are also sensitive to smell. A little goes a long way, so use it sparingly.

· **Serozinc** is a great refreshing mist/hydrator for all skins, not just the oily/combination skin types that it was traditionally marketed for. It's soft, sprays a lovely light mist and is suitable for misting at all times, not just after cleansing.

· **Weleda Skin Food** is still one of my favourites for a face that just wants comfort and/or moisturising. The newer, lighter version is much better for you if you have oily/combination skin. It's a must-have for most skins and most kits, to be honest. It needs warming gently with the fingers before application (an exception to my 'products don't need warming in the hands' rule – page 55).

· **10BALM** by Indeed Labs is a good option for an 'if all else fails, get this on your face STAT' cream, and with good reason. Containing only ten ingredients, all designed to soothe, nourish and calm, you can put this on top of the squalane, or just on its own for immediate relief without feeling too greasy.

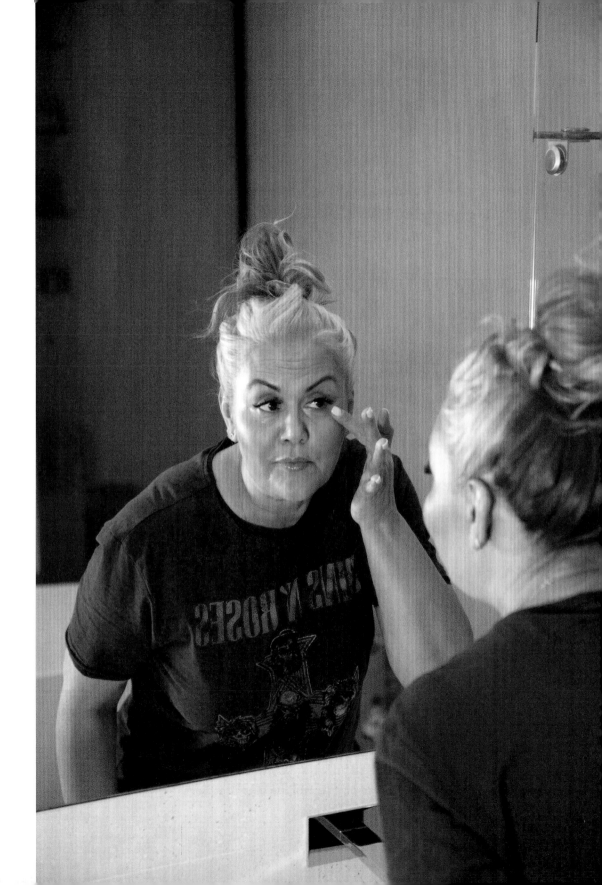

WHEN SHOULD I START USING ANTI-AGEING PRODUCTS?

SPF: technically from birth, but most companies won't advocate using SPF until your baby is 6 months old. Keep them protected from direct sunlight.

VITAMIN A: if you have acne you may be prescribed a retinoid by your doctor. Otherwise, around 30+, depending on lifestyle – if you're a sun worshipper and/or you smoke, you can start earlier.

GLYCOLIC/LACTIC/SALICYLIC ACIDS: again, this depends on lifestyle and skin type. If you have acne you can use salicylic acid topically. The other two can be introduced from the age of 25+ as needed.

VITAMINS C AND E: from the word go. As soon as you start your skincare routine choose something with these in. Good move.

NIACINAMIDE: 25+ ish, again depending on lifestyle and skin type. Acne? Crack on.

The basic thing to remember is that, for women, our collagen production is linked directly to our ovaries. When we are at our most fertile our skin is usually at its best. As you near menopause and go through perimenopause you will notice huge changes in your entire system, not just your skin. Hitting menopause has a direct link to your collagen. It's a bit like someone takes away a little of the scaffolding that supports your facial structure with each passing year.

So, start taking care of your skin when you get your periods, and step it up a notch when you get to 35+ (for example, if you go into early menopause or have a full hysterectomy).

And when you do start using these products, do not forget your SPF.

And if you smoke? Scrap all that advice and use all of the above – now.

SPOTS

Zits. Pustules. Papules. Wheals. Comedones. Milia. There are lots of things that happen to the skin – especially on the face – on a regular basis.

This is purely about SPOTS.

Acne? I'm not talking to you. Blackheads? Nor you. Pustules? Nope. I'm talking about your average spot that pops up occasionally. You know it's coming – you can feel it. It starts with a bump, feels sore, then gets a little red, hurts a little more, then you see a faint hint of something that could be a head. A little white may show underneath.

And then, typically, if you are the average person, you:

- Stab it (leading to scarring)
- Poke it (does absolutely nothing)
- Squeeze it (if you do this too early, the skin will bruise, then potentially scar)
- Load it with tea tree oil (no need – it's probably not bacterial)
- Load it with spot treatment (see above)
- or GOD FORBID – put toothpaste on it (please, no)

Toothpaste. Paste for TEETH. On a spot. **No.**

Next time you feel one of these mothers coming up you will need the following:

- Your hands
- Your moisturiser/a good facial oil
- Your concealer
- Patience

Moisturise the area like it's going out of fashion.

Yes, really. This is particularly good for those big on-the-chin, once-a-month spots. Moisturising it does a few things: it softens the area around the spot – how often have you destroyed the surrounding area of a zit because you treated the area of the said zit so abusively? – and then either makes the spot retreat entirely OR brings it to a head quicker – in which case you have my permission to pop. Pop pop away (see pages 168–171).

WORDS OF WARNING

A 'popable' spot shouldn't really hurt when popping – it should be satisfying.

If it hurts – stop – it's too soon and you will bruise and then possibly scar.

Stop at the first sign of blood – you're about to scar.

Never, ever, ever try to pop milia (see pages 140–141). Get them removed professionally.

The next time you feel Mount Vesuvius brewing under the skin give it a chance, treat it with care, and save the toothpaste for your mouth. Please.

HOW TO POP A SPOT

As much as any dermatologist will tell you not to pop, the fact is that you do. We do. You know you do; I know you do; the industry at large knows that you do, but they pretend that you don't. I know there are some of you that manage to restrain yourselves, but you're in the minority and up there with those people that don't lick their lips when eating a doughnut or chew when eating a fruit pastille. You exist, but the rest of us don't know how you manage it.

I'm a popper. Always have been. There's nothing more satisfying to be honest.

And I know most of you pop because you tell me so – usually with 'don't shout at me' eyes. As if! If it's the right time, I always pop. With that in mind, I offer you *my* way to pop. All risk is your own.

Please bear in mind: **Popping is not picking.** They are two very different things.

How so?

Popping – 'Ooh I see a whitehead! Where did that come from? I think I can get that out. Let me have a go. Yep. Excellent.' *carries on with routine*

Picking – 'Ow. That red lump on my chin is KILLING ME. I must be due on. Bloody hormones. I'm going to get it out.' *attempts to pop red lump for ages*
'OWWW. Ugh. I'll try again later. Ooh there's another one! Maybe that one will come out.' *prods second bump until it bleeds*
'OOWWWW. Ugh. No joy. Why does my skin hate me?'
plays with it all day with dirty fingers, doesn't leave it alone

If you fall into the latter category, you're making the simple mistake of opening the oven door before the cake has risen. A little patience changes the outcome.

A few simple guidelines will give the best result (although do bear in mind that every skin is different) and they will probably go against everything you've read from brands trying to sell you products. Nothing new there, so let's crack on.

WHAT YOU WILL NEED:

'Clean' everything. Clean hands. Clean skin. Clean flannel. Clean tissue. Acids. Cotton pads or a ready-made acid pad. A good-quality (non-mineral oil) facial oil.

- Slipping it into your routine is the easiest way. AM or PM. Not lunchtime in the loo at work.

- Cleanse. With a clean flannel. If the flannel doesn't knock the head off the spot that's your first sign that it may not be ready. If it's sore, it's probably not ready. I steer clear of sore spots. They're still working their way up the dermis food chain and causing inflammation along the way. Soak a cotton pad with acid toner and set it aside (or unpack your ready-made acid pad).

- If you can see white, it's not sore or too tender and everything is clean, take a tissue, rip it in half and wrap it around the forefinger of each hand.

- Finger placement is also crucial. One of the biggest mistakes made when popping is to go straight in from RIGHT NEXT TO THE SPOT. You put your two fingers on the spot and you just push your fingers together, so that you're so close, you literally just get a little teeny whitehead, then everything almost gets pushed back down into the spot. Not good.

- Do NOT use your nails. Use the pads of your fingertips only.

- Put your fingers either side of the spot, as best you can, depending on where it is, obviously. You should be able to SEE the spot. Gently push downwards and then, at a 90-degree angle towards the bottom the spot, start to push upwards. If it's ready, it will come up and out. Gently repeat. When the white stops, and it's spouting pink, STOP. STOP. STOP. STOP.

- If you see blood (it's already too late but...), STOP. You're in scarring territory. Show restraint.

- Now you need to move quickly. Take your pre-soaked acid toner cotton pad, or ready-and-waiting acid pad and apply it firmly to the spot, using a similar pressure as when you've ripped off a plaster or a wax strip. Hard pressure. Hold it down for a few seconds, then turn it over and repeat. There should be no bleeding. If there is, keep the acid on it until it stops. I have been known to walk around making a cup of tea while holding an acid-soaked pad on an overly pronged spot waiting for it to calm itself. The bigger the spot, the longer you hold acid on it.

  Note: this may sting like a MOFO (technical term). Stinging is good. I know I say it all the time, but stinging is good. The acid will be helping to kill the bacteria, helping it heal quicker and making sure the skin is prepped ready for the oil. You'll have a 'Kevin at the sink in *Home Alone*' moment. Embrace it.

- Yes, oil. I don't use drying-out products. If you dry out the spot, you also dry out the area surrounding the spot, causing a ton of inflammation and dehydration and, frankly, making a prime breeding ground for bacteria and scarring. A Juicy Lucy skin is harder to scar. A dried-out, shrivelled-up area will scar easily. Simples.

- Take your acid pad off and put your chosen oil on the area.

- Massage it firmly in. You can't be namby-pamby at this stage. Be firm. Use good, strong pressure, massaging all around the spot and over the spot.

- Depending on the rest of your day/evening, finish your routine, but I try to do this either on mornings that I'm not wearing makeup and am working from home, or in the evenings at teatime.

- It's best to do it when you're at home with a little time afterwards as you're going to repeat the oil application as soon as it has all been absorbed... Apply, wait, absorb, apply, wait, absorb. Repeat at least three times if you can.

- Throughout the day or the next morning, you will find that the spot erupts a little goo, like a mini volcano. Wipe this away with acid and reapply the oil. This sounds time-consuming but I promise we're talking seconds, not hours. And it's worth it if it speeds up the spot healing process and helps prevent scarring.

- If you have a ready spot but you have to go to work, do everything as above, apply your moisturiser over the area, don't avoid it – and then proceed with your makeup. Powder is your friend. Once you get home, cleanse immediately and do it all again. You may find the rest of the spot just throws itself at you willingly, or that it has calmed significantly to be almost invisible. Just don't be tempted to start on it like you're climbing Everest with a pickaxe.

The reason I use oil on spots, rather than drying products, is because in my experience, drying them out doesn't always work and causes more damage. Using oil does one of two things: it either swells up the spot and forces the 'head' of the spot to show up the next morning, or it settles it down and almost disperses the remnants.

> There are, of course, 'extraction tools' available on the market, but you can't use them where you can't see the spot, and you need to know how much pressure is too much.

Freckles are cute. At any age. You will do damage to your skin trying to get rid of them. Leave them alone. Embrace them.

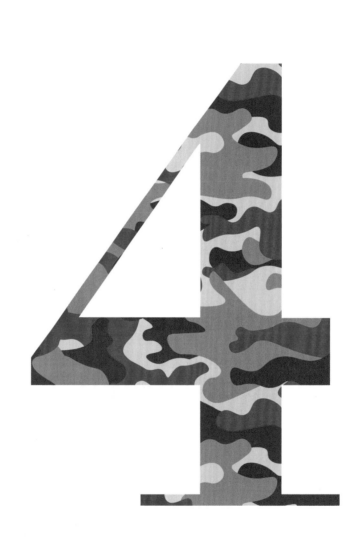

YOUR KIT

"

THE FILLING OF THE SANDWICH IS MORE IMPORTANT THAN THE BREAD

"

WHAT YOU NEED AND WHERE TO START

Now that you know what to do and when to do it, what do you use?

Your skincare kit deserves consideration and a bit of care. Like a bra or a haircut, it's personal to you and is going to see you through the next few months. Its effects are visible every single day, even if they are not obvious.

▌ Skin health – and good skincare – is for life.

Your skin's not a designer handbag. You should be buying products for the formula and the ingredients, not the label, however much you like how the packaging looks. The previous pages should have given you a good idea of the issues you personally have to contend with, and the ingredients that you need to look out for. You should also have a better idea of how to tell if a product is working for you.

When choosing your products, whether you're just starting out in the world of skincare or are a seasoned pro, you need to shop in a way that's financially sustainable; that means not splurging on one 'luxury' product that you then save for 'best'. And on the flip side, you shouldn't be so busy looking to save pennies that you cut corners where you really should be investing. I'll say it again – invest in the middle of your routine where you can. And remember, keep everything (except your cleansing products) out of your bathroom – bathrooms are generally too hot.

This chapter is devoted to your kit. What each product does, where to invest and where you can save if you need to. Follow these rules and you'll soon find that not only are you making the most of every last bit of your product, but you might find you're actually enjoying yourself.

THE ESSENTIALS

Your skincare kit can be as comprehensive or as simple as you want.

I was asked recently what I would take away with me if I could only pick three products. I went with a great balm cleanser, a good retinoid and an SPF50. If I had been asked the same question 30 years ago, I would have said a cleanser, a toner and a thick moisturiser. Your needs change with age; it's impossible to be specific. If you are just starting out and are unsure of what you need, these are the basics.

TEENS – EARLY 20s

- A good eye-makeup remover. This can be from a chemist or a pharmacy brand and doesn't need to be expensive. If you don't wear much makeup, leave this out.

- A good cleanser. This can be your eye-makeup remover if funds are tight, but this age group traditionally embraces heavier makeup, so make sure you are removing it all properly.

- Consider an acid product if you suffer with acne or regular breakouts. Start with a mild lactic or salicylic acid. You do not need to use it every day. Glycolic is not necessary at this stage.

- A moisturiser or light hydrating lotion, depending on your skin type. This can be either a light lotion or a cream formula.

- SPF. Try to find an SPF50 cream that feels comfortable on your skin. SPF30 is the absolute minimum you should go for. Regular use of an SPF at this age will save you time and money in later years.

> **ADD-ON:**
> A decent antioxidant – vitamin C serum is a safe bet. This isn't 100 per cent necessary as a teen, but it stands you in good stead for future years if you start in your early 20s.

20s – MID 30s

- A good eye-makeup remover or first cleanser.

- A second, lighter-textured cleanser for mornings or evenings where you aren't typically removing makeup or SPF.

- Acid toner. Using a gentle acid after your cleansing routine will help keep your skin exfoliated and ensure product penetration. You can introduce glycolic acid here, but lactic and salicylic acid are still helpful.

- A good antioxidant serum. Vitamin C and niacinamide are both good options.

- A multi-molecular-weight hyaluronic acid serum. As you are nearing or entering your 30s, your skin will slowly start to find it more challenging to retain oil and water. Hyaluronic acid is your best friend.

- Eye product. Optional if budget restricts, more necessary if you wear glasses or if your face is regularly exposed to the sun.

- A vitamin A/retinol product. This is not a concern if you are fairly healthy and don't sunbathe/smoke etc., however, if you are the other side of 30 and do, you need a retinoid.

- A moisturiser suited to your skin type.

- SPF. Same as earlier years. Use SPF50, or at least a minimum of SPF30.

ADD-ONS:
A light facial oil if you feel you need it, or in the winter. Apply a couple of drops under your moisturiser in the morning or finish with it in your evening routine. A hydrating hyaluronic-based facial mist. This will keep your hydration levels topped up in the skin without the added weight of a heavier cream.

LATE 30s – EARLY 40s

- A good eye-makeup remover or first cleanser.

- A lighter textured cleanser for your morning cleanse or evenings as a second cleanse, where you aren't typically removing makeup or SPF.

- Acids. Glycolic, lactic or PHA acids can all make an appearance in your kit at this stage, depending on your skin's needs (see pages 189–193).

- A hyaluronic-based facial mist. Your skin finds it harder to retain moisture at this age – this spray replaces that lost moisture. Do not spray plain water over your face: it is not the same thing. Look for 'hyaluronic acid' on the product.

- A good antioxidant serum. Spend your money here. Get a good niacinamide/vitamin C/resveratrol etc., and use it daily.

- A good-quality hyaluronic product. You are more susceptible to trans-epidermal water loss (TEWL) at this age so you will benefit from a daily dose of hyaluronic acid. Do not be fooled into buying a dirt-cheap one: it's likely to be a single-ingredient, heavy hyaluronic acid that won't really penetrate, so it's a false economy.

- Facial oil. Your quickest fix and your best friend.

- Eye product. You will notice the need for these more at this age. Go for lighter textures like gels or light creams. Rich, thicker creams feel luxurious but will make your eyes puffy.

- Vitamin A/retinoid. A must.

- A moisturiser suited to your skin type.

- SPF. Do not forgo this critical step.

40s, 50s, 60s, 70s, 80s & 90s

- A good eye-makeup remover or first cleanser. You may prefer thicker cream cleansers at this point.

- A second, lighter textured cleanser for mornings or evenings where you aren't typically removing makeup or SPF.

- Acids. Glycolic, lactic and PHA acids are all great for older skins.

- A hyaluronic-based facial mist, to replace lost moisture.

- Eye products. Go for gels if you have crepey eyes, or light creams. Richer eye creams are not favourable on an older face.

- Vitamin A/retinoid. An absolute must. Your skin's cell turnover is extremely slow at this age. Vitamin A is your best friend. Jump in.

- Facial oil. A facial oil is essential – it will literally replace the glow on an older face.

- Good antioxidant serums. While these are still important, you may prefer to spend your money 'correcting' issues at this age, and that brings us to...

- A good-quality pigmentation serum/product.

- A good-quality hyaluronic product.

- A moisturiser suited to your skin type. You may want to spend a little more on a moisturiser at this age. There is some merit to a separate night cream for an older skin, but it's more of a 'nice to have' product than a must.

CLEANSERS

A cleanser's job is to gently remove all the makeup, dirt and grime from your face. Cleansers are best chosen with your lifestyle in mind, while also paying attention to your skin concerns.

BALMS OR OILS

These are great for makeup and SPF removal – an oily/acne skin might find them too heavy or problematic to remove. I tend to use these for a first cleanse in the evening.

CREAMS

These do a great job of both removing makeup and cleansing the skin and are made for all skin types.

MILK OR LOTIONS

Traditionally used by French beauty houses, milks are runny, soft, easy to use and remove makeup and SPF and cleanse your skin.

GELS

Popular as a morning cleanse or a second cleanse in the evening (see page 45), gels are the preferred texture for a lot of people with combination/oily skin.

MICELLAR WATER

Micellar waters are a mixture of oil and water that's used as a liquid makeup remover. They should only be used as a first cleanse. Micellar waters are not ideal for regular use, or for cleaning the skin.

TRY THESE...

- Pixi + Caroline Hirons Double Cleanse
- Kate Somerville Goat Milk Cleanser
- OSKIA Renaissance Cleansing Gel
- The Body Shop Camomile Sumptuous Cleansing Butter
- Emma Hardie Moringa Balm
- Joanna Vargas Vitamin C Face Wash
- The Ordinary Squalane Cleanser
- Beauty Pie Japanfusion or Plantastic Balm
- Tata Harper – all her cleansers!
- Clinique Take The Day Off

In general, foaming is what you want washing-up liquid to do, not your cleanser. And a message to the brands: please stop regurgitating the same formulas and recommending them to the same skins. Foaming is NOT best for acne.

SPRITZES

Facial mists and sprays are an easy and affordable way to ensure that your skin stays hydrated without the need for heavier products. They are ideal as either a second tone (spritz) or just your general tone for those of you that don't use acids and/or on days you aren't using acids. Use them alone, after cleansing, under serums, over serums, under moisturiser, over moisturiser, under makeup, over makeup, on an airplane, in your car, at your desk, when it's hot, when it's cold... wherever and whenever. If in doubt, SPRITZ.

Some are water with added minerals such as zinc and magnesium, while others (which tend to be more expensive) have added peptides, rice bran oils, rose oils etc. – just more 'oomph'. Hyaluronic acid and glycerin can usually be found in them, along with other hydrating factors.

They are variously labelled as 'hydrating mists', 'spritzes', 'essences' and 'face sprays'.

TRY THESE...

- La Roche-Posay Toleriane Ultra 8 Face Mist
- La Roche-Posay Serozinc
- Josh Rosebrook Hydrating Accelerator
- Mother Dirt AO+ Mist
- January Labs Restorative Tonic Mist

MICELLAR WATERS ARE A 'PROPER' CLEANSER

I am tagged on Twitter or Instagram on a daily basis whenever there is an article singing the praises about micellar waters, particular cleansers, or wipes (God – always the wipes!), online or in a magazine. I read as many of them as I can: sometimes they make me laugh, sometimes I find I agree with them. But, articles describing micellar water as a cleanser are never one of those times.

Micellar waters were originally designed to be used for those occasional times when you have no access to water, like backstage at fashion shows (hence the huge awareness of Bioderma) or at a festival (see pages 75–78).

Firstly, I will never for the life of me understand why some people think that using these products is 'quicker' than washing your face. If using micellar water is 'quicker' than washing your face, you're using it incorrectly. A quick swipe across the forehead is not going to clean your face. When I have to use them backstage at shows it takes me at least four sets of two separate cotton pads to clean the face of makeup. Using both sides. That's not quick. Add to that the constant rubbing of cotton wool and ingredients that aren't exactly 'softening' and you're setting yourself up for a sore face.

These waters are ingredient-heavy, some contain alcohol and most contain fragrance. Before those of you that have to use micellar waters jump to their defense, as I've already said, do what you have to.

Work situations, new babies, flying, the gym – micellar waters can come in handy. But try to make them a temporary substitute, not a permanent fixture.

WHY I DO NOT LIKE ELECTRONIC CLEANSING BRUSHES

Electronic cleansing brushes, also known as facial brushes, are a so-called 'beauty tool' that have rotating heads and exfoliate and 'deep clean' the skin. Where to begin on why **I'm not a fan**.

- **Because your skin is delicate.** It does not need a sandblaster to cleanse it. You have hands – use them. (If you don't have two hands, obviously do whatever you have to do and ignore this.)

- **Because they are capable of basically destroying your acid mantle.** Do you think your skin is 'purging'? It's not *purging*; it's inflamed. It's shouting at you, begging you to stop whatever it is you're doing to it. Stop it. If you were using a moisturiser that made your face break out into acne you'd be horrified, utterly horrified. And you would, in all likelihood, stop using it immediately and return it, especially if that cream was extortionate. But don't worry! In the case of 'purging', they have a brilliant idea! 'Buy another head'! 'You must just need something a bit more delicate'. Note how they've made it your fault. *Your* problem. And the solution? Spend more money. It's genius, if you think about it.

- **They are often aimed at people with acne.** The fact that these are ever aimed at people with acne is enough to make me feel slightly nauseous. 'Hey, you know what's great for acne? Using a power brush to really make sure the skin is as sore as possible! Brilliant! Let's do that.' No. Please do not.

- **Lack of training when the item is sold.** You can buy the most famous version of these brushes online. Just get it delivered to you, with no human contact from a trained professional advising you on how to use it. Which leads to...

- **People using them incorrectly.** I find, when talking to readers and clients, that these 'tools' are, without doubt, the ones that are most frequently abused.

- **The dirty head.** How many of you wash the brush head properly? Don't tell me 'it dries out and therefore the bacteria die'. Imagine using the same flannel for 2 weeks and never washing it. You can by all means let it 'dry out' between uses if that image makes you feel better, but imagine it. Filth.

- **The cleansers that the original version of these are sold with are 100 per cent horrific.** Horrific. I cannot stress enough how much these should be avoided. I promise you, the thought behind this was, 'How can we make more money?', 'Oh, I know! Let's make our own product! We'll say that it's the only thing people should use with them. OMG that's genius!' This was not a decision made for the benefit of your skin. A foaming, SLS-laden soap with a rotating (oscillating – whatever) power-blaster? In some cases, with grit?

It's like they sat together around a table and said, 'What could we possibly make that could irritate the skin more than say, oh, I don't know, wire wool and washing-up liquid?'.

WHY ARE THEY SO POPULAR?

The popularity of these cleansing brushes is down to numerous factors:

- Because of the timer system, in some cases it will be the first time that some people have thoroughly cleansed their face. If you massaged a cleansing product into your skin with your hands for a full minute and removed it with a flannel after years of splashing off regular milks/gels, your skin would feel the same way.

- If you've never used flannels and acid toners, these brushes will without doubt exfoliate your skin. The first time you use it you will feel like your skin can 'breathe' properly. That's nothing you can't achieve with product and hands (and without sanding your face).

- Marketing. Your mate has one, it's all over the press, you WANT it. 'Oh, look, A PINK ONE!' *man voice* 'OH, LOOK! A black one!'

- And why is it all over the press? Because they make money. BIG, BIG, BIG money for the companies that sell them. Not just the brands; the retailers. If you go into a store and someone tries to sell you this, I promise you they are trying to make their target for the day. They may not have even asked you what skin type you have before they've said, 'Oh, you know what YOU need?!'

BUT: you don't have to listen to me. I know some of you swear by them. Good for you. As I always say, if it ain't broke, don't fix it. And do not stop using something you love on my account. If, however, you have a facial brush sitting in your cupboard that you shelved because it didn't agree with your skin, dig it out. Use it on your feet. Or your bum. Lovely.

I do think that, in years to come, we will see an increase in broken capillaries, stubborn 'bumps' that don't come to a head, and rosacea, and I think this will be related to the use of these 'brushes'.

> If you suffer from eczema, acne or rosacea, for the love of ALL THAT IS SANITY, you have no business blasting your face to kingdom come with these things. No matter what any salesperson says.

You overuse facial tools. A lot of you. You can use them – you're just not meant to use them every time you brush your teeth.

Step away from the trendy facial tool and just wash your face properly.

And while I'm on things I don't like, let me give a special mention to jade rollers (or any type of mineral/crystal rollers). If they make you sit still and chill out while you massage your jawline for 10 minutes, crack on. They won't harm you. But, if you are buying one because the brand says that 'once rubbed onto the skin, it increases circulation and gives a dewy glow' or a 'lift', save your cash.

SKINCARE MYTH

!?#

WAITING LISTS

You know the things. Those long lists that retailers circulate, stating that 'literally thousands' of people are 'eagerly awaiting!' a product. Check out the press most days and you'll see plenty of articles about the latest one.

Here's the thing.

They do not exist. At least not in the way that they are portrayed.

Take it from someone who's spent her life in retail: there is no such thing as a list of thousands of people's names, all of whom are eagerly awaiting whatever product that marketing company is being paid to push that week.

> It's all hype, to make you want the product more and keep up with the Joneses.

In the case of something like the latest iPhone, with 10 million sold in the first weekend of sales, the majority on pre-order (i.e. already bought and paid for), the 'waiting list' is a legitimate claim. It's fact. If a skincare product is sold on pre-order and you pay for it, that's technically a waiting list. The rest is marketing. If a skincare product is really as 'wanted' as that, release it to market, let it genuinely sell out everywhere and spread via word of mouth.

Stop this nonsense.

"

USING ACID TONERS IS LIKE TAKING YOUR FACE TO THE GYM

"

ACIDS

I understand that combining the words 'acid' and 'skin' can potentially be intimidating. Don't be scared! Acids aren't actually that new. One of the first acid toners, P50 by Biologique Recherche, has been going since 1970. I've been banging on about them for ages, and thankfully they've gained in momentum in recent years.

Acids are all about exfoliation, and are derived from professional chemical peels, but are now included in our everyday skincare routines. I originally coined the phrase 'acid toning' to allow readers to easily identify where it goes in their routine i.e. after cleansing – the liquid acid stage basically replaces your traditional toner.

Try to buy two, preferably three, acid products: a strong one for evenings, a lighter one for daytime and one more to mix it up. Different strengths and different acids do different things to the skin, and you'll want to tweak which you use depending on how your skin's feeling.

All acids are available in a variety of strengths, and come in many forms: liquids, pre-soaked pads and gels.

ACIDS OVERVIEW

LACTIC (AHA) – resurfacing, great for dehydrated and dry skin.

GLYCOLIC (AHA) – stimulating for better collagen production, resurfacing.

MALIC (AHA) – resurfacing, good for boosting collagen production.

SALICYLIC (BHA) – best for spots/acne. Surprisingly gentle.

PHAs (POLYHYDROXY ACIDS) – best for those in need of hydration and deep penetration of a product applied afterwards.

There are three main types of acid:

ALPHA HYDROXY ACIDS (AHAs)

These are the most commonly used acids and include glycolic, citric, mandelic, malic, tartaric and lactic. They exfoliate the skin, stimulate collagen and GAGs (glycosaminoglycans) formation. They normalise the stratum corneum (the outer-most layer of the epidermis) and can regulate keratinisation. They are best for targeting signs of ageing.

You need these if your skin is showing signs of ageing.

BETA HYDROXY ACID (BHA)

There is only one beta hydroxy acid – salicylic. It is derived from acetylsalicylic acid, or willow bark. Like AHAs, beta hydroxy acid (BHA) also acts as an exfoliant, increasing the shedding of dead skin cells. BHA is extremely useful for treating breakouts and helps manage keratosis pilaris and other conditions that involve blocked or clogged pores.

You need this if you suffer with blemishes, spots or acne.

POLYHYDROXY ACIDS (PHAs)

The next generation of AHAs, these allow for slower and gradual penetration. The absorption is non-irritating and doesn't sting. PHAs support the matrix around collagen, help restore skin barrier function and protect against collagen degradation. PHAs are probably the most multi-tasking of all acids. Gluconolactone, lactobionic and maltobionic are examples of PHAs. They are best for targeting signs of ageing, and using on sensitive or dehydrated skins.

You need these if your skin is sensitive but you want the effects of acid.

WHAT'S THE MAIN DIFFERENCE BETWEEN THEM?

AHAs are water-soluble and, with the exception of glycolic acid, they do not penetrate deeply beneath the skin's surface. BHA is oil- (lipid-) soluble. This allows the BHA to penetrate oily pores and help to exfoliate the pore itself. This is why salicylic is particularly useful for oily and acneic skins.

PHAs tend to be better for sensitive skins due to their larger molecular size and slower penetration. PHAs are great humectants (they attract moisture to the skin), making them particularly good choices for dehydrated skins.

But that's not the end of it. Within these categories, acids can be broken down into even more types, depending on what they're made from.

GLYCOLIC ACID (AHA)

Containing the smallest molecule in AHAs, glycolic acid is derived from sugarcane and is the most effective AHA due to its ability to penetrate deeply and stimulate fibroblast cells (see Glossary) to aid in collagen production. It exfoliates the skin by increasing cell turnover, helps even out skin tone and builds the support structure in the dermal matrix, which in turn reduces the appearance of wrinkles. It is the only acid that makes you more sun-sensitive.

You need this if you are over 30 or 35 and your main concern is ageing.

LACTIC ACID (AHA)

Historically derived from milk, lactic acid has more recently been synthetically formed to maintain its stability in products. Lactic acid works to dissolve the glue in between cells on the surface, making it good for gently exfoliating. It keeps the skin soft and acts like Pac Man on the surface of the skin, gently eating it away.

You need this if your main concern is dull, dehydrated or dry skin.

MANDELIC ACID (AHA)

Fat-soluble and derived from almonds, this is a good choice for oilier skins, as the molecules can penetrate even the greasiest skin. Mandelic acid is antibacterial and, with regular usage, can reduce oiliness without harshly drying out the skin.

You need this if your skin is on the oilier side, but you don't particularly suffer with spots (can happily be used with a BHA).

CITRIC ACID (AHA)

May help to reverse the signs of photo/sun damage, while also improving the quality of the dermal matrix. It's mostly used at preservative level, just so brands can list it on the ingredients label. Look for specific mentions of citric acid in the descriptions on packaging: if they're not there, it's probably used as a preservative only. You don't need to seek out citric acid especially, but it is used in a lot of formulas.

TARTARIC AND MALIC ACID (AHAs)

Mainly derived from grapes, apples, pears and cherries, these two are gentler on the AHA scale but do act as antioxidants and aid skin respiration. You wouldn't seek these out in particular, as they're not key ingredients.

SALICYLIC ACID (BHA)

Derived from willow bark, salicylic acid is oil-soluble and penetrates and breaks down the 'glue' that causes breakouts and oily, uneven skins. It loosens desmosomes, allowing the cell to let go of the excess sebum that oily skins like to hold on to (think of desmosomes as handcuffs, attaching your cells together – salicylic acid unlocks the handcuffs).

You need this if you suffer from spots. If you live in Europe, this is your alternative to benzoyl peroxide.

GLUCONOLACTONE ACID (PHA)

A largely antioxidant PHA, gluconolactone is the multi-tasker of all acids. It is made of multiple humectant hydroxyls, which hydrate the skin. It also attacks free radicals, protecting the skin from UV damage and strengthening barrier function, allowing the skin to reduce in redness with regular use. Gluconolactone inhibits elastase, the cause of skin sagging, and helps maintain elasticity.

You need this if you have sensitive skin. It plays well with others.

LACTOBIONIC ACIDS (PHAs)

Derived from milk sugars, lactobionic acids are antioxidants. They help prevent and reverse signs of ageing including lines, pigmentation, large pores and uneven skin texture, promote skin firmness and stop the degradation of collagen. A natural humectant, they bind water to the skin.

You need these if you're dehydrated.

MALTOBIONIC ACID (PHA)

The most humectant of acids, maltobionic acid gives antioxidant protection, protects skin from hyperpigmentation caused by sun exposure, and helps prevent collagen degradation. Maltobionic acid can improve skin texture, firmness, clarity and tone, and reduce the appearance of wrinkles. You'll see it in an ingredients list, but don't need to seek it out particularly. It's good if your skin is dry or dehydrated.

THE OTHER 'ACIDS'

Azelaic and hyaluronic acids, although 'acids', are not exfoliating, and so are not in this section. They're just not that kind of acid.

TRY THESE...

- Dr Dennis Gross Alpha Beta Peel (various strengths available)
- Biologique Recherche P50
- First Aid Beauty Facial Radiance Pads
- OSKIA Liquid Mask

- Pixi Glow Tonic
- Kate Somerville Liquid ExfoliKate
- This Works Morning Expert Multi-Acid Acid Pads

ACID MYTHS

!?#

Some of the most frequent questions I am asked concern acids, specifically glycolic acid. So, let's clear a few things up:

MYTH: Glycolic thins the skin.
FACT: Glycolic acid thickens the skin. Glycolic acid exfoliates and thins the outer stratum corneum (the pleasingly named 'horny layer') of your skin, making it more flexible. It also restores the essential components of the skin that are damaged as we age, leading to an increase in collagen fibre density (and therefore thicker skin) that then functions more youthfully. For smoother-textured, softer, younger-looking skin, more evenness of skin tone and clarity, and a fuller, firmer skin with more elasticity and less laxity, use glycolic acid.

MYTH: You must use SPF30 or above if using acids, as AHAs increase sensitivity to UV light.
FACT: Increases in sunburn cell formation have been documented following AHA use, however this effect can be prevented by use of the very lowest level of sunscreen, even as low as an SPF2.

This fact is merely to reassure you that if you use acids, you're not burning your face off when you go outside. It's not to encourage you to cease SPF usage, which you will still need for the usual reasons.

MYTH: AHAs diminish skin barrier function.
FACT: US FDA studies have not shown an increase in the absorption of studied materials, which means that skin barrier function is not decreased. Further studies have demonstrated AHA-related improvements in skin barrier function.

MYTH: AHAs cause skin irritation.
FACT: AHAs are known to occasionally produce transient stinging, especially at higher strengths. The stinging should be fleeting and should not produce excessive redness. Mild irritation can be (but is not always) part of the process.

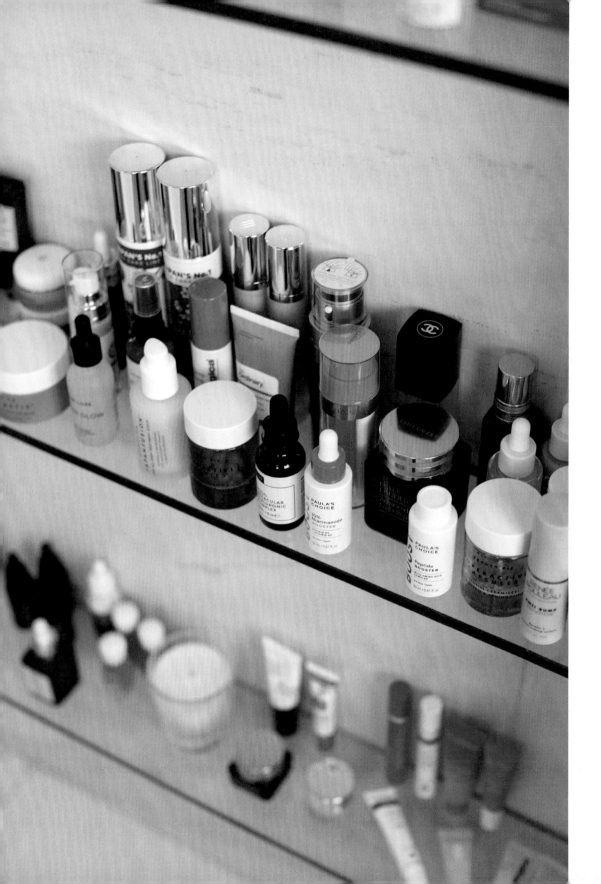

DUPES

Everyone loves a bargain, myself included. Just make sure you are, indeed, getting a bargain and not being 'duped' into thinking that the cheaper version of a product is the same as the original formula. I can promise you that in the majority of cases, it isn't.

Read labels. That will help you find real bargains. Do you need to pay hundreds of pounds for a hyaluronic acid that contains one type of HA? Of course not (unless you want to, obviously). In that case a 'dupe' is indeed a good move.

However, if you're looking at more complicated products like acids and serums, dupes may not be all they seem. Most cheaper brands are purposely making knock-off versions that will include the key ingredient buzzwords from the original higher-priced formulas on the front of the packaging, but minimal amounts of the key ingredient in the product itself.

There are plenty of very affordable brands available on the market without resorting to the 'dupes' that are based on nothing but trying to rip off someone else's idea, piggyback on their success and in turn relieve you of your hard-earned cash for an inferior product.

'Dupes' belong in makeup and nail varnish. There is no 'dupe' for a high-quality, years-of-research-behind-it skincare product. Just because the packaging looks the same, it does not mean the juice is similar.

AN INFERIOR PRODUCT IS A WASTE OF YOUR MONEY, NO MATTER HOW MUCH OF A 'BARGAIN' IT APPEARS

"

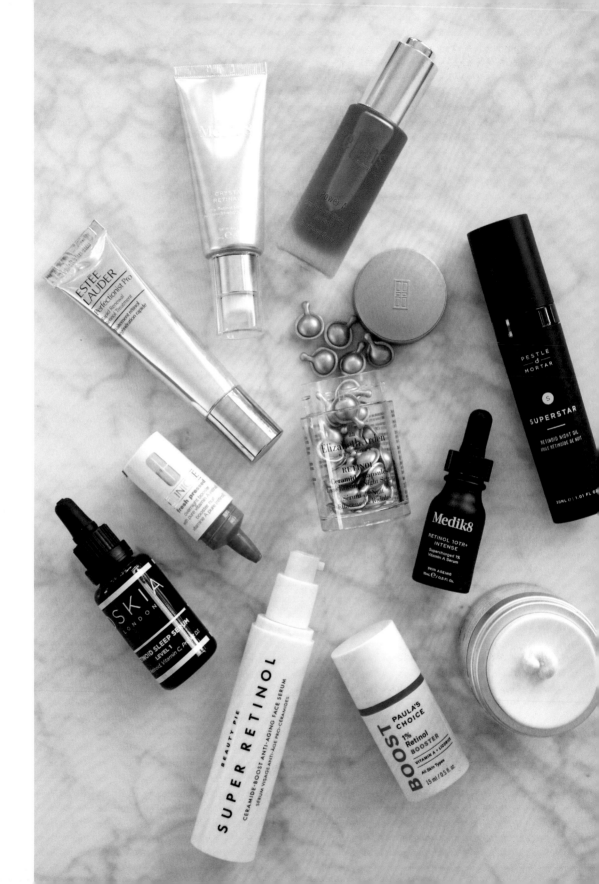

VITAMIN A AND RETINOID PRODUCTS

This is one of the products I'm most frequently asked about, and potentially one of the most confusing. All you need to know is that it's ALL VITAMIN A. In the same way that white sugar, brown sugar and maple syrup are all sugar, retinoid is the family name for any vitamin A product. Other ways you might see this ingredient listed on packaging are: retinol, retinal, retinyl palmitate, tretinoin, retinaldehyde, retinyl retinoate, hydroxypincolone retinoate or adapalene.

> Originally discovered as having beneficial side effects when treating acne, vitamin A is widely considered to be the gold standard of skincare because it is scientifically proven not only to reverse the signs of ageing, but also shown to prevent them.

A lot of people contact me because they're scared to try a vitamin A product, or they used it once, had a bad reaction and are worried about going back to it. There are side effects to using vitamin A products, but with correct usage, there is nothing on the market that gives the same results on the skin.

HOW TO USE

- Use after cleansing, and make sure your skin is dry before you start.

- General guidance is to use vitamin A in the evening, but some newer formulas state that they can be used during the day.

- Always use an SPF (in your morning routine).

- Start with a milder percentage and work your way up. The percentage will vary depending on the type of retinoid (see pages 202–203).

- Generally one full cycle (one tube or jar) of a product is enough to build up resistance and move up to the next strength.

- Less is more. You will be directed to use a pea-sized amount of prescription-strength formulas, however you can use a little more of OTC formulas.

- Avoid the eyes, the area around the nostrils, corners of the mouth and neck (see page 53).

Most people are put off using a vitamin A product because they weren't told how their skin would initially react. Vitamin A, at its core, is designed to resurface the skin, stimulate collagen production and reverse the signs of ageing. This doesn't happen overnight, and might require a bit of a journey. It can be a shock if you were expecting to wake up 10 years younger, but actually you might wake up looking like you've had an allergic reaction, but it is worth it – it just takes a little while to get there.

WHAT TO EXPECT WHEN YOU START

- Redness
- Dryness
- Patches of flaking skin
- Generally irritated skin (in varying degrees, depending on the formula)

I'm really selling it to you, aren't I? This reaction is completely normal and to be expected. To encourage you to keep going, this is what you do while your skin is acclimatising.

- Your first port of call is to buffer the product. This means weakening the formula by adding in a layer of moisturiser either before or after you apply the retinol.

- Avoid foaming products, especially cleansers, as they will be too drying.

- Avoid powders and heavy foundations. They will make the flaking look SO much worse. I refer to my skin as 'sausage roll pastry' when it's at this stage. However, life goes on and if you want to wear makeup, you need a really good moisturiser instead of a primer. I've found Embryolisse Lait-Crème Concentré works really well for me. The mineral oil base, on this occasion, is a plus, as it stops your skin from taking the water from your foundation and going flaky and patchy.

- Oils are your friend. Squalane and jojoba oils are really light and, unlike some heavier oils, won't stop the retinol from working. When I'm using retinols, I have a squalane oil on me at all times and use it throughout the day.

WHAT TO EXPECT ONCE YOUR SKIN ACCLIMATISES

- Smoother skin
- Glowing skin
- Fewer visible lines
- Better skin tone and elasticity
- Plumper skin
- More hydrated skin

HOW OFTEN SHOULD YOU USE IT?

As the great Kate Somerville says, use your vitamin A according to the decade you're in. If you're in your 20s, use it twice a week; 30s, three times a week; 40s, four times a week; and so on.

WHEN WILL YOU SEE THE EFFECTS?

In line with your age, and how much there is to repair, how quickly you'll see results will vary.

- Over 40: 1 month
- 30–40: 2 weeks
- 20–30: strangely longer, as you don't have much to fix

Because the side effects do not show on your skin immediately, you may be tempted to use more than suggested, and apply it more frequently. Do not do this. Seriously. I mean it.

Don't.

HOW DO YOU KNOW IF YOU'VE OVERDONE IT?

- Somebody says, 'Oh my god, what has actually happened to your face?'

- Your normal moisturiser stings.

- Your skin feels burned and is sore. This is beyond dry or uncomfortable. It is literally painful to the touch. A gust of wind would make you wince and you feel like your face is going to fall off.

- It's sore around your nostrils or the corners of your eyes and eyelids.

- Blistering/bleeding (just stop already).

The severity of your reaction, and how long you attempted to use vitamin A for before stopping, will dictate how soon you can try again. Apply a lot of nourishing products while your skin recovers, give it a couple of weeks or longer for your skin to return to normal, then try it again once more, but buffer it and go slowly.

A ROUGH GUIDE TO RETINOIDS

There are plenty of vitamin A derivatives in formulas but these are the main characters you should be inviting to the party:

THE BOSS

Tretinoin (retinoic acid/all trans-retinoic acid), aka 'Tret', is available as prescription-strength products only. It comes in 3 strengths and you will work up from 0.025% to 0.05% and finally 0.1%, guided by your dermatologist. It is suitable for most skin types.
POTENTIAL FOR IRRITATION: high

THE HEAVYWEIGHT

Not the boss but it packs a punch, **retinaldehyde** is the next level down from retinoic acid. It acts quickly on the skin, but can be irritating. It is clinically proven to work up to 11 times faster than retinol. Suitable for older skins that want quick results.
POTENTIAL FOR IRRITATION: medium

THE NEW KID ON THE BLOCK

Retinyl retinoate (RR), less well known than HPR, is the child of retinoic acid and retinol. It's a fairly new addition to the family, and has been shown to be more stable and more active than retinol, causing less irritation. Suitable for sensitive skins.

POTENTIAL FOR IRRITATION: low to medium

THE COUSIN

Related to The Boss but not a direct descendant, **hydroxypincolone retinoate** (HPR) is more of a cousin to its stronger relative. It is sometimes offered in higher percentages because it's an ester (i.e. it's oil-based), and therefore more gentle. Suitable for sensitive skins.

POTENTIAL FOR IRRITATION: low

THE TEENAGER

I call **retinol** the teenager because it's often irritating, in varying strengths. Having said that, retinol is the most widely available vitamin A in over-the-counter products. It is generally available in 0.3%, 0.5% and 1%. It works in the same way as the stronger ingredients above – it just takes you longer to get there. Suitable for all skin types.

POTENTIAL FOR IRRITATION: high, depending on the percentage

THE LINEKER (YEAH, I'M A FOOTBALL FAN)

Adapalene (trade name Differin) plays well with others and has never been sent off, and is available over the counter in the USA. It is mainly used for acne but has proven benefits on signs of ageing on the skin, so is a good pick if you are Stateside and looking for something easy to access that won't break the bank or your skin. Suitable for all skin types, but especially useful for acne or breakouts.

POTENTIAL FOR IRRITATION: fairly low

TRY THESE VITAMIN A BRANDS

- Medik8
- SkinCeuticals
- Paula's Choice
- Murad
- Beauty Pie
- Indeed Labs

SERUMS

YOUR KIT

Serums are one of the most misunderstood and confused elements of the routine. So let's get down to basics. A serum is a product designed to deliver a high concentration of active ingredients directly into your skin. They are the last thing you apply before your moisturiser. And if you're going to spend money anywhere in your routine, it's best spent here.

Think of the serum as the 'treat'ment stage of your routine. The active ingredient you want will depend on the condition that you want to treat. So when buying products, check the label to see if the formula contains the suggested key ingredients for your skin type and condition (see Chapter 2).

Serums can be offered as oils, gels or lotions but are generally water-based. As a rule of thumb, apply the thinnest serums first, however there will always be exceptions, and reading labels is key.

TRY THESE...

These brands all make excellent serums for all skin concerns:

- Beauty Pie
- Medik8
- SkinCeuticals

- Zelens
- Vichy
- La Roche-Posay

- Kate Somerville
- Murad
- OSKIA

MOISTURISERS

This is the final hydrating step in your routine, before you apply SPF, and it's also the product that you don't need to blow your budget on. Moisturisers are generally classed in three categories:

EMOLLIENTS

These add oil to the epidermis and soften and smooth the skin, and are found in products aimed at dry skin.

HUMECTANTS

These attract water from the atmosphere and the epidermis and are found in most moisturisers. They are particularly beneficial for dehydrated and oilier skins.

OCCLUSIVES

These coat the stratum corneum (the outer-most layer of the epidermis) and prevent trans-epidermal water loss (TEWL). They are generally recommended in a professional capacity for people suffering with skin conditions such as eczema or psoriasis.

TRY THESE...

- Kate Somerville Peptide K8 Power Cream
- Jordan Samuel The Performance Cream
- Kate Somerville Nourish
- OSKIA Bedtime Beauty Boost
- Pestle & Mortar Hydrate Moisturiser
- Glossier Priming Moisturiser
- Avène Tolerance Extreme Range
- Murad Hydro-Dynamic Ultimate Moisture
- REN Vita Mineral Daily Supplement Moisturising Cream
- May Lindstrom The Blue Cocoon
- Josh Rosebrook Vital Balm Cream

STEP AWAY FROM THE GLITTER

Glitter in skincare is just a downright nonsense. I don't know who started it. I don't care. It needs to end. And end now.

Glitter is a pain in the arse. It can be nice in an eyeshadow, when applied well. If you're a teen, knock yourself out: now is the time to swim in glitter if you want to. If you're in your 20s and enjoy a glittery face, again, knock yourself out. It's a legal requirement at festivals. I get it.

If, however, you are the rest of us, STOP. JUST MAKE IT STOP.

I mean, I don't know how much any of this needs saying, but there is ABSOLUTELY ZERO BENEFIT TO PUTTING GLITTER IN SKINCARE. If you have less-than-perfect skin, please stay away. It's also bad for the environment and will potentially lead to the next microbead situation (we can only hope brands will be responsible and remove it from their products before that happens).

If you want to take a fun selfie for social media, wearing a glitter mask, that's your call. But DON'T. OKAY? DON'T. JUST DO NOT. I know some of you think it's fun, but the skincare community feels faint with despair at every new launch. And if you are a 'skincare' brand making money selling frigging glitter? Go sit in a dark room and think long and hard about your actions.

MOISTURISER IS YOUR MOST IMPORTANT PURCHASE

I've lost count of the number of times I've had a conversation with people who tell me they are using an incredibly expensive moisturiser, but cleansing (or not) with wipes or a quick wash in the shower.

Your moisturiser is your coat. It's your protection and 'cushion' from the elements.

Of course it's important – and yes, you can find moisturisers that contain all sorts of lovely wonderful things such as peptides, vitamins and other active ingredients, but those ingredients will generally work better for you in a serum where they can more freely penetrate and get to work while your moisturiser stands guard.

There is absolutely no point in buying the latest 'wonder' cream if you've done no prep work. If you spend a fair amount of cash on your cleansing routine, including acid toners, and a bit more on a serum, you can get away with saving your pennies on a moisturiser.

There are, of course, as with anything in life, exceptions. If you are 40+ it is potentially worthwhile using a high-tech moisturiser alongside your serum; one that also contains the 'active' ingredients found in your serum. Attack it from all angles by all means. If you are on a tight budget, prioritise your spending on exfoliating acids and a good retinoid serum and you can get away with cheaper cleansers and moisturisers.

How much time do you spend choosing your coat in the morning compared to picking your outfit?

Your cleanse-acid-serum routine is your 'outfit'. Put the work in and you'll see the results. Just don't forget your coat.

EYE PRODUCTS

There are two camps when it comes to eye products:
- Those who enjoy using it and see the benefits
- Those who think it's unnecessary and a waste of money

I am very much in the former camp. An eye cream or serum has been part of my routine since my 20s. I didn't start earlier because I was pretty healthy – I never smoked, didn't drink much alcohol – but once I was pregnant with my first child (at 22) I changed my mind.

The saying 'the eyes are the window to the soul' is derived from similar medical terms meaning the eyes are *literally* the window to what is going on inside the body. If you are blessed with youth and spectacular health your eyes are, I'm sure, clear and bright, and the skin around the orbicularis oculi area (think panda eye) evenly toned and coloured. However, for *most* of us the above is no longer the case. **Everything** affects your eye area and the health of all of your internal organs is reflected in them...

- Liver problems: yellow eyes
- Problems with your lymph drainage system: puffy, dark circles
- General mild illness: dull eyes
- On medication (especially antibiotics): discoloured, puffy, dull, dehydrated
- Smoking: grey, dehydrated
- Lack of sleep/too much sleep: puffy, dark circles, grey 'tired' eyes
- Bad diet/too much salt, caffeine and alcohol: puffy, dark circles, dehydrated
- Sun damage/ageing: wrinkles, dehydrated

It's a minefield. The bad news is that *any* topical cream would be hard pushed to magically fix the above. What it *will* do, however, especially when used with a concealer, is temporarily mask some of the above. Eye products often contain ingredients such as caffeine, green tea and peptides to target puffiness, dark circles and wrinkles. While we're on the subject – any ethical brand will advise you that the effect of a product will wear off if you discontinue use. **No eye product is a permanent 'fix'.**

I like a separate eye product for a number of reasons but mainly because I am extremely prone to puffy eyelids and dark circles. Both are genetic, and there's nothing I can do to fix them permanently (excluding surgery for the lids), but some things make them much worse, and the heavier formulations of most moisturisers are one of them. For that reason I like thin serums and dedicated formulations for eyes.

If you are young, or have budget concerns, you can skip eye products and take your hydrating serums up to the orbital bone.

A FEW DOS AND DON'TS

- Do not use mineral oil around your eye area. It tends to make the area puffy, which is the opposite of what you want. Use only the lightest of serums on the eyelids, for the same reason.
- Do not be tempted to use more than the advised amount of cream – it's unnecessary, it could cause irritation and is a waste of money.
- If you have eczema or psoriasis in the eye area (which is very common) you can use thicker creams on the lids as you'll need them – depending on the severity of your condition, they may be prescribed by your doctor. Although you might find a nice organic balm somewhere, no skincare brand can legally claim to treat those medical conditions.
- Keep it simple – too much fragrance in a product can really irritate the eye area – your eye product does not need to smell nice.
- Most allergies to eye products and eyeshadows/mineral makeup are caused by an ingredient called **bismuth oxychloride**. It is used to give the shimmer/light-reflective 'glow' and is a big allergen. If you've never been able to use a particular eye cream **or** eyeshadow and had it blamed on 'your eyes' by a brand, check their INCI list: you'll probably see bismuth oxychloride on there. If your mineral makeup makes you itch, check the label.

TRY THESE...

- Kate Somerville Line Release Under Eye Repair Cream
- Sunday Riley Autocorrect Eye Cream
- Paula's Choice Clinical Ceramide-Enriched Firming Eye Cream
- Pestle & Mortar Recover Eye Cream
- Glossier Bubblewrap Eye and Lip Plumping Cream
- OSKIA Eye Wonder Serum

SHEET MASKS

| 'Sheet masks are wipes with holes cut out for the eyes.'

When I tweeted this in 2018, it caused the skincare equivalent of Armageddon.

Some context: I'm not a massive fan of sheet masks, those single-use face-shaped pieces of polyfabric soaked in goodness-knows-what, that promise to saturate your skin with beneficial ingredients. Yes, I've used them, we all have. I've had the Instagram moment with my mum, daughter and I all doing them for the camera, but now I can't be bothered. They're wet, sticky, and do not give you anything you can't get from applying a couple of rounds of hyaluronic acid serum to your face before your moisturiser.

At the risk of completely alienating everyone, I find I am hardly using any masks at all these days. I've got my skincare routine pretty nailed. If you find you need masks regularly, for anything other than pampering and comfort (not to be underestimated by any stretch), look at what needs tweaking in your daily routine as opposed to buying another product that you can only use sporadically in an attempt to fix it.

Now, obviously there are few notable exceptions – times when a mask makes sense:

Travel: I will occasionally use masks when travelling, especially flying (see pages 80–81), but in all honesty I get a better result from a hyaluronic acid serum and a good cream, with a hyaluronic acid mist used sporadically through the journey.

'Glow': I'm all for the occasional resurfacing boost, whether from a gentle exfoliating mask or an acidic mask. Everyone has dull days. But, if you find yourself reaching for them more frequently, you need to check your routine.

Spots: There is nothing more satisfying than putting a clay mask on spots. My teen daughter and her friends are obsessed with masking. They walk around the house with their clay-laden T-zones like they're wearing a badge of honour. As they should be at 18. But I haven't had that kind of skin in a long time. I don't get hormonal spots anymore. It's one of the joys of being closer to menopause than the age I started my periods. If I do get a whacking big red angry spot, I'm far more likely to douse it in acid and oil until it gives in and goes away (see pages 168–171).

Honestly? That's about it. Maybe it's because I'm older. I'm definitely busier, and... I'm pathologically immune to trends.

> Sheet masks aren't going anywhere, and sales of them are booming (considering their effects on the environment, this is not a good thing).

I'm merely suggesting that skincare, especially serums, has evolved to such a degree that you may not need masks. They're at the bottom of my 'kit' list. And if you do use them, bin them. They don't flush.

'ANTI-AGEING' PRODUCTS

'Anti-ageing'. We're all so used to this term that we don't even question it. If a product says it is 'anti-ageing' on the box, then it must be, right?

Wrong.

Remember, old is the goal. I don't like the term anti-ageing – if we're lucky enough, we all get older – but the industry is slow to catch up and still thinks youth is the dream. So, until we come up with a better solution, this is what we're stuck with.

If ever a phrase has been over-used, anti-ageing is the one. Few ingredients are indeed 'anti-ageing', but some are entitled to be called 'ageing prevention' as they do not reverse signs of ageing, but they do help slow them down or prevent them from getting worse.

The next time you pick up a product that claims to be anti-ageing, what you need to look out for is one of these:

SPF

SPF is anti-ageing. It has been proven, undoubtedly, unequivocally. Although if you're younger you could argue that it belongs in the 'prevention' category. It doesn't fix damage that has already been done. That is the job of...

VITAMIN A

Vitamin A is the only other ingredient, along with SPF, that the FDA will legally let manufacturers claim to be anti-ageing in the USA. Vitamin A reverses the signs of ageing. It rebuilds collagen, repairs sun damage and is an all-round good egg. There are various derivatives of vitamin A – if you have previously used a product with vitamin A in it and reacted badly, it may just be that you haven't yet found the right one for you (see pages 199–203).

GLYCOLIC/LACTIC/SALICYLIC ACIDS

Acids used in the right way can be beneficial to the skin. When applied as topical exfoliants they resurface the epidermis, allowing better product penetration and, in the case of some well-formulated AHAs, help rebuild collagen. Glycolic and lactic acids are better for a dryer skin, and salicylic acid is better for oily/combination skin. Don't opt with a very strong product straight away, and do not go mad. Less is sometimes more.

VITAMINS C AND E

These two work well together, as vitamin C is traditionally water-based (newer formulas include oil-based vitamin C) and vitamin E is oil-based, thus protecting both the oil and water parts of the cell. Both are antioxidants, so sit in the 'prevention' category.

NIACINAMIDE

This is vitamin B3 by another name. When used on the skin it has been shown to stimulate the dermis and in turn increase the fatty content of the cells, along with helping the skin retain water. As it is shown to enhance the barrier function of the epidermis (thereby protecting the skin against bacterial attack) it has had good results with acne sufferers.

Other ingredients are beneficial to the skin in other ways, but if anti-ageing is the aim you need some of these in your product (not all of them at once). See page 165 on when you should start using them.

TRY THESE...

- Medik8 Vitamin A range

- Zelens Youth Concentrate

- Alpha-H Vitamin Profiling Kit

- The Ordinary Niacinamide 10% + Zinc 1%

- Paula's Choice 10% Niacinamide Booster

- Kate Somerville + Retinol Vitamin C Moisturiser

- Joanna Vargas Rejuvenating Serum

SKINCARE MYTH

CELLULITE CREAMS WORK

FACT: Cellulite is not caused by trapped 'toxins'. If we were as 'toxic' as some parts of the 'wellness' industry would have us believe, we'd all be dead. A long time ago.

FACT: Cellulite is caused when your underlying fat cells start to push through connective tissue. Connective tissue is weakened by a mixture of things, including hormones, lack of exercise, poor muscle tone, excess fat and poor circulation.

FACT: 90 per cent of women get cellulite, compared to 10 per cent of men. They have stronger connective tissue. They still have fat underneath it, it's just not as easy for it to escape. How rude.

FACT: It gets worse for women as we age. Lack of oestrogen makes it worse.

FACT: It's in your genes. Look at your mum and grandmother. If they have it...

FACT: Some fillers and injectables can help – albeit temporarily – but they only really work on very slim people who have the odd 'dent' rather than full-blown cellulite legs. Think models before catwalk shows/big shoots.

FACT: Lasers, massage (specific for this problem) and radio-frequency treatments can help, but again it will only be temporary. And it takes a ton of sessions. Personally, I think your time would be better spent at the gym/ walking for an hour, rather than lying flat out letting someone pound the area in vain...

FACT: Liposuction does nothing. It's like removing a bit of stuffing from a pillow. It leaves an indentation and doesn't magically spread the fat around nice and neatly.

FACT: Water helps. Eating veg that are water-heavy and drinking a lot of water throughout the day, every day, helps. It doesn't fix it, but it can help.

FACT: Smoking makes cellulite worse, as it weakens connective tissue (collagen). See second point.

FACT: There is not one cellulite cream on the market that gets rid of cellulite. Not one. Either by prescription or over the counter, it makes no difference. They may make your skin feel softer and smoother, but they aren't shifting the fat.

Eat well, move around more, drink plenty of water, take care of your health in general. And even after you've done all that, your genes may well just insist that you keep your cellulite.

Save your money.

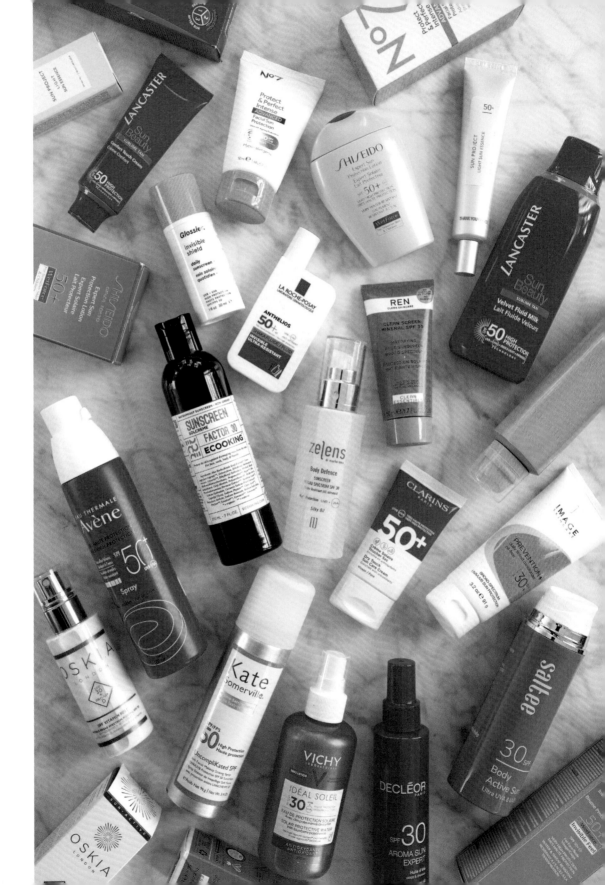

SPF

Gone are the days of my youth, when I'd baste myself with baby oil on a foil suntanning sheet. These days, the sun hits and the SPF gets dragged out of the cupboard quicker than you can say 'lobster'.

> Check for an expiration date – if your SPF doesn't have one, assume it will only last a year. You may need to buy a fresh batch.

How much do you apply? And how high a factor? And WHICH one should you use?

Some very brief and general rules of thumb for sun bunnies and the not-so-keen!

Use broad-spectrum sunscreen – UVA and UVB (think A for ageing, B for burning). UVA rays penetrate deep into the skin, gradually destroying elasticity and causing premature ageing. UVB rays cause skin damage and can alter the structure of skin cells, and ultimately lead to possible skin cancer.

Use either SPF30 or SPF50, nothing lower. Current thinking and medical advice say that using higher than SPF30 can give you a false sense of security, and although studies show that you are much less likely to reapply if you are using a high factor, I prefer a 50, especially on my face. Based on the advice of the Cancer Council in Australia, if you have anything over a SPF30 in your product, you can only call it SPF30+.

TYPES OF SPF: Sun protection usually divides into two camps: Chemical versus Physical (this is where you will find the 'green people'). I personally like an SPF that contains both. I use a broad-spectrum SPF50 on my face and a broad-spectrum SPF30 minimum on my body. I do not use less than a SPF30 on my children. (Well, the ones that I still have some say with!)

WHAT TO ASK WHEN YOU BUY SPF

'What is the SPF?' And, 'Is it a broad-spectrum product?'

There are two main concerns from being in the sun: skin ageing and skin cancer.
UV light causes sunburn and sun damage by damaging cellular DNA.
UVA (long-wave) causes the ageing and **UVB** (short-wave) causes the burning.
Both the US Department of Health and Human Services and the World Health
Organization have identified UV light as a proven human carcinogen.

There is no such thing as a *'safe tan'*. A tan is a sign of DNA damage. It is the
result of a chemical reaction in your body as it tries (and fails) to protect itself
from UV light. Brands selling SPF that use the term 'safe tanning' are at best
misleading and, at worst, clueless.

The appearance of age spots or pigmentation when you're older is down to those
teen family holidays, not the tan you got last year.

'NATURAL' VERSUS 'CHEMICAL'

'Physical' sunscreen (most commonly referred to as 'natural' in marketing
materials) reflects UV light. Traditionally, 'chemical' SPFs absorb the light.
Physical sunscreen, contrary to popular belief, is not 'natural'. Zinc oxide
and titanium dioxide, most commonly used in 'natural' sunscreens have been
shown to potentially be toxic (and I use the word correctly) for fish/sealife –
an estimated 4,000 to 6,000 *metric tons* of sunscreen washes off swimmers'
bodies annually with the potential to cause damage to fragile ecosystems.
Zinc oxide and titanium oxide are not biodegradable and invariably use
nano-technology, which is also being investigated by cancer research bodies
because of its possible links to cancers in humans.

If your preference is to use 'natural' SPF, your closest bet is a 'non-nano' oxide.
Bear in mind it's still technically a chemical, no matter what the 'clean brigade'
say. The term 'non-nano' means nothing to the FDA, but it may be better for you.

"
THE MAJORITY OF SUN DAMAGE IS DONE IN YOUR FIRST 20 YEARS
"

GOVERNMENT GUIDELINES

The US's FDA standards and requirements when it comes to SPF formulas and labelling are different from Europe and Australasia. Following these guidelines can make a difference to a sunscreen's effectiveness. Here's how to make sense of it all, and what to look out for.

> In the USA, SPF labelling is a requirement because the FDA says it is a drug.
>
> In Europe, it is classed as a cosmetic and therefore stating SPF classification is not mandatory, it's just for information.

Having said that, European manufacturers are allowed to use seven proven UVA filters while the FDA in the USA only allows three, technically meaning that a European product has the potential to be more effective than an American-made product.

SPF is only relevant to UVB light. PPD, or Persistent Pigment Darkening, is one way of measuring UVA light, but is now considered out-dated. And the PA++ system, developed in the Far East, is another method used. However, neither of these are allowed when making broad-spectrum claims in the USA. Still with me? No? I don't blame you. It's beyond confusing for the average consumer.

An in vitro test (see page 226) to gauge a critical wavelength is really what a brand should be able to show in order to claim broad spectrum on their packaging in the US and the UK. Critical wavelength tests measure the absorbance of UV light on skin and a critical wavelength of 370nm is what you are looking for on SPF product literature. Not that many brands will bother labelling that information, so do your research or ask them directly if you are looking for a broad-spectrum product (which I highly recommend).

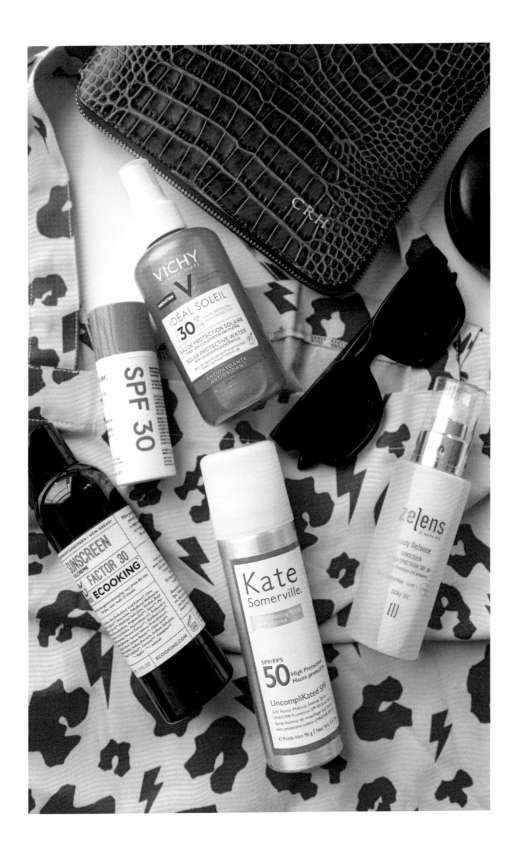

SPF MYTHS

- **'SPF accumulates.'** If you wear a moisturiser, primer and sunscreen you will only have the highest SPF that you are using. You cannot 'add them up'.

- **'Sunscreens can be waterproof.'** No sunscreen is waterproof. Sunscreens can now only be listed legally as 'water resistant'.

- **'SPF60 is twice as effective as SPF30.'** Not true. And while there may only be a 1 per cent difference between SPF30 and SPF50 in theory, there is shown to be a much larger cumulative effect in UVA protection when using a 50. Use SPF50 wherever possible.

- **'Darker skins don't need SPF.'** While darker skin tones are not as vulnerable to UV light because of their built-in SPF of around 13.3, they still need protection from UV damage and should use a minimum of SPF30.

- **'Our SPF is Cruelty-Free.'** Never were more ingredients tested on animals in the skincare industry than those that are used in SPF products. This **does not** mean the final product is tested on animals, so brands that state they are against animal testing and say their products are cruelty-free are not technically *lying*. It means the raw ingredients were, at some point, absolutely tested on animals in a lab to ensure 'efficacy', especially in the USA, where they are classed as drugs. This is true of the entire skincare and health industry, and I mention it not to make you feel bad, just purely to counterbalance the rubbish of 'vegan, animal-friendly, non-toxic SPF50' claims that are, frankly, nonsense. PETA can say there are a wealth of cruelty-free brands, but the reality is that the ingredients were tested on animals at some point. They may be cruelty-free now, but the *ingredients* have probably been tested on animals historically.

> Pre-cancerous moles are either cancerous or they are not. If in doubt, cut it out. A mole is a benign lesion. If you notice any changes, get them checked by an expert.

USE A DEDICATED SPF

I used to get my SPF from my makeup during colder months, but since I've got older and have been using more retinoids, I've stepped up my SPF usage through winter. In the summer I use SPF50 daily: a dedicated sunscreen that gives both UVA and UVB protection. UVC doesn't penetrate the atmosphere so we don't need to worry on that score.

Do not waste your money on a really expensive anti-ageing moisturiser with SPF. SPF is an all-encompassing product that will overtake any active or expensive ingredients in your skincare. SPF is a chemically dominating ingredient and if you load a skin cream with it, that's the sole benefit you'll get from the cream. I would never buy an extortionate anti-ageing moisturiser with SPF – **you're just paying for an expensive SPF**. If you can afford it and you love it, carry on, but you're not getting the best out of your moisturiser. Buy a good moisturiser and a perfectly reasonably priced SPF. Job done.

My problem with SPF in moisturisers is two-fold:

#1 **It gives you a false sense of security.** In the 1920s, when SPF wasn't available, the incidences of melanoma were around 1 in 1,500. In 2013, with years of SPF being available and modern science, the incidences are 1 in 53 – **1 in 53**. Why? Because we apply it once and move on, thinking we're done.

For example, let's say you use a moisturiser containing SPF15 at 8am, and would normally burn after 15 minutes of sun exposure. Technically you should be reapplying your SPF at 11.45am. And that's assuming

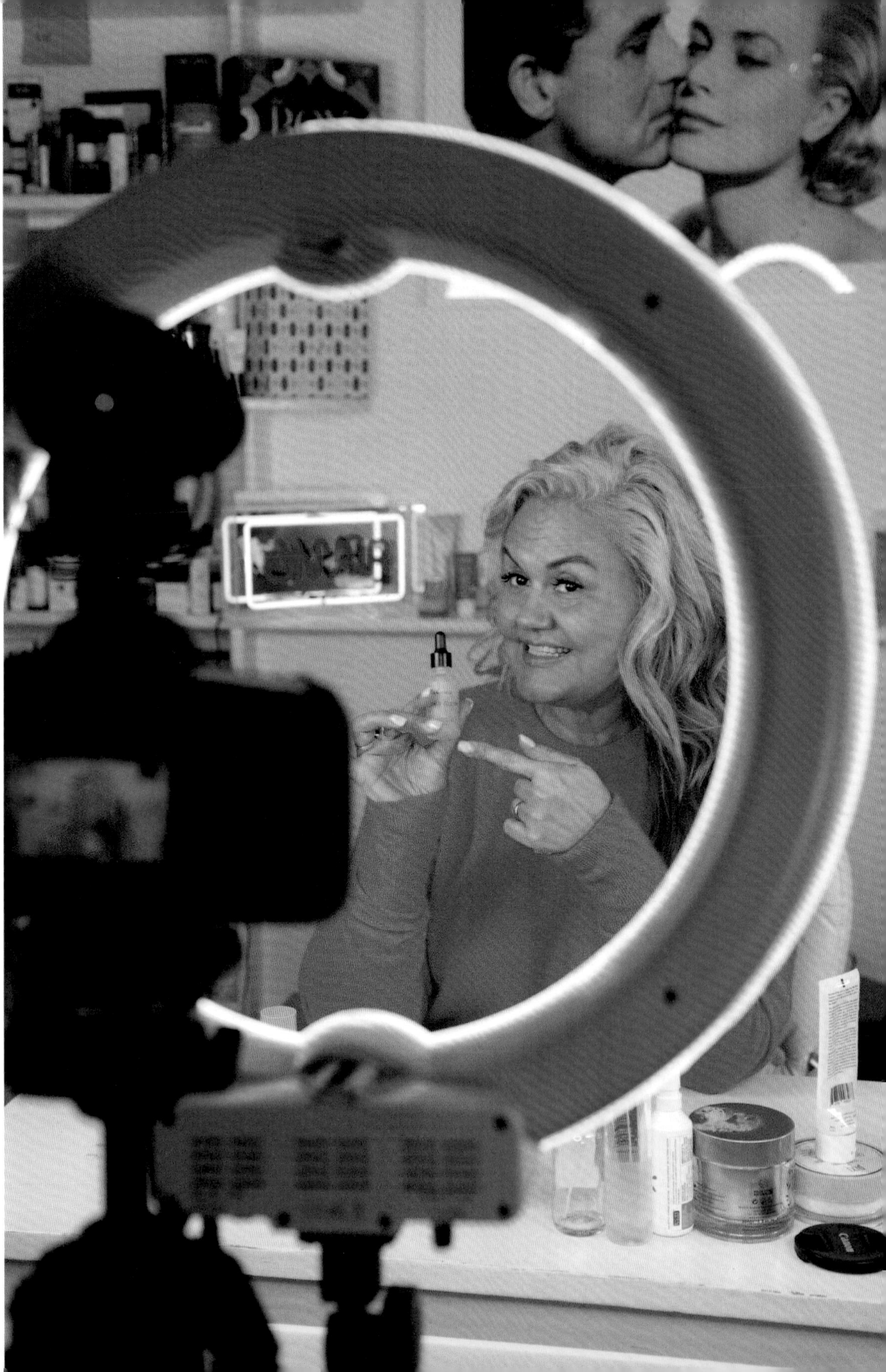

you applied it all over your face – most people leave out areas when moisturising. How are you going to do that without removing your full face of makeup? I know no-one who takes their makeup off halfway through the day to reapply sunscreen.

And if you are sunbathing, to use the recommended amount of sunscreen you would need to use a bottle of that SPF15 moisturiser a day. A DAY.

If you apply your SPF moisturiser religiously every day and think you are protected, you may not be.

#2
A moisturiser containing SPF invariably only protects from UVB – it does not protect you from UVA. So, you won't burn, but your collagen will break down and you'll still get wrinkles. Excellent. Also – SPF moisturisers are less likely to be rub-resistant or water-resistant. If you then apply your makeup with fingers or a brush (everyone) or sweat, it's gone.

If you want proper protection from the sun you need to use a **broad-spectrum sun protectant cream** – a dedicated product that's sole purpose is to protect your skin from the damage the sun does to it.

Companies that add SPF to their general 'anti-ageing' moisturisers are throwing it in there as an 'added benefit' and a sales tool. Sun protection is not an 'added benefit'. It's a critical, proven step to protect skin from ageing. The round UVA symbol, below, can only be shown on packaging of a product that has been proven to provide at least a third of its protection against UVA. Not just UVB.

The EU has also reclassified sun protection ratings:

- Low = 6–14
- Medium = 15–29
- High = 30–50
- Very high = 50+

If you are fair, Caucasian or 'pale' you should be in the **'High'** category. If you are any type of ethnicity that tans easily and rarely burns you can use **medium** as long as you use it wisely. If you are a redhead, however, you are **strictly in the 'Very high'** category. Redheads with freckles have phaeomelanin – as opposed to the rest of us that have eumelanin. They burn easily and quickly, and the damage will be long-lasting. If you use an SPF in the low-medium category you will tan. If you don't want any colour at all you need to use SPF30 and above, and reapply it frequently.

SPF degrades. Buy new SPF products each year.

When we analyse clients' skin, the main areas that nearly *always* show damage are the tops of the ears (ALWAYS the top of the ears), the back of the neck and the tip of the nose. Forewarned is forearmed.

Acne sufferers: while the sun may have a drying effect on your acne; a lot of SPF products are comedogenic. This means they block pores, which can make acne worse. Use oil-free sunscreens if possible.

❚ Enjoy the sun. I LOVE the sun. Just protect yourself.

For tips on using SPF in your daily routine, see page 86.

For tips on using SPF in your daily routine, see page 86.

TRY THESE...

- La Roche-Posay Anthelios
- Ecooking
- EltaMD
- Heliocare
- Evy Technology
- Zelens Daily Defence SPF30

YOUR KIT

WHERE SHOULD I SPEND MOST OF MY MONEY?

So, you now know what's out there and the skincare world is your oyster. What should you spend your hard-earned money on?

The answer is always, always serums.

I always advocate putting most of your money into the **middle** of your routine: serums cost more to make, contain more active ingredients and you can use more than one in your routine. The middle is where you treat/correct/repair, and that is where you should spend the bulk of your budget.

The rise of serums has definitely, in my opinion, bumped moisturisers off the top spot, although moisturisers were never my No.1, more the prevailing thought of the industry back in the early days of Estée Lauder and Elizabeth Arden.

> Spend your money on supplements, skincare, foundation and concealer and scrimp on the rest. You will look fabulous.

Spend up to around £150 (outside the organic market) and you generally get what you pay for (in all circumstances you still need to check the ingredients to see what you are paying for). After that, you're paying for packaging, the rent and payroll and the holiday home of the name on the box. I fully get that the majority of us are on much smaller budgets, but if you can, I would look at the £50–£100 mark for proper hi-tech serums, £30–£50 for moisturisers, and £30–£50 for cleansers, assuming the more expensive ones are pricier because they are larger sizes. Ultimately, buy what you can afford and want to spend. Don't credit-card your skincare.

If you want good-quality skincare and are willing to forgo the hi-tech, you can get amazing quality natural or organic products that are very affordable.

The following lists are organised in terms of cost, with the priciest coming first. I've separated them by age, too, as our skin has different needs as it matures.

TEENS–EARLY 20s

- **Moisturiser.** Younger people tend to wreak more havoc on their skin through their lifestyle – because they can. Their skins need more protection. Younger people are also lazier with their routine (no hate, just an observation) because unless they have a particular concern, they can be. If you're only going to wash your face and slap one thing on, it should be a moisturiser. I would still recommend a separate SPF though.

- **Serum.** Go for a vitamin C product – a good antioxidant. You don't need anything too active or aggressive.

- **Exfoliating acids.** These are generally affordable. Go for something mid-range if you can (see pages 189–194 for more on acids).

- **SPF.** You have youthful, bouncy skin. Keep it that way.

- **Cleanser.** Get into good cleansing habits at this age and you'll be set for life skincare-wise, I promise.

- **Night cream.** Using a dedicated moisturiser for the evening is beneficial if you have particular skin conditions. If you have budget concerns, use a non-SPF moisturiser and you can just buy one and use it day and night. (Just don't forget your separate SPF.)

- **Facial oil.** It's worth investing here – really cheap ones just aren't as good.

- **Eye products.** Not essential at this age – just use your serum if budget is an issue.

- **Face masks.**

- **Scrubs.** These are cheap to manufacture and don't require complex technology.

- **Clay masks.** I could make these at home using a bag of clay and some magnesium. They cost practically nothing to make.

- **Floral water or spritz.** It's basically water.

YOUR KIT

20s–MID 30s

- **Serum.** They contain high-performing ingredients so aren't typically cheap. Within this product category I would include all overnight vitamin A or retinol treatments, hydrating boosters, anti-ageing peptide serums – anything runny that you use underneath a moisturiser or oil.

- **Dedicated night cream.** Emulsions or moisturisers are still fundamentally more expensive to make than cleansers or toners, and if you are under 40 you can still prevent and repair damage before it's too late.

- **Facial oils.** Yes, you can get cheap base oils, but there is a world of difference in my mind between a basic 'face oil' and a sophisticated one made by the likes of doctors, facialists and the leaders of all things face oil, such as French dedicated salon brands.

- **Cleansers.** Go for mid-range.

- **Exfoliating acids.** Affordable, mid-range options are fine.

- **SPF.** Not pricey. Think something you can pick up in a pharmacy.

- **Moisturiser.** Simply opt for a decent product – you don't need to spend a fortune. You can go wild, but ultimately all moisturisers do the same thing.

- **Eye products.** Don't break the bank. If you have a good serum and you are on a budget, you can skip this.

- **Face masks.** If they're hydrating, they predominantly consist of glycerin and hyaluronic acid, and are not expensive to make.

- **Scrubs.**

- **Clay masks.**

- **Floral water or spritz.**

35 AND OLDER

35 and over (or earlier if you are in early menopause for any reason) is the most important age group to me because it's basically ignored by brands, the media, marketing and the medical profession. Any woman who has tried to get HRT recently will know exactly what I'm talking about.

- **Serum/treatments.** Step things up a notch. At this age, the skin needs more peptides, retinols etc.

- **Exfoliating acids.** The best ones cost more, and at our age we need them.

- **Dedicated night cream**

- **Cleanser.** Good balm cleansers can be found at reasonable prices, but the ones I like cost a little more than the average OTC brands.

- **Facial oil.** Again, there is a world of difference between cheap and mid-range.

- **SPF.** A good, dedicated SPF is not extortionate.

- **Moisturiser.** A good hi-tech product for proper hydration and protection (see page 207).

- **Eye products.** I love them and use them religiously, but I also tend to take my serum around the eye area (all of the serums, pretty much, except active ones). Use the thinnest product first. I suffer genetically from droopy eyelids and dark circles because I'm anaemic. I'd be throwing money away on an expensive eye product that I know in my heart won't work. I need one for hydration, to plump up fine lines. That'll do.

- **Face masks.**

- **Scrubs.**

- **Clay masks.**

- **Floral water or spritz.**

HOMEMADE PRODUCTS

Despite what you might read on certain websites, you will find no substitute for good professional skincare in your kitchen. It's wishful thinking. Please do not believe the hype.

The best you can hope for is a temporary softening of the skin (avocado/plain yoghurt) or a very temporary tightening (egg white). The aloe vera that you see listed on a product's INCI list is a world apart from the sticky, clear gel that you get when you cut an aloe leaf. It has to go through a chemical process to even begin to think about penetrating the skin.

There is nothing, I repeat, NOTHING in your larder that can cure acne. I wish there was! But coconut oil, lemon, baking soda, turmeric and the rest all belong in your food, not on your face.

And don't get me started on lemon juice.

'Adding lemon juice to your cleanser will exfoliate your skin!' No, it won't. 'Applying lemon juice to your skin will fix your pigmentation!' No, it won't.

Eat it, by all means. Just don't add it to any product.

Case in point: anyone remember Sun-In from the 80s? Lots of brunette girls going around with orange hair. Nice.

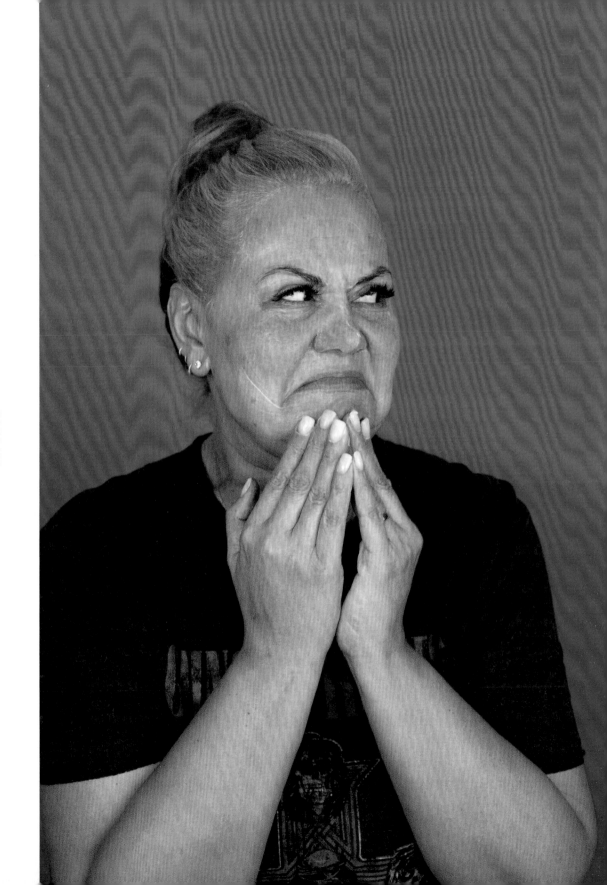

GET IN THE SEA

There are so, SO many products that I would love to throw in the sea (metaphorical sea – remember the environment, people), and brands making them that I would give a good talking to. Whether they're making unproven claims based on the latest buzzword bandwagon or just frightening you into trying to fix a problem you don't have, the skincare industry is rife with repeat offenders. I'm not singling out any particular brands here, but these are the products that have no reason for being on our shelves. Not. A. One.

- **Wipes.** They do not 'clean' your face. They are for Emergencies Only – real emergencies. If you have access to clean water, there *is* no emergency. They're also atrocious for the environment. Remember: Fannies, flights and festivals (see pages 75–79). And NEVER flush.

- **Sheet masks,** aka 'wipes with holes cut out for eyes'. Think of the environment if nothing else.

- **Foaming face washes that contain SLS/SLES** or, more specifically, anything that describes itself as giving you 'squeaky clean' skin. No part of your body should squeak. These products are too drying. Full stop. You may want to also consider removing hair products and toothpaste containing SLS from your routine.

- **Micellar waters.** These are fine for removing eye makeup, or your entire face in an emergency with no access to water, but they're not a one-stop shop for daily use and should be washed off. Use them as a first cleanse only.

- **Pore strips.** I don't care who you see advertising them, no one who works in and on skin and cares deeply about your skin would ever – *ever* – recommend these. Horrible things.

- **Alcohol-laden, old-fashioned 'toners'.** It's time to move on.

- **SPF50 drops** that claim to give you complete SPF coverage, even when mixed with your moisturiser. Righty-ho. How do they do that then? What magical wizardry makes them stay in a pure undiluted form when mixed with another product? Stop it.

233

- **Expensive clay masks.** Clay is one of the cheapest ingredients to put in a product. Don't pay big bucks for it.

- **Harsh scrubs** containing 'husks' or 'shells'. There is no need to be so tough on your skin. It's not 1982. It's the skincare equivalent of using sandpaper to file a beautiful polished table. Actual horror.

- **Cellulite creams.** Cellulite is caused by fat cells pushing through your connective tissue. A cream will not fix it. Use a body brush and a decent body moisturiser. Your skin will feel smoother, but it won't get rid of cellulite. (See also pages 214–215.)

- **Gold in skincare.** Save your money. Wear it on your fingers.

- **Really expensive moisturisers that contain SPF.** SPF overrides any active ingredient in a formula. Don't waste your money. Buy a good, solid moisturiser and a separate SPF instead. Neither needs to be extortionately expensive.

- **Glitter in skincare.** An oxymoron if ever there was one. Why? Exactly. Stop it. This also applies to anything that has a unicorn on the label. Gimmicks have no place in topical skincare (see page 206).

- **Coconut oil.** Although coconut oil has *some* antibacterial properties and can be used as a cleanser, any oil will take your makeup off. It's not the second coming. That's why it belongs here in the GITS list.

- **Products sold using scare tactics.** Don't buy products out of fear. Certain elements of the skincare industry spend their entire marketing budget telling customers what is NOT in their products, and why they should be scared of certain ingredients, as opposed to what their products WILL do for them. Skincare is safe. There is no reason to buy out of fear.

- **Thinking that you have to use everything from the same range.** It's a good selling technique to tell customers that everything 'simply must' come from the same range, but it's not true (see page 237).

- **Any topical skin product made using your own blood.** Taken from the idea of PRP (vampire) facials, founded by Charles Runels, the difference being that once your platelets are mixed in with base ingredients for a skincare product, they become completely inert, and are useless once outside the body. Also: illegal in the EU.[8] Fact.

- **Products that you have never heard of sold via social media ads.** Don't buy these. Remember those black peel-off masks?

- **Silly claims and extortionate pricing.** Brands that produce 'statement skincare', i.e. products that cost silly money for a 30ml of something with a huge claim attached to it, but no clinical trials to back them up. Nothing costs that much in skincare. Nothing. At least be honest and tell people they're paying for the packaging and your mark-up. If you can afford it and enjoy it, great. But if you can't, you're not missing out on anything that you can't get somewhere else for a fraction of the price. If you want leather upholstery and a better sound system in your car, you pay extra, but it doesn't make the car go faster.

- **Excessive layering of products.** I'm the first to hold my hand up and say I will happily layer two – *maybe* three – thin serums on occasion, but I am tagged regularly on Instagram by people/brands posting demonstrations of the application of 5+ serums on a regular basis. Remember, you're talking about penetrating an area literally thinner than this –> ------- <– and only so much will go in. Save your money, use a couple and switch them up on occasion.

- **Cheap dermarollers.** If you insist on doing it yourself at home, buy quality-assured products with short needles, from specialised retailers only. Change it regularly and keep it sterile. Do not buy them online.

- **Skincare fridges.** Fridges do nothing to enhance the efficacy of products. They are completely unnecessary. All OTC products are tested for stability in extreme hot and cold environments before they are sent to market. However, if you like the feeling of something cool on your skin, go ahead – knock yourself out.

- **Celeb- and derm-endorsed products.** Celebs endorsing products in magazines and on TV are being paid. So are dermatologists. Don't believe the hype. Do your research and go with your gut. Anyone saying, 'I only use this product and my skin is amazing!' is usually cashing a cheque somewhere along the way.

- **Mattifying products.** Unless you are a teenager and/or have oily skin, you do not need mattifying products. Healthy skin has a glow.

- **Be aware of dermatologists** recommending *only* La Roche-Posay, Avène, Cetaphil and Vichy (among others) repeatedly, and in isolation. Brands (French pharmacy brands in particular, in the UK) set aside huge marketing budgets every year to target and court dermatologists and pharmacies and win over all their 'affordable' recommendations. It's called '**detailing**' and is literally the skincare equivalent of lobbyists in politics. A full budget dedicated solely to wooing dermatologists, all so that when a magazine asks a derm what affordable product they would recommend they hear the magical, 'Oh, I always recommend XXX in my practice, it's excellent and does exactly the same as professional brands!' We all know it's not true but that's how the cookie crumbles. (That is not to say that these aren't excellent brands – they usually are, but when they appear endorsed by derms everywhere in magazines, someone has been paid.)

- **Botox parties.** Do not, ever, have your botox done at a 'botox party'. No reputable practitioner would provide this service in someone's living room where alcohol is being served.

  The first thing you should ask yourself when having anything done is, 'what would happen if this goes wrong? Can this person treat me for any reaction/ bleeding/burning/bruising/misplacement/damage?' If the answer is not a definitive 'Yes', then don't have the treatment. Simple. Legally, I could give you botox, but I would never do it. Leave it to the medical professionals.

- **Sunbathing.** More specifically, sun 'baking'. We need the sun. It's vital for our vitamin D. But we must respect it. Be sensible. Do not, ever, use sun beds.

- **Pore obsession.** Stop. They are never as big as you think they are.

- **Smoking or vaping.** Stop. The end.

- **Sugar and white carbs.** Avoid these. Junk food is called junk food for a reason.

- **Booze.** Try to lay off the booze, especially if you are menopausal. You will look and feel better without it.

YOU HAVE TO USE EVERYTHING FROM THE SAME BRAND

I'm often asked these two questions:

'Do you use different products every DAY?' and 'Don't you have to use everything from one brand in order for them to really work?'

The answer is 'Yes'. And then 'No'.

Yes, I use different skincare every day, in the same way that I wear different clothes and eat different food, and I always have. Even when wildly restricted by budget, I would have at least two moisturisers and two or three cleansers on rotation. Your skin is different every day. Your products can be, too.

No, you do not have to use everything from the same brand. The only thing to be concerned about is clashing vitamin A products that you get on prescription, but in that case, your doctor would have advised you about what to use/not use when issuing the prescription. Over-the-counter products very rarely 'clash' because the percentages of active ingredients are low – they won't build up or interfere with each other.

What IS important is the order you use items and the formulas themselves. Your serum from XYZ won't know that your moisturiser is from ABC and stop working in protest. That's not how it works, no matter what sales hype you are given from the brands at a beauty counter.

The products I use, as a rule, tend to have peptides, hyaluronic acid and vitamin A (at night) in them. They vary in strength and formulas, though may have similar ingredients. There are thousands of products out there. Embrace them (again, obviously within your budget), and the next time someone tells you that you simply have to use their moisturiser on top of their serum or they won't work, don't buy either of them.

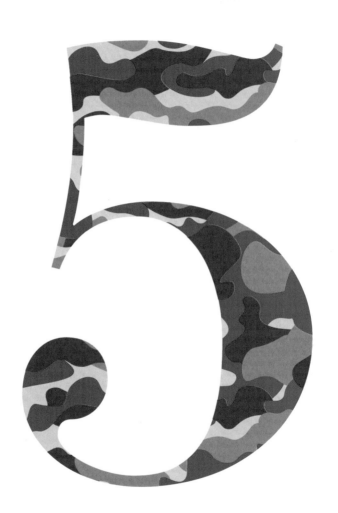

HERE'S THE THING

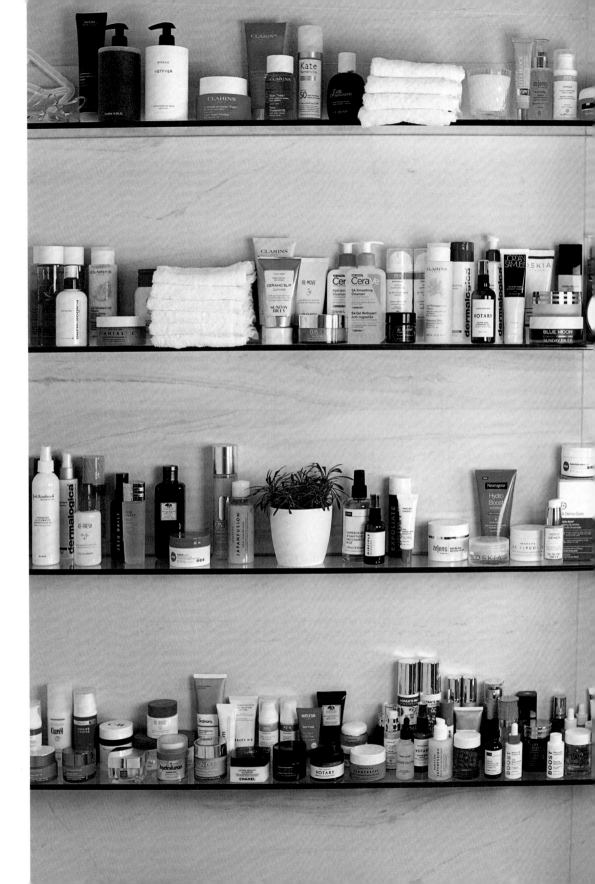

WELCOME TO THE INDUSTRY!

So, by now you should have a better idea what your skin type is, how to treat it, and the products you need. Well, here's the thing. The skincare industry makes a lot of money by confusing you. The more knowledge you have about the products available, the less likely you are to be persuaded to purchase something that you do not need. Whether you're reading packaging or are getting assaulted by social media ads, the terminology is a minefield. So let's break it down Jilly Cooper style and meet the heroes and villains in the world of skincare – the industry jargon – and bust those overused, misused, confusing and downright pointless words and phrases. I want the skincare industry to be taken seriously, and what better way to start than with a healthy dose of reality.

HYPO-ALLERGENIC

Literally means 'should not cause an allergy', which to be honest is a fairly meaningless term. There's no industry or legal standard to back this up, and there are different standards in the USA and EU. Ultimately, this is just **lip service**. What is an extreme allergen to you may be perfectly fine for me.

IS ABSORBED IMMEDIATELY

You will find this claim on products that contain synthetic pushers. These force the product into the skin. Most serums that aren't completely natural or organic contain synthetic pushers. Your skin is highly intelligent – it's not going to absorb anything in a hurry in case it's harmful to you. If it did, we wouldn't need patches for things like HRT and injections for insulin. Its job is to be a barrier. If a product is absorbed straight away, it's not natural (which is fine). (See page 242 for more on what 'natural' means.)

ANIMAL TESTING

Poor animal lovers. Talk about a minefield. Unless a brand categorically states 'against animal testing' or 'no animal testing' on its product, assume it may sell in China and that animal testing is, therefore, a possibility. The Chinese government reserve the right to test any incoming goods on animals, though this law is due to change in 2020. They will get there, I hope. Just because a brand doesn't test its final product on animals, it doesn't mean that all of the ingredients weren't tested on animals in the past. Animal testing is banned in the EU, but sticklers will point to China and say they won't support a brand because the product is sold in China. That is obviously your call, but nothing you put on your face in the UK was tested on an animal in order for you to use it.

If you want to know categorically where a brand stands, you need to ask them: 'Are your ingredients tested on animals *at their source?*', and 'Do you retail in China?' If they don't know, assume they are.

> A brand that cares about animal testing will ensure its standards are met from the very beginning of the production process and will shout it from the rooftops.

NATURAL

The most over-used and abused word in the industry.

> I could take a cup of glue, a sip of aloe vera juice, spit the aloe vera juice into the glue, label it 'natural' and sell it as a skincare product.

There is no legal guideline or industry standard for the word 'natural'. It's all about marketing. If a product is labelled 'natural' you think you're doing yourself some good. Read the label. Educate yourself. There are, *of course*, excellent brands out there that would place themselves in the 'natural' category. There are also some heinous ones. And a word to the wise – the misinformation and scare-mongering is worse when it comes to baby products. Outrageous.

NON-COMEDOGENIC

This literally means 'does not block pores'. Where to start? All evidence that a product is 'non-comedogenic' is anecdotal. It is unproven and untested scientifically. Pure, naturally derived lanolin is supposed to be a 'non-comedogenic' alternative to synthetic lanolin, but if I put any kind of lanolin anywhere near my face it will be covered in huge whiteheads within hours. Use it as a rough guide rather than the word of law.

ORGANIC

This is marginally better than 'natural', as at least there are *some* standards in place, however, the Soil Association, Ecocert and all the numerous international organic certification bodies have different standards between them. You'd need to go directly to their websites to see if your standards match theirs. See page 252.

SHRINKS PORES

> Pores are not doors – they do not open and close.

Nothing opens and closes pores. There is a big fat difference between saying, 'closes pores' and 'minimises the appearance of pores'. One is rubbish and the other is a possibility.

SILKY SMOOTH

Contains silicone. Check the INCI list – anything ending in '...cone' or '...one' is a silicone. I actually don't mind silicones at all, but let's be clear *why* the product is silky smooth.

VELVETY SOFT

See above.

DERMATOLOGIST-TESTED

This has no legal standing or definition. It also does not mean that the product tested 'positively' by a derm, just that it was 'tested'. 'How was it tested?', you may ask? Probably by rubbing a bit on their hand, or on a patient's face, to check for any reaction. It is a genuinely pointless term and I pay no attention to it.

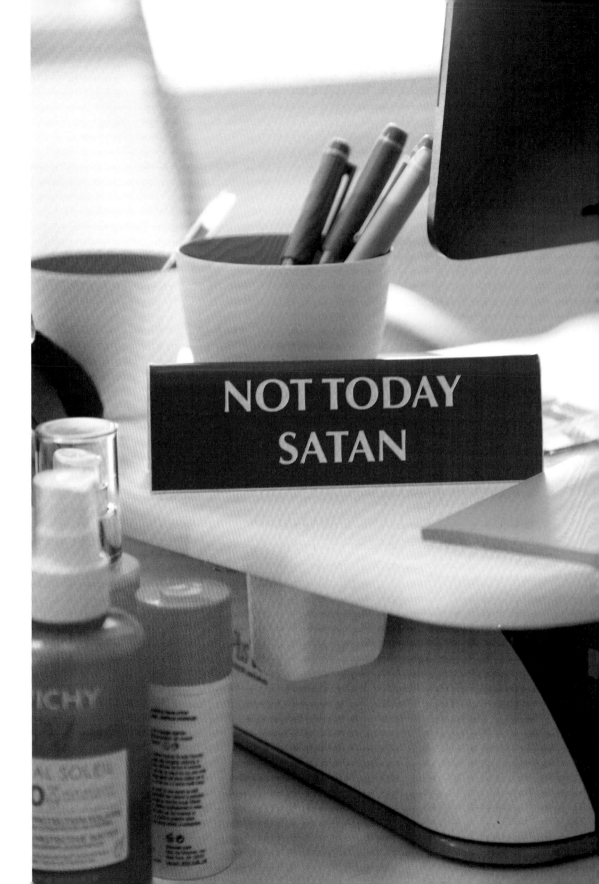

THE DIRT ON 'CLEAN'

The 'clean' skincare and makeup industry is worth a lot of money. Billions.

Over the past decade, skincare brands and retailers have adopted the words 'clean', 'green' and 'detox', and are throwing them around with abandon, to suggest that their skincare is somehow 'purer' and safer for your skin than a 'chemical' product (by the way, ALL products are made of chemicals). It's exhausting. If you know you're going to have an adverse reaction, avoiding certain ingredients is obviously completely valid. But the opposite of clean is dirty, and who wants their diet or skincare to be classed as such? Therein lies the selling power.

Some big brands and retailers have built their business on making you think that the skincare products sold to you can literally cause harm, based not on scientific fact, but the opinion of their founders.

We are now in a situation where the brands in the 'clean' arena use most of their advertising and packaging to tell you what is NOT in their formulas, while seemingly forgetting to advise their customers of what IS in them. As we've seen, you need to know what ingredients are in a product in order to make an informed decision about which will be right for your skin type.

They also bulk out the list of 'forbidden' ingredients by including things that would never be used in skincare in the first place, as if they're doing you a huge favour.

It is the skincare equivalent of saying 'there is no carrot in this yoghurt'.

This has led to the ludicrous outcome of the tail (customers) wagging the dog (the industry). It is both infuriating and upsetting to witness people with real skin concerns being told that they are somehow at fault for choosing to use products that contain the 'suspicious six' or the 'dirty dozen', or any other dramatically named yet arbitrary lists of ingredients.

> 'The good thing about science is that it's true, whether or not you believe in it.'
>
> — **NEIL DEGRASSE TYSON**

Science and scientists are being ignored. Proven, legal safety assessments are being disregarded as if they are meaningless, and retailers are buying into it, heavily.

Sephora now has a 'clean' section. They state that the products in this part of their store and website are 'safe', and that by shopping in this section you are in a 'toxin-free' zone (insinuating, therefore, that the other hundreds of brands on offer in their stores are full of 'toxins'?). This is ironic coming from a retailer that makes the majority of its skincare sales from the prestige, high-tech section.

Allure magazine has the 'Allure Standard'. Credo has the 'Dirty List'. (Yes, really.) Beautycounter have 'The Never List', which excludes nearly 1,500 ingredients from their products, yet they still use essential oils as fragrance — essential oils being one of the biggest-known allergens in skincare.

CAP Beauty store will only consider stocking products that are '100% synthetic free'. They also state: 'High vibrational beauty starts here. Let Mother Nature in and let in the light'. Ahem.

The Detox Market's top-line advertising declares: 'Green beauty brands to detoxify your life', as if we are all bathing in arsenic, while Goop posts articles openly claiming a link between the 'toxic chemicals' found in personal care products to allergies, autism, ADHD and, horrifyingly, cancer, all without linking to scientific papers to back up their opinion.

And they *all* repeatedly state that they have gone down this road because the Environmental Working Group (EWG) told them that 'the FDA have no regulatory control over personal use products'. **This is categorically false and untrue** and repeating something as often as possible **does not make it a fact**.[7]

The 'clean' industry, and it IS an industry, would have you believe that anything man-made is bad for you, and bad for the environment, and that for you and your family to remain safe, and free from 'toxins', you must stick to all-natural ingredients and use as few 'synthetic' ingredients as possible.

The irony is that they also link themselves to sustainability, something that is completely counterproductive to the 'green' and 'natural' movement. There is nothing green and sustainable about pillaging the earth relentlessly for 'natural' ingredients. Palm oil was once considered 'green'. Look where we are now. By all means use products with as few ingredients in them as possible, should you wish. Use products that contain ingredients mostly sourced from plants, should that be your preference. Avoid parabens (see pages 262–263) if you don't want to use them (but short-chain parabens are the safest and most-tested preservatives available). And eliminate all the 'toxins' you see fit from your life. It's 100 per cent your call.

> Just because a product is labelled 'natural' or 'organic' does not mean it is better for you.

Know this:

- The use of the words 'natural', 'clean' and 'green' is completely unregulated.

- Toxicity is dose-dependent. For example, apple pips contain amygdalin, a substance that releases cyanide into your bloodstream when ingested. Apples. Cyanide. Your body disposes of it. THAT'S ITS JOB.

- Every ingredient must go through a chemical process to make it into a product.

- Synthetic fragrances are known to be safer for the skin than 'natural' fragrances such as essential oils. They are also more thoroughly tested.

- OTC skincare (and makeup) sold via reputable brands and retailers **is not 'toxic'.** (I am not talking about 'preservative-free', made-in-the-kitchen-sink products sold independently or on open retailing sites, such as eBay.)

- There is no lead in your lipstick.*

- Deodorant will not give you cancer.

- Water is a chemical.

Charlatans will always try to relieve you of your cash. Do not part with it. You do not have to be 'scared' into buying skincare. Enough with the insanity. I love and use many a product owned by a brand that would place themselves in the 'natural skincare' arena, but I use them *despite* their messaging, not because of it.

*Actually, scientifically, there is the potential for minute trace elements of lead as a by-product to be in your lipstick as a by-product of pigment, but you would need to eat bullets and bullets of lipstick a day in order for lead to register in your system. Please don't worry. Safety assessments are in place, regulations are followed, and no one is trying to hurt you.

"

EVERYTHING IS A CHEMICAL

"

WHEN TO USE 'NATURAL' AND WHEN TO REACH FOR THE 'CHEMICALS'

One of my most-asked questions regarding ingredients is 'Is it natural?', and my answer is always: 'Yes, if that's what you *want*.' It depends how far you want to go, as all products sit somewhere on the spectrum of organic and chemical (and that's why I say a product is '-led'). See also 'Welcome to the Industry!' on pages 241–243.

> Remember – everything is technically a chemical, including water. It's how a product is marketed that makes the distinction.

CHEMICAL-LED: products that contain non-'natural' ingredients – i.e. pretty much anything except a plant.

NATURAL-LED: products that would make the 'natural' consumer happy – they may contain some non-natural ingredients, but the main bulk is natural.

ORGANIC-LED: Products that contain primarily organic ingredients, and usually list a percentage. They could happily be endorsed by the 'clean' brigade.

The best **eye-makeup removers**, such as those by Bioderma, Nars, Clarins and Charlotte Tilbury, invariably contain chemicals. They remove surface junk, so

I don't have a problem with them. If you want to opt for natural, go down the almond oil route, but I find that a tad heavy for my eyes and the residue has the potential to make you very puffy.

Cleansers/second cleansers are at some point going to be used for facial massage, so I steer towards good oils or milk ingredients for that. By their very nature, these contain both.

Acid toners/essences are, by definition, chemical-led. Lovely.

Eye products can be either natural or chemical-led, although I – as an older woman with visible lines etc. – would probably not go 'natural' here. Natural ones feel very nice on the skin, but if you want to fix fine lines, especially in the eye area, you need something made in the lab (which, by the way, all 'natural' products are anyway).

Serums. I nearly always (and happily) use chemical-led serums. Here's why: if you are out of your 20s and have lived any kind of life (I *mean* 'any', I'm not being facetious) you will have signs of ageing on your skin. And I'm sorry, but at a certain point, if you want to reverse those signs of ageing, you need to embrace the chemical. For 'green' reasons, you may decide against that – that's 100 per cent your prerogative, obviously – but I have yet to meet a 'green, organic' product that can actually reverse sun damage, pigmentation and scarring as well as manmade molecules (think retinoids) do. As much as people harp on about rosehip oil for scarring, it has nothing, *nothing* on retinoids available on prescription. It may be marketed as 'a natural alternative to retinol', but in reality, that means that the proof has to be in the pudding, and they are just very, very different ingredients. This also applies to peptides (see Glossary), which are completely manmade in the lab, and are scientifically proven to have a very real effect on the skin.

Your serum is your powerhouse product – it has the biggest job to do. It's the most 'active' product that you will use in your routine. This is when you should embrace the chemical and be a bit more spendy.

There are days when I reach for something more organic in the serum department, usually when I want to get my glow on, just hydrate, or if I am using a particularly silicone-heavy moisturiser.

Moisturisers. This is probably the category where I mix up 'chemical' and 'natural' the most. I love organic/natural-led hydrating, soothing moisturisers. I like how the majority (not all) of them sit under makeup and I tend to use them on days where I am applying self-tan afterwards. The lack of silicone makes for better (fake) tanning.

If, however, I feel my face needs some oomph and a little kick, I would probably use something hi-tech that contains high-performing, active ingredients. For example: a Kate Somerville/Zelens serum under a Tata Harper moisturiser works a treat. Likewise, a Tata Harper serum under a Zelens/Kate Somerville moisturiser is also a good plan. I like to mix it up a little. The reason I invariably mix up the final two stages is silicone. A silicone serum, followed by a silicone moisturiser, followed by either SPF and/or a silicone primer makes for the higher possibility of 'rolling'. And I hate it when my products 'roll' (don't get absorbed and bunch up on the skin's surface); it makes me feel dirty, like I have to do my entire routine again. Weird, maybe, but that's just me.

ORGANIC: IS IT OR ISN'T IT?

I am regularly asked about 'organic' versus 'chemical', and the misuse of the word 'natural' (see page 242). Are the products you are using as 'organic' as they claim, and what does 'organic' mean, anyway?

At the time of writing, there are eight different certification bodies in the UK that give out organic accreditation, and many more worldwide. All of them have different requirements. What is organic for one may not be enough for another. It is as confusing as it is frustrating.

To the questions, 'Is it natural?' or 'Is it organic?', my answer is always: 'Compared to what?'

If organic is important to you, do your research thoroughly. You may be paying for something that came out of the ground or from nature, but if it did so via truly organic channels is open to question. Brands that are obsessively organic will tell you the how, why, when and where behind their products' creation. If there is no trail, I'd ask questions.

DETOX

The definition of 'detox':

detox *informal*
noun
  1. a treatment designed to remove poisonous or harmful substances from your body, especially alcohol and drugs: *'he ended up in detox for three months'*
verb
  2. to rid (the body) or undergo treatment to rid the body of poisonous substances, especially alcohol and drugs: *'he checked into a hospital to detox'*

Despite what the 'clean and green' industry would have you believe, we have our own built-in detox system. It's called your lungs, liver, kidneys and skin. Outside of the medically supervised detox treatment in a hospital or drug-dependency unit, any other use of the word 'detox' is disingenuous at its best, and absolute nonsense at its worst. And it has no business in either the food world or in skincare.

Detox products. Detox creams. Detox teas. Detox pads for your feet. Detox hair straighteners. **Enough.** If your body was 'full of toxins' you would be, at best, very ill and, at worst, dead. Brands: stop hijacking the word to sell more product. If you want to 'keep yourself as healthy as possible', then by all means:

- keep hydrated – with water. Diet Coke doesn't count, people.
- don't smoke
- eat well – at the very least, minimise sugar and white carbs
- exercise (or just go for a bloody walk/have a good regular stretching session)
- get enough sunshine, or supplement with vitamin D

That's all the detox you need.

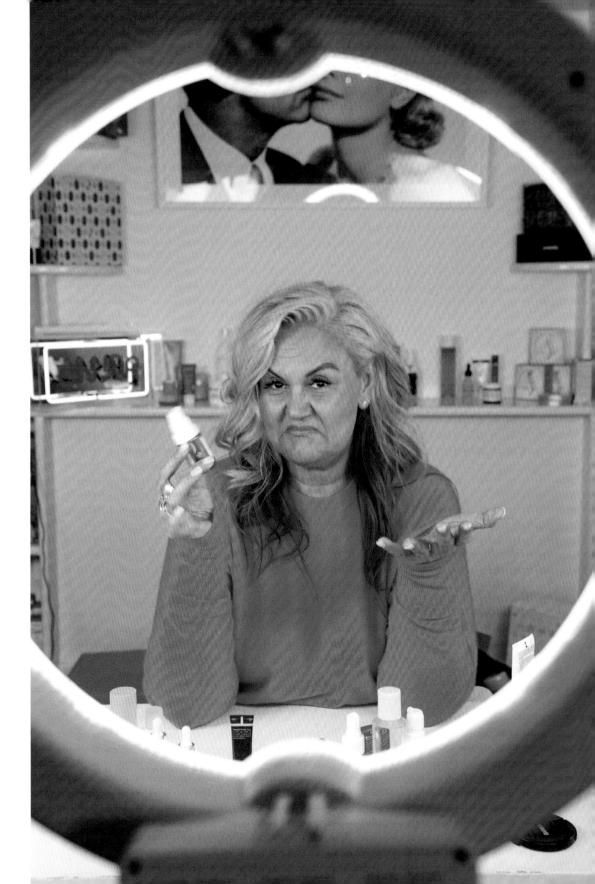

DECODING INGREDIENT LISTS AND CLAIMS

Now that you know all about skincare marketing tactics, let's get down to the formulas and what's in them, so you know what you're spending your money on. A lot of brands don't make it easy, but the ingredients list on any product is in many ways the most important part. Behind all the packaging and marketing, this little list is the science bit – it's essentially what you've paid for. But unless you're a cosmetic scientist or a trained expert, it can be hard to know what you're looking at.

HOW TO READ AN INGREDIENTS LABEL

The first thing to bear in mind is that **the ingredient list is just a guide**. The true breakdown of the ingredients will only be known to the original formulator, the owner of the formula, and the manufacturing lab that makes the products. However, if you learn a few key pointers, reading the list of ingredients on product packaging can still save you a lot of time and effort (and, potentially, money).

Ingredients are legally required to be listed in order, starting with the highest concentrate, until you hit the ingredients that make up less than 1 per cent of the formula. For example, in a moisturising lotion, you'll typically find water ('aqua') first, followed by things like glycerin, hyaluronic acid and, in richer creams, things such as shea butter, squalene and fatty acids. That is easy enough to understand.

The harder part is making sense of what comes in at under 1 per cent, because these ingredients can be listed in any order, and there is no legal obligation to list them in order of descending percentages. This is where brands get creative.

If a brand claims that a product has '25 actives!', I can promise you they will mostly be found under the 1 per cent threshold. This is such common practice that it has its own term – 'Angel Dusting'. Angel dusting is when brands add a miniscule amount of an active ingredient to their formulas in order to make grand marketing claims. From a legal standpoint, the ingredient may have proven clinical results, and it may be in the product, but there is no guarantee that there is enough of the ingredient in the formula to have said effect. That is the aim of the marketing and the assumption of the consumer. There are a couple of key things that you can look out for:

- **Phenoxyethanol or parabens.** Use the appearance of these in ingredient lists as a guide for percentages. Phenoxyethanol, along with parabens, is not allowed to be in formulas at an amount higher than 1 per cent. So, you know that anything listed *after* either of those makes up less than 1 per cent of the product. If a brand is harping on and on about their massively 'active' ingredients and they *all* come after phenoxyethanol or parabens, they may not be that 'active'. There will always be exceptions, such as retinols (frequently used at a strength of 0.3 or 0.5 per cent), but in general, you want peptides, vitamins and the majority of other 'actives' higher than 1 per cent. Mostly. It's not an exact science.

- **Alcohol.** If alcohol is the main ingredient in a product, or in the top three ingredients, I would expect the product to be perhaps an acid or an SPF where it can be necessary to facilitate the formula. You're looking for alcohol denat/denatured alcohol, isopropyl alcohol, SD alcohol or benzyl alcohol. In general, these alcohols are not great for the skin at high concentrations and I tend to avoid them.

FORMULA IS QUEEN – LESS IS SOMETIMES MORE

If you spend any time on social media, you will have noticed competition-level bragging from brands regarding the percentages of ingredients in their formulas. For example, 'contains 25% acid' and 'contains 20% vitamin C': nobody needs a 25% acid or a 20% vitamin C product on their skin on a regular basis. The ever-increasing availability of really high percentages of acids and high-concentration vitamin C products in particular has led to an increase in sensitised skins and the need for medical intervention and stripping back to solid basics.

The rise of single-ingredient formula brands and their marketing, while originally credited with democratising the beauty industry by supposedly talking straight and keeping things simple, in reality has given rise to customers buying multiple products, without proper guidance, and in a lot of cases ending up with 'Status Cosmeticus', aka Cosmetic Intolerance Syndrome.

There are good reasons that professionals would never recommend using a high-percentage acid, followed by a high-percentage vitamin C, followed by another 'active', such as niacinamide or hydroquinone. It's too much. Our skin has evolved over thousands of years into the perfect barrier. It will always win.

> Stronger does not always mean better.
> The formula is what matters.

WHAT DOES 'KEY INGREDIENTS' MEAN?

Key ingredients are the 'actives' added to a formula that have the potential to change the appearance of your skin. They are basically what you are paying for.

ANTI-INFLAMMATORIES
If your skin is red and aggravated, look for products that contain some of these ingredients:

- Aloe vera
- Azelaic acid
- Chamomile
- CoQ10 (Coenzyme Q10 or ubiquinol)
- Feverfew
- Green tea extract
- Licorice extract
- Niacinamide
- Oats
- Pycnogenol
- Zinc

ANTIOXIDANTS
Found in pretty much every product you'll buy (except for cleansers), everyone needs these ingredients because they help protect your skin from external polutants and free radicals.

- Alpha-lipoic acid
- CoQ10
- Green tea extract
- Resveratrol

- Turmeric/curcumin
- Vitamin C
- Vitamin E

HYDRATION

If you are dry or dehydrated, look for moisturisers or facial mists that contain the following at the top of the INCI list:

- Glycerin
- Hyaluronic acid
- Squalane
- Urea

PIGMENTATION ISSUES

These are for brightening dull skin, and in strongest strengths are capable of fading pigmentation damage.

- Hydroquinone
- Kojic acid
- Niacinamide
- Vitamin C

PEPTIDES

If you're looking for an anti-ageing product (though I hate the term) look for the word peptide. Peptides are groups of active ingredients that do everything from aiding collagen production to helping smooth out lines. They are high-tech, not cheap, and you'll usually find them in abundance in serums, which is why serums are more costly.

ANTI-AGEING

Remember, old is the goal, but if you do want to tackle the signs of ageing, look for the following:

- Peptides (see above)
- Vitamin A (retinoids) – these are appropriate for all ages and skin types, but especially for those over 30.
- Vitamin C – this is vital in the skin to support collagen production and help strengthen capillary walls.

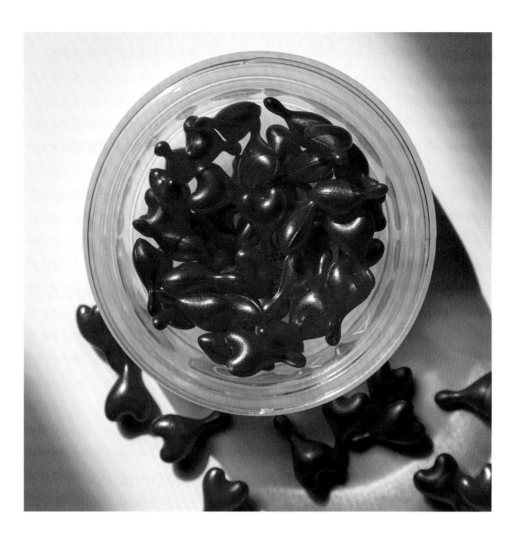

VITAMINS AND MINERALS

These are crucial in skincare so also get their own sub-category, as they can be found in most serums and moisturisers.

- Vitamin A – the aforementioned retinoids, and the gold standard of skincare.
- Vitamin B3 (aka niacinamide) – boosts ceramide production, thus supporting the skin barrier, and helps with post-inflammatory pigmentation.
- Vitamin C – the most commonly known of the vitamins, and the most thoroughly researched antioxidant on the market.
- Vitamin D – think 'defence'. Vitamin D is fortifying, strengthening and supportive of the skin's matrix.
- Vitamin E – used as an antioxidant and also to support and facilitate other ingredients, for example: vitamin A is shown to be more effective when used alongside a vitamin E product.

ACTIVE VERSUS 'INACTIVE' INGREDIENTS

What used to relate purely to ingredients that qualify as drugs is now used as a marketing tool industry-wide, and to say that the terms 'active' and 'inactive' are overused and abused by marketing departments is an understatement.

ACTIVE INGREDIENTS

When used in products that are considered drugs, i.e. SPF products in the USA (see page 220), active ingredients are loosely defined as 'any component of a drug product intended to provide therapeutic and pharmacological activity in direct effect to a diagnosis, cure, mitigation, treatment, or prevention of disease, or to affect the structure or any function of the body of humans.'

Depending on what country you live in, retinoids, acids, and sunscreens like oxybenzone and avobenzone, are all considered 'active', active enough to change the structure of the skin. Take prescription-strength retinoids: in these, the vitamin A will be classed as the drug and therefore 'active', and the other ingredients are 'inactive' because they make up the rest of the formula and do not change the structure of skin. A lot of ingredients considered truly 'active' will have a maximum percentage that they are allowed to be used at in any formula.

WHAT ARE 'ACTIVES'?
'Actives' are ingredients (natural or chemical) that are biologically active and are typically the most potent ingredient in your skincare. They are put in formulas in order to remedy, change or target problems in the skin the product is marketed for.

INACTIVE INGREDIENTS

These are classed as any components of a drug other than the active ingredient. We are now seeing the words 'active' and 'inactive' used on product packaging and marketing material as a selling tool, not just in the case of drugs. A brand will say 'active' ingredients are peptides, vitamin C, seaweed, whale sperm... pick something. Anything. What they actually mean when they say this is, 'this is what we are charging you the big bucks for'.

Inactive ingredients are all too often completely glossed over, ignored or relegated to the very smallest font on the pack, and except in the rarest of circumstances, essentially mean 'the bulk of the product', i.e. water or carrier oils etc.

The potential problems arise when customers who are unaware of the above purchase something and assume that 'inactive' means 'has no effect on the skin'. Just because something doesn't change the structure of the skin (i.e. is 'active') does not mean that it does not affect the skin.

Alcohol, base oils, fragrance and silicones, for example, are all 'inactive' ingredients, yet the ones I am asked about the most by readers. You can bet that a high level of alcohol in a product will be 'active' on your skin in some way.

> If a bacon sandwich was skincare, the bacon would be labelled on the pack as the 'active' ingredient, but the bread would certainly be an active ingredient to someone with a gluten intolerance or a wheat allergy.

Ignore the marketing hype and read the ingredients label. That's where you see what is likely to be an 'inactive' ingredient that could actually be something 'active' for you to look out for.

Some brands have started using bold type for their 'active' ingredients in their INCI lists, in order to make them stand out. Clever, but not if you know what you are looking at.

PARABENS

I am asked on an almost daily basis for my views on parabens, the chemical preservatives used in cosmetic and pharmaceutical products, and am met with outrage by some people who are mortified that I am recommending something that is 'toxic' and can 'give you breast cancer' (erm, no).

In short, my response to the 'outraged' people is always polite and explanatory, but my response to websites spewing out this nonsense is 'bollocks'. They have a lot to answer for. For example, companies that rage about how untrustworthy the skincare industry is because it uses the term 'non-toxic' (because 'non-toxic' means 'absolutely nothing'), and then launch their own range of products described as 'non-toxic'.

I have no problem with short-chain parabens. They are not 'toxic'. I'm not a fan of the way that websites and brands in the 'clean' arena use that word for scare tactics or to make sales.

The word 'toxic' is always dose-dependent.

> If a venomous snake bites you, you could die. If you take a little of that venom and use it to make an antivenom, it could save your life. It's no longer 'toxic'.

In a study of 20 women in 2002,[9] parabens were found to be present in breast cancer tumours. They were also present in breast tissue that had no tumours or cancer present.

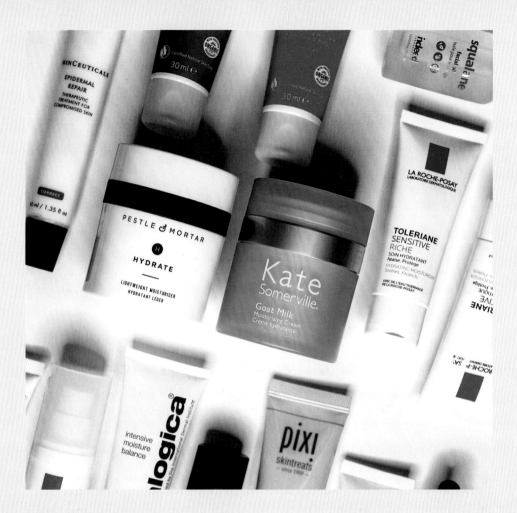

They are mostly present in your wee. That's because you break them down and pee them out.

I'm not a doctor and I'm not a cosmetic scientist but, tellingly, I have yet to work with one who has a problem with parabens in topical formulas.

While it's true that the USA does not do a good enough job of regulating the ingredients of skincare products, the FDA have done research on parabens and found them to be 'completely safe for use in cosmetics'. Similarly, the EU and Canada's governing bodies[10] came to the same conclusion.

If ever there was a case of the tail wagging the dog, this is it. The skincare industry has allowed scaremongering and marketing tactics from the 'clean' movement to lead, when they should have been kicked into touch by science.

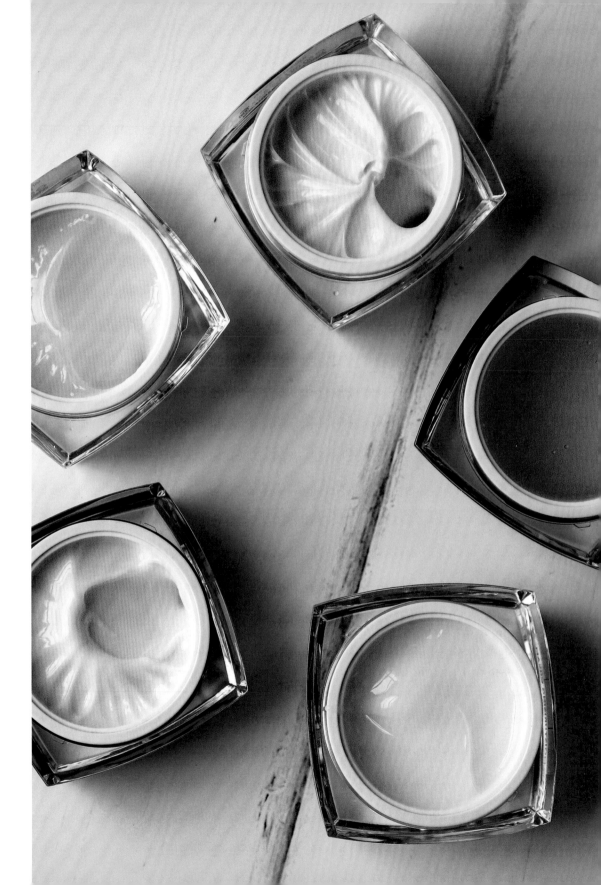

TRIALS AND STUDIES: WHAT DO THEY MEAN?

I am often met with claims of 'clinical trials' and 'independent studies' when reviewing skincare. It's to be expected. Brands want to give the consumer 'evidence' that their product does what it says on the box. The problem arises when they make those claims based on inadequate or irrelevant testing, and put the claims in language that isn't easy for the customer to understand.

So, here's a breakdown of what it all means, in its simplest form:

CONSUMER TRIALS/CONSUMER STUDY

You always see these in the small print on ads. They say something like: 'In a study of 80 women, 67% found that [X] product increased hydration in the skin.'

The major problem with these 'trials' is that you frequently have no idea of the demographic and skin type of those 80 women. If you put a really hydrating moisturiser on a 70-year-old woman who has only ever used soap and water on her face, she may think it's amazing. If you put that same moisturiser on me, I may think it's doing absolutely nothing.

Consumer trials, in a lot of cases, are really just marketing dressed up as facts. It may be a *fact* that '35 out of 50 women found that the product enhanced the firmness of their skin', but what was their skin like before? What is your base level in the group of women? How old are they? Were they wrinkled to begin with? Did they have acne? Did they have sensitive skin? We will never know. These trials are based on the participants feeding back their thoughts on paper, not studied in detail under a microscope in a clinic. That's a consumer trial.

CLINICAL TRIALS

These are, obviously, done in a clinical environment, on people, not petri dishes.

Clinical trials include monitoring the participants before, during and after use of the product and gauging results by scheduling tests, using equipment such as profilometry lasers, and strictly monitoring applications and dosages. During a clinical trial, participants following a protocol are seen regularly by research staff to monitor their results and to determine the effectiveness of the products.

IN VITRO testing ('in vitro' is Latin for 'in glass') is the most common clinical trial. The problem is that testing skincare in a petri dish does not replicate testing it on a live human being. Therefore, I tend to disregard any claims made in connection with in vitro testing. It's basically saying, 'This *might* happen if you use it on your actual skin! Or, you know, it might not.' It's the equivalent of Gordon Ramsay cooking an entire meal for you without tasting the food once during the cooking process. It *should* taste nice, but you don't know if it will until you actually eat it.

IN VIVO testing ('in vivo' is Latin for 'within the living') is the most reliable form of testing as the products are tested on people, not samples in petri dishes. This testing, however, is extremely expensive to perform and understandably not easily available to smaller brands who would struggle to find tens of thousands of dollars to test one product. Most studies conducted in vivo are limited to under 50 people – usually for cost reasons – and take place during a period of 4–12 weeks. For the simple fact that it is testing done on living, breathing human skin, it's still the most reliable form of skincare testing.

So, where does that leave you and I, the consumers who part with their hard-earned cash?

While I always take the results of a full clinical trial seriously, honestly, the only voice I listen to these days is word-of-mouth. If a friend has used something and really rates it, I want to check it out. If another colleague in the industry whose opinion I respect raves about something, I *always* want to check it out.

STEM-CELL PRODUCTS

stem cell
noun
   an undifferentiated cell that gives rise to specialised cells, such as blood cells

There are a lot of 'stem-cell' products around these days. Brands need to be very careful what claims they make when they suggest that a plant stem cell – a PLANT stem cell – can affect the cells in human skin. They can't.

> It's one thing to use peptides to stimulate and give a 'kick' to the skin and collagen; it's another to suggest that those carnations you bought from the petrol garage can reverse ageing and 'wake up' dead cells.

Medical research about stem cells always refers to stem cells that come from human tissue, but plant-derived stem cells are used in skincare products. It is illegal in the EU to use any human-derived tissue or fluid in cosmetics.

Plant stem cells cannot and do not influence stem cells in human skin.

If we could 'wake up' anything 'dead' or 'non-responsive' in the human body, don't you think scientists would use that knowledge to help people who are paralysed? Please.

!?#

'PROFESSIONAL'- AND 'CLINICAL'- STRENGTH PRODUCTS

The current trend of products that are sold in high-street skincare retailers and department stores being marketed as 'professional-strength' or 'clinical' is at best disingenuous, and at worst insulting to the intelligence of both the customer and the trained professional. This claim is mainly used when a product contains stronger active ingredients such as acids and retinoids.

Let's look at peels as an example. True 'professional'- or 'clinical'- grade peels are only sold to qualified, verified and licensed aestheticians and clinics. Those products are not safe in the hands of the untrained consumer. The true professional brands want to see your qualifications, your licence and proof of your liability insurance.

If I perform a modified Jessner peel on a client, the PH is **1.5**. A 10 per cent salicylic peel is **1.8**.

You would never perform that strength of peel three times a week, as is advised with a lot of these products found in traditional beauty hall settings. We find ourselves in a situation where we have brands that do not have any skincare-qualified people at the helm of the company, making 'professional grade' products.

Using 'professional-strength' or 'clinical-strength' on packaging is designed to give customers the impression that they are getting the same product and result that they would receive in a 'professional setting'. They aren't.

The same goes for products called 'facial in a jar', or similar. You cannot replicate a clinic treatment in one application of a cream or serum, and any brands telling you that you can are devaluing our entire professional industry.

THE 500 DALTON RULE

'The what?', I can hear you saying. As a consumer, you have absolutely no need to know about the 500 Dalton Rule. I'm merely sharing this with you because it's outrageous that some brands and websites continue to claim that 60 per cent of what you apply to your skin is absorbed. Cosmetic scientists, pharmacists, aestheticians, dermatologists and doctors all use this as a guideline. I always have the 500 Dalton Rule in my head when reviewing products and recommending what you should put on your face. It's why those of us that work in the industry as qualified professionals are able to collectively roll our eyes at some of the more ridiculous claims that brands make about their products.

The 500 Dalton Rule is the scientific theory that the molecular weight of a compound must be under '500 Dalton' to allow for absorption into the skin.

Our skin is formed of many layers (see pages 12–14) and these layers have worked together perfectly for thousands of years to form the skin and act as a barrier, preventing substances from entering the body, but this barrier is obviously not completely impenetrable.

Arguments for the 500 Dalton Rule are varied but specific:

- Most common contact allergens are found to be under 500 Dalton. Larger molecules are not known as contact sensitisers because they cannot penetrate the skin, so therefore cannot act as allergens in the skin.

- The most commonly used ingredients applied as topical prescription drugs are all under 500 Dalton.

- *All* known topical drugs used in transdermal drug-delivery systems are under 500 Dalton; for example a testosterone patch clocks in at around 288 Daltons. HRT patches work in the same way – they are designed to deliver their component through the skin and into the bloodstream.

- While there are some exceptions to this rule, most researchers would suggest that anything intended to be used for medicinal purposes should be smaller than 500 Daltons to ensure absorption.

Here are the Dalton measurements of some key skincare ingredients:

WATER – 18 Dalton

RETINOL – 286 Dalton

RETINYL PALMITATE – 524 Dalton (This explains why products containing a lot of this ingredient tend to give you a short-term glow, as opposed to really helping collagen and cell turnover etc. It doesn't penetrate the skin.)

MATRIXYL (PEPTIDE) – 578 Dalton

GLYCERIN – 92 Dalton

LACTIC ACID – 90 Dalton

COLLAGEN – 15,000–50,000 Dalton

HYALURONIC ACID – 1–1.5 million Dalton

SUPER-LOW-MOLECULAR WEIGHT HYALURONIC ACID – 10,000 Dalton

ULTRA-LOW-MOLECULAR WEIGHT HYALURONIC ACID – 6,000 Dalton

The 500 Dalton Rule comes into play in the world of skincare in a few ways, but for you, as a customer purchasing products, just bear the following in mind:

- The formula and delivery system is key to the skin's ability to absorb effective ingredients.

- There is a reason most skincare professionals suggest spending the majority of your skincare budget on the 'middle' of your routine (aka serums), and the 500 Dalton Rule gives you some idea as to why: serums tend to contain the largest concentration of ingredients that come in at under 500 Dalton. You do not need to spend a fortune on an expensive moisturiser (unless you want to). While it may 'feel' nice because it is rich in texture and probably occlusive, thereby preventing trans-epidermal water loss (TEWL), ultimately you're paying for the name: the performance levels of a moisturiser do not vary that much across price points.

- The 500 Dalton Rule is a sure-fire way of putting a clear, scientific stop to the constant fear-mongering from the 'green'/'non-toxic' community, such as '60 per cent of what you apply to the skin is immediately absorbed into the bloodstream!' and other such nonsense.

" SKIN IS A BARRIER, NOT A SPONGE "

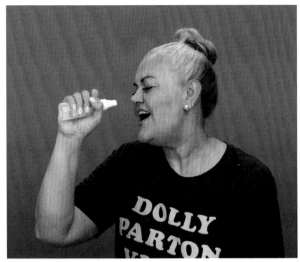

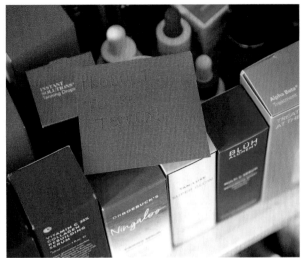

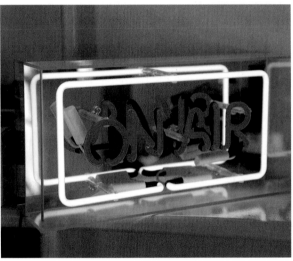

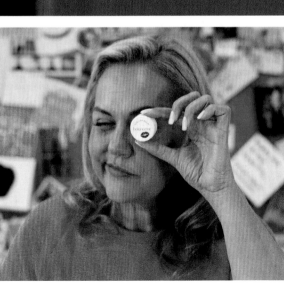

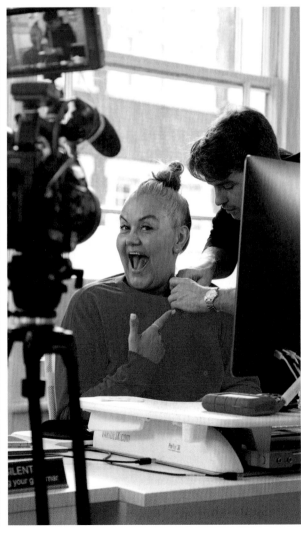

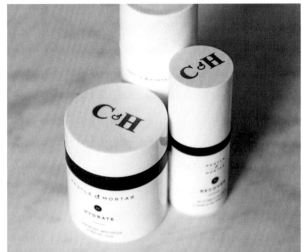

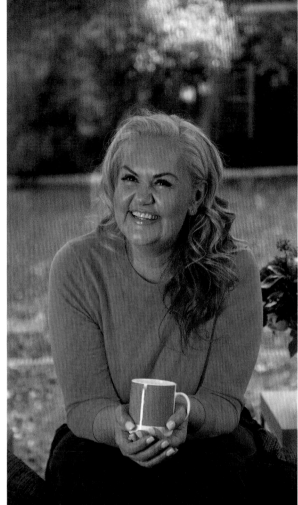

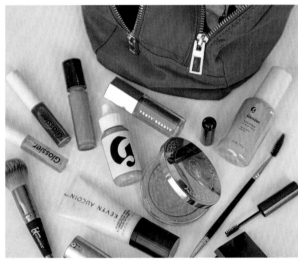

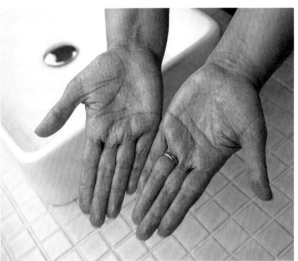

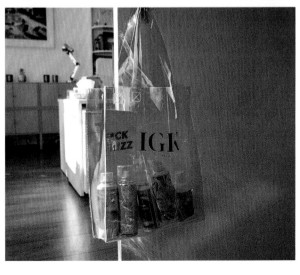

GLOSSARY

Here are a few terms you'll come across as you enter into the world of skincare, along with some of my own favourites.

500 Dalton Rule	The argument that a compound over 500 Daltons cannot effectively penetrate the cutaneous barrier.
acid mantle	Your sebum mixed with your sweat forms your acid mantle, which is a very fine, slightly acidic film on the surface of your skin that gives you extra protection from bacteria and viruses etc.
acne	or 'acne vulgaris' is a skin condition that presents as inflamed skin with pustules, papules and nodules. It is not isolated to teens and not caused by dirt. Hormones, genetics and your environment are the key factors here.
AGEs	Advance glycation end products – proteins and lipids in the skin that have been altered by sugar molecules bonding to them.
AHA	Alpha hydroxy acid (e.g. lactic, glycolic acid) – chemicals used in peels to resurface the outer layer of the epidermis via exfoliation.
alpha-lipoic acid	An enzyme that, applied topically, acts as an antioxidant and is thought to have skin-calming properties.
angel dusting	The highly dubious pratice of brands adding minuscule amounts of active/expensive ingredients to their products to make big claims on packaging.
antioxidant	You'll see this word used numerous times in marketing (and in this book). Antioxidants are molecules that help to prevent oxidation, a chemical reaction that produces free radicals.
astaxanthin	A powerful antioxidant that can also be taken internally via supplementation.
azelaic acid	A fantastic ingredient used as a leave-on exfoliant, with proven benefits for acne skins and treating discolouration and/or scarring. Suitable for all skins.

bakuchiol	A plant-derived product considered a suitable alternative for vitamin A during pregnancy and breastfeeding, as it is shown to have a similar effect on the skin.
barrier function	You will see the term 'skin barrier function' mentioned frequently in this book. The skin barrier resides primarily within the top layer of the epidermis, also known as the stratum corneum or 'horny layer'. A soft, plump skin is a sign of good barrier function. A compromised barrier function will present as dull skin that feels rough and/or dry. Skin barrier function is vital for maintaining the temperature of the skin and protection against environmental aggressors, and maintains proper hydration in the skin.
basal cell carcinoma	The most common form of skin cancer.
BHA	Beta hydroxy acid (e.g. salicylic acid).
bookends	Cleansers and moisturisers in your routine.
benzoyl peroxide	An OTC acne topical treatment, more popular in the US than in Europe.
CIBTAC	A qualfication for beauty therapists: Confederation of International Beauty Therapy and Cosmetologists.
CIDESCO	Comité International d'Esthétique et de Cosmétology – international beauty therapy and aesthetics examination body.
collagen	The scaffolding of the skin and most tissue in the body. A protein that literally gives skin its structure.
comedogenic	Blocks pores.
comedones	Small black or skin-coloured spots caused by sebum blockage. Closed comedones = whiteheads. Open comedones = blackheads.
Cosmelan	An intensive depigmentation chemical peel, that includes an in-clinic treament and follow-up creams.
coQ10/CoEnzymeQ10	Antioxidant.
cosmeceutical	A made-up, non-regulated word that insinuates that the product will alter the biologic function of your skin. Marketing.
cryotherapy	'Cold therapy' originally used in skincare to treat skin cancer, now becoming more popular in clinics as a stand-alone treatment.
D2C	Direct to consumer, avoiding traditional retailers. (See also DTC.)

dermaplaning	A close shave on the face to remove vellous (peach fuzzy) hair, particularly around the jawline and under the ears to allow for better product penetration and give a good glow.
dermatitis	A blanket term for 'inflammation of the skin'. Atopic dermatitis = eczema; contact dermatitis = allergic reaction on the skin.
dermatosis papulosa nigra	Small, benign lesions on the skin, particularly prevalent in darker skins.
dermis	The layer below the epidermis.
DTC	Direct to consumer. Sells online, on sites such as Glossier.
eccrine gland	The most common form of sweat gland, found on all surfaces of the skin.
eczema	Or 'atopic dermatitis', a chronic skin condition that causes itchy, red, flaky skin. Can be genetic but is caused by a mixture of skin barrier dysfunction and your immune system.
elastin	The protein that gives skin its shape.
Endymed	Brilliant, minimally invasive, radio-frequency in-clinic treatment for tightening and contouring skin.
epidermis	The outer layer of the skin, and mainly responsible for a healthy barrier function.
essence	A modern take on toner. Usually a first step in hydration.
EWG	Environmental Working Group – non-charitable organisation. Google it for yourself (it's entertaining).
extrinsic ageing	Skin ageing caused by your lifestyle: diet, environmental factors, smoking and sun exposure.
faradic	Face and body treatment using electrical muscle stimulation.
fibroblast cells	Cells that produce collagen and elastin, among other molecules. Found in the dermis.
fibrosis	When you have an excess of connective tissue, seen most commonly as scarring.
filaggrin	A protein necessary for the healthy barrier function of the epidermis, mutations of which are linked to a lot of cases of eczema and ichthyosis.
flannel	Small face cloth used to remove balm or cleansing oil (first cleanse) and provides mild exfoliation. Called a washcloth in the US.

free radicals	Unstable (altered) atoms that cause damage to DNA, cells and proteins in the skin.
glycolic acid	The mother of all acids, the smallest molecule, able to penetrate the deepest. Used to tackle ageing and acne, among everything else.
galvanic	Electrical treatment to improve skin tone and elasticity.
glutamine	An amino acid that is a building block of protein, among many other uses.
glycation	Occurs when sugar molecules attach themselves to protein or fat in the skin. As collagen is a protein, this can cause the skin to become stiff and lose elasticity.
glycerin	A component found in the skin, glycerin as an ingredient is a must-have humectant that is suitable for all skins and ages.
glycosaminoglycans	The foundation of the extracellular matrix, giving it structure. Key for healing wounds and inflammation.
GMC	General Medical Council (UK)
grip, not slip	How your hands should feel when you're massaging product into the skin.
HA/hyaluronic acid	Found naturally in the body and resides in both the epidermis and the deeper dermis, where it plays a key role in hydration and skin repair. It is able to bind moisture in up to 1,000 times its own weight when topically applied to the skin and also helps the skin heal after injury.
hydroquinone	Used for skin lightening. Percentages vary worldwide, but in the UK it's capped at 4% dosage.
hypertrophic scarring	A raised mass of collagen occuring after damage to the skin i.e. piercings, burns or cuts.
hypo-allergenic	Relatively unlikely to cause an allergic reaction.
ichthyosis	An inherited skin condition that occurs when the skin doesn't shed dead skin cells.
in vitro	'In glass': testing done by scientists, in a petri dish.
in vivo	'Within the living': testing done on living people (organisms).
INCI	International Nomenclature of Cosmetic Ingredients (the list of what's in a product)

intrinsic ageing	The natural course of skin ageing, from the age of approximately 20 onwards (I know), but essentially the depletion of collagen in the dermis.
IPL	Intense Pulsed Light. Mainly used for hair removal, pigmentation and broken capillaries.
ITEC	Qualifications awarded by the International Therapy Examination Council.
J-Beauty	Japanese skincare and makeup.
Jessner peel	Medium-depth in-clinic peel, consisting of a 14g/14g/14g split of resourcinol, lactic acid and salicylic acid in a 95% ethanol base.
Juvederm	Injectable hyaluronic acid dermal fillers.
K-Beauty	Korean skincare and makeup.
keloid scarring	Bulky scar similar to hypertrophic scarring that develops after trauma to the skin. More prevelant in young and darker skins.
keratin	The protein that makes up the outer layer of skin and hair and nails.
keratinocyte	Produces keratin, the primary cell of the epidermis.
kojic acid	Used primarily for tackling pigmentation issues, it has been slowly replacing hydroquinone in OTC formulas.
lactic acid	A great beginner acid, and brilliant for dry skins and treating keratosis pilaris.
Langerhans cells	Your immune cells within the epidermis.
Laser Genesis	Non-invasive heat-based laser with a number of uses (it is mainly used to stimulate collagen).
LLA	L-ascorbic ccid (vitamin C)
MED	Minimal erythema dose – the shortest exposure to UV radiation that produces reddening of the skin.
medical grade	More common in the US, this term actually has no legal standing. The only real 'medical-grade' products are prescription-only.
melanin	The pigment that gives skin, hair and eyes their colour.
melanocytes	The cell that produces and distributes melanin.
melanoma	An area of cancerous cells often caused by excessive exposure to sunlight.
micellar water	Made famous by MUAs backstage, a quick makeup remover.

microbiome	The microorganisms that live on us (and in us). The future of skincare.
microcurrent	Microcurrent electrical neuromuscular stimulator
microneedling	More commonly known by the brand name 'Dermaroller', medical needling is a popular in-clinic treatment that stimulates collagen. Be warned: it only stimulates collagen if you bleed, which usually means in-clinic and using 3mm needles. The at-home kits will not do this.
MLM	Multi-level marketing brands such as Mary Kay, Avon (originally), Tropic, Arbonne, and The Body Shop at Home.
MUA	Make Up Artists
nd:YAG	Laser used predominantly for hair removal and proven safe for darker skins.
niacinamide	Vitamin B3, useful for enhancing skin barrier function and reducing uneven skin tone, lines and wrinkles and dullness.
NMF	Natural moisturising factors including squalane, triglycerides, cholesterol, ceramides and wax esters.
NPD	New product development
occlusive	Blocks your pores.
OTC	Over the counter (i.e. no prescription needed)
parabens	Synthetic chemicals used as preservatives in a variety of products. Successfully ostracised by the 'clean' community, despite being proven safe for use.
PCOS	Polycystic ovary syndrome is a condition in women whereby oestrogen, progesterone and testosterone levels are out of balance. This leads to the growth of ovarian cysts – benign masses on the ovaries.
PD	Perioral dermatitis, or 'irritating red rash around the corners of your mouth and/or nose that won't go away'.
peptides	In their simplest form, peptides are short chains of amino acids that are able to penetrate the skin and tell it how to function.
pH	Potential hydrogen – used to measure acid/alkaline.
PHA	Polyhydroxy acid. A larger-moleculed acid that penetrates more slowly and is thus suitable for most skins, including sensitive.
PIH	Post-inflammatory hyperpigmentation, usually caused by damage to the skin.

Profhilo	A brilliant newer form of injectable hyaluronic acid that not only stimulates your own hyaluronic acid but also has a proven positive effect on skin elasticity and collagen.
PRP	Platelet-rich Plasma, originally used to heal sports injuries on the body, now used in facials. Not proven to be effective and I'm personally not a fan.
psoriasis	Chronic skin condition that produces dry, itchy plaques of skin and normally presents on the elbows, scalp and knees.
pycnogenol	Potent antioxidant derived from the bark of French Maritime pine trees, also proven to be excellent when taken internally.
radio frequency treatment	Uses heat to stimulate collagen, elastin and hyaluronic acid production with the aim of tightening or 'contouring' skin.
Restylane	An injectible hyaluronic-acid filler.
retinoids	Vitamin A derivatives, the gold standard in true anti-ageing skincare.
rosacea	Chronic red, irritated rash with pimples that typically affects the nose, forehead and cheeks.
seborrheic dermatitis	Itchy, red skin found in the sebacious glands, mainly on the face and in the scalp, i.e. dandruff.
sebum	The oily substance containing fat molecules that lubricates and helps waterproof the skin.
silicones	Safe, proven ingredients used to both give slip and carry key active ingredients into the skin. Given a bad rap by the 'clean' brigade, unnecessarily so.
SLS/SLES	Sodium lauryl sulphate/sodium laureth sulfate – foaming agents used in products like shower gels, cleansers and toothpaste. On paper, they're inert and safe. Upon using them on myself and clients, I have found them to be drying and, in the case of SLS, particularly irritating.
squalane	One of my favourite oils, suitable for all skins. Light and nourishing without stickiness.
squamous cell carcinoma	A non-melanoma form of skin cancer.
Status Cosmeticus	Cosmetic Intolerance Syndrome – when you've used too many products and your skin has just had enough.
stratum corneum	The 'horny' layer of the skin, the area most affected by OTC products.

subcision	A surgical procedure using a hypodermic needle quite aggressively under the skin to treat acne scarring.
TEWL	Trans-epidermal water loss
tranexamic acid	Used to brighten the skin and treat discolouration.
triglycerides	Contains a high amount of fatty acids, and is an excellent emollient.
turmeric	Used as an antioxidant and an anti-inflammatory.
ubiquinol	A derivative of CoQ10, an antioxidant that reduces free radicals.
vitamin A	Aka retinoids/retinols.
vitamin B	Niacinamide
vitamin C	One of the most tested and reliable antioxidants.
vitamin D	Actually a hormone, but called the fortifier of the vitamins. Strengthens the skin and in your system is crucial for healthy bones.
vitamin E	The original antioxidant. Makes all the others, especially vitamin C, work better.
vitamin K	Frequently applied after treatments to aid healing and minimise bruising.
vitiligo	A skin disease caused by your immune system destroying the melanocytes in your skin, thus causing large areas of depigmentation.
wax esters	Component of sebum.
500 Dalton Rule	The argument that a compound over 500 Daltons cannot effectively penetrate the cutaneous barrier.

THE BRANDS

Here are some of the brands and products that I am most frequently asked about. The list is by no means exhaustive, and does not include many well-known brands unless I am consistently asked about them (or one of their products). I have distinguished between brands that emphasise the 'clean', plant-based source of their ingredients and those that are science-led and talk more about the product formulas and results, though it's worth remembering that *everything* is a chemical, and everything comes out of a lab. Everything.

WHO	WHAT	WHERE
Alpha-H	Great Australian brand, makers of Liquid Gold. Science- and formula-led.	High street/home shopping/facials
ANR	Advanced Night Repair, an iconic science- and formula-led product from Estée Lauder. Suitable for all skins, especially popular with 35+.	Widely available
Anthelios	A popular pharmacy SPF by La Roche-Posay. Multiple options available. Science- and formula-led.	Widely available
Arbonne	They have an ingredients policy where the first thing listed is 'pure'. Although they use some plant-based ingredients, but not a lot.	Multi-level marketing (see Glossary)
Aveda	The original 'natural' brand, except they really are ethical.	Widely available
Avène	French pharmacy brand that specialises in sensitive skin.	Widely available
Beauty Pie aka BP	A science- and formula-led beauty club with multiple levels of monthly subscription fees.	Online
belif	Korean beauty brand that is a hit Stateside for Sephora. I'm a particular fan of the moisturisers – they're brilliant. They claim they have the 'best' and 'purest' ingredients, which gives the impression they are a 'natural' brand, but this is nonsense. (That's not an insult, just a fact.)	Sephora

Bioderma	French pharmacy brand that makes the most famous micellar water.	Pharmacy
Bioeffect	Founded in Iceland in 2010, Bioeffect is based on an engineered plant-based replica of EGF (epidermal growth factor).	High-end retailers
Biologique Recherche	A French professional brand that makes the iconic P50 and some of the smelliest, yet effective, skincare on the market. Popular with older skins.	Professional/clinic retailers/selected online stores
Caudalie	French spa brand that bases its products on the power of grape seeds as antioxidants. Introduce themselves as 'paraben-free and natural' on their website (rather annoyingly, as I think they are more scientific than the impression this gives).	Space NK/ department store/ specialist retailers
CeraVe	Lauched in the USA in 2006, CeraVe is based entirely on ceramides and replenishing the skin barrier.	Pharmacy
Cetaphil	The infamous cleanser that is still, baffingly, a top seller in the USA. In my opinion, water, three parabens, two alcohols and SLS do not a 'suitable for dry skin' cleanser make. But this doesn't stop it being a bestseller.	Pharmacy
Chantecaille	Luxury family-owned brand. Science- and formula-led, with the levels of 'natural' percentages listed on packaging.	Prestige retailers
Clarins	Family-owned French spa-brand. Science- and formula-led, with plant-based ingredients at the fore on packaging.	Widely available
Clarisonic	Electronic cleansing brushes launched in 2000, now owned by L'Oreal. I'm not a fan (not that that matters – they sell by the shedload).	If you're that desperate for one, do your own research
Clinique	Founded by Estée Lauder in 1968, Clinique are mostly known for the '3-Step', which is a shame because they have far, far better products in their portfolio.	Widely available

Curel	The No.1 selling line in Japan for sensitive skin.	Pharmacy
Darphin	Launched by Pierre Darphin in Paris in 1958, Darphin is one of the brands that first made me fall in love with skincare. Botanical-based, science- and formula-led oils, serums, lotions, milks and creams, all layerable and made bespoke to the individual. Lush.	Professional/clinic retailers/selected department stores/ Space NK
DDG	Created by Dr Dennis Gross, a dermatologist based in New York.	Prestige/department store/Sephora
de Mamiel	Annee de Mamiel is an acupuncturist, aromatherapist and holistic facialist. Her treatments are other-worldly and have to be experienced to be believed. Her science- and botanical-led product line is an extension of this, and it shows. Obsessive about ingredient sourcing (not an insult!).	Prestige/Space NK/ Cult Beauty
Decléor	French-based spa brand owned by L'Oréal. Predominantly plant-ingredient focused.	Prestige/facials
Dermalogica	Founded in 1986 and now owned by Unilever Prestige, Dermalogica is an aesthetician-based brand with an almost cult-like following (not an insult!).	Professional/clinic retailers/selected department stores/ Space NK
Dr Jart+	Founded in 2004, this extremely popular Korean brand is affordable and science-led. I use the Ceramidin line regularly. The brand name stands for 'Dr meets art' – it's not founded by a real doctor. The parent company was aquired by Estée Lauder in 2019.	Sephora/Selfridges/ Cult Beauty
Dr Sam Bunting	Dr Sam's skincare line is based around a simple routine with multi-tasking formulas.	Online
Dr Sebagh	Based in London, Jean-Louis Sebagh specialises in aesthetics and non-invasive treatments. His product line launched in 2006 to huge acclaim. Originally trained as an ENT specialist.	Space NK/ department store/ specialist retailers

Drunk Elephant	Hugely popular US-based brand now owned by Shiseido. Purveyors of the 'suspicious six'. They don't like me because I once gave them construcive feedback on their retinol (not a fan), after positively reviewing 11 of their other products. They call themselves 'clean clinical', so safe to say they place themselves in the 'clean' arena.	Sephora/Space NK/ Cult Beauty
Emma Hardie	Facialist brand. Formula-led. No mention of 'clean' (thankfully).	Prestige/Space NK
ELC	Estée Lauder Companies (Parent companies of brands).	Prestige/department store/Sephora
Elizabeth Arden	This major brand will celebrate its 110th anniversary in 2020.	Prestige/department store
Estée Lauder	The world-renowned brand was founded in 1946.	Prestige/department store
Farmacy	US-based 'farm-to-face' brand that is extremely popular with the Sephora customer in the US. Green. Very green. Take up a lot of internet real estate telling you what is not in their products.	Sephora/Cult Beauty
Foreo	Swedish-based silicone cleansing tool/ applicator that vibrates. A lot. It's literally a vibrator for your face. I'm not a fan. Again, not that this matters – they sell by the shedload.	Various websites and shops
Glossier	Online retailer, offshoot of Into the Gloss. Hugely popular with millenials.	Online
Glow Tonic	One of the original acid toners, now in its 20th year. It's the Pixi product that spawned a multitude of copycat products and the overuse of the word 'glow' on skincare products by brands trying to piggyback on its success.	Mass market/ Sephora/high street/ pharmacy
Good Genes	A hero product from Sunday Riley that uses glycolic acid in the UK and lactic acid in the USA.	Sephora/Space NK/ Cult Beauty

goop	One of the worst offenders for using the term 'non-toxic' in the early days, and then fortuitously launching their own range, which of course is 'non-toxic'. Leaders of the 'clean' movement (that is not a compliment), but in reality their formulas contain high levels of alcohols, essential oils (and their allergen components) and would be classed as 'chemical-based' by anyone in the scientific community.	Online only
GOW	Garden of Wisdom. Ingredient-led, frequently single-ingredient led. Competition for The Ordinary.	Victoria Health in the UK, various stores worldwide
Hada Labo	Good, affordable Japanese range based on the benefits of hyaluronic acid.	Amazon
Helena Rubinstein	The original beauty house. Helena Rubinstein founded her company in 1902, when Elizabeth Arden was 8, and 6 years before Estée Lauder was born. Coined the original three different skin types. Relaunched in the UK in late 2019.	Prestige/department store
Hydraluron	A hyaluronic acid gel by Indeed Labs which is used at the serum stage.	Widely available
Indeed Labs	Makers of Hydraluron, aka 'Hironsluron'.	Widely available
January Labs	Small, independent LA-based brand, focusing on simple yet efficacious formulas.	Niche/smaller retailers
Joanna Vargas	Independent facialist brand. Joanna has clinics in NYC and LA, and specialises in hi-tech facials.	Online/high-end retailers
Josh Rosebrook	Founder of an independent LA-based brand and an absolute gent. Science- and formula-led, with an emphasis on sourcing pristine, active herbs and plants as ingredients. For all skins.	Online/selected independent retailers
Jordan Samuel Skin	Independent Seattle-based brand – Jordan's also a true gent. Jordan and Josh epitomise the new wave of 'customer first' brands.	Online/Cult Beauty UK
Kiehl's	An original true pharmacy brand, now owned by L'Oréal.	Widely available

Kate Somerville	The original celebrity facialist. Still based in LA and now owned by Unilever Presige. One of my favourite people in the industry. Absolutely nothing gets past her – she's the Queen of no BS.	Prestige/facial brand
La Prairie	Swiss brand founded in 1931.	Prestige/department store
Lancer	LA-based dermatologist, founder of the eponymous brand and lover of a facial scrub.	Sephora
Lancôme	Originally launched in 1935, this French beauty house is now owned by L'Oréal.	Department store
LRP/ La Roche-Posay	French-based spa brand owned by L'Oréal.	Widely available
May Lindstrom	LA-based organic brand. May's organic skincare products are properly luxurious. May is also obsessive about ingredient sourcing.	Prestige/selected retailers
Medik8	British-founded brand focusing on CSA: vitamin C and sunscreen in the AM, vitamin A in the PM.	Professional/clinic retailers and selected online stores
Merumaya	Independent British-born brand based on products containing proven active ingredients at affordable prices.	Online/selected retailers
Murad	Dr Howard Murad is one of the most respected dermatologists in the industry. His line is based around proven actives, and his philosophy is to 'eat your water' and reduce your stress as basic self-care for good skin.	Specialist retailers / department store
Neostrata	Originally founded in 1988. NeoStrata and Exuviance, it's slightly more user-friendly diffusion line, were acquired by Johnson & Johnson in 2016.	Professional/clinic retailers and selected online stores with clinics/professional outlets
Obagi	Originally founded by Dr Zein Obagi, a dermatologist in California. Dr Obagi now has nothing to do with the brand, but they still carry through the basic principles, which, in essence, are based on the belief that we over-moisturise the skin.	Doctor/skincare professional

OSKIA	British brand that describes itself as a 'clean, natural brand'. But don't let that put you off. Brilliant products. One of my favourite brands.	Prestige/Space NK
P50	One of the original acids on the market, made by Biologique Recherche, and truly iconic. Notoriously smells of vinegar. You get used to it. And it's worth it.	Professional and clinic retailers/ selected online stores
Paula's Choice	Founded in 1994 by Paula Begoun, Paula's Choice champions a very strict set of guidelines for their products, all of which are based on key, proven ingredients. Paula hates essential oils like I hate wipes.	Online/selected stores
Perricone MD	Originally launched in 1997 by dermatologist Dr Nicholas Perricone, this is now one of the older derm-led brands. Dr Perricone is arguably more known for his anti-inflammatory diet advice and books.	Sephora/Ulta/John Lewis
Pestle & Mortar	Lovely Irish brand that make solid yet simple formulas that are affordable and work. Hard to go wrong here. Also they are lovely people (that is sometimes worth highlighting in this industry).	Online/Irish pharmacies
Pixi	London-born but Swedish-owned. Founders of Glow Tonic. Formula-led with some mention of naturals, but not obsessive.	Widely available
Proactiv	Launched in 1995 and still one of the biggest-selling brands in the USA, mainly through infomercials. Famous for selling kits targeted to acne on a subscription basis. Not a fan – in my opinion their products are too harsh for the skin, especially the skins they are targeted to.	Direct marketing (TV etc.)/Ulta
PTR/Peter Thomas Roth	Eponymous brand founded by PTR, who calls his line 'Clinical Skin Care', despite being neither a dermatologist nor an aesthetician. That annoys me. Can you tell?	Sephora/department store/online

REN	REN were one of the first 'clean' brands on the market (REN means 'clean' in Swedish). Now owned by Unilever. Science- and formula-led, and obsessed with 'naturals'.	Widely available
Renée Rouleau	Texas-based facialist Renée founded her company in 1996 and is known for her '9 Skin Types', giving her consumer an in-depth online diagnosis tool that expands on the traditional 'skin types'.	Online
Rodan + Fields	Multi-level marketing company with the biggest selling skincare line in the USA.	Multi-level marketing only
Sam Farmer	Unisex, non-sexualised formulations for adolescent skin and hair.	Online
Sephora	Founded in France in 1970. Now the largest beauty retailer in North America and owned by LVMH. All-powerful. What they say goes, for most of the brands they carry.	Stores worldwide
Serozinc	A brilliant spray/mist from La Roche-Posay that contains zinc.	High street/French pharmacy
Shiseido	Founded in 1872, Shiseido is now the largest skincare company in Japan and the fifth largest in the world. They own Drunk Elephant, NARS, Laura Mercier and more.	Department store/ Space NK
SK-II	Originally launched in the 1980s and now owned by P&G, SK-II formulas are based around the extract Pitera, derived from yeast. Most famously known for their Treatment Essence and sheet masks.	High-end retailers
SkinCeuticals	Founded by Dr Sheldon Pinnell, possibly one of the most respected and decorated professors of dermatology, who passed away in 2014. The brand is now owned by L'Oréal, who have, thankfully, ensured it has stayed true to its roots and ethos. Extremely science- and formula-led. I pretty much trust anything they say.	Professional/clinic retailers and selected online stores with clinics/professional outlets in bricks and mortar

Skingredients	Young, Irish brand founded by 'The Skin Nerd' Jennifer Rock, based on proven key ingredients and excellent, solid formulas. The future of marketing, branding and messaging. Thank God.	Pharmacy/online
Sisley	French beauty house. Formula is more important than naturals, but they do 'like' a plant: 'The best of plants for the best of cosmetics'.	Prestige/department store
Sunday Riley	Eponymous brand from Sunday Riley, a Texas native with a focus on science.	Sephora/Space NK/ Cult Beauty
Tata Harper	Oh Tata. I love some of Tata's products – her cleansers in particular are amazing – but what I cannot handle is the fact that every product has '100% natural & non-toxic' on the front, as if other skincare lines will kill you. Good products, some of them great, but the messaging is off-putting. Properly 'clean', down to the packaging.	Sephora/Space NK/ Cult Beauty
Tatcha	Founded in 2009 in the USA and now owned by Unilever Prestige. Tatcha is based on Japanese culture and skincare. Claims to offer 'pure' products. In order to get to the ingredients list on the website, you have to first read what 'isn't' in the products: a trend I hope will soon die.	Sephora
The Body Shop	Originally founded by Dame Anita Roddick and now owned by Natura. The Body Shop was one of the first brands to embrace 'giving back', and it remains at the forefront of all issues like sustainability, fair trade, being against animal testing and being a cause for good. Formula-led, although their USP is to base a lot of formulas around key plant-based ingredients.	Own stores
The Blue Cocoon	May Lindstrom's hero product, and one of the most searched products on the blog.	Selected independent retailers
The Inkey List	Launched in 2018 as direct competition to The Ordinary.	Pharmacy/online

The Ordinary	Part of the Deciem group, The Ordinary launched to huge fanfare by offering single-ingredient formulas at cheap prices.	Widely available
Trader Joe's (skincare)	For the most part, excellent, affordable, simple-yet-efficacious products. Always overlooked by the US beauty press. Their USP is to base a lot of formulas around key plant-based ingredients.	Trader Joe's
Tropic	Multi-level marketing range originally founded in the UK by Susie Ma, who sold a 50 per cent share to Alan Sugar after she appeared on *The Apprentice* (UK). The brand mainly talks about what's not in its products, and would absolutely describe themselves as 'green'/'clean'/'natural' (or all of the above). Its reps have a bad marketing habit of talking about their brand positively compared to others, which I am not a fan of, but they listen to feedback, which is more than can be said for a lot of other brands out there.	Online/multi-level marketing
TTDO	Take The Day Off Cleansing Balm by Clinique – an iconic product, known by its acronym in the industry.	
Vichy	Founded in Vichy, France in 1931 and now owned by L'Oréal, the brand's science- and formula-led products are based around the benefits of the thermal spa waters in the town.	High street/French pharmacy
Votary	British natural-led brand founded by Arabella Preston and Charlotte Semler, based on botanicals, predominantly oils.	Space NK/Cult Beauty
Vintner's Daughter	A cult facial oil/serum that contains 22 'nutrient-dense' botanicals. Not cheap, but generally loved once tried. Fully at the front of the 'clean' world.	Space NK/Cult Beauty
Weleda	Launching in Switzerland in 1921 and most well-known for the extremely popular Skin Food moisturiser. Green, plant-based. Science- and formula-led.	Health shops/selected retailers

Zelens	British brand founded by Dr Marko Lens, a consultant reconstructive and plastic surgeon with a PhD from Oxford and Master of Science from Harvard, specialising in skin cancer and skin ageing. Extremely science- and high-performance formula-led, but uses proven plant ingredients in all his formulas. I trust everything he makes. Dr Lens performed my eye surgery.	Doctor/professional/ clinic retailers and selected prestige stores
Zo Skin Health	Newish company founded by Dr Zein Obagi in 2007 (they obviously cannot use his name on packaging). They still hate moisturiser, though (see Obagi).	Professional/clinic retailers and selected online stores

SOURCES

1 British Association of Dermatologists: http://www.bad.org.uk/skin-cancer/sunscreen-fact-sheet#applying-sunscreen

2 Canadian Government Health department: https://www.canada.ca/en/health-canada/services/food-nutrition/healthy-eating/vitamins-minerals/vitamin-calcium-updated-dietary-reference-intakes-nutrition.html

3 Journal of Neuropsychiatry: http://www.jneuropsychiatry.org/peer-review/depression-and-vitamin-d-deficiency-causality-assessment-and-clinical-practice-implications-12051.html

4 NHS: https://www.nhs.uk/news/cancer/vitamin-d-may-reduce-risk-some-cancers/

5 Diabetes.co.uk: https://www.diabetes.co.uk/food/vitamin-d.html

6 NHS: https://www.nhs.uk/conditions/vitamins-and-minerals/vitamin-d/

7 Personal Care Products Council

8 According to EU legislation (Regulations Annexe II, article 416), skincare products containing human-derived ingredients are actually banned in the EU

9 'Concentrations of Parabens in Human Breast Tumours', published in the Journal of Applied Toxicology (Wiley & Sons, Ltd.) and cited on www.dr-baumann.ca: https://www.dr-baumann.ca/science/Concentrations%20of%20Parabens%20in%20Human%20Breast.pdf

10 European Commission's Scientific Committee on Consumer Safety (SCCS) and Canadian Government's Safety of Cosmetic Ingredients

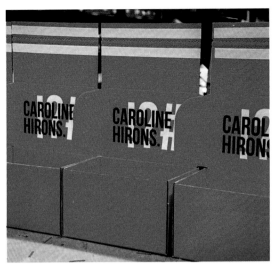

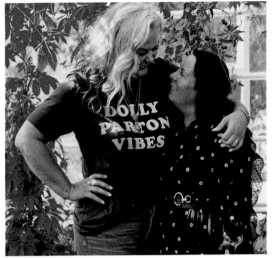

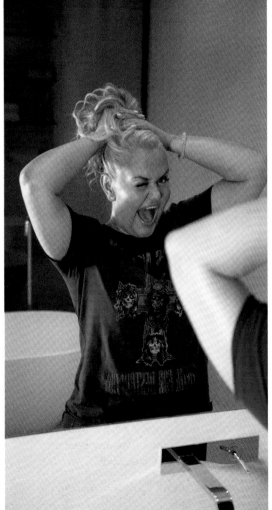

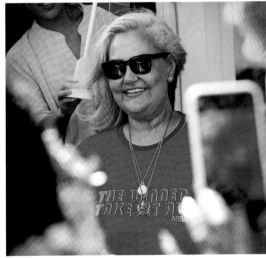

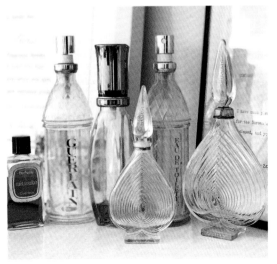

ABOUT THE AUTHOR

With over 120 million views to her blog, Caroline is a fully-trained advanced aesthetician with over 35 years of experience in retail, including 23 in skincare, consulting and advising for retailers and brands in the skincare industry.

Her expert advice talks about the industry she loves, shining an honest light on products that really work, and never sugar-coating her opinion.

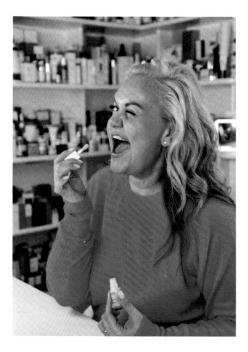

Since starting the blog in 2010, Caroline's no-nonsense approach on what you do and don't need to put on your skin has led her to be named 'The Skincare Queen' by her millions of followers around the world. Her loyal fans refer to themselves as 'The Freaks' and such is the strength of Caroline's knowledge, when she recommends a skincare product, it creates a retail stampede.

Caroline is obsessed with skincare – it's her business as well as her hobby. It's also in her blood as both her mum and nana worked behind beauty counters.

Born and raised in Liverpool and the US, Caroline has lived in London since 1987 with her husband Jim, and their four children.

carolinehirons.com

f CarolineHironsOfficial

🐦 CarolineHirons

📷 CarolineHirons

▶ CarolineHirons

INDEX

299

THANK YOU

This book would not exist without my readers. Thank you, thank you, thank you for trusting me, challenging me and supporting me. A special mention must go to the Skin Freaks group: you're all crazy and I wouldn't have it any other way. And @lizalaska who coined #carolinehironsmademedoit and started a movement that continues to astound me. THANK YOU.

The team at HarperCollins, specifically Lisa Milton, Kate Fox, Laura Nickoll and Louise Evans: thank you for your patience.

Megan Carver: this is kind of all your fault. Thank you for telling me what to do and making it seem not only feasible, but something that I would enjoy. Bev James: thank you for your guidance, support and your calm voice when I'm having a meltdown. Sarah Gordon: thank you for being completely unflappable and keeping me in line. If you were a football team, you'd be LFC. (Jürgen Klopp 'Na Na Na Na Na' #YNWA.)

Contrary to popular belief, I don't want to rock the boat. I don't enjoy it. But sometimes the boat just needs to be knocked off course a little. So, with that in mind, a huge thank you to the brands and retailers that stand on such a strong foundation that they not only don't mind being challenged, they actively encourage it. There are many, but it would be remiss of me not to give a shout out to Alpha-H, Chantecaille, Clarins, Clinique, Dr Dennis Gross, Emma Hardie, Estée Lauder, Medik8, Indeed Labs, Josh Rosebrook, Kate Somerville, May Lindstrom, Murad, OSKIA, Pixi, REN, Sunday Riley, Jordan Samuel, The Body Shop, Votary, Zelens, Debenhams, Harvey Nichols, Harrods, John Lewis, Liberty, Selfridges, Cult Beauty, Cloud 10 and Space NK, all of whom have supported me over the past 10 years. Thank you. And to the PRs that have sometimes been on the receiving end of the rocking and have still become good friends – thank you (and sorry, mate ☺).

Huge thanks also to my excellent doctor friends for their advice and guidance: Dr Marko Lens, Dr Emma Wedgeworth, Dr Sam Bunting, Dr Justine Kluk and Dr Joanna Christou.

My 'keep me put together' team: Josh Wood, Melanie Smith, Daxita Vaghela and Mercedez Mires. I love you all for making me 'look' put together on the outside, even when I don't feel it on the inside.

Thanks to my team at No.39: LouLou, Christopher, Molly, Lucy, Dom, Phil and Alex. The A-Team. May we always drink tea, spend hours talking about lunch options and never be taupe.

Thanks to my family and friends in Liverpool, Warrington, West London and the States, and my girlfriends, both in the industry and outside of it: Amanda Bell, Ateh Jewel, Anna Newton, Dija Ayodele, Charlene Garvey, Joanne Meek, Jen Macrae, Emma Guns, Emily Dougherty, Holly Harper, Emily Jane Johnston, Hannah Martin, Heather McKay, Jamie Klinger, Jennifer Rock, Jini Sanassy, Joanna Vargas, Kate Somerville, Lily Pebbles, Lorna Andrews, Michelle George, Nadine Baggott, Renée Rouleau, Ruth Crilly, Sali Hughes, Teresa Tarmey, Tracy Buchanan, Trinny Woodall, Petra Strand, Stephanie Nicole, Sheila Lund-Pearson, Beatrice Aidin, Lauren Mills, Sarah Coonan, Jo Tutchener-Sharp, Shoshana Gillis, Claire Coleman, Zoe Cook, Holly Brooke, Tracey Woodward, Funmi Fetto, Louise Woollam, Helen Burnham, Jorden Whiffin, Zoe Sugg, Field of Dreams. Thanks, bitches.

And the men: Sam Farmer, Kevin James Bennett, David Kirsch, Dom Smales, George Hammer, Ian Marber, Mark Aldridge, James Lamb, Andy Millward, Tony Oppe, Johannes Bjorklund and Felix Strand – thanks, chaps.

Thanks to my family, all of whom supported me every step of the way: Mum and Steve, Dad and Theresa, Christopher, Michelle, Ethan, James and Heli (who DOES read my blog).

And, finally, thanks to my husband Jim, our four children Ben, Dan, Ava and Max, and Lily too. All of this would be utterly pointless without you all. I love you.

HQ
An imprint of HarperCollinsPublishers Ltd
1 London Bridge Street
London SE1 9GF

First published in Great Britain by
HQ, an imprint of HarperCollinsPublishers Ltd 2020

ISBN 9780008375522
Limited signed edition ISBN 9780008395704
Special edition ISBN 9780008400644

MIX
Paper from
responsible sources
FSC™ C007454

FSC
www.fsc.org

This book is produced from independently certified FSC™ paper
to ensure responsible forest management.

For more information visit: www.harpercollins.co.uk

Editorial Director: Kate Fox
Project editor: Laura Nickoll
Photography: Christopher Oakman
Page design: Louise Evans

Printed and bound in Italy by Rotolito.

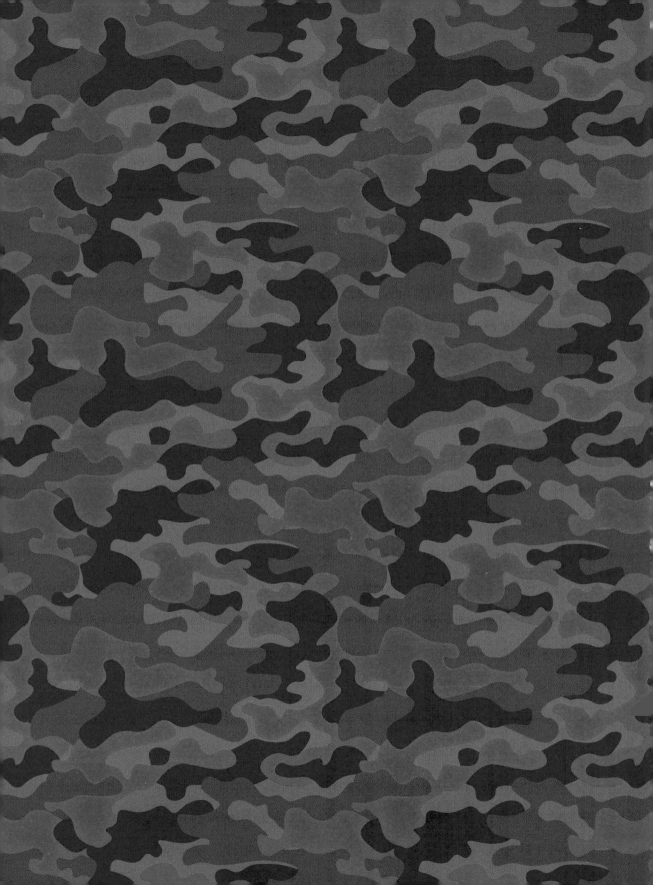